MW00398124

Computed Tomography
of the Spine

Computed Tomography of the Spine

Edited by
M. JUDITH DONOVAN POST, M.D.

Associate Professor of Radiology and of Neurological Surgery
Department of Radiology
Section of Neuroradiology
University of Miami School of Medicine/Jackson Memorial Medical Center
Miami, Florida

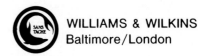

WILLIAMS & WILKINS
Baltimore/London

Copyright ©, 1984
Williams & Wilkins
428 East Preston Street
Baltimore, MD 21202, U.S.A.

Made in the United States of America

Library of Congress Cataloging in Publication Data

Computed tomography of the spine.

Includes index.
1. Spine—Diseases—Diagnosis. 2. Spine—Radiography. 3. Tomography. I. Post,
M. Judith Donovan (Melba Judith Donovan), 1943– . [DNLM: 1. Tomography, X-
ray computed. 2. Spine—Radiography. WE 725 C738] RD768.C653
1984   617′.56   83-3499
ISBN 0-683-06951-9

Composed and printed at the
Waverly Press, Inc.
Mt. Royal and Guilford Aves.
Baltimore, MD 21202, U.S.A.

This book is dedicated to
Kathryn Kirby Post
and to
my husband Tom, my parents Mr. and Mrs. Joseph R. Donovan,
Joe and Molly, Janet, Philip, Chantal, and Alex

Foreword

This monograph prepared under the direction of M. Judith Donovan Post is certainly the most complete and the most documented textbook dealing with pathology of the spine and the spinal cord.

Few great treatises have been devoted to this subject. Until a few years ago, the pathology of the spine and spinal cord was studied by conventional radiographic techniques: plain films, conventional tomography, then myelography with Pantopaque or gas and more recently myelography with metrizamide. A considerable advance in the study of the spine followed the advent of computed tomography (CT).

High-resolution CT obtained after a ScoutView gives very well-localized images. By utilizing a section thickness of 1.5 mm or more, multiplanar reformation, and different window settings, one can be quite sure of the presence of a herniated disc, a tumor, and small calcifications. Analysis of the axial slice allows spinal canal measurements to be made and spinal canal deformities and the abnormal relationships in spondylolithesis or in the "facet syndrome" to be appreciated. This understanding is so important to the study of a patient with back pain. The use of metrizamide with CT allows an accurate assessment of the deformities of the subarachnoid space in cases of intramedullary, intradural-extramedullary, and extradural tumors. In a unique fashion, metrizamide CT scanning also allows the detection and analysis of all the components of spinal cord malformations (myelomeningocele, meningocele, lipoma, diastematomyelia, Arnold-Chiari).

CT obtained after the intravenous injection of an iodinated contrast agent may be helpful in detecting certain lesions such as neuromas, meningiomas, and some vascular bone tumors since these neoplasms may enhance. Intravenous contrast injection may also be helpful in differentiating scar tissue from recurrent disc herniation.

With the availability of CT, what are the indications for conventional radiographic examinations? Certainly very few. Some authors believe that routine plain films are still necessary, augmented by tests in flexion, extension, or in lateral bending. Others feel more confident relying on reformatted CT images. Occasionally conventional tomography is still employed. In the investigation of infectious diseases and bone tumors, radionuclide bone scanning remains appropriate. Spinal angiography also remains useful since it is the only examination which can show the arterial supply and venous drainage of an arteriovenous malformation of the spinal cord. Epidural venography, however, no longer has any indications.

The reader will find in this book all the fundamental principles necessary for understanding what contributes to the quality of a CT image and what causes CT artifacts. The reader will also find discussed the value of the fourth generation CT scan, the importance of a large computer program for multiplanar reformation of the lumbar spine and the technique for performing metrizamide CT scanning as a primary procedure and as a secondary procedure following myelography. A description of various therapeutic procedures performed in conjunction with CT such as chemonucleolysis and facet injection will also be found.

Anatomy is very throughly described and illustrated in this book. Different chapters are devoted to the craniocervical junction, the lumbar spine, and the sacrum.

All of the chapters dealing with pathology of the spinal canal and of the spinal cord are beautifully analyzed and referenced. Very often a multidisciplinary approach is used to study a particular subject. Different authors place emphasis on clinical correlations, on anatomy, on radiology, or on surgical treatment.

The pathology of the spine and of the spinal cord begins with the pediatric age group with excellent discussions on the soft tissues, spinal dysraphism and on syringomyelia and the Arnold-Chiari syndrome.

Many chapters are devoted to disc herniation: at the cervical, thoracic, or lumbar levels. All the different types of disc herniation are well-illustrated. The indications for disc surgery and for chemonucleolysis are very well-analyzed as are the differential diagnosis of disc disease, recurrent disc herniations, postoperative complications, and asymptomatic changes on CT in the postoperative patient.

Stenosis, spondylosis, spondylolithesis, and calcification and ossification of the spinal ligaments are discussed in different chapters.

Very well-documented and attractive works concern primary or secondary tumors of the spine, primary tumors of the spinal cord, and neoplastic infiltration of the epidural space. Radiologic diagnosis and surgical approach are emphasized.

The book has three chapters at the end devoted to infection, trauma, and posttraumatic cysts.

It is a pleasure to congratulate Judith Donovan Post for giving to the neuroradiologic literature such a complete and well-documented textbook. Nothing comparable can be found in this field.

Her own contributions on spinal trauma, spinal dysraphism, and tumors of the spine and spinal cord are superb. The same can be said for all the work presented by her coauthors.

It was for me, before the actual publication of this textbook, a great pleasure to read all these papers which show clearly how neuroradiology is now capable of analyzing such diverse and perplexing diseases of the spine and spinal cord. It is also an honor to write the preface to a book I consider will be a "classic" in the neuroradiologic literature.

All my wishes for the great work of Judith Donovan Post and her coworkers.

With my admiration and my friendship,
G. Salamon
Marseille, June 1983

Preface

The purpose of this book is to demonstrate the diagnostic capabilities of high-resolution CT (HRCT) scanning of the spine and to show the expanded role that CT now plays in the evaluation of spinal pathology. This is done in the hope of benefitting patient care.

The book contains 43 chapters which reflect the experience of many different individuals. It is divided into four major sections:

Section I: Anatomical-Pathological-Computed Tomographic Correlations

Section II: Computed Tomographic Technique: Its Importance to Diagnosis

Section III: Computed Tomography of the Pediatric Spine and of Congenital Anomalies

Section IV: Computed Tomography of the Adult Spine

The questions which these sections address include the following: (1) What information is obtainable from a high-resolution CT of the spine? (2) What is the sensitivity and accuracy of CT in detecting different types of spinal lesions? (3) What role should HRCT be given in the diagnosis of spinal pathology? (4) What role should traditional radiographic studies, such as plain films, conventional tomograms, and myelograms be given now that HRCT is available? (5) What radiographic protocols should be chosen for the investigation of degenerative, congenital, neoplastic, vascular, inflammatory, and traumatic lesions of the spine? (6) What techniques should be chosen to demonstrate these lesions to best advantage? (7) When should noncontrast, intravenously (IV) enhanced and metrizamide CT scans be used? (8) When should metrizamide CT be performed as a primary procedure and when should it be performed following standard myelography? Because CT is still in a state of evolution, it is not surprising to find that some of these questions are answered in different ways by different authors in this book.

Because knowledge of normal anatomy is essential to the recognition of pathological conditions, the book begins with four chapters which describe normal CT spinal anatomy. In the first section, the CT scans of cadaver sections are correlated with the gross specimens. The CT scans of normal live patients are also presented. Emphasis is placed on intraspinal soft-tissue anatomy. However, paraspinal and osseous anatomy is described as well. The normal scans are contrasted with those showing pathology at different spinal levels.

The second section concentrates on CT technique. The nine chapters in this section deal with the physics of CT as well as with the diagnostic capabilities of plain HRCT and of computed assisted myelography. The indications for plain and metrizamide CT are discussed. The value of multiplanar reformation is described in detail. Attention is also drawn to diagnostic pitfalls in CT interpretation.

An extensive review of the use of CT in diagnosing spinal abnormalities in the pediatric age group is presented in the first chapter in Section III. A radiographic protocol for the evaluation of the pediatric spine is also included in this chapter. Attention is focused on spinal dysraphism, congenital syringomyelia, and the Arnold-Chiari malformation in the additional two chapters in this section.

The fourth and largest section of the book contains 27 chapters which include descriptions of CT of disc disease, facet abnormalities and stenosis, inflammatory arthritis, spinal tumors, spinal infection and spinal trauma. Particular emphasis is placed on disc disease since the availability of HRCT has made it possible to establish the diagnosis of many disc herniations noninvasively. Five chapters are devoted to the preoperative CT diagnosis of lumbar, thoracic, and cervical disc herniations and to the differential diagnosis of disc disease. Three chapters discuss the CT findings in the symptomatic and asymptomatic postoperative spine patient. The difficulties encountered in differentiating postoperative changes from recurrent disc herniation are delineated. The criteria found most helpful in distinguishing reherniated discs from scar tissue are described for plain, IV enhanced, and metrizamide CT scans. The subject of chemonucleolysis is presented in three subsequent chapters. The advantage of this procedure over surgery in the treatment of certain lumbar disc herniations and the use of CT to monitor the effectiveness of this procedure are discussed. CT of canine disc herniation and discolysis and its use as a potential diagnostic model for the evaluation of disc disease and discolysis in humans is also described.

The normal and pathological CT anatomy of facet joints and stenosis of varying etiologies are extensively reviewed in nine additional chapters in Section IV. Cadaver specimens with CT correlation are included in this review. Among the various causes of stenosis which are discussed are degenerative facet disease, spondylolisthesis, and ossification and calcification of the spinal ligaments.

Inflammatory arthritis with emphasis on the CT findings in rheumatoid arthritis, spinal tumors and their appearance on plain, IV enhanced, and metrizamide CT scans, and spinal infection and the use of CT in its investigation and follow-up are the subjects of the next five chapters in Section IV. In the final two chapters in the book, attention is focused on CT of spinal trauma. Protocols for the investigation of the acute and chronic spinal injury victim are presented.

The book is divided into these four major sections for organizational purposes and for ease of referral. However, the reader is urged to make liberal use of the index because a certain topic may be discussed in two or more different sections. For example, although CT of spinal tumors is described extensively in Section IV in Chapters 38 through 40, it is also discussed in other sections, such as in Chapters 4, 12, and 14. Normal anatomy is presented not only in the first four chapters of the book but also in many other chapters such as Chapters 12 and 14.

This book should be of interest to all those who are involved in the care of patients with spinal disorders. Radiologists, neurosurgeons, orthopaedic surgeons and neurologists, in particular, should find this book valuable.

Acknowledgments

Gratitude is expressed to the following: Dr. Georges Salamon for writing the Foreword; the contributing authors for their outstanding chapters; the Department of Radiology at the University of Miami School of Medicine/Jackson Memorial Hospital; my colleagues, Dr. Robert Quencer and Dr. Steven Ostrov; Mr. Chris Fletcher for the beautiful photographic work; Paula Garcia, Yolanda Marin, Tamera Johnson, Louise Rhodes, and Maria Gajardo for their excellent secretarial assistance; the CT, Neuroradiology and Fluoroscopy Sections at Jackson Memorial Hospital for their fine technological assistance; and Alice Reid and Jonathan Pine of Williams & Wilkins. Appreciation is also expressed to my mentors in radiology, Dr. Harold D. Rosenbaum, Dr. Jerome Shapiro, Dr. Edward Neuhauser, and Dr. Donald Altman, and in neuroradiology, Dr. Fredie Gargano, Dr. Derek Harwood-Nash, and Dr. Jerome Sheldon. A special word of thanks is extended to my husband and family for their encouragement and support.

M. Judith Donovan Post, M.D.

Contributors

Marie Louise Aubin, M.D., Chef de Service Adjoint, Radiologie, Fondation A. de Rothschild, Paris, France

Vallo Benjamin, M.D., Professor of Neurosurgery, New York University Medical Center, New York, New York

C. V. A. Bowen, M.B., Ch.B., F.R.C.S.(C), Research Fellow in Microsurgery, St. Vincent's Hospital, Melbourne, Australia

Ira F. Braun, M.D., Assistant Professor of Radiology, Emory University Clinic, Atlanta, Georgia

Charles V. Burton, M.D:, Director, Low Back Clinic, The Sister Kenny Institute, Minneapolis, Minnesota

Guillermo F. Carrera, M.D., Associate Professor of Radiology and Orthopedic Surgery, Department of Radiology, The Medical College of Wisconsin, Milwaukee County Medical Complex, Milwaukee, Wisconsin

J. D. Cassidy, D.C., F.C.C.S.(C), Research Associate, Department of Orthopaedics, University Hospital, Saskatoon, Canada

C. Gene Coin, M.D., Cape Fear Valley Neuroscience Institute, Fayetteville, North Carolina, and Moore Memorial Hospital, Pinehurst, North Carolina, and Clinical Associate Professor of Radiology, Bowman Gray School of Medicine, Wake Forest University, Winston-Salem, North Carolina

J. Thaddeus Coin, Ph.D., Duke University Medical Center, Durham, North Carolina

Rosendo D. Diaz, M.D., Assistant Professor of Radiology, Section of Neuroradiology, University of Miami School of Medicine, Jackson Memorial Medical Center, Miami, Florida

Charles C. Edwards, M.D., Associate Professor of Orthopaedic Surgery, University of Maryland School of Medicine, Maryland Institute for Emergency Medicine, Baltimore, Maryland

Frank J. Eismont, M.D., Associate Professor of Orthopaedics and Rehabilitation, Co-Director, Acute Spinal Cord Injury Service, Co-Director, South Florida Spinal Cord Injury System, Attending, Orthopaedic Surgery-Veterans Administration Hospital, University of Miami/Jackson Memorial Medical Center, Miami, Florida

Mokhtar Gado, M.D., Professor of Radiology, Chief, Neuroradiology Section, The Edward Mallinckrodt Institute of Radiology, Washington University School of Medicine, St. Louis, Missouri

J. K. Garrett, D.V.M., Animal Hospital of Fayetteville, Fayetteville, North Carolina

William V. Glenn, Jr., M.D., Private Practice, Multi-Planar Diagnostic Imaging, Inc., Torrance, California

Barth A. Green, M.D., Associate Professor of Neurological Surgery, Co-Director, Acute Spinal Cord Injury Service, Co-Director, South Florida Spinal Cord Injury System, Attending, Neurological Surgery-Veterans Administration Hospital, University of Miami/Jackson Memorial Medical Center, Miami, Florida

Seiko Harata, M.D., Associate Professor, Orthopedic Department, Hirosaki University Hospital, Hirosakishi, Japan

Derek C. Harwood-Nash, M.B., Ch.B., F.R.C.P.(C), Professor of Radiology, University of Toronto, Toronto, Ontario, Canada and Radiologist-in-Chief, Department of Radiology, The Hospital for Sick Children, Toronto, Ontario, Canada

Marvin E. Haskin, M.D., Professor of Radiology, Hahnemann University School of Medicine and Chairman of the Department of Diagnostic Radiology, Hahnemann University Hospital, Philadelphia, Pennsylvania

Victor M. Haughton, M.D., Professor of Radiology and Director, Neuroradiology Research, Department of Radiology, The Medical College of Wisconsin, Milwaukee County Medical Complex and Froedtert Memorial Lutheran Hospital, Milwaukee, Wisconsin

Kenneth B. Heithoff, M.D., Center for Diagnostic Imaging, St. Louis Park, Minnesota

James C. Hirschy, M.D., Hamilton-Hirschy and Abbott, New York, New York and Clinical Assistant Professor of Radiology, New York Hospital-Cornell University College of Medicine, New York, New York

Fred Hodges III, M.D., Professor of Radiology, The Edward Mallinckrodt Institute of Radiology, Washington University School of Medicine, St. Louis, Missouri

Hamilton E. Holmes, M.D., Assistant Clinical Professor of Orthopaedic Surgery, Emory University School of Medicine, Consultant, Spine Clinic, Atlanta V.A. Hospital, Atlanta, Georgia

Goro Irie, M.D., Professor, Department of Radiology, Hokkaido University School of Medicine, Sapporo, Japan

Kinjiro Iwata, M.D., Professor and Chairman, Department of Neurological Surgery, Aichi Medical University, Aichi-ken, Japan

Donald Jacobson, M.S., CT Physicist, General Electric Medical Systems, Milwaukee, Wisconsin

Kiyoshi Kaneda, M.D., Associate Professor, Department of Orthopaedic Surgery, Hokkaido University School of Medicine, Sapporo, Japan

Ronald L. Kaufman, M.D., F.A.C.P., Assistant Professor of Medicine, University of Southern California School of Medicine, Rheumatologist, Ranchos los Amigos Hospital, Downey, California

James W. Keating, Jr., M.D., Assistant Professor, Department of Radiology, Clinical Assistant Professor, Department of Neurological Surgery, Chief, Section of Computed Tomography and Section of Neuroradiology, Tulane University School of Medicine, New Orleans, Louisiana

Charles W. Kerber, M.D., Professor of Clinical Radiology, University of California, San Diego and Consultant in Radiology, V.A. Hospital, San Diego and Director of Neurodiagnostic Center, San Diego, California

W. H. Kirkaldy-Willis, M.A., M.D. F.R.C.S. (E and C), Professor of Orthopaedic Surgery, University Hospital, Saskatoon, Canada

Irvin I. Kricheff, M.D., Professor of Radiology, New York University Medical Center, New York, New York

David L. LaMasters, M.D., Chief, Neuroradiology/Computed Tomography Section, Wilford Hall USAF Medical Center, San Antonio, Texas

S. Henry LaRocca, M.D., Clinical Professor of Orthopaedic Surgery, Tulane University and Clinical Professor of Orthopaedic Surgery, Louisiana State University, New Orleans, Louisiana

Juan-Martin Leborgne, M.D., Neuroradiologist, Section of Neuroradiology and Computed Tomography, Chief, Section of Mammography, Department of Radiology, Mount Sinai Medical Center and Assistant Professor of Radiology, University of Miami School of Medicine, Miami, Florida

Robert M. Lifeso, M.D., F.R.C.S.(C), Chief, Division of Orthopedic Surgery, King Faisal Specialist Hospital and Research Centre, Riyadh, Saudi Arabia, and Consultant Orthopedic Surgeon, Spinal Cord Injuries Unit, Riyadh Central Hospital, Riyadh, Saudi Arabia

Joseph P. Lin, M.D., Professor of Radiology, New York University Medical Center, New York, New York

Ernesto Luciano, Department of Radiology, Tulane University School of Medicine, New Orleans, Louisiana

Leonard I. Malis, M.D., Professor and Chairman, Department of Neurosurgery, Mount Sinai School of Medicine, City University of New York, New York, New York

John R. Mani, M.D., Associate Clinical Professor, Department of Radiology, University of California, San Francisco, California and Chief, Section of Neuroradiology and CT, Ralph K. Davies Medical Center, Franklin Hospital, San Francisco, California

John A. McCulloch, M.D., F.R.C.S.(C), Assistant Professor, University of Toronto, Department of Surgery, St. Michael's Hospital, Toronto, Canada

John D. Meyer, M.D., Assistant Chief of Neuroradiology, Visiting Associate Professor of Radiology, Department of Radiology, Presbyterian-University Hospital, Pittsburgh, Pennsylvania

Kazuo Miyasaka, M.D., Instructor and Head, Section of Neuroradiology and Computed Tomography, Department of Radiology, Hokkaido University School of Medicine, Hokkaido University Hospital, Sapporo, Japan

F. Reed Murtagh, M.D., Clinical Assistant Professor, Radiology Department, Division of Neuroradiology, University of South Florida, College of Medicine and Radiology Department, Tampa General Hospital, Tampa, Florida

Joseph M. D. Nadell, M.D., Associate Professor, Department of Neurological Surgery, Clinical Associate Professor, Department of Pediatrics, Tulane University School of Medicine, New Orleans, Louisiana

Hiroshi Nakagawa, M.D., Associate Professor, Department of Neurological Surgery, Aichi Medical University, Aichi-Ken, Japan

Larry K. Page, M.D., Professor of Neurological Surgery and Chief, Division of Pediatric Neurosurgery, Department of Neurological Surgery, University of Miami School of Medicine, Miami, Florida

Jash Patel, M.D., Instructor, Radiology Department, Neuroradiology Section, The Edward Mallinckrodt Institute of Radiology, Washington University School of Medicine, St. Louis, Missouri

Holger Pettersson, M.D., Associate Professor of Radiology, Department of Radiology, University Hospital, Lund, Sweden

M. Judith Donovan Post, M.D., Associate Professor of Radiology and of Neurological Surgery, Radiology Department, Section of Neuroradiology, University of Miami School of Medicine/Jackson Memorial Medical Center, Miami, Florida

Robert M. Quencer, M.D., Professor of Radiology and Neurological Surgery, Chief, Section of Neuroradiology, University of Miami School of Medicine/Jackson Memorial Medical Center, Miami, Florida

Stephen P. Raskin, M.D., Radiology Department, Bluefield Community Hospital, Bluefield, West Virginia

Wolfgang Rauschning, M.D., Associate Professor, Department of Orthopaedic Surgery, University Hospital, Uppsala, Sweden

Michael L. Rhodes, Ph.D., Director of Research, Multi-Planar Diagnostic Imaging, Inc., Torrance, California

Richard H. Rothman, M.D., Ph.D., Professor of Orthopaedic Surgery, The University of Pennsylvania School of Medicine, Chief of Orthopaedic Surgery, The Pennsylvania Hospital, Philadelphia, Pennsylvania

Stephen L. G. Rothman, M.D., Medical Director, Multi-Planar Diagnostic Imaging, Inc., Torrance, California

Georges Salamon, M.D., Professeur, Service de Radiologie, Hôpital de la Timone, Marseille, France

R. Shannon, M.B., Ch.B., B.A.O., F.R.C.S. (C), Orthopaedic Surgeon, City Hospital, Saskatoon, Canada

Robert Shapiro, M.D., Chairman, Department of Radiology, The Hospital of St. Raphael, New Haven, Connecticut and Clinical Professor of Radiology, Yale University School of Medicine

Jerome J. Sheldon, M.D., Chief, Section of Neuroradiology and Computed Tomography, Department of Radiology, Mount Sinai Medical Center and Associate Professor of Radiology, University of Miami School of Medicine, Miami, Florida

Jan J. Smulewicz, M.D., Director of Radiology, Beth Israel Medical Center, Professor of Radiology, Mount Sinai School of Medicine, City University of New York, New York, New York

S. Tchang, M.D., F.R.C.P.(C), Associate Professor of Diagnostic Radiology, University Hospital, Saskatoon, Canada

J. George Teplick, M.D., Professor of Radiology, Hahnemann University School of Medicine and Director of General Diagnosis, Hahnemann University Hospital, Philadelphia, Pennsylvania

Steven K. Teplick, M.D., Professor of Radiology, Hahnemann University School of Medicine and Chief of Sections on G.I. Radiology and Interventional Radiology, Hahnemann University Hospital, Philadelphia, Pennsylvania

Shuji Tohno, M.D., Professor, Orthopedic Department, Hirosaki University Hospital, Hirosakishi, Japan

Mitsuo Tsuru, M.D., Professor, Department of Neurosurgery, Hokkaido University School of Medicine, Sapporo, Japan

Frans D. J. van Schaik, M.A., Research Associate for Statistics, University of Tilburg, The Netherlands

Jan P. J. van Schaik, M.D., Department of Diagnostic Radiology, University Hospital, Utrecht, The Netherlands

Henk Verbiest, M.D., Ph.D., Professor of Neurosurgery, Emeritus Chairman of the Department of Neurosurgery, University Hospital, Utrecht, The Netherlands

Jacqueline Vignaud, M.D., Chef de Service, Radiologie, Fondation Ophthalmologique, Adolphe De Rothschild, Paris, France

Margaret Anne Whelan, M.D., Neuroradiologist, Department of Radiology, New York University Medical Center, New York, New York

Alan L. Williams, M.D., Professor of Radiology and Chief, Section of Neuroradiology, Department of Radiology, The Medical College of Wisconsin, Milwaukee County Medical Complex and Froedtert Memorial Lutheran Hospital, Milwaukee, Wisconsin

Paul Wozney, M.D., Department of Radiology, University of Pittsburgh, Pittsburgh, Pennsylvania, Formerly Manager, CT Clinical Applications, General Electric Medical Systems, Milwaukee, Wisconsin

Wen C. Yang, M.D., Neuroradiologist-in-charge, Radiology Department, Beth Israel Medical Center, Assistant Professor of Radiology, Mount Sinai School of Medicine, City University of New York, New York, New York

Rosario Zappulla, M.D., Instructor of Neurosurgery, Mount Sinai School of Medicine, City University of New York, New York, New York

Mary Zimmermann, R.T., CT Education Specialist, General Electric Medical Systems, Milwaukee, Wisconsin

Contents

C. Inflammatory Arthritis

D. Spinal Tumors

E. Spinal Infection

F. Spinal Trauma

SECTION I

Anatomical—Pathological—Computed Tomographic Correlations

CHAPTER ONE

Correlative Multiplanar Computed Tomographic Anatomy of the Normal Spine*

WOLFGANG RAUSCHNING, M.D.†

INTRODUCTION

Among the various modern radiographic procedures for evaluation of disorders of the human spine, computed tomography (CT) has a specially promising diagnostic potential (1–13). It presents the spinal soft tissues together with the bony vertebrae and also displays the important axial view of the anatomy, which previously was only obtainable by conventional transverse axial tomography (14–16). Apart from the axial plane, CT also permits visualization of the frontal, sagittal, and any oblique perspective by means of multiplanar image reconstruction. With the present technology, some of the soft-tissue morphology within the spinal canal can be distinguished on noncontrast high-resolution CT scans (17–23). For demonstrating further details, different types of enhancement procedures are used (24–27).

The standard treatises of anatomy contain only few sectional presentations of the spine. Evaluation of CT scans on the basis of these semischematic drawings implies a considerable risk of morphological misconception owing to the wide range of individual anatomical variations. The increasing difficulties presently encountered in the interpretation of CT scans have led to a need for an accurate correlative morphology, as is strikingly reflected

by the large number of radiographic-anatomical atlases that have been issued during the past decade (28–50).

The anatomical material in these works invariably has been based on macrosectioning of postmortem cases. As a rule, decalcified specimens have been sectioned on conventional microtomes, whereas undecalcified, fresh, embalmed, or frozen cadavers have been sliced by means of band saws. In some cases, colored plastic material has been introduced into the vessels and other cavities of the body.

Morphological studies on the human spine constitute a special challenge because of its complex topographic anatomy and the intimate relationship between the supporting skeleton and the contiguous neurovascular elements. Moreover, the multisegmental mobility exerts specific strains on the discs, joint capsules, and ligaments, and in certain positions, affects the spinal cord, the nerve roots, and the dural sheaths. At present, functional-radiographic methods are being increasingly employed in the assessment of spinal disorders (51–52). CT scanning in functional positions is expected to make a major contribution to the diagnostic arsenal in the near future.

The improved resolution and multiplanar image reformatting facilities of modern CT scanners call for accurate anatomical reference material. Rigorous precautions must be taken to ensure the exact coincidence of the plane of sectioning with the plane of scanning. The anatomical images should present without distortion, in natural colors, and in considerable detail.

To obtain anatomical images correlating with multidirectional conventional tomograms of the temporal bone, Rabischong and co-workers (31) developed a technique for milling of frozen specimens. This technique has been utilized by Thompson and Hasso (50) to describe the correlative anatomy of the head and neck.

Based on a new technique for *cryosectioning* of undecalcified human specimens (53), the following method has

* Financial support was received from the Swedish Society of Medical Sciences, the Trygg Hansa Insurance Company and the Swedish Association for Traffic and Polio Injured.
† I want to thank Mr. Agne Lag, Department of Pathology, and Mr. Göran Pettersson, Department of Forensic Medicine for their invaluable help with the cadaver specimens. Peter Pech, M.D., Department of Diagnostic Radiology and Mr. Bjarne Lundholm, Siemens Elema AB are gratefully acknowledged for their assistance in CT scanning of the specimens. Mr. Håkan Pettersson and Mrs. Yvonne Moberg at the Photographic Department, Uppsala University Hospital, and Mr. Chris Fletcher at the University of Miami School of Medicine are acknowledged for their excellent reproduction of the illustrations.

been evolved for studying the normal sectional anatomy of the cervical, thoracic, and lumbosacral spine in different planes and in exact correlation with CT scans obtained from the same frozen specimen.

METHOD

To maintain undistorted topographic anatomy and to prevent drainage of blood and cerebrospinal fluid (CSF) from the specimen, fresh cadaveric spines from persons of various age groups with no known history of any spinal disorder and who apparently were free from anatomically distorting diseases, were deep frozen in situ and cut out with an oscillating saw. In some cases, the CSF was replaced by metrizamide before freezing. After accurate positioning of the specimens in boxes with rectangular and plane-parallel walls under fluoroscopic control for CT scanning in the transaxial, coronal, sagittal, or an oblique plane, the spine segments were freeze-embedded in a semiliquid solution of carboxymethyl cellulose gel. After embedding, the scanning plane was marked on the outer wall of the box.

The specimens were examined on a SOMATOM 2 Siemens whole body scanner. For maximum image resolution, 2-mm thick contiguous slices were chosen. To keep the noise level as low as possible, the highest MAS settings (460 MAS) were used. The specimen was carefully adjusted in the center of the gantry and aligned parallel with the marks on the box using the light beam indicator. Because of the small size of the specimen and for greater ease in visualization, reconstructive zooming with magnification factors of 4X to 6X was employed. The matrix of the scanner measured 265 × 265 mm and the pixel size varied from 0.2–0.4 mm. The raw data from all scans were postprocessed with alternative convolution filters and high-resolution software allowing a spatial resolution down to 0.75 mm.

The specimens were transferred to a cryomicrotome stage with an adjustable ball and socket joint. The undecalcified frozen specimens were sectioned through on a heavy duty cryomicrotome (LKB 2250, Bromma, Sweden) which commonly is used for whole body autoradiography of large experimental animals (54).

Images were obtained by macrophotography of the surface of the block (specimen) at equidistant cutting height intervals of 1 mm during the course of sectioning. Slight thawing of the ice crystals on the cutting surface with a warm cloth soaked in ethylene glycol rendered images with deep natural colors and also prevented recrystallization. A specially designed stable camera stand attached to the knife holder enabled sequential anatomical images with identical magnification to be obtained. A commercial 35 mm SLR camera equipped with flat field macrolenses, and automatic electronic flash units were used. Photographs were taken on Kodachrome 25 ASA color reversal film.

METHODOLOGICAL CONSIDERATIONS

Freezing of cadaveric material is at present the only practical conservation procedure which guarantees that the soft tissues, including fluid-filled cavities, are fixed in their true mutual positions, as well as in their true relation to the supporting skeleton. Freezing also preserves the natural color of the tissues for good photography and prevents drainage of CSF and blood from the specimen, as well as the entrance of air, which causes disturbing CT artifacts. The specific embedding technique employed in this study ensures that CT scanning and sectioning are carried out in identical planes.

As is evident from a comparison of Figures 1.25 and 1.26‡ with the remainder of the figures in this chapter, CT images of frozen material, though still providing sufficient morphological detail, look different from clinical CT scans, apparently owing to distortion of the gray-scale presentation. In some cases, the contrast in the soft tissues was enhanced compared with in vivo CT scans. Commonly, frozen CSF was less radiopaque than CSF in vivo, serving as a natural contrast and permitting demonstration of the spinal cord and the nerve roots on unenhanced CT scans. Thompson and Hasso (50) observed that freezing changes the roentgen-ray absorption characteristics of the brain, making gray matter appear less radiopaque than white. Alfidi and co-workers (33) reported that embalming alters the attenuation of the tissues. Using experimental animals, Wittenberg et al. (55) found significant changes of attenuation values when fresh specimens were frozen. In vivo and in vitro measurements of our own performed on human muscle and fat tissue showed systematic attenuation changes (56). As compared with in vivo values, the density of fat slightly increased in refrigerated and frozen specimens. The attenuation of refrigerated muscle was slightly higher than in vivo, whereas deep freezing decreased the attenuation by an average of 50 HU.

Cryosectioning creates an absolutely smooth cutting surface from which anatomical images with considerable detail and high resolution can be obtained photographically. Photographs can be taken at cutting height intervals exactly corresponding to the CT sections. Irrespective of the unexcelled coincidence of the planes of the CT scans with the planes of the cryosectional images, it is essential to realize that the former represent slices of the specimen, whereas the latter constitute sharp surface images without any extension in depth. In anatomically complex areas of the spine, several anatomical images, therefore, might be required to express all details contained in one CT image, especially when these CT slices are thick. On the other hand, thinner CT cuts permit a more direct correlation of the morphology.

Not all anatomical details observed on the cryosectional images can be distinguished yet on the corresponding CT scans presented in this chapter, but the continuous advances in CT technology may soon allow a better radiographic assessment of the spinal soft tissues. Direct CT scanning of anatomical specimens primarily in other planes than the transaxial one provides less "edgy" images with sharper detail than reformatted images from patients.

---

‡ All figures in Chapter 1 will appear at the end of the chapter on pages 10–57.

Postprocessing of the basic scanning data, however, will permit, in the future, rapid reconstructions of improved image quality (12, 57–59). Such a sequential display poses high demands on the anatomical knowledge of the radiologist because of the unconventional perspectives of the CT scans. Serial cryomicrotomy provides excellent correlative anatomical material for detailed evaluation of CT scans.

GENERAL DESCRIPTION OF THE SPINE§

The spinal column is composed of 24 vertebrae (7 cervical, 12 thoracic, and 5 lumbar), the sacrum, and the coccyx. The vertebrae are conjoined by the intervertebral discs, facet joints, and ligaments. The spine contains the spinal cord with its meningeal envelopes and is surrounded by thick layers of paraspinal muscles and has a richly anastomosing arterial supply and venous drainage. Thirty-one pairs of spinal nerves arise from the spinal cord. The 1st cervical emerges between the occiput and the atlas (Fig. 1.4), and the 8th below the 7th cervical vertebra. Below the 1st thoracic segment, all spinal nerves leave the spinal canal beneath the vertebra with the corresponding number.

The spinal column presents characteristic curves in the sagittal plane:—the cervical (lordotic), thoracic (kyphotic), and lumbar (lordotic) curves. There is also a physiological angulation between the 5th lumbar vertebra and the posteriorly convex sacrum (Fig. 1.32).

Except for the atlas, typical vertebrae consist of anterior elements (the vertebral bodies, intervertebral discs, and longitudinal ligaments) and posterior elements (pedicles, laminae, articular, transverse and spinous processes with intervening joint capsules and ligaments).

Vertebrae

A typical vertebra is composed of a body anteriorly and a neural (vertebral) arch posteriorly, together enclosing the vertebral foramen. The bodies are blocks composed of cancellous bone covered with a thin layer of cortical bone except at the end plates. The cross-sectional shape and dimensions vary greatly. The vertebrae gradually increase in size in the craniocaudal direction. In the cervical spine, the cancellous bone has a fine texture, but toward the lumbar spine it becomes considerably coarser. The vertebrae contain the most voluminous amount of hematopoietic red marrow in the body. Small vascular foramina pierce the cortex of the vertebral bodies. The flat or slightly concave, roughly plane-parallel end plates consist of dense cancellous bone to which the hyaline cartilage end plate is attached firmly. On macerated vertebral specimens, a slightly prominent circular ridge of cortical bone, derived from the united annular apophysis, surrounds this spongy central portion of the vertebral end plate. CT scans

§ The terminology used in this chapter follows the glossary prepared by the Committee on the Spine, American Academy of Orthopaedic Surgeons, Document 675–80 (except for the terms "spinous process" instead, of "spine" and "spinal canal" instead of "vertebral canal").

parallel to the end plate usually exhibit the annular apophysis (Figs. 1.21, 1.28). The vertebral bodies commonly are wider at the end plates and have a waist-shaped narrowing of their intermediate portion. The posterior surface is flat or slightly concave and is pierced by large vascular foramina (Figs. 1.19, 1.20, 1.29, 1.32).

Intervertebral Discs (Figs. 1.2, 1.16, 1.21, 1.22, 1.27, 1.32)

In the undiseased spine, the intervertebral discs have a slightly larger dimension than the contiguous vertebral end plates. They are elastic, biconvex, or wedge-shaped and, functionally, they bulge somewhat into the spinal canal during extension. The intervertebral discs contribute approximately 20–25% of the total length of the cervical and thoracic and 30–35% of that of the lumbar vertebral column. The central and posterior portion of the discs contain the nucleus pulposus, a gelatinous, pulpy substance derived from the notochord. The peripheral part is built up by concentrically oriented lamellae of fibrocartilaginous tissue intermingled with strong collagenous strands forming the annulus fibrosus running obliquely at different angles. These strands are anchored into the annular apophysis and also attach to the vertebral body beyond the end plate blending with the periosteum and the longitudinal ligaments.

Anterior Longitudinal Ligament

The anterior longitudinal ligament forms a flat fibrous band running along the anterior surface of the vertebral column. It consists of deep unisegmental and superficial plurisegmental layers of fibers. From its narrow origin at the base of the skull, it rapidly increases in width covering virtually the whole anterior circumference of the cervical vertebrae. Along the kyphotic curve of the thoracic spine it becomes narrower and in the lordotic lumbar spine it again increases considerably in width and thickness. It is attached to the bodies of the vertebrae by loose areolar tissue, partially filling in their anterior concavities. At the level of the discs, it gets broader and is virtually inseparably interwoven with the fibers of the annulus fibrosus.

Posterior Longitudinal Ligament (Figs. 1.7, 1.17, 1.19, 1.20, 1.22–1.24, 1.29)

The posterior longitudinal ligament consists of a superficial layer extending over several vertebrae and deep unisegmental strands. It extends from the foramen magnum along the posterior surface of the vertebral bodies and intervertebral discs and forms a narrow band behind the vertebral bodies. When their posterior surface is concave, the ligament bridges these concavities in a bowstring fashion from one disc to another. Not infrequently, longitudinal ridges of dense bone project beneath the ligament. Sending obliquely oriented fibers to the vertebral end plates and the annulus, the posterior longitudinal ligament becomes thinner, wider, and less distinct at the disc levels.

Posterior Vertebral Arch

At the upper lateral posterior aspect of the vertebral bodies, a pair of strong pedicles emerges. These conjoin posteriorly to form the laminae. The shallow superior and the deep inferior notches of two adjacent vertebrae, together with the intervertebral disc, form the intervertebral foramen. Pairs of articular processes with cartilage-covered articular facets project cranially and caudally from the pedicles, forming the zygoapophyseal or facet joints. In interaction with the intervertebral discs and the intervening ligaments, these facet joints control the movements between two vertebrae (motion segment unit). These joints are innervated by medial branches of the dorsal rami of the spinal nerves. The laterally projecting transverse processes and the spinous processes (spines) posteriorly mainly constitute lever arms serving for attachments of tendons, ligaments, and muscles. The posterior bony elements are composed essentially of thick cortical bone and contain little red marrow and cancellous bone. Several ligaments act as passive restraints of spinal mobility. The facet joint capsules are elastic, as are the supra- and interspinous ligaments and the ligamentum flavum. The supraspinous ligament runs over the tips of the spinous processes, forming thick fibroelastic strands which also project laterally, transgressing into the coarse thoracolumbar fascia (Figs. 1.20–1.22, 1.24, 1.26). The interspinous ligament, which in the cervical spine is continuous with the heavy nuchal ligament, is considerably thinner, with a loose texture of obliquely crossing fibers leaving holes and defects between them.

The *ligamentum flavum* forms a typical arcade of yellow elastic tissue between the arches of the vertebrae. In the cervical spine, it is a thin membrane, but it gradually increases in thickness in the thoracic spine and becomes thickest (4–5 mm) in the lower lumbar spine. Viewed from the inner aspect of the spinal canal, the ligamentum flavum only leaves a narrow band of cortical bone in the lamina uncovered. It runs from the anteroinferior border of the lamina above to the upper posterior border of the lamina below. This typical insertion of the ligamentum flavum allows the upper and lower portions of a lamina to be distinguished on axial CT scans as well as on anatomical cross-sections, since the lower border of a lamina has the ligamentum flavum at its anterior margin and vice versa. Except for the lower lumbar and upper cervical spine, the ligamentum is not visible from behind, owing to the shingling of the laminae and the overlapping of the spinous processes. Extending laterally, the ligamentum flavum blends with the thick medial and superior portions of the facet joint capsules; the lateral and inferior walls of the joint capsules are thinner.

Spinal Canal (Vertebral Canal)

The spinal canal is composed of osseous elements, the vertebral foramina, and the conjoining ligamentous structures. It is delimited anteriorly by the posterior surface of the vertebral bodies and the intervertebral discs, laterally by the pedicles and the facet joints, and posteriorly by the ligamentum flavum and the neural arch. The spinal canal is covered by a parietal lamina of the dura mater (endorhachis). In the thoracic and upper cervical spine, it is mainly round in cross-section (Figs. 1.1, 1.11, 1.16), whereas in the lower cervical and the lower lumbar spine the configuration is triangular or half-moon shaped (Figs.

1.7, 1.21, 1.27, 1.28). The reiterative sequences of bony and ligamentous elements within one motion segment unit account for the variations in the shape of the spinal canal (Fig. 1.7). It can be divided into a central portion housing the thecal sac and the extradural soft tissues anterior and posterior to the dura. The small, cone-shaped extradural spaces extending anterolaterally from the border of the dura to the medial border of the intervertebral foramen are called *lateral recesses*. As these recesses are occupied mainly by the dorsal and ventral spinal nerve roots contained in the periradicular dural sheath, these recesses also are referred to as the radicular canals or root canals.

The soft tissues in the spinal canal and the intervertebral foramen also may be divided into the saccoradicular and the extradural compartment. The latter contains the epidural fat, the internal vertebral venous plexuses, arteries, nerves, and lymphatic vessels.

Thecal Sac and Spinal Cord

The spinal cord begins at the medulla oblongata where it emerges from the foramen magnum and terminates between the 1st and 2nd lumbar vertebrae where it tapers sharply as the conus medullaris. It is round or elliptical with a greater transverse than anteroposterior (AP) diameter. Its diameters vary considerably at identical levels between different subjects. The spinal cord increases in volume between the spinal levels C4 and T2 (Fig. 1.7) and again between T10 and T12 (Fig. 1.18), where the large nervous plexuses passing to the upper and lower extremities emerge. From side to side, it measures 13 mm at the fusiform thickening of the cervical cord and 8 mm at that of the lumbosacral cord. The thinnest portions of the thoracic cord (diameter 7–8 mm) occupy only a small proportion of the spinal canal (Figs. 1.12, 1.16).

The spinal cord is covered by the pia mater, which laterally conjoins to form the dentate ligament, a suspensory attachment of the cord to the dura. The spinal cord is grooved by longitudinal fissures and sulci, the deepest being the anterior median fissure. The dorsal and ventral spinal roots form from numerous dendritic rootlet filaments emerging from the anterolateral and posterolateral sulcus of the cord (Figs. 1.3, 1.6, 1.7, 1.13). These rootlets merge stepwise to form the ventral and dorsal roots of the spinal nerves, separated by the dentate ligament. As a result of the retardation in growth of the spinal cord in relation to the vertebral column, the rootlets and spinal nerve roots run almost horizontally in the upper cervical spine (Fig. 1.3), then becoming increasingly more oblique, more vertical, and more anteriorly directed at progressively lower levels of the spinal cord (Figs. 1.6, 1.13, 1.18). The lumbosacral spinal roots arise directly from the cord without intermediate rootlets (Figs. 1.18, 1.30) and surround the conus medullaris by four condensations of fibers in the antero- and posterolateral portions of the subarachnoid space. This course of the lumbosacral roots creates a typical X-shaped image on CT scans and anatomical cross-sections (Figs. 1.27, 1.28).

The ventral and the dorsal roots converge somewhat

anteriorly toward the subpedicular gutter, pierce the thecal sac separately, taking along separate sleeves of the arachnoid and dura, and merge after a short distance, forming between them the *interradicular foramen*. In the intervertebral foramen, the dorsal root becomes thickened to form the fusiform dorsal root ganglion (Figs. 1.7, 1.23, 1.24, 1.35). The spinal cord has a thin caudal extension, the filum terminale internum, running caudally together with the nerve roots of the cauda equina. The thecal sac ends at the midsacral level, where it dwindles into the thin filum durae matris spinalis and affixes to the coccyx.

Intervertebral Foramina
(Figs. 1.7, 1.9, 1.14, 1.23, 1.24, 1.33)

The intervertebral foramina are osseofibrous tunnels continuous with the lateral recesses of the spinal canal, through which the segmental nerves and vessels emerge. The spinal nerve roots take an obliquely caudally, laterally, and anteriorly directed course, especially in the cervical spine. In the thoracolumbar spine, intervertebral foramina are directed laterally. In sagittal sections, the intervertebral foramina displays an oval or teardrop configuration, with a greater longitudinal than transverse diameter. The upper (subpedicular) portion is delimited cranially by the notch of the pedicle, anteriorly by the body of the vertebra, and posteriorly by the ligamentum flavum. Especially in the lumbar spine, the lower (discal) portion of the intervertebral foramen is narrower owing to some bulging of the disc. Its narrow floor is the pedicle of the lower vertebra, its posterior wall is formed by the superior articular process of the lower vertebra, and its anterior wall is the variable boundary of the intervening disc. The shape and size of the intervertebral foramen of one individual are subject to considerable variations resulting from specific movements in different positions and from loading of the spine.

The upper portion of the typical intervertebral foramen (Figs. 1.4, 1.7–1.9, 1.14, 1.15, 1.23–1.25, 1.33, 1.35) contains the vaginal extension of the dura with the dorsal root ganglion and the ventral spinal root, the spinal branch of the segmental artery, radicular veins, and the (recurrent) sinuvertebral nerve which arises from the dorsal division of the spinal nerve and re-enters the spinal canal to supply the posterior portion of the anulus fibrosus, the posterior longitudinal ligament, and periosteum of the vertebral body. The lower portion of the intervertebral foramen is occupied by the intervertebral veins and fat tissue. The thoracic spinal nerves are thin and take up a far smaller proportion of the foramina than in the lumbar spine (Fig. 1.14). They are surrounded by wide venous sinuses and some fat tissue and often lie at a distance from the pedicle, whereas the lumbar spinal nerve roots are situated snugly in the lower notch of the pedicle (Fig. 1.33).

Arterial Supply of the Spine

The anterior portions of the spine are supplied by the anterior spinal arteries, which mainly receive their blood from the cervical vertebral arteries (cervical spine), the dorsal branches of the intercostal arteries (thoracic spine), the dorsal branches of the lumbar arteries (lumbar spine), and the dorsal branches of the lateral sacral arteries (sacrum).

The spinal canal and its contents, as well as the major portion of the vertebrae, are supplied by the spinal branches of the cervical vertebral arteries and the dorsal rami or the segmental arteries of the thoracolumbar spine and sacrum. These spinal branches enter the intervertebral foramen where they send off the ventral and dorsal medullary arteries that follow the dorsal and ventral nerve roots to the spinal cord. Here they run in the longitudinal grooves of the cord, covered by the pia mater. The remainder of the spinal branches divide into the anterior laminar arteries (terminating as a delicate arterial network on the inner surface of the posterior arches) and the posterior central arteries (supplying the anterior wall of the spinal canal through nutrient foramina beneath the posterior longitudinal ligament and also forming anastomotic longitudinal plexuses).

Vertebral Veins

The extradural space mainly contains fat and venous plexuses. The venous drainage of the spinal canal and its contents is accomplished by a dorsal and a ventral internal venous plexus. The latter is in continuity with the basivertebral veins, which traverse the central part of the vertebral body and frequently present as V- or Y-shaped figures on CT scans. The basivertebral veins connect the ventral internal veins with the anterior external venous plexuses. Similarly, the less voluminous posterior internal venous plexuses communicate with their external counterparts through longitudinal midline slits in the ligamentum flavum. The intervertebral veins drain the intraspinal blood into the vertebral, intercostal, ascending lumbar, and lateral sacral veins. The spinal veins have no valves and, therefore, reversal of the blood flow may occur.

REGIONAL CHARACTERISTICS OF THE SPINE

The Craniocervical Junction

Unlike the remainder of the vertebrae, the atlas is devoid of a vertebral body. It consists of anterior and posterior arches joined by lateral masses (Fig. 1.1). Cranially, concave articular foveas articulate with the convex condyles of the occiput. Caudally, convex articular facets articulate with the convex superior facets of the axis (Fig. 1.4). The laterally projecting transverse processes have a foramen. The characteristic odontoid process of the axis has true synovial articulation with the anterior arch of the atlas (Figs. 1.1, 1.2). The axis and atlas are anchored to the skull base by several layers of strong ligaments—the apical and lateral alar ligaments. These are covered by the strong cruciform ligament. The lateral bands of the cruciform ligament usually are well demonstrated on CT scans (Figs. 1.1, 1.2). All ligaments are covered by the broad tectorial membrane, an anterior layer of the posterior longitudinal ligament (Fig. 1.2). Posteriorly, the occiput and the atlas are connected by the thin, wide, elastic posterior atlanto-occipital membrane, which is pierced by the vertebral artery and the 1st cervical nerve. Anteriorly, the broad atlanto-occipital and atlantoepistrophic ligaments are partially hidden by the anterior longitudinal ligament.

Cervical Spine from C3 to C7

The vertebral bodies in the cervical spine (Fig. 1.7) are trapezoid in cross-section, about twice as wide from side to side than in AP dimension and with parallel end plates sloping obliquely downward anteriorly. The discs are wedge-shaped, corresponding to the cervical lordosis (Figs. 1.2, 1.5). The upper end plates present sagittal ridges, the uncinate processes, at their lateral or posterolateral margins. Together with corresponding notches in lower end plates of the vertebra above, they form the uncovertebral joints of von Luschka (Fig. 1.7). Osteoarthritic osteophytes arising from these joints may encroach upon the spinal nerve roots. Viewed from the front, the intervertebral joints in the lumbar and thoracic region project behind the pedicles, whereas the cervical facet joints expand laterally behind the vertebrae. Anterior to the facet joints, the transverse processes arise. The transverse foramen houses the vertebral artery and veins and sympathetic nerves. In the deep craniad groove of the transverse process, the spinal nerves and ganglia cross the dorsal border of the artery along with segmental vessels (Figs. 1.4, 1.7). The transverse foramen of the 7th cervical vertebra only contains vertebral veins, not the vertebral artery (Fig. 1.7). Posteriorly broad, V-shaped laminae emerge from the pedicles and conjoin to form short, dwindling, caudally sloping spinous processes, most of which have bifid tips and grooves on their lower surface (Fig. 1.5). Except for the 7th cervical vertebra, the spinous process do not reach the superficial fascia. Their inter- and supraspinous ligaments have a strong midsagittal elastic prolongation, the ligamentum nuchae (Fig. 1.5). The cervical spinal canal is wide, with a round configuration cranially and a more triangular one caudally. Epidural fat tissue is sparse, and wide venous plexuses are present in the lateral parts of the canal surrounding roots and nerves as they leave the intervertebral foramina, forming wide venous sinuses (Figs. 1.1, 1.7–1.9). The sparcity of epidural fat in the cervical canal in contrast to the lumbar canal makes it more difficult to differentiate between the soft tissue structures in the cervical spinal canal on a noncontrast CT scan.

Posteriorly, a number of short unisegmental muscles (rectus capitis superior minor and major, superior and inferior oblique) insert in the atlas (Fig. 1.4). Distal to the atlas, the multisegmental semispinalis and longissimus cervicis muscles constitute the cervical portion of the multifidus. These deep muscles are covered by the thick semispinalis and longissimus capitis, the superficial layer of the splenius capitis, and the trapezius. Laterally, the three scalenus muscles are attached to tubercles at the tips of the transverse processes. Anteriorly, the cervical vertebral column is covered by several portions of the longus capitis and the longus colli and their fascia.

Thoracic Spine

Corresponding to the thoracic kyphosis, the vertebral bodies are slightly wedge-shaped (Figs. 1.12–1.15). The upper thoracic vertebrae are commonly ovoid in cross-section with a larger sagittal than transverse diameter. Progressing caudally, they gradually become larger and broader. Accordingly, the thin discs in the upper thoracic spine get thicker at progressively lower levels. The pedicles are long and the joint facets are oriented in the coronal plane. Down to the 10th thoracic vertebra, the laminae are angulated caudally. Together with the slender, long, obliquely downward-directed spinous processes, they form overlapping osseous shingles (Figs. 1.12, 1.13). Characteristic also are the thick, round transverse processes which run obliquely craniad posteriorly to provide the costotransverse articulations at the level of the intervertebral discs. The ribs also articulate with the two adjacent vertebral bodies and the intervening disc. These costocentral joints have a thick fibrous capsule, the radiate ligament. In addition, the ribs are anchored by several strong costotransverse ligaments (Figs. 1.10, 1.11). The complex bony anatomy of the thoracic spine, together with the ribs, makes it difficult to interpret CT scans from this region. Usually several elements from two segments are displayed on the same image. Because of the length of the pedicles, the spinal canal is round or ovoid in cross-section, with a relatively large AP diameter. A thin layer of epidural fat and veins surrounds the thecal sac fairly evenly. Wide venous sinuses occupy the lateral recesses and intervertebral foramina (Figs. 1.10, 1.11, 1.16).

The thin thoracic spinal roots emerge from the thecal sac, forming short, cone-shaped axillary pouches at the inferomedial border of the pedicles. The periradicular sheaths of the dura are short. The thin thoracic spinal roots occupy a small proportion of the intervertebral foramen and present less readily on CT scans than the thick lumbosacral roots (Figs. 1.14, 1.15, 1.18). The shallow, triangular compartment between the spinous processes and the transverse processes of the thoracic spine, the posterior angles of the ribs, and the thoracolumbar fascia contains the different portions of the sacrospinal muscle (erector trunci). The deepest layer, the multifidus, is posteriorly and laterally covered by the spinalis thoracis, longissimus thoracis, iliocostalis thoracis, and lumborum. The superficial muscles of the thoracic spine form wide and thin muscular plates with mainly obliquely oriented fibers—the serratus posterior inferior, rhomboides major and minor, latissimus dorsi, and trapezius.

Between the ribs, three layers of intercostal muscles (intercostalis externus, internus, and intimus) run in different directions. Anteriorly, the crura of the diaphragm and the large vessels constitute contiguous paraspinal soft tissues.

Lumbar spine (Figs. 1.19–1.33)

The lumbar vertebral bodies are large, round, or elliptical and are wider transversely than in the sagittal plane. The lower lumbar vertebrae are slightly wedge-shaped, in accordance with the lumbar lordosis, as also are the lumbar intervertebral discs. The decided wedge configuration of the L5-S1 disc accounts for the lumbosacral angulation (Fig. 1.32). The lumbar discs are the thickest in the vertebral column (10–15 mm). The pedicles of the lumbar vertebrae are short and strong and the laminae broad and thick. The lower borders of the laminae terminate at the level of the next lower disc. The spinous processes are heavy and more rectangular. The superior articular processes diverge both cranially and dorsally (Figs. 1.21, 1.22, 1.31). Their posterior processes—the mamillary processes—are rounded enlargements for the attachment of muscles (Fig. 1.22). Short accessory processes project from the dorsal inferior surface of the base of the transverse processes. They constitute distinct landmarks on axial CT scans through the lower portion of the pedicles (Figs. 1.19, 1.20).

In cross-sectional displays, the lumbar facet joints frequently assume a biplanar or curvilinear configuration, with the anterior portions oriented toward the coronal plane and the posterior ones more sagittal (Fig. 1.26). The transverse processes are flattened anteroposteriorly and run slightly dorsally and upward. They are conjoined by the intertransverse ligaments which laterally are continuous with the lumbar aponeurosis. The transverse processes of the 5th lumbar vertebra are attached to the iliac crest by the iliolumbar ligaments. Not infrequently these processes articulate or are fused with the iliac bones.

The short pedicles and thick laminae account for the increasingly triangular shape of the lumbar spinal canal toward the lower lumbar spine with the lateral recesses forming rather acute angles at the base of the pedicles. The posterior notch of the posterior arch is deep. The transverse diameter of the canal increases from L1 to L5 whereas the AP diameter decreases. The volume of the thecal sac is related inversely to the amount of epidural tissue and varies within wide ranges. The location of the roots of the cauda equina depends on the position of the patient and does not seem to follow a strict pattern, except for the fact that the roots bound to emergence at the next lower level lie anterolaterally in the thecal sac. A triangular pad of fat with sparse veins of the dorsal internal plexus fills out the acute angle between the two plates of the ligamentum flavum, whereas there is little fat inside the inner notch of the lamina (Figs. 1.19–1.28). The posterior longitudinal ligament may bridge over the posterior concavity of the vertebral body from one disc to another in a bowstring fashion. Owing to this concavity and to the wide venous outlets at the midcorporal level of the vertebra, the spinal canal may assume a diamond configuration (Figs. 1.19, 1.20). In these cases, the posterior longitudinal ligament lies within the spinal canal at a considerable distance from the posterior border of the vertebra. As this ligament is denser than the surrounding tissues, it is often visible on unenhanced CT scans. Together with the retrovertebral venous plexuses, the posterior longitudinal ligament delimits the anterior border of the thecal sac.

Surrounded by connective and fat tissue with fewer veins than in the cervical and thoracic spine, the thick lumbar spinal ganglia occupy the upper portion of the intervertebral foramen (Figs. 1.23–1.25, 1.35). The intervertebral veins are mainly located in the lower portion of the foramen lying between the disc and the ligamentum flavum (Fig. 1.33). The spinal branch of the segmental artery and the sinuvertebral nerve take their course through the upper portion of the foramen.

The dorsal muscle compartment is delimited medially by the spinous processes, anteriorly by the transverse processes and the middle layer of the lumbodorsal fascia, the lumbar aponeurosis, which forms a strong membrane extending from the 12th rib to the iliac crest, and posteriorly by the very coarse posterior lamina of the lumbosacral fascia which distally thickens to form the origin of the sacrospinalis and latissimus dorsi. The transverse processes are connected by three short segmental intertransverse muscles and the intertransverse ligament. The medial intertransverse muscles pass from the mamillary process of the inferior vertebra to the accessory process of the superior vertebra. The muscle strands of the multifidus overlying the posterior arch are separated by layers of fat tissue, which also house the dorsal external venous plexuses, whereas the more superificial layers of the sacrospinalis mainly consist of muscle tissue. In the lumbosacral region, the muscle is homogeneous in cross-section (Fig. 1.34). In the upper lumbar spine, its most lateral portion, the iliocostalis, an intermediate portion, the longissimus, and a medial portion, the spinalis (thoracis) may be distinguished on CT scans (Figs. 1.20–1.28). Occasionally the interspinalis may present on either side of the spinous processes and interspinous ligaments (Figs. 1.22, 1.24). The quadratus lumborum is located anterior to the lumbar aponeurosis. Between the quadratus lumborum and the lumbar aponeurosis and beneath the psoas major, the thick trunks of the lumbosacral nerve plexuses run obliquely downward. The psoas major occupies the grooves on either side of the spinal column and is covered by the anterior layer of the lumbodorsal fascia—the internal abdominal fascia (Figs. 1.19–1.29).

On contiguous CT cuts through the lumbar spine parallel with the end plates of the vertebral bodies, significant reiterative changes of the morphology are observed consistently at different levels within each motion segment unit. The typical landmarks of three such levels are listed below:

1. CT scans through the lower portion of the pedicles (Figs. 1.19, 1.20) show the smallest cross-sectional extension of the vertebral body, the coarse cancellous bone, and large central venous sinuses, and frequently, the typical Y-configuration of the basivertebral vein with its anterior and posterior outlets. They also show the dense cortical bone of the pedicles, the thin upper portion of the lamina with the ligamentum flavum at its posterior border, and the upper portion of the spinous process together with a varying portion of the interspinous ligament posteriorly. Two typical tubercles project dorsally from the pedicle:

the accessory process (lateral) and the base of the upper articular process (medial).

2. CT scans through the intervertebral disc (Figs. 1.21, 1.22, 1.26) and the facet joints demonstrate the maximal circumference of the anulus fibrosus, usually well outlined from the less radiopaque central nucleus pulposus. Toward the adjacent vertebral end plates, a ring of bone, the anular apophysis, may be distinguished from the less dense cartilage end plate in the center, which occasionally shows irregular bony projections. The narrow lower portion of the intervertebral foramen between the disc and the superior articular facet mainly contains veins and fat tissue. The spinal nerves lie outside the spine between the disc and the psoas muscle. Posteriorly, the central portion of the facet joints and the lower portion of the spine of the vertebra above may present as separate portions of bone, conjoined by a Y-shaped ligamentous complex of the ligamentum flavum and the interspinous ligament.

3. CT scans through the lower portion of the vertebral body (Figs. 1.23–1.25) show a greater cross-sectional extension of the vertebral body, and the upper portion of the intervertebral foramen with the dorsal root ganglion. Also seen is the thick base of the inferior articular process, which anterolaterally is covered by the ligamentum flavum constituting the upper portion of the facet joint capsule. The tips of the superior articular processes of the next lower vertebra may be visualized at the anterolateral aspect of the inferior articular processes. Posteriorly the spinous processes usually present in their full length, with the supraspinous ligament extending laterally on either side of their tips.

Sacrum (Figs. 1.34, 1.35)

The sacrum is a thick, curved, triangular bone which has coalesced to form a solid mass from five sacral vertebral segments. Its cranial surface carries the end plate for the lumbosacral disc and the superior articular processes. The thick pars lateralis (ala) bears ear-shaped articular surfaces for the sacroiliac joint anteriorly.

The anterior surface of the sacrum is concave, with transverse ridges indicating the remains of the intervertebral discs. These ridges point at the wide, deeply grooved anterior (pelvic) foramina, the exits of the ventral rami of the sacral nerves. On the convex posterior surface corresponding posterior foramina are found. A median crest of more or less fused spinous tubercles forms a continuation of the spinous processes of the lumbar vertebrae. Less pronounced longitudinal crests on either side of the posterior foramen (exits of the dorsal rami of the sacral nerves) serve as attachments for the sacrospinalis muscle. The sacral canal is narrow in the AP view and triangular in cross-section.

The osseoligamentous space between the spinous crest, the iliac bone, and the thick thoracolumbar fascia houses the multifidus muscle and the origin of the sacrospinalis.

References

1. Hammerschlag SB, Wolpert SM, Carter BL: Computed tomography of the spinal canal. *Radiology* 121:361–367, 1976.
2. Coin CG, Chan YS, Keranen V, et al: Computer assisted myelography in disk disease. *J Comput Assist Tomogr* 1:398–404, 1977.
3. Lee BCP, Kazam E, Newman AD: Computed tomography of the spine and spinal cord. *Radiology* 128:95–102, 1978.
4. Roub LW, Drayer BP: Spinal computed tomography: limitations and applications. *AJR* 133:267–273, 1979.
5. Carrera GF, Haughton VM, Syvertsen A, et al: Computed tomography of the lumbar facet joints. *Radiology* 134:145–148, 1980.
6. Carrera GF, Williams AL, Haughton VM: Computed tomography in sciatica. *Radiology* 137:433–437, 1980.
7. Coin CG: Computed tomography of the spine. In Post MJD. *Radiographic Evaluation of the Spine: Current Advances with Emphasis on Computed Tomography.* New York, Masson Publishing, Inc., 1980, pp. 394–412.
8. Livingston PA, Grayson EV: Computed tomography in the diagnosis of herniated discs in the lumbar spine. In Post MJD: *Radiographic Evaluation of the Spine: Current Advances with Emphasis on Computed Tomography.* New York, Masson Publishing, Inc., 1980, pp. 308–319.
9. Post MJD: CT-update: The impact of time, metrizamide and high resolution on the diagnosis of spinal pathology. In Post MJD: *Radiographic Evaluation of the Spine: Current Advances with Emphasis on Computed Tomography.* New York, Masson Publishing, Inc., 1980, pp. 259–294.
10. Sartor K: Spinale Computertomographie. *Radiologe* 20:485–493, 1980.
11. Williams AL, Haughton VM, Syvertsen A: Computed tomography in the diagnosis of herniated nucleus pulposus. *Radiology* 135:95–99. 1980.
12. Genant HK: Computed tomography. In Resnick D, Niwayama G: *Diagnosis of Bone and Joint Disorders.* Philadelphia, W. B. Saunders, pp. 380–408, 1981.
13. Hirschy JC, Leue WM, Berninger WH, et al: CT of the lumbosacral spine: Importance of tomographic planes parallel to vertebral end plates. *AJR* 126:47–52, 1981.
14. Post MJD, Gargano FP, Vining D, et al: A comparison of radiographic methods of diagnosing constrictive lesions of the spinal canal. Toshiba unit vs. CT scanner. *J. Neurosurg* 48:360–368, 1978.
15. Jacobson RE, Gargano FP, Rosomoff HL: Transverse axial tomography of the spine. Part 1: Axial anatomy of the normal lumbar spine. *J Neurosurg* 42:406–411, 1975.
16. Gargano FP: Transverse axial tomography of the spine. *CRC Crit Rev Clin Radiol Nuclear Med* 8:279–328, 1976.
17. Ethier R, King DG, Melançon D, et al: Development of high resolution computed tomography of the spinal cord. *J Comput Assist Tomogr* 3:433–438, 1979.
18. Haughton VM, Syvertsen A, Williams AL: Soft-tissue anatomy within the spinal canal as seen on computed tomography. *Radiology* 134:649–655, 1980.
19. King DG: Computed tomography of the spine: Resolution requirements and scanning techniques to achieve them. In Post MJD: *Radiographic Evaluation of the Spine: Current Advances with Emphasis on Computed Tomography.* New York, Masson Publishing, Inc., 1980, pp. 366–376.
20. Naidich TP, King DG, Moran CJ, et al: Computed tomography of the lumbar thecal sac. *J Comput Assist Tomogr* 4:37–41, 1980.
21. Bonafé A, Ethier R, Melançon D, et al: High resolution computed tomography in cervical syringomyelia. *J Comput Assist Tomogr* 4:42–47, 1980.
22. Bidgood WD, Scatliff JH: Experimental evaluation of computed tomography of spinal canal contents. In Post MJD: *Radiographic Evaluation of the Spine: Current Advances with Emphasis on Computed Tomography.* New York, Masson Publishing, Inc., 1980, pp. 413–421.
23. Raskin SP: Demonstration of nerve roots on unenhanced computed tomographic scans. *J Comput Assist Tomogr* 5:281–284, 1981.
24. Isherwood I, Fawcitt RA, ClairForbes W, et al: Computer tomography of the spinal canal using metrizamide. *Acta Radiol (Diagn) Suppl* 355:299–305, 1977.

25. Di Chiro G, Schellinger D: Computed tomography of spinal cord after lumbar intrathecal introduction of metrizamide (computer assisted myelography). *Radiology* 120:101–104, 1976.

26. Coin CG, Coin PG: Double-exposure technique in computerized tomography of the spine. *Comput Tomogr* 3:97–99, 1979.

27. Arii H, Takahashi M, Tamakawa Y, et al: Metrizamide spinal computed tomography following myelography. *Comput Tomogr* 4:117–125, 1980.

28. Takahashi S: *An Atlas of Axial Transverse Tomography and its Clinical Application.* Berlin-Heidelberg-New York, Springer Verlag, 1969.

29. Eyclesheimer AC, Schoemaker DM: *A Cross-Section Anatomy.* New York, D. Appleton and Company, 1911, Re-edited by Appleton-Century-Crofts, 1970.

30. Potter GD: *Sectional Anatomy and Tomography of the Head.* New York, 1971. Grune & Stratton.

31. Rabischong P, Vignaud J, Paleirac R, et al: *Tomographie et Anatomie de l'Oreille.* Amsterdam, Art Graphique Lamoth, 1975.

32. Valvassori GE, Buckingham RA: *Tomography and Cross-Sections of the Ear.* Stuttgart, Georg Thieme Publishers, 1975.

33. Alfidi RJ, Haaga J, Weinstein M, et al: *Computed Tomography of the Human Body. An Atlas of Normal Anatomy.* St Louis, C.V. Mosby Company, 1977.

34. Carter BL: Cross-sectional anatomy. Computed tomography and ultrasound correlation (adapted from: Eyclesheimer AC, Schoemaker DM: *A Cross-Section Anatomy,* 1911), New York, Appleton-Century-Crofts, 1977.

35. Gambarelli J, Guérinel G, Chevrot L, et al: Computerized axial tomography. *An Anatomic Atlas of Serial Sections of the Human Body. Anatomy-Radiology-Scanner.* Berlin-Heidelberg-New York, Springer Verlag, 1977.

36. Ledley RS, Huang HK, Mazziotta JC: *Cross-Sectional Anatomy. An Atlas for Computed Tomography.* Baltimore, Williams & Wilkins, 1977.

37. Matsukawa A, Ito T, Kimura K: *Cross-Section Anatomy and Computed Tomography.* Tokyo, Jgaku Tosho Shuppan, 1977.

38. Lyons EA: *A Color Atlas of Sectional Anatomy. Chest, Abdomen and Pelvis.* St Louis, C.V. Mosby, 1978.

39. Matsui T, Hirano A: *An Atlas of the Human Brain for Computerized Tomography.* Tokyo-New York, Igaku-Shoin, 1978.

40. Wyman AC, Lawson TL, Goodman LR: Transverse anatomy of the human thorax, abdomen and pelvis. *An Atlas of Anatomic, Radiologic, Computed Tomographic, and Ultrasonic Correlation.* Boston, Little, Brown, 1978.

41. Kieffer SA, Heitzman ER: *An Atlas of Cross-Sectional Anatomy. Computed Tomography, Ultrasound, Radiography, Gross Anatomy.* Hagerstown, Harper and Row, 1979.

42. Lancourt JE, Glenn WV, Wiltse LL: Multiplanar computerized tomography in the normal spine and in the diagnosis of spinal stenosis. A gross anatomic-computerized tomographic correlation. *Spine* 4:379–390, 1979.

43. Aquilonius SM, Eckernäs SÅ: *A Color Atlas of the Human Brain. Adapted to Computed Tomography.* Stockholm, Esselte Studium, 1980.

44. Bo WJ, Meschan J, Krueger WA: *Basic Atlas of Cross-Sectional Anatomy.* Philadelphia, W.B. Saunders, 1980.

45. Chiu LC, Schapiro RL: *Atlas of Computed Body Tomography. Normal and Abnormal Anatomy.* Baltimore, University Park Press, 1980.

46. Hanaway J, Scott WR, Strother CM: *Atlas of the Human Brain and the Orbit for Computed Tomography,* 2nd ed. St Louis, Green, 1980.

47. Kirkaldy-Willis WH, Heithoff K, Bowen CVA, et al: Pathological anatomy of lumbar spondylosis and stenosis, correlated with the CT scan. In Post MJD: *Radiographic Evaluation of the Spine: Current Advances with Emphasis on Computed Tomography.* New York, Masson Publishing, Inc., 1980, pp. 34–55.

48. Palacios E, Fine M, Haughton VM: *Multiplanar Anatomy of the Head and Neck for Computed Tomography.* New York, John Wiley & Sons, 1980.

49. Peterson RR: *A Cross-Sectional Approach to Anatomy.* Chicago, Year Book Medical Publishers, 1980.

50. Thompson JR, Hasso AN: *Correlative Sectional Anatomy of the Head and Neck. A Color Atlas.* St Louis, Toronto, London, C. V. Mosby, 1980.

51. Thron A, Bockenheimer S: Technik und diagnostischer Wert der lumbalen Funktionsmyelographie beim Bandscheibenprolaps. *Fortschr Röntgenstr* 130:81–84, 1979.

52. Sortland O, Magnaes B, Hauge T: Functional myelography with metrizamide in the diagnosis of lumbar spinal stenosis. *Acta Radiologica (Diagn)* Suppl 355:42–54, 1977.

53. Rauschning W: Popliteal cysts and their relation to the gastrocnemio-semimembranosus bursa. Studies on the surgical and functional anatomy. *Acta Orthop Scand* Suppl 179:1–43, 1979.

54. Ullberg S: The technique of whole body autoradiography. Cryosectioning of large specimens. *Science Tools,* Special Issue, 2–29, 1977.

55. Wittenberg J, Maturi A, Ferruci T, et al: Computerized tomography of in vitro abdominal organs—effect of preservation methods on attenuation coefficient. *Comput Tomog* 1:95–101, 1977.

56. Hemingsson A, Johansson A, Rauschning W: Attenuation in human muscle and fat tissue in vivo and in vitro. *Acta Radiol* (Stockh) 23:149–151, 1982.

57. Ullrich CG, Kieffer SA: Computed tomographic evaluation of the lumbar spine: Quantitative aspects and sagittal-coronal reconstruction. In Post MJD: *Radiographic Evaluation of Spine: Current Advances with Emphasis on Computed Tomography,* New York, Masson Publishing, Inc., 1980, pp. 88–107.

58. Herman GT, Coin CG: The use of three-dimensional computer display in the study of disk disease. *J Comput Assist Tomogr* 4:564–567, 1980.

59. Glenn WV Jr, Rhodes ML, Altschuler EM: Multiplanar computerized tomography of lumbar disc abnormalities: The proponent's viewpoint. In Post MJD: *Radiographic Evaluation of the Spine: Current Advances with Emphasis on Computed Tomography.* New York, Masson Publishing, Inc., 1980, pp. 108–138.

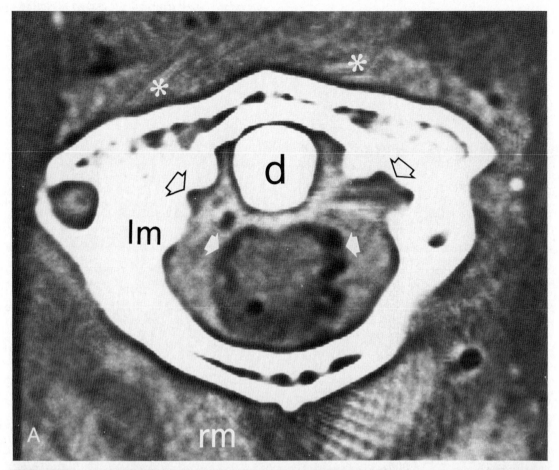

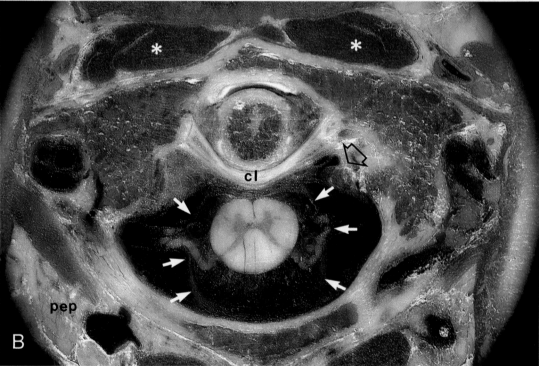

Figure 1.1. Axial CT scan (A) and anatomical section (B) through the upper portion of the atlas. Note the synovial joint between the dens (*d*) and the atlas and the lateral bands of the cruciform ligament (*cl*) inserting in deep notches (*open arrows*) in the lateral masses (*lm*). The vertebral artery is seen in the right transverse foramen. The subarachnoid space with the cord and root filaments is well outlined (*solid arrowheads*). The attentuation of the CSF is low, its dark color on the anatomical section is caused by hemorrhage (*white arrows*). The thecal sac is surrounded by wide homogeneous blood sinuses (*rm* = rectus capitis major, *pep* = posterior external venous plexuses; * = rectus capitis anterius and longus capitis).

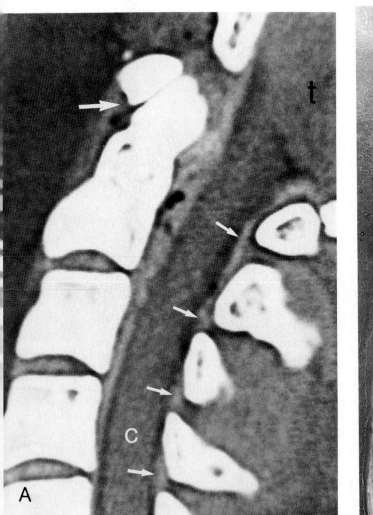
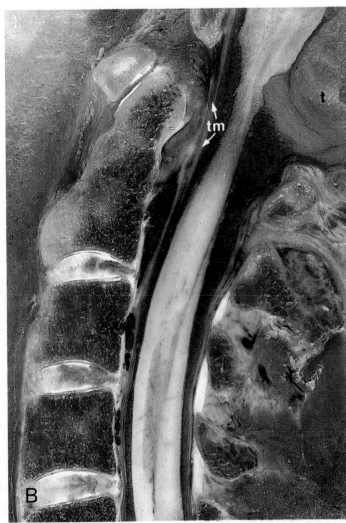

Figure 1.2.   Sagittal, slightly paramedian CT scan (A) and anatomical section (B) through the upper cervical spine. Note the tonsil of the cerebellum (*t*), the spinal cord (*c*), arthritis in the joint between the dens and the atlas (*arrow*). The tectorial membrane (*tm*) covers the transverse bands of the cruciform ligament. Note the absence of epidural fat. The ligamentum flavum is well outlined (*small arrows*).

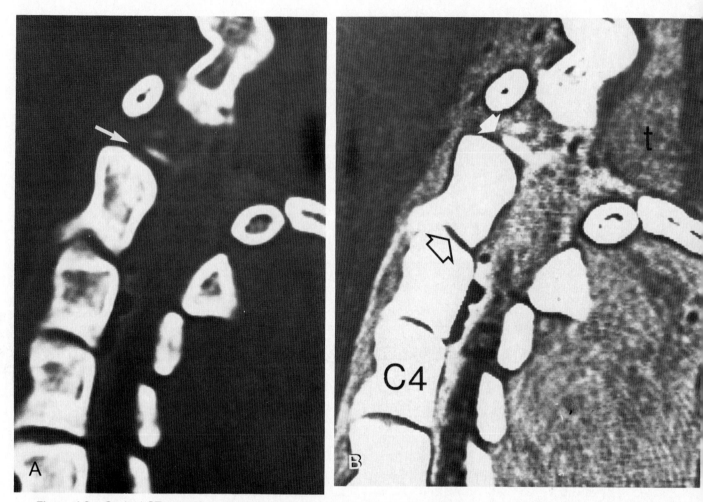

Figure 1.3.   Sagittal CT scan (A = osseous image, B = soft-tissue image) and anatomical section (C, D = detail) through the lateral recesses of the upper cervical spine. Note the tonsil of the cerebellum (*t*), the medial border of the atlantoaxial joint (*filled arrow*), the uncovertebral joint between C2 and C3 (*open arrow*). The thin cervical nerve roots (*white arrows*) are surrounded by wide venous sinuses. At C4 and C5, the subarachnoid space is opened exposing the dorsal and ventral rootlet filaments (*r*). The CSF is frozen to ice (*oi* = obliquus capitis inferius, *sc* = semispinalis capitis).

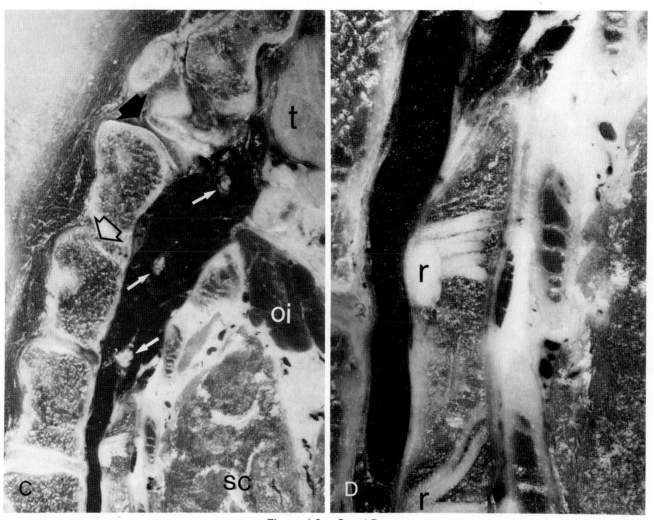

Figure 1.3.   C and D.

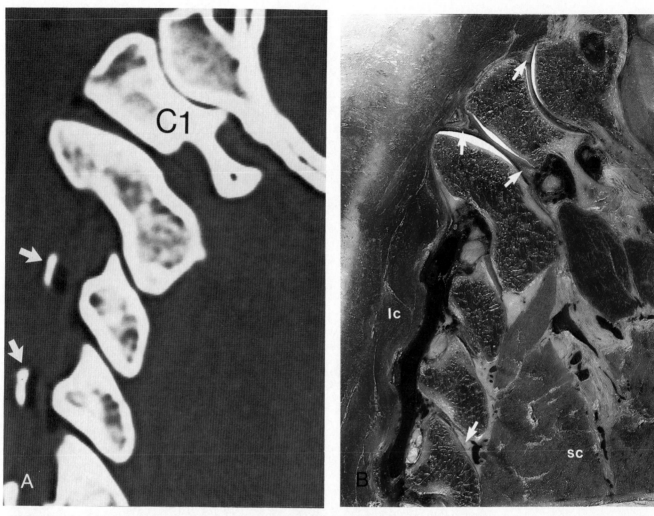

Figure 1.4.   Sagittal CT scan (A), anatomical section (B), and anatomical details (C and D) through the facet joints and the vertebral artery of the upper cervical spine. Meniscoid synovial folds project into the atlantoaxial joint and the facet joints (*arrows*). At this level, the crossway of the vertebral artery (*va*) and the spinal nerves (*sn*) and ganglia is seen. *Arrows* indicate the transverse processes on the CT scan. (*hy* = hypoglossal canal and nerve, *lc* = longus colli, *oi* = obliquus capitis inferius, *sc* = semispinalis cervicis).

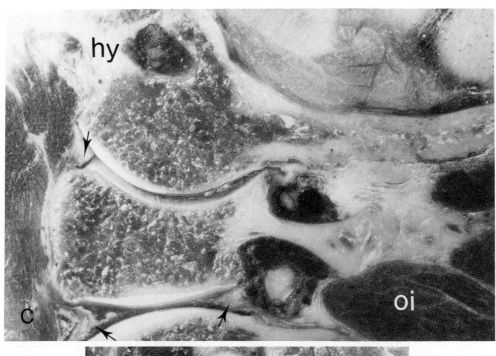

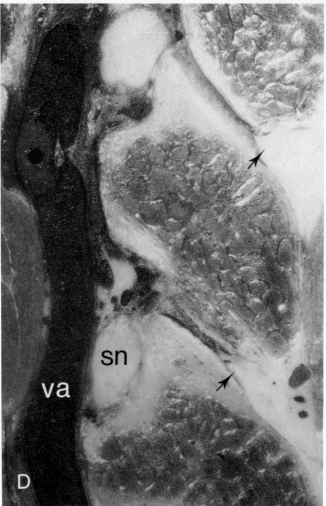

Figure 1.4.   C and D.

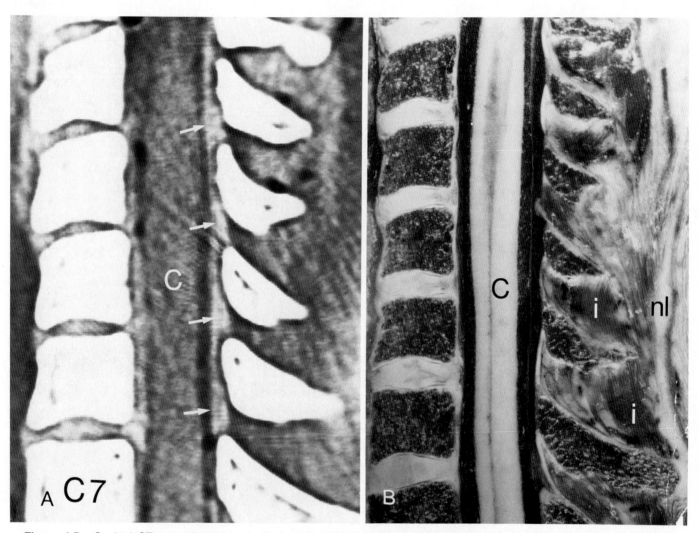

Figure 1.5.   Sagittal CT scan (A) and anatomical section (B) through the lower cervical spine. The spinal cord (*c*) and the ligamentum flavum (*arrows*) are well demonstrated on the CT scan (*nl* = nuchal ligament, *i* = interspinalis muscle).

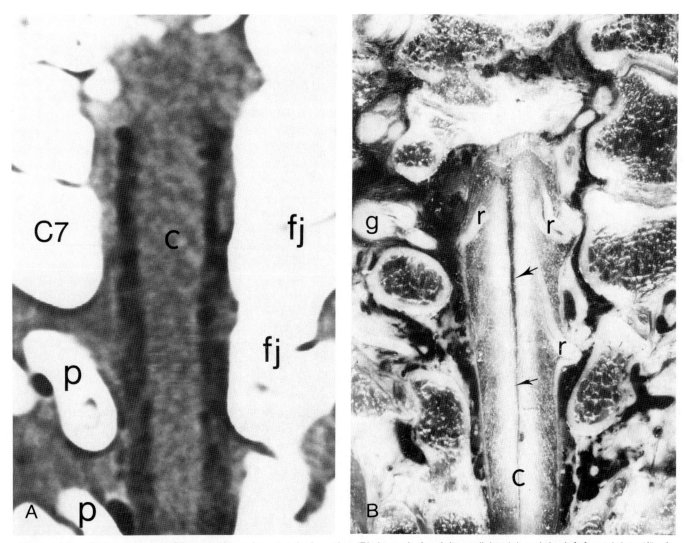

Figure 1.6.   Oblique coronal CT scan (A) and anatomical section (B) through the right pedicles (*p*) and the left facet joints (*fj*) of the lower cervical and upper thoracic spine. The spinal cord (*c*) is exposed showing the ventral longitudinal spinal artery (*arrows*) and obliquely caudad running ventral nerve rootlets (*r*). Venous sinuses surround the nerve roots and ganglia (*g*) in the lateral recesses and the intervertebral foramina.

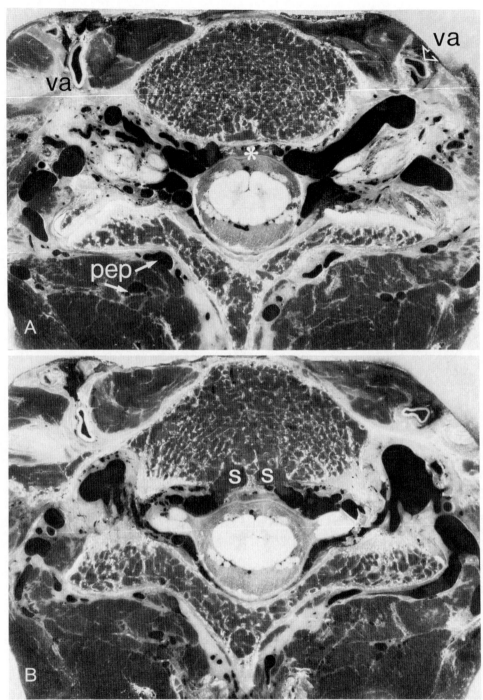

Figure 1.7.   Sequence of axial anatomical sections progressing from C7 to C6 and with 3 mm between the cuts. The vertebral artery (*va*) runs through the transverse foramen of C6 (in Fig. 1.7G) but outside the C7 transverse foramen (Fig. 1.7A). The posterior longitudinal ligament (*) is well outlined on all sections. It covers the sinoid venous outlets (*s*) of the C7 vertebral body (Fig. 1.7B). Note the triangular shape of the spinal canal and the marked lateral recesses on Figure 1.7C. Figure 1.7D shows the upper border of the lamina and the upper cartilaginous end plate of C7. A small protrusion (*arrow*) is seen in the C6–C7 disc (Fig. 17E) as well as the thin ventral spinal nerve root and the dorsal root ganglion (*g*) crossing the vertebral artery. Note also the uncinate process (*up*) of C7. Figure 1.7G shows the lower body and lamina of C6 and the preganglionic spinal nerve roots. Wide posterior external venous plexuses (*pep*) cover the vertebral arches posteriorly.

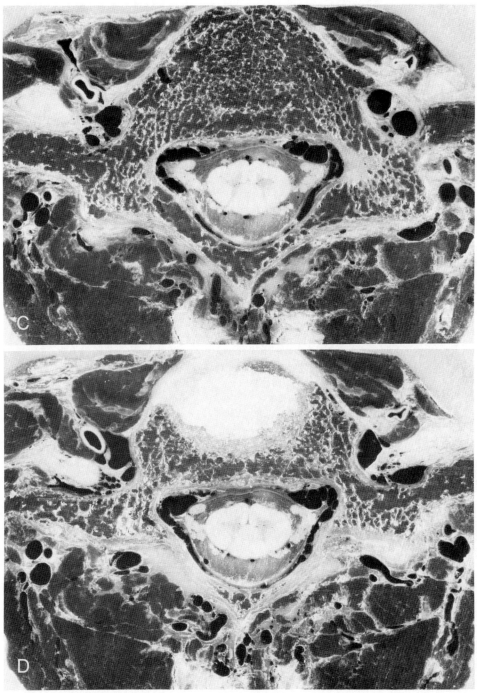

Figure 1.7. C and D.

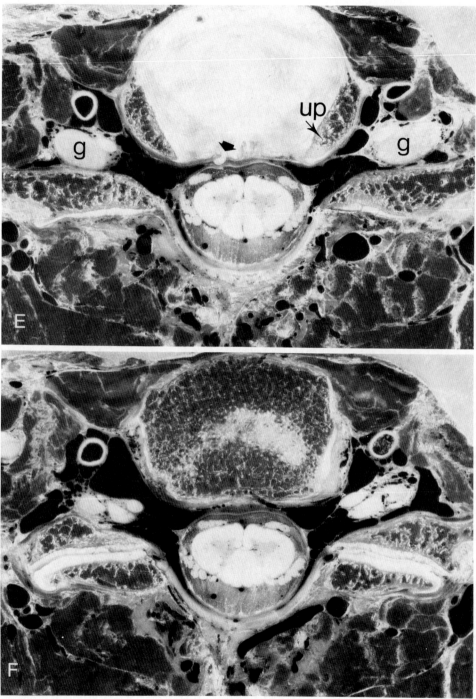

Figure 1.7.   E and F.

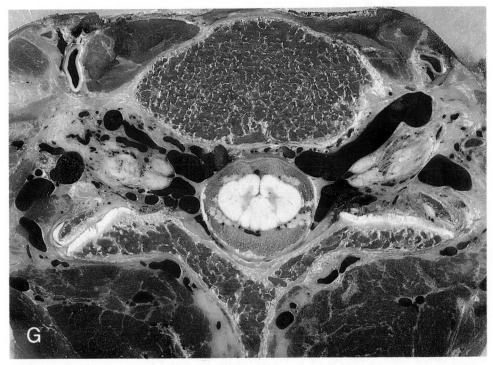

Figure 1.7.   G.

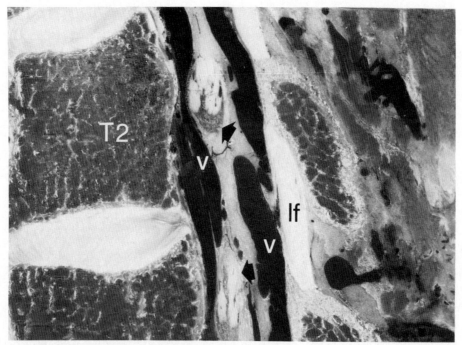

Figure 1.8.   Sagittal anatomical section through the lateral recess of the upper thoracic spine. The ventral and dorsal internal venous plexuses (*v*) surround vaginal extensions of the thecal sac with the spinal nerve roots (*arrows*). A narrow septum of fat tissue extends longitudinally between the root sheaths. (*lf* = ligamentum flavum.)

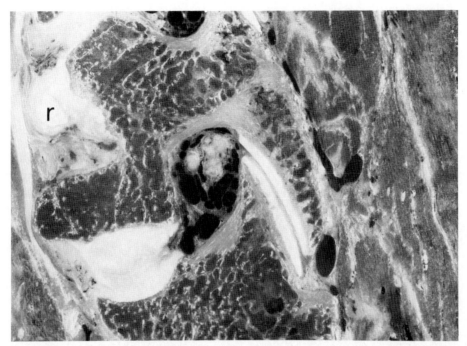

Figure 1.9.   Sagittal anatomical section through the lateral portion of the T1–T2 intervertebral foramen. Note the location of the spinal nerve roots in the subpedicular gutter of the foramen. The vertebral body articulates with the first rib (*r*).

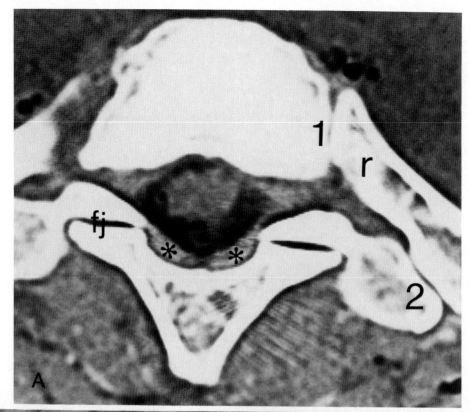

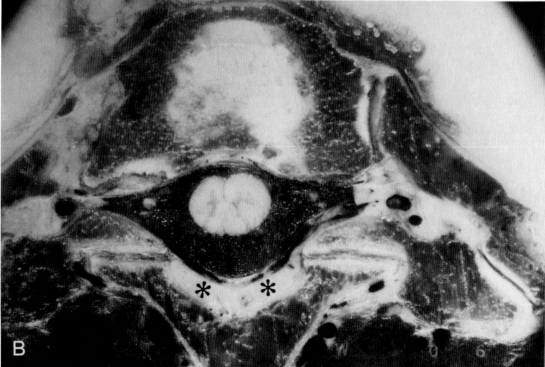

Figure 1.10.   Axial CT scan (A) and anatomical section (B) through the upper end plate of T3. Note the inferior portion of the T2 lamina with the ligamentum flavum anteriorly (*). The facet joints (*fj*) are oriented in the coronal plane. The costocentral (*1*) and the costotransverse joints (*2*) articulating with the third rib (*r*) are clearly outlined on the left side.

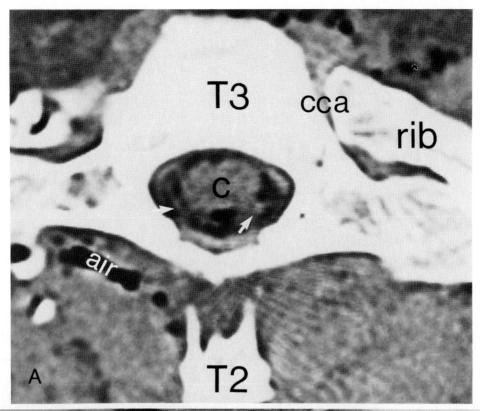

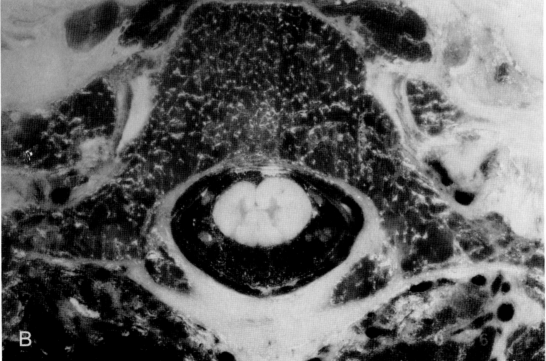

Figure 1.11.   Axial CT scan (A) and anatomical section (B) through the pedicle and the upper border of T3. Posteriorly the spinous process of T2 projects. The thecal sac is evenly surrounded by a thin layer of internal venous plexuses but no epidural fat. Air-filled veins are seen dorsal to the right lamina. The spinal cord (c) and rootlets (*arrows*) are visible on this unenhanced CT scan (*cca* = costocentral articulation).

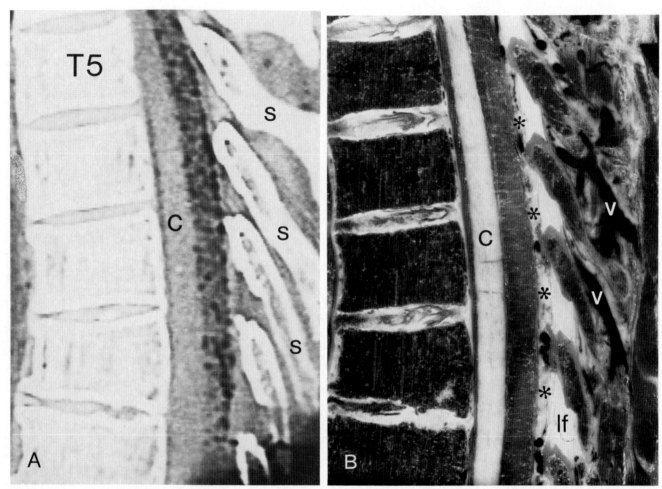

Figure 1.12.   Sagittal, slightly paramedian CT scan (A) and anatomical section (B) through the midthoracic spine. The CSF of this specimen contains small air bubbles which sharply delineates the spinal cord (*c*) in the anterior portion of the subarachnoid space. Note the wedge shape of the vertebral bodies and the shingling of the spinous processes (*s*). No extradural fat is seen ventrally. Posteriorly fat pads (*) occupy the inner border of the thick ligamentum flavum (*lf*). Note also the relationship of the wide posterior venous plexuses (*v*) to the laminae and spinous processes.

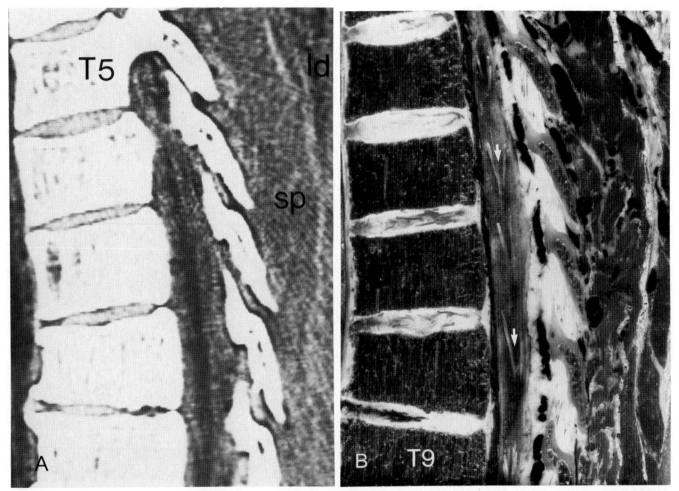

Figure 1.13.   Sagittal CT scan (A) and anatomical section (B) through the lateral resesses of the midthoracic spine. Laterally in the thecal sac the ventral and dorsal roots (*arrows*) conjoin towards the intervertebral foramina (*sp* = sacrospinalis, *ld* = latissimus dorsi).

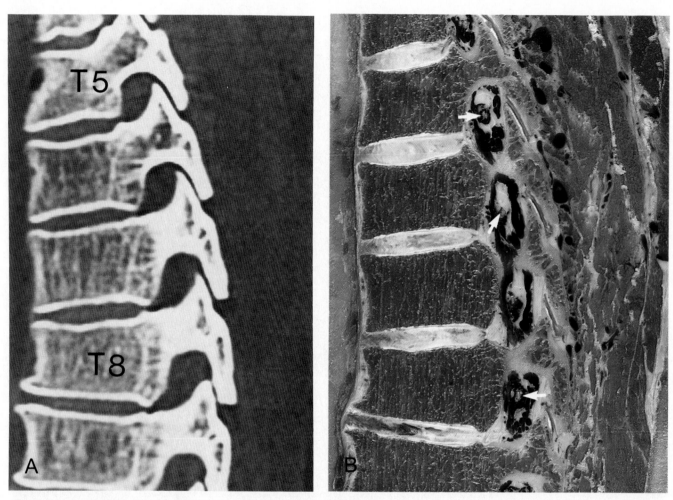

Figure 1.14.   Sagittal CT scan (A) and anatomical section (B) through the intervertebral foramina and facet joints of the midthoracic spine (T4–T9). The pedicles are long. Only a small proportion of the large, oval foramina is occupied by the thin thoracic nerve roots (*arrows*). Note the voluminous segmental venous plexuses and the relative sparsity of fat in the foramina. The T8 disc is degenerated.

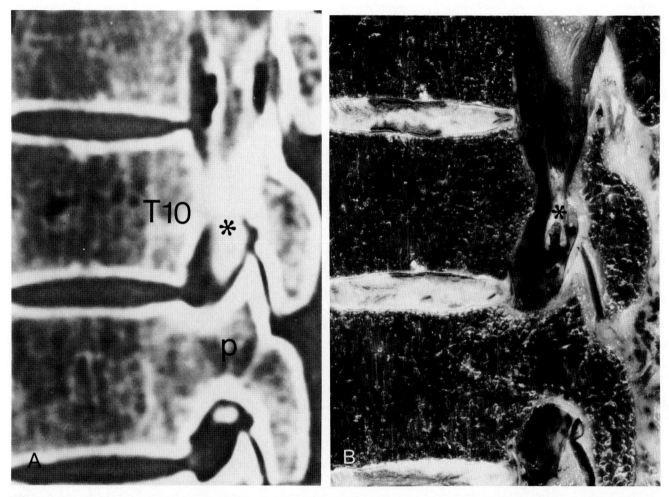

Figure 1.15. Contrast enhanced sagittal CT scan (A) and anatomical section (B) through the lateral recess of T10 and the intervertebral foramen of T11 showing the relationship of the short thoracic root sleeve (*) to the pedicle (*p*).

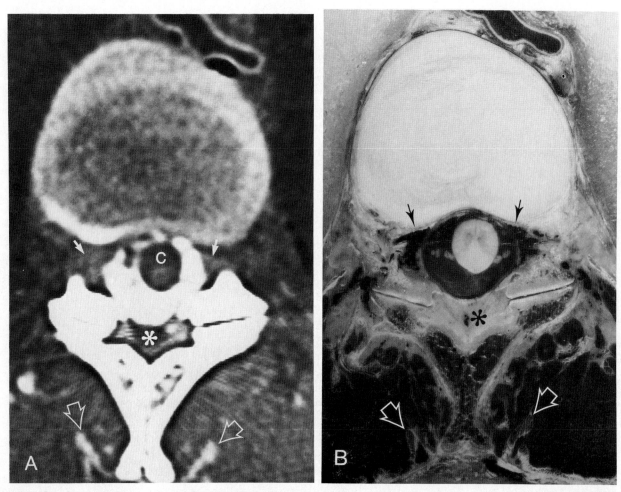

Figure 1.16.   Contrast enhanced axial CT scan (A) and anatomical section (B) through the T6–T7 disc. The thecal sac is almost round. The spinal cord (*c*) and some nerve roots are seen. The ligamentum flavum and a triangular fat pad fill the notch of the T6 lamina (*). Extradural venous plexuses (*filled arrows*) lateral to the dura can be distinguished from epidural fat. The anulus fibrosus and the anular apophysis are denser than the nucleus pulposus. Note the tendons adjacent to the tips of the spinous process (*open arrows*).

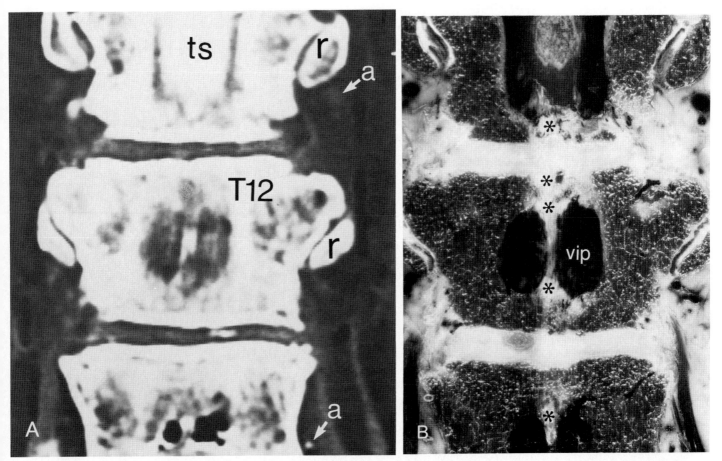

Figure 1.17.   Contrast enhanced coronal CT scan (A) and anatomical section (B) through the posterior border of the vertebrae of the thoracolumbar junction. The 11th and 12th ribs (*r*) articulate with the vertebral bodies. The spinal canal is opened anteriorly at the concavity of the vertebrae exposing the posterior longitudinal ligament (*) and the contiguous retrovertebral venous plexuses (*vip*) and the thecal sac (*ts*). Note also the outline of the segmental arteries (*a*).

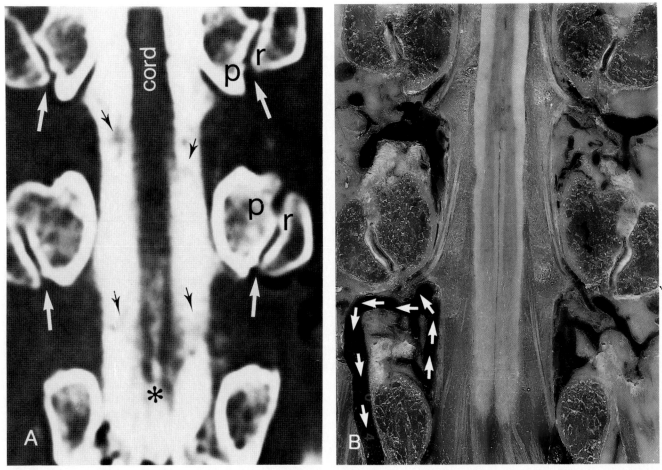

Figure 1.18. Contrast enhanced coronal CT scan (A) and anatomical section (B) through the pedicles at the thoracolumbar junction. Note the termination of the spinal cord (*). The spinal roots are faintly seen (*black arrows*). The ribs (*r*) also articulate with the base of the pedicles (*white arrows*). The (dorsal) nerve roots in the lateral recesses snugly follow the inner contour of the pedicles (*p*) piercing the thecal sac by short, strut-formed sleeves of the dura. Wide venous sinuses intermingled with epidural fat border the dura laterally. The course of the segmental vein in the right T12 intervertebral foramen is well demonstrated on the anatomical section (*white arrows*).

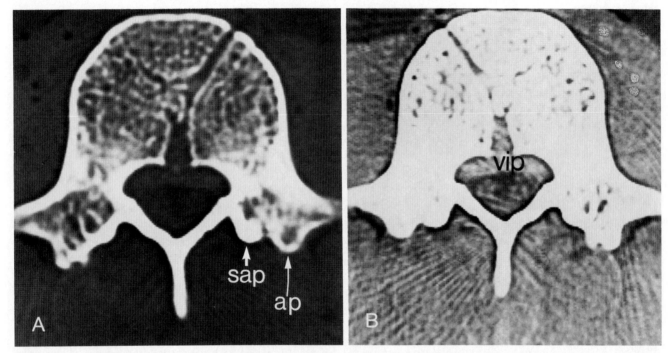

Figure 1.19.   Axial CT scan (A = bone window, B = soft-tissue window) and anatomical section (C and D = detail) through the pedicle of L4 (Specimen P 33). The coarse spongiosa of the vertebral body is transgressed by the basivertebral vein which communicates with the ventral external and internal venous plexuses (*vip*). The posterior longitudinal ligament covers the wide sinusoid outlet of the *vip* and also delimits the thecal sac anteriorly. The vaginal extensions of the dura with the spinal nerve roots (*curved arrows*) lie in the lateral recesses [*ap* = accessory process, *sap* = base of the superior articular process, *i* = interspinalis muscle, *s* = sacrospinalis (thoracis), *l* = longissimus (thoracis), *p* = psoas major].

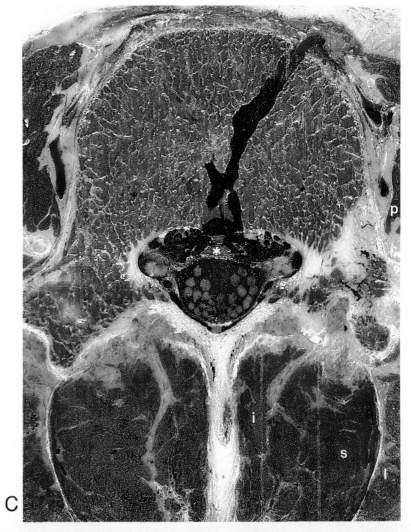

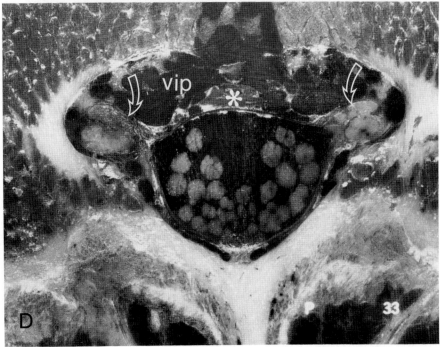

Figure 1.19. C and D.

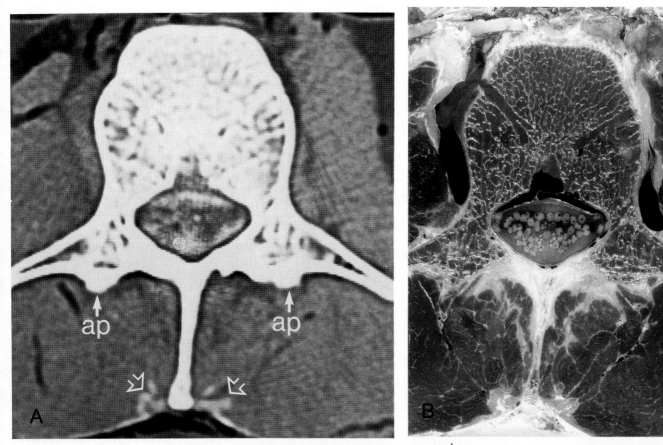

Figure 1.20.   (cf Fig. 1.19).   Contrast enhanced axial CT scan (A) and anatomical section (B) through the lower portion of the pedicle of L4 (Specimen V 30). Note the diamond-configuration of the spinal canal and the width of the thecal sac (*white arrows*). The ventral external venous plexuses communicate with the basivertebral vein. The spinous process is displayed at its whole length with strong portions of the supraspinous ligament on either sides of its tips (*open arrows*) (ap = accessory process).

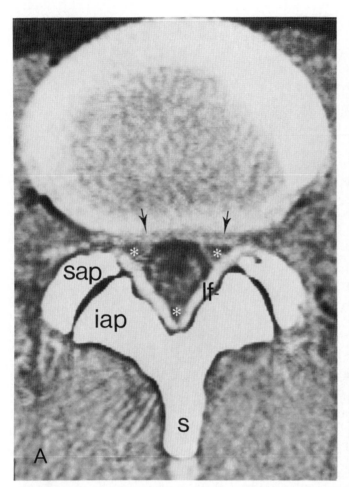
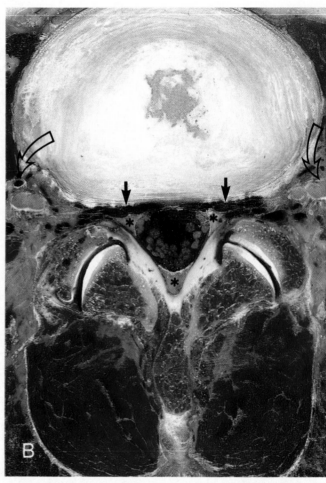

Figure 1.21.   Axial CT scans (A and C = detail) and anatomical sections (B and D = detail) through the L3–L4 disc (Specimen P 33). Sections A and D are slightly more craniad than B and C. Note the structure of the disc, the dense retrodiscal venous plexuses (*filled black arrows*), the triangular fat pads in the lateral recesses and the posterior angle between the laminae (*). Sagittal grooves on the lower aspect of the lamina "separate" the inferior articular processes (*iap*) from the spinous process (*s*) of L3. The ligamentum flavum (*lf*) forms a thick arcade at the ventral aspect of the superior articular processes (*sap*) of L4. The posterior capsule of the facet joints is thin. The facet joints are filled with synovial ice. Note the wide synovial recesses beneath the ligamentum flavum (*lf*). The spinal nerves lie outside the intervertebral foramen (*curved open arrows*) together with the spinal branches of the segmental arteries.

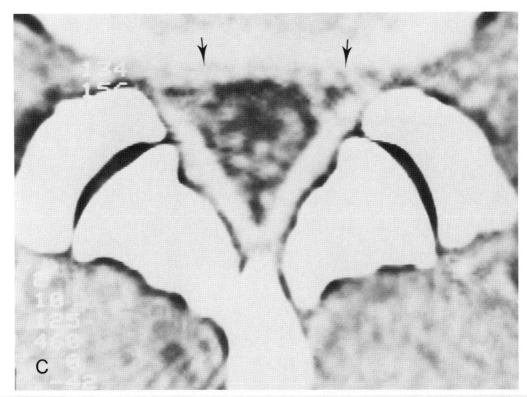

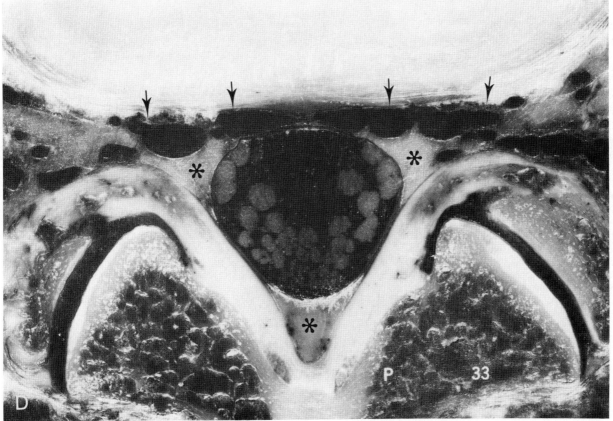

Figure 1.21.   C and D.

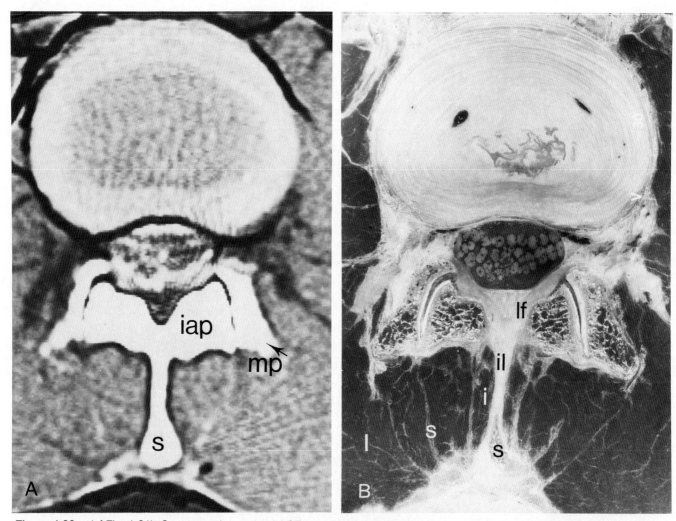

Figure 1.22.   (cf Fig. 1.21). Contrast enhanced axial CT scan (A) and anatomical section (B) through the L3–L4 disc (Specimen V 30). The thecal sac is much wider than in Figure 1.21. Round mamillary processes (*mp*) project posteriorly from the superior articular processes. The inferior articular processes (*iap*) and the lower border of the L3 spinous process (*s*) are ''connected'' by a Y-shaped ligamentous complex of the interspinous ligament (*il*) which anteriorly blends with the two portions of the ligamentum flavum (*lf*) [*i* = interspinalis, *s* = spinalis (thoracis), *l* = longissimus (thoracis)].

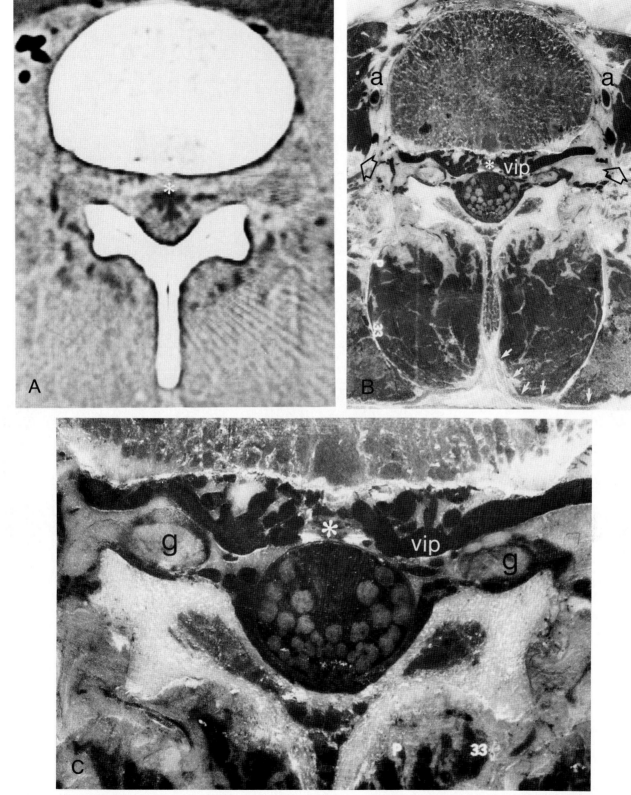

Figure 1.23.   Axial CT scan (A) and anatomical sections (B and C = detail) through the lower body (upper foramen) of L3 (Specimen P 33). Note the segmental arteries (*a*) between the vertebral body and the psoas major. The thick and narrow posterior longitudinal ligament (*) divides the ventral internal venous plexus (*vip*) into a right and a left portion. The dorsal spinal root ganglia (*g*) fit snugly into scalloping of the subpedicular portion of the pedicle. The continuity of the inter- and supraspinous ligaments with the thoracolumbar fascia is indicated by *white closed arrows*. *Black open arrows* point at the L2 spinal nerves.

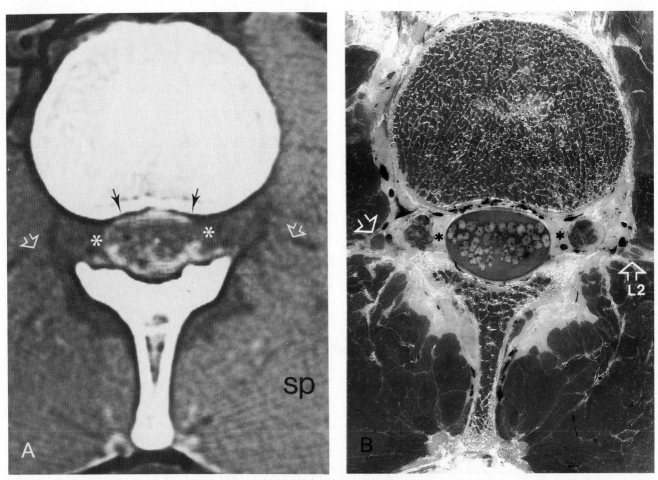

Figure 1.24.   (cf Fig. 1.23). Contrast enhanced axial CT scan (A) and anatomical section (B) through the lower body (upper foramen) of L3. (Specimen V 30). Note extradural fat pads (*) in the (axillary) angles between the thecal sac and the vaginal extensions of the dura housing the spinal nerve roots. The ventral internal venous plexuses (*arrows*) are less voluminous than in Figure 1.23. *Open white arrows* mark the second lumbar spinal nerves. (sp = sacrospinalis.)

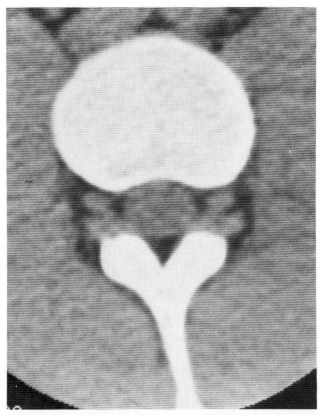

Figure 1.25.   (cf Figs. 1.23 and 1.24).   In vivo axial CT scan from a patient (Courtesy Dr. J. M. Leborgne, Mount Sinai Hospital, Miami Beach) through the lower body of a lumbar vertebra. The low attenuation of the fat tissue contrasts well with the thecal sac, the spinal ganglia, and the ligamentum flavum. The paraspinal muscles appear more homogeneous. The roots of the cauda equina are faintly visible.

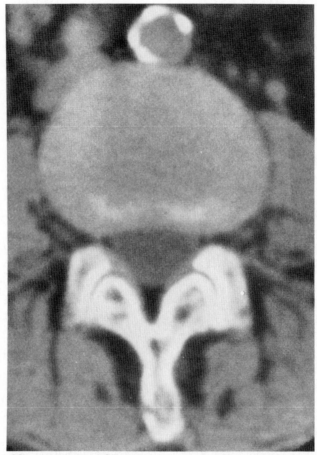

Figure 1.26.   (cf Figs. 1.21 and 1.22).   In vivo axial CT scan from a patient (Courtesy Dr. J. M. Leborgne, Mount Sinai Hospital, Miami Beach) through a lumbar intervertebral disc. Note the high density of the in vivo CSF. The muscle strands are more sharply outlined than on the CT scans from frozen specimens.

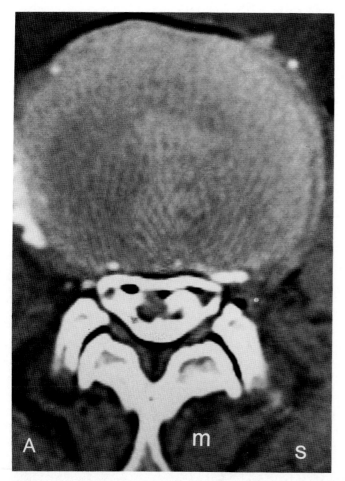
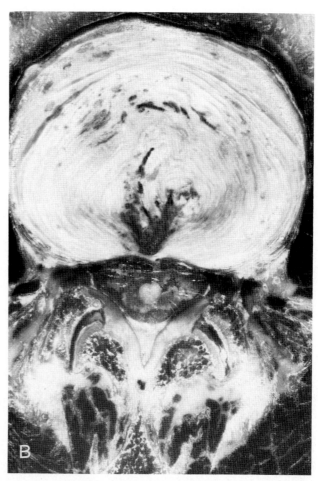

Figure 1.27. Contrast enhanced axial CT scan (A) and anatomical section (B) through the lower portion of the L1–L2 disc. Note the degeneration of the disc and the osteophytes on its right border and the incongruency of the facet joints. The conus medullaris together with bundles of spinal nerve roots in the antero- and posterolateral quadrants of the thecal sac cause an X-shaped image of the neural structures. In this frozen specimen the muscle layers are fairly well outlined [*m* = multifidus, *s* = spinalis (thoracis)].

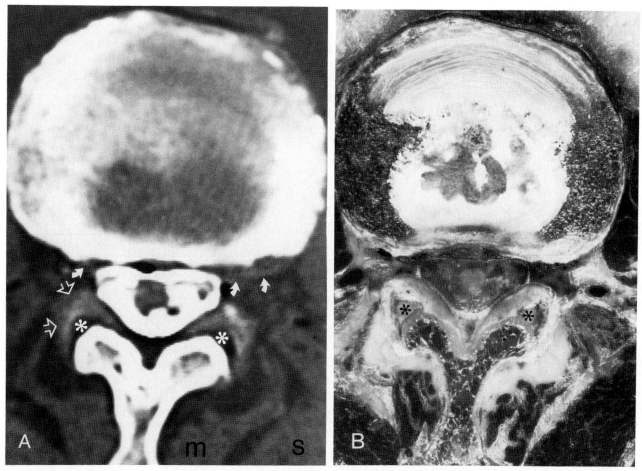

Figure 1.28. Same specimen as in Figure 1.27. CT scan (A) and anatomical section (B) through the lower end plate of L1. The normal posterior anulus of the disc seemingly protrudes beyond the osseous border of the vertebra (*filled white arrows*). The thick curved portions of the upper ligamentum flavum form the upper capsule of the facet joints (*open white arrows*) and enclose conicshaped articular fat pads (*). The ligamentum flavum also encroaches upon the width of this intermediate portion of the foramen [*m* = multifidus, *s* = spinalis (thoracis)].

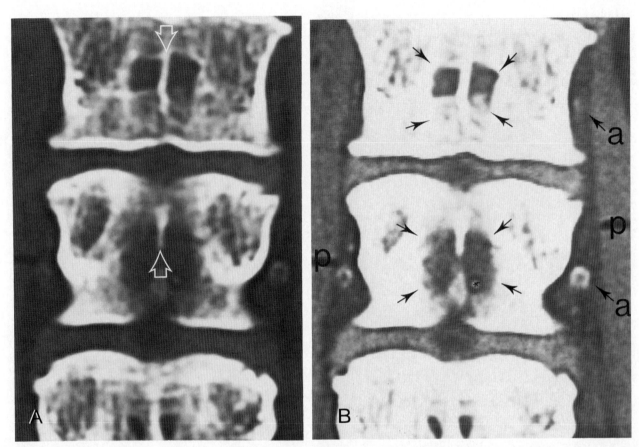

Figure 1.29. Coronal CT scan (A = bone window, B = soft-tissue window) and anatomical sections (C and D = detail) through the posterior border of the three upper lumbar vertebrae. The spinal canal is opened at the concavity of the midvertebral bodies exposing the ventral internal venous plexuses (*black arrows*) and a longitudinal median bony crest subajcent to the posterior longitudinal ligament (*open white arrows*). The discs, the psoas major (*p*), and the segmental arteries (*a*) are well demonstrated on the CT scan. Figure 1.29D shows at higher magnification the posterior longitudinal ligament (*pll*) crossing over the L2–L3 disc.

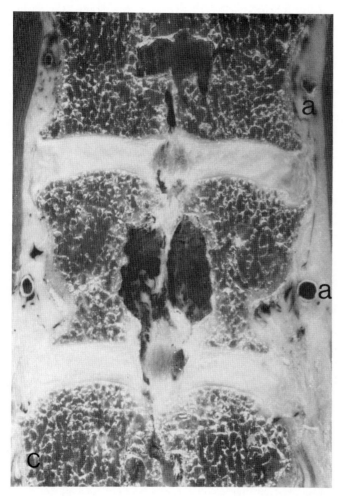
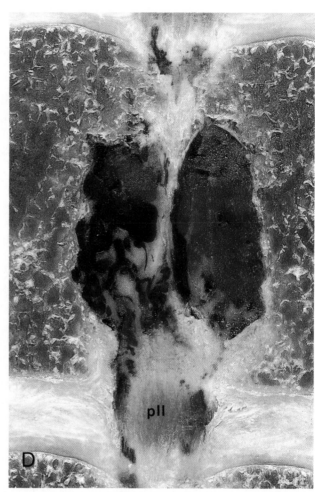

Figure 1.29.   C and D.

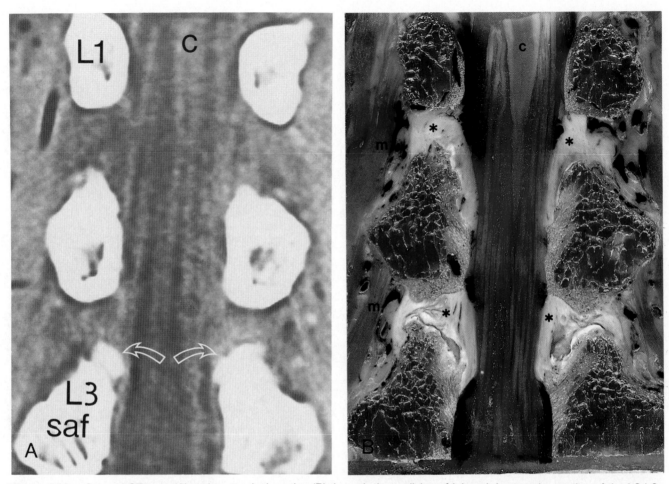

Figure 1.30.   Coronal CT scan (A) and anatomical section (B) through the pedicles of L1 and the anterior portion of the L2-L3 facet joints (*saf* = superior articular facet). Note the conus medullaris (*c*) and the posterior nerve roots of the cauda equina. The ligamentum flavum (*) causes hourglass-shaped narrowing of the thecal sac posteriorly (m = muscle strands of the multifidus). The anterior tips of the inferior articular processes are indicated by *curved open arrows* in Figure 1.30A.

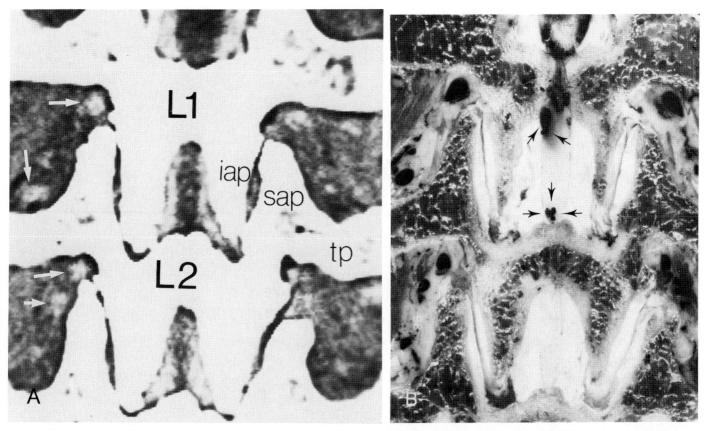

Figure 1.31.   Coronal CT scan (A) and anatomical section (B) through the posterior portions of the L1-L3 facet joints. Note the more sagittal orientation of the joint spaces posteriorly. The ligamentum flavum conjoins posteriorly, anastomotic veins pierce the ligament in the midline (*black arrows*). The segmental blood vessels are visible on the CT scan (*tp* = transverse process, *iap* = inferior articular process, *sap* = superior articular process).

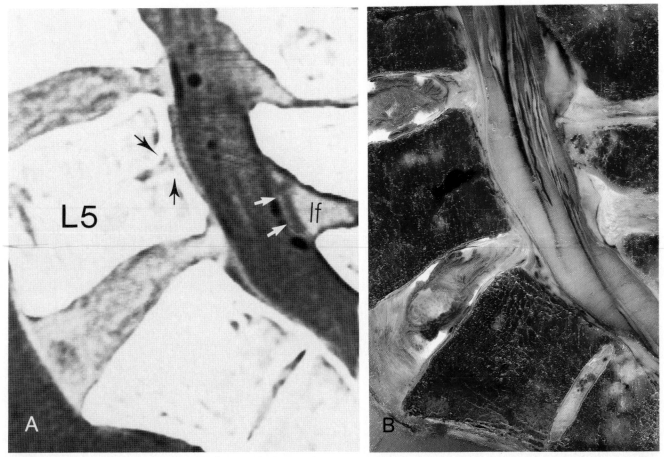

Figure 1.32. Midsagittal CT scan (A) and anatomical section (B) through the lumbosacral spine. The CT scan shows the cloudy structure of the nucleus pulposus and the dense, slightly bulging anulus fibrosus. The outlet of the basivertebral vein in L5 is marked by *black arrows*. The ligamentum flavum (*lf*) can be distinguished from the epidural fat overlying it anteriorly (*white arrows*). The spinal nerve roots are faintly seen.

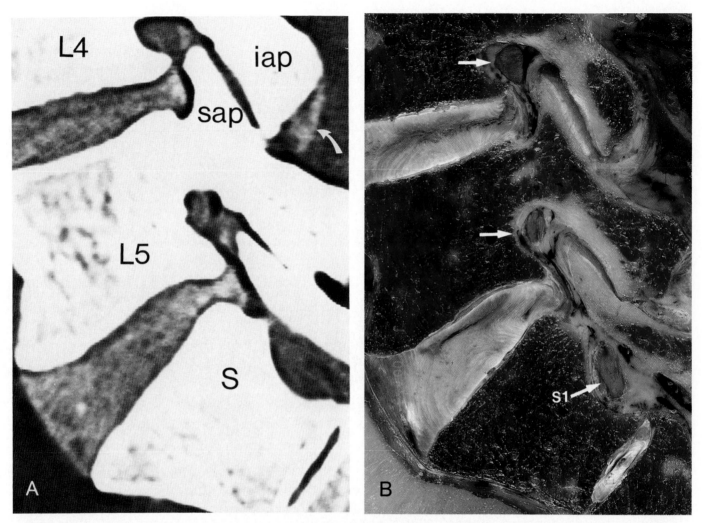

Figure 1.33.   Sagittal CT scan (A) and anatomical section (B and C = detail) through the intervertebral foramen and facet joints of the lumbosacral spine. Note the wedge shape of the lumbosacral disc. The dorsal root ganglia and the ventral spinal roots lie in the subpedicular notch (*arrows*). The lower portion of the foramen is narrow. The S1 ganglion is seen in the wide pelvic sacral foramen. The posterior capsule of the facet joint is faintly outlined (*curved white arrow*) (*iap* = inferior articular process, *sap* = superior articular process).

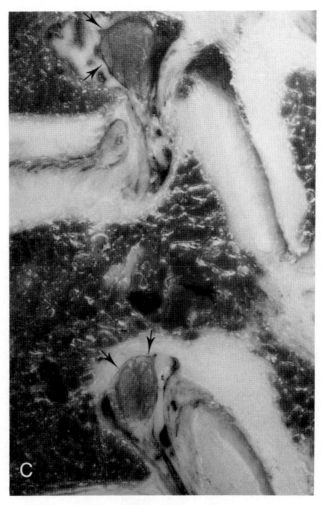

Figure 1.33.   C.

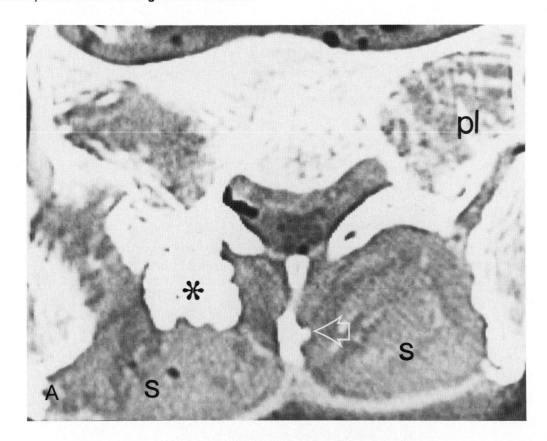

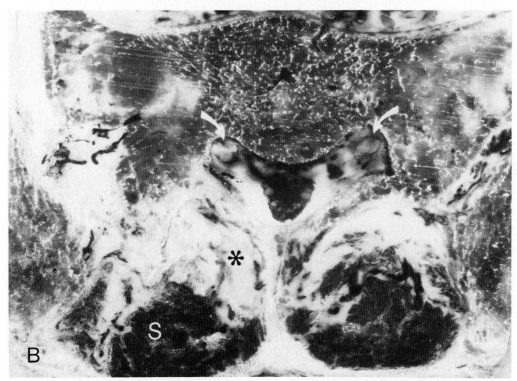

Figure 1.34. Axial CT scan (A) and anatomical section (B) through the upper sacrum. Note the arthritic right inferior articular process of L5 (*). The inferior tip of the L5 spinous process (*arrow*) is continuous with the intra- and supraspinous ligament which blend posteriorly with the lumbosacral fascia. The bone in the central portion of the sacrum is denser than in the pars lateralis (*pl*). *Curved white arrows* mark the S1 spinal nerve and ganglion (*s* = sacrospinalis).

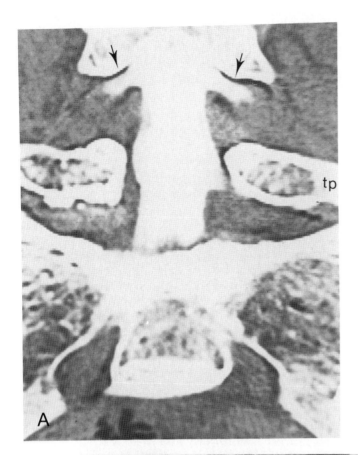

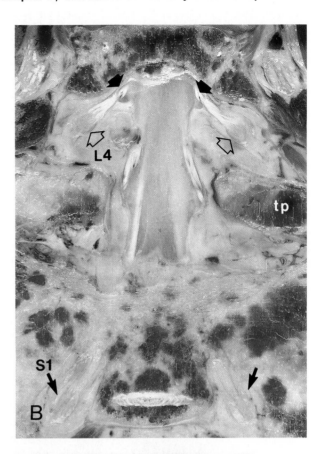

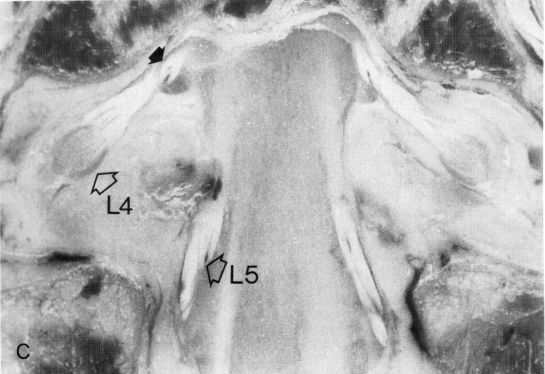

Figure 1.35.   Contrast enhanced coronal CT scan (A) and anatomical section (B and C = detail) through the anterior lumbosacral spinal canal. Note the sheaths of the L4 roots on the CT scan (*black arrows*), the dorsal root ganglia of L4 (*open arrows* in Fig. 1.35B) and the right ventral root of L4 (*solid black arrow*) in Figure 1.35C. The S1 root ganglia present in the pelvic sacral foramen (S1) (*tp* = transverse process of L5).

CHAPTER TWO

Computed Tomography of the Craniovertebal Junction

DAVID L. LaMASTERS, M.D.*

INTRODUCTION

The craniovertebral junction is a complex anatomical region, functionally distinct from the lower cervical spine. Mass lesions, dysplasias, malformations, and other processes arising at this level produce a perplexing clinical picture with extremity weakness, suboccipital pain, paresthesias, ataxia, and stereoanesthesia (1, 2). Delayed diagnosis or misdiagnosis is common (3). Symptoms often will be attributed to cervical spondylytic disease or "multiple sclerosis" (4). Coexistence of the former with a lesion at the craniovertebral junction further complicates the clinical assessment (5).

The advent of computed tomography (CT) has greatly simplified the radiographic evaluation of clinically suspect lesions at the craniovertebral junction. CT allows simultaneous evaluation of the bony canal and neural elements. The contents of the upper spinal canal and foramen magnum are poorly demonstrated on noncontrast scans. When signs of medullary or upper cervical cord impairment or compression are present, the use of an intrathecal contrast agent such as metrizamide is required to visualize the intraspinal contents. The routine use of multiplanar reformations (MPR) with metrizamide CT cisternography allows perception of spatial relationships between lesion and neural canal. Intravenous contrast has utility in assessing the enhancement pattern of vascular lesions such as glomus jugulare tumors, occasional neuromas, angiofibromas, arteriovenous malformations, and chordomas.

Before the CT era, Pantopaque cisternography was the procedure of choice in excluding an upper cervical or foramen magnum process. Although good opacification of the posterior fossa and upper cervical cisterns can be achieved with this technique, both prone and supine examinations are required. Care must be taken to avoid permanent deposition of Pantopaque into the middle fossa cisterns.

Vertebral angiography remains necessary in instances where encasement of the vertebral artery is considered possible, usually with extramedullary tumors such as meningioma, chordoma, and nasopharyngeal carcinoma. The opposite vertebral artery also should be studied to assess flow and patency in case the involved vertebral must be sacrificed at surgery.

Complex motion tomography (CMT) has little role at present in evaluation of craniovertebral pathology. Current generation CT with edge-enhancement techniques provides superior resolution of osseous detail (6, 7). Derangements of the adjacent soft tissues and neural elements may be assessed simultaneously with CT, an advantage not shared by conventional tomography. The radiation dose delivered with CT is significantly less than with CMT (8). The dose delivered per axial high-resolution CT (HRCT) is approximately 4.0 rads whereas 1.0 rad is delivered per section with CMT (9). However, dosage with CMT is cumulative, thus, if 20 are required the total dose is roughly 20.0 rads whereas a comparable number of CT slices results in a total dose of only 4.0 rads.

TECHNIQUE

Metrizamide CT cisternography is a simple technique with little clinical morbidity and should be the primary radiographic procedure when neurological signs of a craniovertebral process exist. It can be performed as an adjunct to cervical myelography or as a primary procedure. As a primary exam, 4–5 cc of a 190 mg/ml (I) metrizamide is injected into the lumbar subarachnoid space under fluoroscopic control. The patient is tilted 45° Trendelenburg, both prone and supine for a total of 4 minutes and then transferred to the CT suite. When CT cisternography follows cervical myelography, a 4- to 6-hour delay is imposed to avoid untoward side effects from immediate deposition of high concentrations of metrizamide into the basal cisterns. During this period, the patient is kept in the semiupright position and fluid intake is encouraged.

A large aperture scanner with gantry tilt capability is preferable. The latter feature is helpful in angling the axial sections so as to avoid teeth fillings and other metalic objects often present in planes through C1 and C2. Axial scans are obtained from C2 through the 4th ventricle. Collimation of 5.0 mm with table motion of 3.0 mm (2.0 mm overlap) is generally adequate and allows generation of MPR images.

ANATOMY-MULTIPLANAR REFORMATIONS

The use of sagittal, coronal, and oblique reformatted images often helps clarify the spatial relationships between normal neural or osseous structures and pathological lesions, particularly tumors. The normal anatomy of the foramen magnum region as seen on axial CT sections has been described in the radiographic literature (10).

* The author wishes to express his appreciation to Michael Brant-Zawadski, M.D. for his significant contributions to this chapter and to Professor Jack deGroot for permission to reproduce the anatomical specimens.

Reformatted images from metrizamide CT cisternograms are less familiar and will be discussed briefly.

A reformatted image in the midsagittal plane displays the contour of the brainstem (Fig. 2.1 A, B). The neuroaxis is narrowest at the cervicomedullary junction, gradually widening in the medulla, and abruptly so at the belly of the pons. The basilar artery may be identified as a negative defect anterior to the pons in the basal cisterns. The 4th ventricle normally fills with contrast on cisternographic studies. In the sagittal plane, the long axis of the 4th ventricle parallels the brainstem, its apex is directed posteriorly, projecting into the vermis. Displacement of the 4th ventricle may be measured directly from the refor-

matted image by the method of Twining (11). The midpoint of Twining's line should fall along the 4th ventricular floor. The folia of the cerebellar vermis, posterior and above the 4th ventricle are usually well defined, outlined by contrast in the superior cerebellar cistern and cisterna magna. At the level of the foramen magnum, the cisterns surrounding the lower medulla reach their greatest dimensions, wider posteriorly where the cervical subarachnoid space merges with the cisterna magna.

Parasagittal and coronal reformations best define the position of the cerebellar tonsils (Figs. 2.2 and 2.3). The tonsils are rounded, hemispheric projections extending from the medial and inferior aspect of each cerebellar

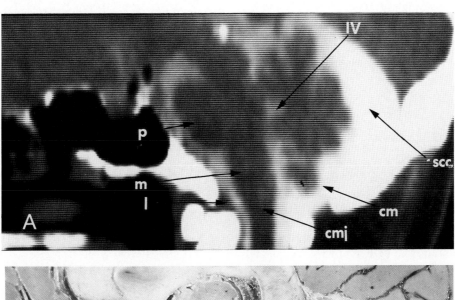

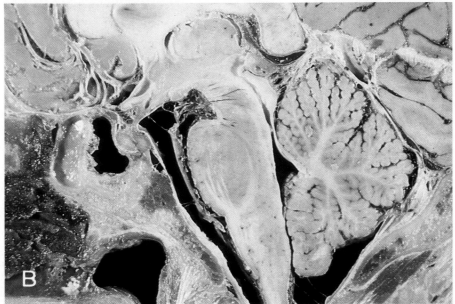

Figure 2.1.   Midline Sagittal Section—Brainstem: The CT reformatted image A and gross specimen B demonstrate the midline relationships at the craniovertebral junction. The medulla (*m*), pons (*p*) and mesencephalon ascend through the posterior fossa at 75–80° to the axial plane. The 4th ventricle (*IV*) and basal cisterns are normally opacified. The transverse, alar, and cruciate ligaments (*l*) lie anterior to the cervicomedullary junction (*cmj*). The cisterna magna (*cm*) and superior cerebellar cistern (*scc*) are prominent in this patient. (This CT section as well as all the other illustrations in this chapter except for Figs. 2.21 and 2.22 were obtained with 5-mm collimation with a 3-mm table motion.)

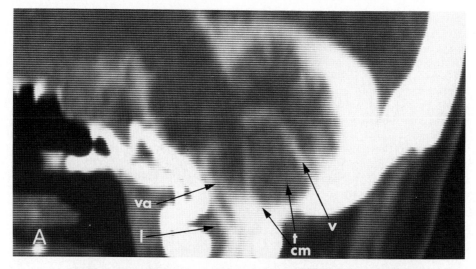

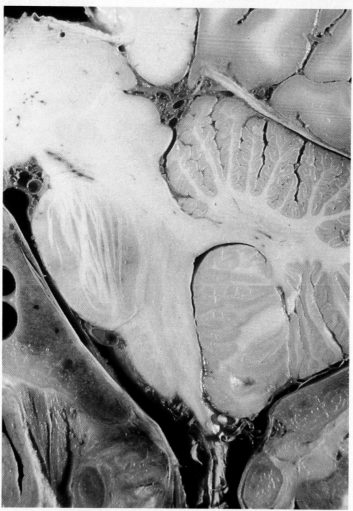

Figure 2.2. Parasagittal Section—Cerebellar Tonsil: The reformatted parasagittal CT section A, and corresponding cadaver specimen B show the normal position of the cerebellar tonsil (*t*). Contrast in the vallecula (*v*) surrounds the anterior, superior, and posterior aspects of the tonsil, whereas the cisterna magna (*cm*) covers the inferior surface. The vertebral artery (*va*) passes lateral to the medulla and ascends to the level of the pons. Again, the ligaments (*l*) joining the clivus, C1, and C2 are noted.

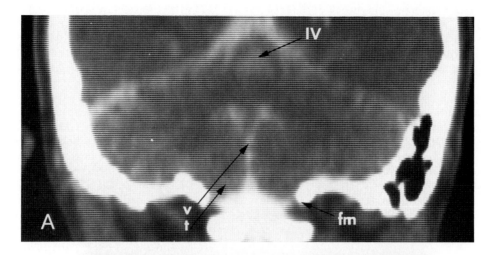

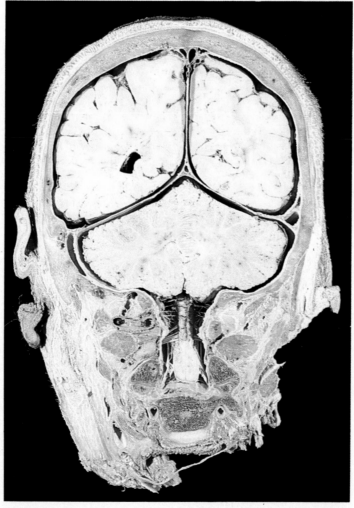

Figure 2.3.   Orthogonal Coronal Section—Tonsils: The coronal CT reformation A, taken 90° to the axial plane again shows the normal position of the cerebellar tonsils (*t*) above the outer table of the foramen magnum (*fm*). A similar relationship is noted on the cadaver section B taken at a slightly different obliquity. The vallecula (*v*) in this view lies above and between the tonsils. The 4th ventricle (*IV*) is opacified.

hemisphere. The superior and medial surface of the tonsil is defined by contrast in the vallecula, while the cisterna magna covers the posterior and inferior aspects. Although the tonsils may be within or above the foramen magnum, extension below the outer table is abnormal and indicates herniation (12).

The orientation of the brainstem is such that coronal sections orthogonal to the axial plane fail to display the entire neuroaxis. An oblique coronal angled at 75–80° to the anthropological base line parallels the longitudinal axis and permits assessment of the entire brainstem on a single image (Fig. 2.4). In this projection, the medulla, pons, and midbrain are seen in ascending sequence. The middle cerebellar peduncles diverge laterally from the pons into the cerebellar hemispheres. The hemispheric folia are surrounded by contrast in the superior cerebellar cistern.

Although in most instances the foramen magnum lies in the plane of axial CT sections, on occasion it does not. The orientation of the foramen magnum depends upon the length of the clivus. When the later is foreshortened, the foramen magnum may be angled 5–15° to the axial plane (13). A para-axial reformation, however, allows for assessment of the foramen magnum on a single image (Fig. 2.5). The foramen magnum is roughly oval in contour, trapezoidal in its anterior one-third, and elliptical posteriorly. In a series of 25 patients without craniovertebral pathology, the foramen magnum measured by electronic cursor from axial CT sections was 3.73 cm in AP diameter with a range of 3.36–4.0 cm. The dimension in lateral greatest width at the posterior portion of the occipital condyles was 3.09 cm with a range of 2.80–3.44 cm. This differs from the data of Coin and Malkasian (14) who reported somewhat smaller dimensions in dried human skulls.

PATHOLOGICAL CONDITIONS

Unlike the lower cervical spine, the craniovertebral junction is an uncommon site for degenerative or spondylytic disease. More typical of this region are congenital and acquired conditions such as the Chiari malformation, basilar invagination, achondroplasia, and atlantoaxial dislocation. Tumors also occur and may be either extramedullary or intramedullary. The former encompasses malignant and benign lesions including meningioma, neuroma, chordoma, plasmacytoma, chondroma, metastases and contiguous invasion from nasopharyngeal carcinoma whereas the latter includes tumors of the cervical cord and medulla; ependymoma, astrocytoma, and syringomyelia. Several dysplasias of bone also affect the foramen magnum including Paget's disease, Von Buchem's, fibrous dysplasia, osteopetrosis, craniometaphysial dysplasia, and Engelman-Camurati (progressive diaphyseal dysplasia).

CONGENITAL CONDITIONS
Chiari Malformation

Characterized by a varying degree of downward tonsillar herniation and deformity of the medulla, vermis, and 4th ventricle, the Chiari malformation may be subdivided into two major types. In type I, the cerebellar tonsils are displaced downward through the foramen magnum usually to the level of C1 (Fig. 2.6). The tonsils are deformed and have a trapezoid or rectangular shape, closely applied to the upper cervical cord. The brainstem and 4th ventricle are normal. Onset of symptoms is in adolescence or young adulthood, characterized by suboccipital pain. A variable association with syringomyelia also is found (15). The mechanism of injury is believed to be chronic trauma, and compression of the lower brainstem, as the cisterns which normally cushion the upper cord and medulla are compromised by tonsillar tissue (16, 17).

The Chiari II malformation is more extensive. The medulla, pons, 4th ventricle, cerebellar vermis, tonsils, and hemispheres are displaced through an enlarged foramen magnum (Fig. 2.7). The tonsils are elongated and ribbon-like extending into the lower cervical spine. Other associated intracranial findings demonstrable on CT include deformity of the tentorium with upward herniation of the cerebellum, clival and petrous scalloping, tectal beaking, hydrocephalus, enlargement of the massa intermedia, and hypoplasia of the falx (18–20). Some form of spinal dysraphism, usually a myelomeningocele is present. Syringomyelia, tethered cord, and lipoma may also be found.

Metrizamide CT cisternography is the simplest method for assessing the craniovertebral abnormalities present in the Chiari malformation. Without intrathecal enhancement, the position of the tonsils cannot reliably be ascertained (Fig. 2.6A). The presence of an associated syrinx can be documented with delayed CT scans (Fig. 2.6D). Reformations are helpful in demonstrating the level to which the tonsils extend (Fig. 2.7B). In both Chiari I and II, the cisterns at the foramen magnum are attenuated. The 4th ventricle usually is not opacified in the Chiari II malformation due to kinking of the outlet foramina. On axial CT sections, the upper cord and medulla are flattened rather than round or elliptical.

ACHONDROPLASIA

Achondroplasia is an autosomal dominant condition characterized by defective endochondral bone formation leading to rhizomelic dwarfism. Intracranial manifestations include megalencephaly with or without hydrocephalus and a small, stenotic foramen magnum (21). The dens usually protrudes through the foramen magnum further compromising the neural canal (Fig. 2.8A and B). The jugular foramen may be stenosed as well, producing elevated venous pressure (Fig. 2.8C) (22). The latter is believed to be an etiological factor in the development of hydrocephalus, since cerebrospinal fluid (CSF) resorption is related inversely to intracranial venous pressure.

ATLANTOAXIAL SUBLUXATION

Atlantoxial subluxation may be either congenital or acquired. In the former, it is associated with "floppy infants" (Down's syndrome) in which the transverse, cruciate, and alar ligaments are lax. As an acquired condition,

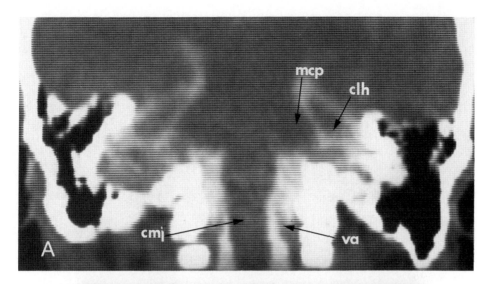

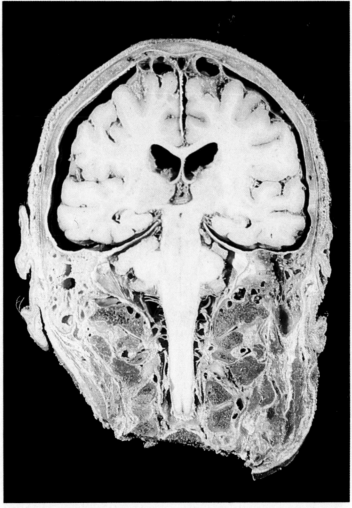

Figure 2.4. Oblique 75° Coronal Section—Brainstem: A second view of the entire neuroaxis can be obtained by a reformatted image angled at 75–80° to the axial plane A. The neuroaxis is narrowest at the cervicomedullary junction (*cmj*) and widens abruptly at the pons, where the middle cerebellar peduncles (*mcp*) diverge into the cerebellar hemispheres (*clh*). The vertebral arteries (*va*) pass laterally around the lower medulla.

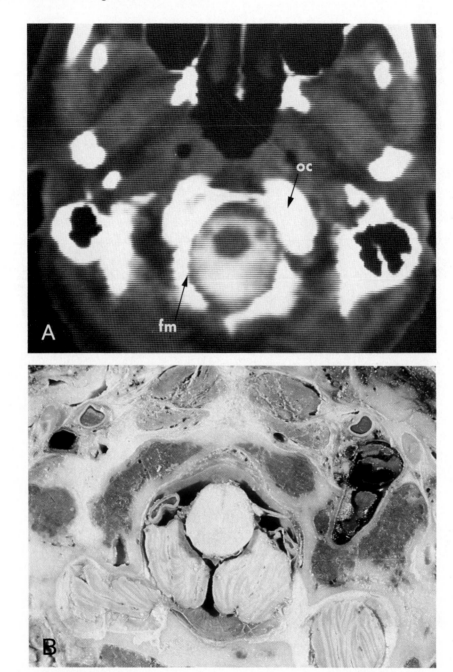

Figure 2.5. Para-Axial Section—Foramen Magnum: The true contour and size of the foramen magnum (*fm*) may be appreciated in a para-axial CT reformation taken tangent to the outer table A. Normally, the anterior one-third of the foramen magnum is trapezoidal bounded laterally by the occipital condyles (*oc*); whereas the posterior two-thirds is round to ellipsoid in shape. The tonsils should not be seen at this level.

dislocation occurs with inflammatory states, pharyngitis, cervical adenitis, rheumatoid arthritis, and severe trauma (23, 24). With weakening or rupture of the transverse ligament, the skull and atlas slip forward on the axis increasing the atlanto-odontoid space. With severe rotation, the articular facets of C1 and C2 may override and lock, fixing the inferior facet of C1 anterior to the superior facet of C2 (Fig. 2.9).

FORAMEN MAGNUM TUMORS

Metrizamide CT cisternography has greatest utility in the diagnosis of both intramedullary and extramedullary mass lesions at the craniovertebral junction. Cervical myelography with metrizamide is inadequate in excluding a foramen magnum tumor, as one cannot opacify the basal cisterns without significant clinical morbidity. CT

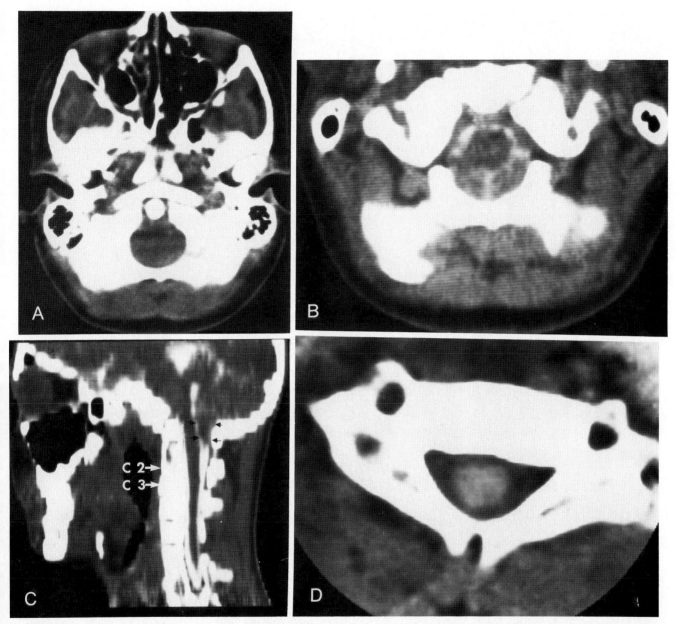

Figure 2.6.   Chiari I Malformation: A. Noncontrast CT scan through the foramen magnum fails to define the tonsils. The contour and size of the foramen magnum is normal. B. Metrizamide CT cisternogram at the same level demonstrates the tonsils which are abnormally shaped and closely applied to the dorsal surface of the cord. C. Sagittal reformation with the tonsils extending below the outer table of the foramen magnum (*black arrows*). The bodies of C2 and C3 are fused (*white arrows*) in this patient who has a known Klippel-Fiel deformity. D. Delayed scan at 6 hours documented the presence of an associated syrinx.

without intrathecal enhancement cannot define intraspinal contents routinely, thus, even large lesions may be missed (Fig. 2.10).

EXTRAMEDULLARY TUMORS

Meningioma

Meningiomas are the most common benign mass lesion arising at the foramen magnum. Yasuoka et al. (25) in a review of 57 benign craniovertebral tumors, found 37 meningiomas. Most are located anterior or anteromedial and produce symptoms by direct cord compression. Meningiomas are most commonly intradural, extramedullary in location, and on metrizamide CT cisternograms an acute angle with the contrast column may be identified (Fig. 2.10B) (26). Frequently, meningiomas achieve significant size before diagnosis, as the capacious nature of the upper cervical cisterns and cisterna magna allow large tumors with little cord compromise (Fig. 2.11A) (27). Reformatted images are useful in showing the degree of cord displacement; and a cleavage plane between tumor and cord (Figs. 2.10C and D, and 2.11B).

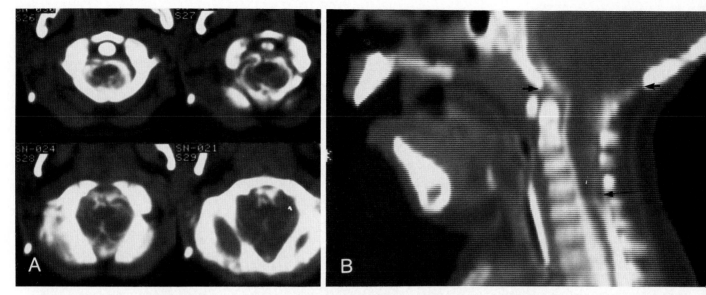

Figure 2.7.   Chiari II Malformation: A. Multiple axial sections at the foramen magnum after injection of metrizamide show herniation of cerebellar hemispheric tissue to C2. The cerebellar folia are outlined. The foramen magnum is enlarged. B. The tonsils are compressed to a ribbon-like band and extend to C5 (*long arrow*). The width of the foramen magnum is readily apparent on the sagittal reformation (*short arrows*). The 4th ventricle is not opacified.

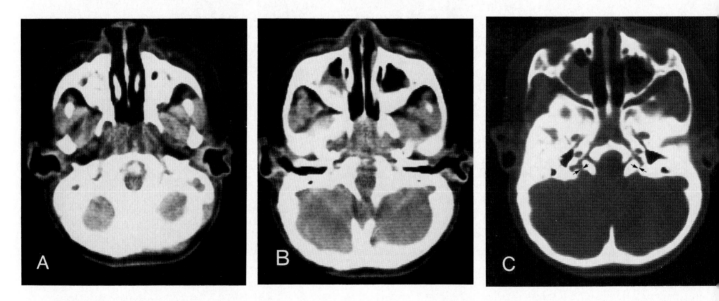

Figure 2.8.   Achondroplasia: A, B. The foramen magnum is small and stenotic. The dens protrudes cephalad further compromising the neural canal. C. The jugular fossa is compromised severely on the left and moderately so on the right (*small arrows*). The hypoglossal canals (medial) are normal.

Neurinoma

Neural sheath tumors affecting the craniovertebral junction may arise from the lower cranial nerves (IX-XII) or the upper cervical spinal nerves (C1, C2). Enlargement of the adjacent neural foramina is common and the tumor may extend beyond the spine into the paravertebral region. Both schwannomas and neurofibromas occur; the latter, in association with neurofibromatosis are often multiple (Fig. 13A). In distinction to meningioma, neuromas arise in a more lateral location (Fig. 2.12). As with meningiomas, neuromas are often quite large at the time of diagnosis (Fig. 2.14). Neuromas may be either intradural, extramedullary, or entirely extradural, the last being most common (28). When located extradurally, the interface between tumor and contrast-filled subarachnoid space is smoothly indented; acute margins are not seen (Fig. 2.12A).

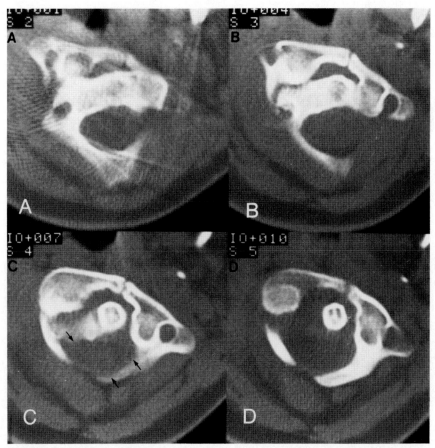

Figure 2.9. Down's Syndrome—Rotatory Atlantoaxial Subluxation: A, B. Axial CT sections at the body of C2 show anterior displacement of the right lateral mass of C1 on C2. The inferior facet of C1 has overridden the superior facet of C2 and locked. C, D. Although C1 has rotated 30–35° on the dens, the spinal canal is compromised only mildly (*small arrows*). No neurological deficit was present upon exam.

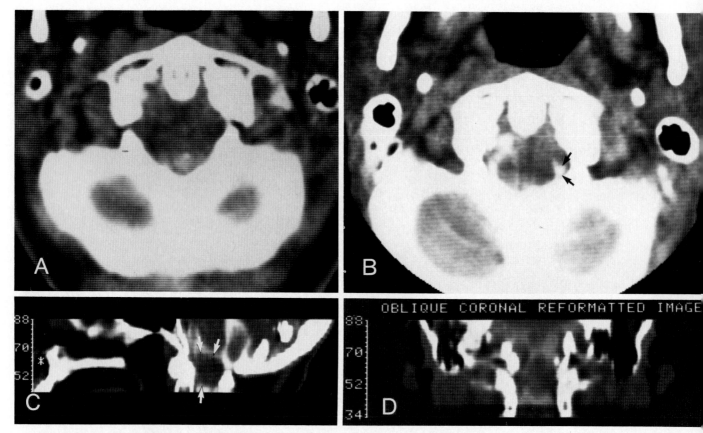

Figure 2.10.   Foramen Magnum Meningioma: A. Axial CT scan at C1 and the foramen magnum is normal. No hyperostosis was identified. B. Metrizamide CT cisternogram clearly defines a mass lesion anteriorly to the left of midline apparently continuous with spinal canal and cord. The cord is displaced posteriorly. The mass has acute margins with the contrast column suggesting an intradural-extramedullary process (*arrows*). C. Left parasagittal reformation with the mass outlined with contrast (*arrows*). D. Oblique coronal section shows the mass en face, displacing the cord away. At surgery, an intradural-extramedullary meningioma was excised.

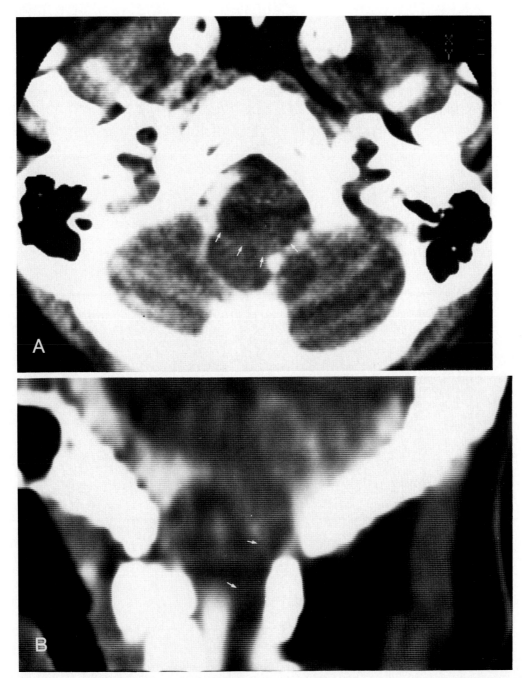

Figure 2.11.   Meningioma: A. Axial CT section with metrizamide shows a large mass (*arrows*) displacing the cord posterior and to the right. B. Midline sagittal reformation demonstrated the severe displacement of the cord (*arrows*). The cisterna magna is obliterated. The tumor occupies the anterior half of the foramen magnum.

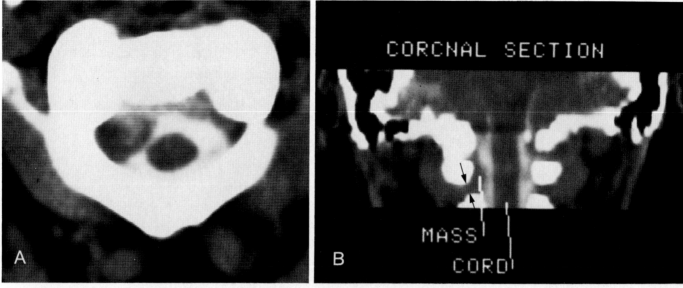

Figure 2.12. C1, C2 Neuroma: A. CT cisternogram obtained 6 hours after metrizamide myelography defines an extraaxial mass. The cord is neither displaced nor compressed. B. Orthogonal coronal demonstrates the mass protruding from a slightly enlarged intervertebral foramen (*arrows*). At surgery, an entirely extradural neuroma was removed from the right C2 spinal nerve.

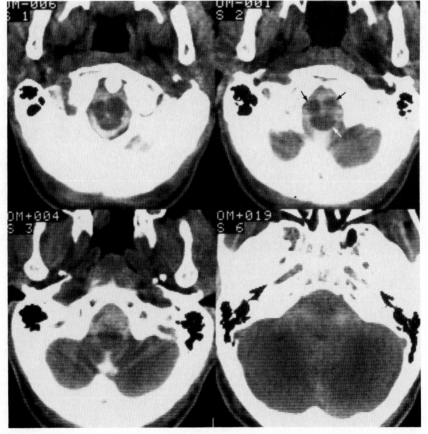

Figure 2.13. Neurofibromatosis: Multiple axial CT scans obtained at the foramen magnum after metrizamide myelography demonstrated an apparent C5, C6 complete block. Two masses are seen anterior to the cord at C1 (*black arrows*). The cord is flattened and slightly atrophic (*white arrow*). The block in the lower cervical spine was caused by dumbbell neuromas. The masses at the foramen magnum are presumed bilateral C2 neuromas.

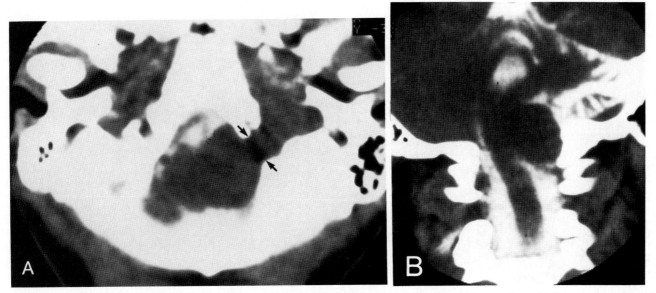

Figure 2.14. Hypoglossal Neuroma: A. Cisternographic study at the foramen magnum with an enlarged left hypoglossal canal (*arrows*) and a large extra-axial mass displacing the lower medulla. B. Coronal section: The mass extending from the hypoglossal canal both compresses and displaces the medulla.

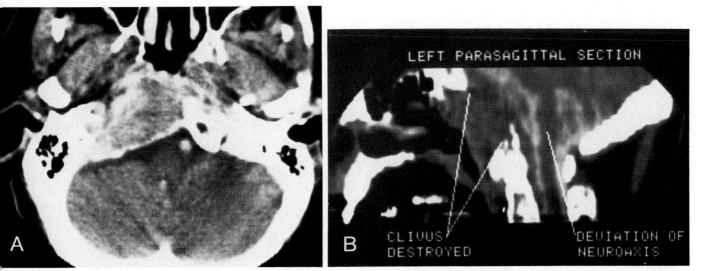

Figure 2.15. Clivus Chordoma: A. Axial intravenously enhanced scan: A large enhancing mass fills the preclival space and nasopharynx. The clivus and right petrous apex have been destroyed. B. Sagittal reformation: metrizamide CT cisternogram. The soft-tissue mass attenuates the basal cisterns displacing the neuroaxis posteriorly. There is, however, no frank invasion of the brainstem.

Chordoma

Chordomas arise from remnants of the primitive notochord. In the craniovertebral region, the clivus is the most common site of origin, although the upper cervical vertebrae may be affected. Chordomas are malignant, aggressive tumors which are locally invasive. With time, chordomas may traverse the dura and directly invade the brainstem (29). HRCT with edge enhancement best demonstrates the extent of bony destruction; however, metrizamide CT cisternography better defines transgression of the dura and involvement of the cord and brainstem (Fig.

2.15). Calcification is stated to occur in 30–70%. The soft-tissue component to these tumors is often substantial, filling the nasopharynx, sella, sphenoid, and preclival spaces (Fig. 2.15B).

NASOPHARYNGEAL CARCINOMA

The role of CT in evaluation of nasopharyngeal tumors which invade the craniovertebral junction usually is limited to defining the extent of lesion. Most nasopharyngeal carcinomas are diagnosed clinically before radiological

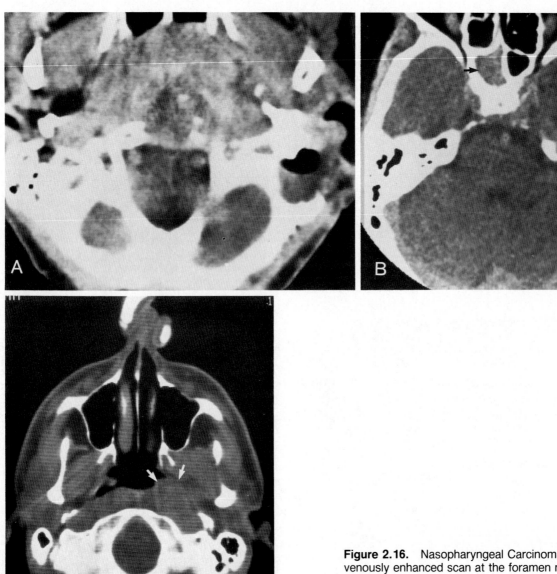

Figure 2.16. Nasopharyngeal Carcinoma: A, B. Axial intravenously enhanced scan at the foramen magnum: The anterior rim of the foramen magnum has been destroyed. A bulky soft-tissue mass fills the nasopharynx and extends anterior to the pterygoids and cephalad into the sphenoid sinus and prepontine cistern. C. Axial scan—Müeller maneuver: The left pharyngeal recess is nondistensible (*arrows*) in this patient with an isodense pharyngeal tumor. This technique is useful when overt signs of bone destruction or mass effect are minimal or absent.

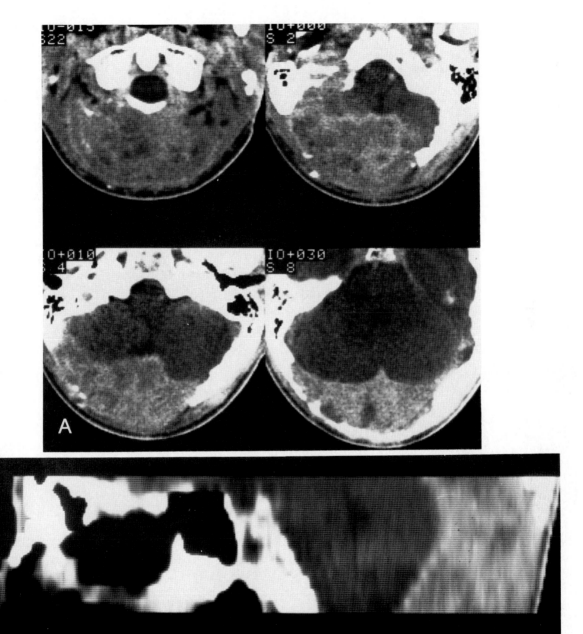

Figure 2.17. Plasmacytoma—Occiput: A. Multiple intravenously enhanced sections through the occiput. The occipital squamosa has largely been destroyed and replaced by a large enhancing soft-tissue mass. B. Midsagittal reformation: The cerebellar vermis and 4th ventricle are displaced anteriorly.

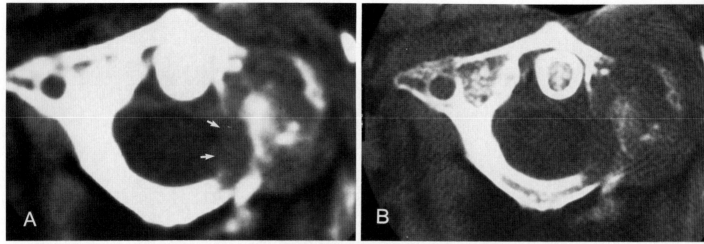

Figure 2.18.   Breast Metastasis to C1, C2: A. The left lateral mass and lamina of C1 are permeated and destroyed. The soft-tissue component extends into the spinal canal (*arrows*) and the paravertebral region. B. Edge-enhanced image better defines the degree of osseous destruction.

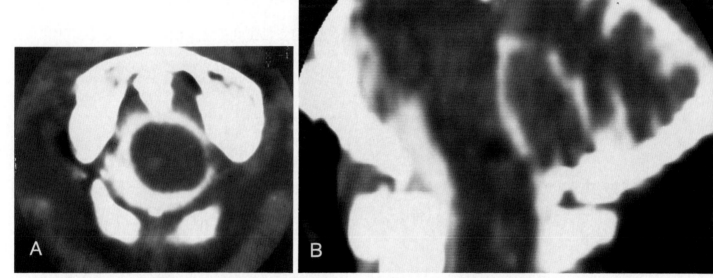

Figure 2.19.   Cervical Ependymona: A. Metrizamide CT cisternogram is at the level of the occipital condyles. The upper cord is expanded eccentrically to the left. B. Sagittal reformation medulla: Both cord and medulla are involved. The epicenter of the tumor approximates the foramen magnum.

evaluation. Unfortunately, these tumors often have reached an advanced state before diagnosis and treatment (30). In roughly 35% of malignant nasopharyngeal tumors, bone destruction is present with involvement of the basiocciput in 25% (31). HRCT allows definition of the degree of osseous destruction and soft-tissue extent (Fig. 2.16). Further definition of parapharyngeal invasion can be documented by scans obtained with the patient performing the Müeller maneuver (Fig. 2.16C).

MULTIPLE MYELOMA

Although solitary plasmacytoma and multiple myeloma are more common in the cranial vault, the skull base and

craniovertebral junction also are affected (32, 33). Skull base plasmacytomas are invariably destructive and are associated with both an exocranial and endocranial soft-tissue component. The brainstem, 4th ventricle, and cerebellum are displaced and distorted as these tumors enlarge (Fig. 2.17). Angiographically, plasmacytomas tend to be moderately vascular, supplied by meningeal vessels (34). CT scans with intravenous contrast may show moderate enhancement (Fig. 2.17A). The presence of Bence-Jones protein in the urine establishes the diagnosis.

METASTASES

Metastases to the craniovertebral junction are uncommon. Invasion of the skull base occurs most frequently

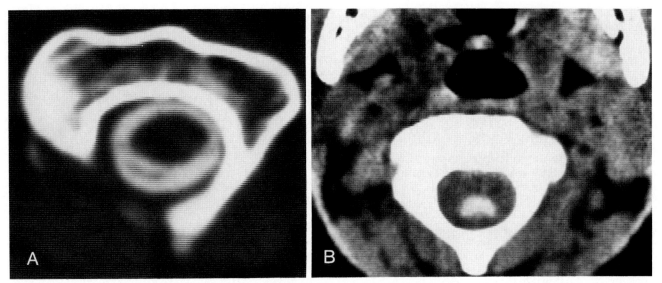

Figure 2.20 Syringomyelia: A. Metrizamide CT cisternogram at 10 minutes after injection. The cord is slightly enlarged but no central cavity is defined. B. Six-hour delay scan: Metrizamide has been absorbed largely from the subarachnoid space, but is concentrated densely in the central cavity.

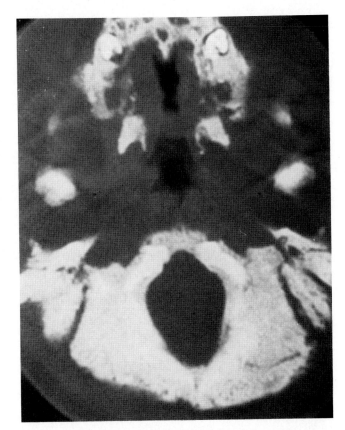

Figure 2.21. Osteopetrosis: Edge-enhanced axial 1.5-mm section: The density of the basiocciput is increased. No diploic space is seen. The pterygoids and maxilla also are affected.

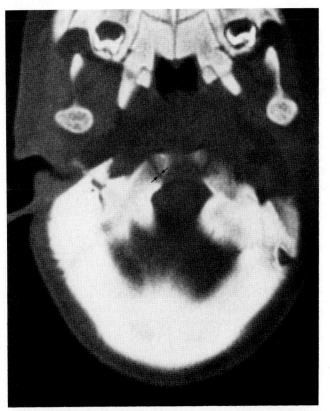

Figure 2.22. Craniometaphyseal Dysplasia; Edge-enhanced axial 1.5-mm section: The overall bone density is increased. The skull is thickened and the diploe obliterated. The hypo-glossal canals are stenosed (*arrows*).

with breast carcinoma although metastases from lymphoma, lung cancer, and head and neck malignancies also occur (35). Bone destruction with a soft-tissue mass is the usual CT finding (Fig. 2.18). The CT appearance, however,

is nonspecific as other lesions such as infection, myeloma, and primary bone tumors are indistinguishable. Multiple lesions, though, favor metastases or myeloma. Metastatic disease produces local pain and cranial nerve deficits, especially when the clivus and anterior aspect of the foramen magnum are involved.

INTRAMEDULLARY TUMORS

Glioma

Ependymoma is the commonest primary tumor arising from the spinal cord. Although the filum terminale and conus medullaris are the most frequent sites of origin, they can occur at the craniovertebral junction (Fig. 2.19). The cord is expanded in a fusiform fashion with extension longitudinally over several cord segments (36). A cystic cavity within the tumor may be demonstrated with CT cisternography. Unlike syringomyelia, the cord may appear somewhat lobulated on axial sections (Fig. 2.19A). Astrocytomas occur with slightly less frequency than ependymomas and are radiographically indistinguishable.

SYRINGOMYELIA

Syringomyelia like primary cord tumors produces fusiform dilitation of the cervical cord. The central cavity may extend above the foramen magnum into the medulla. Metrizamide CT cisternography has proven highly successful at demonstrating both cord size and the presence of a central cavity (39). The cyst cavity often is unopacified when scans are obtained immediately after metrizamide injection. However, delayed scans (6 hours) usually define the syrinx (Fig. 2.20). The cord more frequently is normal to small in diameter; thus, opacification of the central canal is essential for diagnosis. With scans taken 12, 24, and 48 hours after injection, the concentration of contrast in the subarachnoid space diminishes whereas the opacification of the cyst increases suggesting transneural passage of metrizamide (38).

BONY DYSPLASIA

Osteopetrosis

Osteopetrosis may be inherited as an autosomal dominant or recessive trait; the latter form is more severe with death in childhood usually from severe anemia. The disease is characterized by an overall increase in bone density caused by a failure in resorption of the primary spongiosa. Radiographically, the diploic space and marrow cavities are obliterated and the neural foramina are stenosed (39). HRCT with edge enhancement is the procedure of choice in evaluating compromise of the basal foramina canals (Fig. 2.21). The foramen magnum, hypoglossal canal, and jugular fossa invariably are involved, with associated palsies of the lower cranial nerves. Hydrocephalus occurs with stenosis and occlusion of the jugular canal, as CSF resorption diminishes with increased venous pressure.

Craniometaphyseal Dysplasia (Pyle's Disease)

Like osteopetrosis, craniometaphyseal dysplasia is characterized by sclerosis of the skull base with associated stenosis and eventual obliteration of the basal foramina

(Fig. 2.22). The metaphyses in the appendicular skeleton are undertubulated with a typical "Erlenmeyer flask" appearance (40).

CONCLUSION

HRCT is capable of defining most lesions affecting the skull base and upper cervical spine. The role of CT cisternography lies in the evaluation of intraspinal processes which may go undetected when studied by conventional CT alone. HRCT with edge-enhancement technique is most useful in assessing the osseous spinal canal and defining primary bone lesions of the skull base.

References

1. Taylor AR, Byrnes DP: Foramen magnum and high cervical cord compression. *Brain* 97:473–480, 1974.
2. Blom S, Ekbom KA: Early clinical signs of meningiomas of the foramen magnum. *J Neurosurg* 19:661–664, 1962.
3. Howe JR, Taren JA: Foramen magnum tumors: Pitfalls in diagnosis. *JAMA* 225:1061–1066, 1973.
4. Aring CD: Lesions about the junction of medulla and spinal cord, commentary. *JAMA* 229:1879, 1974.
5. Bull J: Missed foramen magnum tumors, editorial. *Lancet* 2:1482, 1973.
6. Schaffer KA, Valz DJ, Haughton VM: Manipulation of CT data for temporal bone imaging. *Radiology* 137:825–829, 1980.
7. Winter J: Edge enhancement of computed tomography by digital unsharp masking. *Radiology* 135:234, 1980.
8. Becker H, Grace H, Hackler H, et al: The base of the skull: A comparison of computed and, conventional tomography. *J Comput Assist Tomgr* 2:113–118, 1978.
9. Maue-Dickson W, Trefler M, Dickson DR: Comparison of dosimetry and image quality in computed and conventional tomography. *Radiology* 131:509–514, 1979.
10. Drayer BP, Rosenbaum AE, Higman HB: Cerebrospinal fluid imaging using serial metrizamide CT cisternography. *Neuroradiology* 13:7–17, 1977.
11. Hilal SK, Tookoran H, Wood EH: Displacement of the aqueduct of Sylvius by posterior fossa tumors. *Acta Radiol (Diag)* 9:167–182, 1969.
12. Wickbom I, Hanafee W: Soft tissue masses immediately below the foramen magnum. *Acta Radiol* 1:647–658, 1963.
13. McRae DL: Craniovertebral junction. In Newton TH, Potts DG: *Radiology of the Skull and Brain*. St. Louis, C. V. Mosby, 1971, vol. 1, book 1, pp 260–274.
14. Coin CG, Malkasian DR: Foramen magnum. In Newton TH, Potts DG: *Radiology of the Skull and Brain*. St. Louis, C. V. Mosby, 1971, vol 1, book 1, pp 275–286.
15. Banerji NK, Millar JHD: Chiari malformation presenting in adult life—its relationship to syringomyelia. *Brain* 97:157–168, 1974.
16. Appleby A, Foster JB, Hankinson J, Hudgson P: The diagnosis and management of the Chiari anomalies in adult life. *Brain* 91:131–140, 1968.
17. Saez RJ, Onofrio BM, Yanagehara T: Experience with the Arnold-Chiari malformation 1960–1975. *J Neurosurg* 45:416–422, 1976.
18. Naidich TP, Pudlowski RM, Naidich JB, et al: Computed tomographic signs of the Chiari II malformation. Part I: Skull and dural partitions. *Radiology* 134:65–71, 1980.
19. Naidich TP, Pudlowski RM, Naidich JB, et al: Computed tomographic signs of the Chiari II malformation. Part II: Midbrain and cerebellum. *Radiology* 134:391–398, 1980.
20. Naidich TP, Pudlowski Rm, Naidich JB, et al: Computed tomographic signs of the Chiari II malformation. Part III: Ventricules and cisterns. *Radiology* 134:657–663, 1980.
21. Langer LO, Baumann PA, Gorlin RJ: Achondroplasia. *AJR*

100:12–26, 1967.

22. Yamada H, Nakamura S, Tajima M, et al: Neurological manifestations of pediatric achondroplasia. *J Neurosurg* 54:49–57, 1981.

23. Shapiro R, Youngberg AS, Rothman SLG: The differential diagnosis of traumatic lesions of the occipitoatlanto-axial segment. *Radiol Clin North Am* 11:505–526, 1973.

24. Martel W, Tishler JM: Observations on the spine in mongolism. *AJR* 98:630–638, 1966.

25. Yasuoka S, Okazaki H, Daube JR, MacCarty CS: Foramen magnum tumors. *J Neurosurg* 49:828–838, 1978.

26. Lombardi G, Passerini A: Spinal cord tumors. *Radiology* 76:381–391, 1961.

27. Stein BM, Leeds NE, Taveras JM, et al: Meningiomas of the foramen magnum. *J Neurosurg* 20:740–751, 1963.

28. Slooff JL, Kernohan JW, MacCarty CS: *Primary Intramedullary Tumors of the Spinal cord and Filum Terminale.* Philadelphia-London, WB Saunders, 1964.

29. Firooznia H, Pinto RS, Lin JP, Baruch HH, Zausner J: Chordoma: Radiologic evaluation of 20 cases. *AJR* 127:797–805, 1976.

30. Bertelsen K, Andersen AP, Elbrond O, et al: Malignant tumors of the nasopharynx. *Acta Radiol* 14:177–186, 1975.

31. Miller WE, Holman CB, Kockerty MB, et al: Roentgenologic manifestations of malignant tumors of the nasopharynx. *AJR* 106:813–823, 1969.

32. Fujiwara S, Matsushima T, Kitamaru K, et al: Solitary plasmacytoma in the cerebellopontine angle. *Surg Neurol* 13:211–214, 1980.

33. Trolard J, Phelps PD: Plasmacytoma of the skull base. *Clin Radiol* 22:93–96, 1971.

34. Kutcher R, Ghatak NR, Leeds NE: Plasmacytoma of the calvaria. *Radiology* 113:111–115, 1974.

35. Vekram B, Chu F: Radiation therapy for metastases to the base of the skull. *Radiology* 130:465–468, 1979.

36. Traub SP: Mass lesions of the spinal canal. *Semin Roentgol* 7(3):240–259, 1972.

37. Bonafe A, Manelfe C, Espagno J, et al: Evaluation of syringomyelia with metrizamide computed tomographic myelography. *J Comput Assist Tomogr* 4(6):797–802, 1980.

38. Aubin ML, Vignaud J, Gordin C, Bar D: Computed tomography in 75 clinical cases of syringomyelia. *AJNR* 2:199–204, 1981.

39. Yu JS: Osteopetrosis. *Arch Dis Child* 46:257, 1971.

40. Carlson OH, Harris GBC: Craniometaphyseal dysplasia. *Radiology* 103:147–151, 1972.

CHAPTER THREE

Computed Tomographic Anatomy of the Lumbosacral Spine

ROBERT SHAPIRO, M.D.*

The application of high-resolution CT to the lumbar spine has sparked a renewed interest in the anatomy of this region. Whereas myelography visualizes only the subarachnoid space and its contents, CT visualizes the dura, epidural space and anterior epidural veins, the spinal nerves and dorsal root ganglion, the ligamentum flavum, the intervertebral discs, the facets and interfacet joints, and the bony canal. A thorough knowledge of the normal CT anatomy of the lumbar spine is indispensable for the recognition and understanding of various pathological processes.

VERTEBRAE

The lumbar vertebral bodies are oval in shape with their long axis oriented transversely (Fig. 3.1). The short pedicles, laminae, and spinous processes are fairly thick whereas the longer transverse processes are more slender. The vertebral bodies and their appendages have well-defined cortical margins surrounding a trabecular spongiosa.

BONY SPINAL CANAL

In the upper lumbar region, the bony canal is oval at the level of the pedicles but tends to become triangular more caudally (Fig. 3.2). Approximately 10–20% of normal spinal canals at L5 have a trefoil shape (Fig. 3.3). The anterior wall of the spinal canal is formed by the posterior margins of the vertebral bodies, the intervertebral discs, and the posterior longitudinal ligaments. The posterior wall is formed by the ligamentum flavum and the laminae dorsal to the ligament (Fig. 3.4). The lateral walls are formed by the pedicles and laminae. All of these structures are visualized routinely by CT with the possible exception of the posterior longitudinal ligament. Although the latter can be recognized when it is calcified, it cannot normally be separated from the annulus at the level of the intervertebral disc. Haughton and Williams (1) indicate that the normal posterior longitudinal ligament occasionally may be identified at the level of the midvertebral body. The normal ligamentum flavum is 2–4 mm thick at its attachment to the inner aspect of the laminae and articular processes; laterally, it dips into the intervertebral foramen (Figs. 3.5 and 3.6).

*The author is deeply grateful to Terry Ostrander, Chief CT Technologist, for her invaluable assistance.

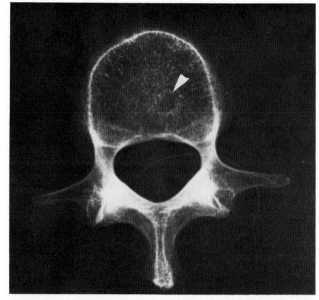

Figure 3.1. Frontal radiograph of a dried specimen of L2 demonstrating the oval shape of the vertebral body and the bony canal. Note that the largest diameter of the canal is directed transversely. Note the Schmorl's node (*arrowhead*).

The sagittal (anteroposterior) and transverse (interpediculate) diameters of the spinal canal are measured easily by placing a cursor on the appropriate points and reading the distance directly from the monitor (Fig. 3.7). Accurate measurements are made best with a bone window setting. A sagittal diameter less than 15 mm is suggestive of central spinal stenosis.

LATERAL RECESS

Axial sections through the pedicles demonstrate the lateral recess (nerve root canal) on either side. The recess is funnel shaped and varies somewhat in length (Fig. 3.8). In the upper lumbar spine, the lateral recess is insignificant due to the short intraspinal segment of the corresponding lumbar nerves. At these levels, because the theca is related intimately to the medial wall of the pedicles, the nerve root exiting from the lateral margin of the theca immediately enters the intervertebral foramen. At L4, L5, and S1, however, the lateral recesses are longer. Therefore, a hypertrophic superior articular process, a lateral bulging disc, or a posterolateral vertebral osteophyte can narrow the lateral recess (Fig. 3.9). The lateral recess

78

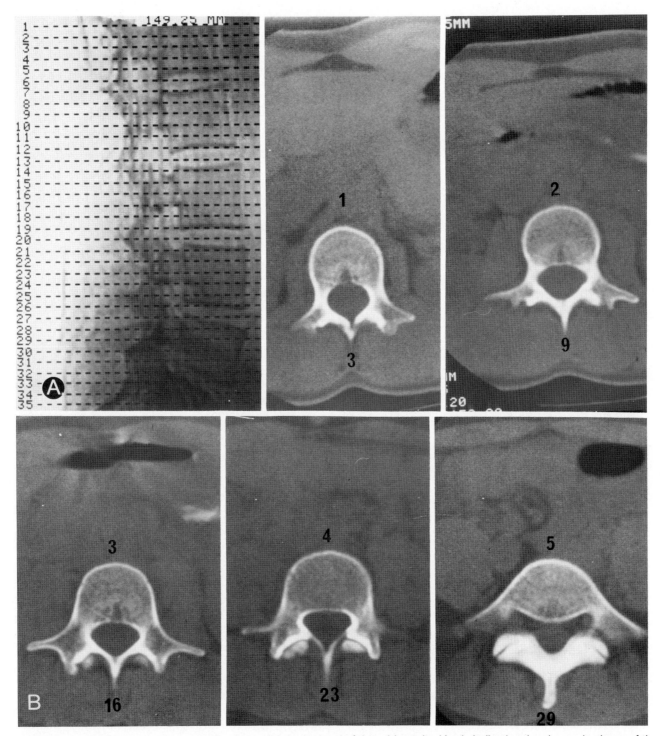

Figure 3.2.   Axial CT scans of a normal lumbar spine at the level of the midvertebral body indicating the change in shape of the bony canal from an oval in the upper lumbar region to a triangular configuration distally. The numbers above the vertebral bodies indicate the vertebral number. The numbers below the spinous processes indicate the level of the slice on the scout film.

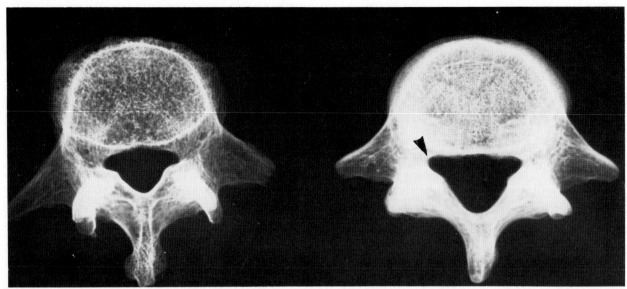

Figure 3.3. Frontal radiographs of two dried specimens of L5 with a trefoil-shaped bony canal. Note the ample space of the canal on the reader's right and the reduced space of the canal on the reader's left. One can readily appreciate how hypertrophy of the laminae or superior articular processes, or vertebral osteophyte formation can compromise the smaller canal on the left. The lateral recess is identified by an *arrowhead.*

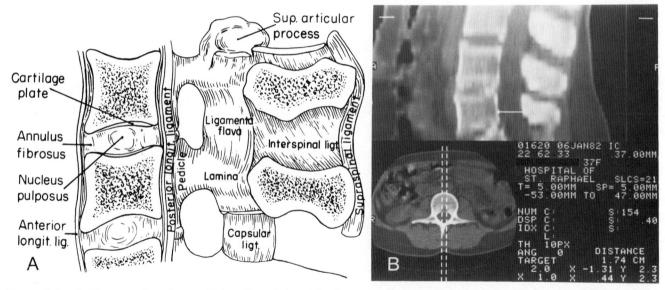

Figure 3.4. A. Diagram of median sagittal section of the midlumbar spine depicting the structures which border the bony spinal canal. B. Sagittal reconstruction of the lower lumbar spine demonstrating the anteroposterior diameter of the bony spinal canal.

contains the segmental nerve root after it leaves the thecal sac before it passes below the pedicle, to exit through the intervertebral foramen. The lateral recess is bounded anteriorly by the posterolateral aspect of the vertebral body, posteriorly by the overhanging shelf of the superior articular process, and laterally by the medial wall of the pedicle. The shortest height of the lateral recess should be measured, i.e., at the superior aspect of the pedicle where the superior articular process slopes anteriorly (Fig. 3.10). A height of 5 mm or more excludes lateral recess stenosis; a height of 3 mm or less strongly suggests spinal stenosis.

INTERVERTEBRAL FORAMEN

The intervertebral (neural) foramen is shaped like an inverted tear drop or trumpet. Anteriorly, the foramen is bounded by the posterior surface of the corresponding two vertebral bodies and intercalated disc. Posterosuperiorly, the foramen is bounded by the proximal inferior articular process and its pedicle; posteroinferiorly, it is bounded by the distal superior articular process and its pedicle (Fig. 3.11). The intervertebral foramen contains a short, thin segment of ligamentum flavum medially, epidural fat, the

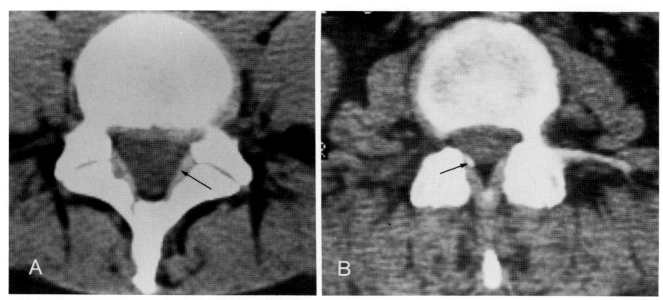

Figure 3.5. A. Axial scan through the body of L4 showing the normal ligamentum flavum (*arrow*). B. Similar section in another patient with calcification of the right ligamentum flavum (*arrow*).

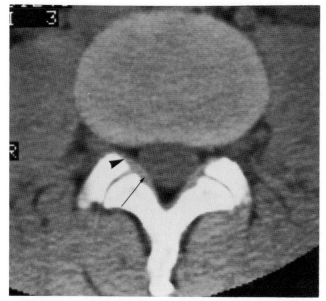

Figure 3.6. Axial scan through the L3–L4 intervertebral disc. Note the ligamentum flavum (*arrow*) and its lateral attachment in the intervertebral foramen (*arrowhead*).

radicular vein, the spinal nerve, and the dorsal root ganglion. All of these structures can be visualized by CT. The foramen also contains the sinuvertebral nerve and artery just ventral to the spinal nerve but these structures are too small to be imaged by CT. It is important to recall that the spinal nerve occupies the upper one-half of the intervertebral foramen. Hence, lesions which constrict only the lower half of the foramen do not compress the spinal nerve at this level.

FACET JOINTS

The diarthrodial facet (zygapophyseal) joints lie between adjacent superior and inferior articular processes on either side (Fig. 3.12). The joints in the lumbar region (particularly lower down) tend to be oriented coronally. They are fairly symmetrical at a given level and have flat or slightly curved surfaces. The joint surface of each articular process is capped by a 2- to 4-mm layer of hyaline cartilage and innervated by the posterior ramus of the spinal nerve. The joints have a synovial lining and a fibrous capsule. The anterior margin of the lamina medial to the facet joint is notched at the site of insertion of the facet joint capsule.

EPIDURAL SPACE

The epidural space contains a varying amount of fat within the spinal canal and the neural foramina. The fat (−100 HU) provides excellent contrast for delineation of the higher density nerve roots and intervertebral veins (30–60 HU), dural sac (30 HU), and intervertebral discs (70–130 HU). Usually there is little or no epidural fat anterior to the thecal sac at the level of the L3–L4 and L4–L5 discs (Figs. 3.13 and 3.14). This makes it difficult to delineate the anterior margin of the thecal sac and the nerve root sheaths as they arise from the lateral thecal margins. The anterior epidural space is usually most capacious at the lumbosacral level where the dural sac begins to taper (Fig. 3.15). In some patients, however, there is little or no anterior epidural fat at the lumbosacral interspace (Fig. 3.16). In the absence of anterior epidural fat, it is important not to be misled by a transverse or slightly oblique band of decreased attenuation due to an artifact from the zygapophyseal joint (see Fig. 3.16B). This artifact, which is seen most often at L5–S1, may give the

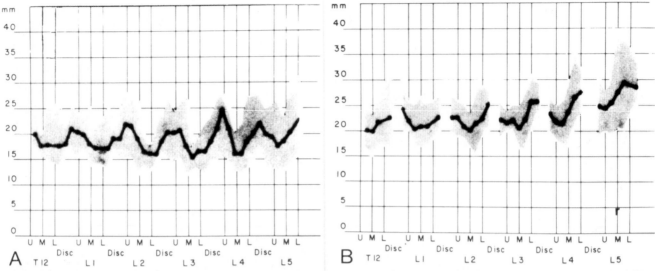

Figure 3.7. Diagram of the normal anteroposterior (sagittal) diameter (A), and transverse (interpediculate—IP) diameter (B) at the various lumbar spinal levels. (Reproduced from Ullrich et al. *Radiology* 134:137, 1980.)

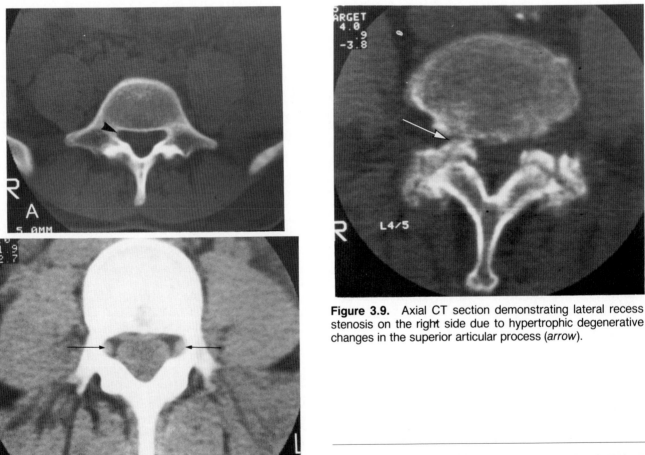

Figure 3.9. Axial CT section demonstrating lateral recess stenosis on the right side due to hypertrophic degenerative changes in the superior articular process (*arrow*).

Figure 3.8. A. Axial section through the pedicle of L5 demonstrating the lateral recess (*arrowhead*). B. Similar scan in another patient through the pedicle of L4 showing the nerve root in the lateral recess (*arrows*).

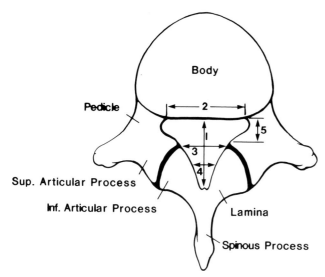

Figure 3.10. Schematic diagram of the bony spinal canal showing the lateral recess and its measurements along with other important spinal measurements. (*1*) sagittal (AP) diameter, (*2*) interpediculate (transverse) diameter, (*3*) interfacetal distance, (*4*) interlaminar distance, (*5*) depth of lateral recess.

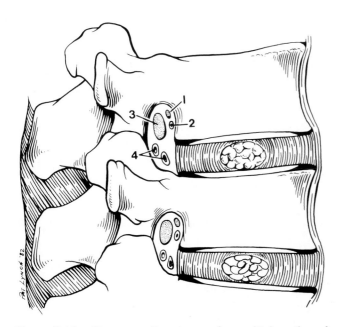

Figure 3.11. Diagrammatic schema of a sagittal section of the midlumbar spine showing the intervertebral foramen, its boundaries and contents. (*1*) sinuvertebral nerve, (*2*) sinuvertebral artery, (*3*) segmental spinal nerve, (*4*) radicular veins.

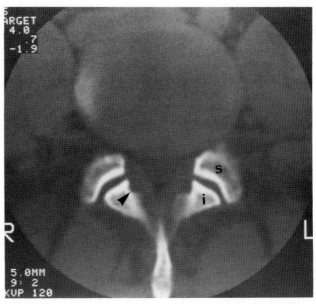

Figure 3.12. Axial CT section showing normal facets and facet joints at L3–L4. Note the congruence of the opposing surfaces of the superior (*s*) and inferior (*i*) articular processes. Note also the notch for insertion of the joint capsule (*arrowhead*). The subchondral bone on each side of the joint is homogeneous and sharply defined.

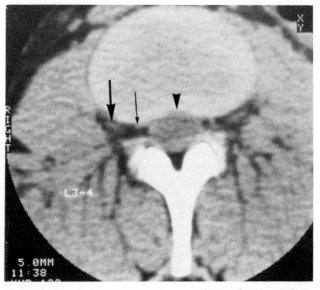

Figure 3.13. Axial CT scan of a normal L3–L4 intervertebral disc. At this level, the posterior aspect of the disc has a shallow central concavity (*arrowhead*) with the thecal sac closely approximated to the disc. Note the absence of epidural fat anterior to the thecal sac. Note also the lateral position of the anterior epidural vein (*thin arrow*). The anterior surface of the dural sac cannot be identified. The posterior aspect of the thecal sac is well defined by epidural fat. The nerve root (*thick arrow*) traversing the intervertebral foramen is seen clearly because of the surrounding epidural fat. Note the symmetry of the epidural fat deposits in both foramina.

erroneous impression of a disc protrusion when in fact the real disc-thecal interface is anterior to the artifact. Whenever necessary, the anterior surface of the thecal sac can be identified clearly by rescanning after the injection of metrizamide (4 ml of 60 mg·I/ml) into the distal lumbar subarachnoid space). At times, a thin membranous epi-

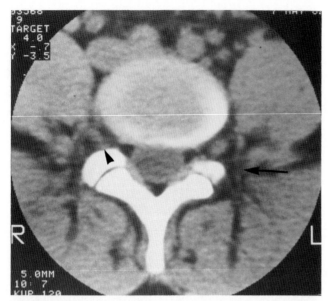

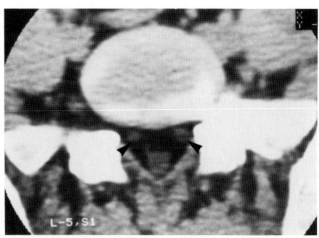

Figure 3.15. Normal axial CT scan at the level of the lumbosacral disc in a patient with abundant epidural fat anterior to the thecal sac. In such patients, the entire thecal sac, including the anterior surface is well defined. Note the symmetrical S1 nerve roots (*large arrowheads*).

Figure 3.14. Normal axial CT scan at the L4–L5 intervertebral disc level demonstrating a straight or flat posterior disc margin and no anterior epidural fat. Note the nerve root (*arrowhead*) in the intervertebral foramen and the segmental lumbar vein (*arrow*).

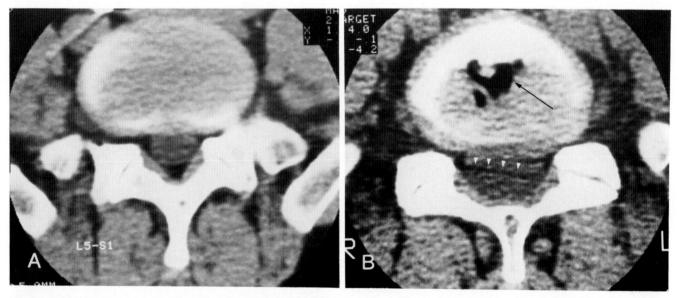

Figure 3.16. A. Normal axial CT scan of the lumbosacral disc in a patient with no anterior epidural fat. B. Similar scan showing an interfacet artifact (*arrowheads*) and a degenerated bulging lumbosacral disc with a vacuum phenomenon (*arrow*).

dural plica extends from the anterior aspect of the thecal sac to the posterior surface of the vertebral body (Fig. 3.17).

THECAL SAC AND NERVE ROOTS

The upper lumbar thecal (dural) sac is round or tubular in shape with well-defined margins (Fig. 3.18). The thecal sac tapers from the level of L3 down. At the level of L4–

L5 and L5–S1, the anterior surface of the sac often is flattened (Fig. 3.19). The dural-leptomeningeal interface and the individual nerve roots in the cauda equina cannot be distinguished routinely without subarachnoid metrizamide. When metrizamide is used to opacify the subarachnoid space, the latter is surrounded by a thin radiolucent rim representing the composite subdural-epidural space (Fig. 3.20A). At each interspace, the anterior and posterior nerve roots are visualized as two radiolucent

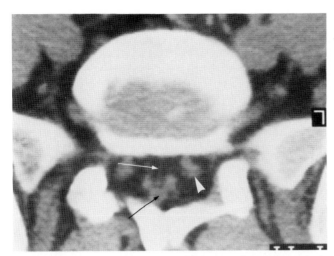

Figure 3.17. Axial scan at L5–S1 in a patient with an epidural plica (*white arrow*) connecting the anterior surface of the thecal sac to the posterior vertebral body. Note also the large symmetrical S1 roots (*arrowhead*) and thecal sac (*black arrow*).

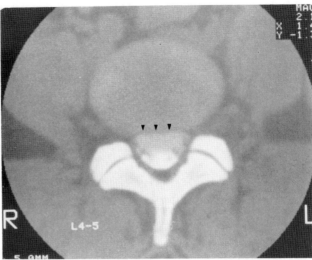

Figure 3.19. Supine axial metrizamide CT scans of the same patient at the level of the L4–L5 disc. Note the relatively flat configuration of the anterior surface of the thecal sac (*arrowheads*).

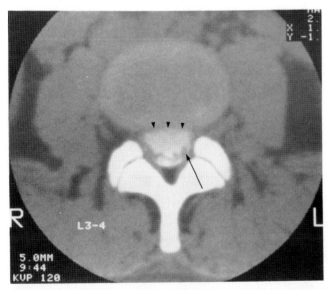

Figure 3.18. Supine axial metrizamide CT scan of a normal L3–L4 disc. The convex anterior thecal surface is well delineated (*arrowheads*). The contrast is denser in the most dependent portion of the thecal sac. Note the individual nerve roots (*arrow*).

Figure 3.20. A. Axial metrizamide CT scan at the lumbosacral interspace photographed with a soft-tissue window to show the thin radiolucent line representing the interface between the subarachnoid space and the composite subdural-epidural space (*arrows*). B. Same patient photographed with a bone window setting demonstrating the anterior (*thin white arrow*) and posterior (*thick white arrow*) L5 roots beginning to exit through the intervertebral foramen. Note the comparable roots of S1 (*black arrows*) in the lateral gutter of the thecal sac.

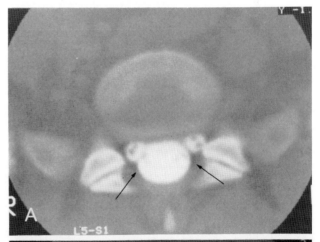

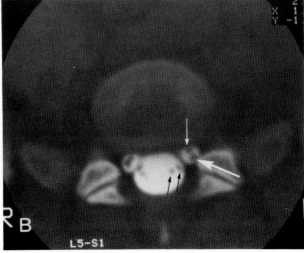

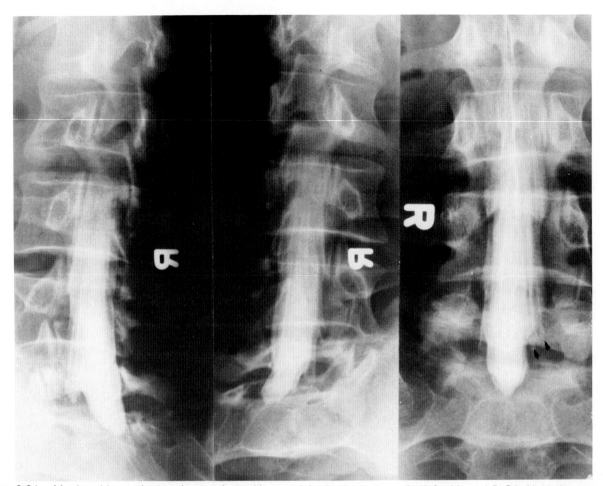

Figure 3.21. Metrizamide myelogram in a patient with a conjoint nerve root on the left side at L5–S1. Note the two roots contained in the same sleeve (*arrowheads*).

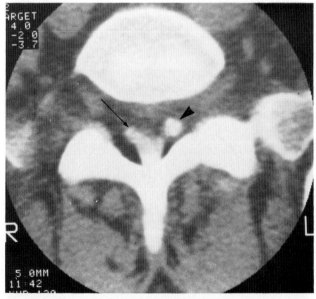

Figure 3.22. Axial metrizamide CT scan in the same patient at the level of the L5–S1 intervertebral foramen showing the metrizamide-filled large conjoint axillary sleeve on the left side (*arrowhead*) and the normal smaller sleeve on the right (*arrow*).

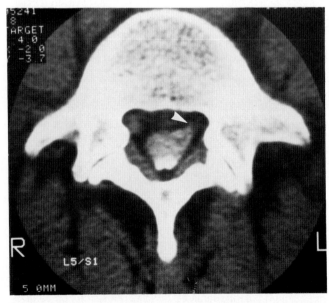

Figure 3.23. Axial section at the level of the lower border of the body of L5 adjacent to the disc showing the metrizamide-filled large conjoint root sleeve on the left (*arrowhead*).

dots in the opaque contrast column of the nerve root sleeve (Fig. 3.20B). Occasionally, there may be a conjoint nerve root with enlargement of the root sleeve containing the two roots for adjacent levels, i.e., L5, S1 (Figs. 3.21–3.23). In such cases, four radiolucent dots may be recognized within the opacified sleeve, representing the anterior and posterior roots of the conjoint nerve. A conjoint nerve root

may be suspected on a plain scan if there is an asymmetrical soft-tissue density not surrounded by fat in one lateral recess. The suspicion can be confirmed by a metrizamide CT scan at the appropriate level.

Normally, the unopacified nerve roots are visualized as 2- to 3-mm circular densities surrounded by symmetrical

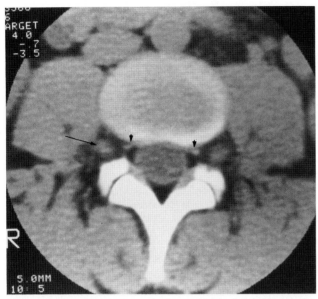

Figure 3.24. Axial CT scan at the level of the L3–L4 disc demonstrating the dorsal nerve root ganglion (*arrow*) in the intervertebral foramen. Note also a single epidural vein on either side (*arrowheads*).

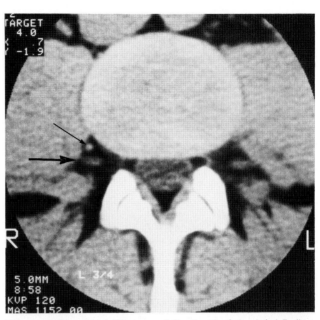

Figure 3.26. Axial CT scan at the level of the L4–L5 disc. The horizontal course of the radicular vein in the intervertebral foramen is clearly shown (*thick arrow*). Note the L4 nerve root in the intervertebral foramen (*thin arrow*).

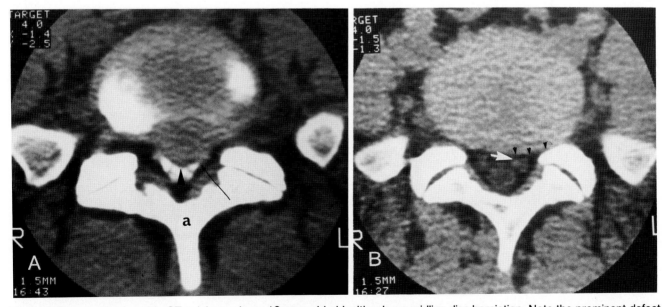

Figure 3.25. A. Metrizamide CT axial scan in an 18-year-old girl with a large midline disc herniation. Note the prominent defect on the opacified anterior theca (*arrowhead*) and the slight posterior displacement of the left nerve root (*arrow*) compared to the right due to greater extent of the herniation to the left of the midline. B. Axial CT scan in another patient at L5–S1 showing mild bulging of the disc on the left (*arrowheads*) with some posterior displacement of the ipsilateral nerve root (*arrow*).

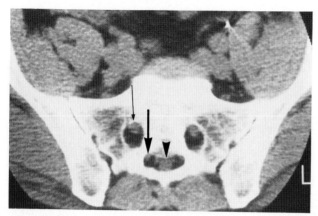

Figure 3.27.   Axial scan demonstrating symmetrical S1 (*thin arrow*) and S2 (*thick arrow*) roots in their respective foramina along with the tapered dural sac (*arrowhead*).

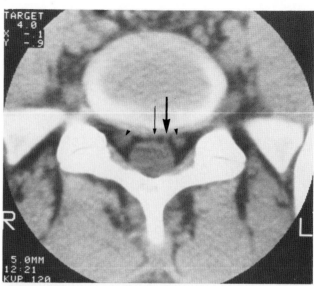

Figure 3.28.   Axial scan demonstrating normal asymmetry of the S1 nerve roots (*arrowheads*). The right S1 nerve is larger than the left because of dilatation of the right S1 nerve root sleeve. This can be confirmed by metrizamide. It is important to differentiate this normal variant from edema of the nerve secondary to pressure from a herniated disc at the lumbosacral interspace. Note the medial (*thin arrow*) and lateral (*thick arrow*) anterior epidural veins.

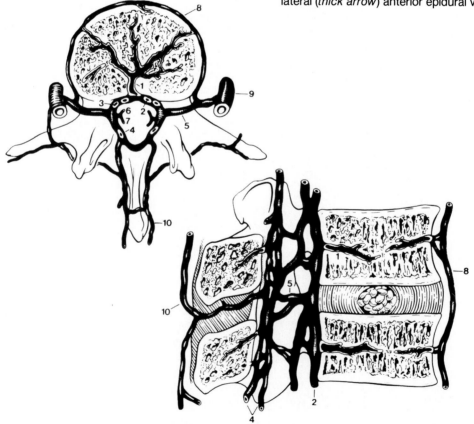

Figure 3.29.   Artist's sketch of the lumbar vertebral plexus in the axial and midsagittal projections. (*1*) basivertebral vein, (*2*) medial anterior epidural vein, (*3*) lateral anterior epidural vein, (*4*) posterior epidural vein, (*5*) intervertebral vein, (*6*) anterior radicular vein, (*7*) posterior radicular vein, (*8*) anterior external vertebral vein, (*9*) ascending lumbar vein, (*10*) posterior external vertebral plexus.

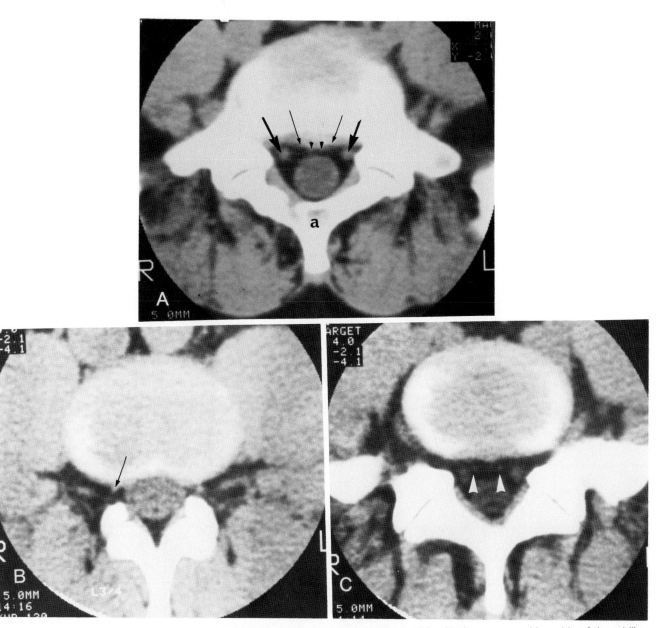

Figure 3.30.   A. Axial CT scan at the lumbosacral interspace. Note the paired epidural veins, one on either side of the midline (*arrowheads*). Note also the symmetrical S1 nerve roots (*thick arrows*) and the ample epidural fat completely outlining the thecal sac. Visualization of a variable segment of the L5–S1 disc (*thin arrows*) behind the body of L5 is due to the angulation of the x-ray beam with respect to the plane of the disc. The amount of disc visualized depends on the degree of angulation. The normal disc does not compress the thecal sac or nerve roots. B. Axial CT scan in another patient showing the lateral position of the anterior epidural veins at L3–L4 (*arrow*). C. A more medial position at L5–S1 (*arrowheads*) is shown.

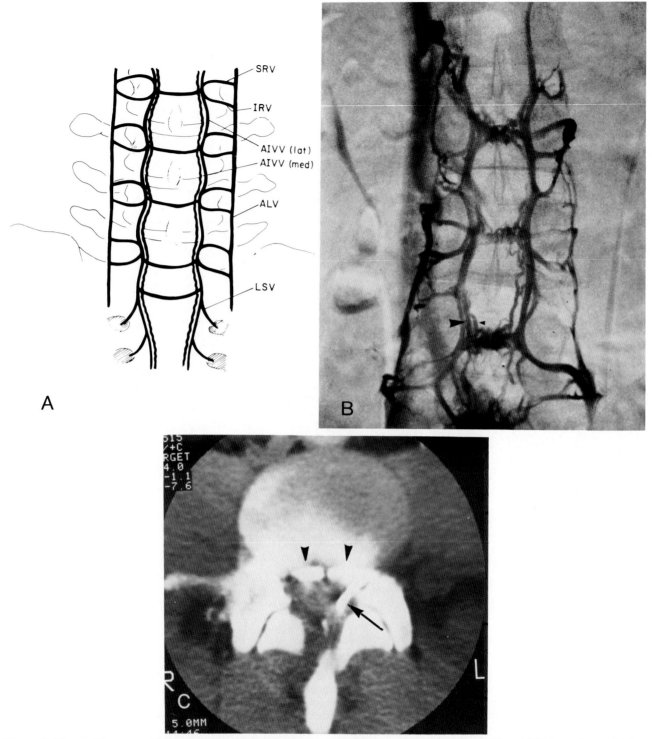

Figure 3.31.   A. Diagrammatic schema illustrating the significant epidural venous anatomy. *SRV* and *IRV*, superior and inferior radicular veins; *AIVV* (med) and *AIVV* (lat), anterior medial and lateral epidural veins; *ALV*, ascending lumbar vein; *LSV*, lateral sacral vein. B. Epidural venogram demonstrating paired medial (*thin arrowhead*) and lateral (*thick arrowhead*) anterior epidural veins on either side of the midline. C. Axial CT scan at L4–L5 in a patient with bilateral catheters in the lateral sacral veins. The scan was performed during the injection of contrast medium with the patient straining. Note the normal position of the anterior epidural veins (*arrowheads*) and the intervertebral vein (*arrow*).

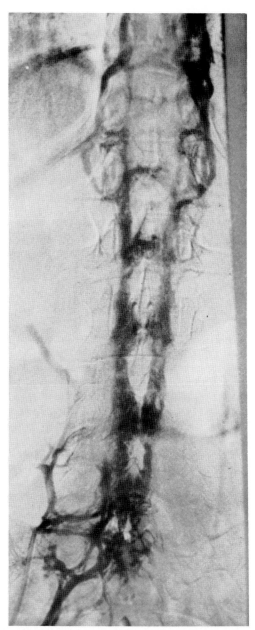

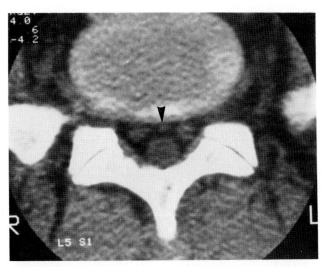

Figure 3.33.   Axial CT scan at lumbosacral interspace in a patient with a central racemose anterior epidural vein pattern (*arrowhead*).

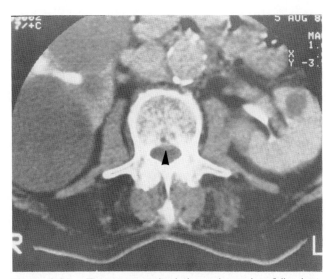

Figure 3.34.   The retrovertebral plexus (*arrowhead*) lies just behind the center of the vertebral body. It is often capped by a small bony mound.

Figure 3.32.   Epidural venogram showing racemose pattern of anterior epidural veins instead of a single or double pair of veins on each side of the midline.

epidural fat anterolateral to the thecal sac (see Fig. 3.15). The upper lumbar nerve roots tend to arise more or less horizontally whereas the lower roots, i.e., from L3 down, come off at a more acute angle from the lateral thecal margin. The dorsal ganglion also can be seen as a rounded density in the intervertebral foramen (Fig. 3.24). The nerve roots are usually symmetrical as they come off the antero-lateral aspect of the thecal sac and lie in the same plane. Posterior displacement of one nerve root compared to its opposite mate is an important finding in the diagnosis of a small disc herniation or a free fragment (Fig. 3.25). Within the neural foramen, the anterolateral course of the

nerve roots distinguishes them from the more transverse orientation of the radicular veins (Fig. 3.26). Occasionally, asymmetry of the S1 roots in the first sacral foramina occurs as a normal variant due to dilatation of the nerve root sheath, i.e., perineural sacral cyst (Figs. 3.27 and 3.28).

EPIDURAL VEINS (FIG. 3.29)

The anterior epidural veins lie more medially and are smaller than the nerve roots. In some patients, only one set of paired veins can be recognized (Fig. 3.30). In other patients, paired medial and lateral veins can be distin-guished on either side of the midline at the level of the intervertebral disc (Fig. 3.31; also see Fig. 3.28). At the lumbosacral level, the veins may be, at times, racemose rather than paired (Figs. 3.32 and 3.33). Even when they are prominent, the veins should not be confused with a bulging disc because of their lower attenuation value (30 HU) compared with that of the disc (70–130 HU). The anterior internal vertebral (epidural) veins anastomose with the external vertebral plexus via the intervertebral veins (see Fig. 3.29). The retrovertebral venous plexus lies just behind the center of the vertebral body (Fig. 3.34). It connects the anterior internal vertebral veins with the basivertebral plexus draining the vertebral body. The junction of the basivertebral veins with the retrovertebral plexus often is capped by a small bony spur anterior to the retrovertebral plexus (Fig. 3.35). The bony cap may project slightly into the spinal canal.

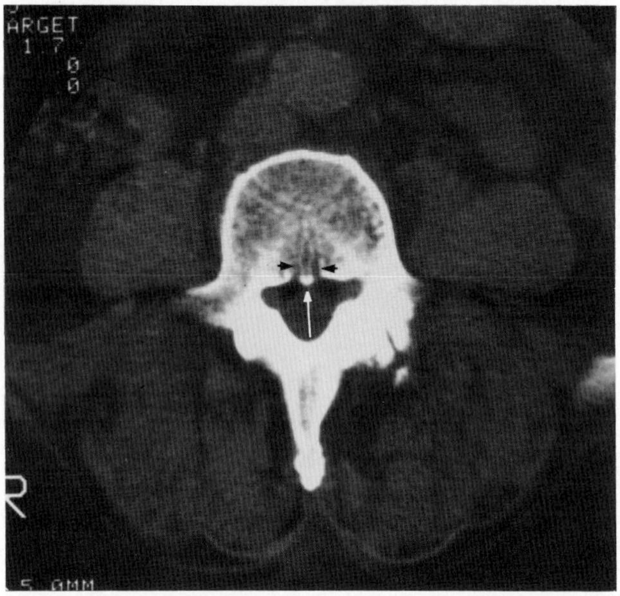

INTERVERTEBRAL DISC

The posterior margin of the normal intervertebral disc from L1–L2 to L4–L5 has a shallow concavity (see Figs. 3.13, 3.14, 3.18, and 3.19). The posterior aspect of the lumbosacral disc is straight or slightly convex (see Figs. 3.15, 3.16, and 3.20A). With aging and some degeneration, it is common to find some convexity to the posterior margins of the disc at several interspaces. As long as these minimal diffuse anular bulges do not compress or displace the epidural fat, theca, or nerve roots, they are not considered to be clinically significant (see Fig. 3.30). The intervertebral disc has a greater attenuation value than the thecal sac; the nucleus pulposus and the anulus have an equal density.

Not uncommonly, a portion of the nucleus pulposus herniates through a fissure in the vertebral end plate into the body of the vertebra, i.e., Schmorl's node. The latter always is related closely to the disc. Axial scans close to the end plate visualize the intrabody nuclear herniation as a focal area of decreased attenuation often surrounded by a zone of sclerosis (Fig. 3.36A). Calcification of the anulus is readily visible (Fig. 3.36B).

Figure 3.35. Bony projection (*arrow*) capping the retrovertebral plexus. Note the basivertebral vein (*arrowheads*).

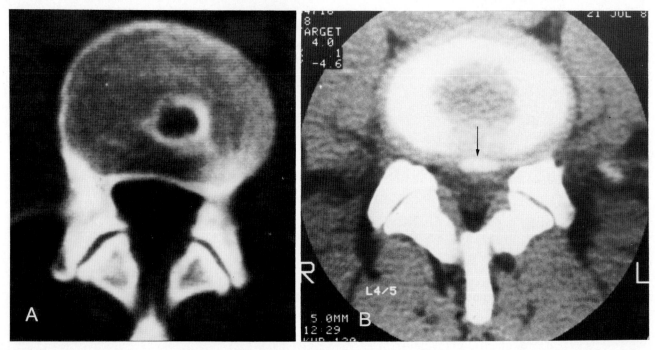

Figure 3.36. A. Axial scan demonstrating a Schmorl's node (*arrow*). Note the sclerotic rim surrounding the area of decreased attenuation which represents the intrabody nuclear herniation. B. Axial scan through the L4–L5 interspace showing calcification of the annulus (*arrow*).

THE ILIOLUMBAR LIGAMENT AND SPINAL MUSCLES (FIGS. 3.37 AND 3.38)

The iliolumbar ligament extends from the lateral aspect of the transverse process of L5 to the medial margin of the ilium (Fig. 3.37).

The psoas major muscle, which attaches to the entire lumbar spine, is seen as a slender structure at the level of L1. It becomes progressively larger as it courses distally in the lumbar gutter to reach its maximal size at the lumbosacral level.

The quadratus lumborum is a flat muscle which arises from the iliac crest and inserts into the medial aspect of the 12th rib. It has a transverse orientation in the paravertebral gutter and merges medially with the psoas major.

The sacrospinalis dorsi (erector spini) arises from the iliac crest, the posterior sacroiliac ligament, and the dorsal aspect of the lumbar and upper sacral spines. It separates into two parts, the larger medial segment comprising the longissimus dorsi and the smaller lateral iliocostalis segment. The iliocostalis inserts into the angle of the lower six ribs whereas the longissimus dorsi inserts into most of the ribs and into the thoracic transverse processes and upper lumbar accessory processes.

The semispinalis and multifidus muscles occupy the vertebral furrow below the sacrospinalis muscle. They are separated from one another incompletely; the multifidus

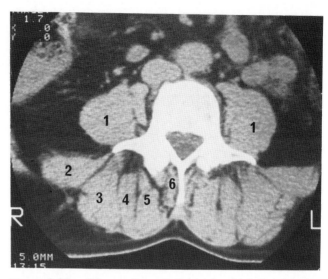

Figure 3.38. CT scan through the body of L4 showing the posterior spinal musculature. (*1*) psoas major, (*2*) quadratus lumborum, (*3*) iliocostalis, (*4*) longissimus dorsi, (*5*) multifidus, (*6*) interspinalis.

is placed more deeply than the semispinalis. Both muscles extend obliquely upward from the transverse to the spinous processes. The interspinalis muscles are made up of short fasciculi that correct the inferior surface of the proximal spinous process to the superior surface of the adjacent spinous process below.

Bibliography

1. Haughton V, Williams AL: *Computed Tomography of the Spine.* St. Louis, C. V. Mosby, p. 102, 1982.
2. Carrera GF, Williams AL, Haughton VM: Computed tomography of the lumbar facet joints. *Radiology* 134:145–148, 1980.
3. Dorwart RH, de Groot J, Eberhardt KS: Computed tomography of the lumbosacral spine: normal anatomy and variants. In Genant HK, Chafetz N, Helms CA: *Computed Tomography of the Lumbar Spine.* San Francisco, Univ. of Calif. Printing Dept., 1982.
4. Haughton V, Syvertsen A, Williams AL: Soft tissue anatomy within the spinal canal as seen on computed tomography. *Radiology* 134:649–655, 1980.
5. Heithoff KR: High-resolution computed tomography in the differential diagnosis of soft-tissue pathology of the lumbar spine. In Genant HK, Chafetz N, Helms CA: *Computed Tomography of the Lumbar Spine.* San Francisco, Univ. of Calif. Printing Dept., 1982.
6. Kaiser JA, Mall JC: Pitfalls in computed tomography of the lumbar spine. In Genant HK, Chafetz N, Helms CA: *Computed Tomography of the Lumbar Spine.* San Francisco, Univ. of Calif. Printing Dept., 1982.
7. Williams AL, Haughton VM, Daniels DL, et al: Recognition of lateral lumbar disk herniation. *AJNR* 3:211–213, 1982.

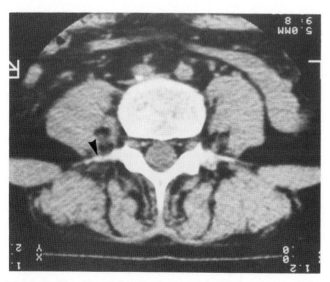

Figure 3.37. The iliolumbar ligament (*arrowhead*) runs from the transverse process of L5 to the medial surface of the ilium.

CHAPTER FOUR

Computed Tomography of the Sacrum

MARGARET ANNE WHELAN, M.D.

INTRODUCTION

The curved surface of the sacrum ideally lends itself to evaluation by computed tomography (CT). Plain films of the sacrum, even with tomography, can be difficult to evaluate and may not either identify the abnormality or fully clarify the etiology of a lesion once it has been detected by conventional techniques. High-resolution CT is not only the most accurate means of evaluating the sacrum, but analysis of the alteration of the various sacral components, central canal, foramina, bony matrix, and perisacral soft tissues adds specifity to the CT diagnosis.

NORMAL GROSS ANATOMY

Before analyzing the pathological processes which affect the sacrum, it is necessary to have a working knowledge of the normal anatomy of the sacrum. The sacrum lies at the upper posterior portion of the pelvic cavity. It is a triangular bone formed by the fusion of the five sacral vertebrae. These five vertebrae begin to fuse with each other from below upward at about the 17th or 18th year; fusion being complete by the 23rd year. There are five sacral surfaces; namely, pelvic, dorsal, lateral, superior (base), and inferior (apex). Within this bony sacrum are the dorsal midline canal, four ventral sacral foramina, and four dorsal sacral foramina. The midline dorsal canal contains the five pairs of sacral nerve roots which descend from the conus medullaris. The first four sacral nerve roots exit through their respective foramina whereas the 5th nerve root exits between the sacrum and the coccyx. Because all the major nerve roots exit anteriorly, the ventral foramina are much larger than the dorsal foramina which carry only minor cutaneous nerve roots. The large ventral foramina begin medially and dorsally near the central canal travelling laterally, anteriorly, and inferiorly to end at the ventral surface of the sacrum. Thus, the ventral portion of the sacrum displays the four pairs of sacral foramina which communicate with the central sacral canal through intervertebral foramina. On this ventral surface, the area between the right and left sacral foramina is composed of the flattened pelvic surfaces of the bodies of the sacral vertebrae, whereas the ventral portion lateral to the sacral foramina is formed by the costal elements which unite with one another and then fuse with the vertebrae.

The convex dorsal surface of the sacrum is composed of multiple longitudinal crests. Starting from the midline and moving laterally there is the median sacral crest, the intermediate sacral crest, the dorsal foramina, and the lateral sacral crest. In the midline, the median sacral crest represents the fused spines of the sacral vertebrae. Along this crest, there are either three or four spinous tubercles whereas beneath the lowest tubercle, there is a gap in the posterior wall of the sacral canal called the sacral hiatus. This sacral hiatus results from the failure of the lamina of the 5th sacral vertebrae to fuse in the midline. The intermediate crests form at the lateral surface of the fused sacral laminae and consist of a row of four small tubercles representing the fusion of the articular processes. The sacroiliac ligaments are attached at this level. The inferior articular processes of the 5th sacral vertebrae project downwards at the sides of the sacral hiatus forming the sacral cornua, to which are attached the intercornual ligaments linking the sacrum to the coccyx. The four small sacral foramina on the dorsal surface communicate with the central sacral canal through the intervertebral foramina. The lateral sacral crests formed by the fusion of the transverse processes are the most laterally placed crests on the dorsal sacral surface. These lateral crests consist of a row of tubercles called the transverse tubercles. The lateral surface of the sacrum is formed by the fusion of the transverse processes with the costal elements. The broad, superior, auricular surface articulates with the ilium, whereas posterior to this surface a number of ligaments attach to the sacrum. Below the articulation with the ilium, the lateral surface narrows abruptly and curves medially to form the inferior lateral angle.

The superior surface or base of the sacrum is composed of the upper surface of the 1st sacral vertebra. The large convex anterior border of this 1st sacral vertebra is called the sacral promontory. At this level, the central sacral canal is triangular in shape due to the short pedicles. The large superior articular facets of S1 project dorsomedially to articulate with the inferior articular facets of L5. The transverse processes and costal elements of S1 then fuse to the body forming the lateral portion of the upper sacrum or alae.

The inferior surface or apex of the sacrum consists of the inferior surface of the body of S5. At its most inferior aspect, this S5 body widens to form a broad oval facet for articulation with the coccyx.

CONVENTIONAL RADIOLOGY

Before the introduction of CT scanning, suspected problems in the lumbosacral region were evaluated by a routine lumbosacral series consisting of anteroposterior (AP), lateral, both obliques at 45°, and a coned down view of L5-S1. With this conventional view, however, the curved sacral surface was foreshortened making evaluation of the sacrum difficult. To overcome this problem, an AP sacral view with the x-ray tube angled 15–20° cephalad could be performed. Although this view could compensate for foreshortening of the sacrum, this area was still difficult to evaluate because of overlying bowel gas and fecal material. Conventional tomograms could overcome these problems largely but provided a high-radiation dose to the pelvis and were still unable to evaluate the surrounding soft tissues fully. Thus, CT was easily adapted to the evaluation of this anatomic area (1).

NORMAL CT ANATOMY

In order to analyze the normal anatomy of the sacrum on CT, it is necessary to visualize the sacrum in an axial plane. In this regard, the central sacral canal and the four paired ventral and dorsal sacral foramina become the most important anatomical points. On CT, the S1 level is easily distinguished by the convex promontory (Fig. 4.1). The central sacral canal at this level is triangular and connects to both the ventral S1 foramina and dorsal S1 foramina through the intervertebral foramina located in the lateral wall of the central sacral canal (Fig. 4.1). Both the ventral and dorsal foramina begin posteriorly and medially near the sacral canal. The smaller dorsal foramina travel laterally to end shortly below their origin whereas the larger ventral foramina course laterally, anteriorly, and inferiorly ending at the ventral surface of the sacrum. The longest foramina is S1, generally measuring 10–15 mm in length (Fig. 4.2). As the S1 foramina ends, the S2 nerve

root can be identified close to the central sacral canal. Again the ventral S2 canals travels anteriorly, laterally, and inferiorly ending approximately 10 mm below their origin (Fig. 4.3). At the S3 level, there is a marked diminution in both the size of the AP diameter of the sacrum as well as the sacroiliac joint (Fig. 4.4). Because the S3 and S4 nerve roots are much smaller than the S1 and S2 nerve roots, their respective canals are shorter. Therefore, both the ventral and dorsal foramina of S3 and S4 can be seen frequently on the same CT section. Although the level of the sacral hiatus varies with the individual, it can generally be seen at or below the S4 level (Fig. 4.5). Finally, the tip of the sacrum can be demonstrated on CT by identifying the broad, flat oval facet which articulates with the coccyx. Just behind the oval facet are the caudal ends of the sacral cornua which form a ligamentous attachment to the coccygeal cornua (38–42).

PATHOLOGY

The lumbosacral region is the most common site of congenital anomalies in the spine (2). These developmental problems include spina bifida, dysraphism, meningocele, meningomyelocele, lipoma, dermoid, tethered cord, dural ectasia, arachnoid cysts, and sacral agenesis.

Isolated S1 spina bifida is the most common bony anomaly of the sacrum occurring in up to 20% of the population (2). More extensive fusion anomalies of the sacrum are associated more commonly with lesions such as meningocele, lipoma, and tethered cord. Frequently, however,

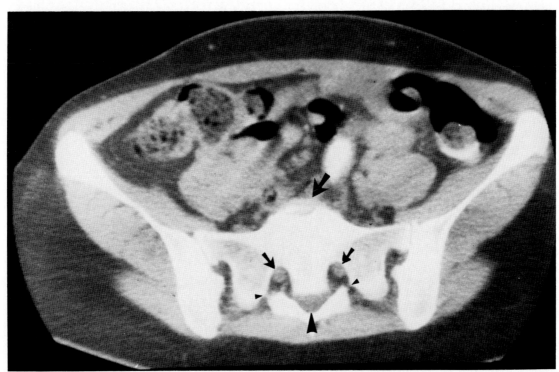

Figure 4.1.   Upper Sacrum: CT scan demonstrates the upper sacrum with the promontory anteriorly (*large arrow*). The central canal (*large arrowhead*) is seen dorsally with the proximal ventral S1 canals (*small arrows*) and the dorsal S1 foramina (*small arrowheads*) laterally.

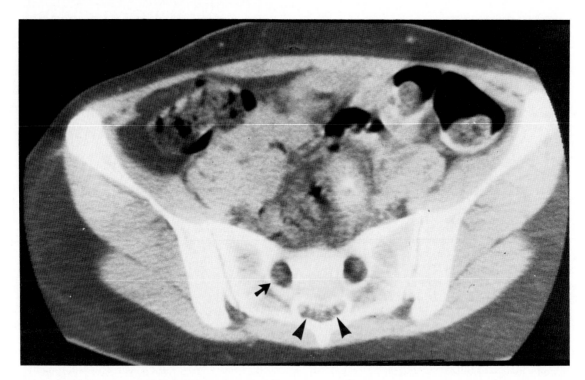

Figure 4.2.   S1–S2 Level: CT scan demonstrates the distal end of the S1 canal (*arrow*) containing the ventral S1 nerve root. The dorsal central sacral canal (*large arrowheads*) contains the sacral nerve roots, S2–S5. The sacraoiliac joints are large at this level.

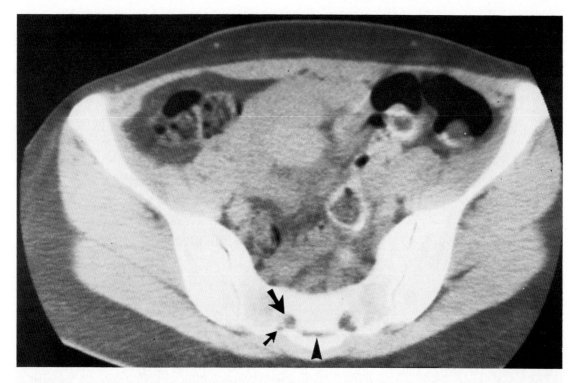

Figure 4.3.   CT scan demonstrates the proximal end of the ventral S2 foramina (*large arrow*) as well as the smaller dorsal S2 foramina (*small arrow*). At this level, the central canal (*arrowhead*) has assumed a more elliptical shape. The sacroiliac joints remain prominent at this level.

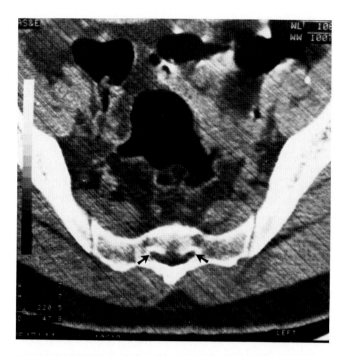

Figure 4.4.   S3 Level: CT scan reveals marked diminution in the size of the sacroiliac joints at this level. The S3 canals (*arrows*) containing the ventral S3 roots are seen forming at the anterolateral margins of the central canal.

the bony sacral anomalies may be difficult to appreciate due to overlying bowel gas and foreshortening of the sacrum on the conventional lumbosacral series (3). CT allows accurate evaluation of the bony sacrum in suspected cases of spinal dysraphism (4–8), as well as providing information as to the presence of a meningocele or lipoma.

Meningoceles represent extrusions of the leptomeninges through a developmental defect in the dura matter (9). As previously noted, there frequently are associated bony abnormalities. They occur in the lumbosacral and suboccipital areas. A meningocele may be simple, filled with cerebrospinal fluid (CSF), or complex, containing elements of the spinal cord or cauda equina (meningomyelocele) in addition to the CSF. Deposits of fat are found commonly in association with meningoceles.

Sacral meningoceles may project dorsally, anteriorly, or laterally as well as remaining totally within the sacrum, so-called occult meningoceles. The dorsal lesions are the most common and generally the easiest to detect, in that there is usually a superficial swelling under the skin.

Anterior meningoceles are much less common (10). They may be felt on rectal exam displacing the bowel forward, and are associated with a defect in the anterior vertebral body. It is important to determine the presence of an anterior meningocele in that an anterior approach could lead to infection of the sac and meningitis.

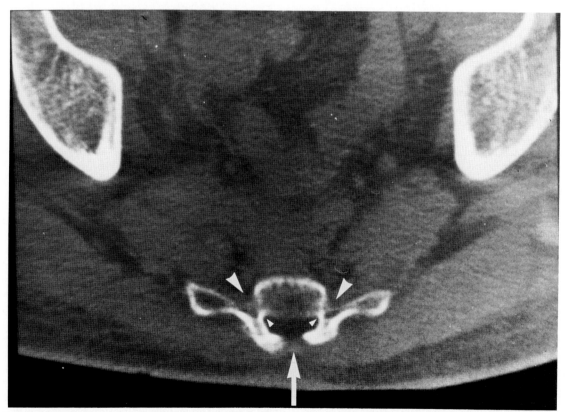

Figure 4.5.   S4 Level: CT scan demonstrates the sacral hiatus dorsally (*arrow*). The ventral S3 roots (*large arrowheads*) have exited, whereas the S4 canals are about to form in the anterolateral margins of the central canal (*small arrowheads*).

Lateral meningoceles are again much less common than the dorsal variety, and may be mistaken for paraspinal neoplasms on conventional plain films (9).

Occult meningoceles are outpouchings of the arachnoid within the sacrum just above the termination of the dural sac. These lesions are generally small and of no clinical significance. However, like all meningoceles, they may enlarge and eventually erode bone.

High-resolution CT scan is the single most valuable study in the evaluation of these lesions, especially when combined with the introduction of a water-soluble contrast agent, such as metrizamide, into the subarachnoid space. On CT, meningoceles cause primary expansion of the central sacral canal (Fig. 4.6) (3). The extent and location of the arachnoid protrusion can be determined easily, while the exact level of the site of extrusion can be visualized, thus, facilitating surgical repair (Fig. 4.6). In addition to outlining fully the meningocele, metrizamide allows identification of the conus, which is usually abnormally low in these situations (Fig. 4.7). CT alone cannot make this determination.

As previously mentioned, these meningoceles commonly are associated with lipomas. The low-density numbers characteristic of these fatty neoplasms are easily detected by CT scan (Figs. 4.7 and 4.8) (9). Again, there is primarily expansion of the central sacral canal with relative sparing of the sacral foramina (3). Similarly, dermoids which contain both calcium and fat can be identified easily by CT scan.

Meningoceles, lipomas, and dermoids commonly are associated with tethered cord. In this condition, the conus ends below the L2 level (11). Although this developmental defect generally is diagnosed in childhood, there is a growing number of reports of adult presentation of tethered cord (12). Various degrees of neurological dysfunction are attributed to this anomaly, including bowel and bladder dysfunction, spastic gait, lower extremity weakness, scoliosis, pes cavus, and impotence. Although tethered cord may be an isolated finding, it frequently is associated with cutaneous, dural, and vertebral anomalies. Although clinical examination may reveal the superficial abnormal marker (hemangioma, hair tuft, or sinus tract) and CT may demonstrate the dural and vertebral anomalies, the determination of the position of the conus requires myelography. It is preferable to perform this study with a water-soluble substance such as metrizamide, in that this allows combination of the myelogram with CT and avoids the necessity of contrast removal which is more dangerous in low conus situations (3).

Congenital dural ectasia generally is seen in neurofibromatosis. Here there is a weakness of the dura allowing dilatation of the subarachnoid space which with the passage of time may continue to increase in size, resulting in bone erosion. In these cases, CT shows uniform expansion of the central canal (Fig. 4.9). CT combined with metrizamide will allow the documentation of the dural ectasia as well as the detection of any associated neurofibromas on the roots within the canal.

Anomalies of the subarachnoid space also may involve the root after leaving the central canal and range from the commonly seen dilated root sleeve to the less frequent root diverticulum, root cyst, and perineural cyst (9). Root cysts generally occur in the lumbosacral region. They have narrow necks and may enlarge to result in sacral bone erosion, or may become totally isolated secondary to inflammation. The perineural cyst or Tarlov cyst occurs beyond the arachnoid sleeve and does not connect with the subarachnoid space. Both lesions may cause compression of the nerve root mimicking herniated disc (13–15). Again, CT can identify widening or asymmetry of the sacral foramina secondary to these cysts, whereas combined with metrizamide the connection of the cyst with the subarachnoid space can be established.

Sacral agenesis may be partial or complete, and may have varying associated findings including gluteal skin dimpling, loss of the gluteal fold, myelomeningocele, sacral lipoma, tethered cord, as well as orthopaedic and anorectal anomalies (16). There is usually a neurogenic bladder and varying degrees of neurological deficit with the motor deficit exceeding the sensory one. Additionally, sacral agenesis is reported as being more common in infants with diabetic mothers or with a strong family history of diabetes (17, 18). Although complete agenesis usually is confirmed on plain films, partial agenesis may be difficult to diagnose (19, 20). CT allows an accurate noninvasive means of establishing both the degree of sacral agenesis as well as related anomalies such as meningocele, lipoma, and tethered cord (Fig. 4.10).

NEOPLASMS

Neural

The neoplasms of neural origin occurring in the sacrum include neurofibroma, neurinomas, chordoma, and ependymoma of the filum terminale.

Both *neurofibromas* and *neurinomas* are nerve sheath tumors. The primary difference is that neurofibromas have nerve fibers passing through them, and are associated more commonly with Von Recklinghausen's disease (7). In addition, histologically, neurofibromas have a higher connective fiber content with a more irregular pattern as compared to the neurinoma (9). Neurofibromas may result in erosion of the vertebral bodies or pedicles. Such plain film changes may also be seen with neurinomas. Neurinomas, also referred to as schwannoma and neurilemomas, arise from the nerve sheath cells of Schwann and occur throughout the spine. They occur with equal frequency in both men and women, most commonly in the 3rd and 4th decade.

Neurofibromas and neurinomas in the sacrum are best evaluated with CT scan. With these lesions, there is selective expansion of the sacral foramina by a soft tissue lesion (Figs. 4.11 and 4.12) (3). Because these lesions are slow growing, the bony margins are sharp and well corticated. In cases of neurofibromatosis, however, the detection of smaller intradural neurofibromas within the spinal canal

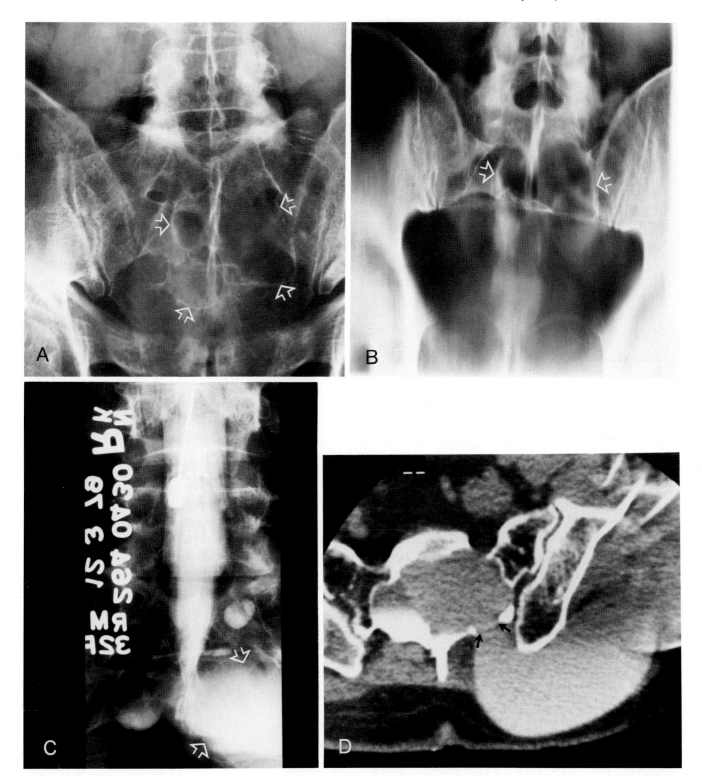

Figure 4.6. Adult Meningocele: AP of the sacrum (A) demonstrates lucent region with a well-corticated margin (*arrows*). Tomography (B) clearly defines the well-circumscribed sacral lucency (*arrows*). Metrizamide myelography (C) reveals the meningocele sac filled with contrast (*arrows*). The metrizamide CT scan (D) shows expansion of the central sacral canal by the contrast filled sac. The dorsal bony dehiscence (*arrows*) is outlined clearly on CT scan.

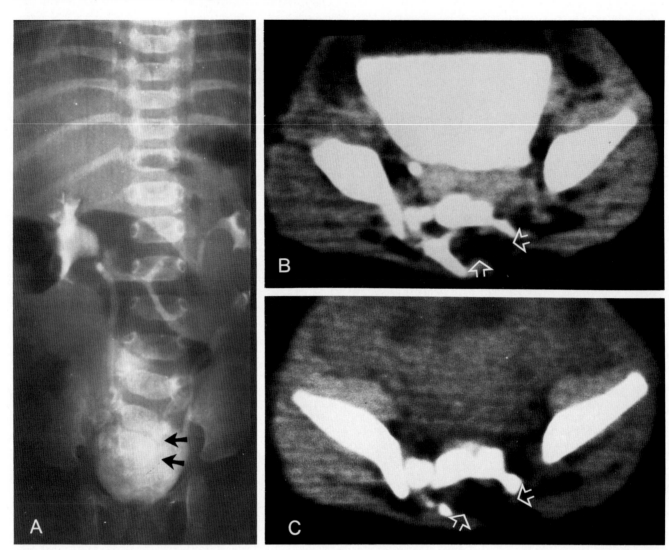

Figure 4.7. Sacral Lipoma with Tethered Cord: AP film, A, demonstrates anomalous sacral hemivertebrae (*arrows*) with evidence of a double-collecting system in the left kidney. Noncontrast CT scans, B and C, demonstrate congenital absence of the dorsal sacrum as well as a central canal widened by a lipoma (*open arrows*) which extends into the superficial dorsal soft tissues. Metrizamide myelography, D and E, further reveals a tethered cord (*arrowheads*) leading into the lipoma (*arrows*) as well as a small meningocele (*white arrowheads*) at the distal end of the sac.

requires contrast in the subarachnoid space. Again, the use of a water-soluble agent allows the combination of the myelogram with CT.

Chordomas are rare malignancies arising from remanants of notochord. They occur primarily at either end of the vertebral column (21–23) and represent the most common primary neoplasm of the sacrum (24). In a series of 91 primary sacral neoplasms, chordoma accounted for almost one-half the cases (25). These lesions are twice as common in men and generally occur in the 3rd and 4th decades. Chordomas are relatively low malignancy lesions. Initially, they are encapsulated, but later they break through the capsule, invading the adjacent bone and soft tissues. Chordomas do not metastasize distally with the exception of those located in the sacrum where there is a

5–10% incidence of metastasis (9). The most common presenting symptoms of sacral chordomas are bowel and bladder dysfunction and impotence. Before the availability of CT scan, these tumors were diagnosed by plain film, and conventional tomography. Chordomas characteristically revealed sacral bone destruction with calcifications representing either fragments of destroyed bone or a degenerative change in the tumor itself (26, 27). With CT scan, both the bone and soft-tissue changes can be outlined. Similar to the conventional tomographic findings, sacral chordomas demonstate bone destruction with a large soft-tissue mass containing calcification (3, 26) (Fig. 4.13). These calcifications most probably represent bony debris from the destructive process. CT clearly delimits both the ventral and dorsal soft-tissue components (Fig.

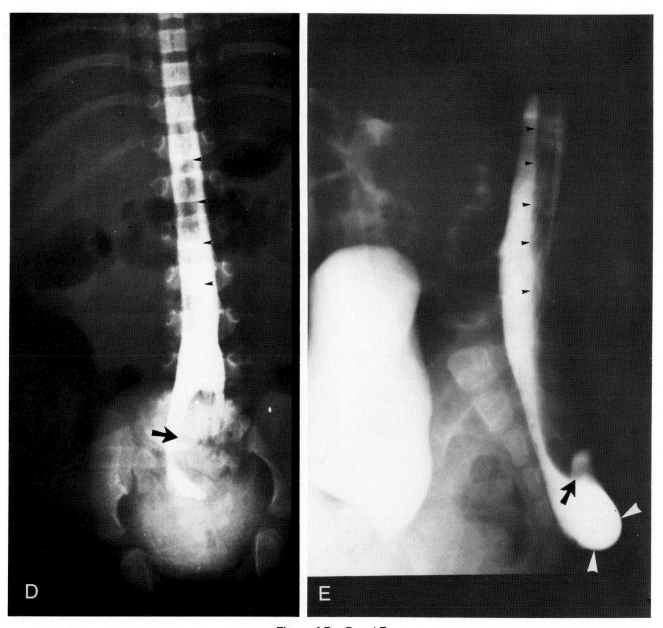

Figure 4.7. D and E.

4.14), thus facilitating the surgical approach. Furthermore, CT provides an easy, accurate means of following both the response of tumor to chemotherapy and/or radiation and the detection of recurrent tumor.

Ependymomas comprise approximately 65% of intramedullary spinal tumors (2). Because the largest amount of ependymal tissue occurs in the region of the conus medullaris and filum terminale (2, 9), it is understandable that 60% of ependymomas are found in these areas. These neoplasms are slow growing and may show widening of the spinal canal on plain films. Myelography demonstrates classic intramedullary widening. Similarly, CT will demonstrate widening of the central sacral canal by a soft-tissue mass with densities greater than CSF.

OSSEOUS LESIONS

Sacral neoplasms affecting the bone are relatively uncommon. Chordoma, the most common primary sacral neoplasm in the adult population has been discussed previously under neoplasms of neural origin. In the adult, giant cell tumor is the second most common lesion (24, 25), accounting for approximately 13% of the Memorial series (25), whereas in the pediatric population, teratoma represents the most commonly seen primary sacral neoplasm (28–30).

The remainder of cases include a variety of primary bone tumors, namely, Ewing's sarcoma, fibrosarcoma, chondrosarcoma, osteogenic sarcoma, reticulum cell sar-

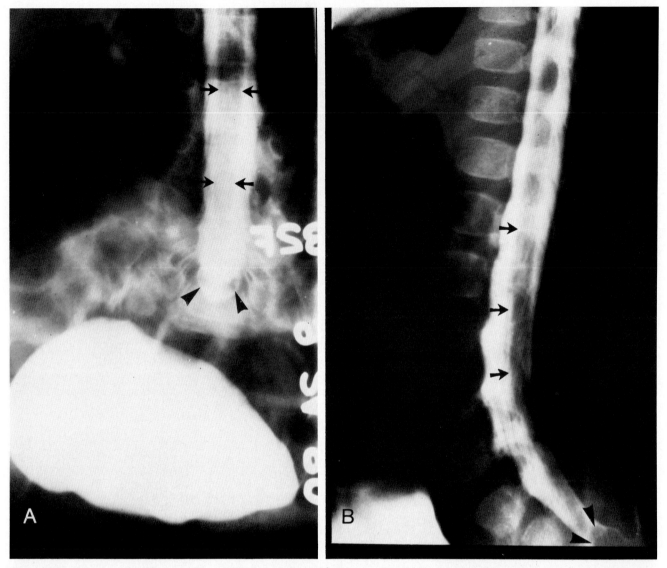

Figure 4.8.   Lipoma with Meningocele and Tethered Cord: Myelogram, A and B, demonstrates a tethered cord (*arrows*) in a patient with neurogenic bladder. A filling defect (*arrowheads*) appears at the distal end of the metrizamide column. CT scan, C, D, and E, performed after myelography reveals the low density lipoma (*large arrowheads*), as well as the small meningocele (*small arrowheads*) protruding dorsally through the dysraphic sacrum.

coma, lymphoma, plasmacytoma, aneurysmal bone cyst, benign osteoblastoma and osteochondroma as well as metastatic lesions (31–33).

Giant cell tumors consist of multinucleated giant cells within a fibroid stroma. Although the majority of these tumors are benign, as many as 50% may recur after initial treatment; while approximately 10% may be malignant on initial presentation. Giant cell tumor may rarely metastasize to the lungs (34). However, it is difficult to predict at presentation which tumor will behave aggressively making management difficult.

The prognosis of giant-cell tumor of the sacrum is much worse than giant-cell tumors in other sites, in that the recurrence and death rates are much higher (25). A factor in this poorer prognosis is a greater delay in diagnosis of

tumors in the sacrum, so that the giant-cell tumors in this area tend to be larger when detected, than tumors in the more common sites.

As with most sacral lesions, there are frequently nonspecific symptoms such as low back pain and pelvic pressure. Early diagnosis is difficult in that plain film findings may be subtle. Radiographically, these lesions are characteristically lucent. Similarly, on CT scan, giant-cell tumors appear as osteolytic, expanding, frequently eccentric lesions, generally with a subarticular location (25, 32) (Fig. 4.15). CT enables earlier detection of these lesions, as well as accurate determination of the extent of the neoplasm. Finally, CT provides a means of follow-up care in evaluating patients for recurrent tumor.

Teratomas of the sacrococcygeal region arise from the

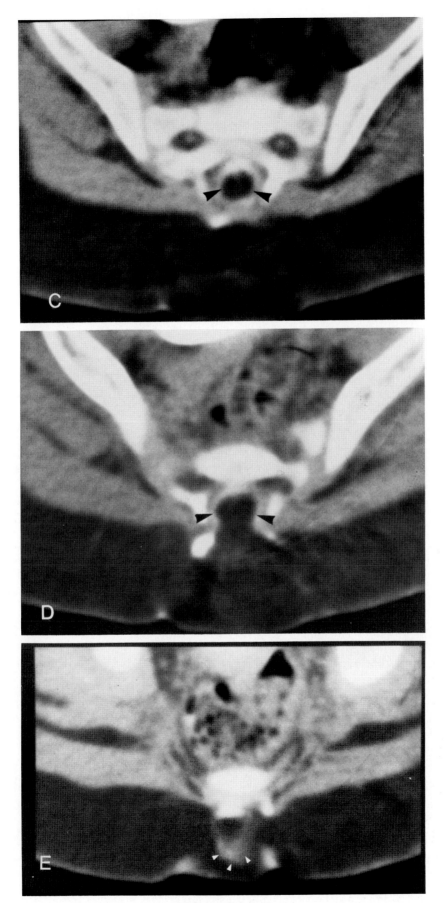

Figure 4.8. C–E.

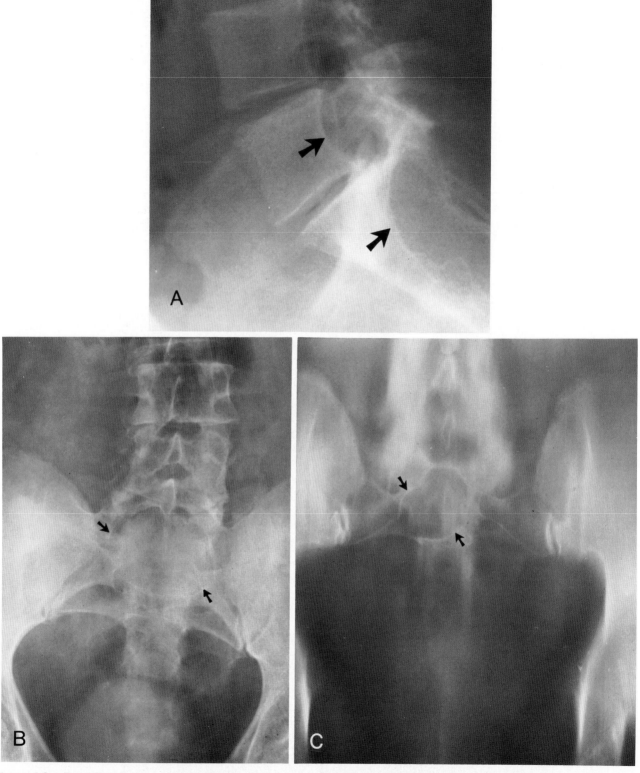

Figure 4.9. Dural Ectasia in a patient with neurofibromatosis: Lateral view of the sacrum, A, demonstrates scalloping of the posterior border of the vertebrae (*large arrows*). AP view, B, reveals a sclerotic rim seen to better advantage on tomography, C. CT scans, D–G, show expansion of the central sacral canal with relative sparing of the foramina. The sacral nerves can be distinguished on E and F (*white arrowheads*) whereas on G, the soft-tissue mass is seen extruding ventrolaterally into the pelvis (*open arrows*). Metrizamide myelography, H, confirms the presence of an ectatic dura.

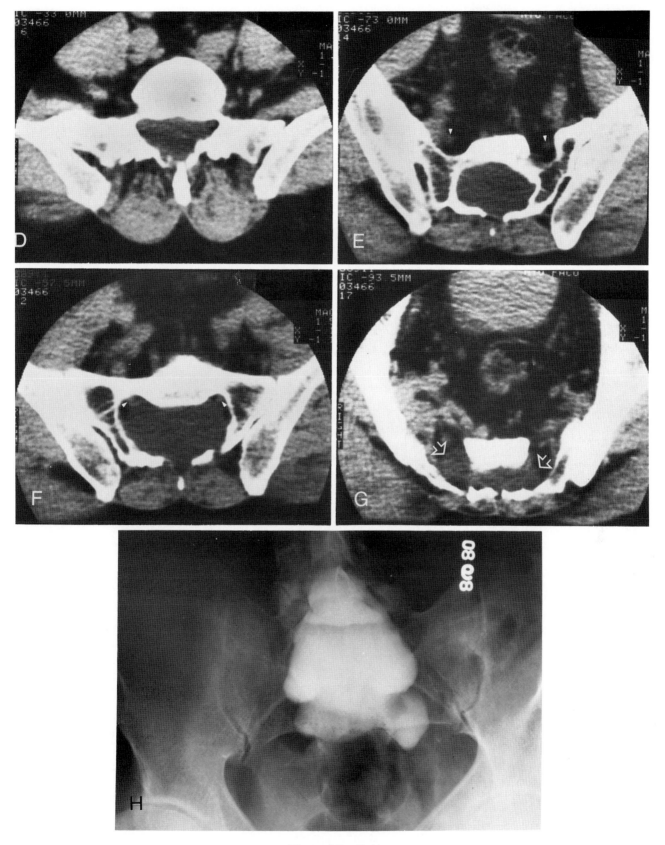

Figure 4.9.   D–H.

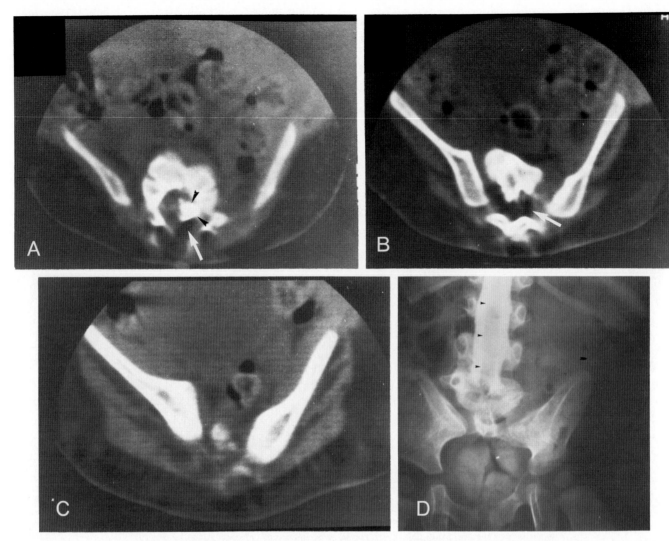

Figure 4.10. Sacral Agenesis: Noncontrast CT scans, A–C, demonstrate malformation of the L5 vertebra with absence of the sacral elements. There is fat density within the sacral canal at the L5-S1 level on A and B (*arrows*) as well as a bone fragment within the canal on A (*arrowheads*). The metrizamide myelogram, D, reveals a tethered cord (*arrowheads*) with an abrupt end to the dural tube at the L5 level.

pluripotential cells of Hensen's node within and anterior to the coccyx (35). Approximately 75% of cases occur in females (28, 29). These tumors generally present as an external mass over the sacrum. Teratomas are usually benign, but about 10–13% are malignant and are uniformly fatal (28, 29). It has been suggested that the frequency of malignancy in these teratomas increases with age (36), and that benign neonatal lesions which are undetected may undergo malignant degeneration. Radiographically, these lesions present as soft-tissue masses (Fig. 4.16). Calcification is seen in about 35% of lesions (28). Histologically, these soft-tissue lesions are both solid and cystic. Frequently, the fluid within the teratoma is of CSF density, not secondary to a connection to the subarachnoid space, but due to the choroid plexus within the tumor mass (28). Thus, CT may demonstrate a soft-tissue lesion with cystic areas and calcification. CT provides a useful

means of distinguishing these lesions from the more commonly seen neonatal lesions, meningocele and lipoma.

Ewing's sarcoma is a malignant, round cell tumor usually occurring in patients between 5 and 14 years of age (37). The patients commonly have malaise, fever, leukocytosis, and elevated sedimentation rate, as well as pain and local tenderness. The pelvis is the second most common site after the femur (37). Radiographically, these lesions are usually osteolytic, although they may exhibit bone production and lamellated periosteal reaction. Visualization of the sacrum and pelvis on plain film, especially in children, is often difficult due to overlying bowel gas and feces. CT scan, however, obviates these problems by clearly visualizing both the bony destruction as well as associated soft-tissue masses with these lesions (Fig. 4.17).

Fibrosarcoma is a malignant fibroblastic neoplasm of

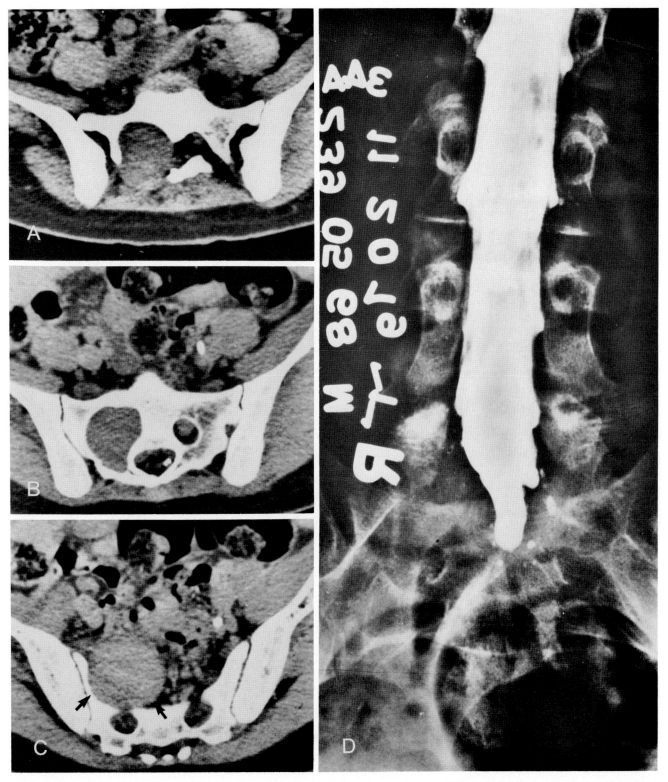

Figure 4.11.   Sacral Neurofibroma: Axial CT scans, A–C reveal selective expansion of the right S1 foramen and canal by a large soft-tissue mass which projects into the pelvis (*arrows*). The myelogram, D, demonstrates an extradural defect at S1 secondary to the large neurofibroma.

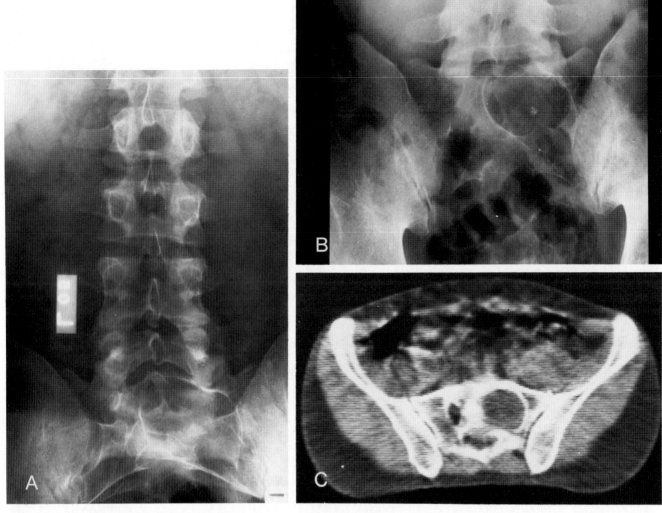

Figure 4.12. Sacral Neurofibroma: AP view from the lumbosacral series, A, demonstrates a lucency with a sclerotic margin. Routine sacral view with the tube angled cephalad, B shows the lesion to better advantage. Noncontrast CT scan, C, reveals selective uniform expansion of the ventral S1 foramina by the neurofibroma.

bone which does not form osteoid or chondroid matrix (37). There is a wide age range from the 2nd–7th decade with the pelvis being the most common site of involvement. Radiographically, there is generally a large soft-tissue mass associated with an osteolytic bone lesion. Fibrosarcomas also may demonstrate sequestration, a rare finding in bone neoplasms. Similar changes also may be seen with CT scan (Fig. 4.18). Again, CT scan provides the best modality for evaluating these lesions, in that the soft-tissue mass as well as the bony lesion can be visualized.

Chondrosarcoma is the third most commonly seen primary bone malignancy after myeloma and osteogenic sarcoma. (37). These tumors may occur in the center of the bone or along the periphery. Chondrosarcomas may develop from exostosis, enchondromas, or in areas affected by Paget's disese. These tumors usually present in middle-

aged adults with a chronic history of dull pain. Central chondrosarcomas may occur in the sacrum. Radiologically, these lesions are osteolytic without well-defined sclerotic margins. They usually contain characteristic "punctate", "snowflake" calcifications. On CT scan, there is a similar osteolytic appearance. However, identification of the characteristic calcifications as well as the soft-tissue component is facilitated (24). This feature is especially useful in determining malignant degeneration in Paget's disease (Fig. 4.19).

Osteogenic sarcoma is a malignant primary bone neoplasm arising from primitive, undifferentiated mesenchyme. It is twice as common in men, and occurs primarily in young adults with 70–80% of the cases occurring between 10–30 years of age (37). Most osteosarcomas in the older age group are secondary to previous bone conditions

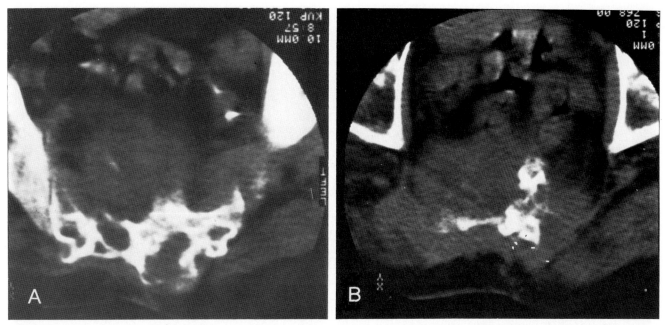

Figure 4.13. Chordoma: Noncontrast CT scans, A and B, reveal marked destruction of the sacrum associated with a large soft-tissue mass. This highly lytic lesion obliterates both the central canal as well as the sacral foramina.

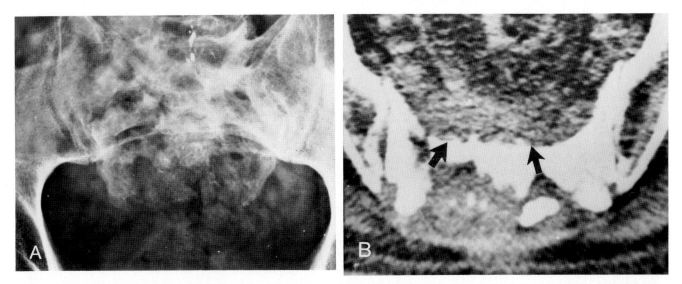

Figure 4.14. Sacral Chordoma: AP films of the pelvis shows destruction of the inferior margin of the sacrum (A). Axial CT scan B, however, clearly demonstrates both the extensive bony destruction as well as the soft-tissue component both dorsally and ventrally (*arrows*).

such as Paget's disease. After myeloma, osteosarcoma is the most common primary neoplasm of bone. Although the most common site is the metaphysis of long bones, osteogenic sarcoma may occur in any location including the pelvis. In patients with sarcomatous degeneration of Paget's disease, the pelvis is a more common location than in the young adult. These tumors were classically diagnosed by their roentgenographic appearance, namely, periosteal new bone formation, generally sunburst or on-

ion-peel in appearance, associated with a soft-tissue mass. The affected bone may show increased density, or destruction change. CT allows visualization of both the soft-tissue mass as well as the bone changes. Recent reports also indicate that CT scan can be used accurately to determine the extent of the true intramedullary bone involvement, which may be difficult on either plain films or conventional tomography (32). Additionally, lung metastases which commonly occur with this lesion may be deter-

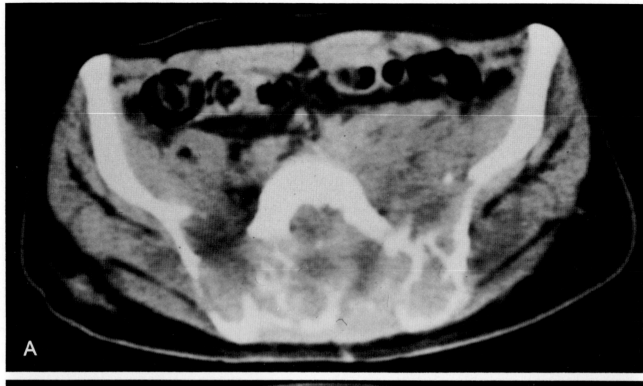

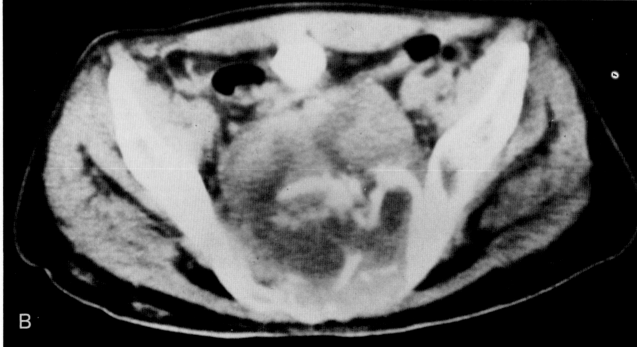

Figure 4.15. Giant Cell Tumor: Axial CT scans, A and B, reveal extensive destruction of the sacrum extending across both sacroiliac joints. There is an associated nonhomogeneous ventral soft-tissue mass.

mined at the same time using the CT scan.

Primary reticulum cell sarcoma of bone and *lymphoma* may rarely affect the sacrum. Reticulum cell sarcoma of bone affects all ages and has a male predominence (37).

These patients are generally well, even when the local disease is extensive. Radiographically, it affects the marrow of tubular bones and becomes extensively permeated in the medullary cavity before destroying the cortex.

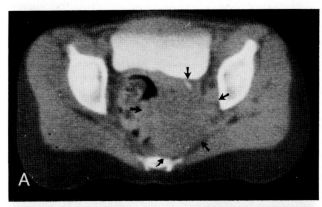
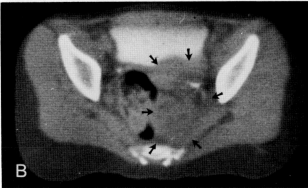

Figure 4.16. Sacral Teratoma: Axial CT scans, A and B, reveal a large presacral soft-tissue mass (*arrows*) pushing the rectal air to the right and identing the posterior wall of the contrast-filled bladder. As with most teratomas, the predominant feature is a soft-tissue mass with no demonstrable effect on the bony sacrum. (Case courtesy of Dr. Deck of Memorial Sloane-Kettering.)

There is frequently a large, associated soft-tissue mass (37). On CT scan, the extent of the permeative bony lesion as well as the soft-tissue component is evident (Fig. 4.20). The sacrum rarely may be affected with generalized lymphoma. Here, again CT scan accurately defines both the extent of the nodal involvement as well as the bony change (Fig. 4.21).

Multiple myeloma is the most common primary malignancy of bone. It arises from hematopoietic elements in the bone marrow, generally occurring between the ages of 40–70, and being twice as common in males (37). Myeloma primarily involves red marrow, with prime locations being pelvis, ribs, skull, spine, and mandible. Although myeloma is generally a diffuse process, these abnormal cells may proliferate locally resulting in tumorlike plasmacytomas. These lesions may be located in the sacrum.

Classically, myeloma appears as multiple osteolytic lesions scattered throughout the skeleton. There is generally no periosteal reaction. Plasmacytomas are classically very destructive lesions, usually with a bubbly appearance, which expand the bone and then break through the cortex resulting in a soft-tissue mass (24). The CT appearance of myeloma is similar to that seen on conventional radio-

graphs. However, the ability of CT to detect these lesions, especially a solitary plasmacytoma of the sacrum is increased.

Aneurysmal bone cysts are benign lesions consisting of blood-filled, honeycombed spaces frequently lined by granulation tissue, osteoid and multinucleated giant cells. The spine is a common location with occasional involvement of the sacrum (24). Aneurysmal bone cyst usually affects young adults and can arise from pre-existing bone lesions, such as chondroblastoma, and giant cell tumor (37). These lesions are purely osteolytic and balloon out the bone. The margins may be sclerotic or ill-defined, whereas the size of the lesion may progress rapidly over a short period of time. These lesions may break through the cortex causing soft-tissue hemorrhage. Similar changes may be appreciated on CT scan, but again with sacral lesions, CT will make the character and extent of the bone change easier to delineate, while also outlining the soft-tissue component.

Metastases may result from hematogenous or lymphatic spread, as well as direct extension. In the adult, the most common primary carcinomas are lung, prostate, breast, and kidney, whereas in the pediatric age group, neuroblastoma is the most common source of metastasis. These bony metastases are characteristically lytic, with the exception of prostate carcinoma which usually results in blastic lesions. Radiographically, these lesions are generally ill defined. The CT findings are similar to the plain film changes, but with varying degrees of soft-tissue mass (Figs. 4.22 and 4.23).

INFLAMMATORY LESIONS

Sacral inflammation may be the result of hematogenous spread, but more commonly is the result of decubitus ulcers or extension from pelvic infections. Again, the early changes of sacral osteomyelitis may be difficult to appreciate on plain films. With CT scan, however, both the bone destruction as well as the soft-tissue lesion may be delineated. On CT scan, sacral abscess may demonstrate air fluid levels, spread across the sacroiliac joints as well as disruption of the soft-tissue planes (Fig. 4.24). Patients with abscesses in this region are classically difficult to examine radiographically. CT provides an efficient means of documenting the extent of the lesion as well as facilitating surgical drainage and monitoring the response to antibiotic therapy.

TRAUMA

The evaluation of the extent of pelvic trauma is difficult with conventional radiographic techniques. Additionally, positioning for various radiographs may increase fracture fragment displacement. Using CT scan, the injured patient may be examined for both soft-tissue and bone injury without undo manipulation. Furthermore, a body cast which seriously degrades routine radiographic images, provides no problem with CT scan. CT easily outlines the size of fracture fragments as well as their displacement

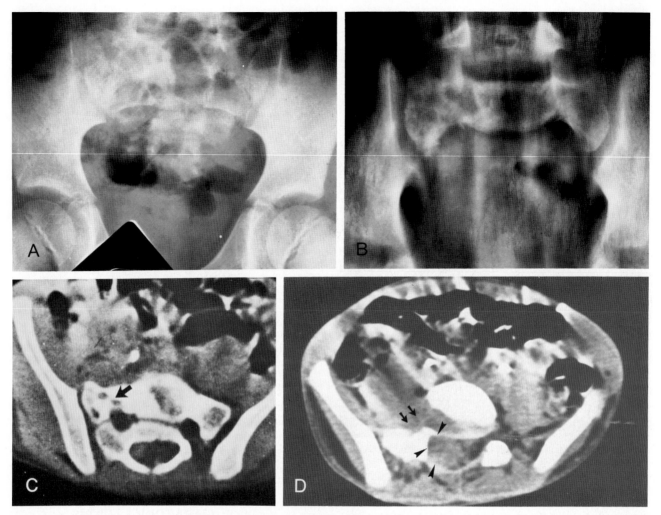

Figure 4.17. Ewing's Sarcoma: Plain film, A, suggests mottling of the right sacral ala, which is confirmed on tomography, B. D, Axial CT scans, C and D, show both the bony abnormality, C (*arrow*), as well as the soft-tissue component, both inside (*arrowheads*, D) and outside (*arrows*, D) the spinal canal. Note that the normal epidural and paraspinal fat planes are lost on the right.

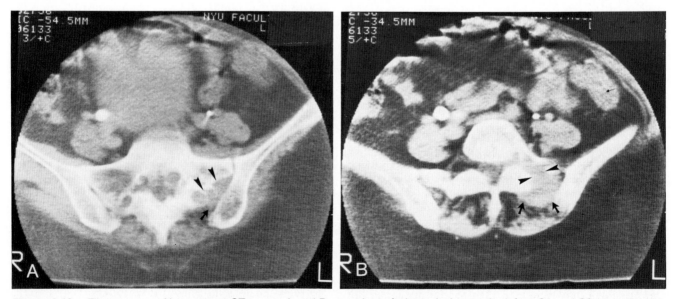

Figure 4.18. Fibrosarcoma: Noncontrast CT scans, A and B, reveal a soft-tissue lesion on the left at S1 and S2 (*arrowheads*) in association with an area of bony destruction (*arrows*). Note that on B, the soft-tissue lesion has not crossed the joint space.

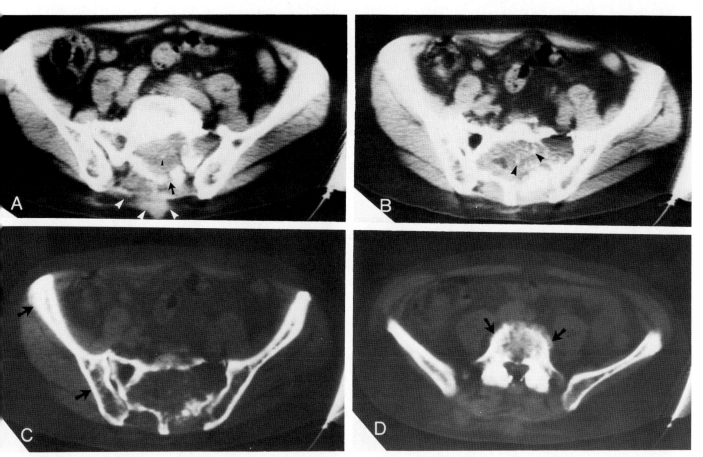

Figure 4.19. Chondrosarcoma with Paget's Disease: Axial CT scans are done at soft-tissue, A and B, and bone, C and D, windows. There is destruction of the sacrum by a large soft-tissue mass containing calcifications, A and B (*arrowheads*). The borders of the lesion are irregular and there is disruption of the dorsal cortex, A, (*black arrow*) with extension into the soft tissues, A, (*white arrowheads*). In C and D, there is expansion of the right iliac bone and L5 vertebra with thickened tabeculae and cortex secondary to Paget's disease (*arrows*). (Case courtesy of Dr. Deck of Memorial Sloane-Kettering.)

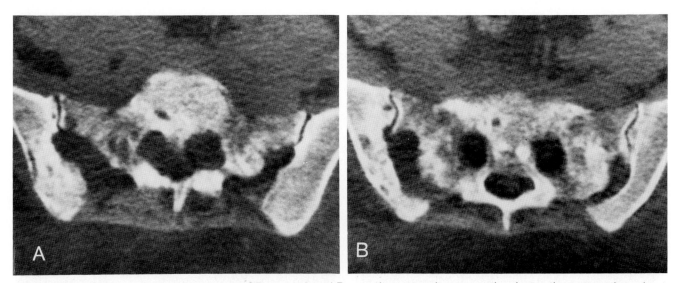

Figure 4.20. Sacral Lymphosarcoma: Axial CT scans, A and B, reveal an extensive permeative destructive pattern throughout the sacrum with evidence of nodal soft-tissue masses anteriorly.

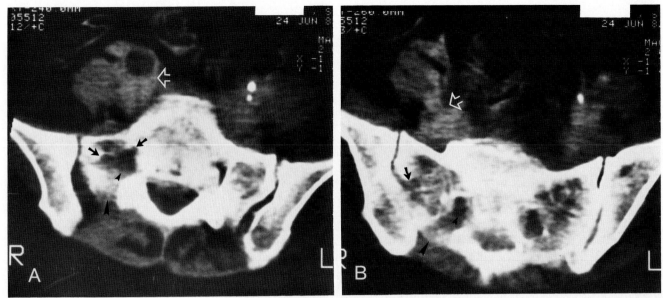

Figure 4.21. Histiocytic Lymphoma: CT scans done after intravenous contrast, A and B, reveal a lytic defect in the right sacral ala (*arrows*). The dorsal cortical margin of the sacrum is disrupted (*large arrowheads*) and the posterior margins of the sacral foramina are destroyed (*small arrowheads*). Enlarged lymph nodes (*open arrows*) are seen obstructing the right ureter. (Case courtesy of Dr. Naidich of New York University Medical Center.)

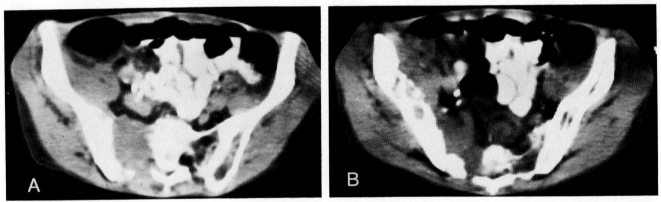

Figure 4.22. Lung Metastasis to Sacrum: Noncontrast CT scans, A and B, demonstrate destruction of the sacrum and iliac bone in association with a soft-tissue mass.

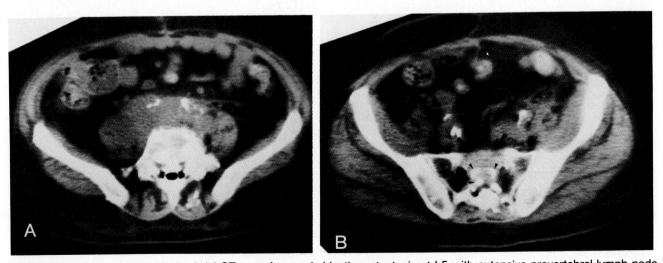

Figure 4.23. Prostate Metastasis: Axial CT scan A, reveals blastic metastasis at L5 with extensive prevertebral lymph node involvement. On B, the sacrum demonstrates both the dense bone of blastic metastasis (*arrowheads*) as well as a lytic component anteriorly replaced by a soft-tissue mass (*arrows*). (Case courtesy of Dr. Deck of Memorial Sloane-Kettering.)

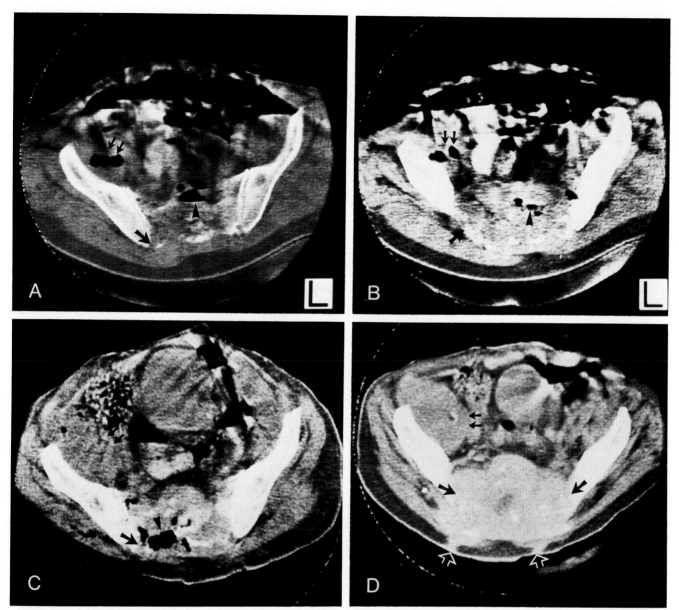

Figure 4.24. Sacral Abscess S/P Bowel Resection: CT scans, A and B, demonstrate destruction of the sacrum by a soft-tissue mass containing air-fluid levels (*arrowheads*). The abscess is crossing the sacroiliac joints (*arrows*) as well as involving the iliacus muscle (*double arrows*) Follow-up CT scan done 2 weeks, C, and 6 weeks, D, after the initial scan show continued sacral and sacroiliac joint destruction. The latest scan, D, reveals a larger mass containing bony debris and spreading dorsally to affect the superficial soft tissues (*open arrows*). (Case courtesy of Dr. Megibow of New York University Medical Center.)

and relationship to the major sacral foramina (33) (Fig. 4.25). Sacroiliac joint diastasis can be determined accurately, while the extent of pelvic hematoma can be defined. Furthermore, the use of intravenous contrast allows evaluation of the genitourinary tract on the initial CT scan. Finally, CT provides a reliable method of evaluating the results of orthopaedic procedures in these cases of sacral trauma.

METABOLIC DISEASES

Although the sacrum may be affected by metabolic

problems such as Paget's, anemia, and parathyroid disease, these entities remain primarily plain film diagnoses. It is generally not necessary to employ CT scan to establish involvement of the sacrum. However, in those instances, where a patient with Paget's disease is suspected of developing a sarcoma, CT can be of great use in determining the presence of a secondary neoplasm.

SUMMARY

The extreme usefulness and accuracy of CT scan in detecting sacral lesions is evident. It is preferable to scan

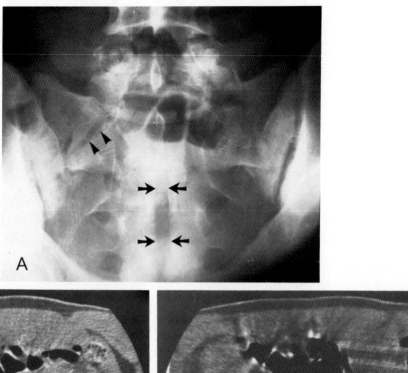

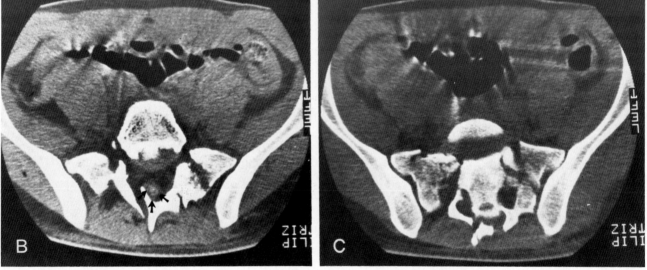

Figure 4.25. Sacral Trauma: AP sacral view, A, demonstrates a longitudinal midline fracture (*large arrows*), as well as an oblique fracture line on the right at S1 (*arrowheads*). Axial CT scans, B-E, however, reveal the true extent of the trauma with fractures through the lamina, sacral alae, and sacral body. The deformities of the sacral foramina and central canal can be appreciated. At the level of L5-S1 (B), an intracanalicular hematoma (*small arrows*) can be seen in addition to the fractures through the L5 lamina and sacral alae. Metrizamide myelography, F, demonstrates the extradural defect caused by the hematoma (*arrowheads*).

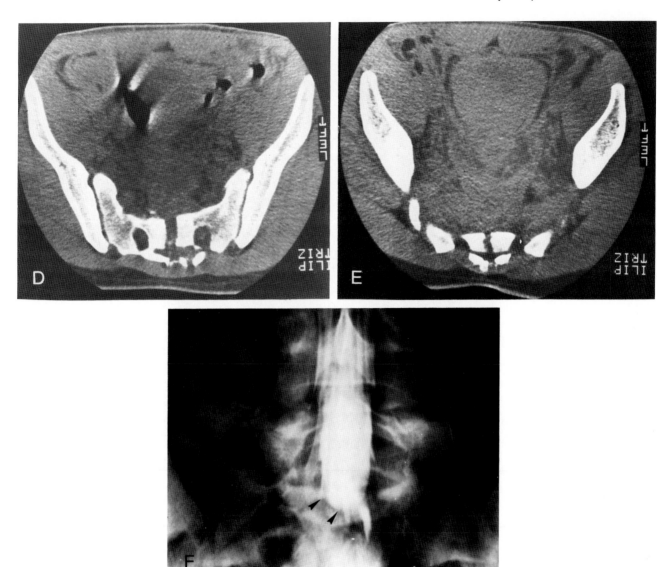

Figure 4.25.   D-F.

the sacrum on the later generation scanners using 5-mm sections. No angulation of the gantry is generally needed. The sections should be imaged with both soft-tissue and bone windows. It is not necessary to administer intravenous contrast, unless it is desired to determine the effect of the sacral lesion on the ureters and bladder.

Although certain CT features, namely, selective expansion of the central canal and sacral foramina lend a specificity to the CT diagnosis, it is difficult to distinguish the various sacral neoplasms by CT alone. Thus, clinical history is important in the accurate interpretation of these lesions. Furthermore, whereas abscess may be indicated by fluid levels and involvement of the S1 joint, aggressive tumors may mimic infection. Again, history is important in narrowing the differential possibilities. It is clear, however, that high-resolution CT scan, has established itself as the modality of choice in the work-up of patients with a suspected sacral lesion.

Bibliography

1. Naidich D, Freedman M, Bowerman I, et al: Computerized tomography in the evaluation of soft tissue components of bony lesions of the pelvis: Skeleton. *Radiology* 3:144–148, 1978.
2. Peterson HO, Kieffer SA: *Introduction to Neuroradiology.* 1st ed., New York, Harper and Row, 1972.
3. Whelan MA, Hilal SK, Gold RP, et al: Computed tomography of the sacrum. Pathology. *AJNR* 3:555–560, 1982.
4. Hammerschlag, BS, Wolpert SM, Carter BL: Computed tomography of the spinal canal. *Radiology* 121:361–367, 1976.
5. Lee BCP, Kayam E, Newman AD: Computed tomography of the spine and spinal cord. *Radiology* 128:95–102, 1978.
6. Scatliff JH, Bridgood WD, Killebrew K, et al: Computed tomography and spinal dysraphism. Clinical and phantom stud-

ies. *Neuroradiology* 17:71–75, 1979.

7. Weinstein MA, Rothner AD, Duchesneau P, et al: Computed tomography in diastematomyelia. *Radiology* 117:609–611, 1975.

8. Wolpert, S. M., Scott, R. M., Carter, B. L.: Computed tomography in spinal dysraphism. *Surg Neurol* 8:199–206, 1977.

9. Taveras JM, Wood EH: *Diagnostic Neuroradiology*, 2nd ed., Baltimore, Williams & Wilkins 1976.

10. Baleriaux-Waha, Osteux M, Terivinghu G, et al: The management of anterior sacral meningocoele with computed tomography. *Neuroradiology* 14:45–46, 1977.

11. Fitz CR, Harwood-Nash DC: The tethered conus. *AJR* 125:515–523, 1975.

12. Kaplan JO, Quencer RM: The occult tethered conus syndrome in the adult. *Radiology* 137:387–391, 1980.

13. Crellin RQ, Jones ER: Sacral extradural cysts, a rare cause of low backache and sciatica. *J Bone Joint Surg* 55B:20, 1973.

14. Janecki CJ, Nelson CL, Dohn DF: Intrasacral cyst. Report of a case and review of the literature. *J Bone Joint Surg* 54A:423, 1972.

15. Luken MG, Michelson IW, Whelan MA, et al: Sacral holes: The diagnosis of sacral lesions. *Surg Neurol* 15:377–383, 1981.

16. Moriani, AJ, Stern J, Khan AV, et al: Sacral agenesis: An analysis of 11 cases and review of the literature. *J Urol* 122:684–686, 1979.

17. Sarnat HB, Case ME, Graviss R: Sacral agenesis, neurologic and neuropathologic features. *Neurology* 26:1124, 1976.

18. Passage E, Lenz W: Syndrome of caudal regression in infants of diabetic mothers: Observations of further cases. *Pediatrics* 37:672, 1966.

19. Korobkin M, Novick HP, Palubinskas AJ: Asymptomatic sacral agenesis with neurogenic bladder in a 42 year old man. *AJR* 115:611, 1972.

20. Lourie H: Sacral agenesis: Case report. *J Neurosurg* 38:92–95, 1973.

21. Wood EH, and Himadi GM: Chordomas. A roentgenological study of 16 cases previously unreported. *Radiology* 54:706–716, 1950.

22. Horowitz T: Chordal ectopia and its possible relation to chordoma. *Arch Pathol* 31:354–362, 1941.

23. Dahlin DC, and McCarthy CA: Chordoma. A study of 59 cases. *Cancer* 5:1170–1178, 1967.

24. Turner ML, Mulhern CB, Dalinka MK: Lesions of the sacrum: Differential diagnosis and radiological evaluation. *JAMA* 245:275–277, 1981.

25. Smith J, Wixom D, Watson RC: Giant cell tumor of the sacrum. *J Assoc Canad Radiol* 30:34–39, 1979.

26. Firooznia H, Pinto RS, Lin JP, et al: Chordoma. Radiologic evaluation of 20 Cases. *AJR* 127:797–805, 1976.

27. Firooznia H, and Pinto RS: "Chordoma." In Dlethelm L, et al: *Encyclopedia of Medical Radiology*. Berlin, Heidelberg, New York, Springer-Verlag, 1977.

28. Ein SH, Adeyemi SD, Mancer K: Benign sacrococcygeal teratomas in infants and children. *Ann Surg* 191:382–384, 1980.

29. Valdiserri RO, Yunis EJ: Sacrococcygeal teratomas: A review of 68 cases. *Cancer* 48:217–221, 1981.

30. Smith Wl, Stokka C, Franken EA: Arteriography of sacrococcygeal teratomas. *Radiology* 137:653–655, 1980.

31. Berger JF, Kuhn JP: Computed tomography of tumors of the musculoskeletal system in children. *Radiology* 127:171–175, 1978.

32. De Santos LA, Bernardino ME, Murray JA: Computed tomography in the evaluation of osteosarcoma. Experience with 25 cases. *AJR* 132:535–540, 1979.

33. Gilula LA, Murphy WA, Tailor CC, et al: Computed tomography of the osseous pelvis. *Radiology* 132:107–114, 1979.

34. Storgardter FL, Cooperman LR: Giant cell tumor of sacrum with multiple pulmonary metastases and long term survival. *Br J Radiol* 44:976–979, 1971.

35. Donnellan WA, Swenson O: Benign and malignant sacrococcygeal teratomas. *Surg* 64:834–846, 1968.

36. Altman RP, Randolph JG, Lilly JR: Sacrococcygeal teratoma: American Academy of Pediatrics surgical section survey. *J Pediatr Surg* 9:389–398, 1974.

37. Edeiken J, Hodes PJ: *Roentgen Diagnosis of Diseases of Bone*. 2nd ed., Baltimore, Williams & Wilkins, 1973.

38. Caffey J: *Pediatric X-ray Diagnosis*. 5th ed, Chicago, Normal Vertebral Column, Medical Publishers, Inc., 1967.

39. *Cunningham's Textbook of Anatomy*. 12th ed., Romanes GJ: Oxford, Toronto, New York, Oxford Medical Publications, pp. 98–100, 1981.

40. Anderson JE: *Grant's Atlas of Anatomy*. 7th ed., Williams & Wilkins, Baltimore, London, 1978.

41. Williams, Warwick: *Gray's Anatomy*. 36th British ed., Philadelphia, WB, Saunders pp. 279–282, 1980.

42. Whelan MA, Gold RP: Computed tomography of the sacrum—normal anatomy. AJNR, 3:547–554, 1982.

43. Burrows FGO: Some aspects of occult spinal dysraphism: A study of 90 cases. *Br J Radiol* 41:496–507, 1968.

44. Lichtenstein BW: "Spinal Dysraphism": Spina bifida and myelodysplasia. *Arch Neurol Psychiatry* 44:792–809, 1940.

45. Till K: Spinal dysraphism. A study of congenital malformations of the lower back. *J Bone Joint Surg (Br)* 51:415–422, 1969.

46. Stanley JK, Owen R, Koff S: Congenital sacral anomalies. *J Bone Joint Surg* 61-B: 401–409, 1979.

47. Harwood-Nash DC, Fitz CR, Resjo M, et al. Congenital and cord lesions in children and computed tomographic metrizamide myelography. *Neuroradiology* 16:69–70, 1978.

48. Sostrin RD, Thompson JR, Rouke SA, et al: Occult spinal dysraphism in the geriatric patient. *Radiology* 125:165–169, 1977.

49. Pool JL: Spinal cord and local signs secondary to occult sacral meningoceles in adults. *Bull NY Acad Med* 28:655–663, 1952.

50. Dahlin DC, Cupps RE, Johnson EW: Giant cell tumor. A study of 195 cases. *Cancer* 25:1061–1070, 1970.

51. Goldenberg RR, Campbell CJ, Bonfiglio M: Giant cell tumor of bone. An analysis of 218 cases. *J Bone Joint Surg* 52A:619–664, 1970.

52. Johnson EW, Gee VR, Dahlin DC: Giant cell tumors of the sacrum. *Am J Orthop* 4:302–305, 1962.

SECTION II

Computed Tomographic Technique: Its Importance to Diagnosis

A. IMAGE PRODUCTION

CHAPTER FIVE

A Systems Approach to Computed Tomographic Image Quality*

PAUL WOZNEY, M.D., DONALD JACOBSON, M.S., and MARY ZIMMERMANN, R.T.

INTRODUCTION

There are many events between the decision to obtain a computed tomographic (CT) image of a patient and the diagnostic report placed in the chart. Each event may affect the final result, and an understanding of the critical factors improves the reliability of the diagnosis. This chapter delineates those factors associated with the CT equipment itself which most impact the final image quality. Principal focus is on the rotate-rotate (so-called third generation) CT scanner. We will identify the components which produce a CT image, examine their effect on image quality, and suggest actions which can optimize the final image. Of necessity, this discussion must be brief and eclectic. For the interested reader who desires a more detailed development of these concepts, several excellent papers are available (1,2).

At the outset, it must be acknowledged that there is much written and little known concerning the final and most critical stage in imaging: human evaluation. Psycho-perceptual studies have emphasized some important facts, so obvious that they are easily ignored; these include the training of the observer and the conditions under which the image is evaluated. We all have had the experience of recognizing familiar objects or images more easily than those which are unfamiliar.

Less often recognized are the effects of the surrounding environment on image interpretation. Ambient lighting has a profound effect: high light levels render subtle contrast differences more difficult to see on a video monitor or film image, although making a reflective image clearer. Other factors, more poorly understood, include the source of light, color, and level of surrounding activity.

To make the discussion of image quality more precise, the concepts of spatial resolution and contrast discrimination must be considered. Spatial resolution relates to the smallest object separation visible independent of contrast level, whereas contrast discrimination describes the ability to resolve subtle differences in object densities. These two properties are inter-related because to visualize an object, it must differ from its surroundings. The smaller the object, the greater that difference must be for the object to be visible. One need think of only two illustrative examples: in a coal bin, a small bright light is easily visible, whereas a large black cat is not.

Detection of a structure depends on it differing from its environment. There are numerous components in the imaging chain which affect this detectability. These may be grouped into those associated with basic system design, and those which are determined by the fashion in which the machine is operated, including calibration and maintenance.

SYSTEM DESIGN

A CT system consists of both the physical parts (hardware) and the computer instructions (software). Although the software is intangible, it is a major component of the system, constituting up to 25% of the total system design cost. For convenience, the following analysis treats each component in isolation, but in reality final system performance is only partially predictable from the component

* A complete list of individuals whose thoughts have contributed to this discussion would exhaust the reader and authors. Special appreciation, however, is extended to the following: Donald Volz, Ph.D. for the image comparisons shown in Figures 5.5, 5.7, 5.10, 5.11, 5.13, 5.14, and 5.15; Alan Williams, M.D. for providing the clinical material and original impetus for the image comparison illustrated in Figures 5.19 and 5.20; Donna Lake, R. T. for the technical assistance in Figures 5.19 and 5.20; William Hand, M.S., Jean-Pierre Georges, Ph.D., Patricia Layzell, DCRR, and Norbert Pelc, Ph.D. for technical review; and Laurie Gronitz for secretarial support.

design. There are many interactions and design compromises that only become apparent when the total system is evaluated (Fig. 5.1). The formation of a CT image involves three essential steps: data acquisition, image processing, and image display (Fig. 5.2). Each of these, in turn, involve various components of hardware and software.

X-Ray Generation

Data acquisition includes generation and collimation of the x-ray beam; transmission through the patient; and detection and digitization of the beam exiting the patient (Fig. 5.3). X-ray generation begins when the generator applies high voltage to the tube, producing an electron current which hits the anode and creates the output radiation. The resultant x-rays are shaped into a beam by the collimator, modified in intensity and spectrum by the filter, and attenuated as they pass through the patient. The attenuated beam is collected by the detector array, then amplified and converted to digital data by the data acquisition system (DAS) (Fig. 5.4.).

The generator-tube subsystem determines the character of the original x-ray beam. The beam is polyenergetic (containing a range of energies). The highest energy equals the peak voltage applied (KVP), but the average energy is considerably lower, and is dependent on KVP and beam filtration. For example, for one commercial scanner with KVP equal to 120, the effective beam energy is 73 KEV. The process of measuring x-ray attenuation and assigning CT numbers depends on the x-ray spectrum being constant and the effective energy reliably known. This requires that the generator have KVP stability and accuracy.

The generator energy is delivered to the x-ray tube, which produces the x-rays. This is an inefficient process: over 99% of the energy from the generator goes into heat rather than x-rays. Because excessive heat damages tube components, the energy delivered to each component must be limited to maintain an acceptable temperature throughout the tube. There are four temperatures of concern: that of the anode, the focal spot track, the bearing, and the overall tube casing. The instantaneous focal spot temperature limits the power (MA × KVP) that can be applied to the tube. This affects both the basic design of the tube and the operation of the scanner.

The anode receives the bulk of the energy, and is designed to absorb and dissipate it efficiently. The anode temperature is a result of the anode heat capacity and the rate at which it dissipates heat. Rotation of the anode spreads the heat out on the circular focal track, increasing instantaneous power capacity. A smaller focal spot is required for higher spatial resolution, however, this focuses more energy into a smaller area on the anode, raising the local temperature. This forces a design compromise between focal spot size and energy delivered to the tube. During CT operation, the tube current (MA) is limited principally by the anode temperature. As the tube anode, casing, and bearing heat up, increased time is required between scans for cooling. This limits the scan repetition rate and the technique per scan. In addition, tubes in CT may be subjected to over 70 times the stress encountered

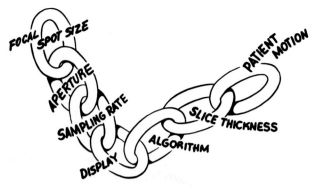

Figure 5.1. Image quality is determined by a complex interaction of many factors.

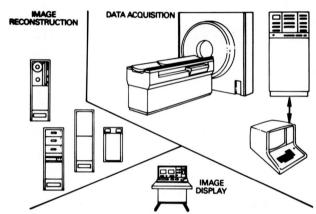

Figure 5.2. The components of a CT system may be grouped into those related to data acquisition, image reconstruction, and image display.

in angiography. Although techniques vary, the MAS per CT slice may be equivalent to an entire angiographic study. A busy angiographic suite may perform six studies daily, while an average CT site performs 300 slices daily. Lower techniques reduce the stress on the tube, but also lower the dose, thus, decreasing the tissue contrast discrimination due to increased image noise.

The energy spectrum of the radiation has a complex effect on image quality. At a higher effective energy, more radiation passes through the patient and a smaller fraction of the photons are attenuated differentially, resulting in lower contrast discrimination for a given photon flux to the detector. However, at low energy, the dose required to image anatomy adequately may be prohibitive because so many of the low energy photons are absorbed within the patient. A final consideration is that at higher KVP considerably more x-rays are produced for the same tube current. The setting of KVP, thus, involves a compromise between x-ray tube emission and differential absorption.

The tube current may be either pulsed or continuously on and there are advantages to each design. When sampling at a slow to moderate rate, it is technically feasible to turn off the x-ray current and beam between samples and still obtain sufficient photon flux during each pulse. However, at the high data rates (approaching 1000 Hz) desirable in fast scanning, the tube must be on continuously to maintain optimal beam intensity, and the detector output must be measured continuously.

This has important design considerations for the generator and DAS as well as the tube. In a pulsed system, the generator requires a pulse bias tank, and the tube a grid, to generate the bursts of tube current. With a continuous-on system, the design of the tube is simplified and cost reduced. The DAS, however, calibrates itself in a pulsed system during periods devoid of x-ray flux; a more sophisticated and expensive design is required to achieve the necessary stability in a continuous-on system.

From the tube the x-ray beam passes through a collimator, which limits it to a prescribed slice thickness, between about 1.5–10 mm. A high-quality collimator ensures that all of the dose delivered to the patient falls on the detector and contributes to the image, resulting in lower patient dose for contiguous slices. Advantages of thinner slices include more frequent sampling perpendicular to the scan plan, better reformatted images in non-axial planes (Fig. 5.5), and reduction of partial volume artifacts (3). However, examinations composed of thin slices stress the tube more, for the following reason. Because less of the output radiation passes through the collimator to irradiate the patient and contribute to the image, the resultant signal-to-noise ratio is lowered. Technique is increased to maintain a desired ratio.

On many CT scanners, the beam also passes through a compensating filter which shapes the beam intensity. The purpose of the filter is to produce a beam intensity and spectrum profile which, when coupled with the approximately round shape of the patient, produces a more uniform spectrum and field of radiation to the detection system. This allows the detection electronics to sample the output with a high degree of precision by reducing the dynamic range requirements. It also results in more uniform noise properties. Filtration also reduces patient dose by eliminating low energy photons which would not contribute to the image.

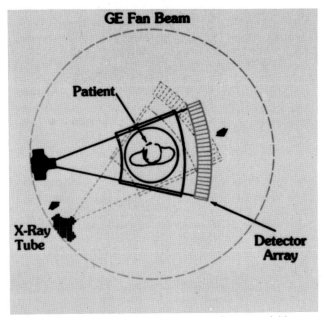

Figure 5.3. The essential elements to data acquisition are the generation of x-rays by the tube and detection by the detection array.

DAS DYNAMIC RANGE

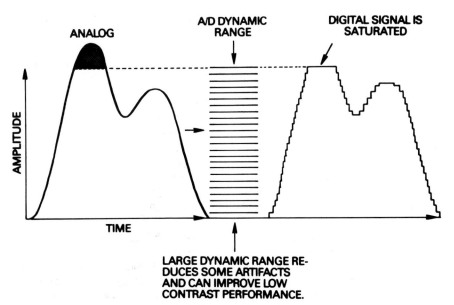

Figure 5.4. The DAS converts the electrical current (analog signal) into numbers for the computer (digital output). The dynamic range is the range of current over which the digital output accurately tracks the current.

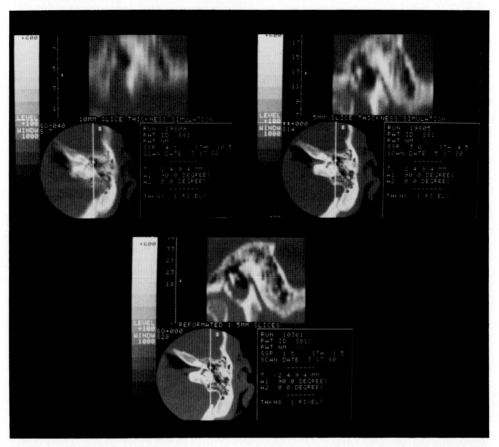

Figure 5.5. Effect of slice thickness on reformatted image quality. The three sagittal images are produced from nominal 1.5-mm, 5-mm, and 10-mm slice series. The 5-mm series is overlapped 2 mm and the 10-mm series is overlapped 5 mm.

X-Ray Detection

After collimation and filtration, the x-ray beam passes through the patient, is differentially attenuated, and detected by the detection subsystem. This subsystem consists of a detector array and the DAS. The detector array consists of many individual detector elements, each of which converts incident x-rays to an electrical current which the DAS records, measures, and digitizes.

Accurate photon detection and measurement is a complex inter-relation of detector efficiency, detector stability, and DAS performance. In order to optimize total performance, the components must be matched to produce optimal performance of the subsystem as a unit.

The detector array generally is composed of individual cells of detector material spaced at uniform intervals. The x-ray photons are detected by interacting with the detector substance. Currently available materials are either gaseous (high pressure xenon) or solid (cesium iodide, cadmium tungstate, bismuth germanate). The very fact that several different substances are in widespread use confirms the suspicion that none is ideal.

A detector array using xenon is stable over time and detects the x-ray photons reproducibly and reliably. It produces a high-quality signal that is digitized accurately by the DAS. The principal theoretical disadvantage is that because xenon is a gas, it is less efficient per unit length at stopping x-ray photons than a denser solid substance. The currently available solid-state materials present different problems. Cesium iodide changes its character as it is irradiated, and requires frequent normalization and calibration. Cadmium tungstate and bismuth germanate emit a low signal for each photon detected. This signal must be amplified by the DAS, and noise is added in the process. This is analogous to tuning in a weak radio station; when the volume is increased there is static noise present with the signal.

Two design features of the detector array are the effective detector aperture size and sampling distance (Fig. 5.6 and 5.7). The effective aperture size is equal to the physical width of each detection element divided by system magnification. The detector sampling distance is the spacing between adjacent rays within a view. In a rotate-rotate system, this is equal to the detector spacing divided by the system magnification. By aligning the detector array one-quarter of a sample off center during a 360° scan, the effective spacing can be halved (4). Spatial resolution of the scan data is dependent on the focal spot size, effective

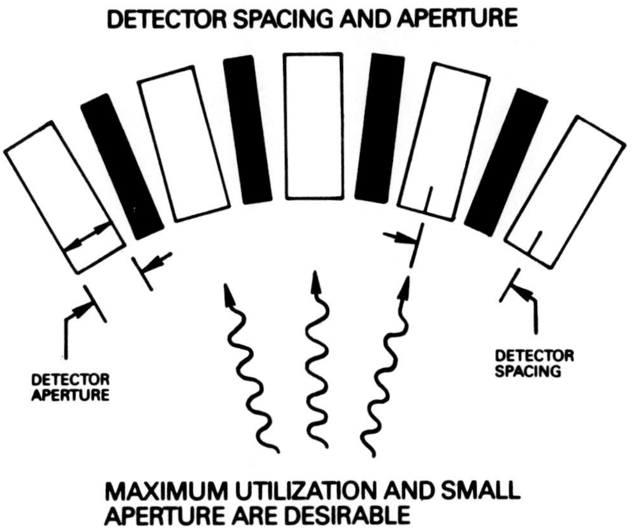

DETECTOR SPACING AND APERTURE

MAXIMUM UTILIZATION AND SMALL APERTURE ARE DESIRABLE

Figure 5.6. The detector array is made up of individual detector elements. The detector aperture is a critical element in determining the limiting spatial resolution of the system. More widely spaced detectors result in poorer dose utilization and lower resolution in the SPR mode.

aperture width, and detector sampling distance. It is not sufficient to have only a narrow aperture; a small focal spot is required to create a sharp shadow on the detector array.

The signals which are produced by the detector are relayed to the DAS which performs preprocessing on the signals, usually including amplification, time integration, and analog to digital conversion (Fig. 5.4). The DAS samples the detector array at specified intervals; each sample is called a view. The angular coverage of each view is determined by the integration time of the DAS multiplied by the rotational speed of the x-ray tube in a rotate-rotate system. The more total views obtained, the more information that is available for reconstruction of the image. A given number of views may be obtained by sampling slowly over a long period of time, or more rapidly over a short time. The complete story is still more complex, for each set of view data consists of the reading from each detector element. The data rate is, therefore, the product of the rays per view times the number of views per second. Technology has improved the data rate capacity of the DAS dramatically: only 30,000 samples per second were available with technology in 1975, whereas 740,000 sam-

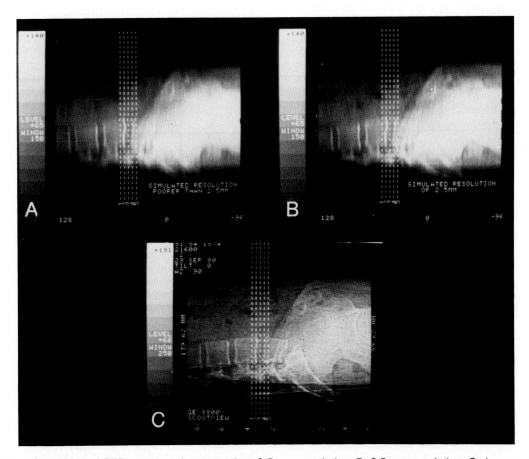

Figure 5.7. Simulation of SPR systems: A, poorer than 2.5-mm resolution; B, 2.5-mm resolution; C, 1-mm resolution.

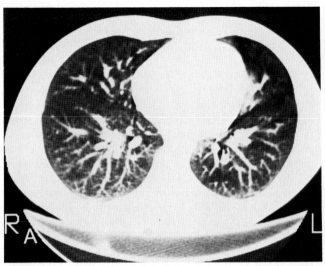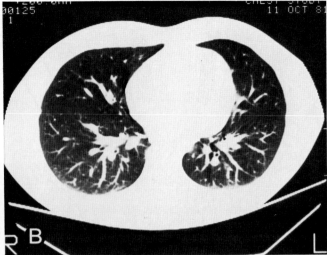

Figure 5.8. Illustration of DAS sampling effects on image quality. A. CT 8800 4.8-second scan with 288 views. DAS rate = 60 views per second. B. CT 9800 2-second scan with 1000 processed views obtained at 984 scan views per second. The radial streaks ("view aliasing") in A result from the lower view number.

ples per second were achieved in 1981. The practical effect is illustrated in Figs. 5.8A and B. The CT 8800 image was obtained with a 60-Hz DAS and a 4.8-second scan: a total of 288 processed views was obtained. The CT 9800 was produced with a 984-Hz DAS and a 2-second scan: 1968 scanned views were obtained. The increased sampling eliminates view-associated artifacts.

Ideally, the DAS should translate the detector current accurately into specific numbers for the computer (Fig. 5.4). This requires low electronic noise and accurate analog-to-digital (A-D) conversion. The A-D conversion consists of assigning the current from the detector a specific number, and is described by considering the dynamic range of the DAS. This is that range of current over which the DAS accurately translates the current into a number. The number of discrete steps which the DAS can assign to the output current is generally expressed in binary terminology: 16 bits (2^{16}) means there are 65,000 (approximately) discrete steps. Twenty bits of data provide more discrete steps (over 1,000,000). With more steps, it is possible to divide the range of current into smaller steps, providing greater precision. It also is possible to increase the range over which the current is measured.

As mentioned previously, the detector array-DAS subsystem must be considered as a unit, and evaluated for its overall ability to translate the x-ray beam emerging from the patient into numbers fed to the computational subsystem. Both the detector and DAS have a dynamic range; the overall range is the smaller of the two.

There is a lower threshold below which no photons are detected nor any current is produced, and an upper limit above which the signal is saturated or over-ranged. At low dose rates (at the detector), the electronic noise can be the limiting factor because the signal is small. This can be due to low dose from the tube, an obese patient, or thin (1.5-mm) slices. Low intrinsic noise in the detector and DAS

is desirable. At high doses, the range may be limited by DAS or detector saturation. As described previously, increasing the DAS dynamic range can expand this range.

Table-Gantry Subsystem

The placement of the x-ray tube and the detector about the center of rotation (isocenter) often is referred to as system geometry. The actual spatial resolution of the system is determined by the relationship of the focal spot to the detector element aperture. The distance from the x-ray tube focal spot to the detector, divided by the distance between the focal spot and the isocenter is the magnification of the system. The magnification determines the effective aperture and effective focal spot size in the scanned volume. A high magnification results in a small effective detector aperture but requires a small focal spot to achieve higher resolution.

The geometric arrangement of the detectors, their construction, and the fundamental mechanism for data collection determine the scatter susceptibility. High scatter rejection is desirable for accurate x-ray attenuation measurement for high-fidelity CT imaging. Rotate-rotate systems employ narrow detectors focused at the tube focal spot providing quite good scatter rejection. Stationary detector systems require detectors with a wide (up to 35°) radiation acceptance angle. However, scatter rejection can be achieved by placing the detectors farther from the scan field.

Localization

The preceding discussion assumes that the anatomy of interest actually is located within the scan plane. In the early days of CT, slice prescription was limited to positioning the scan plane by reference to external anatomical landmarks. This method was reasonably accurate, but a major improvement was the addition of scanned projec-

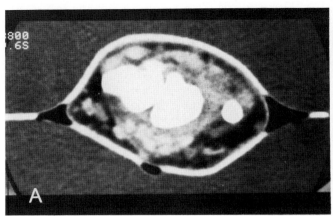 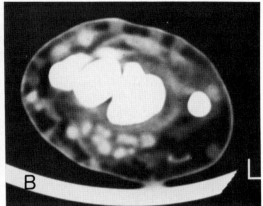

Figure 5.9. Illustration of the combined effects of increased resolution, increased view sampling, and expanded dynamic range. The tendons and superficial vessels are sharper in the right image (Fig. 5.9B). Note that the bolus bag of water, necessary in Figure 5.9A, is absent in Figure 5.9B, because the dynamic range has been expanded from 65,000 to 1,000,000. A. CT 8800 9.8-second, 576 view image; resolution 1.0 mm. B. CT 9800 4-second image; 3936 scan views processed into 1000 display views, resolution 0.7 mm.

tion radiography (SPR) to CT scanners. This allowed slice prescription by reference to internal bony landmarks (5).

Important design criteria for SPR include image resolution and accurate table positioning. The image resolution is dependent on the projection of the anatomy on the detector array, the beam width, the incrementation of the table between each sample of data collected, and the algorithm employed in image construction. The more closely spaced the detection elements, the higher the spatial resolution (Figs. 5.6 and 5.7).

The clinical value of SPR is dependent principally upon high-quality images (Fig. 5.7), table positioning accuracy, and patient immobility. There is no intrinsic connection between the SPR and the axial images; they are only related by the measured position of the table. Commercial scanners show considerable variation in table incrementation and repositioning accuracy; they range from better than 0.25 mm, to 5 mm, or worse. Patient motion may be of any magnitude—including leaving the table entirely. Clearly, if there is patient motion or there are table errors, the slice prescribed may not be at the location desired.

Image Processing: Scan Data Reconstruction

The x-ray attenuation measurements, referred to as digital scan data (or raw data), are sent to the computer for processing. The first stage in image processing involves offset correction, calibration, and normalization of the scan data. Offset correction accounts for the fact that even in the absence of x-rays, a signal may be produced by each channel of the detector array and DAS. Calibration references the measured x-ray attenuation of an individual detector to a standard attenuation profile obtained from a calibration phantom, made of water, plastic, or air. Normalization adjusts the output data to reflect tube output variations, recorded by reference detector elements. After these steps, corrections for beam-hardening are applied to the data. Beam-hardening refers to the change in spectrum

of the x-ray beam emerging from the patient relative to the entering beam. Lower energy photons are preferentially attenuated, shifting the spectrum to higher ("harder") energies.

The next step in image formation is the mathematical filtration of the projection data. The frequency spectrum of the mathematical filter determines the noise and resolution properties of the final image. A lower frequency cut-off will result in an image with lower noise, but less resolution capability, while passing higher frequencies into the image increases the noise but affords a higher capability for resolution. This fundamental concept bears repeating: higher resolution means sharper definition of all details including noise and artifacts, other factors being equal. Other system parameters such as x-ray tube focal spot size, detector aperture, sampling distance, or display pixel size also may impact system resolution.

Low contrast detectability in clinical imaging involves a subtle combination of resolution capability and noise characteristics of the image. These are nearly impossible to quantify, because the human eye-brain system has the capability of "seeing through" noise and picking out structures, particularly if edges are detectable in the image. This is relevant in defining reconstruction algorithms. In actual practice, empirical comparisons have been employed for such definitions.

The next step in image formation is back-projection of the filtered profiles into the reconstruction pixel matrix. During back-projection, the values deposited in each pixel are summed to determine the attenuation value for each pixel in the reconstruction matrix. From the attenuation value, the CT number then is calculated using the following familiar relationship.

$$\text{CT Number (HU)} = \frac{\text{attenuation (tissue)} - \text{attenuation (water)}}{\text{attenuation (water)}} \times 1000$$

In order to achieve CT number accuracy, care must be taken in the production of the x-ray attenuation data and in the amplification, digitization, normalization, offset correction, calibration, filtration, and back-projection of the scan data.

Almost all scanners used today employ a scale which assigns a CT number of −1000 HU to air and 0 to water (some earlier machines used a value of −500 for air, 0 for water). The upper limit varies among different scanner models. Originally, +1000 HU was common, however with the discovery that temporal bone may be as dense as +2500 HU, the CT scale has been extended on many scanners to +3000 HU.

The image now exists in the computer as numbers in the reconstruction matrix. Typically, the 16-bit (or more) raw data has now been processed to 11 or 12 bits (approximately 2000 or 4000 values) of display data.

Image Processing: Display Data Manipulation

After the scan data has been reconstructed into the display data, further manipulation is possible. The most common manipulation is magnification combined with smoothing; the latter eliminates the appearance of discrete blocks of enlarged pixels. Reformatting is another significant manipulation of display data. Because anatomy frequently is not axial, visualization in a nonaxial plane may aid diagnosis. This may be accomplished by having the computer stack several slices together, then reslice the stack of pixels along a nonaxial plane (Fig. 5.5). This is particularly important in evaluation of the spine, where the anatomical curves make it difficult to slice consistently through the intervertebral space (6).

Image Display

The matrix of CT numbers residing in the computer is then displayed, usually on a video monitor for viewing and diagnosis. This conversion takes place in a device called a display controller. This device takes the CT numbers in digital form from the computer and translates this information into a video signal which is sent to the display monitor. The conversion from digital to analog presents fewer technical difficulties than the reverse process at the DAS. Care must be taken in the engineering design to assure that the display accurately and reproducibly reflects the internal digital data.

One must now consider the characteristics of human vision. Under optimal conditions, only 20–50 levels (4 to 6 bits) of gray are perceptible. The stored image has a range nearly 100 times that, (11 or 12 bits). Clearly, these all cannot be seen at once. The window width and level settings on the CT console allow the viewer to select the CT numbers to be displayed as shades of gray. The window width control determines the range of CT numbers, whereas the level determines where this range is centered. Manipulation of these controls dramatically alters the appearance of an image. A wider window width means each shade of gray represents a wider range of CT numbers, resulting in an image with reduced contrast. Conversely, a narrower range enhances subtle CT number

differences, providing better visualization of low contrast areas. Both wide and narrow window width and level settings may be employed to display all the stored digital information.

The use of color displays for CT images is an area which can generate strong emotions; however, certain qualities of color displays are clear. Despite the fact that colors vary uniformly in frequency, they are not perceived as a continuous spectrum as are shades of a color (or shades of gray). Colors are perceived as discontinuous steps. This makes it difficult for the eye to "see through noise" and pick out a structure from the color confetti of noise. A U.S. military reconnaissance group, with more than a casual interest in image analysis, found in one study that in 90% of the cases, monochromatic photos were more reliably analyzed than color ones. The effect of colored noise in obscuring information is probably a major factor in this result (7).

A fundamental property of a digital image is the pixel size, which is the amount of anatomy represented by one pixel. Because each pixel is uniform (has only one shade of gray), the smaller the pixel, the more closely the display represents the anatomy. Pixel size can be a limiting factor in the resolution presented in the displayed image. Pixel size, field of view (FOV), and matrix size are related simply as illustrated in the equation shown.

$$\text{Pixel Size (mm)} = \frac{\text{Field of View (mm)}}{\text{Matrix Size}}$$

For example, if the FOV is 550 mm and the matrix is 256 × 256 pixels, the pixel size will be approximately 2 mm, whereas for a 250-mm FOV, the pixel size for the same matrix is approximately 1 mm.

A feature available on many CT systems today allows the user to choose the FOV, which alters the pixel size and eliminates the display limitation to resolution. With this capability, it is possible to have exactly the same resolution in a 256-matrix image as in a 512-matrix image. The difference will be that the FOV for the 512-matrix image will be twice as large as for the 256-matrix. Variable FOV is a significant improvement over simple magnification because the original scan data are employed for a new reconstruction. There is no pixel interpolation which can degrade the image. One drawback, however, is that the scan data must be saved, and additional reconstruction time may be necessary.

The ultimate resolution in a video display is related to the size of the scanning electron beam spot, the number of video lines which produce the image, and the video band width (8). Although it is feasible to display 4000 spots across each of 4000 lines, such displays rely on slow scan rates and are not practical for clinical application in CT.

The display matrix size available on CT machines has increased gradually from 80 × 80 on the first units to 512 × 512 on the most recent ones. This matrix represents a practical compromise of reconstructive time, memory storage capacity, and system resolution as well as video refresh rate. The CT image display also provides many capabilities which enhance the diagnostic potential of the CT image, such as region of interest calculations (with CT number mean and standard deviation), distance/angle measurement between two points, histograms, the option of selecting black or white bone, and image rotation.

Image Recording

Images may be stored either as digital data or as hard copy on paper or film. Magnetic tape and floppy discs are the two forms of digital data storage separate from the CT system itself. Magnetic tape is superior for storage longer than a few months; floppy discs are suitable only for interim storage. Even when the diagnosis is made directly from the video display, a permanent (hard-copy) record generally is made for future reference. Such a record always is made when primary diagnosis is not made from the CT console. The most widely employed method remains photography from the monitor on silver halide film, although alternate methods are available (9). This transfer from monitor image to film image is an involved process, and requires care to optimize.

A proper match of video monitor and film, in addition to careful adjustment of monitor and level controls, is necessary for optimum hard-copy production. Factors which can offset the fidelity include video cable losses and noise susceptibility, the monitor phosphor, display controller look-up (gamma) table for conversion of the digital data to scanning spot intensity, film speed, film quality (10), and processor quality (11).

System Performance

The final image quality results from the synergistic interaction of the foregoing system components. To understand this interaction better, we will consider spatial resolution and contrast discrimination in slightly greater detail; a more rigorous but still accessible discussion is found in Blumenfeld (1). Fundamental to a discussion of spatial resolution is an understanding of sampling theory. There is a theorem which states that any complex object can be broken down into a set of periodic structures with different spacings. The different spacings also can be expressed as different frequencies; these are the frequencies of which we speak in technical discussions. The sharper an edge, the more high frequency (closely spaced) components are present. We are interested in determining the minimum spacing detectable with a given sampling aperture. It is clear that if we use a narrow aperture the edges of the structure can be well defined. The output signal then consists of the record of what each detector element has seen. Now, if we gradually increase the aperture size,

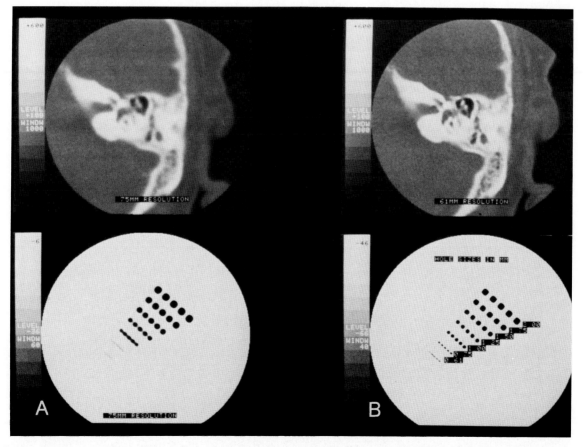

Figure 5.10.   Improvement in spatial resolution by increasing kernel roll off beyond the Nyquist frequency. Although this results in an increase in aliasing and noise, it is not evident at this wide window. A. 0.75-mm resolution. B. 0.61-mm resolution.

we get an increasingly unclear signal until finally there is no signal when the detector spacing equals the object spacing. Intuitively, one also can see that if very few samples were taken, there would not be enough information to define the object at all.

We now arrive at the fundamental law of information theory, known as the Nyquist theorem. It specifies that the minimum object spacing detectable by a given sampling interval is twice that interval. If, however, there are frequency elements within a structure that are higher than the Nyquist frequency, they will produce aliasing. This is an artificial response, created by the inability to generate adequately spaced samples. Higher frequencies, caused by sharper edges, are processed incorrectly by the imaging system as lower frequency elements, resulting in artifacts (Fig. 5.10).

Several of the previously discussed components affect the system resolution. The focal spot size, system geometry, and detector element aperture determine the ultimate resolution. This may be compromised by any element in the data acquisition, reconstruction or display processes. These include the reconstruction algorithm, the convolution filter, the pixel size for back projection, the type of back projection interpolation, and the matrix size of the display.

Contrast discrimination is a function of object size, background contrast, and noise (Fig. 5.11). Noise may be added at every stage in the imaging chain. There may be uncompensated variations in tube output, electronic noise in the detector and DAS, and algorithm noise. In a well-designed CT system, these, however, are typically less important than photon noise and image artifacts.

In order to quantify the interaction of these components, a contrast-detail-dose (CDD) curve is employed, which illustrates the fundamental interrelation of contrast and spatial resolution (12, 13). Figure 5.12 shows the CDD curves for a representative CT scanner. Contrast values corresponding to two tissue interfaces, muscle-bone (800 HU) and gray-white matter in the brain (5 HU) may be identified. The overall curves show that in order to see objects that differ little from their surroundings, they must be relatively large. A higher dose provides more information and improves the imaging of low contrast objects (Fig. 5.14). For high-contrast interfaces, however, dose does not make a significant difference (Fig. 5.13).

Partial Volume

The previous discussion has ignored an important interaction: the relationship between slice thickness and the thickness of the imaged object. When the object is thicker than the slice thickness, a thicker slice will always produce a less noisy image, because it has, in effect, been interrogated by more photons. However, when the structure is small, a thinner slice can produce a higher contrast

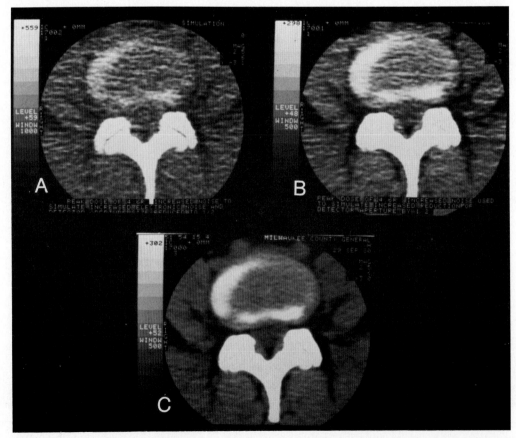

Figure 5.11. Effect of noise on contrast discrimination. Increasing amounts of noise (A, B) are added to the original image (C). This noise could result from electronic noise, reduced dose, or system nonlinearities.

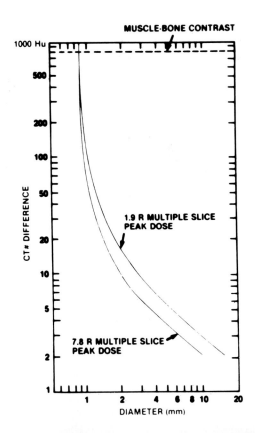

(Fig. 5.15) image through decrease or elimination of the partial volume effect. This also reduces the interpetrous artifact for a similar reason (3). A thinner slice also may increase sharpness by imaging overlapping structures in separate slices.

SYSTEM OPERATION

Proper operation of the CT system can affect the resultant image dramatically, overshadowing the design factors previously discussed. There are five facets to optimal image production with a particular CT unit: patient handling, machine calibration and technique selection, image viewing, and finally, hard-copy production.

Patient Handling

Although often neglected in image quality discussions, clearly an essential element of a clinical scan is the patient. A successful scan requires the patient's cooperation and the operator's attention to detail. An explanation of the study and the steps of the procedure reduce patient anxiety, discomfort, and resultant motion. Because motion of high-density material causes artifacts, objects such as

Figure 5.12.   This contrast-detail dose curve illustrates the inter-relation of these parameters. The vertical scale is the contrast; the horizontal is object diameter. A set of curves for different doses describes the relationship.

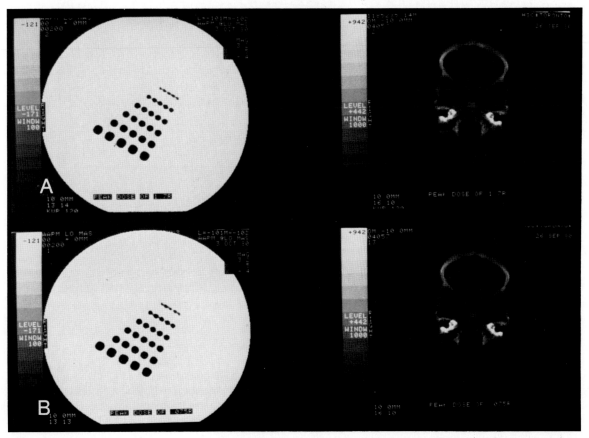

Figure 5.13.   For high-contrast objects, the spatial resolution is independent of dose. The upper images are produced with a 1.7-R dose, the lower with 0.075 R.

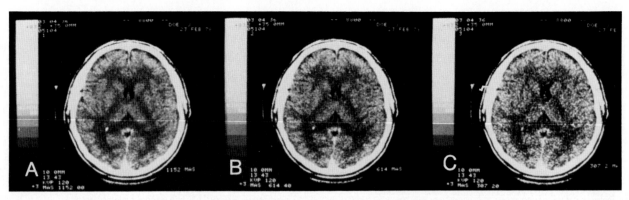

Figure 5.14. Illustration of the effect of increasing dose on contrast resolution. The three slices were produced with 1152 MAS, 614 MAS, and 307 MAS (A, B, and C, respectively). As the technique is decreased, the gray matter-white matter delineation becomes increasingly more difficult to identify. These images correspond to three of the family of increasing dose curves on the CDD graph in Figure 5.12.

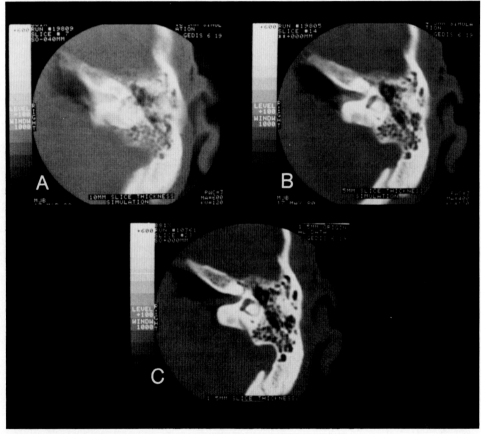

Figure 5.15. Effect of slice thickness on scan plane resolution for small anatomical structures. Each image was generated from contiguous 1.5-mm (A, C) slice thickness scans. A. The 10-mm slice is generated from seven slices, the 5-mm (B) from three slices.

hair pins, rings, and snaps should be removed. If residual barium is present in the bowel, postponement of the study may be advisable.

Controlling patient motion can scarcely be overemphasized, because motion results in streaks and blurring within the scan plane (Fig. 5.16–5.18). It may be caused by involuntary factors such as bowel motion, hiccups, or patient disorientation. In pediatric patients, swaddling and security are keys to obtaining diagnostic images (14). Short scan times are particularly useful in minimizing motion artifacts.

A frequent cause of motion artifacts is patient respira-

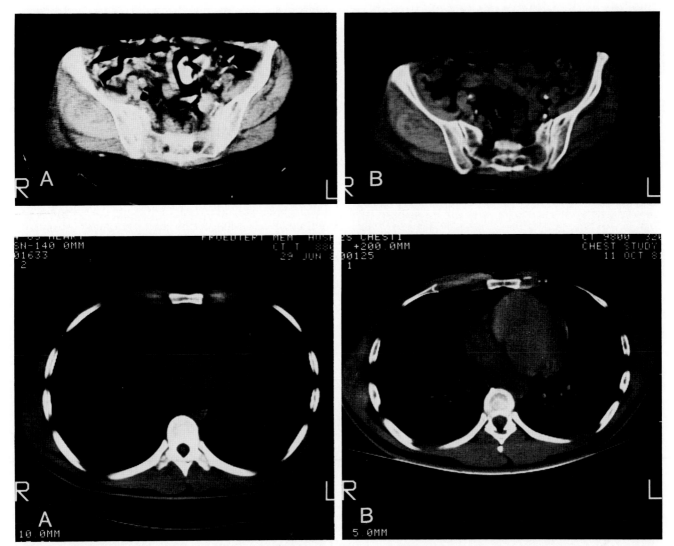

Figures 5.16 and 5.17.   Comparison of temporal resolution on motion artifacts. Figures 5.16A and 5.17A are 4.8-second scans; Figures 5.16B and 5.17B are 2.0-second scans in the same patients, at the same anatomical levels, and at the same techniques. Notice the prominent peristaltic streaks (Fig. 5.16A) and cardiac motion streaks (Fig. 5.17A) reduced at the more rapid scan times. A contributing factor is also the greatly increased sampling rates (60 Hz vs. 984 Hz).

tion, particularly when imaging the neck, chest, and abdomen. A few minutes of rehearsal of the patient breathing technique yields patient understanding, relaxes the patient further, and is amply repaid in artifact-free scans. Although controversy exists regarding the ideal method, the most reproducible scans are obtained by imaging at end-tidal volume. The patient is instructed to breathe in, breathe out, and relax. The elastic recoil of the lungs returns the chest to a reproducible resting position. The patient then holds his breath until the scan is completed.

In addition to the obvious artifacts from motion, correlations between the localization SPR and axial slices prescribed from it depend on a lack of patient motion, as previously discussed. When prescribed slice location and actual location fail to correspond, a common cause is patient motion during the elapsed time between the two

scans, which may be as great as 45 minutes for the final slices in a series. This problem may be ameliorated by taking an additional SPR after the axial series to confirm slice location.

Positioning

In order to obtain an optimal scan series, the patient must be positioned correctly. This involves the table linear location, gantry tilt, and table elevation. Initial positioning is aided greatly by alignment lights associated with the CT gantry and table; the lights define the scan plane. The gantry may be tilted to correspond to external landmarks, or to match structures seen on the SPR. The ability of the SPR to define the scan plane in relation to internal bony landmarks extends and refines the localization capability of the external lights.

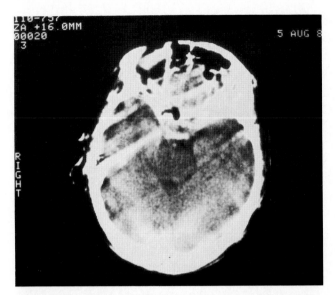

Figure 5.18. Motion artifact: patient moved head during scanning, and produced the broad, diagonal streaks.

Centering the patient within the scan field is important. The external localization lights also aid in positioning the table elevation. Alternately, when the first slice is obtained, a grid may be displayed which graphically indicates the location of the patient within the scan field. The table may then be raised or lowered as necessary or the patient may be repositioned.

There are two principal reasons for proper patient centering. The first is to avoid blocking the reference detectors. These detectors are employed to monitor x-ray tube output, and may be located on the outside edge of the detector array. When an object is in the path between the x-ray source and these detectors, the reference channels will detect the difference in attenuation values. This may result in a shift of CT number values, due to improper normalization. In addition, if the patient is off-center, certain detectors may be overexposed, producing saturation or over-ranging of the DAS. This may result in an advisory message to the operator on the alphanumeric screen, and cause the operator to reduce technique inappropriately. If the proper technique was chosen originally, recentering of the patient often will resolve this problem. A wider dynamic range greatly reduces this problem, because over-ranging of the DAS is less likely. The second reason for accurate centering is to match patient shape to the calibration phantoms better; this improves CT number accuracy.

Centering should be checked periodically when scanning, particularly in patients with a barrel chest and small AP abdominal diameter. The initial chest scan may be centered, but, as scanning progresses toward the feet, the patient contour changes, resulting in the patient being too low in the scan field. This can be adjusted by raising the table to the proper height. When this is done, however, the SPR may no longer be reliable for slice prescription if the gantry is tilted. An additional SPR should be taken if

slice positioning is critical. Changing the table height would also distort reformations of the display data. It is also important to specify a scan field which includes the entire patient. The reconstruction algorithm generally assumes that there is no material outside the specified scan field; if there is, image quality may be compromised (Figs. 5.19 and 5.20).

Calibration and Technique

The CT scan must be calibrated: referenced to an external standard. Water, plastic, and air commonly are employed as reference materials. The necessity and effect of calibration varies dramatically between CT models, but, all machines will perform at their optimal level only when calibrated according to the manufacturer's instructions. Lack of calibration may result in shading, an increase in noise, CT number inaccuracy, and other artifacts such as rings.

Choice of technique is a complex topic beyond the scope of the current discussion, and is related closely to a particular CT model and the clinical objective of the study. Appropriate choice of technique has a major impact on contrast resolution, as previously discussed. Higher technique results in greater photon flux, decreased noise, and increased contrast discrimination. Thicker slices (5 mm rather than 1.5 mm) often yield better images of disc herniation because more photons contribute to the image.

Image Recording

All the care taken in maximizing the information in the final CT image can be negated by improperly exposed or processed film. This is an especially important concern in departments where diagnosis is done from film. Proper density and contrast in a CT image film, necessary for transferral of maximum information, requires proper camera maintenance, film selection, film handling, and film processor control. Film is available which is designed by the film manufacturers to record the video image faithfully, however, the unique features of photographing the video display must be addressed (8). The camera should be adjusted initially to match the characteristics of the film used, and the gray scale should span the linear portion of the film. The film stock should be rotated, protected from heat, light, and ionizing radiation, and developed in a well-maintained processor. Film handling is also important. Use of outdated film, or storing film in areas of high temperature, may result in a diffuse increase in background gray level in the image (fogging). Creasing the film will result in a distinct crescent-shaped artifact.

The multiformat camera requires attention weekly to monitor electronic drift in the circuits. This drift may distort the image by changing the horizontal or vertical dimension of the image. This is particularly important when measurements are made from the image, as in stereotaxis or treatment planning. Drift also may modify the gray levels subtly.

Rapid film processing is quite sensitive to chemical strength, chemical temperature, proper replenishment, and circulation. Because any of these parameters can

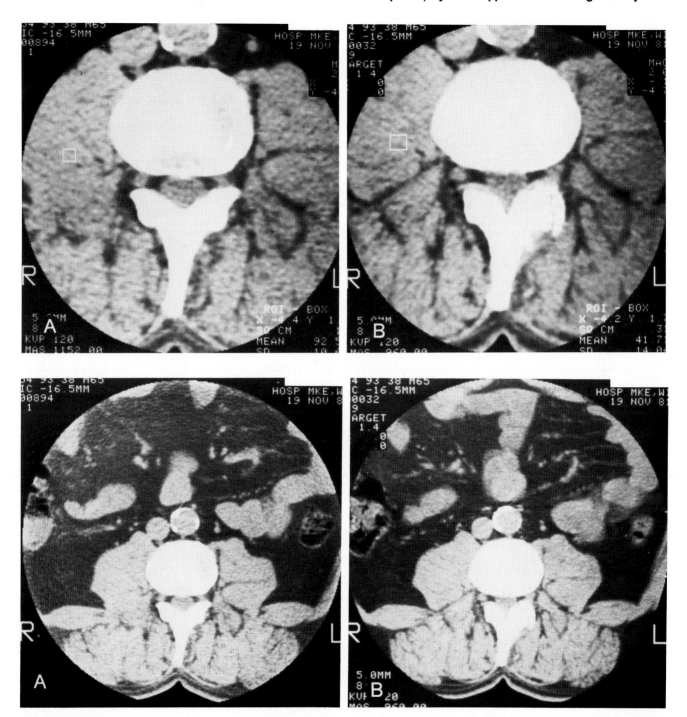

Figures 5.19 and 5.20. Effect of inaccurate identification of anatomical extent to the reconstruction algorithm. Figures 5.19A and 5.20A specify no material outside the field. In Figure 5.19A, the CT number is calculated incorrectly at 92 HU. In Figure 5.20A, increased noise is apparent near the periphery.

change over a short period of time, the processor is the most variable segment in the imaging chain and should be monitored continuously. A control program should be in place for every processor (11). This can be done conveniently by measuring the density of selected steps on the gray bar present on the images from most CT scanners.

A more accurate method is to expose a film each day with a sensitometer. After processing, a densitometer should be employed to measure densities on the film. It is recommended that the film speed should be monitored at the center of the step wedge where the optical density is approximately 1.5. Adjacent steps also should be monitored for average gradient. These parameters along with film base and fog can be plotted to monitor the performance of film production facilities effectively. Further degradation is unavoidable in transfer to reflective media; the maximum image detail reproducible in print is 85% of the original (15).

SUMMARY: STRENGTHENING THE LINKS IN THE CHAIN

High-fidelity image quality is achieved through the cooperative interaction of the CT manufacturer, the service organization, and the CT owner-operator. Each group controls specific elements in the imaging chain and communication between them is essential for production of optimal images.

The basic system is designed by the engineering department in cooperation with the manufacturing department. Because the tolerances for building a high-performance CT system are stringent, rigorous adherence to manufacturing standards is required. Two examples are the CT detector and the DAS. High-fidelity CT imaging demands detector manufacturing precision at the level of 1/10,000th of an inch, and exceptionally stable and noise-free electronic circuitry in the DAS. It is only with refinements in manufacturing processes, and strict supervision by the quality control department, that CT scanners can be produced commercially in large quantities.

One important component provided by the manufacturer is the set of image reconstruction algorithms. These may be defined in software, dedicated hardware, or a combination of the two. The more flexible the configuration, the more easily image improvements generated from basic research can be incorporated into systems. Selection of desirable algorithms is accomplished best by the manufacturers and medical community working closely together. Although numerous objective measurements of image quality have been developed which provide useful guidelines, experience has shown that the clinical value of new developments can only be determined by using the system in a clinical setting.

As discussed, proper system operation and maintenance ensure that the CT system meets its design objectives in actual clinical use. Patient motion, technique selection, and image manipulation affect the diagnostic value of a CT study. In addition, routine preventive maintenance of the CT system, multiformat camera, and film processor reduces downtime while contributing to the production of consistently high-quality images.

Bibliography

1. Blumenfeld SM: Physical principle of high-resolution CT with the General Electric CT/T 8800. In Post MJD: *Radiographic Evaluation of the Spine: Current Advances with Emphasis on Computed Tomography.* New York, Masson Publishing, Inc. 1980, p. 4–33.
2. Newton TH, Potts DG: *Technical Aspects of Computed Tomography, Radiology of the Skull and Brain.* Vol. 5. St. Louis, C.V. Mosby, 1981.
3. Glover GH, Pelc N: Nonlinear partial volume artifacts in x-ray computed tomography. *Med Phys* 7:238–248, 1980.
4. Brooks RA, Di Chiro G: Slice geometry in computer assisted tomography. *J Comput Assist Tomogr* 1:191–199, 1977.
5. Foley WD, Haughton VM, Lawson TL, et al: The advantages of computed generated digital radiography in CT. Paper 9, 64th Annual Scientific Assembly and Annual Meeting, Radiological Society of North America. November 28, 1978.
6. Hirschy JC, Leue WM, Berninger WH, et al: CT of the lumbosacral spine: Importance of tomographic planes parallel to vertebral end plates. *AJR* 126:47–52, 1981.
7. Biberman LM: *Perception of Displayed Information.* New York, Plenum Press, 1973.
8. Schwenker RP: Technical considerations in displaying and photographing digital data in medical imaging. *Appl Opt Instrum Med* 173:199–201, 1979.
9. Lee KR, Dwyer SJ, Anderson WH, et al.: Continuous image recording using gray-tone, dry-process silver paper. *Radiology* 139:493–496, 1981.
10. Schwenker RP: Film selection for computed tomography and ultrasound video photography SPIE. *Appl Opt Instrum Med* 173:7, 1979.
11. Lamel DA, Brown RF, Shaver JW, et al: Correlated Lecture Laboratory Series in Diagnostic Radiological Physics, U.S. Government Printing Office, Washington, DC, 1981.
12. Cohen G: Contrast-detail-dose analysis of six different computed tomographic scanners. *J Comput Assist Tomogr* 3:197–203, 1979.
13. Cohen G, DiBianca FA: The use of contrast-detail-dose evaluation of image quality in a computed tomographic scanner. *J Comput Assist Tomogr* 3:189–195, 1979.
14. Harwood-Nash D: Computed tomography of the pediatric spine: A protocol for the 1980's. *Radiol Clin North Am* 19:479–494, September 1981.
15. Williams & Wilkins: Illustration preparation. Baltimore, Williams & Wilkins, 1979, p. 1.
16. Brooks RA, Glover GH, Talbert AJ, et al: Aliasing: a source of streaks in computed tomograms. *J Comput Assist Tomogr* 3:511, 1979.
17. Burgess AE, Wagner RF, Jennings RJ, et al: Efficiency of human visual signal recognition. *Science* 214:93–94, 1981.
18. Coin CG, Coin JT: Computed tomography of cervical disk disease: Technical considerations with representative case reports. *J Comput Assist Tomogr* 5:275–280, 1981.
19. Foley WD, Lawson TL, Scanlon GT, et al: Digital radiography of the chest using a computed tomography instrument. *Radiology* 133:231–234, 1979.
20. Fullerton GD, Blanco E: Fundamentals of computerized tomography (CT) tissue characterization of the brain. Proceedings of SPIE—The International Society for Optical Engineering, Vol. 273, March 22–24, 1981.
21. Genant HK, Boyd D: Quantitative bone mineral analysis using dual energy computed tomography. *Invest Radiol* Nov/Dec, 1977.
22. Glover GH, Eisner RL: Theoretical resolution of CT systems. *J Comput Assist Tomogr* 3:85–91, 1979.
23. Haughton VM, Syvertsen A, Williams AL: Normal and pathologic anatomy of the spine: a CT study. Paper 46, 64th Annual Scientific Assembly and Annual Meeting, Radiological Society of North America, November, 28, 1978.
24. Hounsfield GN: Some practical problems in computerized tomography scanning. In Ter-Pogossian MM, Phelps ME, Brownell GL, et al: *Reconstruction Tomography in Diagnostic Radiology and Nuclear Medicine.* Baltimore, University Park Press, 1977.
25. Stockham CD: A simulation study of aliasing in stationary detector systems. Paper 418, 65th Annual Scientific Assembly and Annual Meeting, Radiological Society of North America, Chicago, December 1, 1978.
26. Trefler M, Haughton VM: Patient dose and image quality in computed tomography. *AJNR* 2:269–271, 1981.
27. Yester MV, Barnes GT: Geometrical limitations of CT scanner resolution. Proceedings of the Society of Photo Optical Instrumentation Engineering 127, "Applications of Optical Instrumentation in Medicine VI." Boston, MA, 1977, p. 296–303.

B. THE DIAGNOSTIC CAPABILITIES OF PLAIN HIGH-RESOLUTION COMPUTED TOMOGRAPHY AND MULTIPLANAR REFORMATIONS

CHAPTER SIX

An Overview of Lumbar Computed Tomography/Multiplanar Reformations: What Are Its Elements and How Do They Fit Together?

WILLIAM V. GLENN, Jr., M.D., STEPHEN L. G. ROTHMAN, M.D., MICHAEL L. RHODES, Ph.D., and CHARLES W. KERBER, M.D.

INTRODUCTION

Multi-Planar Diagnostic Imaging, Inc. (MPDI), in Torrance, CA, is a spine-dedicated CT scanning operation for the greater Los Angeles area. With three high-resolution General Electric scanners doing 85% spine CT, it is the largest and busiest spine CT clinical practice in the world. The number of spine patients scanned per month is approximately 750. The computer sciences group affiliated with MPDI, and resident to its facility, has done extensive research to perfect and streamline CT examinations of the spine in order to maximize the transfer of information to the referring physician. One manifestation of that effort is a shared central data processing service for a network (38 on August 15, 1983) of data-connected GE scanners. The number of cases processed per month over the network (and interpreted by radiologists at each network site) is approximately 3000.

This writing presents the findings and conclusions of an outpatient spine practice with the scientific resources to do whatever seemed best, whether that meant modifying the scanning equipment, software, film formats, or anything else, without dependence on a manufacturer.

PROS AND CONS OF COMPUTED TOMOGRAPHY/MULTIPLANAR REFORMATIONS (CT/MPR) VS. TILTING-GANTRY, AXIAL-ONLY SPINE EXAMINATIONS

Today, two basic methods of CT spine evaluation are popular: the tilting-gantry, axial-only technique, and the three-axis evaluation using routine axial, sagittal, and coronal views. The latter uses image reformatting by computer to create the additional views. How do these two methods differ? What are the advantages and disadvantages of each?

Most spine CT exams are attempted by scanning with a tilted gantry, producing slices paralleling (or nearly paralleling) the disc spaces. Scans often are taken only within the disc spaces. This approach is known as the tilting-gantry, axial-only method, or as simply the "transaxial" method.

In the second approach, the scanning plane remains vertical, or untilted. The patient moves through the scanner incrementally, with each axial slice slightly overlapping its neighbor. The sequence of slices is continuous through disc spaces and vertebral body segments alike. Figure 6.1 illustrates some of the different scanning techniques (slice spacing, angles, etc.) in the two methodologies.

For the second approach, once the axial images have been created they then pass back into a computer, where additional images are derived for both sagittal and coronal planes of view. Both the image size and image spacing of these reformatted views **match** the size and spacing of the original axial slices (Figure 6.2). This careful spatial matching and integration of three sets of views is critical to the true "CT/MPR" examination. It is important to note that CT/MPR does not mean spine images that are located randomly, spaced arbitrarily, and of different size relative to axial images. CT/MPR, as described in this Chapter, therefore, is distinct from other less rigorous uses of reformation capabilities.

Until 1981, spine CT reformation seldom was used. The images were difficult to produce, "stairstepped", grainy, and of generally poor technical quality. Reformation also increased the scanning computer's workload and reduced the system's throughput by preventing simultaneous patient scanning.

The following section lists the pros and cons of each methodology that are presented most often by the proponents.

Tilting-Gantry Axial-Only

Pro: 1. Fast—less than 30 minutes per patient for 15–18 slices.
2. No added computational overhead is involved

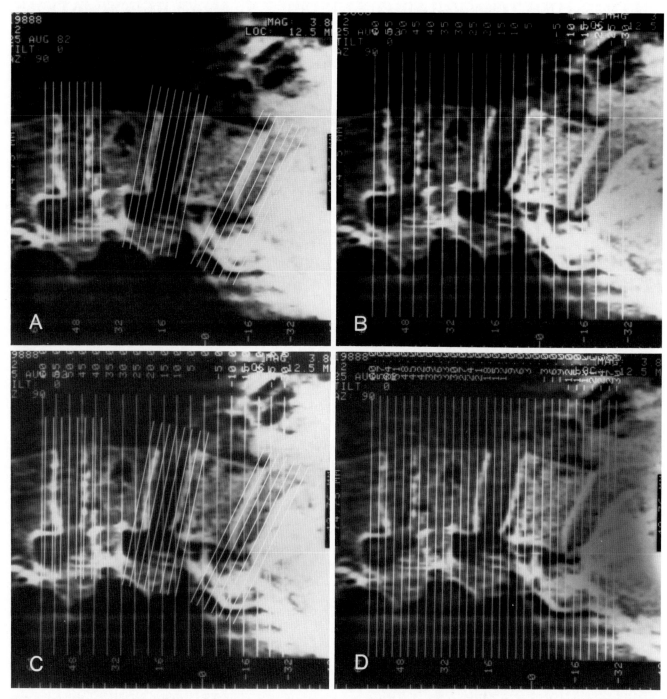

Figure 6.1. Some of the currently used scanning techniques: A. Illustrated are tilted axial scans taken at the interspaces only, thus, leaving scanning gaps at the vertebral body segments. B. Shown are nontilted parallel axial images taken with 5.0-mm slice thicknesses and 5.0-mm spacing. The images are adjacent. C. A combination of A and B is shown. In D, the 5.0-mm thick nontilted images are similar to B but with closer 3.0-mm spacing. This is the scanning technique routinely used for lumbar CT/MPR studies (see text).

for after-hours work.

3. No special software is needed for the scanner.
4. No extra training is required for either technologist or radiologist.
5. The examination can be offered at a lower price than a true CT/MPR examination.

Con: 1. Parts of every spine are missed when only the interspaces are scanned. Disc fragments are missed in the nonimaged areas.
2. Center-field or targeted images used in tilted-gantry scans do not display the full slice of the body actually scanned; peripheral pathology is

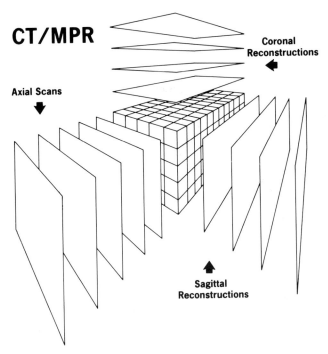

CT/MPR

Axial Scans

Coronal Reconstructions

Sagittal Reconstructions

Figure 6.2. CT/MPR schematic: This drawing illustrates the equal image spacing in three different projections. For lumbar work, the image intervals are 3.0 mm; for cervical, the intervals are 1.5 mm; and for temporal bone CT/MPR work, the intervals are 1.0 mm in each of the three projections. The schematic illustrates nothing more than polytome technique applied to CT images: small localized regions of interest in multiple projections at equal image spacing; one film typically has a composite grouping of images in the same orientation in numbered sequence.

missed as a result.

3. Peak entry skin dose to the patient often rises above the "doubling" level of overlapped non-tilted slices, due to the foldback effect when the gantry angle changes. One needs only to look at a typical lateral ScoutView and note where the scan lines produced at different levels overlap.
4. Referring physicians often find the films confusing and, therefore, may not fully achieve a complete three-dimensional understanding of the patient's anatomy.
5. Interspaces, especially the L5/S1 space, frequently lie at angles that cannot be reached by a tilting gantry. Estimates range from 15–30% of patients.
6. Radiologists who see a limited number of spines find the axial-only cases more difficult to interpret and tend to over-read disc/anulus abnormalities.
7. Each examination must be slightly different, many requiring judgment by the technologist or the radiologist while the patient is on the scanning table.

8. Follow-up exams are difficult to duplicate precisely.

CT/MPR

Pro: 1. CT/MPR standardizes examinations. Uniform performance of the scan prevents faulty judgment during the scanning process.
2. Follow-up exams are easy to duplicate.
3. All parts of the spine region under study are visualized in three planes of view. There are no skipped areas over the vertebral body segments.
4. Views of the entire abdomen allow the radiologist to see additional or unsuspected pathology outside the spine centerfield.
5. Peak entry skin dose to the patient does not rise above the doubling level of overlapped slices.
6. Each case can be presented in a prone (surgical) orientation with sagittal and coronal views that are familiar to the surgeon who has worked from myelography in the past. This improves transfer of information to the referring physician.
7. Interpretation is easier for the radiologist who sees a limited number of spine cases. The additional views offer an easy method for confirming suspected pathology.
8. Film format is tidy, presenting many images near each other, consecutively numbered, with cross-referencing that allows the reader to determine precisely a data point in question on all three views.
9. Soft-tissue windowed images are presented in true-to-life size; measurements from film are direct.

Con: 1. CT/MPR requires extra training for radiologists and technologists.
2. After-hours computer time is needed for reformatting of the transaxial images.
3. There is an increase in cost per patient, and hence the amount that must be charged for the examination.
4. The scanning process takes longer; a typical exam may take 15 minutes longer (from 34–45 minutes) due to more slices and x-ray tube cooling time.
5. There is more (up to double) storage space required for images on magnetic tape, due to the higher number of slices and more segments covered per examination. This also increases film usage.
6. CT/MPR is not essential in diagnosing every spine case.

SUGGESTED MINIMUM STANDARDS FOR BOTH METHODOLOGIES

Many of the 13,000 spine patients examined in the past 18 months at MPDI had already been examined by CT, both by tilting-gantry and reformation techniques. Many of these prior studies are clearly unsatisfactory. Certain standards for spine examination are needed, both to ensure a minimum standard of medical care and to allow third-party carriers to respond logically. The following minimum criteria are suggested:

FULL-FIELD IMAGES (Same for Both Exams)

A complete set of full-field images should be presented for interpretation. These images show anatomy throughout the region irradiated in covering the specified spine segments. The space between the filmed slices should not exceed 6.0 mm. The purpose is to avoid overlooking peripheral pathology outside the immediate vicinity of the spine, which occurs in 3–5% of cases.

DOSAGE

Tilting-Gantry, Axial-Only

One-time slice overlaps in subsequent tilted images within the interspaces so that the peak entry skin dose in a rescanned region never rises above three times the transaxial dose level.

CT/MPR

Peak entry skin dose for the examination should not exceed two times the peak entry skin dose from the transaxial images themselves. This limits overlaps to not more than one-half the slice thickness used in the study.

RESOLUTION

Slice Thickness (Same for Both Exams)

Slice thicknesses should not be more than 5.0 mm for any region of the spine being examined. Slice thicknesses above 3.0 mm should be avoided for cervical cases.

Partial Volume (CT/MPR)

Scan spacing should not be more than 3.0–4.0 mm in lumbar/thoracic regions and not more than 1.5–2.0 mm in the cervical spine.

IMAGE REGISTRATION

Axial (Same for Both Exams)

Slices taken should be numbered and indexed to both AP and lateral CT localizer films of the region examined. The axial slice numbers should be presented clearly on the films.

Sagittal and Coronal (CT/MPR)

Sagittal and coronal images, computed from the original image data, should have spacing identical to the spacing of the original transaxial slices in the study.

BONE-DETAIL AND SOFT-TISSUE IMAGES (Same for Both Exams)

Images in the study should be filmed twice with consistent level and window values, one series for bone detail and one series for soft tissue.

REPORT CUES AND IMAGE ANNOTATION (Same for Both Exams)

During the interpretation process, the films for every case should be marked by the radiologist and these marks referenced in the dictated text. For outpatient referrals, these films should be sent to the referring physician along with the report.

QUANTIFY ABNORMALITIES (Same for Both Exams)

The referenced pathology should be quantified in the report, i.e., disc bulges measured in millimeters.

TECHNICAL DETAILS FOR LUMBAR CT/MPR

Two types of reformation exams currently are being performed in the United States. The first is interactive (e.g., GE ARRANGE) and requires the technologist or radiologist to sit at the CT display console and create individual coronal and sagittal images. Examples are shown in Figure 6.3. The second type of reformation, shown in Figure 6.4, is noninteractive (e.g., network CT/MPR). This requires no computer expertise and no physician's console manipulation. The radiologist works only from filmed images at the view box, as in Figure 6.5.

Types of Lumbar Exams

The recommendation of the CT/MPR spine exam described here is based on 13,000 cases scanned and on careful consultation with more than 100 spine surgeons and their neurological colleagues. Three distinct lumbar spine examinations are ordered routinely by these referring physicians (Fig. 6.6). Each type of exam is divided into a high-detail portion for the vertebral bodies and interspaces of primary interest plus a survey portion for additional interspaces. The high-detail, or CT/MPR, portion requires a series of closely spaced, parallel, overlapping images obtained with no gantry tilting. Slice thickness is 5.0 mm; scanning interval is 3.0 mm, producing a 2.0-mm overlap. The survey portion of each examination (covering the remaining upper lumbar interspaces) is limited to interspaces only and is performed with two axial slices at 5.0-mm intervals obtained with the gantry tilted to the angulation of the interspace.

As indicated in Figure 6.6, a limited study covers from the 1st sacral segment through the pedicles of L4. This normally requires 18–24 axial slices for the CT/MPR portion and six slices to survey the upper three lumbar interspaces. A standard study covers from the 1st sacral segment to the midbody of L3 (25–34 slices) and an additional four survey images through the upper two lumbar interspaces. An extended study covers the S1 segment to the pedicles of L2 (40–45 slices) plus two additional tilted survey images for the L1/2 interspace. From the first 8000 spine CT/MPR cases, the frequency of each type of study was: 8.5%, limited exams; 69%, standard exams; 22.5% extended exams.

SUGGESTED LUMBAR PROCEDURE

The patient is placed in the scanner (GE 8800) feet first with knees supported comfortably in a flexed position. The patient position within the scanning aperture should result with the spine in the center of the scanning field (Fig. 6.7A). A guide or test slice preceding the overlapped

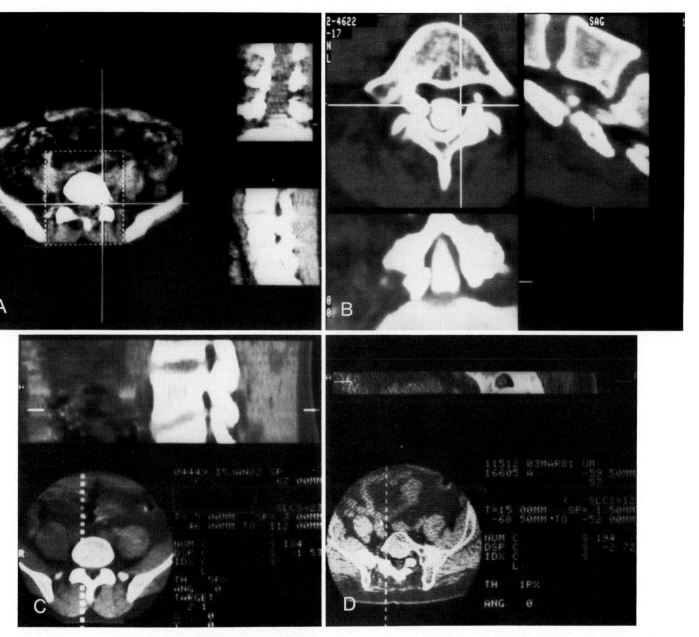

Figure 6.3. Examples of currently available manufacturer-supplied interactive reformation software. A is from Pfizer scanner. B was created by a Picker scanner. Both C and D came from GE scanners. D shows a very short sagittal image because the axial scans were taken *only* at the interspace.

sequence may be helpful. The spine should be in the center of the field of view with the spine's sagittal and coronal planes parallel with the table.

The iliac crest is a good landmark for taking the AP and lateral localizing scans, i.e., GE ScoutViews. A suggested starting index is 200, with a 0 location at the iliac crests and −80 for the end position (Fig. 6.7B). After viewing the ScoutViews, the technologist chooses beginning and ending locations for the scans (Fig. 6.7C), locating the first slice through the midbody of S1 (Fig. 6.7D) and the last slice at the lower margin of the L3 pedicle (Fig. 6.7E). The

reason for starting caudally is because patients who do move usually move later in the exam. As most lumbar abnormalities occur in the lower two interspaces, image degradation, therefore, would occur in an area of relatively low disease incidence. Significant movement occurs in very few lumbar spine CT cases.

DOSE AND SCAN-TIME CONSIDERATIONS

The overlapping sequence of 5.0-mm thick axial images taken every 3.0 mm produces a 2.0-mm overlap, in which the peak skin dose corresponds to the levels shown in

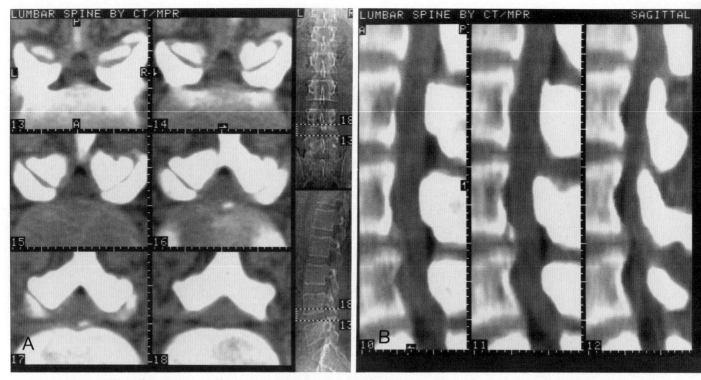

Figure 6.4. MPDI's CT/MPR image format: A. A composite axial image representing one image file and one button push on the camera. It consists of six sequential axial images plus a PA and lateral ScoutView with the position and orientation of each axial image noted. B. A composite sagittal image containing three sagittal planes numbered from left to right, with an image interval that matches the original axial slice spacing shown in the composite axial in A.

Figure 6.8. The recommended dose and technique factors are illustrated in Figure 6.9. For a medium adult with a 32″–37″ waistline, 480 mAs (tube current × scan time) results in a peak skin dose of 5.4 rads, including the dose contributed by the overlapped image sequence. By following the technique factors recommended in Figure 6.9, an average patient mix allows 45-minute scheduling intervals without undue stress. Large patients will lengthen extended studies to one hour. The low mA settings reflected in Figure 6.9 represent a deliberate attempt to run the scanner below commonly used mA settings in order to minimize radiation to the patient and to extend the life of the x-ray tube.

Because the reformatted sets of coronal and sagittal images offer additional opportunities to detect abnormalities, the individual axial images can be of slightly lower dose, and therefore slightly less contrast resolution, without sacrificing the overall diagnostic accuracy of the CT/MPR exam. A simple modification to the scanner and the tube's warmup procedures will extend the life of the tube to more than 30,000 exposures on the average.

Film Organization and Case Reporting

It is important for the CT/MPR cases to be photographed and presented to the radiologist and referring physician in an easily understood format. For spine cases, the CT films should be presented so that all physicians can correlate it easily with routine spine films and myelography.

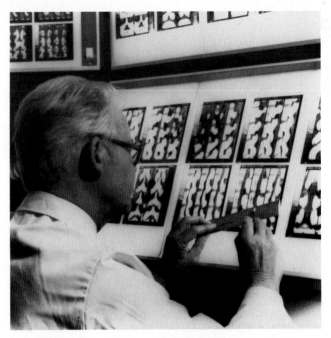

Figure 6.5. Life-size CT/MPR films on viewbox.

An attempt should be made to condense the CT examination onto the fewest possible films without unduly reducing the image size. This perhaps is accomplished best

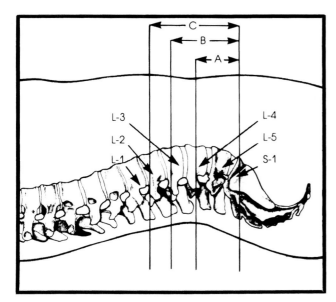

Figure 6.6. Types of CT/MPR lumbar studies (high-detail portion): limited exam (A); standard exam (B); and extended study (C). For the survey portion (remaining upper lumbar interspaces) of each type exam, two contiguous 5.0-mm thick axial images are taken at each interspace. The detailed portion of each exam uses a vertical, nontilted gantry. For the upper lumbar survey levels, the gantry is tilted to conform to the angulation of each interspace.

by magnifying the area of interest and removing extraneous anatomy from the final film image. To exclude the possibility of missing significant nonspinal lesions causing back pain, small full-field axial images should be presented as well. Highly targeted small-diameter fields of view eliminate this possibility.

Finally, the filming format should be complete enough to allow the radiologist to interpret the case thoroughly, accurately, and without the necessity of using the scanner's console to take more pictures. This degree of completeness and organization also ensures that the referring physician who does not have the luxury of a CT console will get the necessary information.

Figure 6.10 illustrates the film format currently in use in many spine scanning centers. The three rows represent axial, sagittal, and coronal perspective, in that order. Each row contains four boxes. The first box on the left is a schematic drawing of the CT images within the region of interest, which is set within the full-field image by the technologist. This region of interest creates a rectangular three-dimensional block of data from which the complete series of axial, sagittal, and coronal images is derived. The second box in each row shows the appearance of a single 14″ × 17″ film. The third box shows one quadrant of that film and the fourth box a detailed blowup of one specific image from that quadrant. From any one of these blowup pictures it is possible to predict the image that contains that same anulus calcification (see Fig. 6.10) in either of the other two perspectives. This is done by use of the tick-mark localization strategy described below, which allows three-plane correlation without using a console and com-

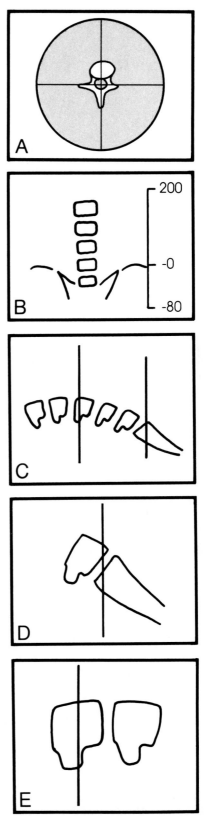

Figure 6.7. Centering the patient and setting exam limits. A. Spine location within the scan field. B. ScoutView obtained between −80 and 200, using the iliac crests as the 0 location. C-E. The initial (S1) and ending (midbody L3) locations for the high-detail portion of a standard three-level lumbar exam.

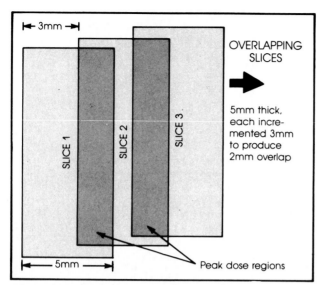

Figure 6.8. Slice thickness and overlap. For the high-detail portion of lumbar CT exams, slice thickness of 5.0 mm and a scanning interval of 3.0 mm is recommended.

PATIENT TYPE	WAIST (INCHES)	TUBE mA	NO. VIEWS	TOTAL mAS	PEAK ENTRY SKIN DOSE (RADS)
Large Adult	38-44	320	576	614	7.3
Medium Adult	32-37	250	576	480	5.4
Small Adult	26-31	200	576	384	4.1
Child	N/A	320	288	307	2.1
Infant	N/A	250	288	240	1.6

Figure 6.9. Suggested lumbar CT/MPR technique factors for GE 8800.

puter. It must be remembered that the referring physician does not have a console and computer, and therefore, the films must transmit all possible and available information the first time.

From "slice" image data contained within the region of interest, all of the axial, sagittal, and coronal images are computed and organized into composite groups. The composite axial image, which represents one button push on the camera and one storage file on the disk, usually contains six small, numbered axial images plus a postero-anterior ScoutView and a lateral ScoutView along the right margin (Figs. 6.4 and 6.10). The position of each axial image is marked clearly on these ScoutViews. The prone orientation of the axial images is shown, but the more

familiar supine body format is possible also. Sagittal and coronal composites usually contain three and two images, respectively, as in Figure 6.10. When photographed in 4-on-1 quadrant format using the large 14″ × 17″ film, the composite images in each perspective are life-size, which facilitates direct measurements on the films with a simple ruler. If these measurements from film are not considered important, the 14″ × 17″ films can be exposed in 12-on-1 format, thus saving approximately two films per case.

DETAILED LOCALIZATION STRATEGY INHERENT IN CT/MPR FILMS

Tick marks located along the top or bottom of an axial image (see Figure 6.10, *top right corner*) represent individual sagittal images counted from left to right. Tick marks located along the side of an axial image represent the coronal image series counted from posterior to anterior. Every fifth tick mark is large. The distance between any two tick marks is 3.0 mm, an interval that is determined automatically by the couch increments specified at the time the original axial scans were obtained. For lumbar spine cases, these intervals are 3.0 mm. For cervical cases, the intervals are 1.5 mm. For sella and temporal bone work, the same life-size CT/MPR processing adjusts to 1.5-mm or 1.0-mm scanning intervals. As shown schematically in Figure 6.2, a true CT/MPR examination, when filmed, should present a complete series of coronal and sagittal images at intervals that match axial scan intervals.

The focal disc or anulus calcification shown in blowup axial image 16 in the first row of Figure 6.10 illustrates the important localization and verification function provided by the tick marks. By counting along the bottom tick marks of blowup axial image 16, the focal calcification should be visible on blowup sagittal 11 in the second row of Figure 6.10. Likewise, by counting along the left margin of axial image 16, the calcification should be seen on blowup coronal image 10 in the third row of Figure 6.10. The same localization scheme also works in reverse, i.e., by *starting* with either sagittal 11 or coronal 10 instead of axial 16. A finding on one image of one orientation can lead to that same finding on a specific image in each of the other two orientations.

SAMPLE LUMBAR REPORTING FORM

Figure 6.11 is the front side of MPDI's lumbar CT reporting form. The top half is for summarizing the objective findings. The bottom half is for supporting details, which include graded findings at each lumbar level, specification of key images showing the major abnormalities, and miscellaneous notations. The graded findings are organized so that each lumbar level is represented by a horizontal row of blanks. Each column of blanks indicates a specific structure (e.g., left facet) at the different lumbar levels. The columns are organized so that left-sided structures are toward the left of the form and right-sided structures are toward the right side of the form. This conforms with the prone axial-image orientation favored by our referring surgeons so that left-sided structures are on both the left side of the form and the left side of the films. This left/right orientation is maintained within the three columns

Schematic Diagram	14" x 17" Film Layout	Film Quadrant	Detailed Blow-Up

AXIAL

Axial scans are taken every 3 mm.

Each axial image has coronal tick marks on the side and sagittal tick marks on the top or bottom. Arrows indicate the counting direction.

Axial images are numbered from inferior to superior and viewed from below.

See also sagittal #11 and coronal #10.

SAGITTAL

Sagittal images are produced every 3 mm from left to right.

Each sagittal image has axial tick marks on the side and coronal tick marks at the bottom. Arrows indicate the counting direction.

Sagittal images are numbered left to right and viewed from the left.

See also axial #16 and coronal #10.

CORONAL

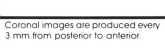

Coronal images are produced every 3 mm from posterior to anterior.

Each coronal image has axial tick marks on the side and sagittal tick marks at the bottom. Arrows indicate the counting direction.

Coronal images are numbered from posterior to anterior and viewed from posterior.

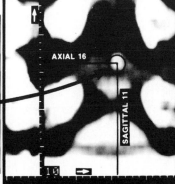

See also axial #16 and sagittal #11.

Figure 6.10. Summary of the MPDI CT/MPR lumbar film format: Images in each sequence have standardized intervals corresponding to the original scanning interval used for the axial images. *Arrows* on the detailed blowup pictures (*4th box in each row*) indicate the counting direction for the localization tick marks, which correspond to the numbered images in the other two image perspectives. Compare detailed blowup images of axial 16, sagittal 11, and coronal 10 (see text).

that constitute the "tri-joint complex" and "central canal", as shown in Figure 6.11.

The reverse side of the lumbar reporting form also is divided into top and bottom halves. The top half is the organizational detail (Figure 6.10) of axial, sagittal, and coronal sequences of images, and the inter-relationships

SPINE EXAMINATION REPORT

Patient Name   Date   X-Ray/Tape No.

Summary:

SEE REVERSE SIDE FOR FILM ORGANIZATION AND EXAMPLES ILLUSTRATING 1-5 GRADING SYSTEM

Graded Findings and Abbreviations:

1 = Normal (1MM)	**4** = Moderate (5MM)	**VC** = Vacuum Change
2 = Slight (2MM)	**5** = Severe (>6MM)	**OR** = Osteophytic Ridging
3 = Mild (3MM)	**★** = Soft Tissue	**PD** = Pars Defects

FH = Flavum Hypertrophy	**Sp** = Spur	**IJ** = Irregular Joint
LAM = Laminectomy	**F** = Fused	**DN** = Degenerative Narrowing
HL = Hemilaminectomy	**NF** = Not Fused	**SL** = Sublux

	TRI-JOINT COMPLEX			CANAL				OTHER	
	LEFT FORAMEN	LEFT FACET	DISC/ ANNULUS	RIGHT FACET	LT. LAT. RECESS	CENTRAL	RT. LAT. RECESS	RIGHT FORAMEN	
L1-L2	_____	_____	_____	_____	_____	_____	_____	_____	_____ L1-L2
L2-L3	_____	_____	_____	_____	_____	_____	_____	_____	_____ L2-L3
L3-L4	_____	_____	_____	_____	_____	_____	_____	_____	_____ L3-L4
L4-L5	_____	_____	_____	_____	_____	_____	_____	_____	_____ L4-L5
L5-S1	_____	_____	_____	_____	_____	_____	_____	_____	_____ L5-S1
	_____	_____	_____	_____	_____	_____	_____	_____	

Miscellaneous Findings

Lumbar Segments _____ Transitional Segment _____
Residual Pantopaque: _____ Few Drops; _____ Several CC's

Radiologist

_____
(Typed Name)

_____
(Signature)

Key Images

	Lifesize	Non-Lifesize
Axial	_____	Bone Density Axial _____
Sagittal	_____	Bone Density Sagittal _____
Coronal	_____	Bone Density Coronal _____
Other	_____	Reduced Full Field
	_____	Supine Images _____

Figure 6.11. MPDI's lumbar CT/MPR reporting form: *Top half* is for case summary and *bottom half* is for supporting details, i.e., graded findings, notation of key images, and so on. Form can be filled out with either regular typewriter or from sprocket-driven computer printer following CRT entry of information.

that are inherent in this film format for localization purposes. The bottom half of the reverse side shows the grading system used for key components of the lumbar spine (Fig. 6.12). This is discussed in Chapter 7.

CT/MPR Data Processing Strategy Via High-Speed Network Computer Communication

The key problem, i.e., time element, in routine clinical use of CT reformations has been solved. Until recently, the primary deterrent to reformatting spine cases (or sellas, orbits, etc.) has been the console time required of technologists and radiologists. As the reformatting effort becomes more meticulous, personnel time rises sharply. So too does time away from patient scanning, because the CT computer is tied up. These disadvantages are reflections not of reformatting, per se, but of the interactive, console-based software (see Fig. 6.3) now available from CT manufacturers.

GRADING SYSTEM EXAMPLES

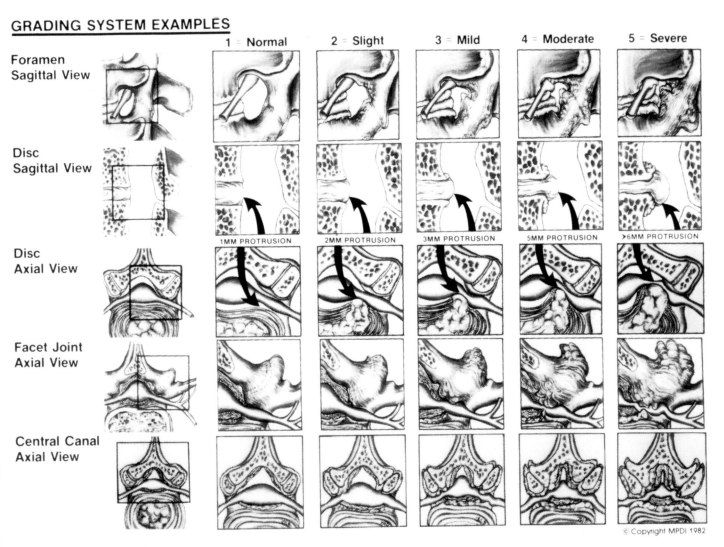

Figure 6.12. Schematic anatomic drawing for five-point lumbar spine grading system. Division between "normal" and "abnormal" is between grade 3 (mild) and grade 4 (moderate). These schematic drawings are on the reverse side of the CT/MPR lumbar form shown in Figure 6.11.

NETWORK CONCEPT

There is now another way to accomplish very detailed reformatting with minimum time overhead and no interruption of the daytime scanning schedule. Nor do the technologists and radiologists have to stay late. The solution is to have all reformations performed by a shared computer facility late at night when the scanner normally is not running. CT/MPR photography is deferred until the following morning when the time requirement is simply 13–15 minutes of photography for each case. During the preceding night shift (12:00 AM–6:00 AM), each CT/MPR case was reformatted automatically by a processing service that conducts a late-night dialogue with the CT scanning computer over high-speed digital communication lines. This is an automatic, noninteractive approach to the reformatted methodology. It is based on an image process-

ing service that is simple to use and requires no special computer training. Only a short time is needed at the console to photograph results.

Currently, a group of 38 GE 8800 scanners around the country are using this network concept. The first 27 locations are shown in Figure 6.13. GE participated in the site selection as well as required network installation and warranty extension. Each site interprets its own cases. All sites share in a standard scanning technique and film format. Software improvements or interesting teaching cases can be distributed easily to all sites via the network the same night. All benefit quickly from improvements originating at individual network sites.

Figure 6.14 illustrates connection of a standard GE 8800 scanner (Data General S/200 or S/140 Eclipse) to the CT/MPR processing network, requiring General Electric field service installation of a Data General Universal Line Mul-

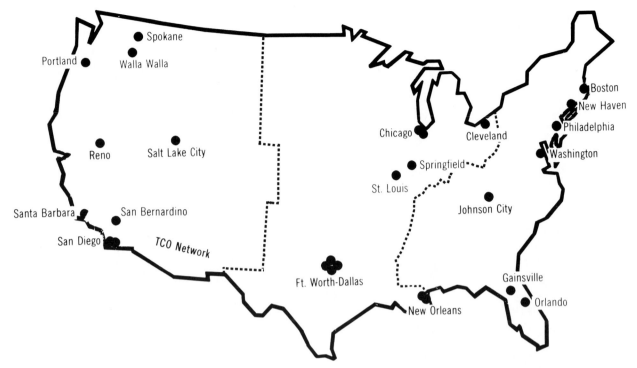

Figure 6.13. The first 27 CT/MPR network locations as of January, 1983.

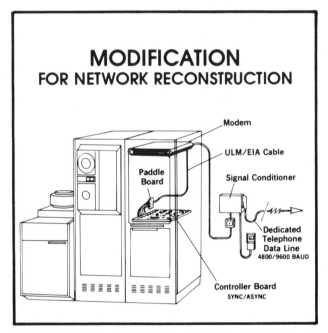

Figure 6.14. Minor additions to CT computer for network connection.

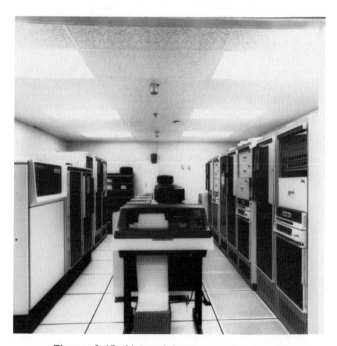

Figure 6.15. Network host computer system.

tiplexor board (ULM Model 4242). The addition of 13 wires from the ULM board to the computer's central processing unit usually takes about three hours. Standard cable connections are made from the ULM board to a 4800-baud modem.

The network host computer facility in Figure 6.15 is made of three Data General S/200 computers, a Data General S/140, and a 32-bit Data General MV/8000 located in Torrance, CA. The MV/8000 computer system has six million bytes of main memory, a virtual memory operating system (AOS/VS), 16 9600-baud digital communication channels, and 1800 megabytes of disk storage. This initial minimum configuration is designed to grow with network demand in a modular fashion in terms of additional central processing units, processing lines, and disk storage.

NETWORK OPERATION

From an operational standpoint, the CT technologist at a remote site begins a CT/MPR processing connection by initiating the "CTNET" program just before leaving at night. This usually requires about 30 seconds of technologist time per case. The CTNET program requests run numbers of cases to be network processed and then simply enters a wait state until signaled by the host computer facility. Network processing accepts a mixture of CT/MPR cases (lumbar, cervical, sella, orbit, etc.) with differential axial image spacing and circles of reconstruction (one case to another). The host computer searches for processing work by sequentially checking the scanner systems of network members. The primary host computer automatically establishes processing connections with those sites found in wait status. Once the processing connection is initiated, the remote CT scanner computer and the host computer facility conduct a high-speed dialogue involving extensive data compression of CT image data transmitted between the remote and the host computers. CT/MPR processing and image reformatting are distributed between both computer systems. Every CT/MPR submission is processed, in part, at the host computer. There is also, necessarily, image processing that takes place at each remote site. For example, remote computers allocate file space for network-processed images. Region-of-interest box setting is done at the central processing computer by experienced staff.

The computing burden for a life-size CT/MPR case is large and, therefore, time-consuming for several reasons. First, each gantry-produced axial image is adjusted for size in order to ensure that the composite axial, composite coronal, and composite sagittal images will be perfectly life-size when photographed in the 4-on-1 film format. Second, a sophisticated low-distortion algorithm not only eliminates the expected steps along bone edges but also produces a complete series of sagittal and coronal images within the predetermined region-of-interest box. Finally, composite groupings of reduced, full-field, supine-orientation images also are created and stored on the disk.

Because filming and interpretation are preserved completely at the local site, the deferred batch processing is a totally transparent operation to network members. As of Sept 1, 1983, over 24,500 CT/MPR examinations had been reformatted via network processing.

How reliable is the network connection? What happens when there is a failure? Four possible failures may occur:

1. The GTE lines go dead.
2. The modem linking the scanner's computer to the network line fails.
3. The scanner's computer goes down.
4. One of the large network computers fails.

Network reliability for the first 24,500 cases has increased from 92% in August 1981 to over 98% in Sept 1983. All failures are logged and investigated. GTE lines are the weakest link. They occasionally go dead just as a regular phone line will. A prompt call by network personnel to a central number gives 24-hour troubleshooting; usually the service is back in 2–4 hours.

Rarely, the modem fails. This has, over all sites, happened only twice. The modem either is replaced or repaired. This has taken one day at one site, and two days at the other site. Modem failure is tolerable because it does not interrupt scanning, and the vast majority of spine work is not emergent. If the scanner's computer fails, local GE engineers respond. The network has never caused failure of scanner-computer hardware at any site connected. The fourth potential failure is the central network host computing facility itself. To date, no significant problems have been encountered.

If the scanner is needed for an emergency scan during a late-night network dialogue, simple interrupt procedures will take the local CT computer "off the air." When the emergency scans are finished, network restart is simple and the processing dialogue continues from the point of interruption.

QUESTIONS AND ANSWERS

Questions for Referring Physicians

A pair of four-hour spine CT reading tutorials were conducted at MPDI for 75 Los Angeles referring physicians, who filled out questionnaires. Their specialties were: orthopaedic surgery (62%), neurology (22%), neurosurgery (10%), and internal medicine/rheumatology (6%). All physicians had referred patients to a spine CT facility (MPDI) utilizing the CT/MPR film format. Twenty-four percent of physicians were classed as lightly exposed to CT/MPR in that they had referred 0–5 cases, 35% had referred 5–15 cases (medium exposure), and 41% had more than 15 cases. The questions and their answers are valuable to anyone interested in offering spine CT examinations.

QUESTION

Do you want to receive case films for your own review?

RESPONSE

One hundred percent said yes, but later questions showed that not all actually looked at the films.

QUESTION

Which views do you look at?

RESPONSE

When a CT/MPR case report is *abnormal*, 95% of physicians review the films themselves vs. 57% who review the films for a normal report. Five percent indicated they reviewed axial images alone; 90% said they used the axials in combination with either sagittal or sagittal plus coronal images; 5% had no opinion. For orientation of only the axial images, 2% preferred supine images, 25% had no preference, and 73% preferred the prone axial-image orientation.

QUESTION

What type of reports are preferred?

RESPONSE

Only 3% of referring physicians preferred an unstructured, freeform, descriptive report. Ninety-two percent favored a structured report form that incorporates a section for graded findings (see Sample Lumbar Reporting Form, p. 144). When asked about developing an analogous cervical report form, 93% were in favor, 5% had no opinion, and 2% preferred the unstructured descriptive reporting format.

QUESTION

Do you prefer uniformity in CT exam performance, interpretation, and film format?

RESPONSE

In this three-part question, there was overwhelming endorsement for the concept of standardization. One element was the manner in which the actual scans are taken and what anatomy is covered or possibly skipped. For this, 87% indicated the exam performance variables should be tightly defined: slice thickness, scan interval, number of spine levels covered, tilting gantry, nontilting gantry, interspace-only scans vs. interspace plus vertebral body levels, acceptable radiation dose thresholds, etc. Uniform interpretive criteria were endorsed positively by 85%, and a set of uniform film organization and format criteria (image orientation, size, windowing, etc.) were favored by 87%.

QUESTION

What is your tendency to order myelography?

RESPONSE

Given an unequivocally positive lumbar CT exam and a symptomatic patient, 33% of referring physicians would recommend or perform myelography on more than 50% of these patients. Given a negative CT exam, 16% would recommend or perform a myelography on more than 50% of their patients. However, when the CT exam was negative, 59% of physicians indicated they would be willing to stop the radiographic workup (no myelography) and simply wait until further workup was mandated by continued or increasing symptoms.

QUESTION

What do you believe is the relative diagnostic accuracy of CT/MPR vs. axial-only lumbar methodology?

RESPONSE

When asked for a personal preference with regard to CT spine examination philosophy, 3% specified axial only, 5% had no opinion, and 92% preferred the CT/MPR approach. When asked to estimate the overall diagnostic accuracy of CT/MPR vs. axial only, 87% indicated they believed the diagnostic accuracy of CT/MPR to be approximately 75% or greater, whereas 5% thought CT/MPR exams were accurate 50% of the time or less. For axial-only spine exams, 46% believed the accuracy to be 75% or better, whereas 40% believed these exams were accurate 50% of the time or less. No opinion was expressed

in 8% and 14% for the two parts of this question, respectively.

Referring physicians prioritized the CT/MPR advantages as follows (highest priority first): direct measurements from life-size films, better spatial or three-dimensional perception, more appropriate surgical orientation, more complete exam, and finally, added information on sagittal and coronal images.

CHECK ON FORMAT-EXPOSURE BIAS IN THE PHYSICIAN GROUP ANSWERING THE QUESTIONNAIRE

Questionnaires from the 15 "lightly exposed" referring physicians (24%), with 0–5 prior case referrals to MPDI, were tabulated separately to expose any prejudice that more frequent use of MPDI's CT/MPR format might have introduced. Surprisingly, these results were more polarized than the overall totals. As in the overall results, 100% wanted films sent to their offices. In the question of film use, 94% reviewed abnormal cases, whereas 73% reviewed normal case films. The preferred combination of views was: 80% relied on coronal and/or sagittal as well as on the axial images. For axial orientation, 47% had no preference, 53% preferred prone axial images, and none requested supine axial orientation. All 15, or 100%, wanted a structured lumbar report form, with a grading system; 93% favored development of a structured, graded form for cervical studies.

On the question of standardization of exam performance, interpretive criteria, and film organization, the affirmative preferences were 100%, 100%, and 87%, respectively. When asked about personal preferences regarding the axial-only methodology vs. CT/MPR methodology, this group preferred axial only 7%, CT/MPR 80%, and no preference in 13%. For overall diagnostic accuracy, 100% of these 15 physicians believed CT/MPR was 75% accurate or better, whereas only 67% believed the axial-only methodology was 75% accurate or better. Conversely, none believed CT/MPR was less than 50% accurate, whereas 33% indicated that level of confidence for the axial-only approach.

Questions for Radiologists

QUESTION

Are detailed multiplanar films required for diagnosis in every spine CT case?

RESPONSE

The answer is, obviously—no. Then why do we suggest that this approach should be used routinely in all spine cases? One reason is because it is a more complete examination that is better understood by the referring physician. It is impossible to know, a priori, which cases need only a limited study. Another reason is the speed and efficiency that result from the CT/MPR standardization—first in making the images and later when interpreting them. Having precisely the same film sequence each time makes it easier to put the case up for viewing. Once the films are on an alternator, each reader develops an efficient and precise search pattern.

How often do the additional reformatted images help? In our practice, a conservative estimate is 75% of cases, which can come about in five distinct ways:

1. Key finding(s) seen *only* in reformatted image.
2. Key finding(s) seen *first* in reformatted image, then retrospectively in original axial images.
3. Suspicious but inconclusive observation from axial images confirmed or ruled out with additional coronal or sagittal perspective.
4. Finding(s) best understood by referring physicians when the reformatted images are available.
5. Case interpretation accomplished more quickly and more accurately with multiple views than with axial views alone.

QUESTION

If a finding is not present on axial images, will it exist on reformatted images?

RESPONSE

Strictly speaking—no. But *perception* of abnormality is the issue. The question would be more relevant if it were stated, "Can a thing be perceived from the reformatted images that was not perceived from the axial scans?" The answer to this is a resounding yes. Some structures are displayed optimally in axial planes; others are not. A basic radiological rule states: get additional views. It is a good rule, and applies as well to CT as to plain films.

QUESTION

Can images similar to CT/MPR images be created using the manufacturer-supplied interactive capabilities at the physician's viewing console?

RESPONSE

Yes, to a great degree. Similar reformatted images can be made with any interactive reformatting software (e.g., GE ARRANGE). Usually, few reformatted images are created because reformatting requires interruption of patient scanning. Duplicating the CT/MPR format on a scanner's computer is most time-consuming. Images are created and photographed one at a time. Duplicating a network-processed CT/MPR standard lumbar exam with ARRANGE requires twice as many films (15–16), 675 keystrokes at the console, over at least 90 minutes. An inexperienced operator would take longer.

QUESTION

Why are axial composite views displayed in the prone position in the MPDI format when scans are done supine?

RESPONSE

We advocate and use prone images, quite simply, because the referring physicians—largely spine surgeons—prefer it. Supine axial images also are available. The original and the more recent surveys show that the referring physicians want images oriented to match the patient on the operating table. Dorsal is up, ventral is down, and

the left side of an axial image corresponds to the patient's left side. The life-size format makes comparisons in the operating room easy and also facilitates direct measurements from the films, which referring physicians enjoy doing themselves. The film format was created for the consumer, the referring physician, instead of being designed to suit a particular scanner's computer capacity or some radiologist's preconceived idea of what the referring physician wants.

QUESTION

Why don't all authorities recommend routinely reformatting spine cases?

RESPONSE

Until very recently, the resolution of reformatted images was generally poor. As a rule, those speaking against reformation have either little admitted experience or an exposure that is entirely limited to the tedious interactive approach. Some have no experience with high-quality reformatted images. Conclusions thus drawn do not apply necessarily to modern CT/MPR. No one would deny the necessity for lateral chest radiographs even though the majority of abnormalities are clearly visible on frontal films. The nature of the practice also has an effect. Those that are very consumer-oriented view network CT/MPR with enthusiasm. In situations where radiologists are not plentiful and the spine CT demand is high, the economies and image detail furnished are keenly appreciated. Average added cost per case over the network is $46.00: The amount is less as volume increases.

Questions About CT/MPR Network Processing

QUESTION

Since network-based CT/MPR is described as not one but a whole series of interdependent optimizations, what is the big picture? How do the pieces fit together?

RESPONSE

The best way to obtain a clear and accurate overview is to list each component in the entire process and indicate how that piece of equipment or that person is affected. The components are listed in sequence, with the two most important (referring physician and patient) being last.

Component	Benefit
Gantry	There is an average tube life of 32,000 exposures with modified break-in and warmup procedure. Routine spine CT/MPR avoids high mA settings (400 and above). Throughput of patients is predictable and uniform due to standardized CT/MPR scanning protocol.
Computer	By late-night processing connection to a large host computer, the CT computer accomplishes much more in a given 24-hour period (Fig. 6.16). The late-night processing is performed automatically, thus, requiring no local attention or

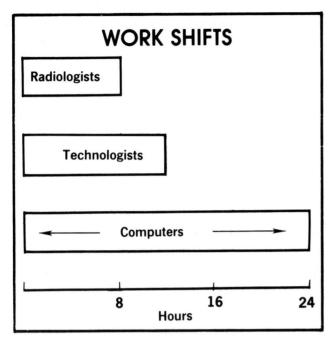

Figure 6.16. CT computer works three shifts.

monitoring technologist. The use of the third shift does not compete with routine daily scanning. The data compression used in CT/MPR network processing has been adapted to a new tape archiving program that provides 90% better utilization of magnetic tape for image archiving.

Technologist   Minimum time requirements in postprocessing (e.g., reformatting) and photographic duties: 30 seconds required to submit case to network; 13–15 minutes required to photograph each case the next morning. In the near future, two new camera modifications will eliminate film exposure and cassette changing and, therefore, will reduce technologist time to near zero (see below).

Radiologist   There is no need to monitor spine examinations; no need to spend considerable time at CT display console (which is fun, but generally unproductive). Structured CT/MPR reporting form aids fast reading and recovery from interruptions. Grading system yields uniformity of interpretation among different film readers. Film format (see below) also adapts very easily to other free-form styles of reporting.
Useful film format: lots of visual cues for the beginner; quick reading because of complete ordered sequences, which have standardized matching image inter-

vals and images sized for direct measurements from film. Films are comprehensive, thus, obviating the need to return to the technologist or console for more pictures. Interpretive accuracy is high because of multiple views at right angles and easy cross-referencing between views, as well as the routine availability of soft-tissue photographs, bone-window photographs, and full-field axial views for nonspine incidental findings.

Camera/Film   Nearly 50% better film utilization when images are recorded in composite groupings rather than individually as with interactive reformation programs. The CT/MPR methodology has focused attention on the photography step (13–15 minutes per case) as the next "bottleneck" to overcome.
Near future: camera will have simple, adaptable magazine loader and computer control, thus, eliminating time now spent setting windows, exposing films, and changing film cassettes.

Referring Physician   Maximum film understanding from prone (surgical) orientation of axial images. Complete set of familiar sagittal views. Easy measurements from life-size images. Uniform format.

Patient   The most thorough possible exam at the lowest possible x-ray exposure, with a total of 5 lumbar levels covered. CT/MPR scanning technique leaves no scanning gaps between interspaces mid-L3 to upper S1 in the standard lumbar examination. Interspace-only survey slices taken at L1-2 and L2-3 in the standard lumbar examination. Low mA setting, routinely used restricts dose. Film organization and format is designed for no cognitive gaps by radiologist, who must interpret the case accurately, and referring physician or surgeon, who must understand the images and the interpretation accurately to act in the patient's best interest.

QUESTION

What type of CT facility gains the most from performing network CT/MPR cases?

RESPONSE

A caricature of the "ideal" network site would be a description of six important characteristics. Few sites have all, but many facilities have at least four.

1. *Need efficiency boost.* This applies to most hospital and private-practice settings with rapidly growing spine demand and patient schedules already near capacity. In fact, the entire network concept originated within a pri-

vate practice with strong motivation for efficiency in scanning and film reading. Such scanners rarely operate beyond 9:00 PM and infrequently are used for late-night emergencies. This makes for smooth network operation, even though emergency interrupt procedures are simple to use and are exercised routinely at some of the large hospitals with network links.

2. *Standard GE 8800 system (no separate IPDC) configuration.* The standard single-gantry, single-computer combination represents not only the vast majority of GE 8800 installations (more than 80%) but also the configuration most in need of network aid.

3. *Relative shortage of physician personnel.* This often means no available residents or fellows. All ancillary CT image processing and routine photographic requirements usually fall upon the CT technologist and the system's single computer. In those practices, the same technologist and the same computer are needed to run the gantry to scan patients. A heavy scanning schedule is typical.

4. *Outpatient setting that may not be adjacent to either a hospital or a medical office building.* A private-practice outpatient CT setting does not enjoy the advantages of the 1-on-1 interaction between the physician who ordered the examination and the radiologist who interpreted the results. In such a free-standing CT clinic, one generates a set of films, which are forwarded routinely to the referring physician. The organizational structure of these films must be simple and unambiguous so the referring physician may review them by himself with confidence and understanding.

5. *Philosophy to delegate as much of the scanning and filming to CT technologists as possible.* Network-based CT/MPR maximizes the opportunity and safety margin for such delegation. Because all patients are scanned in exactly the same fashion, decisions by the radiologist regarding where to start, where to stop, how much gantry-tilt, etc., may be avoided. This means that the radiologist need not be in the scanning suite, but rather can devote more time to reading cases or doing other radiographic procedures. Because all cases are filmed in exactly the same way, the radiologist need not concern himself with setting window-width or window-level parameters.

Conveniently, neither the radiologists nor the technologists are required to do the actual software reformatting themselves. This is delegated to the network. This leaves only the photographic step, which currently requires 13–15 minutes per case and represents the most time-consuming step in doing CT/MPR by network. This, too, soon will have a solution with two adaptations to the standard GE camera: the first is a pair of 100-film magazines for exposed and unexposed film, and the second is network software control of film exposure, selection of window-width/window-level settings, and selection of 12-on-1 vs. 4-on-1 format. The goal is that the first technologist to arrive each morning will simply head for the dark room with the magazine of already-exposed CT/MPR films.

6. *Attention to needs of referring physicians.* This is more intangible but perhaps most important of all. Because the CT/MPR film format was devised by a panel of physicians who do mostly spine surgery, every attempt was made to optimize the film format for their needs: life-size images, prone orientation in the axials, and tick-mark localization on each view allows cross-referencing of alternate planes of view while working from films. Thor-

ough understanding of film format reinforces understanding of the clinical results—if CT is to replace myelography as a primary spinal diagnostic tool, this understanding is critical. Anything that minimizes variation in scanning technique, film format, and interpretive criteria from case to case also reinforces the understanding and enthusiasm of the referral base.

QUESTION

Who developed and provides the network processing concept?

RESPONSE

Development and implementation of the CT/MPR network capability would not have been possible without the close cooperation of the GE Medical Systems Division in Milwaukee. The network capability was developed by MPDI, a California corporation founded with backing from private investors. MPDI has three missions: (1) to provide the highest quality private outpatient CT scanning as a service to local physicians; (2) to develop and make available to other practicing radiologists computer processing of locally generated images so that body parts may be examined expeditiously and carefully, producing uniform, easily read, and high-quality images for maximum patient benefit; (3) to do basic research development and teach advanced computer graphics as applied to all medical imaging modalities.

For its own clinical use, MPDI has three GE CT scanners operating in the Torrance headquarters facility plus a sister site in Costa Mesa.

The Torrance facility also houses large network computer systems; there the high-speed phone links end. In addition to scan processing, the system transmits data packages back to the sites. Such data packets consist of new or expanded computer programs (updates are normal and continuous) and cases for teaching or consultation.

Finally, a team of physicians and full-time engineers and computer scientists continues to pursue new developments. No federal funding is used; private and individual monies support the individual projects. Work in progress includes CT-guided stereotactics, three-dimensional picture processing, GE camera modifications, CT-aided individualized hip prostheses, etc.

QUESTION

Does life-size magnification degrade image quality? More importantly, does network processing lower spatial or contrast resolution?

RESPONSE

The answer is clearly and firmly—no. Some confusion has arisen when authors compared 12-on-1 with 4-on-1 axial photographs. There also has been some artifact introduced by varying, for publication, the amount of photographic magnification. When patients are scanned using large fields of view, scanner images show anatomy much smaller than life-size. Magnification of these axial images enlarges the quantum mottle, creating optical degradation in the resultant images. When smaller fields of view are chosen (i.e., small-diameter target reconstruction), the raw CT data produce images close to life-size, then the incremental magnification to actual life-size introduces *no* discernible degradation. In principle, the more a digital image is magnified the more it is degraded optically, but if life-size processing is applied to images that are already close to life-size, one cannot distinguish optical differences. The table of choices, costs, and results (Table 6.1) compares a 30-slice lumbar spine study for an average adult. For the times listed, no other computer interrupts were allowed during scanning or reconstruction, that is, no independent physician's console images were viewed.

Table 6.1 illustrates three important points: first, when regular or nonlife-size output is taken from network processing, there is absolutely *no* difference in image quality from gantry data. Second, for the highest quality LIFE-SIZE™ network-processed images, target factors that increase axial images to "just below" life-size will produce imperceptible differences. Third, time-to-scan, radiation, and patient throughput (tube cooling, reconstruction time) all must be considered. Thus, we recommend that target factors above 2.1 should be avoided in busy CT sections. The second technique listed appears to be the best compromise: 320 mA, with a prospective target factor of 2.1.

QUESTION

From a technical viewpoint, what are the key advantages to a network of computers? How do they apply to CT image processing?

RESPONSE

Many large computationally powerful computer systems have emphasized distribution of their power to users. In university and large business environments computer access has taken the form of terminals distributed to hundreds of students or employees. This type of access can allow all users to share the central computer, all its programs, all its disk memory, and all its peripheral devices (i.e., printers, plotters, card punchers, display devices). Such large systems can execute programs extremely quickly, giving the appearance to any one user that the entire computer system is at his sole disposal.

The characteristic that makes such large distributed systems so attractive is the concept of program and device *sharing*. All users can share the power of a single computer.

Using digital networks, the concept of sharing has been extended from many terminals as users of a shared computer to many computers as users of a larger shared computer. In this new type of collaboration, interaction takes place on a level of speed and volume that only computers can maintain. At this level of discourse, entire files of hundreds of thousands of characters are transmitted in the time one terminal user could type a single line of text. The benefits to any one computer so connected to other network computers similarly are extended. Now, computer programs, libraries of data, and computer devices can be shared between computer systems.

During the last decade, the Advanced Research Projects Agency of the Department of Defense funded pioneering efforts to design, implement, and measure a network to interconnect computer systems. This network allowed computers of different manufacturers to communicate and share resources. Among the several benefits of the project, protocols for computer dialogue (i.e., X.25, X.75), automatic error detection and correction, and message-switched communications strategies resulted. Using these

Table 6.1.
Choices, Costs, and Results

Scan Technique	Scan Time	GE Recons Time	GE Image Quality	Network Image Quality	
				Nonlife-size	LIFESIZE™
320 mA target factor: 1.7	40 min	55 sec/slice 28 min total	Standard FOV: 25 cm Full perimeter anatomy surveyed	No change, same image data that gantry delivers	Subtle blur due to image magnification
320 mA target factor: 2.1	40 min	55 sec/slice 28 min total	Improved FOV: 20 cm Loss of some perimeter anatomy	No change, same image data that gantry delivers	Identical bone edges, no difference in soft tissue
320 mA target factor: 2.8	40 min	105 sec/slice 53 min total	Best resolution FOV: 16 cm No perimeter anatomy viewed, center on spine critical	No change, same image data that gantry delivers	Absolutely no difference when compared to nonlife-size

results, proven analytically and in practice for nearly 15 years with over 100 computers connected, commercial networks recently have offered similar services. One such service, offered by GTE Telenet, is used by MPDI for its CT/MPR network.

Scanner systems connected to the CT/MPR network are given access to the programs, memory, disk drives, and essentially all of the resources of MPDI's central 32-bit computer system. In addition to the added computional power extended to the remote scanner systems, the convenience of updating all connected scanners to new improved program features cannot be overstated. Now, any time a program feature is added to demonstrate patient anatomy in CT better, improve diagnosis, aid referring physician image understanding, or help CT technologists scan, the improvement is distributed instantaneously to all network scanners.

The approach is simply *sharing*—sharing computer resources on a scale and convenience until only recently possible.

DISCUSSION AND SUMMARY

As a general rule, the utilization of CT in the U.S. is 60–70% head CT and 30–40% body CT. Use of CT for spine diagnosis, although growing steadily, is a small component of body CT and an even smaller portion of overall CT utilization. It reasonably follows that CT manufacturers would deliver CT systems with performance characteristics and special features addressing the dominant utilization patterns; considerably less emphasis would be given to a new and still emerging clinical application such as the spine. Any unique spine data-processing requirements (e.g., reformatting, interactive display, etc.) simply reinforce this tendency.

The detailed CT/MPR methodology presented in this chapter represents a combination of several optimizations: scanning technique, a unique film format organized for efficient understanding, and a computer network approach that fully addresses the anticipated high national demand for CT spine diagnosis. Our total control over critical aspects of image processing and display software has enabled new capabilities to evolve naturally, based on day-to-day clinical needs. Earlier concepts emphasizing extensive radiologist interaction with the CT display console have given way to the more appropriate and acceptable strategy of reading cases entirely from a standardized film format.

The key issue in optimal CT spine diagnosis is not as simple as locating a CT scanner that can make high-resolution transverse images. The challenge now is to transfer efficiently to film the image data required for easy and complete understanding by the referring physician and radiologist. The majority of CT scanners frustrate that goal, as they have one gantry, one computer, and no freestanding off-line display console with a separate computer and camera.

Whether the referring physician chooses a CT scan or a myelographic exam, he should be able to go to the patient's film jacket and place either set of films on the view box with equal ease and equal understanding of the pathology. A spine CT case becomes tedious when treated as a lengthy series of individual pictures rather than as a coherent unit or sequence of carefully registered and cross-referenced images. No physician should have to integrate a lengthy series of axial images mentally in order to imagine what the myelogram would probably look like. Our format presents that image right on the film, for every case, and for every location in the region of interest.

More spine CT may be a mixed blessing. Will detailed images of insignificant or irrelevant pathology lead to unnecessary surgery? Remember, about one-half of patients undergoing cervical myelography have "abnormal" lumbar myelograms. What will happen when surgeons see clinically silent bone spurs, laminar thickening, disc/anulus bulging, facet hypertrophy, or foraminal encroachment? To fulfill our professional obligation as radiologists, we must present CT's morphological details in a cognitively standardized and extremely complete fashion so that the surgeon himself can totally understand each situation. Only then can he or she make precise correlations with patient history, neurological exam, and other diagnostic information.

We contend that the ultimate role and extent of spine CT utilization will be determined by referring orthopaedic surgeons, neurosurgeons, and neurologists. These are the physicians who order most myelograms. If safe CT supplants myelography, these referring subspecialists must feel comfortable and competent in their understanding of CT images and cases. It is our job as radiologists to do everything we can to enhance our referring physician's grasp and appreciation of the images themselves.

Referring physicians will play a key role in spine CT's clinical impact, and we radiologists should listen carefully to the requests made by these referring physicians. Informal surveys, as discussed on p. 147, should be viewed simply as a first step. Periodic updates are also important. It is unlikely that the referring physicians answering our questionnaire were oriented too heavily toward the CT/MPR methodology to be representative for two reasons. First, 24% of those physicians were lightly exposed to the CT/MPR lumbar format. Their answers to key questions showed the same strong preferences as physicians with more exposure to the same approach. Second, Los Angeles referring physicians are quite familiar with several different spine CT approaches. It is estimated conservatively that 20,000 reformatted spine CT exams have been performed on high-resolution, rotating-geometry scanners in the Los Angeles area since 1980. The reformatted approach (in whatever form) represents 25–50% of the spine CT exams being done. Over 55 GE 8800 scanners in the Greater Los Angeles area account for 175–225 CT spine scans per day, as determined by a recent telephone survey. Many other types of high-resolution scanners are also in operation. Given these facts, it is clear that Los Angeles area referring physicians (orthopaedists, neurologists, neurosurgeons, etc.) have been well exposed to a wide variety of spine CT.

For spine work, CT/MPR and the axial-only, tilted-gantry methodologies both are clinically valid and proven approaches. The axial-only approach represents a subset of CT/MPR attributes. Because both will be widely used, it is important that there be consensus on minimal criteria for exam performance, exam interpretation, case organization on films, and cost. The most logical participants in that consensus should be referring subspecialities, radiologists, and third-party payors. Reaching a consensus will not be easy, but the ultimate benefactor will be the patient with a backache.

CHAPTER SEVEN

Lumbar Computed Tomography/Multiplanar Reformations, A Reading Primer

CHARLES W. KERBER, M.D., WILLIAM V. GLENN, Jr., M.D., and STEPHEN L. G. ROTHMAN, M.D.

Imagine the surprise and delight felt by that first radiologist who realized—quite incidentally—that the body scanner showed not only abdominal organs but also the intervertebral *disc*. And imagine the thrill she* felt when the scanner made the first image of a herniated nucleus pulposus. Finally, we could evaluate the disc nonintrusively. Refinements in technique led to greater resolution. Better resolution gave greater diagnostic accuracy; few disc herniations were missed, and there was talk of the obsolete myelogram. But a mental set developed. Enthralled with our ability to diagnosis soft-tissue infringement upon a root, we (relatively) ignored the other causes of radiculopathy, and the many "failed backs" continued to fail to find relief of their pain. Still the original accomplishment was a significant one. We do not denegrate it—but we do hope to make you aware that there are other causes of back pain and radiculopathy, and that a complete understanding of the back's altered biomechanics and pathological anatomy is necessary to plan rational, successful treatment.

The spine scanning techniques which evolved followed logically from the body scan format. Superb images were produced. But there was some dissatisfaction with the way the images were presented. This dissatisfaction came not from radiologists, but from the consumers—the spine surgeons. What do you think would happen if you assembled 30 spine surgeons in a room and told them they could not leave until they had reached a consensus about the spine format they wanted? Would they care that spine scanning evolved from body scans? Would they care about the radiographic convention of viewing bodies from below? Would they care about the workload imposed upon the hapless programmer who must write their difficult presentation? You guessed right. They finally did devise a format, modified it, revised it, and revised it again. After eight permutations, they said:

A total body scan on the left contains all of the needed data. It contains too much in fact. If we simply magnify the area of interest, window for soft tissue, and take as many large pictures as our consumers wish, we might need 20 14 × 17 films. Think of the time spent. Let us rather cone down to the area of interest right away. We'll get an overview later. By the way, ignore the abnormal neural arch ... if you can.

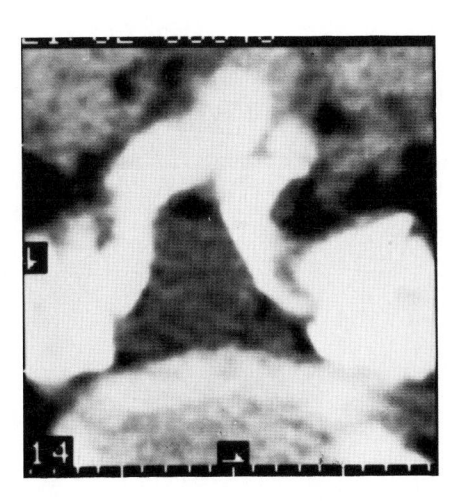

* No sexism in this chapter—especially with an editor named Judy!

Next, they said, occasional views are inadequate. Give us close overlapping cuts and no skip areas. Consecutively number the images and off to the side, put both frontal and lateral digital radiographs, clearly marked to show where each slice was taken. Place numbers on the digital radiographs to correspond to the numbers in the lower left-hand corner of the axial images.

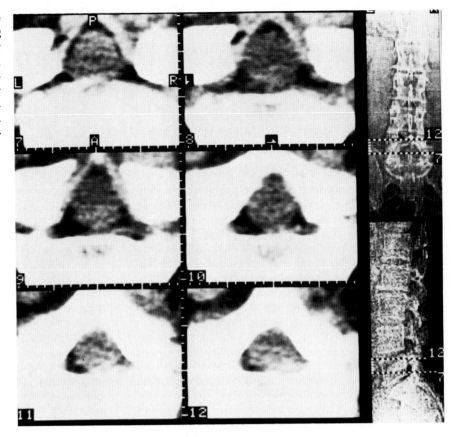

Now, for reformatting. Again, no skip areas. These sagittal (or lateral) views 3 mm apart progress from the left neural foramina, through midline, and across to the other side. Consecutive numbering allows no mistaking the location. This patient has a tight left L5-S1 neural foramen (slice 4), a calcified disc at L5-S1 (slices 7,8,9), a soft disc, and probably a free fragment over the body of L5 (see slice 11 and count up 10–12 tick marks) and a tight neural foramen between L4–5 on the right (see slice 15).

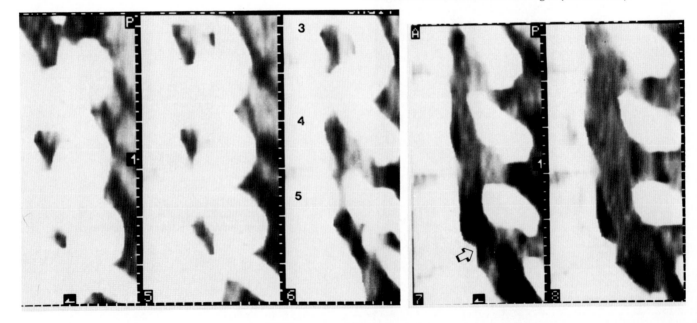

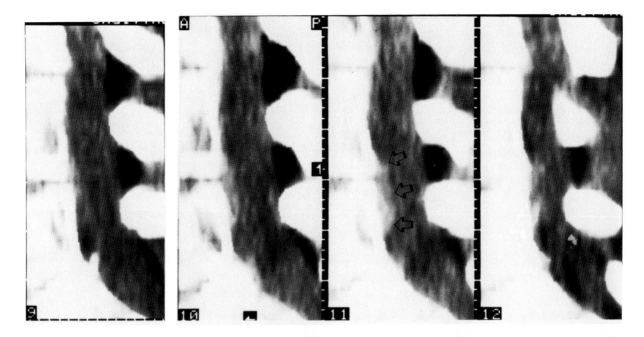

The numbers in the lower left part of the picture ensure that the slices are consecutive.

They insisted upon markings which permitted precise cross-correlation of findings from one view to another. Look at slice 11. The soft disc is obvious. Count up 11 or 12 marks (the computer arrow on slice 10 shows the direction to count. It's not a numeral 1). Now go back to axial 11 and 12 and see the absence of fat on the right (harder to see it on the axial? Yes. Sagittals are generally better to perceive disc herniations).

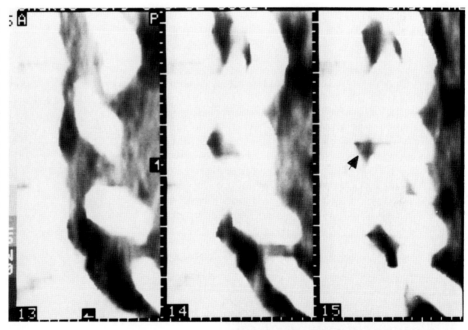

Let's not forget labels and orientation. Left is left, dorsal is up, ventral or anterior is down, just as it is at the operating table. Note the tick marks and the unambiguous labeling at the bottom and along the sides. In the lumbar spine, these small marks are 3 mm apart.

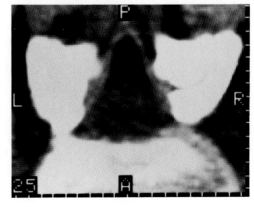

As most surgeons work about 18–24″ from their eyes without an operating microscope, they want images life-size. They can measure directly from the scans, correlating the scan findings with the findings seen at the operating table.

Coronal soft-tissue views round out this portion of the examination. Because the coronals were normal in this case, we omitted them to save space, and will show examples later. Please note that all soft-tissue windowed images are made life-size.

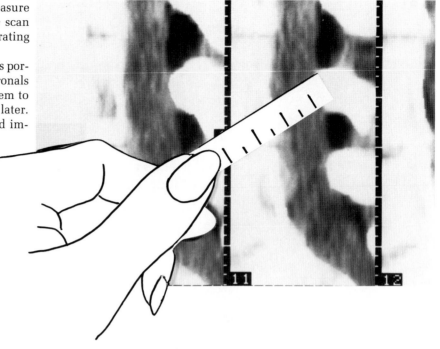

But soft-tissue windows would not be enough. Remember, bony abnormalities are frequently the cause of the complaint. As a complete series of images in three projections is already available, they may now be windowed best to show the bone abnormalities. This patient has encroachment upon her L5-S1 neural foramina by bony osetophytes. To save space in this chapter, we have not included all of the sagittal reconstructions and have have stopped at her midline. To save space and film on an everyday basis, we can make these bone images smaller than life-size. These views show the neural foramina, apophyseal joints, and vertebral body alignment.

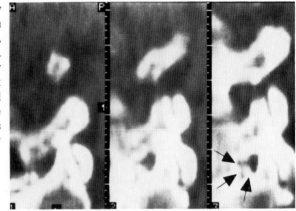

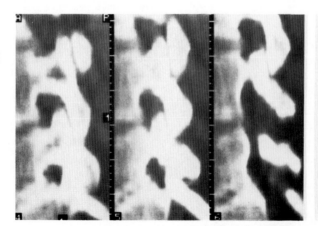

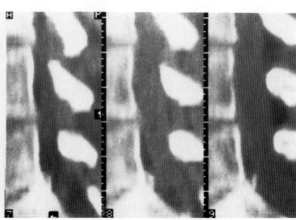

Coronal views show the apophyseal joints to good advantage. The upper joints are narrow (*arrows, right image*), the lower joints ankylosed (*open arrows, left image*). Coronal views also show scoliosis and laminectomies. Axial bone windows complete the spine portion but are not demonstrated here to save space.

All that remains now is a minified overview of the abdominal organs (see below).

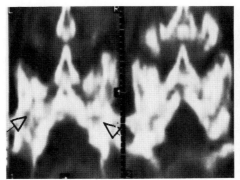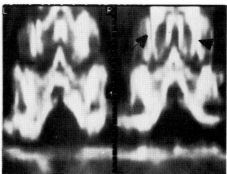

That's all there is to it. Six or seven 14 × 17 films on the viewbox give the big picture, with all the images presented in a tidy, logical format. If you interpret these reasonably and accurately, it will be you who understands the patient's whole problem. As an added benefit, you have gotten all of these pictures without slowing patient throughput.

If you do not know the basic organization of this format or its rationale, those six films containing about 140 images appear overwhelming. Without background knowledge, one's mind tends to turn off. With a little practice though, the efficiency of the system becomes evident.

To summarize, there are seven subsets of images, each image consecutively numbered, each able to be compared quickly and accurately to any other image. The first subset produced by the computer is a series of life-size axial views, windowed for soft tissues. Then come sagittal and coronal soft-tissue reconstructions, also life-size. Next, smaller images, windowed for bone: again axial, sagittal, then coronal views. Finally, minified whole body images ensure that nothing outside the narrow field of the spine is missed.

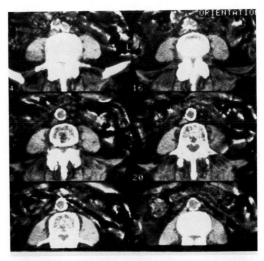

Is there a best reading sequence? For you, yes, and you will develop your own style as you gain experience. The standard reporting form is a help (see below) because it acts as a checklist, ensuring that you will not forget something significant after an interruption. To program your own internal computer though, you need a system. Try the following reading sequence as we go through this sample case. Note please that the sequence is the reverse of that used by the computer to produce the films. We have experimented teaching both ways, and find that this gives the fastest learning curve.

First, examine the whole body scans; her muscle mass is small and she has a small abdominal aortic dilatation.

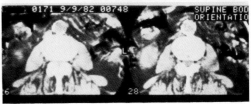

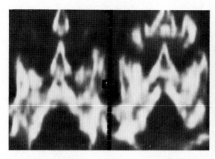 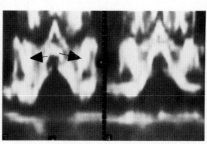 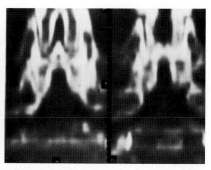

Now let's look at the bone-windowed coronals. The most dorsal or superior are on the left, the most ventral have been omitted. On the left, note the spinous processes and the degenerated apophyseal joints (*arrows*).

The sagittal bone windows come next. We have included only the foramina and midline cuts to save space. The L4-5 foramina are elongated in an AP direction (look at the normal one on the last case above), and the midline cuts show that she has, as a result of the slippage, a pseudospondylolisthesis. Remember, the bone windows undercall foraminal encroachment. No normal apophyseal joints are visible (compare with the center images on page 165).

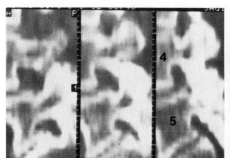 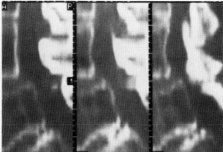 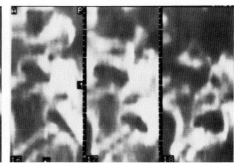

Next, examine the axial views (also windowed for bone). We start out caudally and then move higher. Here is another view of the degenerative hypertrophic change that has occurred around the apophyseal joints. It is difficult to see any joint space at the lower two levels. The partial volume effect seen on slice 15 is explained easily by cross-referencing back to the sagittal view. The degenerative arthritis plus calcifications of the ligamentum flavum makes her canal small both centrally and in the lateral recess, but these judgments are made best on the soft-tissue window views. The coronal soft-tissue images did not help so we have omitted them.

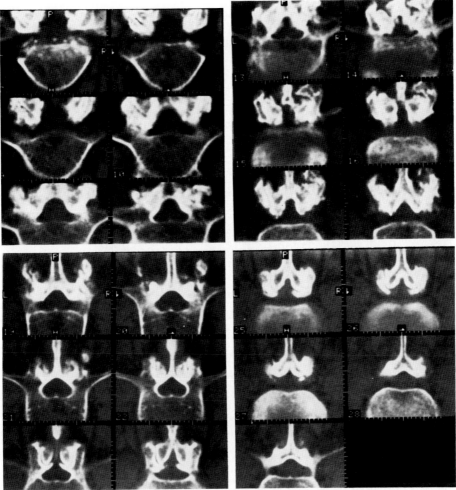

As a general rule, the sagittal soft-tissue views give more information than the others, and these bear more than casual study. Her degenerative disease has severely narrowed the left L5-S1, foramen (*closed arrows*, view 5). As we progress medially, the lateral recesses come into view (slices 8,9). Slices 10 and 11 show the severely narrowed central canal, and calcification of the ligamentum. Progressing further to the right, we see the L4–5 foramen occluded by soft tissue and bony spur (*arrow*, slices 15,16).

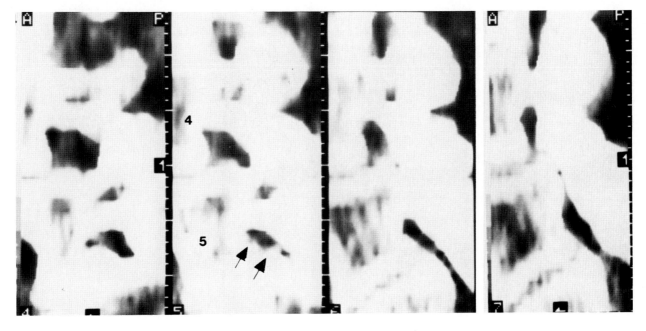

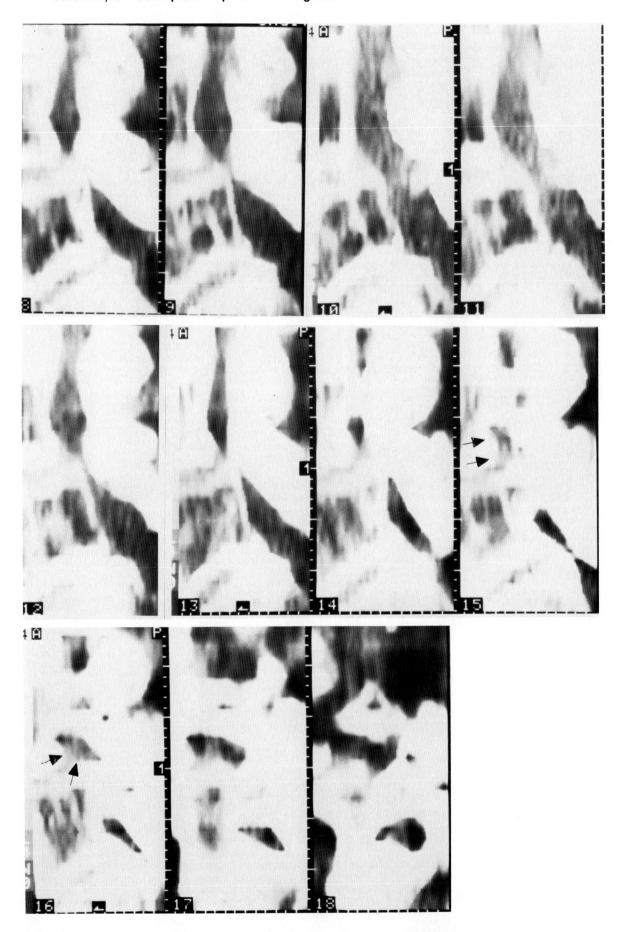

Finally, we read the soft-tissue windowed axial views. Correlation with the sagittals and coronals yields a complete understanding of her altered anatomy. She has severe stenosis secondary to apophyseal joint and disc degeneration, with pseudospondylolisthesis, bony overgrowth, and ankylosis of the apophyseal joints, severe narrowing of the left L5-S1 foramen, and severe narrowing of the right L4–5 foramen. With these data, rational treatment plans can be presented to her.

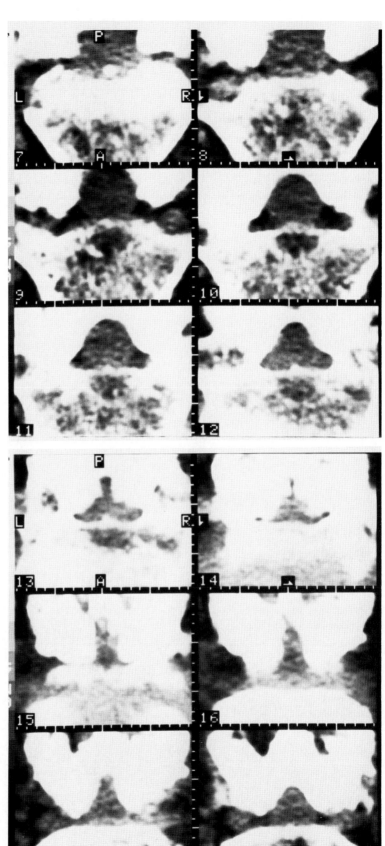

The pathological changes then may be graded with some objectivity using this standardized chart, and entered on the form. The reporting form also contains space for a narrative summary. A close second in importance to the standardization is the form's function as a checklist. After the inevitable phone interruption, the radiologist can find his place easily and resume his reading sequence.

SEE REVERSE SIDE FOR FILM ORGANIZATION AND EXAMPLES ILLUSTRATING 1-5 GRADING SYSTEM

Graded Findings and Abbreviations:

1 = Normal (1MM)	**4** = Moderate (5MM)	**VC** = Vacuum Change
2 = Slight (2MM)	**5** = Severe (>6MM)	**OR** = Osteophytic Ridging
3 = Mild (3MM)	**★** = Soft Tissue	**PD** = Pars Defects

FH = Flavum Hypertrophy	**Sp** = Spur	**IJ** = Irregular Joint
LAM = Laminectomy	**F** = Fused	**DN** = Degenerative Narrowing
HL = Hemilaminectomy	**NF** = Not Fused	**SL** = Sublux

	TRI-JOINT COMPLEX			CANAL				OTHER	
	LEFT FORAMEN	LEFT FACET	DISC/ ANNULUS	RIGHT FACET	LT. LAT. RECESS	CENTRAL	RT. LAT. RECESS	RIGHT FORAMEN	
L1-L2	___	___	___	___	___	___	___	___	___ L1-L2
L2-L3	___	___	___	___	___	___	___	___	___ L2-L3
L3-L4	___	___	___	___	___	___	___	___	___ L3-L4
L4-L5	___	___	___	___	___	___	___	___	___ L4-L5
L5-S1	___	___	___	___	___	___	___	___	___ L5-S1

Miscellaneous Findings

Lumbar Segments _____ Transitional Segment _____

Residual Pantopaque _____ Few Drops; _____ Several CC's

Radiologist

_____

(Typed Name)

_____

(Signature)

Key Images

	Lifesize	Non-Lifesize	
Axial	_____	Bone Density Axial	_____
Sagittal	_____	Bone Density Sagittal	_____
Coronal	_____	Bone Density Coronal	_____
Other	_____	Reduced Full Field Supine Images	_____

GRADING SYSTEM EXAMPLES

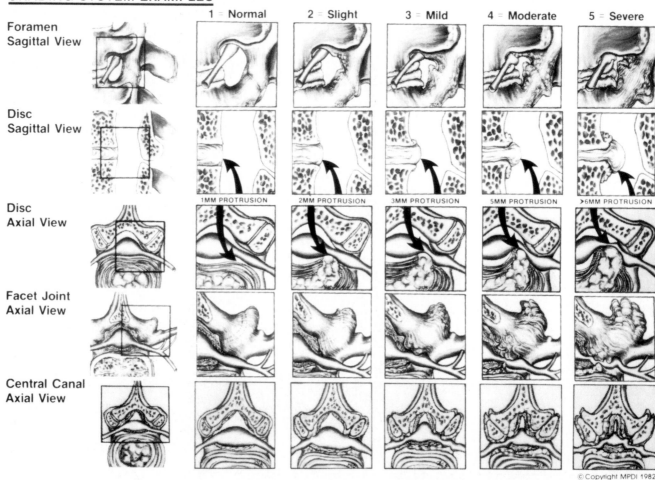

	1 = Normal	2 = Slight	3 = Mild	4 = Moderate	5 = Severe
Foramen Sagittal View					
Disc Sagittal View	1MM PROTRUSION	2MM PROTRUSION	3MM PROTRUSION	5MM PROTRUSION	>6MM PROTRUSION
Disc Axial View					
Facet Joint Axial View					
Central Canal Axial View					

That's all there is to it. Let's try a few cases now to develop your proficiency. We will omit irrelevant views to save space.

These coronal bone-window views show us the lamina and apophyseal joints. A nice example of normal.

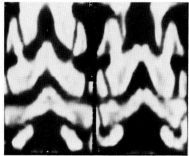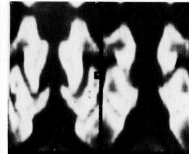

Next, the sagittal reconstructions show us the pedicle height, the condition of the neural foramina, and the quality of the apophyseal joints. They are all normal. He has a slightly accentuated lumbar lordosis.

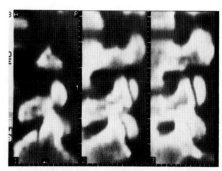

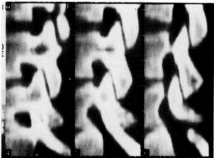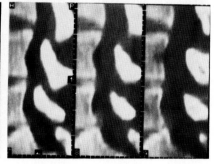

Now look at the soft-tissue window sagittals.

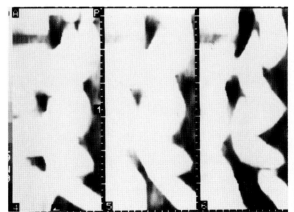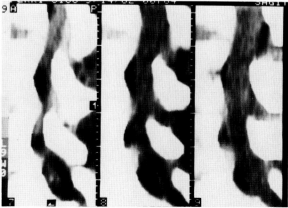

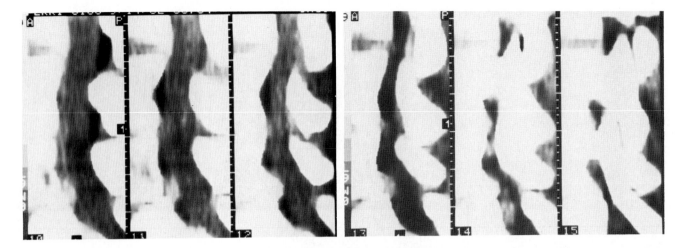

These show a large, soft disc protruding back into the central canal (count up 6–8 ticks on cuts 10 and 11). It extends also into the lateral recess.

Additionally, his left L4–5 and L5-S1 foramina are moderately narrowed. Compare the highest (normal) foramina on slices 4 and 5 with the lower two foramina.

The axial views show the herniation too—or do they? Would you be sure on that single slice 9 given the disc's appearance above and below?

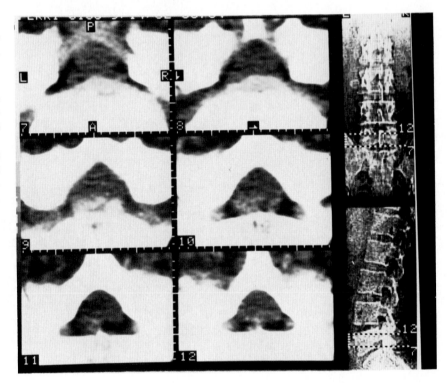

Data to be reconstructed must be on the axial views. Data *presence* is not the problem; *perception* is. And that's where the additional views help. Incidentally, this disc was visible on the coronals too. We will show you more below. Take a moment now to go back over this case to program your own internal computer for normal. Ask yourself specific questions about each joint and foramen. Fill out the sample report (see page 164).

Now, let us try a more difficult one. The coronal view shows a scoliosis. Anything else? Look again before going to the axials. Now look at the axials. Is that a soft disc in the right foramen on cut 17? Now go through the sagittal sequence.

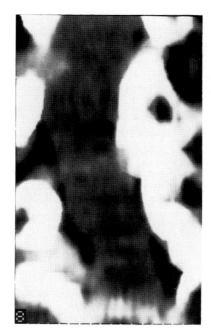

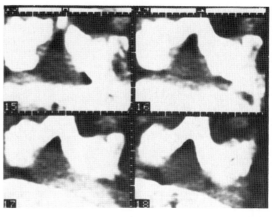

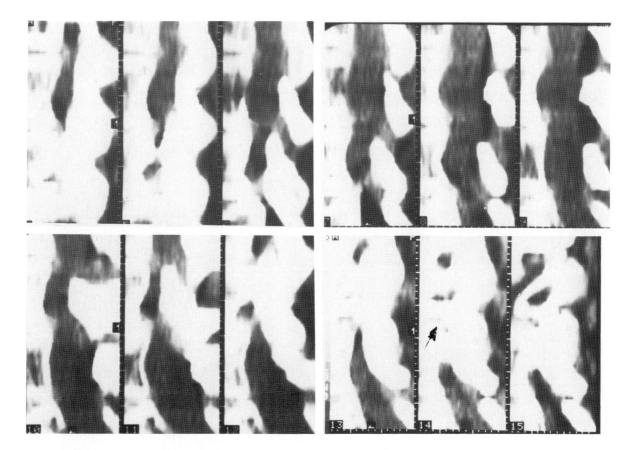

Both bone and soft tissue fill the L5-S1 foramen. Look back at the coronal. Did you see it before? While you are looking at the coronal, do you notice the soft tissue at the left L3–4 foramen too? It's not visible on the sagittal because of the scoliosis. Continue through the sagittals, and note the disc bulge at L4–5 (upper far right) and the complete occlusion of the right L4–5 foramen (*arrow*), also predictable from the coronal view.

Try another difficult case. Bone window sagittals, from left through right foramina show bilateral pars interarticularis defects (*white arrows*), and a grade 1 spondylolisthesis (*white open arrow*). The dorsoventral elongation of the foramina is characteristic of this disease. Secondary degenerative changes often close off the foramina. The axial views show the lysis (*arrowhead*), and extra peculiar bone over the lamina. He has had a fusion.

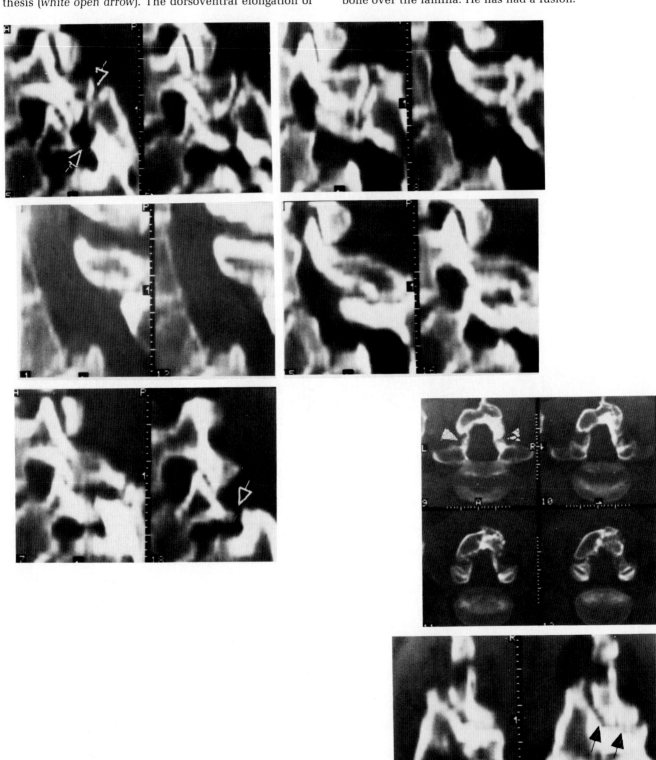

It is not until we look at the coronal view though that we see the pseudarthrosis through the fusion (*arrows*).

Now try an easy one. If you saw slice 10 on a standard body presentation, would you wonder about a disc herniation? The side by side format though encourages the perception of forward shift of the upper vertebral body. Slices 13 and 14 show a bony defect (*arrow*).

The sagittals show the defects to best advantage, show the elongation of the foramina, and show the degree of slippage and the reactive sclerosis of the vertebral endplates. They also show an unsuspected and severe foraminal stenosis at the level above.

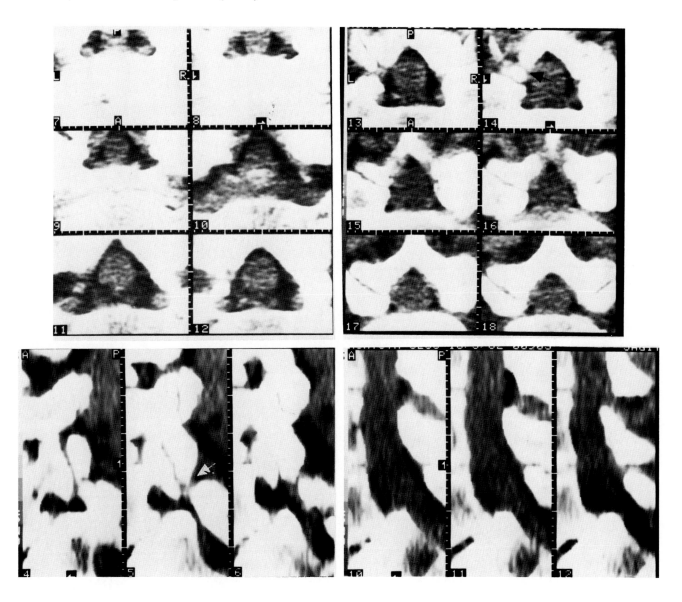

CT/MPR has no peer when evaluating the postoperative spine. Note the absence of laminae on these coronals (*arrows*). Now examine the sagittals. Can you explain his recurrent back pain?

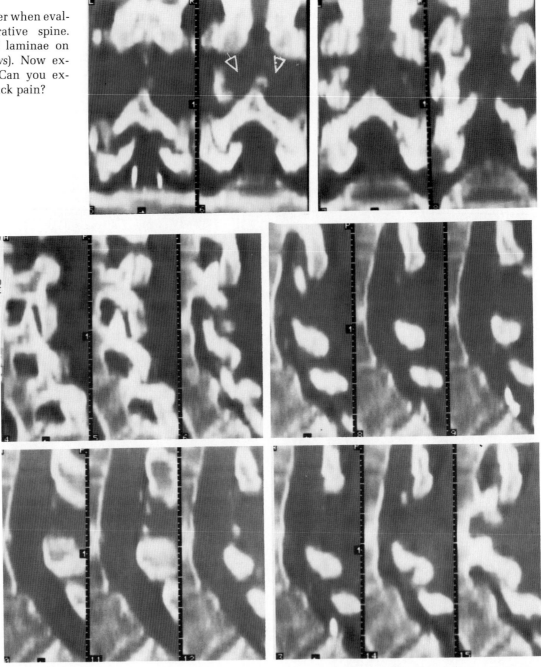

The sagittals show his laminectomy, normal foramina, and a good decompression. They also show an unsuspected pedicle fracture (see enlargement at right). The surgeon was doubtful enough to explore.

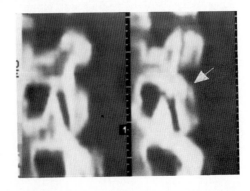

This is the same patient. Can you see the fracture on his axial views?

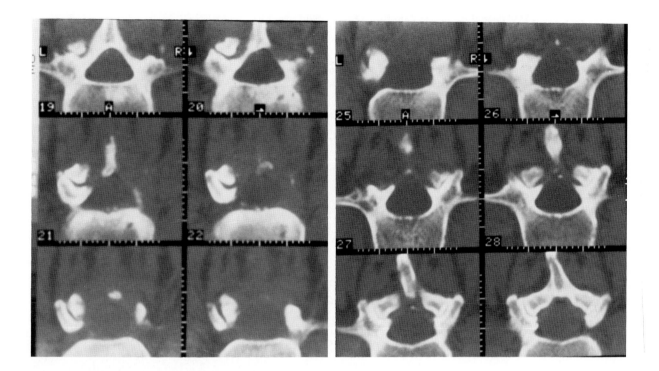

Our next patient also has recurrent low back pain treated with multiple operations and finally, fusion. He still hurts. Why?

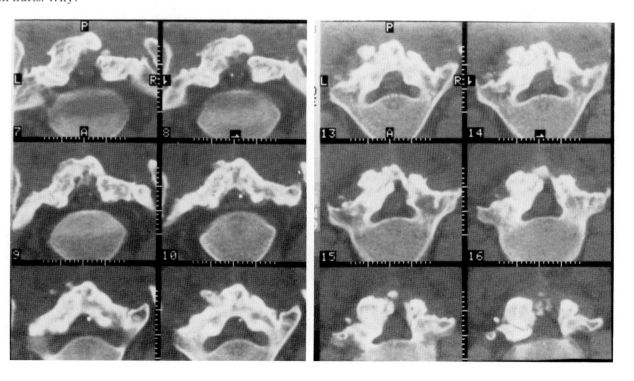

The sagittal reconstructions show a good fusion mass, but unfortunately there is a pseudoarthrosis in its center (*arrows*). Another cause of failed back.

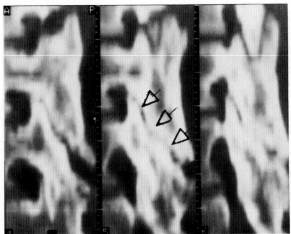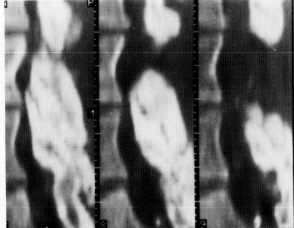

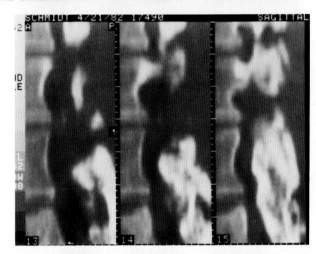

This is the most important case you will examine here. The patient is a vigorous 54-year-old male who is in pain. He has had multiple operations. How do you read his scan?

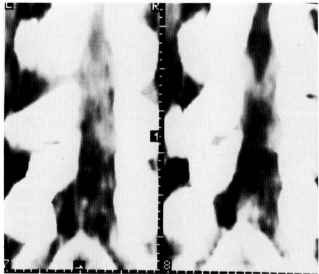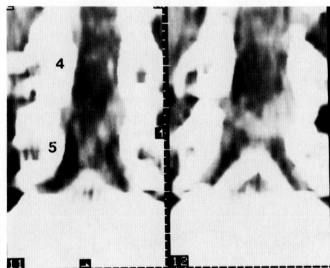

First, the coronal views. Cuts here through the pedicles show *no* fat at L4–5. Is there space for a healthy nerve? Not likely. The changes are similar at L5-S1. Again, there is no space.

Now, let us look at selected sagittal slices. Note that the left L4–5 and L5–1 foraminal cuts confirm the coronal findings. No fat is present; there is severe foraminal encroachment.

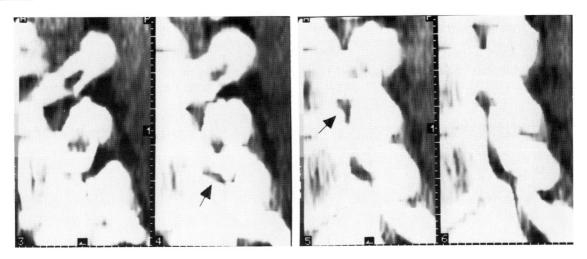

Skip a few slices to the midline. Note the adequacy and extent of his decompressive laminectomy. We will continue to the right foramina, and again, note the terribly severe narrowing (*arrows*).

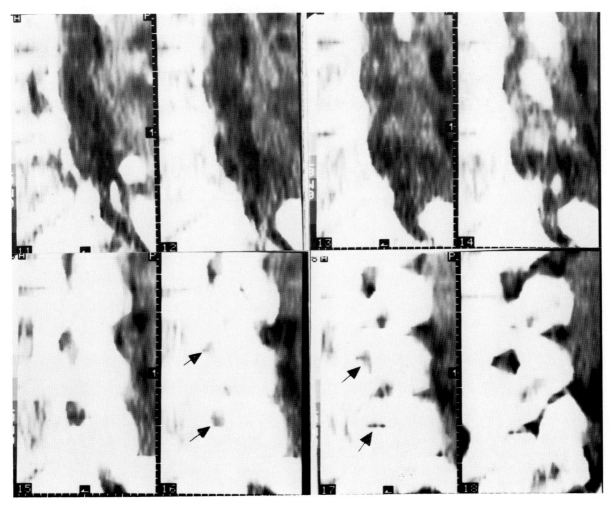

This patient illustrates the most common constellation of changes seen in the postoperative failed back syndrome. Despite operative notes to the contrary, his foramina are still stenotic. Are new operations needed? Perhaps; follow-up clinical and radiographic studies will prove (or disprove) this contention. Until then, we can at least alert our colleagues to the complete findings and hope that an adequate and correct operation will be performed.

You have looked at some difficult cases using this new format and have seen pathology we only dreamed of visualizing a few years ago. By the way, did you notice that you did not even need the axials on this last postoperative case?

We do not recommend omitting any views—axials included. We do hope to communicate our enthusiasm for this format though, and to show you that it is a logical, reasonable presentation which is well accepted by our clinical colleagues. CT/MPR affords economics and efficiencies in performing the exam, in presenting the images, and in reading the films. Most importantly, it allows us to develop an integrated, clear, and complete mental image of both bony and soft-tissue spine pathology. With that understanding, better patient care must result.

CHAPTER EIGHT

High-Resolution Multiplanar Reformatting

JAMES C. HIRSCHY, M.D.

Multiplanar reformatting (MPR) of the spine after axial examination by computed tomography (CT) is a most useful diagnostic modality. It is like the axiom every radiologist learns early in training: when in doubt, take another radiograph. The body is three-dimensional, and requires more than one projection for evaluation.

In the examination of the spine by plain roentgenograms, anterior-posterior and lateral views are the bare minimum, with oblique and tilted projections often necessary to appreciate the three-dimensional form of the vertebral column. Axial CT has simplified the evaluation of the spine, its contents, and surrounding structures. However, it was not until Glenn et al. (1) developed a technique to reformat data already acquired during axial scanning that a three-dimensional evaluation could be obtained without "taking another projection!" MPR is, in essence, manipulation of data from multiple axial scans stored in the computer to provide sections that differ from the scanned plane. The reformatted images are particularly useful to demonstrate the solidity of a fusion, to evaluate stenosis of the canal, or to locate a tumor or extruded disc that is pressing on a nerve root.

Early reformatted images were of poor quality because the slices were thick (10–12 mm). Improved reformatted images could be obtained by overlapping two slices which markedly increased the patient's radiation dose. The thick slices also had a pronounced partial volume effect that created false images. The early examinations also were limited by inaccurate or inconsistent table motion and indexing (2). Now reformatted images of a quality and clarity approaching that of the axial slices are possible on most computed tomographic equipment. By using a scan 5 mm or less in thickness, overlapping is not required. This reduces the patient's total irradiation dose and the thinner slices give greater clarity, reduce the partial volume effect, and permit sharp and detailed reformatted images which are as good in quality as the axial slices (Fig. 8.1). The thinnest slices available, 1.5 mm and 2 mm, produce the best detail (3) but are often impractical because too many slices and too much time are necessary to cover the usual volume of tissue.

This chapter addresses itself to the clinical application and usefulness of computer reformatting of the axial data. Since Rhodes et al. (4) described the extraction of oblique planes from serial CT sections, most manufacturers now offer this as either standard equipment or as software options. The new software programs allow sagittal or coronal images to be rotated and tilted. By being able to rotate and tilt the image, the spines of patients who are unable to lie flat, are scoliotic, or have prominent lordosis, ky-

phosis, or tilt can be evaluated with ease. No body motion during the entire scanning procedure is essential for successful reformatting. This has not been a problem except in rare cases when the patient is either extremely jittery or in such severe pain that he is constantly moving. In such situations, a reformatted image is a jagged conglomeration of individual slices that were made in different positions, and the image becomes useless (Fig. 8.2).

In viewing an axial image, the horizontal plane represents the X axis. The Y axis is represented by the vertical direction. By rotating either the X or Y axis of these images, one can develop an oblique paraaxial image. The Z plane represents the third dimension which is equivalent to the region in front of or behind the axial image. If multiple single axial slices are taken in a contiguous fashion and a sagittal coronal reconstruction is developed, the new image represents the Z axis of the axial slices.

All of the illustrated cases were scanned on a GE 8800 utilizing a preproduction version of ARRANGE software. By using fast tube cooling, careful selection of technique, and batch processing, a total spine examination consisting of a digital radiograph ("Scout View") for localization, and 24 or 25 axial images is performed in 12–15 minutes. Five minutes is more than adequate to position and prepare the patient before scanning and to assist the patient from the scanning room when the examination is completed. It is possible to schedule a new patient every 30 minutes throughout the working day and have little or no patient waiting time delay.

In the preproduction version of ARRANGE, 4–5 minutes is required for data manipulation, reformatting of the images, and filming. It is necessary to do this while "off line", because immediate reformatting precludes the ability to scan another patient simultaneously. With newer versions of ARRANGE, reformatting can be done while other patients are being scanned.

Using MPR, clinical examples of the lumbar, thoracic, and cervical regions are described. Because of their normal anatomical configurations, each of these three sections of the spine presents a different problem in scanning and in data manipulation.

The use of contrast material is usually not necessary in evaluation of the spine with CT. However, there are exceptions. Suspected intrathecal tumors require intravenous (IV) contrast material in order to identify those lesions which are of an enhancing nature. When such a tumor is suspected, scanning commences when approximately half of a 42-g iodine IV drip has been administered. The rest of the IV contrast medium is given as the scanning continues.

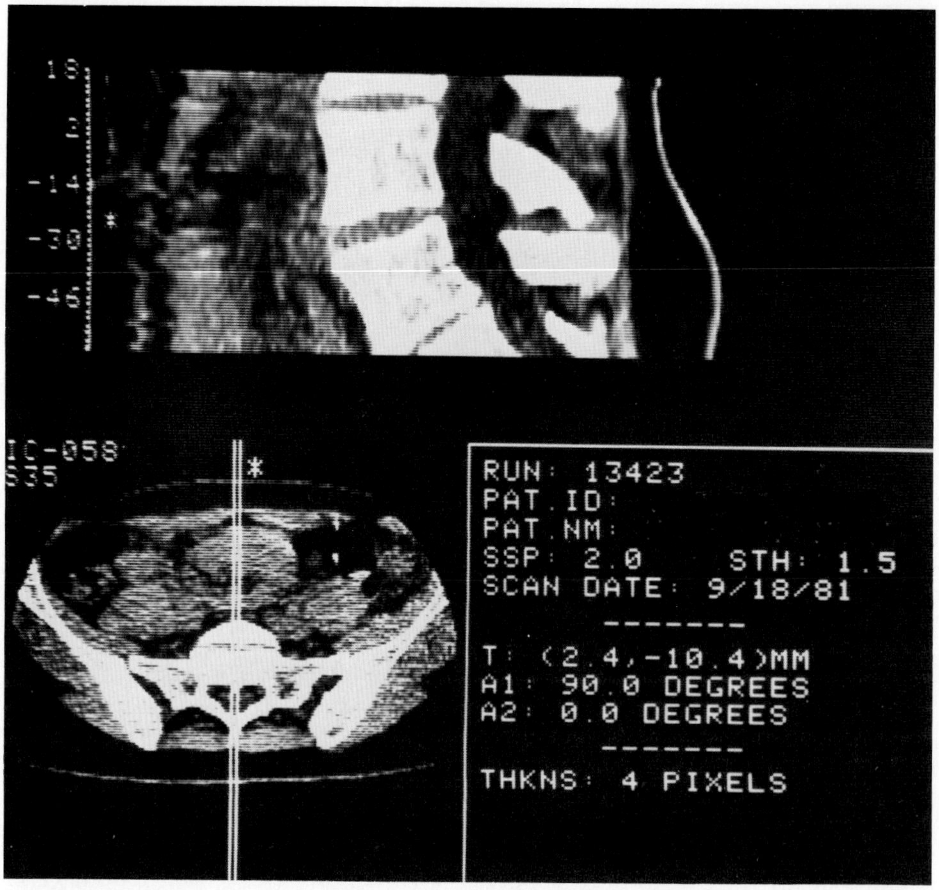

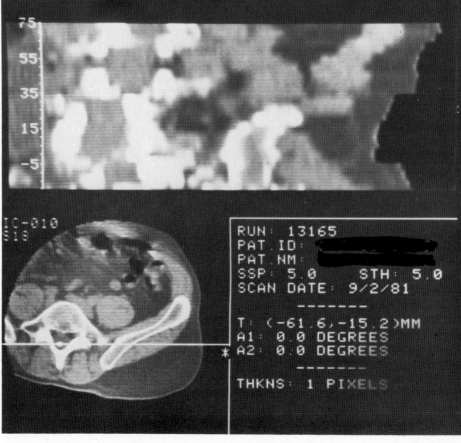

Figure 8.1. In a high-resolution sagittal view of the lumbar spine, disc space narrowing is observed at the L5–S1 level. There is excellent visualization of the posterior vascular canal of the L5 vertebral body.

Figure 8.2. A coronal reformatted image is distorted and unreadable because of extensive patient motion. The patient moved in the mediolateral direction between individual scans. This results in the coronal reformatted image being displaced at several levels so that the neural canal has a jagged edge.

Intrathecal administration of metrizamide is sometimes useful for identifying small extruded discs and is necessary for identification of small tumors of the filum terminale. Administration of 5 ml of metrizamide diluted to one-fourth of the recommended strength for myelograms allows excellent visualization of the contrast without artifact formation. If the density of the contrast is too great, the scan can have streaks. By using a small amount of low-concentration contrast material, the procedure can be done safely on an out-patient basis.

LUMBAR SPINE

Scanning technique

Using a digital radiograph for positioning, a 1.5- or 5-mm thick axial slice (depending on individual physician's preference) is taken through the center of each individual intervertebral disc space from L1–S1. The level from L3–S1 is then rescanned with 5-mm thick contiguous slices. The technique used in the angled images is 120 KV, 400 MA, pulse width of 3, and a scan time of 9.6 seconds. This is equal to 768 MAS. Five scans are taken, one through each disc space. The 5-mm thick slices taken in a contiguous unangled fashion utilize 120 KV, 320 MA, pulse width of 2, and 9.6-second scan time. This is equal to 409.6 MAS. If either the pulse width or MA is increased, increasing tube cooling time can occur after the 10th slice. By

using the factors given, a slice can be taken and completed every 28 seconds. Nineteen to 22 of the unangled 5-mm slices usually covers the area from the mid-L3 level to the bottom of the L5–S1 disc space.

Most CT examinations of the spine are of the lumbar region where spinal stenosis or herniated disc is very common, and can cause low back and radicular type leg pain (5–7). A normal CT examination without contrast and with reformatting frequently can demonstrate the nerve roots within the thecal sac (8) (Fig. 8.3). A small amount of fat usually surrounds the thecal sac and nerve root sheaths (Fig. 8.4). When small amounts of metrizamide are used in conjunction with the CT examination, the nerve roots can be identified routinely and evaluated (Fig. 8.5). If an intrathecal lesion or tumor of the cauda equinae is suspected, IV contrast or intrathecal metrizamide must be given in order for the CT study to be of diagnostic value.

If the patient has a prominent lordosis and the axial CT images are not absolutely parallel to the disc or vertebral end plates, a soft-tissue mass that apparently protrudes into the neural canal is visualized due to the partial volume effect. The "soft-tissue mass" is actually the posterior aspect of the normal unextruded and nonbulging disc (Fig. 8.6). To the unwary, this soft-tissue density can be confused with a herniated disc (8) (Fig. 8.7A). Reformatting in both sagittal and oblique axial projections (Fig.

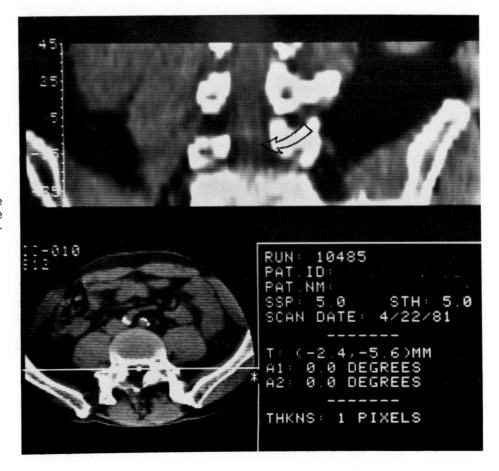

Figure 8.3. The individual nerve roots in the lower thecal sac are frequently identified as in this coronal reformatted image (*arrow*).

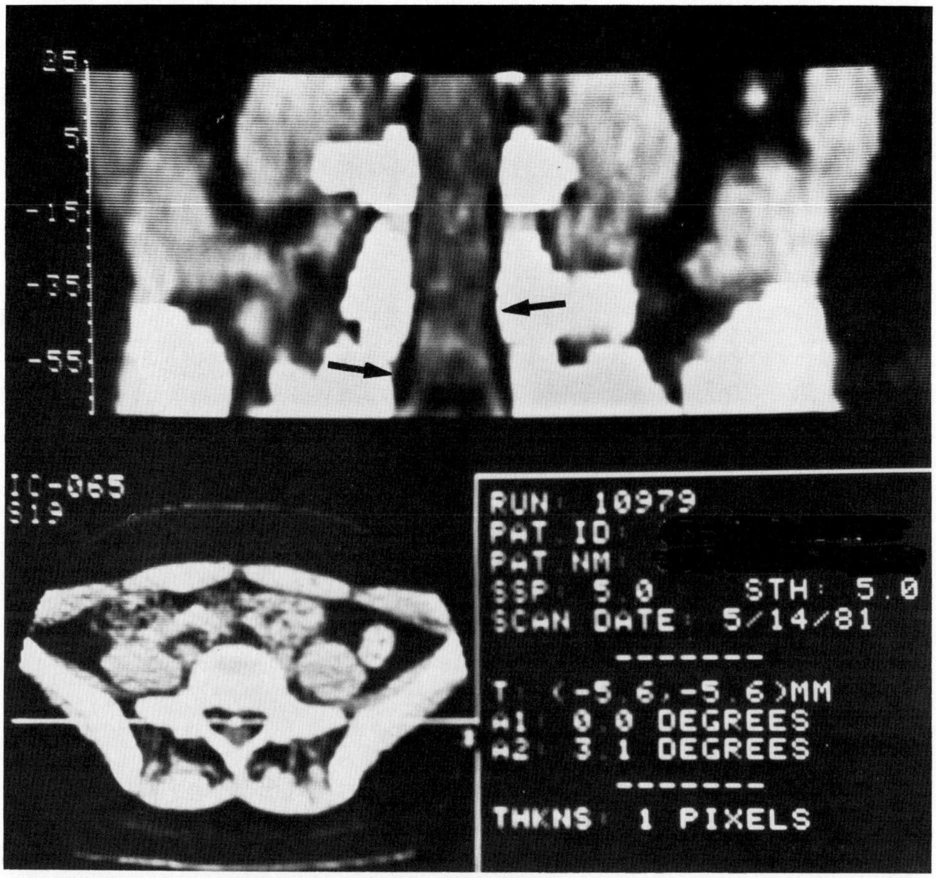

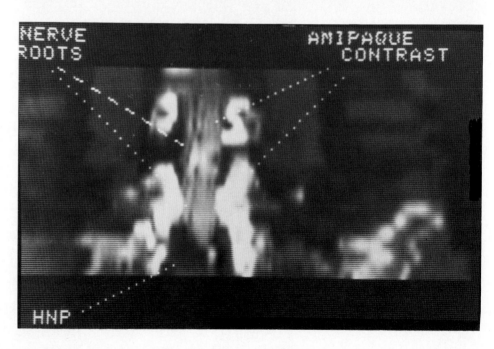

Figure 8.4. The perineural fat on the lateral aspects of the thecal sac should be clearly defined (*arrows*). Obliteration of the fat suggests a filling defect, mass, or stenosis.

Figure 8.5. Small amounts of metrizamide demonstrate the nerve roots very well. Only minute amounts of contrast are necessary, or artifact formation can occur. There is a large extruded disc on the right at the L5–S1 level.

8.7B) shows that there is no evidence of disc disease. Many times, an extruded disc can be visualized best on the sagittal or coronal reformatted image (Fig. 8.8). The size and location of the lesion also is delineated more accurately on a reformatted image. Multiplicity of herniated disc is not unusual (Fig. 8.9), and because of this, the spine is routinely scanned from L3–S1 to cover the entire area where herniated discs are most common. Reformatting is also an important aid in evaluation of spinal fusions. A reformatted image is similar to a linear tomogram taken through the posterior elements of the spine without the disadvantage of having superimposed tissues which need to be blurred. By tilting the reformatted coronal image, the entire fusion can be seen in a single plane. Even with meticulous positioning, it is unlikely that the plane of the spinal fusion would be parallel to the film in standard linear tomography.

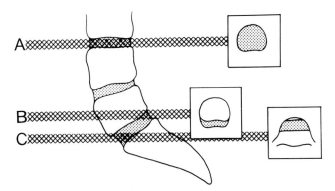

Figure 8.6. Axial CT slices of lumbosacral spine can give images of normal lumbosacral spine that have different appearances depending on where the slice is made in relation to the spinal curve. Cross-hatch lines represent various slices and boxes represent axial images. Slice A represents a normal disc. Slice B mimics herniated disc. Slice C shows disc material between two bones.

Case 1: A 47-year-old woman with a spinal fusion from L2–S1 presented with persistent back pain. CT examination with reformatting showed the spinal fusion to be solid (Fig. 8.10). Individual axial slices cannot show the extent of or solidity of the fusion. A small bulging disc at L5–S1 accounted for the patient's symptoms.

Case 2: A similar example is a 30-year-old male physician with spondylolisthesis who underwent a spinal fusion six months earlier. Back pain with associated sciatica persisted. Myelography (Fig. 8.11A) was reported as normal. CT examination showed a bulging disc at L4–5 (Fig. 8.11B), and also showed that the fusion was not yet solid (Fig. 8.11C). Because of the spondylolisthesis, the thecal sac was lifted off the posterior margin of the neural canal, resulting in lack of pressure from the extruded disc and accounting for the "normal" myelogram. Displacement of the left nerve root was seen with the CT examination and the herniated disc is seen to good advantage on the sagittal reformatted image.

Case 3: An active 83-year-old man with a history of disc disease and spinal fusion from L3 downward experienced progressively greater back pain and increased difficulty in walking. CT reformatted images showed a soft-tissue density in the posterior aspect of the neural canal at the L2–3 level (Fig. 8.12A). Introduction of metrizamide showed a partial blockage at the L2–3 level by a posterior mass (Fig. 8.12B). Most of the contrast remained below the L3 level with little above L3. CT after the myelography (Fig. 8.12C) shows that there is some contrast above the location of the incomplete spinal block which helps delineate the nerve roots. Although there was a herniated disc anteriorly at the L2–3 and L4–5 levels, there was also a pronounced hypertrophy of the ligamentum flavum which was the primary factor in the extrinsic pressure and blockage of the thecal sac (Fig. 8.12D). Hypertrophic changes

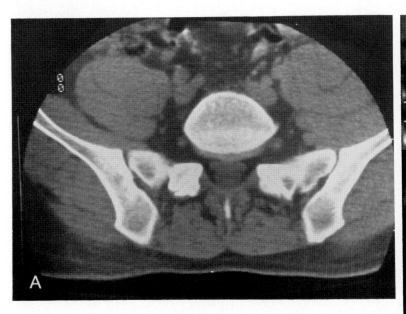

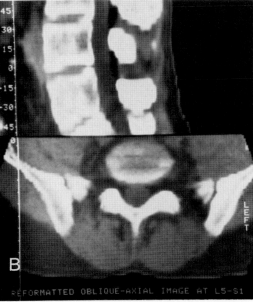

Figure 8.7. A. A posterior extension of a soft-tissue mass which apparently protrudes into the neural canal represents a "pseudodisc." This is the posterior projection of the nonherniated disc as demonstrated in Slice B of Figure 8.6. B. A reformatted sagittal image fails to reveal a posterior protruding disc. The oblique-axial image is reformatted to be parallel to the L5–S1 disc space and vertebral end plates. It also fails to demonstrate a herniated disc.

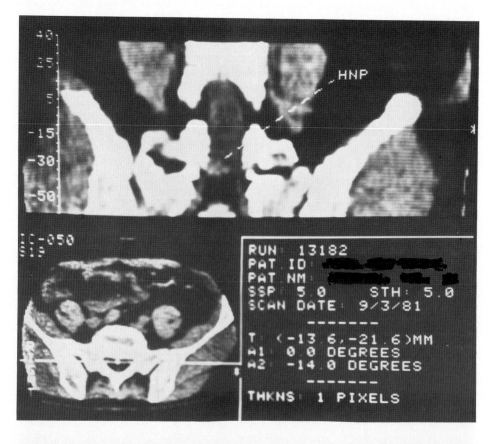

Figure 8.8. A coronal view shows an extruded disc on the right at the L5–S1 level. Multiple images demonstrating the pathological findings are helpful in confirming the diagnosis.

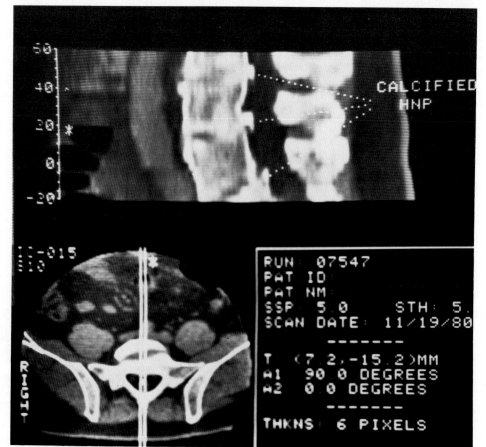

Figure 8.9. The lumbar spine is routinely scanned from L3–S1 because of frequency of multiple findings. In this sagittal reformatted image, three densely calcified herniated discs are identified.

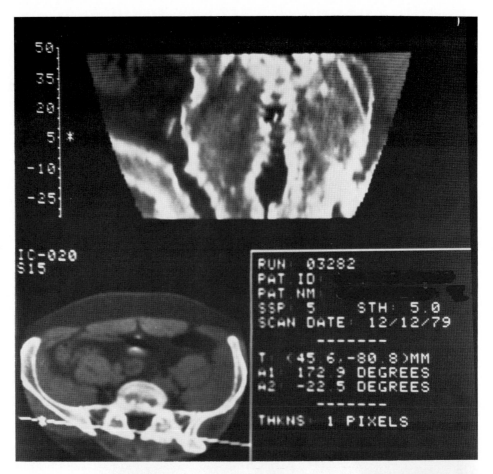

Figure 8.10. A solid spinal fusion is observed on this tilted coronal reformatted image. Reformatted images give as much information, if not more, than linear tomography and require much less radiation.

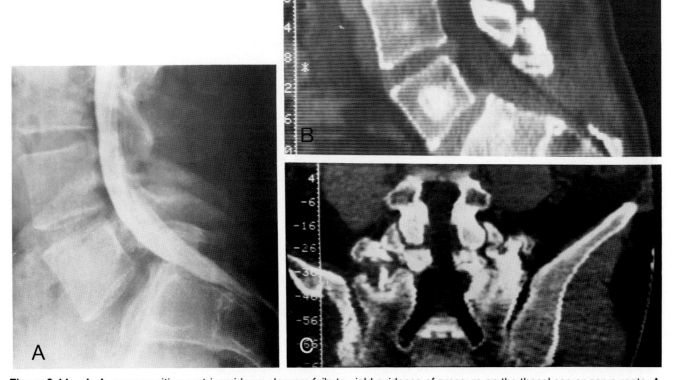

Figure 8.11. A. A prone position metrizamide myelogram fails to yield evidence of pressure on the thecal sac or nerve roots. A spondylolisthesis at L5–S1 lifts the lower thecal sac off of the posterior margins of the L4–5 vertebral bodies. A large extruded disc could be present at either L4–5 or L5–S1 and not detected. B. A sagittal reformatted image of the same patient demonstrates a large extruded disc at L4–5. Although there is prominence of the posterior margin of the disc at the L5–S1 level because of the spondylolisthesis, there is no herniation. A large bone island is visible in the midportion of the L5 vertebral body which is seen on the plain films only in retrospect (see Fig. 8.11A). C. A posterior spinal fusion at L5–S1 for spondylolisthesis is demonstrated to be ununited.

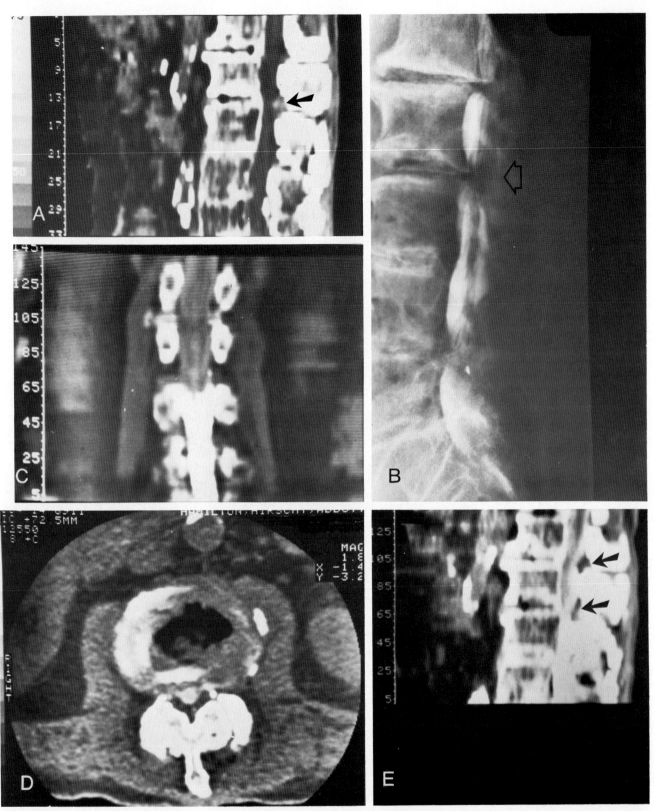

Figure 8.12.   A. On the sagittal reformatted image of a patient with a spinal fusion from L3 downward, a large soft-tissue mass (*arrow*) protrudes posteriorly at the L2–3 level, and pushes the thecal sac forward. A protruding disc is seen at the L4–5 level. B. A prone myelogram examination shows the posterior pressure on the lower thecal sac at the L2–3 level (*arrowhead*). C. A coronal reformatted image shows a partial block of the contrast at the L2–3 level. A dense white metrizamide column remains in the lower portion, while the diluted contrast above the L2–3 level clearly outlines the nerve roots. D. An axial image at the L2–3 disc space shows cystic degeneration of the disc, and a marked thickening of the ligamentum flavae which results in anterior displacement of the constricted and narrowed thecal sac. E. The sagittal reformatted image after the metrizamide myelogram demonstrates the soft-tissue mass projecting anteriorly from the posterior elements at both the L2–3 and L1–2 levels (*arrows*). This represents stenosis secondary to hypertrophy of the ligamentum flavae.

also contributed to the patient's spinal stenosis. The reformatted sagittal images done both before and after administration of intrathecal metrizamide (Fig. 8.12E) give a much more accurate demonstration of the source of the back pain and its complex etiology.

Case 4: Back and leg pain can also be caused by a sacral cyst, as illustrated by a 56-year-old man whose roentgenograms of the spine were interpreted originally as normal, but on retrospect showed widening of the diameter of the sacral canal (Fig. 8.13A). CT showed the dilated thecal sac

extending into the sacral canal where it expanded the canal and eroded through the anterior wall of the sacrum (Fig. 8.13B and C). Reformatted images are dramatic in visualizing the extent of the cyst.

Case 5: A 38-year-old man with impotence was referred by his urologist who suspected that a herniated L1–2 disc was the cause. CT examination with reformatting showed bony spurs at D12–L1 (Fig. 8.14) that narrowed the anterior posterior diameter of the neural canal to 10 mm. The normal mean value of the neural canal at the D12–L1 level

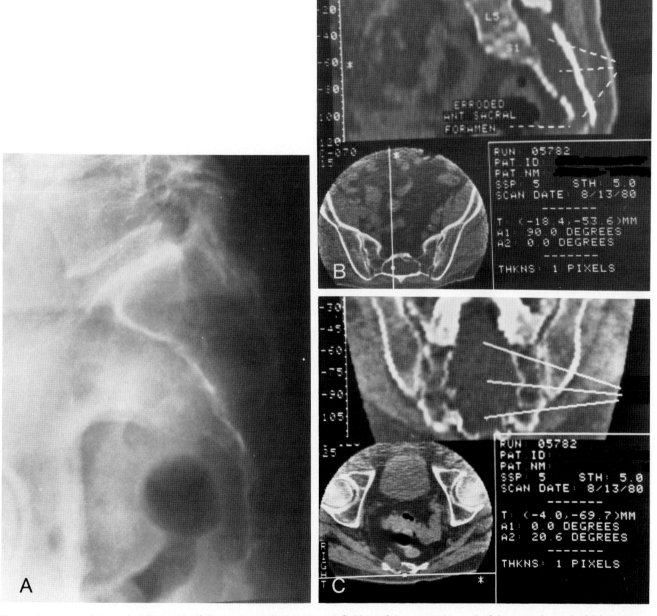

Figure 8.13.   A. A lateral radiograph of the sacrum shows poor definition of the posterior wall of the sacral canal which appears to be demineralized or eroded. B. A sagittal reformatted image shows a large sacral cyst or occult sacral meningocele (Tarlov cyst) which is widening the entire sacral canal and has eroded the anterior sacral foramen in the lower sacrum. C. A tilted coronal reformatted image shows the lateral extent of the bone destruction and erosion caused by this occult sacral meningocele. Notice on the axial image the protrusion of the cyst through the right lower sacral canal.

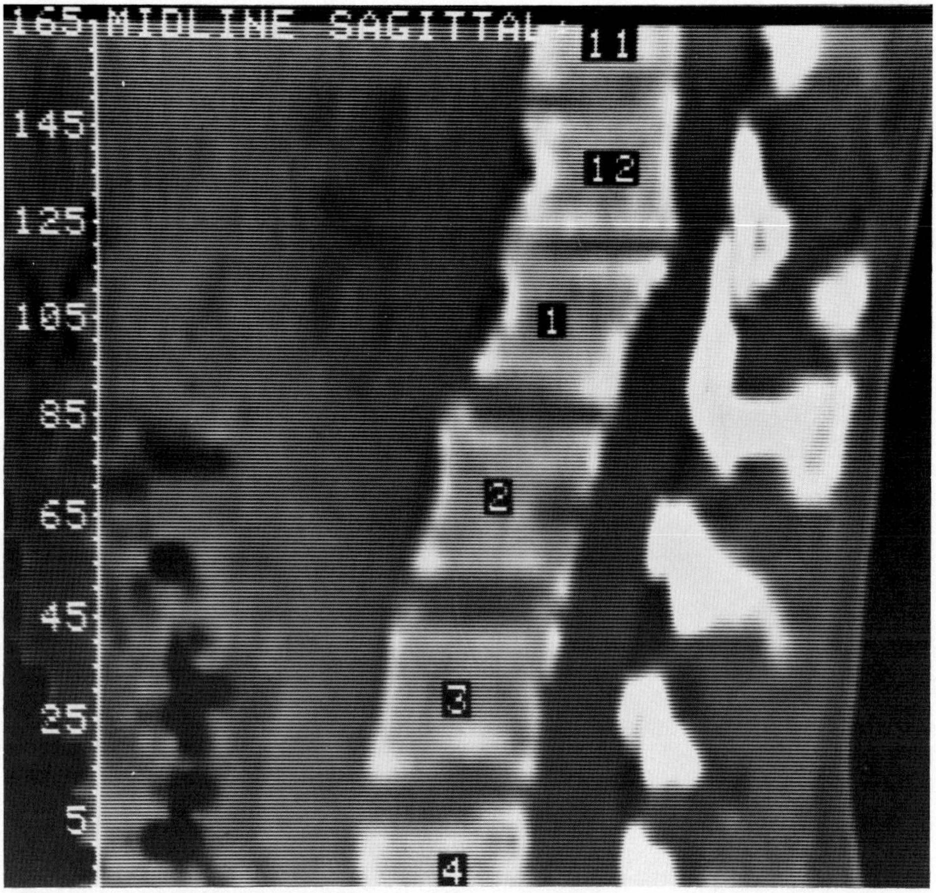

Figure 8.14. A midline sagittal reformatted image taken through the lower thoracic and upper lumbar region shows narrowing of the canal at the D12–L1 level secondary to degenerative changes and hypertrophic spurs. This secondary spinal stenosis resulted in sexual impotency.

is 20 mm (10).

Case 6: A 53-year-old male with known cutaneous neurofibromatosis presented with low back pain. Initial roentgenograms showed some erosive changes in the L5 pedicle (Fig. 8.15A). CT evaluation of this area showed a large soft-tissue mass with erosion of the left sacral neural canal. The mass displaced the thecal sac to the right and the nerve root posteriorly. The mass measured 2.5 cm in its greatest cross-sectional area. The reformatted images showed the sharply defined margin of the mass as well as the erosion of the adjacent bone (Fig. 8.15B and C). The findings are consistent with the patient's neurofibromatosis.

Case 7: A 57-year-old male was being evaluated for possible extruded disc or spinal stenosis because of nerve impingement symptoms. Axial CT images showed a collection of perithecal gas outlining the vertebral vein and displacing the thecal sac posteriorly (Fig. 8.16A). It has been reported that gas collections in the neural canal are rare and that it represents pieces of extruded disc containing central gaseous degeneration (11). In the case illustrated, there is no evidence of extruded disc material. It is thought that the cystic degeneration in neighboring disc spaces has produced the gas which is loculated within the neural canal. The reformatted images show the precise position of the gas adjacent to the thecal sac (Fig. 8.16B).

Case 8: A 73-year-old female was referred for evaluation of back pain and sciatica. The CT images showed a marked

rotatory scoliosis (Fig. 8.17A). Reformatted true coronal views were possible by rotating the Z plane so that the neural canal could be viewed directly en face (Fig. 17B). The pronounced dextroscoliotic curve could not be straightened with reformatting computer techniques but could be evaluated segmentally (Fig. 8.17C and D). A herniated disc is seen at L4–5 on one of the sagittal views.

DORSAL SPINE

Scanning technique

Because of the length of the dorsal spine, it is impractical to scan the entire distance with 5-mm thick slices. If symptoms are vague or of a nonlocalizing nature, 10-mm thick contiguous images are obtained from D1–12. Unfortunately, this survey approach results in less smooth reformatted images with reduced detail and spatial resolution. If a disc or other lesion is suspected clinically at a specific level, that area can be scanned with thinner axial slices and that will result in cleaner, more detailed reformatted pictures.

Technical factors remain similar to those used in scanning the lumbar spine: 120 KV, 320 MA, and a pulse width of 2. The slices are either 5 or 10 mm in width. If the wider slice is selected, the pulse width can be increased to 3 without delay for tube cooling.

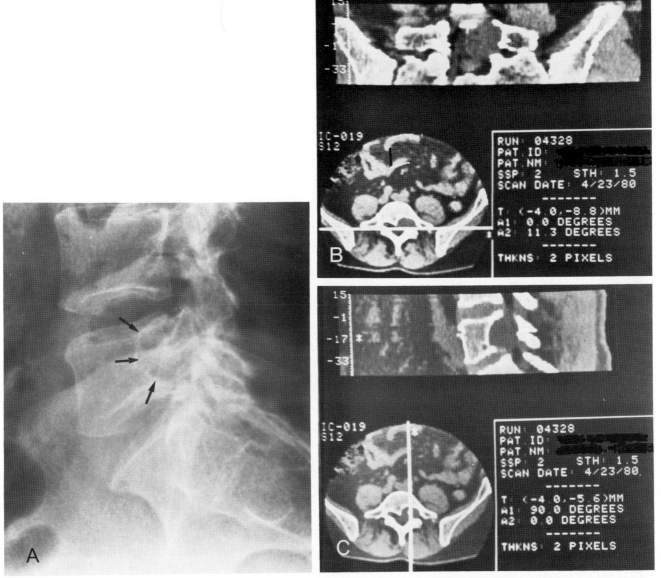

Figure 8.15. A. A lateral radiograph of the lumbosacral region shows a sclerotic erosion involving the posterior aspect of the L5 vertebral body (*arrows*) in a patient with cutaneous neurofibromatosis. B. A coronal tilted reformatted image with high-resolution scanning shows the soft-tissue mass and associated displacement of the lower thecal sac and nerve roots to the right. There is bone erosion involving the lateral wall and pedicle of L5 on the left. C. A parasagittal reformatted image through the area of sacral destruction clearly demonstrates this neurofibroma which is eroding into the posterior margin of the L5 vertebral body.

Case 9: A 52-year-old male physician complained of progressive leg weakness and muscle spasm. CT of the dorsal spine was performed to evaluate for possible herniated disc. The examination showed a dural or epidural lipoma that was displacing the spinal cord forward and to the right (Fig. 8.18A). The extent of this large lesion was appreciated best by sagittal reformatting (Fig. 8.18B). Because of the chronicity of his symptoms and the apparent benign nature of the lesion, the patient elected not to have surgery.

Case 10: Acute low thoracic back pain caused a 78-year-old male to seek medical help. CT examination showed a paraspinal mass (Fig. 8.19A). MPR showed that the mass was extremely long and paraspinous in position (Fig. 8.19B). Because of the destruction of the 12th thoracic vertebral body and paravertebral mass, metastatic disease was suspected. Biopsy showed that this represented a chordoma.

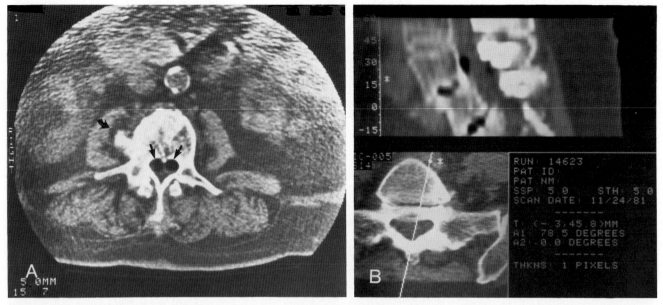

Figure 8.16. A. An axial scan through the midportion of the L4 vertebral body shows a collection of well-defined gas (*arrows*) in the neural canal. The gas pushes the thecal sac posteriorly and clearly outlines the posterior venous plexus as it arises from the vertebral body. A bursa has formed around a large osteophyte arising from the right lateral margin of the vertebral body (*curved arrow*). B. A sagittal reformatted image shows the collection of gas in the neural canal with no evidence of an associated soft-tissue mass. The gas is most likely from the cystic degeneration at the L4–5 disc space. There is also cystic degeneration at L5–S1.

CERVICAL SPINE

Scanning technique

For an adequate examination of the cervical spine even with specific localized symptoms it is best to scan the entire cervical region from C1–D1. Technical factors should be KV 120, MA 320 when scanning through the mandibular region and base of skull. The MA can be reduced to 250 MA in the midcervical area and then, because of the greater volume of tissue in the upper chest, increased to 320 or 400 MA in the lower cervical and upper thoracic spine. Positioning the cervical spine and shoulders in the center of the gantry minimizes artifacts.

Case 11: A 72-year-old male physician had slowly progressive arm weakness and paresthesias over the past 10 years. Radiographs showed evidence of extensive diffuse idiopathic senile hyperostosis (DISH) with associated ossification of the posterior spinal ligament (Fig. 8.20A). On CT, the axial slices showed a marked narrowing of the neural canal and pressure on the spinal cord (Fig. 8.20B). On a single reformatted image, the extent of the ossification of the posterior spinal ligament, and its protrusion into the neural canal, and related displacement of the spinal cord were demonstrated (Fig. 8.20C). MPR was able to show the entire extent of the ossification on a single view rather than on the multiple axial slices. The patient thought that he could live with his condition and has refused surgery.

Case 12: A 52-year-old woman with known cutaneous melanoma presented with neck and right arm pain. Plain films were equivocal. Linear tomography showed destruc-

tion of the lamina and enlargement of the neural foramen on the right at the C3 level (Fig. 8.21A). A CT examination showed tumor invading the C2 vertebral body with bone destruction (Fig. 8.2) and a soft-tissue mass extending into the neural canal and displacement of the spinal cord (Fig. 8.21C). The lesion was treated with radiation therapy (Cobalt 60) and the patient has had marked improvement in her symptoms. Reformatting (Fig. 8.21D) allowed the entire cervical spine to be seen in more than one projection and facilitated a more accurate three-dimensional evaluation.

Case 13: A 20-year-old man presented with six months of progressive arm weakness and muscle wasting. The neurological examination suggested a cervical cord tumor. Myelography was inconclusive but suggestive of minimal widening of the midcervical cord (Fig. 8.22A). CT examination with use of IV contrast showed an area of increased uptake and enhancement at the C5 level (Fig. 8.22B). MPR clearly shows the area of tumor enhancement and its relationship to surrounding structures (Fig. 8.22C and D). The reformatting allows clear positioning of the tumor in relationship to the neural canal and its location at the C5 level. The size and volume of the lesion in relationship to the cord can be appreciated. Surgery proved the lesion to be a low-grade astrocytoma.

Case 14: A 67-year-old woman presented with neuresthesia of both upper and lower extremities with vague weakness and muscle twitching of the right leg during sleep. The symptoms had been slowly progressive for 7 years after an automobile accident. Radiographs of the cervical spine showed degenerative changes plus a flexion deformity in the midcervical spine with anterior subluxation of C5 in relation to C6 and disruption of the posterior

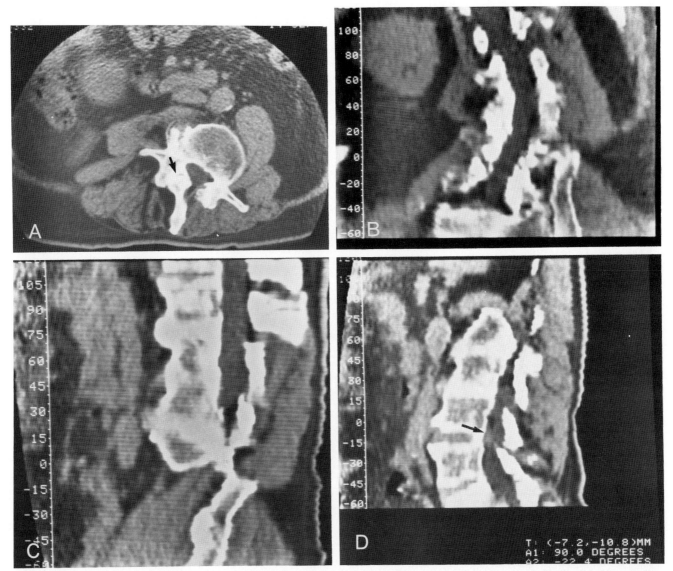

Figure 8.17.   A. An axial image taken through the midlumbar region shows a marked rotatory scoliosis of the spine and degenerative changes involving the apophyseal joints, which are narrowed and sclerotic (*arrow*). B. An oblique tilted coronal reformatted image is able to compensate for the scoliosis allowing the neural canal to be viewed en face. C. A tilted sagittal image was reformatted through the upper part of the spine. Because of the degree of the lateral scoliosis, the entire neural canal cannot be evaluated in any single plane. D. A tilted sagittal reformatted image for evaluation of the lower portion of the neural canal shows a well-defined extruded disc (*arrow*) at the L4–5 level.

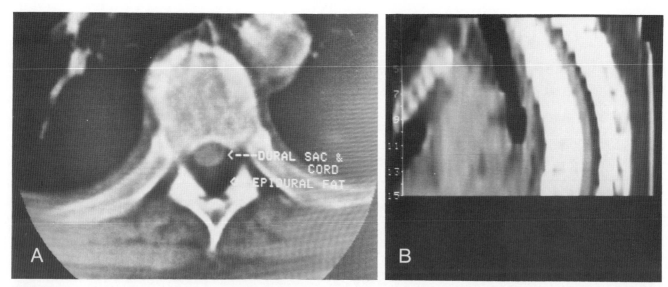

Figure 8.18. A. An axial slice taken through the midthoracic region shows a large collection of epidural fat displacing the dural sac and spinal cord anteriorly and slightly to the right of the midline. B. The sagittal reformatted image shows the large extent of the epidural lipoma extending throughout the entire midthoracic region. The thoracic region is the most common location for epidural lipomas and they frequently are large and encompass several vertebral levels.

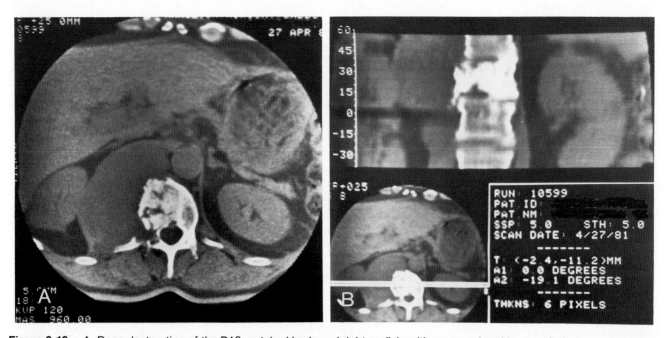

Figure 8.19. A. Bone destruction of the D12 vertebral body and right pedicle with an associated large soft-tissue mass is seen on an axial reconstruction. Although initially thought to be lymphoma or metastatic disease, biopsy showed it to be a primary chordoma. B. The extent of the soft-tissue mass is demonstrated best by a tilted coronal reformatted image. The soft-tissue mass extends both above and below the origin of the chordoma.

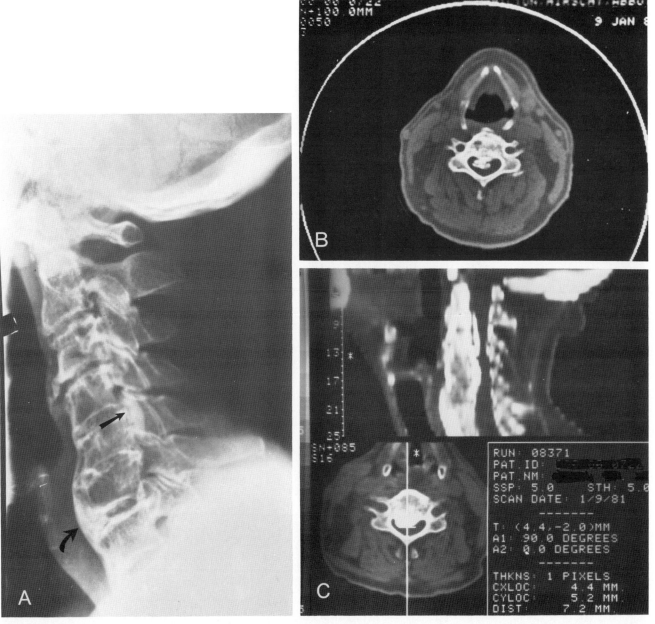

Figure 8.20.   A. Extensive degenerative changes in the cervical spine represent DISH. There is ossification of the lower anterior spinal ligament (*curved arrow*). Ossification of the posterior spinal ligament is also identified at the C4–5 level (*arrow*). B. An axial image taken through the lower cervical spine demonstrated ossification of the posterior spinal ligament. The ossification reduces the anterior-posterior dimension of the neural canal to less than one-half of its normal size and results in posterior displacement of the spinal cord. C. The sagittal reformatted image shows the extent of the ossification of the posterior spinal ligament. The reformatted image helps to demonstrate the pathology in a single view, rather than analyzing numerous axial slices. The anterior-posterior dimension of the neural canal is 7.2 mm, whereas the normal dimension is 15–20 mm in this region.

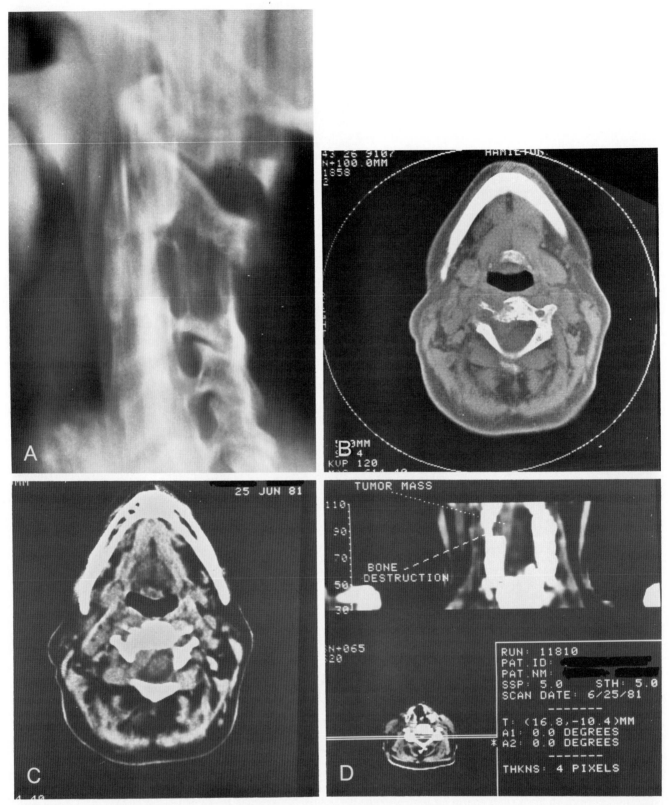

Figure 8.21. A. A lateral linear tomogram of the cervical spine shows a large destructive lesion involving C3. It is metastatic involvement of the bone from a cutaneous melanoma. B. An axial slice taken through C3 shows the destruction of the vertebral body. The bone window setting used to demonstrate the osseous involvement burns out the soft-tissue component. C. An axial slice using a soft-tissue window taken 5 mm above the slice in Figure 8.21B demonstrates the soft-tissue mass arising from the tumor. The mass is displacing the cervical cord to the left. D. A coronal reformatted image shows the extent of the soft-tissue mass and bone destruction from the melanoma. The reformatted image helps locate the pathology.

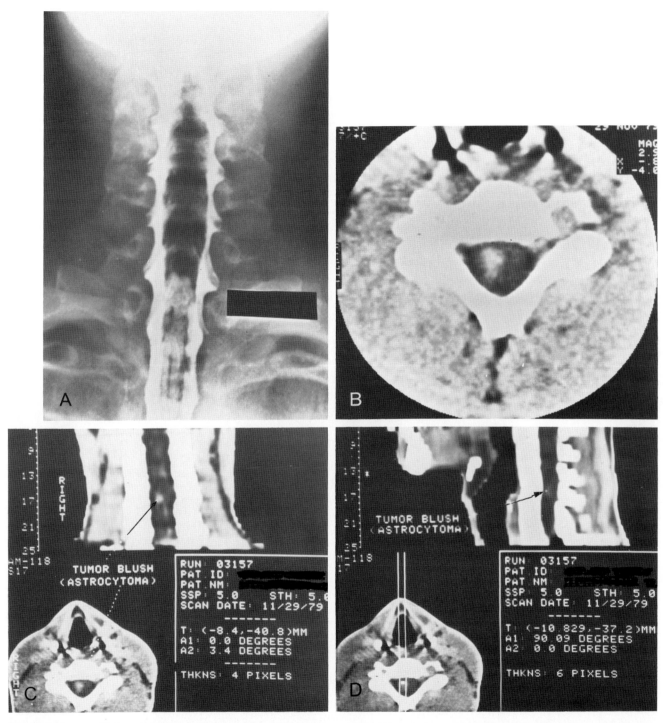

Figure 8.22.   A. Slight widening of the lower cervical cord is seen on a Pantopaque myelogram. The findings were equivocal and the patient was suspected to have a cervical cord tumor. B. An axial image after injection of IV contrast material shows a tumor blush in the lower cervical cord. It was shown to be a low grade astrocytoma. C. The lateral reformatted image shows the location of the astrocytoma at the C5 level (*arrow*). D. The coronal reformatted image also shows the tumor blush in the cervical cord (*arrow*). The reformatted images were very helpful in determining the precise anatomical location of this neoplasm.

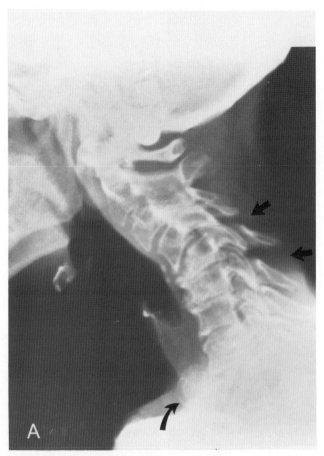

Figure 8.23. A. A lateral radiograph of the cervical spine shows a subluxation at both the C4–5 and C5–6 levels. Widening of the interspace between the spinous processes (*arrows*) indicates disruption of the interspinous ligament. An incidental finding was a large calcified nodule in the thyroid gland (*curved arrow*). B. A sagittal reformatted image from 5-mm thick slices shows a large tumor mass at the C2 level. The tumor is causing posterior displacement of the upper cervical cord. C. After administration of IV contrast material, the tumor mass at C2 showed increased blush. The axial image showed a feeding vessel of a cervical meningioma passing through the right neural foramen. D. Sagittal reformatted image using 1.5-mm thick slices taken at 2-mm intervals shows the C3 meningioma to excellent advantage and, when compared with Figure 8.23B, demonstrates increased resolution. E. A tilted coronal reformatted image of the cervical spine shows the meningioma in the neural canal and its precise cephalad and caudad extension.

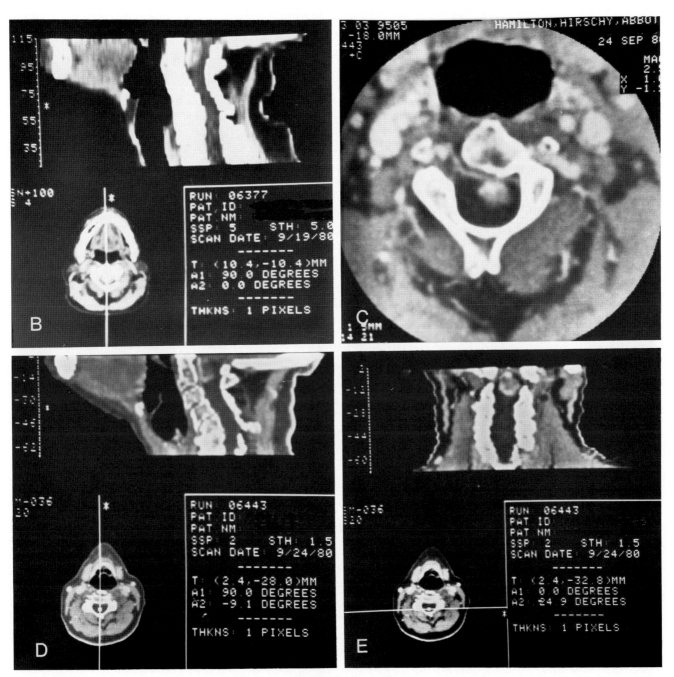

Figure 8.23. B–E.

spinal ligaments (Fig. 8.23A). These findings were thought to be responsible for the patient's symptoms. A spinal fusion was recommended but the patient desired further consultation. A CT scan of the midcervical spine was recommended for more complete evaluation of this area to determine the degree of suspected spinal stenosis and spinal cord compression. On a scan of C1–D1, a large extrathecal tumor was discovered at the C2 level. This was best seen with sagittal reformatting (Fig. 8.23B). Rescanning the spine after the administration of IV contrast material showed increased contrast in the lesion, suggesting a meningioma. The feeding vessel was demonstrated on one axial slice (Fig. 8.23C). Reconstructions showed the exact location of the tumor in relation to the spinal cord, its length, and position (Fig. 8.23D and E). The reconstructions also demonstrated subluxation of the C5–6 vertebral bodies and posterior displacement of the spinal cord at this level. All symptoms were relieved after surgical removal of the meningioma and posterior wiring of the spinous processes at the C5, C6 levels.

Bibliography

1. Glenn Jr. WV, Johnston RJ, Morton PE, et al: Further investigation in initial clinical use of advanced CT display capability. *Invest Radiol* 10:479–489, 1975.
2. Pevsner PH, Kreel L, King DC, et al: Technical note: Multiple axis reconstruction from axial transverse data. *J Comput Assist Tomogr* 3:279–281, 1979.
3. Coin CG, Coin JT: Computed tomography of cervical disc disease: Technical considerations with representative case reports. *J Comput Assist Tomogr* 5:275–280, 1981.
4. Rhodes ML, Glenn WV, Azzawi YM: Extracting oblique planes from serial CT sections. *J Comput Assist Tomogr* 4:649–657, 1980.
5. Fetterly MP, Moss AA, Margolin FR: Role of computed tomography in patients with "sciatica." *J Comput Assist Tomogr* 4:335–341, 1980.
6. Nadich TP, King DG, Moran CJ, et al.: Computed tomography of the lumbar thecal sac. *J Comput Assist Tomogr* 4:37–41, 1980.
7. Williams AL, Haughton VM, Syvertsen A: Computed tomography in the diagnosis of herniated nucleus pulposus. *Radiology* 135:95–99, 1980.
8. Raskin SP: Demonstration of nerve roots on unenhanced computed tomographic scans. *J Comput Assist Tomogr* 5:281–284, 1981.
9. Hirschy JC, Leue WM, Berninger WH, et al: CT of the lumbosacral spine: Importance of tomographic planes parallel to vertical end plate. *AJNR* 1:551–556, 1980.
10. Ullrich CG, Kieffer SA: Computed tomographic evaluation of the lumbar spine: quantitative aspects and sagittal-coronal reconstruction. In Post MJD (Ed): *Radiographic Evaluation of the Spine: Current Advances with Emphasis on Computed Tomography.* New York, Masson Publishing USA, 1980.
11. Austin RM, Bankoff MS, Carter DL: Gas collections in the spinal canal on computed tomography. *J Comput Assist Tomogr* 5:522–524, 1981.

CHAPTER NINE

Pitfalls and Artifacts in Computed Tomographic Scanning of the Spine

JAMES C. HIRSCHY, M.D.

Continued experience with thin-slice high-resolution scanning of the spine has led to the discovery of some pitfalls, including artifacts that can confuse accurate diagnosis and mimic disease. Knowing where to look for them keeps false-positive and false-negative diagnoses to a minimum.

The pitfalls are: misinterpretation of normally exiting lumbar nerve roots, pseudodisc herniations secondary to spinal tilt and scoliosis, pseudofractures due to venous channels, and misdiagnoses of spinal stenosis. Thick slices can obscure a small protruding or bulging disc. High-density materials like retained Pantopaque or metallic surgical devices can result in streak artifact formation leading to misinterpretations. Streaking is also the result of edge effect. Limited (selective) scanning of the spine can result in false-negative diagnoses.

In the lower thecal sac, the nerve roots exit via the nerve sheaths in the anterior or volar location, rather than laterally as they do in the region of the spinal cord. As the nerves exit, it is not uncommon to see a pronounced soft-tissue density approximating the anterior aspect of the thecal sac. This soft-tissue density consists of the layers of the dural sheath and nerve roots. It is often of greater density than the cerebrospinal fluid within the sac because of superimposition of the dural layers, and can mimic an extruded disc (Fig. 9.1A). The confusion is resolved easily by observing the contiguous axial slice immediately caudad to the area on which the mass or masses may be recognized as well-defined nerve roots anterolateral to the thecal sac (Fig. 9.1B). Confirmation that there is no herniated disc is made by utilizing a sagittal reformatted image (Fig. 9.1C) and an oblique-axial image (Fig. 9.1D).

In addition to the pseudodisc protrusion, (described in the Chapter 8 on High-Resolution Multiplanar Reformatting), commonly encountered at the L5-S1 level, a pseudodisc can be seen at other levels in patients with a lumbar tilt or scoliosis. It appears to be a lateral or posterolateral herniation mimicking a protruded disc (Fig. 9.2A). A similar shadow can occur in patients with spondylolisthesis (Fig. 9.3A) when the neural axis of the vertebral bodies in the area of the defect are not perpendicular to the axial CT slices. By using MPR, it is possible to acquire a true coronal or sagittal view of the spine (Figs. 9.2B and 9.3B). With these reformatted images, an axial image that is parallel to the vertebral end plates can be generated (Figs. 9.2C and 9.3C). The new axial images show no evidence of herniated disc.

When thin slices are taken through the vertebral body and they are parallel to the basivertebral veins, the veins can mimic a bi- or tri-radiate fracture (Fig. 9.4A and B). The presence of the posterior midline drainage of the veins into the venous plexus covered by the osseous cap which is located in the midportion of the vertebral body confirms the fact that there is no fracture.

In the evaluation of spinal stenosis, a thin (1.5-mm) slice can give the impression that the neural canal is larger than it actually is if the scanning angle is not absolutely perpendicular to the long axis of the neural canal (Fig. 9.5A–C). The phenomenon is similar to slicing a salami diagonally (Fig. 9.6). The resulting slice has an oval shape that is larger than a true cross-section. Thicker axial slices (10 mm) are self-correcting because of the partial volume effect at the margin of the neural canal (Fig. 9.7). If the scanning angle were absolutely perpendicular to the axis of the neural canal, varying slice thickness would have no effect and the absolute measurement would remain constant.

The diagnosis of spinal stenosis may be missed in individuals who have marked hypertrophy of the ligamentum flavum. With a wide or bone window setting, the actual size and dimension of the canal can be normal (Fig. 9.8A). By narrowing the window to a soft-tissue setting and increasing the contrast, the soft tissues are demonstrated clearly and any constriction or stenosis of the neural canal is apparent (Fig. 9.8B).

The selection or use of axial slices greater than 5 mm thick can result in a partial volume effect that obscures pathology (Fig. 9.9A–C). The average normal adult disc space is slightly greater than 5 mm. An 8-, 10-, or 12-mm thick slice would include one or both vertebral end plates in the scan volume (Fig. 9.10). The vertebral end plate predominates and can obscure soft tissues.

Retained contrast from Pantopaque myelography is a common source of artifacts (Fig. 9.11). Metallic high-density surgical material can produce odd shadows which project into the spinal canal. Surgical clips in the neutral canal can create bizarre patterns (Fig. 9.12).

A metallic surgical device in the spine called a disc expander, briefly used in the 1950s, is another cause of streaking (Fig. 9.13). Usually seen at the L5-S1 level, the metallic rods or spheres were inserted into the disc space to replace an excised nucleus pulposus in order to maintain normal intervertebral disc height. Many of the disc expanders fractured through the vertebral end plates; the technique was discarded quickly in favor of spinal fusion.

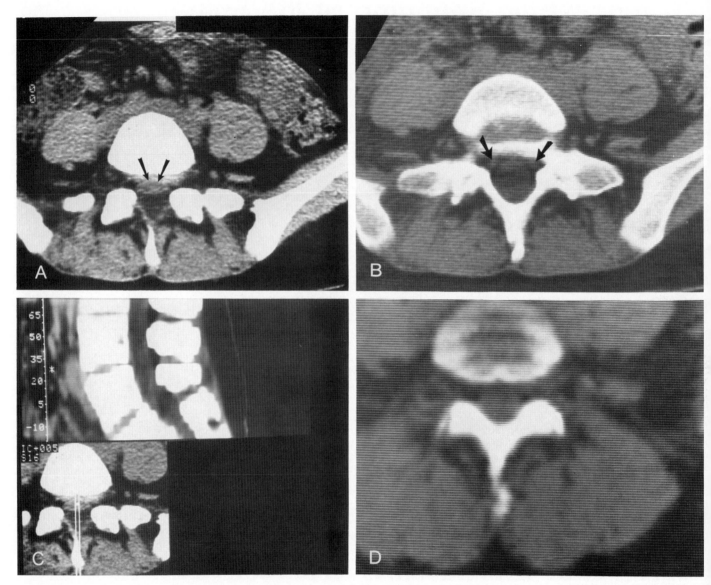

Figure 9.1.   A. A 5-mm axial slice taken through the region of the L5-S1 disc space shows a pronounced soft-tissue density located between the body of the L5 vertebra and the fluid-filled thecal sac. The finding is suspicious for a large centrally herniated disc (*arrows*). B. An axial slice taken immediately caudad to the image shown in Figure 9.1A. The L5 nerve roots are defined clearly immediately anterolateral to the thecal sac (*arrows*). C. The sagittal reformatted image fails to reveal any suggestion of increased soft-tissue bulging around the intervertebral disc space. D. A reformatted oblique-axial image through the disc space at L5-S1 shows normal nerve roots and no evidence of a herniated disc.

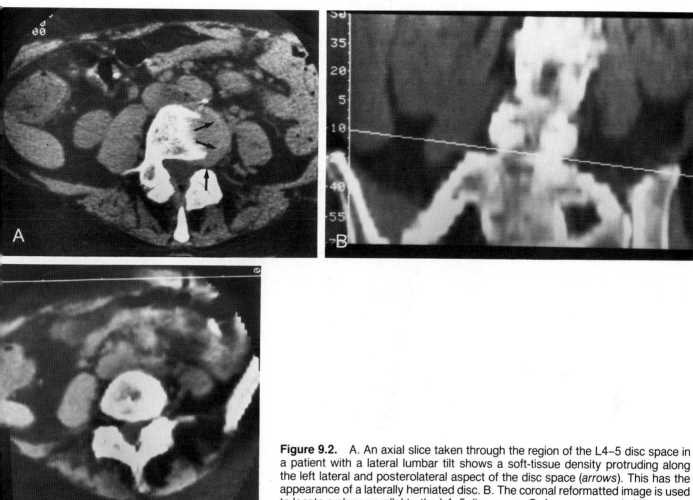

Figure 9.2.   A. An axial slice taken through the region of the L4–5 disc space in a patient with a lateral lumbar tilt shows a soft-tissue density protruding along the left lateral and posterolateral aspect of the disc space (*arrows*). This has the appearance of a laterally herniated disc. B. The coronal reformatted image is used to locate a plane parallel to the L4–5 disc space. C. A reconstructed oblique-axial image adjusting for the patient's lumbar tilt and lordosis shows that there is no evidence of lateral or posterolateral protrusion of disc material.

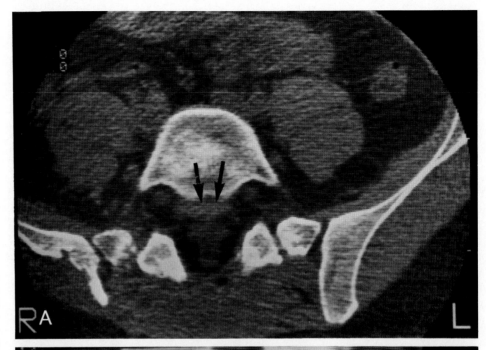

Figure 9.3. A. In individuals with a spondylolisthesis, it is not uncommon to see a large soft-tissue density mimicking a herniated disc (*arrows*). B. The sagittal reformatted image fails to reveal evidence of disc material protruding into the neural canal at the level of the spondylolisthesis. A herniated disc is seen at L4–5 (*arrow*). C. Using 1.5-mm axial slices at 2-mm intervals, a reformatted oblique axial image parallel to the intervertebral disc space at L5-S1 shows no herniated disc.

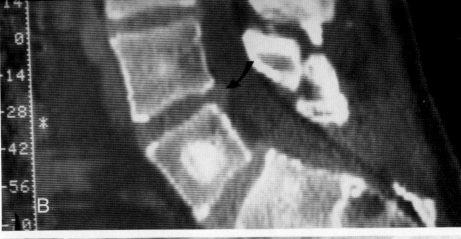

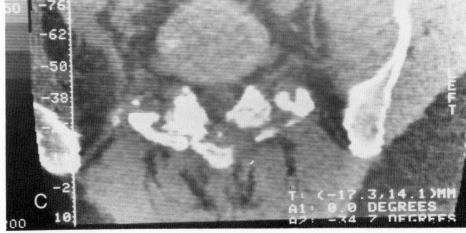

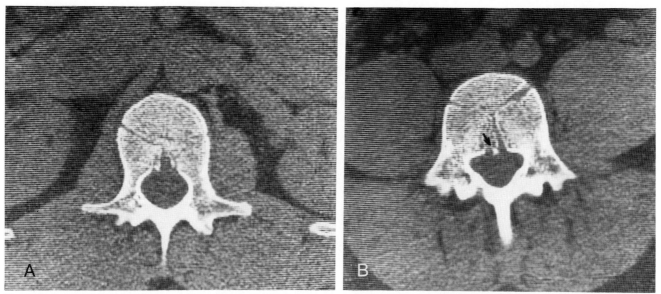

Figure 9.4. A. A 1.5-mm thick axial slice taken through the midportion of a lumbar vertebral body shows what appears to be a biradiate fracture on the right side, extending into the central venous channel. These lines represent a normal basivertebral vein. B. A 1.5-mm thick axial slice taken through the midportion of a lumbar vertebral body shows an apparent triradiate fracture. This represents the normal basivertebral veins that are in the same plane as the axial slice. The central posterior extension into the region of the bony cap (*arrow*) confirms that this is a normal anatomical finding and should not be diagnosed as a fracture.

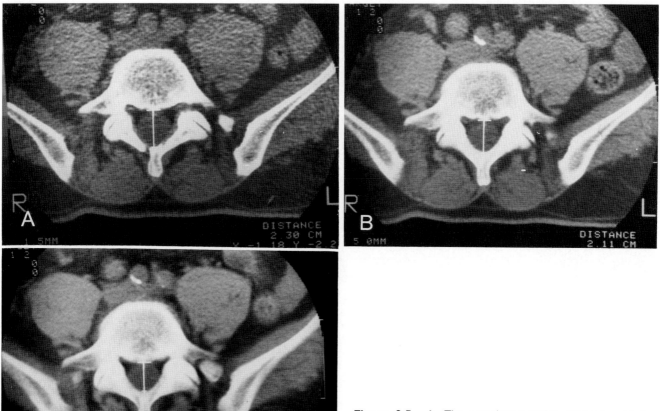

Figure 9.5. A. The anterior-posterior dimension of the neural canal at L5 using a 1.5-mm thick slice is 23 mm. B. By increasing the slice thickness to 5 mm, the anterior-posterior dimension of the neural canal becomes 21.1 mm. C. By increasing the slice thickness to 10 mm, the anterior-posterior dimension of the neural canal becomes 18.6 mm.

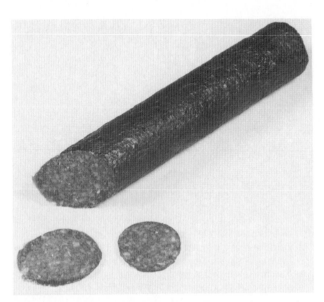

Figure 9.6. The diameter of a slice of salami varies according to the degree of obliquity of the slice.

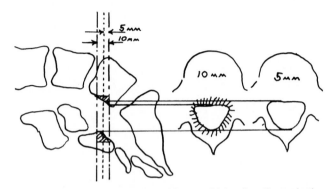

Figure 9.7. A 5-mm and a 10-mm thick slice through the same tilted vertebral body demonstrates that the neural canal appears to be smaller on the thicker slice due to a partial volume effect.

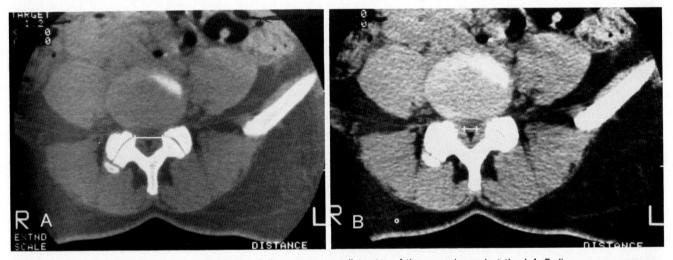

Figure 9.8. A. If a bone window setting is used, the transverse diameter of the neural canal at the L4–5 disc space measures 18.6 mm, which is normal. B. By using a soft-tissue window setting, marked hypertrophy and thickening of the ligamentum flavum is identified, reducing the transverse diameter of the neural canal to 7.7 mm, indicative of spinal stenosis.

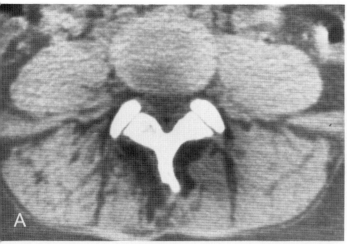

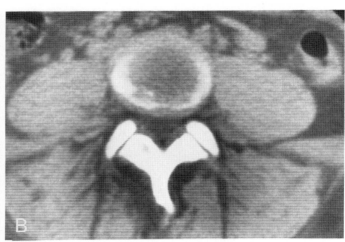

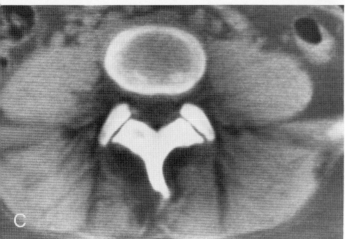

Figure 9.9.   A. A 1.5-mm thick axial slice taken through the central portion of an L4–5 disc. The anulus is of greater density than the central nucleus pulposus. No evidence of bone is identified, indicating that the axial slice is taken parallel to the intervertebral disc. B. A 5-mm thick slice taken at the same level and angle shows a portion of the vertebral end plate projecting in the region of the anulus. C. A 10-mm slice includes more bone in the vertebral end plate so that it is more difficult to determine whether or not the scan goes through the disc space. Although the image shown is less grainy due to a higher photon flux, a thick slice can obscure pathology due to partial volume effect.

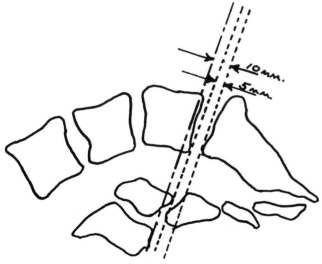

Figure 9.10.   Increased slice thickness through an intervertebral disc space can include the vertebral end plate. As the bone is of higher density, it predominates on the final reconstructed image.

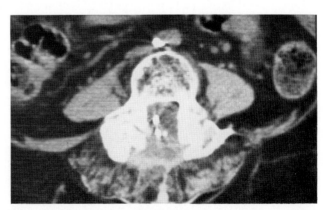

Figure 9.11.   Retained Pantopaque from a myelogram results in streak artifacts that are projected into the right margin of the neural canal. The streaking should not be confused with herniated disc material.

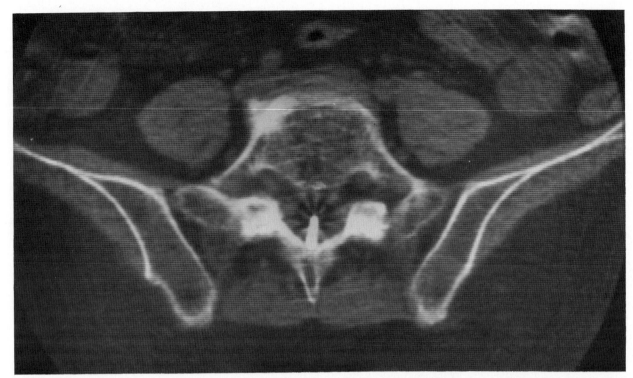

Figure 9.12.   A metallic surgical clip on one of the nerve roots results in a star artifact formation. Heavy metal can obscure a minimally herniated disc.

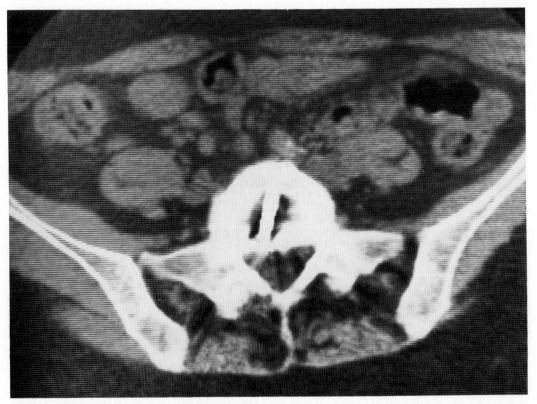

Figure 9.13.   A disc expander located at the L5-S1 disc space results in artifact formation projecting into the region of the right lateral recess. The streak artifacts mimic a herniated disc.

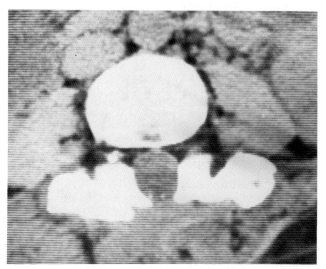

Figure 9.14.   The edge effect of the facet joints can result in aliasing or streak artifacts that can give a soft-tissue density that can mimic a centrally herniated disc.

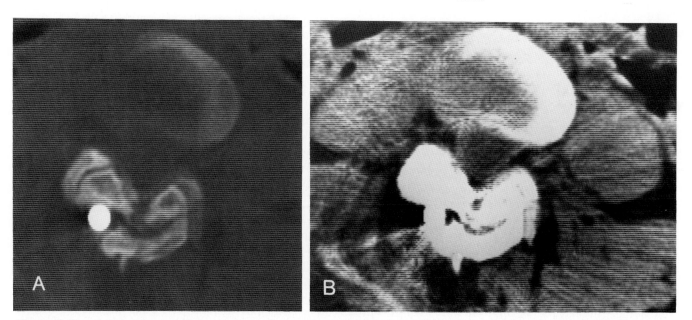

Figure 9.15.   A. By using a wide or bone window setting, an axial slice taken through a Harrington rod shows no artifact formation. The osseous elements of the spine are easy to evaluate. B. Using a soft-tissue window setting on the computer slightly increases artifact formation but the resulting image is still adequate for evaluation of possible herniated disc material.

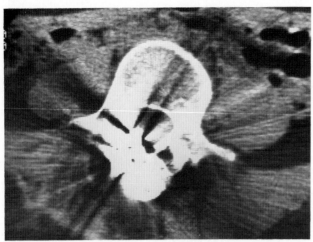

Figure 9.16.   Images taken through the high-density metal hook of a Harrington rod result in pronounced artifact formation which can obscure all soft-tissue density and make evaluation of a disc in this region impossible.

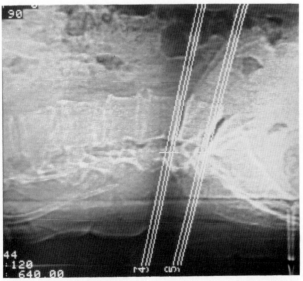

Figure 9.17.   A lateral digital radiograph indicates the location of slices through the L4–5 and the L5-S1 disc spaces.

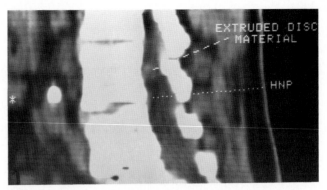

Figure 9.18.   A reformatted sagittal image demonstrates a large collection of extruded disc material which had migrated cephalad to the midportion of the L4 vertebral body. The extruded material would have been missed if only the disc spaces were scanned as in Figure 9.17.

Streak or aliasing artifacts can occur when the density of the organ differs markedly from the surrounding tissues. These artifacts are encountered in brain scanning in the area of the posterior fossa between the petrous ridges. In the abdomen, they are seen when there is an air-fluid interface in the stomach or intestines. In the spine, the facet or apophyseal joints can cause these streaks (Fig. 9.14) which can mimic a herniated nucleus pulposus. This edge effect is caused by a sudden change in the density of an organ or object and its surrounding tissues as measured electronically in the Data Acquisition System (DAS) of the scanner.

Harrington rods should not be an obstacle to or contraindication for scanning. By using a wide window or extended range on the viewing console of the computer, most streak artifacts can be minimized (Fig. 9.15A and B). A minimally herniated or protruding disc would be difficult to evaluate by using the extended range, but bone detail and some pathology can be assessed. The metallic mass of the hooks at the ends of the rods increases the aliasing streaks and artifact formation (Fig. 9.16) and can make interpretation of pathology in this region impossible.

In order to save time and increase patient throughput, some scanning centers limit their axial slices to the disc spaces and adjacent areas where pathology is suspected (Fig. 9.17). This procedure can detect most bulging or herniated discs, but may miss an extruded disc or nucleus pulposus that has migrated to the level of the midvertebral body (Fig. 9.18). Multiple contiguous axial slices through a volume of tissue following by MPR can minimize the number of false negatives.

Avoiding pitfalls in diagnosis depends on appropriately planned scanning, with close attention to the reformatted image. Reformatting is an integral part of the examination and can resolve many ambiguous findings. By manipulating collected data, looking at adjacent slices, and using computer controls to alter densities, most pitfalls can be avoided and accuracy of CT diagnosis improves.

CHAPTER TEN

Fourth Generation Computed Tomographic Scanning of the Spinal Cord

JAMES W. KEATING, Jr., M.D., JOSEPH M. D. NADELL, M.D., and ERNESTO LUCIANO

INTRODUCTION

The spinal cord has been a difficult region to image with the technique of CT. With fourth generation technology, however, the imaging of the region is accomplished with more confidence (1–3). The Picker "Synerview 600" CT scanner is one of the first fourth generation CT scanners that has been available for clinical practice in this country. The Radiology Department of the Tulane Medical Center installed this fourth generation CT scanner in November, 1978. This present analysis represents the clinical experience of over 100 cases examined because of suspected spinal cord disorders. The work-up of these patients with suspected spinal cord disorders has changed significantly at Tulane Medical Center because of the improvement in CT technology. A concise description of the technical aspects of the fourth generation system will be included in addition to the presentation of the clinical material with an outline of updated radiographic work-ups of the more common major disorders of the spinal cord. The cases described represent examples of the spectrum of spinal cord pathology that currently may be diagnosed more accurately with a more noninvasive and less expensive means. These disorders include syringomyelia, spinal cord masses, atrophy, traumatic laceration, anomalies, and gross alteration of the bony spinal architecture.

TECHNICAL CONSIDERATIONS

The CT examination of the spinal cord will be described. It is useful to know before the procedure if there is a known lesion at a specific site because the examination may be custom tailored to that particular part of the spinal cord. The patient is positioned supine on an examining table with the use of a board to support the head. A headrest produces undesired artifacts in the cervical studies. Waterbags about the neck may be of value (as used in angiography) to equalize the volume of tissue studied in a large field size if the examination includes both the neck and the thorax. A "pilot" scan (comparable to a "scout" view) is a planar densitograph which looks like a conventional radiograph. A pilot scan is accomplished first in the lateral projection. The first "cut" is then positioned just above the foramen magnum. A slice thickness is chosen which is 6 mm. This represents a compromise between increased spatial resolution, e.g., thin section cuts (2 mm) and contrast resolution, e.g., larger slices (1 cm). In addition, there are practical limitations to slice thickness which must be considered in a busy department where computer scheduling time is precious. A 6-mm slice thickness with a 4-mm table index (amount of distance the table moves after each exposure) provides a reasonable compromise. If artifacts, such as tooth fillings, degrade the image of the upper cervical cord, this may be obviated by tilting the gantry cephalad by as much as 20° or the chin may be raised to position the metal fillings more cephalad in relation to the cord. It is possible to choose a small field size or reconstruction diameter, e.g., 12 cm. This proves more effective for studying the spinal cord.

It is critical that the neuroradiologist design the CT scan in a patient with a suspected spinal cord disorder to image the structures deemed clinically important in that specific case best. This may require altering technical factors to achieve the appropriate spatial and contrast resolution. Contrast resolution is a measure of an imaging system's ability to discriminate structures of different attenuation values against a uniform and homogeneous background. It may be expressed as the smallest visable object size at a given contrast difference using a special low contrast phantom designed to vary simultaneously the size and contrast of objects in a uniform background (e.g., 4 mm/0.3%). Spatial resolution, on the other hand, is a measure of a scanner's ability to discriminate objects of similar attenuation values a small distance apart against a uniform background. One method of measurement uses a line pair phantom and expresses performance as MTF (Modulation Transfer Function) e.g., 5 line pair/cm (4).

To achieve maximum contrast resolution, a radiographic technique is employed using a relatively low KVP (100–130) and a high MAS. In order to limit motion artifacts, a short scan speed is chosen which produces an exposure time of approximately 4 seconds. The MA chosen will range from 5–200. An image reconstruction algorithm is a software mathematical function that can vary the amount of spatial or contrast resolution acquired in a CT image. At present, with the Synerview 600 CT scanner, about six possible algorithms are available to the technician. A compensator is a filter which absorbs low energy x-rays and reduces the patient skin dose by approximately 40%. It produces a more uniform beam. Contrast resolution may be enhanced by its removal.

Certain technical options improve both spatial and contrast resolution. The scan angle is the amount of rotation of the x-ray tube relative to the stationary detectors. One may elect 230°, 360°, or 398° scan angles. The 398° scan angle produces the highest resolution but necessitates a longer exposure time. A small field size puts only the spine on the matrix display which allows a faster sampling rate which results in more measurements per unit of tissue examined, therefore, increasing both spatial and contrast resolution.

Some options improve spatial contrast only. The matrix size is the number of points across the diameter of the image used in its reconstruction. For each pixel, a unique CT number has been calculated. A 512 × 512 matrix increases the amount of pixels per image and increases spatial resolution. A new "Spot Scan" update is used primarily for 2-mm thin-section imaging of small structures such as lumbar discs, inner ears, and orbits where spatial resolution is the prime objective. The Spot Scan employs a smaller collimation or detector aperture of the Bismuth Germinate crystal of 2.8 mm instead of the usual 4-mm size. For routine screening examinations of the spinal cord, because contrast resolution is more important than spatial resolution, the routine 4-mm detector aperture is selected instead of the Spot Scan option with the smaller 2.8-mm size. The 4-mm collimation gives a less "noisy" image than the 2.8-mm one.

There are multiple computer updates or accessories that may offer visual adjuvants to the viewer. These include a density measurement cursor, reversed images, annotation capability, zoom, track cursor, histograms, isodensity highlights, multiformat display, and instant sagittal and coronal reconstruction and update. The value of these accessories for purposes of diagnosis is not clearly established. They are of considerable benefit, however, in displaying the scan to physicians unfamiliar with the anatomical views in the usual axial format.

Contrast agents in general use include intravenous iodinated diatrizoate and iothalamate compounds and in-

trathecal water soluble contrast agents such as metrizamide (Amipaque). A metrizamide CT myelogram (MCTM) may be accomplished after a routine metrizamide myelogram. The presence of the high-density iodinated contrast agent in the subarachnoid space decreases the contrast resolution of the cord substance, particularly with the high dosages needed for adequate routine myelography. If only a CT examination is required, much smaller volumes with weaker concentrations of iodine afford better results. It may be necessary to perform the scan 3–12 hours after the myelogram to avoid the blurring effect on the central cord tissue or the computer artifacts noted with high concentration metrizamide. The MCTM is most useful in demonstrating the size and shape of the cord, particularly in the thoracic area. The plain CT scan evaluates cord tissue homogenicity to much better advantage. Intravenous contrast enhancement can demonstrate very vascular lesions such as a large AVM, but it has not been routine for screening purposes at this institution because of its projected low yield and the prospect of contrast reactions.

CLINICAL MATERIAL
Case 1: Astrocytoma

This 14-year-old male (Figs. 10.1–10.3) presented with a 3-year history of severe back pain and a normal neurological examination. There was a kyphosis and a slight scoliosis. A total myelogram demonstrated enlargement of the entire spinal cord. The conus was more enlarged than the proximal cord. The patient had a subtotal resection of the tumor and drainage of a cyst in the conus with a stint (Fig. 10.3). The patient received postoperative radiation. A follow-up metrizamide CT myelogram 20 months after surgery showed some decrease in size of the thoracic cord. The child has remained neurologically intact.

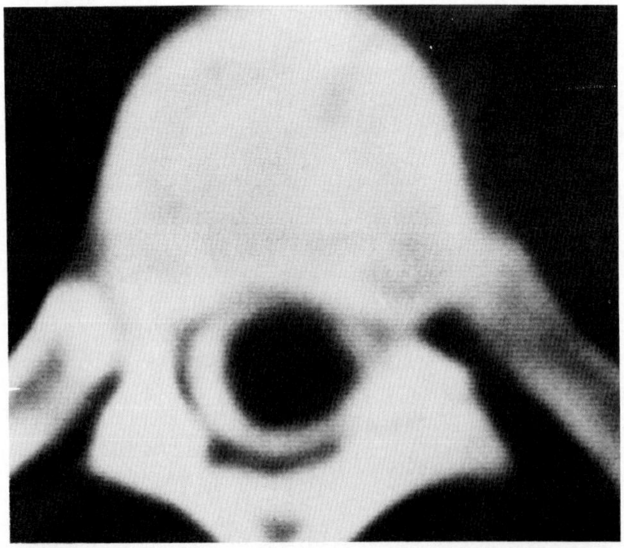

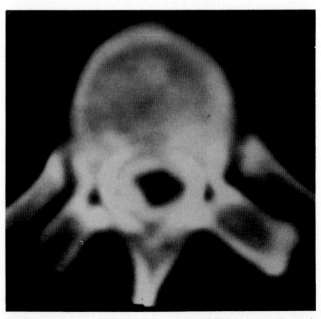

Figure 10.1. Case 1: Astrocytoma. In this patient with an astrocytoma of the entire spinal cord, the postoperative MCTM shows a markedly enlarged thoracic cord with a rounded configuration at a level above the operative site.

Figure 10.2. Case 1: Astrocytoma. MCTM at lower thoracic level in area adjacent to site of surgery demonstrating abnormal "diamond" configuration of spinal cord.

Case 2: Syringomyelia

This 43-year-old female presented with a long history of progressive signs of cervical myelopathy. A posterior fossa exploratory craniotomy was accomplished at age 35 which was negative. A recent repeat myelogram showed some interval widening of the cervical cord. An 8-hour delayed MCTM demonstrated a syrinx with passage of contrast into a central cavity (Fig. 10.4). The syrinx was surgically drained into the subarachnoid space, and the patient has had no progression of disease.

Case 3: Diastematomyelia

This 5-year-old female had a severe congenital scoliosis and dysraphism of the cervical spine. At age 14 months, a posterior cervical spine exploration was accomplished, but a fusion was not attempted. At age 5, a MCTM demonstrated a widened canal and a split cervical cord (Fig. 10.5).

Case 4: Metastasis

This 29-year-old male had a 2-year history of progressive paralysis of the lower extremities. A neurological examination demonstrated motor and sensory findings compatible with a T-5 level lesion. However, a limited myelogram was said to be negative. After several months, a MCTM was accomplished, and a fusiform intramedullary lesion with a small adjacent posterior arachnoid cyst was identified (Fig. 10.6). A laminectomy was done and the biopsy report described an intramedullary round cell tumor of unclear etiology and an adjacent arachnoidal cyst. Two weeks later, the patient died suddenly. At autopsy, a glioblastoma multiforme of the brain was found. The lesion in the thoracic cord then was thought to represent a metastasis or "seed" from the primary brain tumor.

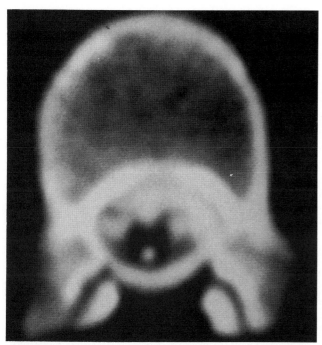

Figure 10.3. Case 1: Astrocytoma. MCTM at level of conus showing decompression of the tumor cyst. Notice also the stint in the conus posteriorly. Its patency is documented by virtue of the fact that it is filled with metrizamide.

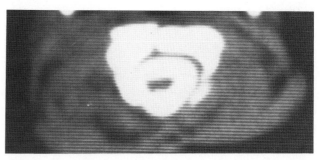

Figure 10.5. Case 3: Diastematomyelia. MCTM shows a "split cord" in the cervical area in a patient with spinal dysraphism and a severe scoliosis.

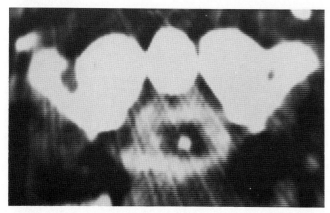

Figure 10.4. Case 2: Syringomyelia. A delayed MCTM shows contrast agent within a syrinx of the upper cervical spinal cord. The image is degraded by teeth artifacts.

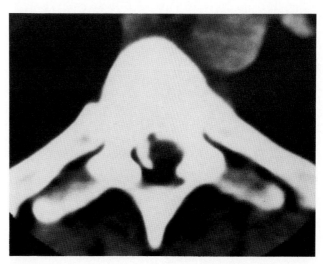

Figure 10.6. Case 4: Metastasis. MCTM demonstrates an enlarged cord at the T5 level with an adjacent low density posterior arachnoidal cyst. The intramedullary lesion was diagnosed at autopsy as a metastasis.

Case 5: Diastematomyelia

This 17-year-old female was born with a meningomyelocele which was surgically closed at birth. A thoracolumbar fusion was performed at age 5. However, the patient recently had progression of the scoliosis. A myelogram and a MCTM demonstrated a diastematomyelia (Figs. 10.7–10.9). At surgery, a large prominent spur was encountered in the lumbar area. In addition, a split cord was observed. The right cord was smaller and tethered in

the scar of the remnant meningomyelocele. The cord was released. Postoperatively, the child noted increased movement in her right distal foot.

Case 6: Arteriovenous Malformation

This 38-year-old male presented with a 1-year history of urinary retention and a 3-year history of left foot numbness. A neurological exam demonstrated a spastic, ataxic gait with clonus at the knees and ankles. The myelogram and MCTM showed a fusiform swelling of the cord at T4 (Fig. 10.10). A thoracic laminectomy was performed, and a thrombosed AVM with areas of necrosis was encountered. Postoperatively, the patient had improvement in bladder function as well as in gait.

Case 7: Syringomyelia

This 21-year-old female presented with a 2-year history of progressive motor and sensory deficits of all four extremities and abnormal Babinski reflexes. The myelogram showed widening of the entire spinal cord and bony spinal canal. The CT showed the cord to be enlarged and of mixed density (Fig. 10.11). A cervical laminectomy was performed and a myelotomy accomplished of a large cystic cavity with a tube. Postoperatively, the gait has improved, but there has been no change in the sensory loss.

Case 8: Ependymoma

This 8-year-old male had a 3-year history of progressive quadriplegia. At 6 years of age, an ependymoma involving the entire cord had been diagnosed at surgery. Spinal radiation resulted in some improvement of strength and movement of the extremities. A recent myelogram showed a block at T9 and interval expansion of the cord. A MCTM was accomplished with instillation of contrast via a C1–C2 approach into a large cyst that extended to the upper thoracic area (Fig. 10.12). A cervical laminectomy was done and the necrotic tumor cavity debrided. During the recovery process, the patient died of Pneumocystis carinii.

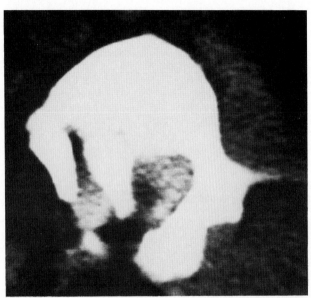

Figure 10.7. Case 5: Diastematomyelia. MCTM demonstrates a bony spur and a large "left cord" in the lumbar spine. The "right cord" was smaller and tethered in the scar of a remnant meningomyelocele.

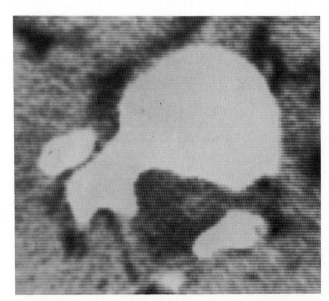

Figure 10.8. Case 5: Diastematomyelia. Noncontrast CT of such high resolution that the spinal cord can be distinguished in the lower thoracic spinal canal.

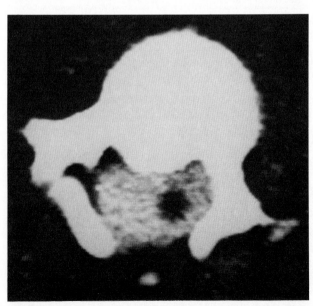

Figure 10.9. Case 5: Diastematomyelia. MCTM at same level as Figure 10.8 documents position of the spinal cord.

Case 9: Post-Traumatic Cyst

This 39-year-old acquired a C7-T1 fracture dislocation from injury sustained in a motor vehicle accident. It caused a partial quadriparesis. A posterior cervical fusion was accomplished, and he experienced some improvement in strength and could ambulate with crutches. Eight months after surgery, he had the onset of weakness and loss of temperature sensation in his right hand. A myelogram demonstrated a block at C7. A cervical discectomy and interbody fusion at C7-T1 was accomplished. However, the patient's neurological status continued to deteriorate. A CT scan showed a cyst in the entire cervical cord (Fig. 10.13). The patient refused further surgical intervention and continues to become progressively quadriplegic.

Case 10: Ossification of the Posterior Longitudinal Ligament

This 66-year-old male had a 1-year history of numbness in both hands. The original diagnosis was a carpal tunnel syndrome, but the nerve conduction studies were normal. Physical examination demonstrated a wide-based, unsteady gait and weakness of both arms. Plain films of the cervical spine showed a bony structure in the cervical canal. The myelogram revealed an increased anteroposterior diameter of the cord secondary to ventral cord compression. The CT scan demonstrated that the bone structure was ossification of the posterior longitudinal

ligament and that the cord was being displaced posteriorly by this structure (Figs. 10.14 and 10.15). The patient had a posterior cervical laminectomy from C2–C6 with decompression of the cord. Postoperatively, the patient had significant improvement in his coordination, strength, and gait.

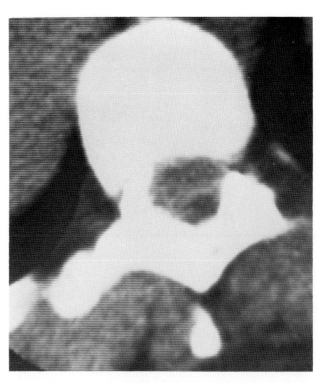

Figure 10.11. Case 7: Syringomyelia. The cord is widened considerably and its substance is of abnormal texture and density. The spinal cord fills the entire bony canal. There is residual Pantopaque in the subarachnoid space.

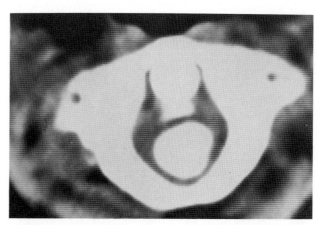

Figure 10.12. Case 8: Ependymoma. Direct needle puncture for metrizamide endomyelography of a large cyst-like chamber in the cervical region in a patient with tumor infiltration of the entire spinal cord. This axial projection shows the contrast filling the cystic and necrotic portion of the tumor.

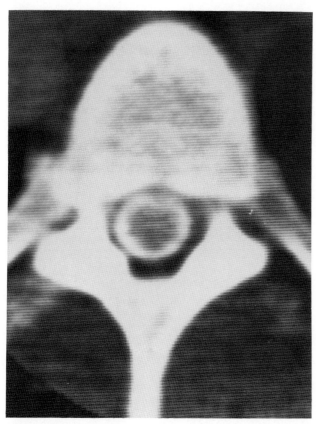

Figure 10.10. Case 6: Arteriovenous Malformation. MCTM shows fusiform swelling of thoracic cord at level of T5 found at surgery to be a focal AVM.

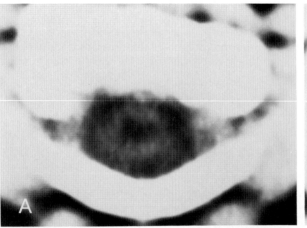 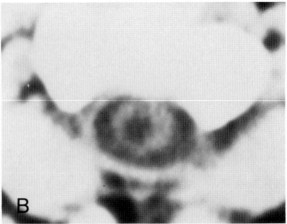

Figure 10.13. Case 9: Post-Traumatic Cyst. Noncontrast CT scans (A and B) at level of C2 show a central area of low density in a patient with previous upper thoracic cord injury and progressive ascending paraplegia.

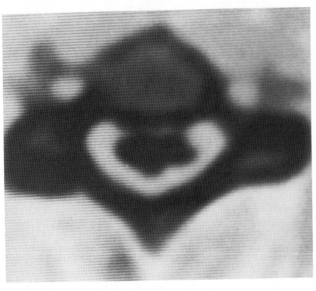 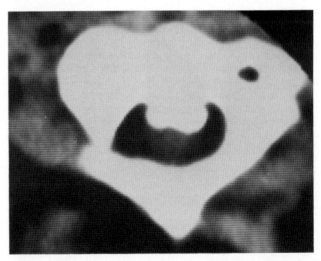

Figure 10.14. Case 10: Ossification of the Posterior Longitudinal Ligament. CT with reversed images at bone settings showing exuberant ossification of the posterior longitudinal ligament in the upper cervical spine which is causing considerable narrowing of the spinal canal.

Figure 10.15. Case 10: Ossification of the Posterior Longitudinal Ligament. CT at a narrow window demonstrating that the spinal cord is being compressed and displaced posteriorly by the ossified posterior longitudinal ligament.

Case 11: Fracture of the Odontoid

This 19-year-old female was involved in a motor vehicle accident. She presented with pain localized to the base of the occiput and a normal physical examination. Cervical spine films and CT showed an odontoid fracture with rotary subluxation of C1 on C2 (Fig. 10.16). The patient had a posterior cervical fusion of C1 and C2 and postoperatively has remained neurologically intact.

Case 12: Laceration of the Cord

This 3-month-old male was born at 30 weeks of gestation by a difficult breech delivery with forceps. The child sustained a fracture of the humerus. He was lethargic with no spontaneous movement of the extremities. After birth,

a myelogram and a MCTM revealed laceration of the cord and avulsion of the brachial plexus bilaterally. The child subsequently was admitted to the hospital with pneumonia and died of a respiratory arrest.

PHYSICAL PRINCIPLES OF FOURTH GENERATION CT

CT is a radiological method in which a large number of x-ray attenuation measurements are generated by a precise geometric scanning device and transformed by advanced computer programs into an accurate cross-sectional anatomical image that can be interpreted visually. As in any other conventional geometric unit, CT irradiates sectional anatomy with a moving x-ray tube assembly mounted in a gantry which rotates around the patient

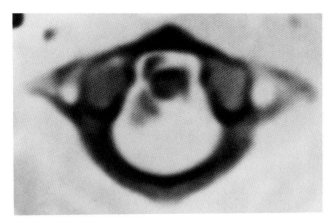

Figure 10.16. Case 11: Fracture. CT of odontoid with reversed images at bone settings shows fracture, rotary subluxation of C1 on C2, and bone fragments, displaced into the spinal canal.

lying in an axial plane. As the tube rotates, an x-ray beam is generated. The beam is measured by an array of detectors. The CT computer system then assigns spatial orientation to each of these measurements and stores them into the computer memory. An axial tomographic section is obtained from the stored information. Furthermore, an entire set of axial images can be assembled into "stacks" of data which can be further "reformatted" into sagittal (lateral), coronal (frontal), or oblique projections or reconstructions (5, 6).

The method of data acquisition in a fourth generation CT scan can be illustrated as follows: an x-ray tube of conventional design is energized through a potential difference in the range of 100–140 KVP with a tube current between 5 MA and 200 MA. The beam of photons is collimated to a fan-shaped geometry. This beam crosses the patient transversely and after further collimation, the portion of the beam which exits from the patient impinges upon a scintillation detector composed of a luminiscent Bismuth Germinate crystal optically coupled to a photomultiplier tube. As the x-ray photons hit the crystals, they scintillate or give off photons of visible light which are detected further by a photomultiplier tube capable of converting this signal into direct current. The computer system then amplifies the signal, converts it from analog to digital form, and stores it into its memory. The relative brightness at a given point in the final image reflects the degree of x-ray absorption by the sample tissue (6). A brief review of the evolution of the four generations of CT scanners may be of interest to the reader.

The first generation CT technology required a single roentgen tube to generate a pencil-shaped beam collimated to a rectangle 3.0 × 3.0 mm in width and about 13 mm long. The beam passed through the patient and was recorded by a crystal detector. The x-ray tube-detector assembly was then translated across the object under examination to complete a scan. After each scan, the assembly rotated 1° about a perpendicular axis in order to project another scan, and each produced 160 readings

(projection profiles). This process was repeated for 180° so that a sufficient number of projections (160 × 180 = 26,800) were recorded. Because both the x-ray tube and the detector moved in this scanner, scan times were very slow, averaging 4–5 minutes. As a result, motion artifacts due to patient movements produced a marked degradation of the final image (6–8).

The second generation in scanning hardware resulted from the necessity to reduce scanning time for each cross-section. The second generation scanner reduced scanning time to about 15–20 seconds, which is about the limit of breathholding time for a healthy individual. This improvement in scanning efficiency was due largely to the utilization of a narrow fan-shaped beam and an increased number of detectors (10–30) and increased rotation to 10° rather than 1°, yet keeping the "rotate-translate" technology of the first generation system. The faster scanning times in the second generation system also were associated with more rapid computation of data aiding patient thruput and making possible body scanning (6, 8).

The introduction of pure rotary scanners gave rise to a third generation of CT systems. Rotary motion scanners produce an image of higher quality (contrast plus spatial resolution) than the older systems. The third generation system utilizes a much wider fan beam and a large array of detectors. Both the x-ray source and the xenon gas detectors rotate synchronously 180 or 360° around the patient, thus, reducing scanning time to about 4–10 seconds. Moreover, this scanner is able to angle the gantry, therefore, allowing a wider range of anatomical planes to be examined. The software improvements accompanying this system included better capabilities for sagittal and coronal reconstructions. Patient thruput also was improved somewhat due to the availability of scout views (planar densitograph) which allow for better and more precise localization of scanning planes (5, 8).

The fourth generation scanning system relies upon a rotary x-ray source and a stationary array of 600 Bismuth Germinate detectors which are fixed in the gantry. The x-ray source emits a collimated fan-shaped beam while rotating as much as 398° within the gantry. As it rotates, each detector views the x-ray as it passes through the detector's field of view (detector fan) which corresponds to the scan field diameter. Because the patient does not completely fill the scan field diameter, the x-ray source is seen by each detector initially through empty space (air), followed by the cross-section of the body and finally again through air. Therefore, this system is capable of calibrating itself relative to the known constant density of air, before and after the collection of data from the object under examination. Via these calibration values, each detector assembly (crystal plus photomultiplier and analog circuits) is monitored. Thus, each data profile is normalized by computer software minimizing any possible attenuation drift. This innovation is termed "Constant Calibration."

DISCUSSION

The spinal cord has proved a difficult target for CT scanning with early generation models. With the evolution of high-resolution technology, the cord may be studied accurately and reliably. In our opinion, the fourth generation technology represents the most sophisticated CT scanning system to date and provides the most reliable and precise images of the spinal cord. Routine standard physical measurements of spatial and contrast resolution comparing third and fourth generation machines are not impressive. The superiority of the fourth generation system is probably multifactorial. It is related to such factors as short exposure time, decreased noise, linearity of CT numbers, improved edge enhancement, and software updates such as special algorithms that maximize contrast resolution (8–10). Another attraction of fourth generation technology is speed and convenience of the system to manipulate data such as instant acquisition of coronal and sagittal reconstructions and instant updates of the original reconstruction.

The spinal cord is imaged quite accurately in the cervical spine with fourth generation CT technology. Its size and shape often can be determined without the assistance of artificial contrast agents, e.g., metrizamide (Fig. 10.17). High-resolution CT reveals that the cervical cord is round at C1–C2 and oval in the lower cervical spine. It shows that its widest diameter is at about C6 but that the cervical enlargement extends from approximately C3–4 to T2.

CT also shows that the thoracic cord is smaller and more round in configuration than the cervical cord and that it progressively decreases in size until about the T9 level. It demonstrates that from approximately T9–T12 the cord widens again because of the lumbosacral cord enlargement which is associated with innervation of the lower extremities. In contrast to the cervical cord, however, the thoracic cord is not reliably imaged on a plain CT scan. The CT computer has more difficulty in depicting a concise image of the thoracic cord. Intrathecal metrizamide is needed before an accurate assessment of the size and shape of the thoracic spinal cord can be made.

In addition to determining the size and shape of the spinal cord, fourth generation CT technology also can assess its texture and density. The texture and density (attenuation coefficient) of the spinal cord can be evaluated best on a noncontrast CT scan. The presence of metrizamide in the subarachnoid space causes enough "computer overshoot" so that the cord appears homogeneous on a MCTM when it may not be.

Because CT can assess the size, shape, and texture of the spinal cord, it can detect pathological conditions which affect it. For example, because CT can recognize cord enlargement, it can discern cord neoplasms (Fig. 10.1). Similarly, when the cord is small, it can diagnose cord atrophy. After trauma, CT can detect cord swelling, intramedullary hemorrhage, and even cord laceration. CT also can identify hypodense lesions within the cord, such as syringomyelia and post-traumatic cord cysts (Figs. 10.4 and 10.13). After a terminal ventriculostomy or stint placement for permanent cyst decompression (Figs. 10.2 and 10.3) CT can discern irregularity of the spinal cord.

CT's evaluation of the spinal cord, however, may be hindered occasionally by various artifacts which degrade the CT image. Residual Pantopaque often will present as a white area with black periphery. This is due to overshoot which implies a change in attenuation so high that it cannot be handled by the computer. A "herring-bone" pattern presents over the whole image if the shoulder is scanned with the same technical factors employed for the neck. If the headrest is not removed, there are characteristic artifacts seen in the upper cervical spine. Dental fillings may be a source of streak artifacts (Fig. 10.18). The use of an algorithm intended for high spatial resolution produces a "grainy" texture to the image due to the inherent noise. Bone, metal, and even high concentrations of metrizamide cause artifacts which might be considered computer overshoot. This is seen frequently in the spinal cord behind the odontoid process in normal patients. The artifact looks like a small intramedullary cyst (Fig. 10.19). There are sometimes artifacts at the level of C1 and the foramen magnum (Fig. 10.20) and at the shoulder which must be discounted which look like large black bands and

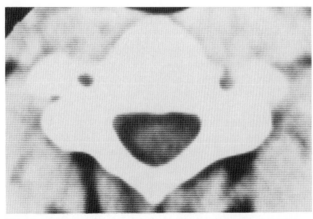

Figure 10.17. Noncontrast CT showing normal size of lower cervical cord.

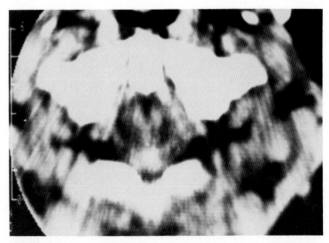

Figure 10.18. Streak artifacts at level of C1 caused by dental fillings and large triangular artifact posterior to odontoid caused by computer overshoot.

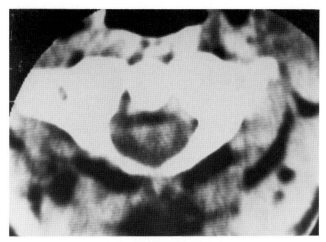

Figure 10.19.   Noncontrast CT at C1 showing frequent artifact that simulates a small low density syrinx.

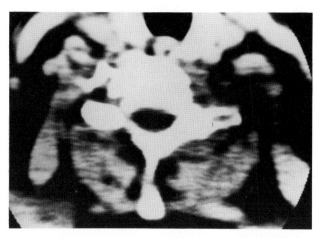

Figure 10.21.   Noncontrast CT at level of shoulder with large black artifacts obscuring all detail of the intraspinal contents.

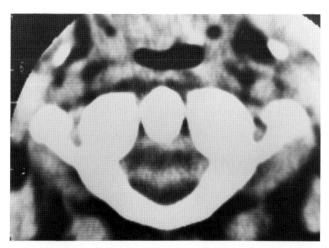

Figure 10.20.   Noncontrast CT at level of C1 and the foramen magnum showing band-like artifacts that degrade the image of the spinal cord.

are due to computer overshoot (Fig. 10.21).

Because artifacts degrade the CT image, caution must be used in evaluating the spinal cord when they are present. Caution also must be employed in determining the appropriateness of a particular CT examination. Because there are values and limitations to each type of CT study, it is important to chose the procedure which will evaluate a particular type of spinal pathology best. For example, plain high-resolution CT can assess adequately the size and configuration of the cervical spinal cord. It also can detect such entities as spinal stenosis, fractures, bony anomalies, ossification of the posterior longitudinal ligament, degenerative joint disease, and lumbar disc herniations. However, it cannot detect certain normal structures such as the dentate ligaments, the septum posticum, and the thoracic cord.

It, therefore, is useful to employ intrathecal metrizamide to evaluate the spinal cord and to detect certain cord lesions. Placing the window level between the mean density of the cord and the cerebrospinal fluid space affords the most accurate presentation of cord size as measured in phantom models. Varying window width has little or no effect on the accuracy of cord measurements. Wider window settings, however, provide a more aesthetic image but decreased contrast resolution (12).

It often is necessary to do the MCTM after a standard myelogram so as to avoid two separate invasive procedures. The amount of contrast needed for a conventional metrizamide myelogram greatly exceeds the optimal dosage for MCTM. Sequential or delayed scanning is then mandatory to demonstrate small lesions or to avoid computer artifacts because high volume contrast increases the partial volume phenomenon (13). As little as 5 ml of 170 mg %/ml I may be more than adequate for a MCTM whereas some neuroradiologists may use from 5–16 ml of metrizamide at 170–300 mg I/ml for routine myelograms. Frequently, screening thoracic myelography is not done in some institutions in the supine position with large volumes of contrast. Therefore, many small lesions can be missed in the thoracic canal and remain undiagnosed until they become so large that they obstruct the canal (Case 4). However, if MCTM is employed, these lesions can be detected when they are small. MCTM also can identify structures not visible on conventional myelography such as pronounced median fissures, dentate ligaments, and the septum posticum.

MCTM is the procedure of choice with a combination of plain films for evaluation of spinal dysraphism in infants and children (14). It provides accurate delineation of complex bony abnormalities, displays the relationship of associated intraspinal and paraspinal masses to the cord, and visualizes the cord (or cords) itself (Figs. 10.7–10.9) (15). MCTM is an excellent means of diagnosing focal fusiform intramedullary enlargement of the cord often missed on routine myelography (Case 4). In our series, there was a case of a focal AVM (Fig. 10.10), a focal transverse myelitis, and a focal metastasis in the thoracic cord (Fig. 10.6) not appreciated by conventional myelography but demonstrated on MCTM.

MCTM is also the best radiographic study to completely evaluate syringomyelia and post-traumatic cord cysts. Although plain high-resolution CT can detect some hypodensities within the spinal cord, it may not delineate the entire extent of the syringomyelic cavities and post-traumatic cord cysts. In contrast, because metrizamide can enter a syrinx or a cyst, a delayed MCTM can demonstrate the longitudinal extent of these lesions without the use of direct cyst puncture. In post-traumatic syrinxes, lesions which may develop years after focal cord injury and which may cause progressive neurological deficits (16), also can determine whether there are one or more cysts. The demonstration during metrizamide CT scanning of syrinx cavities or cord cysts is especially important because conventional myelography may show in a significant number of patients only normal sized cords (17). Another advantage to metrizamide CT scanning is that it may be able to determine whether there is a communication with the fourth ventricle and syringohydromyelia. This information is important to the neurosurgeon because a terminal ventriculostomy may be considered if there is no connection to the fourth ventricle whereas a ventriculoatrial shunt may be employed if there is a communicating hydrocephalus and a communication with the fourth ventricle.

In addition to MCTM there are other types of enhanced CT scans of the spine which can be used to evaluate certain spinal lesions. Intravenous contrast enhancement of the cord with diatriazoate and iothalamate compounds has been recommended by some authors to separate vascular from avascular lesions. Some researchers even employ spinal angiography. Xenon enhancement has even been tested by Pullicino and his associates (18). Xenon may increase the attenuation of the cord substance sufficiently to improve detection of intramedullary cysts. Coin et al. (19) reported that acute lesions of multiple sclerosis are seen as low or isodense lesions which enhance with intravenous contrast agents. In our experience, however, the use of such intravenous or intra-arterial agents to enhance the cord plays a minor role in the work-up of the usual patient with a suspected spinal cord lesion and probably will be limited to selected, known lesions where there are special considerations such as the feasibility of therapeutic embolization techniques for AVMs.

CONCLUSION

The workup of neuroradiological problems changes with the advent of new technology. Fourth generation CT scanning offers a new geometry capable of improved imaging of the spinal cord. The use of intrathecal contrast agents is not required in all cases because of the reliability of the newer systems. Each examination must be custom tailored for the suspected disorder when possible. This can afford greater contrast resolution and may eliminate the need for traditional parts of the work-up such as myelography. A variety of technical hardware and soft-

ware options are available to the technologist depending on the requirements of the individual case. Tissue homogenicity of the cord is best visualized without the use of metrizamide. There are several techniques such as Xenon enhancement which are presently primarily at an experimental state of development. A thorough examination of the cord is possible in the average clinical setting with the usual materials and methods if a fourth generation scanner is available. The geometry of the CT scanner has improved considerably in the last decade. The first generation geometry was designed for the study of the brain, but now the fourth generation system can image more difficult targets such as the spinal cord and lumbar discs.

References

1. Thijssen HOM, Keyser A, Horstink MWM, et al: Morphology of the cervical spinal cord on computed myelography. *Neuroradiology* 18:57–62, 1979.
2. Nakagawa H, Huang YP, Malis LI, et al: Computed tomography of intraspinal and paraspinal neoplasms. *J Comput Assist Tomogr* 1:377–390, 1977.
3. Ethier R, King DG, Melancon D, et al: Development of high resolution computed tomography of the spinal cord. *J Comput Assist Tomogr* 3:433–438, 1979.
4. McCullough EC, Payne JT, Baker HL, et al: Performance evaluation and quality assurance of computed tomography scanners, with illustrations from EMI, ACTA, and Delta scanners. *Radiology* 120:173–188, 1976.
5. Raskin SP: Introduction to computed tomography of the lumbar spine. *Orthopaedics* 3:1011–1023, 1980.
6. Weisberg LA, Nice CM, Katz M: *Cerebral Computed Tomography*. Philadelphia, WB Saunders, 1978, pp. 10–28.
7. Ter-Pogossian MM: Basic principles of computed axial tomography. *Semin Nucl Med* 7:109–127, 1977.
8. Joseph PM: The influence of gantry geometry on aliasing and other geometry dependent errors. *IEEE Trans Nucl Sci* NS-27:1104–1111, 1980.
9. Joseph PM, Spital RD, Stockham CD: The effects of sampling on CT images. *Comput Tomogr* 4:189–206, 1980.
10. Roub LW, Drayer BP: Spinal computed tomography: limitations and applications. *AJR* 133:267–273, 1979.
11. van der Tas C: Importance of computer-assisted myelography in diseases affecting the vertebral column. *Diagn Imaging* 48:71–79, 1979.
12. Seibert CE, Barnes JE, Dreisbach JN, et al: Accurate CT measurements of the spinal cord using metrizamide: physical factors. *AJR* 136:777–780, 1981.
13. Arii H, Takahashi M, Tamakawa Y, et al: Metrizamide spinal computed tomography following myelography. *Comput Tomogr* 4:117–125, 1980.
14. James HE, Oliff M: Computed tomography in spinal dysraphism. *J Comput Assist Tomogr* 1:391–397, 1977.
15. Resjö M, Harwood-Nash DC, Fitz CR, et al: Computed tomographic metrizamide myelography in spinal dysraphism in infants and children. *J Comput Assist Tomogr* 2:549–558, 1978.
16. Shannon N, Symon L, Logue V, et al: Clinical features, investigation and treatment of post-traumatic syringomyelia. *J Neurol Neurosurg Psychiatr* 44:35–42, 1981.
17. Bonafe' A, Ethier R, Melancon D, et al: High resolution computed tomography in cervical syringomyelia. *J Comput Assist Tomogr* 4:42–47, 1980.
18. Pullicino P, du Boulay GH, Kendall BE. Xenon enhancement for computed tomography of the spinal cord. *Neuroradiology* 18:63–66, 1979.
19. Coin CG, Hucks-Folliss A. Cervical computed tomography in multiple sclerosis with spinal cord involvement. *J Comput Assist Tomogr* 3:421–422, 1979.

CHAPTER ELEVEN

The Practical Present and the Anticipated Future of Computed Tomography

CHARLES V. BURTON, M.D.*

THE PRACTICAL PRESENT

Innovation in medicine typically has been a process fraught with frustration, grudging acceptance, and a period of abuse of the concept in its initial phase of use. There are those happy occasions when a creative step forward occurs in a political and sociological environment consistent with its consideration and acceptance. W. Konrad Röentgen was fortunate to experience this when he announced his discovery of x-ray in 1896. Ingnaz Philipp Semmelweis encountered the reverse when he showed scientifically that the devastating rampages of puerpual fever could be avoided by the simple act of physicians washing their hands between the autopsy and delivery rooms. Röentgen advanced to acclaim and renown. Semmelweis died in 1865, a broken man in an asylum, never having had the opportunity of seeing his pertinent recommendations being put into use.

We now exist in a political and sociological environment which recognizes the horrendous escalation of health care costs and is attempting (through the continuation of illogical thinking) to extricate itself by persisting in self-destructive policies. As a close observer of the passing scene, the author continues to image the vision of a hunter who has stepped into his own spring trap, and rather than by separating the jaws chooses to amputate his leg. It is amazing to realize that in the United States total health care expenditures are presently about $235 billion ($1059 per capita and 9.3% of Gross National Product) (1). Like the hunter, much of the responsibility for present unnecessary cost rests with government, particularly in the area of unneeded restrictive drug and device regulation, "red tape" and paperwork, and the plague of unmeritorious malpractice claims which have created the practice of "defensive" medicine. In the corporate area, the escalation of product liability cases and associated litigation cases have created a "siege" mentality which has produced much greater cost and dramatically decreased innovation and risk-taking in the marketplace. The other reality is the much-needed move to cost containment. This collision course is only too readily apparent given maintenance of present philosophy. "The key to growth in this era of cost containment and maturing markets will continue to be new technology", believes John M. Ketteringham of Ar-

thur D. Little (2). Whereas certain areas, such as hospital materials management (representing about 42% of the average hospital's budget) will be a target for cutting costs, we certainly can expect future containment of cost for diagnosis and treatment. It is here that technology, particularly CT, digital, ultrasonic, nuclear magnetic resonance (NMR), and positron-emission tomography (PET) imaging may serve as a means to allow better care, at lesser cost, than presently available.

It is healthy occasionally to step aside and reflect on a situation from a different point of view. Biomedical instrumentation in the Soviet Union serves well as this point of reference. Their system inherently limits technological advancement, but is rapidly advancing by copying and emulating technology from other countries. At the same time, this country, in fact, is progressively creating a system which inherently limits technological advancement (3) and is adopting the worst attributes of the Soviet system.

The most dramatic case study of our attempt to suffocate highly valuable and cost-effective new technology in the United States has been the saga of CT scanning. CT was born in England in the 1970s and entered upon the American medical scene in 1973. CT appeared to be "heaven sent" as a scapegoat for designation by health care planners as "expensive and unnecessary new technology" under the provisions of the 1974 Federal Health Planning Act. These planners assumed that their role was to limit and restrict CT and embarked on a program to prove this point (4). Despite this mind-set, CT imaging now has been clearly documented to have established new diagnostic and therapeutic dimensions and also has been cost-effective in this regard. At this time, there has not only been a complete governmental turnaround (prompted in part by lawsuits by patients who were denied this quality of care) but also an awareness of government that they also hold responsibility to "promote" effective health care.

To say that CT has revolutionized the practice of neurosurgery is an understatement. CT has offered more and uniquely different information regarding head anatomy. This information is not only immediately available and noninvasive, but also allows the success of treatment to be monitored in a serial and measurable manner. The inherent information limitations of angiography and air studies caused many patients to require exploratory surgery (particularly in trauma cases). Because of CT the need for this is now quite small. Surgery is now often carried out to address well-localized (and well-appreci-

---

*The author would like to express his personal appreciation to his associates, Drs. Kenneth Heithoff, Charles Ray, Alex Lifson, and Harvey Aaron for their professional assistance and intellectual stimulation in the preparation of this chapter.

215

ated) areas of pathology. CT's imaging capabilities in regard to the accurate diagnosis of brain disease was (despite the opposition of the regulators) quickly appreciated by the medical community (5). This has not been, until recently, true for other body applications when lumbar CT (of the high-resolution soft-tissue differentiation variety) was shown to have a high level of diagnostic and therapeutic potential by Glenn et al. (6), Heithoff (7), Meyer et al. (8), and Burton et al. (9) based on the predictive anatomical studies of Verbiest (10), Crock (11), Farfan (12), Kirkaldy-Willis et al. (13, 14), Epstein et al. (15, 16), Ehni (17), and Choudhury and Taylor (18).

High-resolution CT scanning of the lumbar spine is a particularly pertinent aspect of imaging to focus on because it has brought a poorly understood anatomical structure, the lumbar spine, to objective review and measurement. It has allowed the documentation of disease entities only recently suspected, and has begun to explain why our society has a 25–30% failure rate in back surgery. By allowing an appreciation of lateral spinal stenosis as a pathological entity CT has assisted in identifying it as the major cause of failed back surgery syndrome. The economic import of back pain alone in regard to health care costs is staggering.

It has been estimated that 80% of the population experiences significantly incapacitating low back pain at some time. Back pain alone accounts for 26% of all time lost from work (this can be as high as 46% in the transportation industries). In 1978, the National Safety Council estimated the occurrence of 400,000 disabling occupational back injuries (representing about 20% of all compensable work accidents). By 1979, the figure increased to 460,000, a 15% increase in a single year (20)!

An approximation of the magnitude of the low back problem can be derived from the information that in 1980 the cost of workers' compensation alone to industry in the state of Minnesota was about $500 million. Whereas low back cases represented 30% of the diagnoses, they alone represented *60% of all monies spent* (21).

In 1975, 100 consecutive "failed back surgery cases" from our institution were reviewed. The average patient had experienced 3.6 back operations and 2.8 myelograms and had spent an average of $75,000 in direct medical costs to achieve a totally incapacitated state in which thousands of dollars were being spent annually for continuing medical care and drugs.

Best's Review recently documented a typical failed back surgery case which started in 1976 as an "acute back sprain." After the fourth operative procedure (a fusion) in 1979 the insurance carrier had already expended $89,711 in compensation and medical expenses and was estimating a final liability on their part of $955,880 (20).

The reason why back problems account for such an inordinate share of the health care dollar unquestionably is due to the inefficiency of effective treatment based on accurate diagnosis. As a neurosurgeon whose organization "salvages" over 500 failed back surgery cases each year through the process of comprehensive rehabilitation, this has become painfully evident. A recent interinstitutional

study on failed back surgery patients (19) has shown that of the primary organic reasons for failure of surgery, the presence of unrecognized lateral spinal stenosis (57–58%) was the main reason for failure. Iatrogenic problems such as adhesive arachnoiditis (6–16%) and epidural fibrosis (6–8%) were also contributory. Although most arachnoiditis can be avoided by ceasing to employ iophendylate as a diagnostic medium and epidural fibrosis by the surgical use of full-thickness autogenous fat grafts, lateral spinal stenosis clearly could be addressed surgically if appreciated by lumbar CT scanning. There is little argument at this time that quality high-resolution CT scans beat myelography for accurate lumbar spine diagnosis (22).

When one considers the frustrating waste of health care resources in the low back area at this time, CT emerges not only as an important objective noninvasive tool, but it also emerges as a potential means of substantially *decreasing* health care costs in this area while also decreasing much human suffering.

With experience gained through performing over 16,000 lumbar CT scans since 1977 at our institution (7), it seems clear that this test will become the dominant means of documenting pathology and treatment modalities involving the lumbar spine in the future. It also is likely that it will serve as an effective means of identifying, in asymptomatic individuals, their future *risk* of having problems. For a society unduly focused on "treatment," "prevention" represents a new and *very* cost-effective new vista.

ADDITIONAL CONSIDERATIONS REGARDING CT

CT is not inexpensive: The range of cost seems to be between $250–1000 per study, depending more on geographic location than quality. While radiation is significant, it is usually less than a cerebral arteriogram or lumbar myelogram. At our institution, the measured skin dose for a lumbar scan is about 2.2 Rads. As in any new technology we must concern ourselves with potential abuse. There is quite simply a great deal of poor-quality imaging being passed off as high state-of-the-art technology. Perhaps this is one of the prices that must be paid for advancement, but it could be minimized by professional action.

At this point in time, CT imaging is capable of producing anatomical data never before seen. The question must be asked as to whether the information being presented is optimal for observer comprehension. New data reconstruction techniques and two- and three-dimensional display systems are now being pioneered (23, 24).

At the Lawrence Livermore National Laboratory, the present research program with x-ray lasers (the x-raser) may provide an exciting new means of producing holographic biological images (25).

When one combines these advances with the ability to serially monitor patients, we can expect an ever-heightened understanding of the natural history of the disease entities being observed.

THE FUTURE

A recent science fiction film took place on a futuristic mining community located on Io, a moon of Jupiter. The medical dispensary scene showed a trauma victim being wheeled into a tube containing rotating lights and being scanned in toto. Within moments, a comprehensive viewing of bones and soft tissues was initiated on a screen. A computer also analyzed a blood sample for all usual and unusual substances.

I do not expect to see the colonization of Io in my lifetime, but I fully expect to see imaging and computer analysis of this type and even more sophisticated applications. In my mind, the individual will lay "spread-eagled" on the white surface of a table top. Imaging will be performed by interaction between nonionizing radiation and electromagnetic fields. In this set-up, the imager would not only survey bones, organs, and other soft tissues, but also would assess dynamic functions such as cardiopulmonary, peripheral blood flow, etc., as well as provide blood cell and chemistry readout with tissue metabolic determinations. These data will be monitored by computer to compare normal values, identify variations present, and *predict* potential problems. All effort ultimately would be directed toward prevention rather than treatment. With the exception of traumatic injury, most other potential disease (infectious already eliminated by inoculation) could be identified and prevented. Health care would be of a minor concern as most needs would have been anticipated and avoided. The greatest future frustration would belong to government trying to match Social Security benefits to dramatically lengthened longevity.

Is there a realistic expectation that the scenario predicted can occur? In regard to the computer, Dr. Carl Sagan [26] recalled that in 1960 the typical processor boasted about 100 active components/cm³; this is now 10 million components/cm³, and he expects density to increase another thousand-fold by 1990. While density is now doubling about every 14 months, the *cost* of circuitry is being halved every 2 years. This trend also is present on the random-access memory front, where it is now conceivable that the entire contents of a University Medical Library can be available on a single hard computer disc. The amount of information storage possible combined with rapid access may well be a means by which human beings will potentiate the extremely low usage of the 20 billion intracranial neurons with which we all start life.

Although CT as we know it has far from reached its zenith, its inherent limitations for technical advancement and its present need for ionizing radiation remove it as the only contender in the imaging field by the futurist. This author believes that the greatest potential lies in a marriage of CT with NMR and an alliance, to some degree, with a modification of PET.

Although the true potential of PET is not limited to only radioactive substances, its present use requires this. By "tagging" substances and following their fate in the body through isotope decay monitoring, it has shed new light on many physiological processes which could not be studied as effectively in any other way. With the release of a positive electron (positron) during decay, there is almost immediate combination with an electron and mutual annihilation by the emission of two divergent gamma rays which are recorded by a circular array of detectors [27]. PET remains an exciting and expensive research tool at this time, awaiting technology to potentiate its value.

NMR has been a well-recognized means for chemists to determine molecular structure for many years. In the past 10 years, efforts have been made to apply it to body imaging, and whereas NMR is only now coming into reasonable clinical use, its vistas seem theoretically to be unlimited and, for this reason, the modality deserves careful consideration. In NMR, ionizing radiation is replaced by high-intensity electromagnetic fields used to align molecular atomic nuclei to this field. All nuclei with an odd number of protons or neutrons act like small magnets, and when influenced by a strong direct current magnetic field, align themselves with the field and spin (precess) in this field at a resonant frequency related to the strength of the applied field. This axis of rotation can be flipped or turned around with imposed alternating magnetic fields (radio waves) of exact energies related to the magnetic field at the nucleus and a NMR signal produced. In returning to the normal state, a flipped nucleus can radiate back these radio waves or dissipate the energy thermally by coupling it to paramagnetic atoms in surrounding tissue. The latter property allows the observation of a NMR absorption spectrum for an object. Because hydrogen is the most abundant odd mass number nucleus in animals, NMR is ideally suited to map hydrogen densities [28] (as opposed to x-ray which reflects differences in electron densities). It is not, however, theoretically limited to producing similar images on protons alone, and recent work with other nuclei clearly demonstrate the potential for the dynamic detailed imaging of the *physiological* state of an organ or body part [29]. When one recognizes that NMR can provide a dynamic monitoring of physiochemical phenomena on a continuing basis and that CT provides a static image of anatomical tissue density differences, the complementary nature of this information becomes evident.

It used to be that the press reported the news and did not create it. The basic idea is a good one and is applicable to imaging. The technique is charged with reporting the status of the human body and not changing it in the process. The latter concern is still a major one because our true understanding of the biological effects of ionizing radiation and high-intensity magnetic fields is primitive.

NMR is unlikely to threaten CT in the near future. Its high-resolution and technical limitations (at this time) and high cost ($2,000,000 to $3,000,000 per unit) [30] will see to that. It is, however, a veritable "Pandora's Box" of possibilities leading ultimately to profound potential changes in the philosophies and practice of medicine as we now know it. Future medical students may do well to recognize that they will be entering a changed world in which their technical knowledge may very well be the means of achieving their value to our society.

References

1. Gemple PA: Arthur D. Little Health Impact Study. Quoted in *Ortho Today* Vol. 2, 1981.
2. Ketteringham JM: Arthur D. Little Health Impact Study. Quoted in *Ortho Today* Vol. 2, 1981.
3. Burton C, Gardner RM: Biomedical instrumentation in the Soviet Union. *Med Instrum* 11:124–126, 1977.
4. Burton CV: Neuroradiology and computerized tomographic scanning. In Laufman H: *Hospital Special-Care Facilities* New York, Academic Press, 1981.
5. French BN, Maass L: Revolution in neurodiagnosis: Computed tomography of the brain. *J West Med* 127:231–4, 1977.
6. Glenn WV Jr., Rhodes ML, Altschuler EM, et al: Multiplanar display computerized body tomography applications in the lumbar spine. *Spine* 4:282–352, 1979.
7. Heithoff KB: High-resolution computed tomography of the lumbar spine. *Postgrad Med* 70:193–213, 1981.
8. Meyer GA, Haughton VM, Williams AL: Diagnosis of herniated lumbar disc with computed tomography. *N Engl J Med* 301:1166–1167, 1979.
9. Burton CV, Heithoff KB, Kirkaldy-Willis W, et al: Computed tomographic scanning and the lumbar spine: Part II: Clinical considerations. *Spine* 4:356–363, 1979.
10. Verbiest H: A radicular syndrome from developmental narrowing of the lumbar vertebral canal. *J Bone Joint Surg* 36:230–237, 1954.
11. Crock HV: Isolated lumbar disc resorption as a cause of nerve root canal stenosis. *Clin Orthop* 115:109–115, 1976.
12. Farfan HF: Pathologic changes with intervertebral joint rotational instability in the rabbit. *Can J Surg* 14:71–79, 1971.
13. Kirkaldy-Willis WH, Paine KWE, Cachoix J et al: Lumbar spinal stenosis. *Clin Orthop* 99:30–50, 1974.
14. Kirkaldy-Willis WH, McIvor GWD: Symposium: Spinal stenosis. *Clin Orthop* 115:1–144, 1976.
15. Epstein JA, Epstein BS, Rosenthal AD, et al: Sciatica caused by nerve root entrapment in the lateral recess: The superior facet syndrome. *J. Neurosurg* 36:484–489, 1972.
16. Epstein JA, Epstein BS, Lavine LS, et al: Lumbar nerve root compression at the intervertebral foramina caused by arthritis of the posterior facets. *J Neurosurg* 39:362–369, 1973.
17. Ehni G: Significance of the small lumbar spinal canal: Cauda equina compression syndromes due to spondylolysis. Parts 1–4. *J Neurosurg* 31:490–512, 1969.
18. Choudhury AR, Taylor JC: Occult lumbar spinal stenosis. *J Neurol Neurosurg Psychiatry* 40:506–510, 1977.
19. Burton CV, Kirkaldy-Willis WH, Yong-Hing K, et al: Causes of failure of surgery on the lumbar spine. *Clin Orthop* 157:191–9, 1981.
20. Antonakes JA: Claims cost of low back pain. In: *Best's Review* (Property/Casualty Insurance Edition) 82:36–129, 1981.
21. Burton CV: Conservative management of low back pain. *Postgrad Med* 70:168–183, 1981.
22. Melamed JL: CT beats myelography for lumbar spine diagnoses. *JAMA* 246:22,1981.
23. Glenn WV: Image generation and display techniques for CT scan data: Thin transverse and reconstructed coronal and sagittal planes. *Invest Radiol* 10:403, 1975.
24. Glenn WV: Further investigation and initial clinical use of advanced CT display capability. *Invest Radiol* 10:479, 1975.
25. Robinson AL: X-ray holography experiment planned. *Science* 215:488–490, 1982.
26. Sagan C: Quoted in *Computerworld*, March 30, 1981, p. 37.
27. Ter-Pogossian MM, Raichle ME, Sobel BE: Positron-emission tomography. *Sci Am* 243:171–181, 1980.
28. Crooks LE, Grover TP, Kaufman L, et al: Tomographic imaging with nuclear magnetic resonance. *Invest Radiol* 13:63–66, 1978.
29. Marx JL: NMR opens a new window into the body. *Science* 210:302–305, 1980.
30. Reported in *Radiology Today* 3:1, 1981.

C. THE DIAGNOSTIC CAPABILITIES OF METRIZAMIDE COMPUTED TOMOGRAPHY

CHAPTER TWELVE

Computed Tomography of the Spine with Metrizamide

MOKHTAR GADO, M.D., FRED HODGES III, M.D., and JASH PATEL, M.D.

INTRODUCTION

The most important advance in CT of the spine was the improvement in spatial resolution of the CT image with preservation of contrast discrimination allowing the visualization of soft tissues as well as bony structures. It, therefore, is possible to outline the dural sac distinct from the surrounding low-density epidural fat. It also is possible to visualize the nerve root and ganglion in the foramen as well as the borders of the intervertebral disc and the ligamenta flava.

However, because of the limited inherent contrast between the cord or nerve roots on the one hand and the cerebrospinal fluid (CSF) on the other hand, visualization of intradural structures without intrathecal contrast material has been limited by the relative size of the cord or cauda equina roots to the size of the surrounding CSF space. For example, at the level of the craniocervical junction, the abundance of the CSF space in relation to the small size of the cord enables us to visualize that part of the cord consistently by plain CT without intrathecal contrast material (Fig. 12.1A). On the other hand, in the lower cervical and in the thoracic region, the visualization of the spinal cord by plain CT is not achieved with the same consistency (Fig. 12.1B). Furthermore, in the lumbar region, the roots of the cauda equina rarely are visualized on plain CT. Opacification of the CSF by a water-soluble iodinated contrast material results in enhancing the contrast between the CSF and the cord or roots, and enhances the visualization of all these intradural structures (Fig. 12.1C and D). In addition, the outer border of the contrast column determines the configuration of the dural sac and enables us to determine the size and shape of the dural sac. Furthermore, the space between the contrast column and the bony spinal canal appears as a negative space which represents the epidural space. The size and shape of this space is a valuable observation in radiological diagnosis.

Metrizamide CT (MTZ/CT) may be referred to as CT myelography as distinct from conventional myelography. CT metrizamide myelography has the advantage over conventional myelography in two respects: 1. A smaller dose of metrizamide produces on CT a density sufficient to obtain a diagnostic image, unobtainable by conventional myelography unless a much higher concentration

is used. 2. The cross-sectional display which is an inherent feature of the CT image provides, in many instances, the clues to a diagnosis that could not be made by the projections of conventional myelography.

Technique

PUNCTURE

In the vast majority of the cases, MTZ/CT myelography can be obtained by lumbar puncture. We believe that the lateral cervical puncture should be reserved to those cases in which complete block in the spinal canal prevents the arrival of contrast material from the site of the lumbar puncture to a region above the level of the block. The lumbar puncture is performed under fluoroscopic control with the patient in the prone position as in conventional myelography. In those cases in which a cervical lateral puncture is required, the patient may be in the prone position, to allow pooling of the contrast material in the cervical region, and the puncture is performed under fluoroscopic control using a horizontal x-ray beam. If pooling of the contrast material in the cervical region is not required, the patient may be kept in the lateral decubitus position and the puncture is performed under fluoroscopic control using the vertical beam with the x-ray table tilted to allow gravitation of the contrast material away from the craniocervical junction, toward the region of interest.

INJECTION OF CONTRAST MATERIAL

It is advisable to inject the contrast material under fluoroscopic control to ascertain the intra-arachnoid location of the injected matrial. Extra-arachnoid contrast material has a characteristic appearance on CT which shows a radiodense rim surrounding the cauda equina (Fig. 12.2). Metrizamide in a concentration of 170 mg/ml and a volume of 7 ml is adequate for CT myelography. If the examination is limited to the lumbar region, the contrast material is injected with the table tilted to allow gravitation of the contrast column to the bottom of the dural sac. After the needle is removed, the table is tilted in the opposite direction to allow the spreading of the contrast material up to the thoracolumbar junction. The patient should be kept in the prone position while being transferred to the CT suite. At the time of CT scanning,

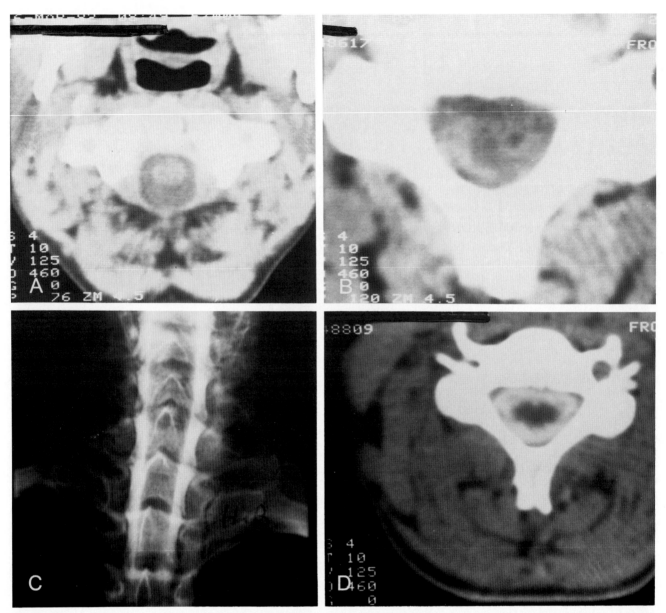

Figure 12.1. The value of MTZ/CT. A. Plain CT at the level C1–2. Th small size of the cord in relation to the surrounding subarachnoid space allows good visualization of this part without contrast material. B. In the lower cervical region, the larger size of the cord in relation to the surrounding CSF may result in poor visualization. In this case, the appearance suggested swelling of the cord and nonuniformity of its density (false-positive). C. AP view of a metrizamide myelogram shows normal appearance of the cord and subarachnoid space. D. MTZ/CT of the lower cervical region shows normal appearance of the cord. The findings on plain CT were artifacts caused by the small size of the subarachnoid space and the relatively large size of the cord.

the patient is turned in the supine position to allow mixing of the contrast material and avoid layering.

For examination of the thoracic region, the patient is kept in the decubitus position while tilting the table to allow the contrast material to flow from the lumbar region to the thoracic region. The patient then is turned supine. This allows the contrast material to pool in the hollow of the thoracic spinal curvature. The patient should be kept in the supine position while being transferred to the CT

suite. At the time of CT scanning, the patient is turned prone and then supine to allow mixing of the contrast column and avoid layering, as mentioned above.

For examination of the cervical region, the table is tilted "head down" before injection is started. The injected contrast material, thus, will gravitate to the cervical region. The head of the patient should be kept extended and supported by soft pads to allow pooling of the contrast column in the cervical curvature. After injection, the table

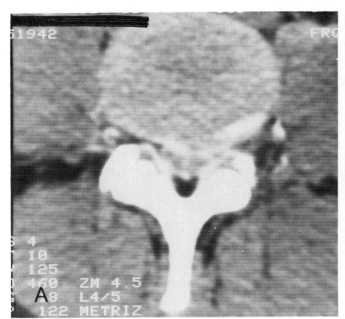 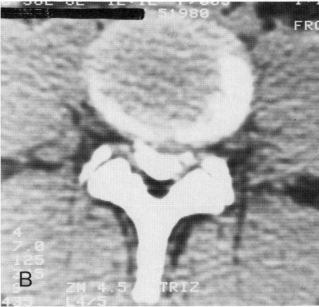

Figure 12.2. Subdural injection of contrast material. A. Extra arachnoid injection. The contrast material in the subdural space follows precisely the contour of the dural sac and is surrounded with epidural fat. Within this rim of enhancement, the contents of the dural sac contain no metrizamide. The portion of contrast material in the epidural space is seen lining the anterior surface of the ligamentum flavum and also in the fat in the foramina bilaterally. B. Repeat injection on the next day. The contrast material was delivered successfully into the subarachnoid space. There is no trace of the water-soluble contrast material in the extra-arachnoid spaces from the previous injection. This is an advantage to the use of water-soluble media.

is returned to the horizontal position. The patient should be kept in the prone position while being transferred to the CT suite. At the time of CT scanning, the patient will be turned supine and this will allow mixing of the contrast column and avoid layering as mentioned above.

SCANNING

Contiguous 4-mm thick slices are obtained without overlap or with 1-mm overlap. Alternative methods include 2-mm thick contiguous slices or 5-mm thick slices with 2-mm overlapping. When the contrast density is high enough, one may resort to alternative methods of image processing which provide edge enhancing. Such methods show sharp definition of the borders of the structures of the nervous system appearing as negative shadows within the contrast column.

Reformatting of the images in the sagittal and coronal projections are most helpful in determining the degree of encroachment upon the cord or the cauda equina by extradural or intradural lesions. At the craniocervical junction, reformatting is indispensable in demonstrating the relationship of the ectopic tonsils to the junction between the cord and medulla.

SIDE EFFECTS

Unlike plain CT, MTZ/CT myelography is an invasive technique. Side effects may occur in patients who have history of a seizure disorder or allergy to iodinated contrast material. Injection of metrizamide in the subarachnoid space may cause headache, nausea and vomiting, backache, and muscle spasms (1).

Table 12.1.
Normal CT Spinal Cord Measurements in mm

Level	Transverse	Sagittal
C1	8–12	6–8
C5	12–15	5–7
C7	7–10	6–8
T1 through T10	7–9	5–7

Less common complications are a confusional state or rarely a generalized seizure. The likelihood of these side effects is reduced by using the low concentration mentioned above.

Normal Anatomy

THE SPINAL CORD

The spinal cord extends from the foramen magnum down to the level L1–2. The size and shape of the cord varies from one region to the other. The absolute measurements of the anteroposterior (AP) and transverse diameters are affected strongly by the window level or centerpoint of the window setting on the scanner. Setting the level one-half way between the value of the metrizamide-enhanced CSF and the value of the cord substance results in apparently accurate measurements by ruler or by computer software (2). There are some useful generalizations regarding measurements by CT in adults (Table 12.1). The cervical cord is fairly constant in its AP diameter from C1 to C7 measuring 6–8 mm, slightly less in the midcervical region (corrected for variable enlargement or

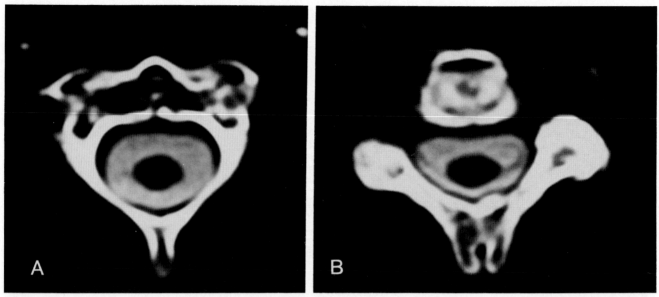

Figure 12.3. A, B. Normal MTZ/CT. In the upper cervical region, the size of the cord is small in relation to the surrounding subarachnoid space. The cord appears rounded or slightly oval in configuration. The dorsal and ventral roots may be visualized extending from the cord to the lateral corners of the subarachnoid space.

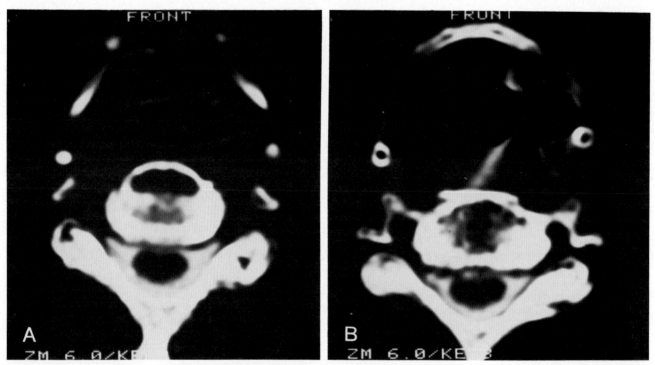

Figure 12.4. A, B. Normal MTZ/CT. At the level of the cervical enlargement of the cord, there is an increase in the AP and lateral diameters of the cord. The anterior midline fissure of the cord is obvious. The root sheath extends into the foramen and is visualized as a horizontal extension of the subarachnoid space.

minification produced by the imaging system). The corrected transverse diameter is 8–11 mm at the level of C1 (Fig. 12.3) and 7–10 mm at C7, T1 (Fig. 12.5). It widens gradually to a maximum of 12–15 mm at the level of C5

(Fig. 12.4).

The thoracic cord is slightly ovoid. Its sagittal diameter is slightly less than the transverse diameter. It gently narrows from T1 to T7 (Fig. 12.6) and becomes then

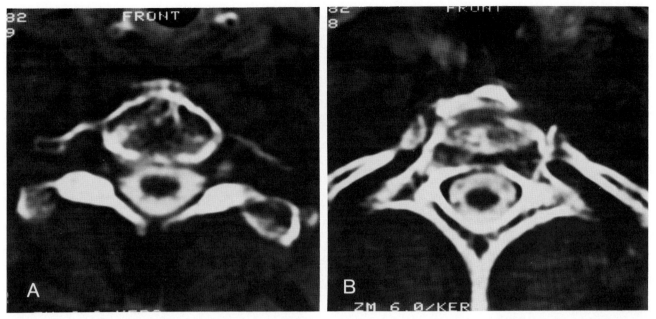

Figure 12.5. A, B. Normal MTZ/CT. At the cervicothoracic junction, the cord becomes smaller in size in relation to the surrounding subarachnoid space.

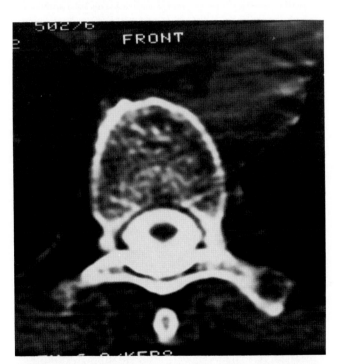

Figure 12.6. Normal MTZ/CT. In the midthoracic region, the cord is at its smallest size.

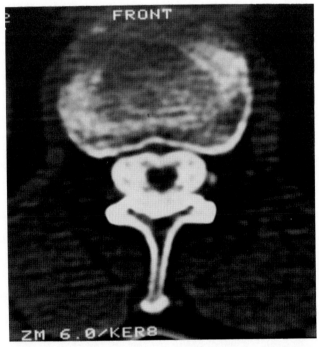

Figure 12.7. Normal MTZ/CT. At the level of the conus, there is an increase in the size of the thoracic cord. Note the arrangement of the ventral and dorsal roots as they emerge from the cord at this level.

gradually wider from T9 to the conus medullaris as a result of the lumbar roots arising in it at these levels (Fig. 12.7). From T1 to T9 or 10, it measures about 7 mm in its sagittal dimension and 9 mm in its transverse dimension. Normal limits are not known but the range is probably not much more than 2 mm (Table 12.1).

It is obvious that a precise determination of abnormal cord enlargement or atrophy is not possible. There is a range of normal that is not precisely defined and there is some uncertainty of actual measurement accuracy. Fur-

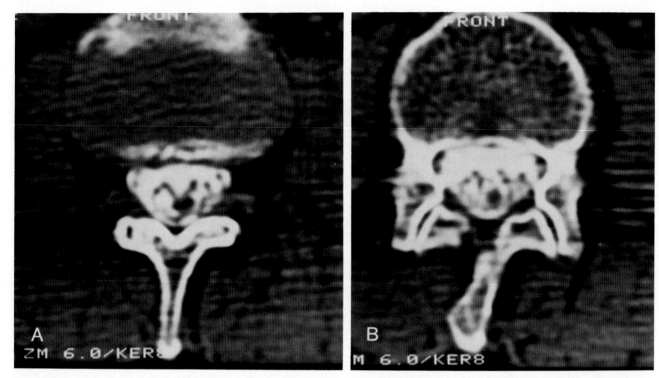

Figure 12.8.   A, B. Normal MTZ/CT. The tip of the conus is significantly smaller in size. The lumbar roots surround the tip of the conus.

thermore, distortion may result readily from dural impingement by disc, ligament, or bone. Nevertheless, gross enlargement is detected readily as it is with standard myelography. At the level of each interspace, two roots emerge one from the dorsolateral aspect of the cord and one from the anterolateral aspect (Fig. 12.3B). These dorsal and ventral roots on each side converge toward the lateral border of the contrast column and may be identified as they enter the root sheath when the latter is visualized (see below). There are, therefore, two pairs of roots at the level of each intervertebral foramen. In the thoracic region, the visibility of these roots is less consistent because the roots describe a slanting course caudad. The slant increases with the lower level of the thoracic segment in question. The group of roots that arise from the lumbar enlargement of the cord appear as a group of small circular negative shadows surrounding the tapering end of the conus medullarus (Fig. 12.8).

THE CAUDA EQUINA

The upper end of the cauda equina surrounds the tapering end of the conus medullarus (Fig. 12.8). Below the level of the tip of the conus, the cauda equina appears as a large number of small, rounded filling defects in the contrast column (Fig. 12.9). These negative shadows represent each a nerve root. Obviously, there are for each segment a dorsal and a ventral root, but the distinction of these is not possible. The negative shadows are distributed uniformly within the dural sac. The filum terminale which lies in the central part of the dural sac is indistinct from the roots of the cauda equina. The cauda equina

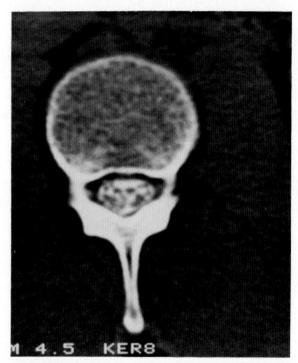

Figure 12.9.   Normal MTZ/CT. The roots of the cauda equina appear as rounded filling defects inside the dural sac.

extends in the dural sac from the level L1–2 down to the lower end of the cul-de-sac. This usually lies at the level of S1–2.

THE DURAL SAC AND THE ROOT SHEATH

The dural membrane is lined by the thin arachnoid. There is no demonstrable space between these two membranes and they can be considered, for radiological purposes, as one membrane. This membrane separates the subarachnoid space filled with metrizamide from the extradural space. The contour of the contrast column, therefore, can be considered as descriptive of the dural sac itself. The space between the contrast column and the bony spinal canal is the extradural space. At the level of each intervertebral foramen, a root sheath is seen resembling a sleeve-like extension of the subarachnoid space into the intervertebral foramen. The root sheath contains the dorsal and ventral roots of that level. In the cervical region, the root sheath can be seen extending in a trans-

verse direction from the dural sac into the foramen (Fig. 12.4). The same is true in the upper thoracic region. In the lower thoracic region however, the root sheath follows a slanting course and, therefore, is not visualized in the plane of one CT slice. In the lumbar region, the root sheath can be followed in a series of contiguous slices from the point where it originates from the dural sac at the level of the upper disc plate of a vertebra (Fig. 12.10). In the next slice below, the root sheath appears rounded, contrast-filled lying in the lateral gutter and separated from the dural sac by a short space filled with epidural fat. In this location, the contrast-filled root sheath lies at the medial border of the pedicle. In the next slice caudad, below the level of the pedicle and within the intervertebral foramen, the arachnoid sheath blends with the perineureum and the subarachnoid space ceases to exist and, therefore, no

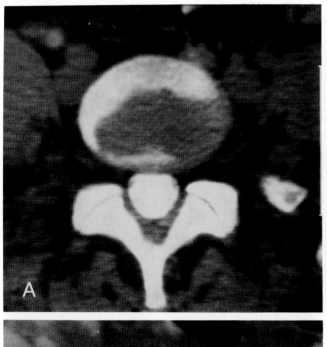

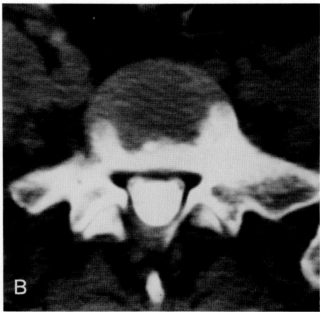

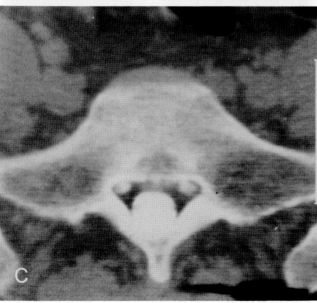

Figure 12.10. Normal MTZ/CT, lumbar region. A. At the level of the L5-S1 disc, the nerve root appears as a filling defect at the lateral angle of the contrast column. B. At the level of the disc plate of S1, the root sheath takes off from the dural sac. C. At a lower level, the root sheath appears separate from the dural sac against the medial border of the lateral mass of the sacral segment.

contrast-filled sheath may be identified.

Below the lower end of the cul-de-sac, the sacral and coccygeal root sheaths may be filled with metrizamide for a short distance within the bony spinal canal of the sacrum. Beyond a certain limit, these root sheaths appear as soft-tissue shadows with no contrast within.

CLASSIFICATION OF INTRASPINAL LESIONS
Radiological Classification

As described above, there are two concentric interfaces discerned on a CT myelogram image. The inner of these two interfaces separates the contrast column from the substance of the cord and outlines the surface of the cord. The outer one separates the contrast material from the epidural space and, therefore, outlines the contour of the dural sac. Therefore, a convenient CT myelographic classification of three lesions by morphology would be as follows:

1. Intramedullary Lesions: These are lesions that lie within and distort the inner interface, i.e., within the cord material.

2. Intradural Extramedullary Lesions: As mentioned before, the dura and arachnoid for radiological purposes are considered as one and the same membrane. Therefore, intradural extramedullary lesions are located between the inner and outer interfaces. These lesions lie within the subarachnoid space and may arise from the meninges, the nerve roots, or the blood vessels.

3. Extradural Lesions: These are lesions that lie and arise outside the outer interface, i.e., between the dura and the bony spinal canal. They may arise from bone or soft tissue outside the dural membrane.

Pathological Classification

At any of the above described morphological locations, lesions could be classified pathologically by their etiological nature. These lesions, therefore, could be described as: 1. congential, 2. inflammatory, 3. traumatic, 4. neoplastic.

INTRAMEDULLARY LESIONS
Intramedullary Neoplasms

These lesions cause enlargement of the cord which may be symmetrical (Fig. 12.11) or nonsymmetrical (Fig. 12.12). Focal and nonsymmetric enlargement of the cord is appreciated more readily than diffuse enlargement, especially if it is of a slight degree. Asymmetrical or unilateral focal deformity and enlargement may indicate exophytic growth of an intramedullary lesion or an applied abnormality on the surface of the cord, i.e., an extramedullary lesion.

The largest group of intramedullary neoplasms are the gliomas (Fig. 12.11). These include astrocytoma, oligodendroglioma, ependymoma, and glioblastoma. Intramedullary metastatic disease (Fig. 12.12), presumably hematogeneously spread, formerly considered extremely rare, now is being reported more frequently (4, 5).

Cystic formation within a tumor may not be demonstra-

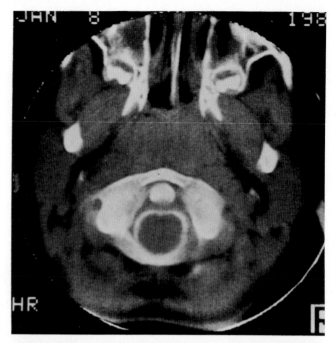

Figure 12.11. Astrocytoma of the upper cervical cord. Widening of the cord is shown by thinning of the contrast rim at the level C1.

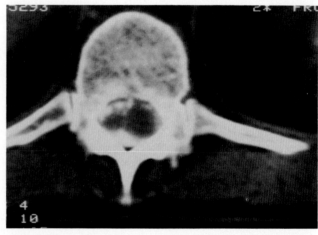

Figure 12.12. Metastases. Irregular intramedullary metastases at the level T12.

ble by plain CT because the presence of high protein content or desquamated material may elevate the attenuation. An important consideration is the effect of metrizamide upon the cord and abnormalities within the cord such as a cyst. The spinal cord, like the brain, will increase in attenuation when surrounded with metrizamide, but the relationship between concentration, duration of exposure, and the increased attenuation has not been worked out. Therefore, cystic tumors are not necessarily opacified with metrizamide more than the surrounding cord.

In syringomyelia and hydromyelia, however, the cyst

becomes denser with time after intrathecal injection of metrizamide. The contrast material migrates into the cyst either directly when the cyst is in communication with the subarachnoid space or over a long time across tissue barriers when the syringomyelia is not communicating (6, 7). Syringomyelia is a condition where cavitation occurs in the spinal cord extending over many segments. When the cavity is a distended central canal, the condition is known as hydromyelia. It is a congenital anomaly and is usually associated with Chiari type I malformation (8). These two conditions may be difficult to differentiate even at necropsy (9). We, therefore, will use the term syringo-hydromyelia. The condition may cause expansion and swelling of the spinal cord encroaching upon the contrast column (10). When the cavity is decompressed by surgery establishing a free communication with the subarachnoid space, the cord appears flattened, i.e., atrophic. In some cases, the cord containing the cavity may be normal in size. The diagnosis then will depend only on the demonstration of contrast material within the cavity of the cyst. The contrast material may appear within the cavity immediately after injection in the subarachnoid space or it may take a few hours. It usually clears completely from the cavity within 24 hours.

Intramedullary Inflammatory Lesions

These may resemble true neoplasms. Granuloma, tuberculosis, or sarcoid (11) abscess and the swollen cord of viral transverse myelitis or multiple sclerosis (12) may be impossible to differentiate from neoplasm. Clinical features and follow-up scanning may be helpful.

Trauma

Swelling of the cord after trauma due to contusion or

an intramedullary hematoma resembles neoplasm (Fig. 12.13). The history of trauma and the presence of associated density change on plain CT or associated bony changes help in making the diagnosis. The outline of the swollen cord may be smooth or asymmetrical if the swelling is not uniform. The presence of irregularity of the contour of the cord in cases of trauma may be produced by the presence of a blood clot on the surface of the cord.

Atrophy of the Cord

This may occur as a result of trauma (Fig. 12.14) previous surgery, after shunting of the syringohydromyelic cavity (Fig. 12.15) or as a result of advanced spondylosis (Fig. 12.16). The cord is decreased particularly in its AP diameter. The transverse diameter is not reduced to the same degree because the cord is held by the ligamentum denticulatum. The anterior median fissure is widened. The thickness of the cord may not be uniform and the cord may give the appearance of "rosary beads."

Congenital Anomalies of the Cord

The term spinal dysraphism covers developmental anomalies that arise from cutaneous, mesoderm, or neural derivatives of the median dorsal region in the embryo. It includes tethered cord (Fig. 12.17), diastematomyelia, neurenteric cysts. Meningoceles and myelomeningoceles (Fig. 12.18) are also a part of this entity but will be described separately in the section of extramedullary lesions.

CT myelographic findings of the tethered cord include low position of the conus medullarus and increased thickness of the filum terminale which lies in a more dorsal location. The association of tethered cord and the Arnold-Chiari malformation has been reported. MTZ/CT myelography is essential for the exact definition of the anatomical

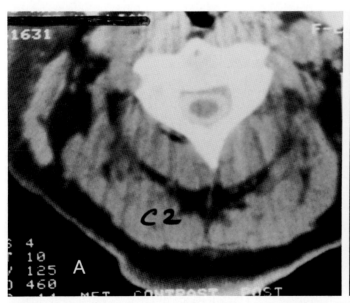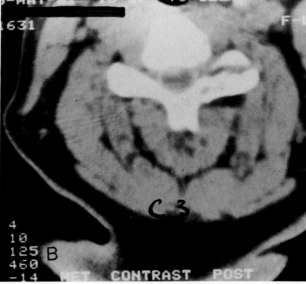

Figure 12.13. Post-traumatic swelling of the cervical cord. A. Normal appearance of the cord and subarachnoid space at the level C2. B. At the level C3, there is fracture of the lateral mass of C3 and the lamina on the left side. This was visualized by plain CT. The swelling of the cord shown here by metrizamide could not be demonstrated by plain CT. The cord is increased in size and the subarachnoid space filled with metrizamide appears as a thin rim.

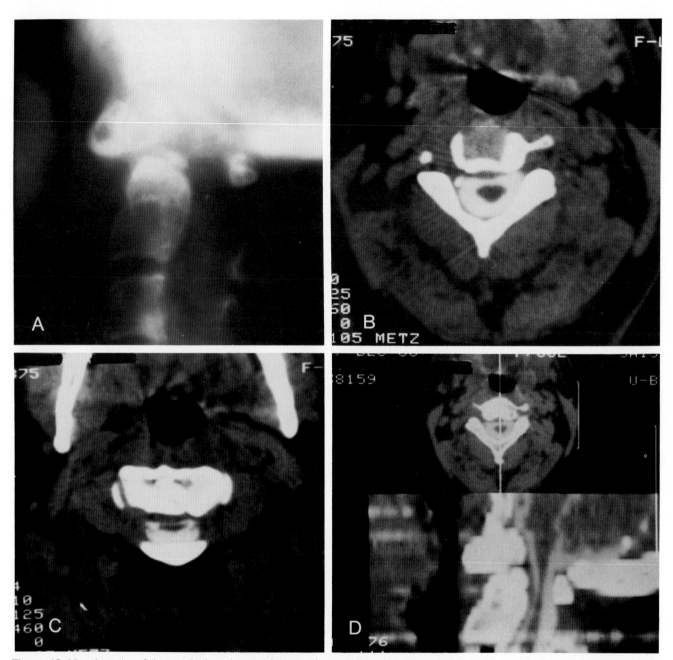

Figure 12.14. Atrophy of the cervical cord secondary to atlanto-axial subluxation. A. Lateral polytome shows separation of the odontoid (congenital or traumatic). There is some displacement resulting in narrowing of the space available to the cord at the C1–2 level. B. At the level C2–3, MTZ/CT shows normal appearance of the cord. C. At the upper level of C2, MTZ/CT shows severe atrophy of the cord. D. Sagittal reformatting of MTZ/CT shows severe atrophy of the cord at the level C1–2.

structures and the correct diagnosis of these anomalies (Figs. 12.17 and 12.18). Plain CT should be done before lumbar or lateral cervical puncture in order to identify the size of the subarachnoid space around the cord in the lumbar region or in the craniocervical junction, when the Chiari malformation is associated.

In diastematomyelia, the spinal canal is divided by a bony septum, spicule, or a fibrous septum in approximately 70% of the cases (13). More importantly, the spinal

cord may be divided into two hemicords. Diplomyelia is, however, a condition of segmental duplication of the entire cord including gray and white matter (13, 14). The nerve roots arise only laterally in diastomatmyelia in contrast to diplomyelia where the spinal cord roots arise from both aspects of each cord.

MTZ/CT myelography demonstrates the hemicords or duplication of the spinal cord by showing these as two negative shadows (15). The fibrous septum in diastematomyelia may not be visualized by plain CT and will be demonstrated only by MTZ/CT myelography. This technique demonstrates also any associated meningocele or meningomyelocele in the same patient.

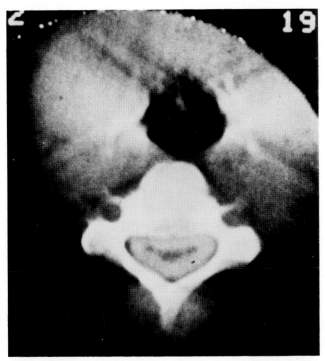

Figure 12.15. Cord atrophy. Case of hydromyelia which was treated by shunt of the cord cyst to the subarachnoid space. MTZ/CT at the level C3 shows flattening of the cord.

The presence of tonsillar ectopia in Chiari malformation may be demonstrated in some instances by plain CT, when there is sufficient contrast difference between the cerebellar tonsils and the surrounding CSF. In other instances, however, contrast difference is not sufficient (Fig. 12.19A). In these cases, opacification of CSF by metrizamide allows the diagnosis to be made readily (Fig. 12.19B and C).

INTRADURAL EXTRAMEDULLARY LESIONS
Neoplasms

The great majority of these tumors are either meningiomas or schwannomas and the familiar features shown by metrizamide CT myelography are those of a filling defect. At times, multiple schwannomas may be demonstrated in cases of von Recklinghausen's Disease (Fig. 12.20). "Drop metastases" and metastases that are blood borne such as melanoma and carcinoma as well as rare lesions may all present as filling defects in the intradural extramedullary space (Fig. 12.21).

Inflammatory Conditions

Arachnoiditis causes variable disruption and distortion of the subarachnoid space (Fig. 12.22). It may produce an appearance suggesting either intramedullary or extramedullary tumor. Another appearance in arachnoiditis is the formation of multiple loculi of contrast material separated by irregular spaces (Fig. 12.23). A third appearance is the paucity of roots of the cauda equina, presumably due to their adhesion to the inner surface of the arachnoid, and clumping (Fig. 12.24).

Granulomas, focal infection, and subdural empyema cannot be differentiated from an epidural condition. A

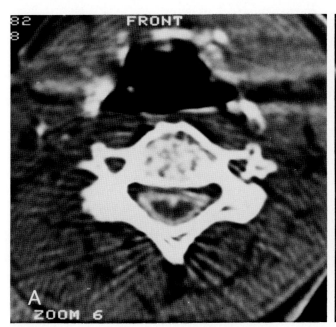
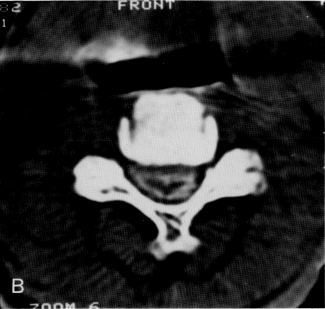

Figure 12.16. Atrophy of the cord secondary to spondylosis. A. MTZ/CT at the level C3 shows normal appearance of the cord. B. MTZ/CT at the level of C3–4 shows bar formation and severe atrophy of the cord.

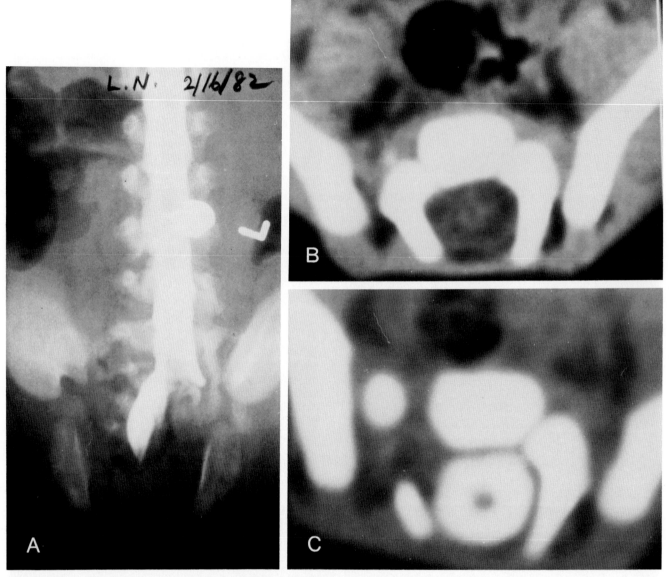

Figure 12.17. Dysraphism. A. Lumbar myelogram shows tethering of the cord and expansion of the contrast column caudally. B. Plain CT at the level of the first sacral segment suggests tethering of the cord. C. MTZ/CT confirms the diagnosis.

hematoma in the subarachnoid space may simulate an intramedullary disease and present as an irregular increase in the size of the negative shadow of the cord.

Congenital Anomalies of the Intradural Extramedullary Structures

Arachnoid cysts or intrasacral meningoceles represent developmental anomalies with the formation of CSF-filled spaces. The communication with the subarachnoid space varies in patency and, therefore, the lesion may fill instantly with contrast material at MTZ/CT myelography or it may appear as a negative shadow resembling a solid mass. In the latter case, the correct diagnosis may be made if CT scanning is repeated after several hours (Fig. 12.25). At this time, contrast material appears within the cyst and

establishes the correct diagnosis. These lesions may cause expansion of the bony spinal canal indistinguishable from that seen in slow-growing tumors such as a neurofibroma (Fig. 12.26). The lesion may not be identified by conventional myelography if the communication with the subarachnoid space is narrow enough to prevent a high concentration of contrast material within the cyst. CT myelography is often successful where conventional myelography is unsuccessful in detecting these lesions (Fig. 12.25).

Meningocele and meningomyelocele are congenital malformations of the neural arch of the vertebral body with protrusion of the meninges through the congenital defect outside the confines of the spinal canal (16). The contents of this sac may consist only of CSF (meningocele)

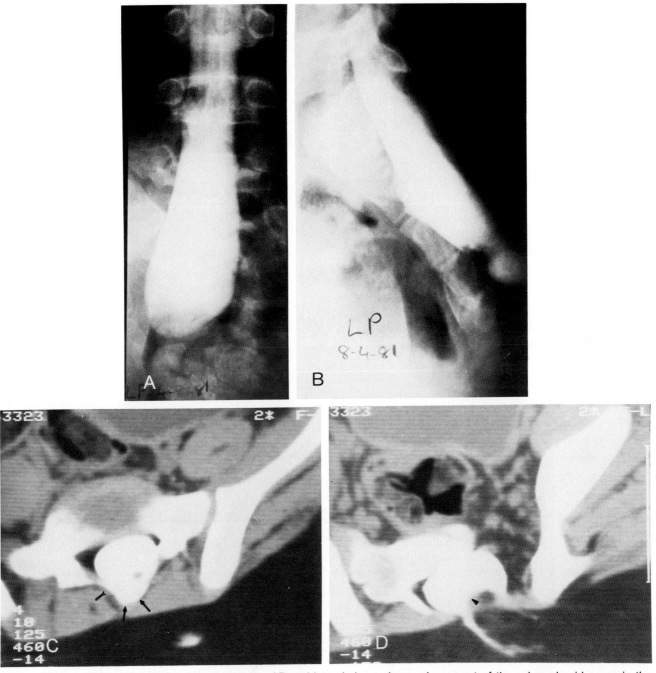

Figure 12.18. Lipomeningocele. A, B. Myelogram AP and lateral views show enlargement of the subarachnoid space in the sacral region but offer no information about the soft-tissue anomaly. C. MTZ/CT shows a meningocele (*arrows*) and a thickened filum terminale (or cord) appearing as a filling defect within the contrast column. D. The exact relationship of the lipoma to the subarachnoid space (*arrowheads*) is shown by MTZ/CT.

or neural elements as well (myelomeningocele) or fat along with CSF (lipomeningocele) (Figs. 12.17 and 12.18). The MTZ/CT myelogram opacifies the CSF component of the lesion and this may outline the other contents of the sac. Meningoceles are most common in the sacral region and in the lumbosacral junction but may be seen also in the cervical region. The anomaly may be associated with

tethered cord, which appears as a rounded defect within the contrast-filled subarachnoid space in the lumbar region.

The conjoined sheath anomaly usually involves the 5th lumbar and 1st sacral roots. The anomaly consists of a common origin of two root sheaths (17). Each root lies within its own arachnoid space but both are within one

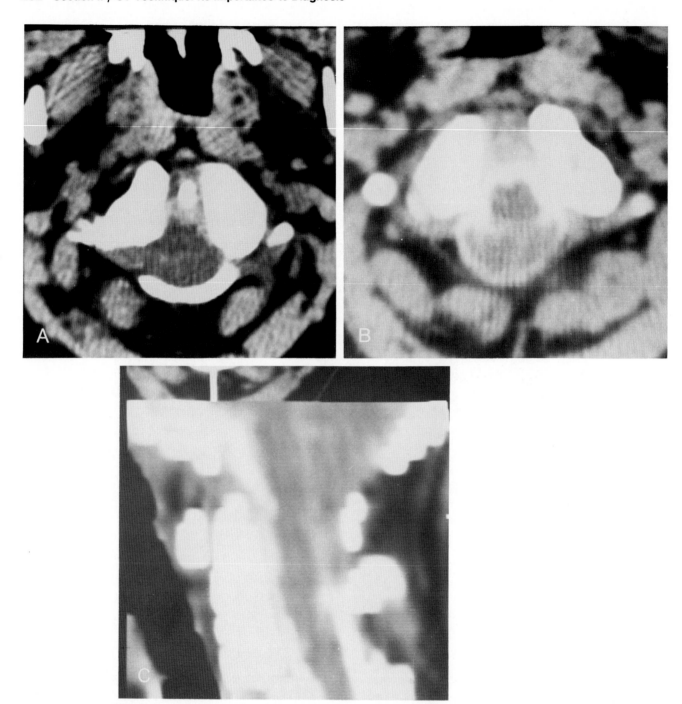

Figure 12.19. Chiari malformation. A. Plain CT below the foramen magnum shows no distinction between CSF and soft tissues. B. MTZ/CT at approximately the same level shows the cerebellar ectopia behind the medulla below the foramen magnum. C. Sagittally reformatted MTZ/CT image shows severe degree of cerebellar ectopia. The cerebellar tonsils reach almost to the lower border of the neural arch of C2.

dural sheath. As a result, the contrast-filled arachnoid space of the conjoined sheath appears larger in size than the normal side (Fig. 12.27). Furthermore, the site of origin of the conjoined sheath is usually intermediate between the sites of origin of each of the two component arachnoid sheaths. This anomaly has been reported in association with disc rupture or spinal stenosis. It is claimed that the anomaly itself is not the cause of symptoms but rather the anomalous location of the roots increases their vulnerability to compression by disc protrusion or spinal stenosis. It is, therefore, essential to recognize the anatomy of these roots before surgery.

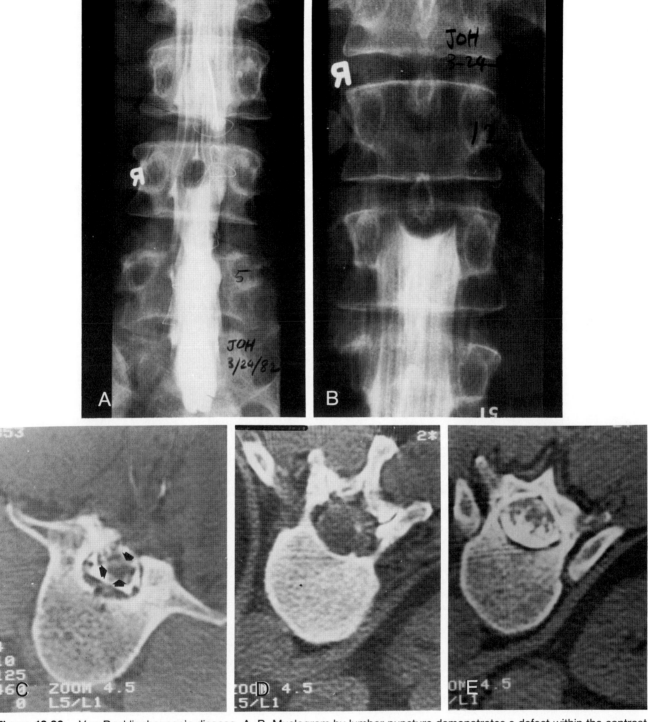

Figure 12.20.   Von Recklinghausen's disease. A, B. Myelogram by lumbar puncture demonstrates a defect within the contrast column at the level L4. There is also complete block at the level L1. Conventional myelography shows no contrast material above the level of the block. C–E. MTZ/CT (in prone position) shows the lesion at L4 as a defect (*arrows*) among the numerous roots of the cauda equina in C and A. Complete block with no metrizamide at L1 in D. At the level T12, just above the block, the conus and surrounding roots of the cauda equina are seen in E. Metrizamide allows the determination of the upper limit of the block which often is not determined by conventional myelography.

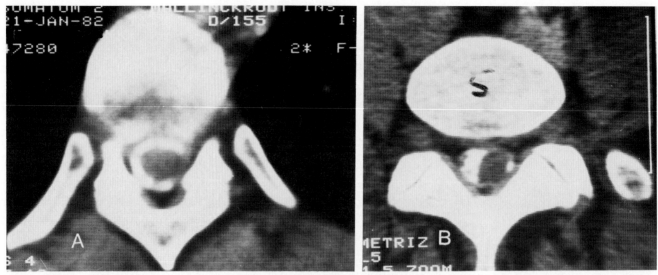

Figure 12.21.   A, B. Multiple hemangioblastomas. CT with metrizamide shows expansion of the cord at T9 in A and a well-defined defect at L5 in B.

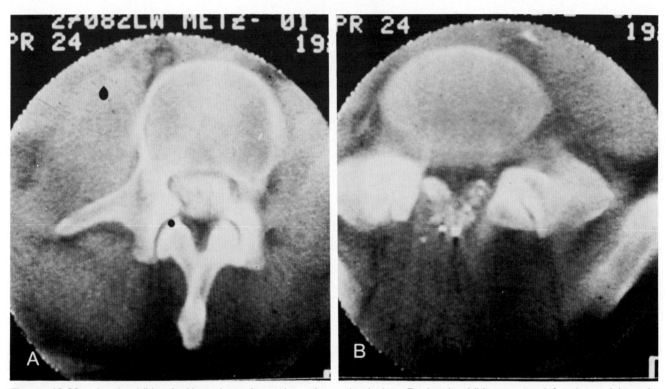

Figure 12.22.   Arachnoiditis. A. Normal cauda equina, above the lesion. B. Arachnoiditis causes deformity and irregular disorganization of the contrast column at L5-S1.

EXTRADURAL LESIONS

The most important group of disease conditions in this section is degenerative disese. They include degenerative changes both in the intervertebral joint and in the posterior articular joints. The radiological findings in this group include changes in the configuration of the dural sac as well as the individual root sheaths on both sides.

Intervertebral Disc Degeneration

The diagnosis of herniated lumbar intervertebral disc is made by plain CT in the majority of cases and is discussed elsewhere. The role of MTZ/CT myelography is limited to those cases in which the diagnosis could not be made by plain CT. Diffuse bulge is the earliest stage of disc degeneration. It is the result of tears or cracks in the

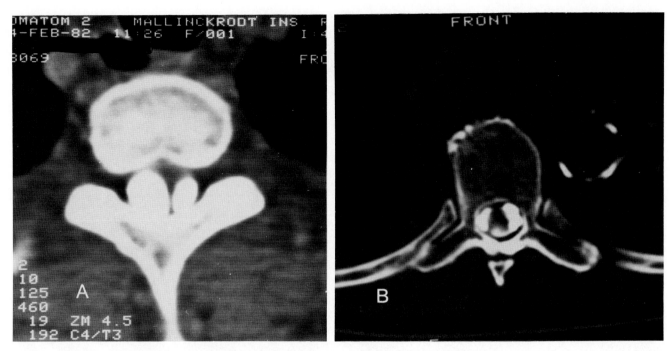

Figure 12.23. Arachnoiditis in two different patients. The subarachnoid space is separated into two compartments or loculi, filled with metrizamide. In A, the compartments are separated by a band. In B, the loculi are wide apart.

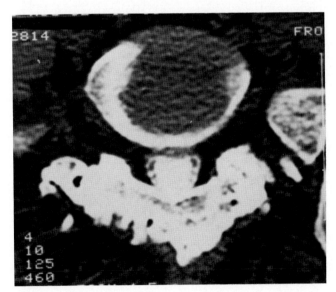

Figure 12.24. Arachnoiditis. On MTZ/CT, the roots are sparse presumably due to being adherent to the wall of the subarachnoid space.

anulus. The bulging is uniform. This appears on CT myelography as a uniform impression on the anterior aspect of the contrast column. There is usually no obliteration of the root sheath on either side. When rupture of the anulus and herniation of disc material take place, the identation is "focal." This focality is illustrated best by CT myelography which displays the entire contour of the contrast column in the axial projection. According to the site of

the focal indentation of the contrast column, the disc rupture may be described as central, paracentral, or lateral. The indentation appears as a "defect" in the contrast column. Central disc rupture is illustrated best by CT myelography (Figure 12.28). Therefore, it should be done in all cases in which there is any doubt about the diagnosis in plain CT or in conventional myelography. In assessing central disc herniation by CT metrizamide myelography, one has to keep in mind the normal variations in the configuration of the anterior border of the contrast column in the axial projection. In the upper lumbar region, the anterior border of the contrast column is curved with a forward bulge conforming with the configuration of the posterior border of the vertebral body. In the midlumbar region, the anterior border of the contrast column is straight. In the lower lumbar region, the border shows a gentle curve of concavity. When this concavity is seen in the midlumbar region or when it is exaggerated in the lower lumbar region, the diagnosis of central disc herniation may be made.

When disc rupture is posterolateral, the diagnosis is easier than when it is central, because there is no normal variation that could resemble the appearance. The normal configuration of the lumbar dural sac in the axial projection has two anterolateral angles. "Amputation" of the lateral angle occurs in posterolateral disc herniation (Fig. 12.29). This usually is associated with obliteration of the root sheath at its takeoff from the dural sac. The latter finding is elicited easily by comparing both sides. When the herniated fragment is large in size or when it has migrated away from the site of the rupture, the deformity of the contrast column appears at a location away from

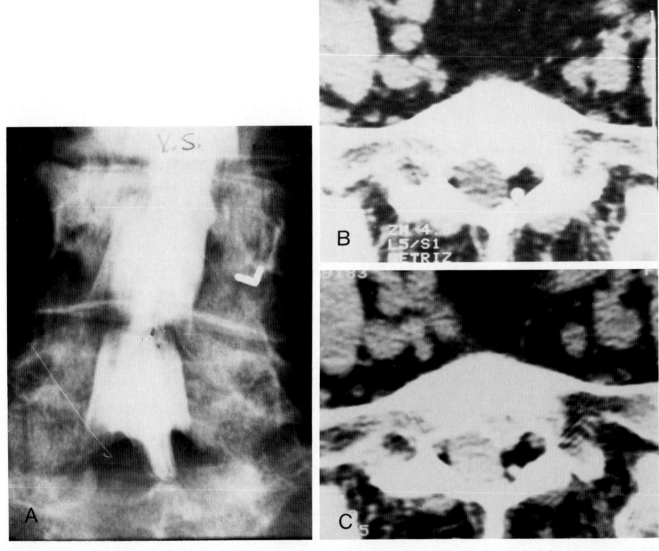

Figure 12.25. Intrasacral meningocele. A. Myelogram shows a short dural sac ending at the level L5-S1. No demonstrable filling of a cyst. B. MTZ/CT soon after myelography shows a root sheath cyst on the right side with no entry of the contrast material into the cyst. Note erosion of the posterior border of the sacral body at that level. C. Three hours later, a scan at approximately the same level shows the cyst (intrasacral meningocele) filled with metrizamide. Delayed CT may confirm communication with the subarachnoid space and distinguish this condition from a tumor.

the disc level itself. It, therefore, appears at the level of the body of the vertebra below and less commonly, the vertebra above (Fig. 12.30). This is particularly true in cases of disc extrusion. The fragment in these locations causes also obliteration of the root sheath which lies at the medial and inferomedial border of the pedicle.

At the lumbosacral junction, the dural sac is small in size and the epidural fat is abundant. As a result, one may encounter a situation in which the herniated fragment does not cause deformity of the contrast column. In these cases, the signs of root compression are those of "displace-

ment" of the contrast-filled root sheath on that side compared to the opposite side or "obliteration", i.e., nonfilling of the root sheath, in which case the shadow of the root sheath is indistinct from the herniated disc mass (Fig. 12.31). Displacement and obliteration are both signs of compression of the nerve root.

Postoperative changes after surgery for excision of herniated disc fragment have been described on plain CT (18). On CT myelography (Fig. 12.32), the most conspicuous finding is the eccentric position of the dural sac as a result of removal of bone and soft tissue in the process of

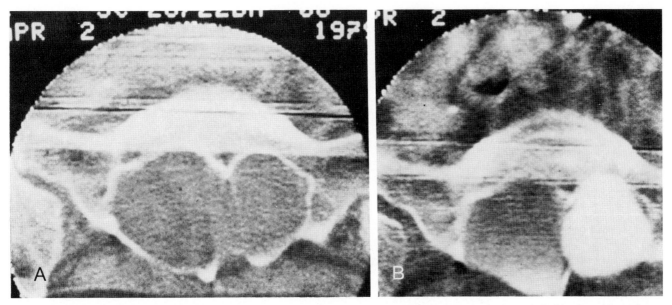

Figure 12.26. Intrasacral meningocele. A. Plain CT shows erosion of the wall of the bony spinal canal. B. Metrizamide outlines the cysts that caused the erosion.

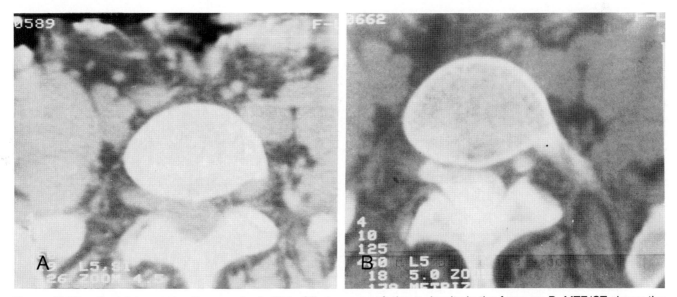

Figure 12.27. Conjoint root sheath anomaly. A. Plain CT shows a soft-tissue density in the foramen. B. MTZ/CT shows the conjoint sheath filled with contrast material.

partial or complete hemilaminectomy as well as the formation of scar at the site of surgery. Besides the eccentric position, the contour of the dural sac itself is asymmetrical due to focal bulging at the site of the defect in the bone or soft tissue. These changes are normal postoperative findings and do not imply complications. Surgical complications detected by CT myelography include CSF leak and arachnoiditis. The cause of CSF leak is usually a tear in the dura and arachnoid. This may involve the root sheath or the dural sac itself. The condition is demonstrated best by CT myelography. Plain CT does not provide this diagnosis. The patients are suspected to have this condition

when a soft-tissue mass can be palpated, is reducible, and is pulsatile with coughing. The contrast material outlines the sac which resembles a meningocele (Fig. 12.33). The site of communication with the dural sac or the root sheath, therefore, is demonstrated and can be treated surgically. In more advanced cases, the meningocele extends into the soft-tissue planes all the way out to the skin (Fig 12.33). In less advanced cases, the lesion may appear only as a contrast-filled space within the muscle planes around the spine.

The development of arachnoiditis after surgery or after Pantopaque myelography is detected by MTZ/CT myelog-

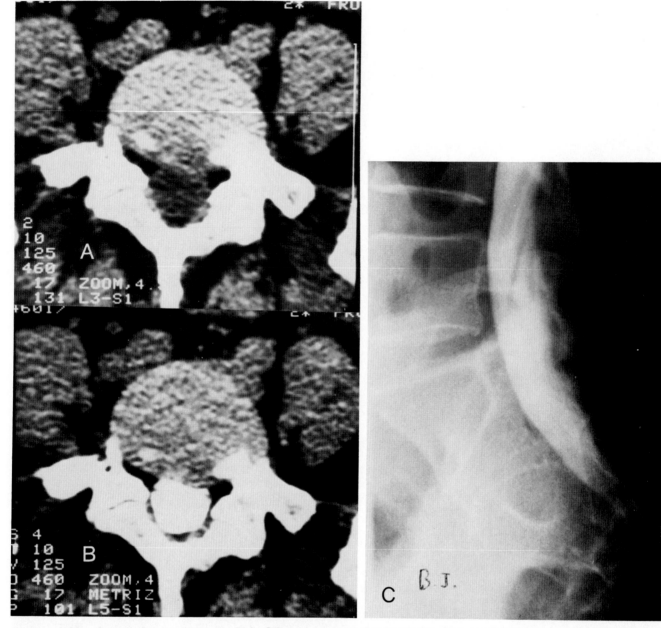

Figure 12.28. Central disc herniation. A. Plain CT shows central disc herniation. The exact interface between the disc and dural sac may be questionable. B. Myelogram shows normal appearance. C. Postmyelogram CT is very helpful in demonstrating that the indentation of the dural sac is slightly off central.

raphy by demonstrating the CT findings previously mentioned in the section of inflammatory disease in the intradural extramedullary space (Figs. 12.22–12.24). These include deformity of the contrast column, loculation of the contrast material, and the adherence of the roots to the wall of the subarachnoid space resulting in "paucity" of roots within the contrast column and the presence of "clumping" of the nerve roots.

Degenerative Spinal Stenosis

This condition is the result of degenerative changes in the posterior articular joints. The changes include hyper-

trophy of the ligaments as well as bony structures. The superior and inferior articular processes are both involved. There may be also an element of idiopathic developmental spinal stenosis which affects the orientation and thickness of the laminae and results in decrease of the midsagittal diameter. Lateral spinal stenosis refers to the encroachment upon the lateral gutter of the bony spinal canal by hypertrophy of the superior articular process of the vertebra below. Central spinal stenosis refers to the encroachment upon the central part of the canal by the hypertrophied inferior articular process and the lamina of the vertebra above (19, 20).

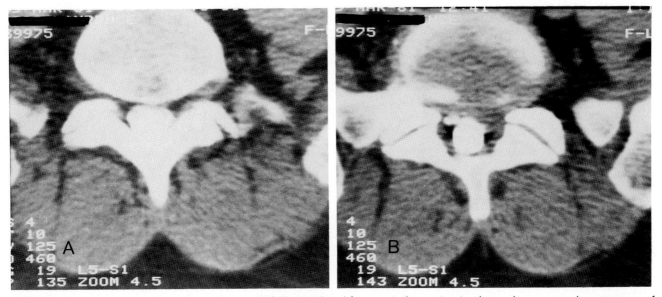

Figure 12.29. Herniated disc. A. Above the level of the herniated fragment, the contrast column shows normal appearance of its two lateral angles. B. There is a defect encroaching upon the lateral angle of the contrast column on the left side. The left root sheath is not filled.

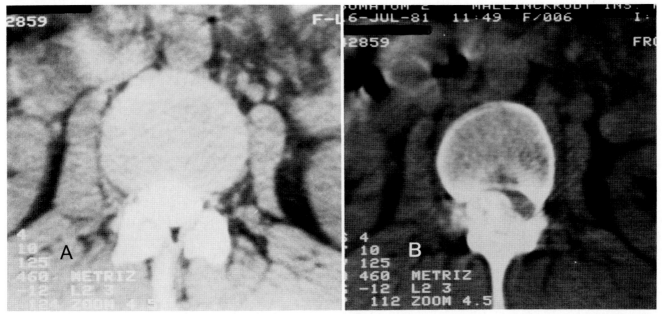

Figure 12.30. Migration of herniated fragment. A. At the level of the intervertebral disc, the contrast column is not deformed. B. At the level of the pedicle above the disc, the herniated fragment encroaches upon the contrast column.

The earliest change in spinal stenosis is decrease in size of the contrast column at the level of the articulation compared to the levels of the bodies of the vertebrae above and below (Fig. 12.34B). This is due to the encroachment upon the spinal canal by the elements of the posterior articulation and also by the disc plates when degenerative changes in the articular intervertebral articulation is associated as is often the case.

At a later stage, the density of the contrast column is reduced at the level of the intervertebral articulation as compared to the levels of the bodies above and below. This is the result of paucity of contrast due to "crowding" of the roots together due to further decrease in the available subarachnoid space (Fig. 12.34B). In more severe cases, there is virtual "interruption" of the contrast column at the level of articulation (Fig. 12.34C). This indicates a significant compression of the cauda equina. The contrast material will be absent in the CT slice at the level of the intervertebral articulation while the density of the material and the appearance of the dural sac are normal

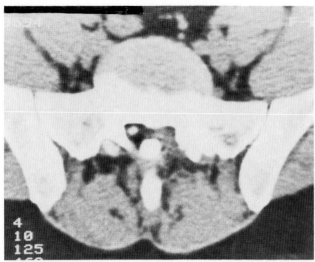

Figure 12.31. Herniated disc at L5-S1. The dural sac is often small in size at this level and the epidural space is abundant. In this case, the herniated disc mass does not impinge upon the contrast column but displaces the root sheath on the left side and prevents its filling.

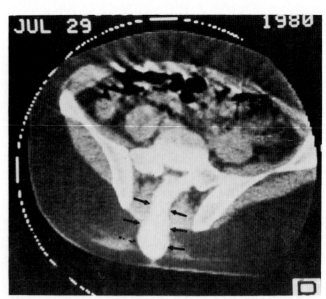

Figure 12.33. Postoperative false meningocele. MTZ/CT shows a column of contrast material (*arrows*) extending from the dural sac to the skin.

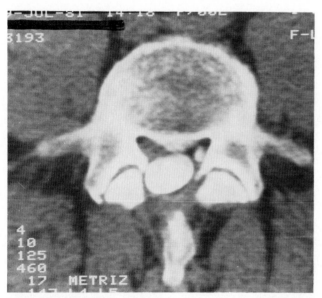

Figure 12.32. Postoperative changes after disc surgery. Note the eccentric position of the dural sac and bulging of its posterior border on the right side which was the side of the laminectomy.

proximal to the block.

In cases of spinal stenosis, the examination should include the entire lumbar region from L1 through S1, because the stenotic process may involve two levels with an intervening normal level.

Evaluation of postoperative cases after decompression of spinal stenosis demonstrates removal of the spinous process and the laminae as well as medial partial facetectomy on both sides. The *effect* of decompression, however,

can be evaluated only by MTZ/CT myelography. In these cases, the dural sac is displaced dorsally away from the body of the vertebra. The configuration of the dural sac also is altered. Focal bulging of the dural sac at the decompression level is seen and the root shadows show sufficient metrizamide to indicate the absence of crowding of the roots. Depending on the degree of lateral extension of the bone decompression procedure, the dural sac may or may not show an hour-glass configuration. This is due to constriction of the midportion of the contrast column by the borders of bone resection. Eccentric configuration of the dural sac indicates asymmetry of bone decompression. If complications arise such as false meningocele or arachnoiditis, the signs will be as previously described in the section of Disc Herniation.

Traumatic Lesions

In acute trauma, the bony spinal canal may be encroached upon by one of three factors: 1. subluxation, 2. displaced fragment of a fracture, 3. epidural hematoma. MTZ/CT myelography in all cases demonstrates the width of the subarachnoid space around the cord or the cauda equina.

A displaced bone fragment (Fig. 12.35) pushes the dura away from the rest of the bony wall on the side of the fragment against the bony wall on the opposite side. Compression of the cord is indicated by narrowing of the subarachnoid space containing the contrast material as well as deformity and displacement of the spinal cord itself. The epidural space between the displaced fragment and the contrast column is narrowed whereas on both sides of the fragment, the space is widened. In cases of severe compression of the cord, the subarachnoid space may be obliterated completely and no contrast material appears at the level of the displaced fragment as opposed

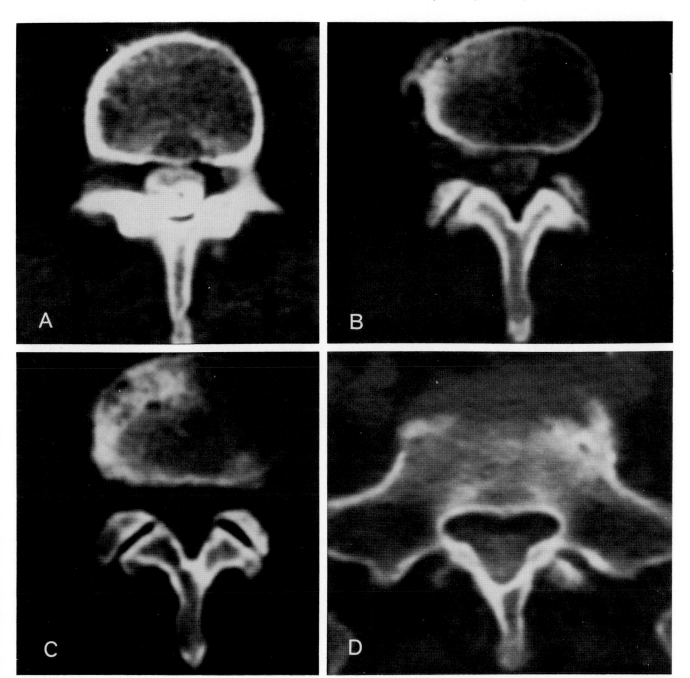

Figure 12.34. Spinal stenosis at L4–5. A. The slice just above the level of the stenosis shows normal appearance of the contrast column. B. The next slice below shows a smaller contrast column. Note also the lower density of the contrast column. C. At the next level below, there is complete absence of contrast material, indicating severe stenosis and compression of the cauda equina. D. Normal appearance returns at the level L5-S1.

to the appearance proximal to the fracture level. In cases of such degree of block, a small amount of contrast material may still appear in low concentration distal to the level of the block. The absence of contrast material around the cord at the site of trauma is an indication of severe compression of the spinal cord. The appearance of epidural hematoma (24) on MTZ/CT myelography is indistinguishable from the appearance of epidural empyema or infiltrating tumor in the epidural space.

Another complication of trauma which can only be diagnosed by CT metrizamide myelography is swelling of the cord previously discussed (Fig 12.13).

Neoplasms

The most common neoplasm in the epidural compartment is metastases and lymphoma, usually a part of sys-

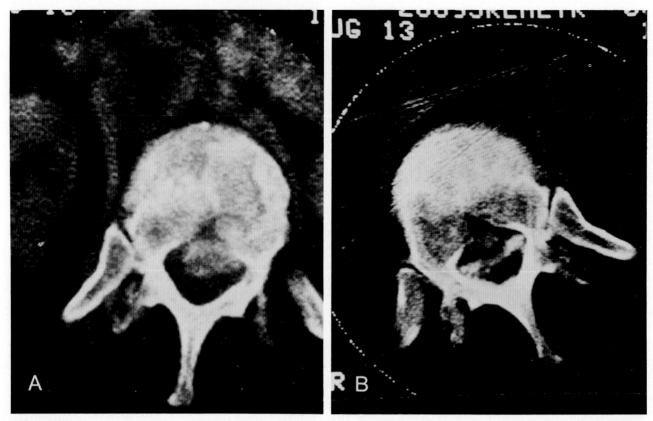

Figure 12.35. Fracture of the 12th thoracic vertebral body. A. Plain CT shows a fragment of the fractured vertebra driven into the bony spinal canal. B. MTZ/CT shows the effect of the displaced bone fragment. There is widening of the epidural space, narrowing of the space filled with contrast material and displacement and deformity of the cord against the posterior wall of the spinal canal.

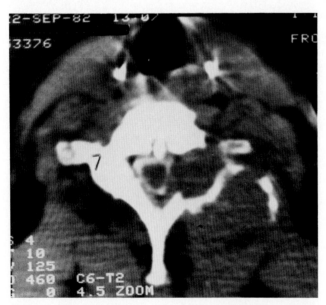

Figure 12.36. Metastatic carcinoma of the prostate. There is bone destruction and widening of the epidural space at the expense of the subarachnoid space. The contrast column and the cord are displaced to the opposite side.

temic disease. Primary intraspinal extradural neoplasms are uncommon. They may arise from lymphoid tissue, vascular tissue, adipose tissue. Tumors of the primitive notocord or from nerve tissue also may occur. Examples of these are neurolemmoma (21), neurofibroma, ependymoma (22), and paraganglioma (23). Tumors also may arise from connective tissue such as fibroma, synovioma, and of course, tumors of bone and cartilage.

Tumors may invade the spinal canal from outside the spine such as developmental or congenital lesions or later developing neoplasm as neuroblastoma, rhabdomyosarcoma, solitary myeloma, medulloblastoma (from the posterior fossa), etc. Metastatic tumors from outside the spinal canal may be carried within the canal by the bloodstream or by lymph channels.

The MTZ/CT myelographic picture of epidural tumor is indistinguishable from hematoma or infection. The extradural space is increased in width at the expense of the contrast-filled subarachnoid space. The contrast column appears deformed and is displaced by the tumor. The cord and the cauda equina also are displaced within the contrast column (Figs. 12.36 and 12.37). The differentiation between extradural and intradural extramedullary tumors should be made by the sharp angle at the border of

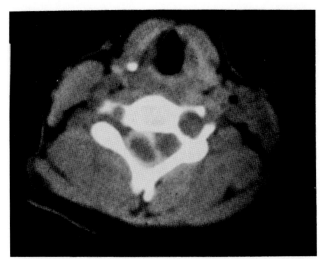

Figure 12.37. Neurofibroma. The widening of the epidural space and the displacement of the contrast column and cord are similar to the case in Figure 12.36 but the bony changes are different.

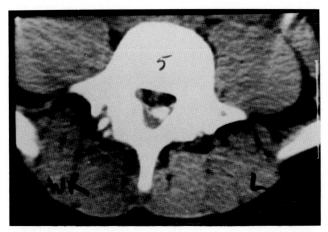

Figure 12.38. Epidural empyema. There is widening of the epidural space behind the body of L5 and under the right ligamentum flavum at L5-S1, with displacement of the contrast column.

the defect caused by intradural lesion (Figs. 12.20 and 12.21) as compared to the obtuse angle of the defect caused by the extradural tumor (Figs. 12.36 and 12.37).

Difficulty in diagnosis may be caused in cases of extradural tumor with an intradural component such as occurs sometimes in neurofibroma.

The lesion in lymphoma may be localized or diffuse involving a region corresponding to several vertebrae and it also may surround the entire circumference of the dural sac.

Inflammatory Conditions

An epidural abscess (epidural empyema) causes widening of the epidural space with displacement and deformity of the dural sac (Fig. 12.38). A diffuse picture similar to diffuse infiltrative lymphoma may be produced by the

condition of chronic hypertrophic pachymeningitis.

The similarity, therefore, between an epidural neoplasm, hematoma (24), or abscess should be re-emphasized. The correct diagnosis may be helped by keeping the possibility of this similarity in mind and paying particular attention to the clinical history, the presenting symptoms and signs, and the nature of the bony changes.

References

1. Baker RA, Hillman BJ, McLennan JE, et al: Sequelae of metrizamide myelography in 200 examinations. *AJR* 130:499–502, 1978.
2. Siebert CE, Barnes JE, Dreisbach JN, et al: Accurate CT measurement of the spinal cord using metrizamide: physical factors. *AJNR* 2:75–78, 1981.
3. Shapiro R: *Myelography*, 3rd Edition. Chicago, Year Book Publishers, Inc., 1975.
4. Moffie D, Stefanko SZ: Intramedullary metastasis. *Clin Neurol* 82:199–202, 1980.
5. Smaltino F, Bernini FP, Santoro S: Computerized tomography in the diagnosis of intramedullary metastases. *Acta Neurochir* 52:299–303, 1980.
6. Aubin ML, Vignaud J, Jardin C, et al: Computed tomography in 75 clinical cases of syringomyelia. *AJNR* 2:199–204, 1981.
7. Resjo IM, Harwood-Nash DC, Fitz CR, et al: Computed tomographic metrizamide myelography in syringohydromyelia. *Radiology* 131:405–407, 1979.
8. Forbes W St. C, Isherwood I: Computed tomography in syringomyelia and the associated Arnold-Chiari Type I malformation. *Neuroradiology* 15:73–78, 1978.
9. Hughes JT: Diseases of the spine and spinal cord. In: Blackwood W, Corsellis JAN: *Greenfield's Neuropathology*. 3rd Edition. London, Edward Arnold Publishers, 1976, pp 668–670.
10. Bonafe A, Manelfe C, Espagno J, et al: Evaluation of syringomyelia with metrizamide computed tomographic myelography. *J Comput Assist Tomogr* 4:797–802, 1980.
11. Kanoff RB, Rubert R: Sarcoidosis presenting as a dorsal spinal cord tumor: report of a case. *J Am Osteopath Assoc* 79:765–767, 1980.
12. Coin CG, Hucks-Folliss A: Cervical computed tomography in multiple sclerosis with spinal cord involvement. *J Comput Assist Tomogr* 3:421–422, 1979.
13. Arrendondo F, Haughton VM, Hemmy DC, et al: Computed tomographic appearance of spinal cord in diastematomyelia. *Radiology* 136:685–688, 1980.
14. Scatliff JH, Bidgood WD, Killebrew K, et al: Computed tomography and spinal dysraphism: Clinical and phantom studies. *Neuroradiology* 17:71–75, 1979.
15. Scotti G, Musgrave MA, Harwood-Nash DC, et al: Diastematomyelia in children: Metrizamide and CT metrizamide myelography. *AJNR* 1:403–410, 1980.
16. Harwood-Nash DC, Fitz CR: Computed tomography and the pediatric spine: Computed tomography metrizamide myelography in children. In: Post MJD: *Radiographic Evaluation of the Spine: Current Advances with Emphasis on Computed Tomography*. New York, Masson Publishing, 1980, Chapt. 1, pp 4–33.
17. Keon-Cohen B: Abnormal arrangement of the lower lumbar and first sacral nerves within the spinal canal. *J Bone Joint Surg* 50-B:261–265, 1968.
18. Gado MH, Hodges FJ III, Patel JP: Spine. In: Lee JKT, Sagel SS, Stanley RJ: *Computed Body Tomography*. New York, Raven Press, 1982, pp 415–452.
19. Lancourt JE, Glenn WV, Wiltse LL: Multiplanar computerized tomography in the normal spine and in the diagnosis of spinal stenosis: A gross anatomic-computerized tomographic correlation. *Spine* 4:379–390, 1979.
20. McAfee PC, Ullrich CG, Yuan HA, et al: Computed tomography in degenerative spinal stenosis. *Clin Orthop Rel Res*

161:221–234, 1981.
21. Yang WC, Zappulla R, Malis L: Neurilemmoma in lumbar intervertebral foramen. *J Comput Assist Tomogr* 5:904–906, 1981.
22. Siegel RS, William AG, Mettler FA Jr, et al: Intraspinal extra-dural ependymoma: Case report. *J Comput Assist Tomogr* 6:189–192, 1982.

23. Nakagawa H, Mallis LI, Huang YP: Computed tomography of soft tissue masses related to the spinal column. In: Post MJD: *Radiographic Evaluation of the Spine: Current Advances with Emphasis on Computed Tomography.* New York, Masson Publishing, 1980, pp 320–352.
24. Post MJD, Seminer DS, Quencer RM: CT Diagnosis of spinal epidural hematoma. *AJNR* 3:190–192, 1982.

CHAPTER THIRTEEN

High-Resolution Computed Tomography in the Diagnosis of Intraspinal Soft-Tissue Lesions

HIROSHI NAKAGAWA, M.D., KAZUO MIYASAKA, M.D., and KINJIRO IWATA, M.D.*

The advent of high-resolution CT (HRCT) has resulted in a further increase in the role of CT in the evaluation of intraspinal pathology.

With second generation scanners, some intraspinal tumors such as calcified meningiomas, lipomas, osteoblastomas, and schwannomas with bony erosion could be diagnosed with reasonable certainty (1–5). However, the spinal cord and the subarachnoid space were poorly visualized by these scanners.

By using third or fourth generation CT scanners with better contrast and spatial resolution, the normal anatomy of the intraspinal contents is delineated much more routinely (6–8).

The visibility of the cord is affected mainly by the relative size of the cord and the subarachnoid space and often is disturbed by artifacts which are not infrequently caused by cardiac or laryngeal motions.

As reported by Taylor et al. (9), the thoracic cord was well-visualized in 33% of the 67 images on plain CT.

Recently, Xenon has been employed as an inhaled gas or intrathecally for contrast enhancement of CT of the spinal cord (10, 11), but the future of its clinical use is not certain.

The water-soluble contrast metrizamide, on the other hand, has been established as an easily used and reasonably safe material for intrathecal injection (12). Therefore, metrizamide CT after myelography now is performed routinely with few serious complications. Because metrizamide CT clearly demonstrates the cord and the subarachnoid space in a transverse axial plane, its use has increased the diagnostic value of CT in the evaluation of intraspinal disease greatly.

MATERIAL AND METHODS

As shown in Table 13.1, in the last 16-month period, 480 cases of various spinal disorders were studied with Somatom 2 by Siemens and TCT-60A by Toshiba. Contiguous slices of 4 or 5 mm were used routinely. However, 2-mm thick slices or overlapping cuts were employed in selected cases such as in cervical soft-disc herniations. Sagittal or coronal reconstructions were obtained when necessary.

---

* We would like to thank Drs. A. Takahashi, K. Sahashi, and S. Goto for referring their patients. We are also grateful to Miss C. Hiraoka for secretarial work.

Table 13.1.
Cases of Spinal Pathology Examined by HRCT from April 1981 to July 1982

		Plain or enhanced CT	Metrizamide CT	Both
Discogenic disease	190			
Cervical	110	59	28	23
Thoracic	4	1	3	0
Lumbar	76	63	4	9
Ligamentous ossification	31	21	4	6
Trauma	28	20	4	4
Congenital anomalies	61			
Scoliosis, block vertebrae	20	19	1	0
Syrinx, Arnold-Chiari	19	4	2	13
Spina bifida	12	9	1	2
Spondylolysis	9	6	3	0
Atlantoaxial dislocation	23	10	7	6
Tumors	65			
Intramedullary	8	2	2	4
Intradural	21	9	3	9
Extradural	28	20	5	3
Primary bone tumors	8	7	0	1
Infections	10	9	1	0
Others	21	15	3	3
Normal	42	28	10	4
Total	480	305 (64%)	77 (16%)	98 (20%)

Of the 480 cases, 40% represented discogenic disease including soft disc herniations, spondylosis, and canal stenosis; 14% tumors; 13% congenital anomalies; 9% normal; 7% spinal ligamentous ossification or calcification; 6% trauma; 5% atlantoaxial dislocation; 2% infection; and 4% miscellaneous.

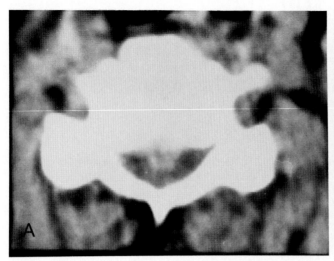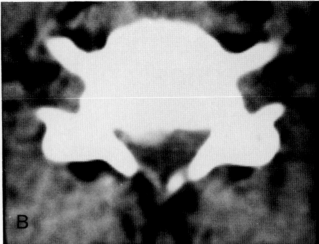

Figure 13.1. Cervical disc protrusions demonstrated on thin section (2-mm) plain CT scans. A. Central disc at C4-C5. B. Posterolateral disc at C5-C6 on the right.

Metrizamide CT was performed after myelography in 36% of patients, 16% of whom also were studied by plain CT.

While reviewing our material, we asked ourselves the following questions:

How accurate is plain or enhanced CT in the delineation of soft-tissue lesions in the spinal canal?
What is the limitation of HRCT scanners?
What is the relationship between myelography and metrizamide CT in the diagnosis of intraspinal lesions?

Our case material which will be presented in the pages to follow provide answers to these questions.

RESULTS AND DISCUSSION

CT anatomy of the lumbosacral canal using late generation CT scanners was studied in detail by Haughton and his colleagues (7).

The dural sac, nerve root sheath, ganglion, ligamentum flavum, retrovertebral plexus, and anterior internal vertebral veins all can be demonstrated without intravenous (IV) contrast enhancement. The diagnosis of lumbar disc herniation and associated spondylotic changes is made quite easily and comfortably with plain CT as will be discussed in other chapters in this book.

The spinal cord at C1 and C2 almost always is visible because of the wide subarachnoid space. As a result, plain CT is of considerable diagnostic value at this level (13). On the other hand, the visibility of the cord in the mid- and lower cervical and thoracic regions is not yet good enough for definitive diagnosis even with late generation CT scanners, although the cord in the midthoracic area is seen in one-third of the cases (9). This is particularly true in the presence of cord compression by an intraspinal mass where the subarachnoid space is obliterated or narrowed. Therefore, metrizamide myelography followed by

metrizamide CT is still valuable in the diagnosis of intraspinal pathology.

Cervical Soft Disc Herniations

Although a large midline cervical disc may be delineated by second generation scanners (4, 14), direct visualization of relatively small cervical discs which often are associated with spondylotic spurs is still difficult and not entirely reliable using contiguous 5-mm CT slices.

Lateral digital radiography and thin section (1.5-mm or 2-mm) HRCT, however, have increased dramatically the diagnostic accuracy of this disease (15, 16). Central and centrolateral discs of various size now are visualized directly by plain CT. They appear as soft-tissue masses adjacent to a disc space level (Fig. 13.1). Nevertheless, intrathecal injection of metrizamide is still mandatory in order to delineate the compressed cord and the shifted anterior median raphe (Fig. 13.2).

Whereas a central disc protrusion may be overlooked or visualized poorly because of a block on conventional myelography, metrizamide CT is able to demonstrate the midline disc and the compressed cord directly (Fig. 13.3). It also provides critical information concerning surgical approach. When midline cervical disc herniations are detected by metrizamide CT (15, 16), an anterior approach is chosen.

Tumors

INTRAMEDULLARY TUMORS

The diagnostic accuracy of the current CT scanners in evaluating intramedullary tumors when no intrathecal contrast is used is still controversial, because delineation of the cord is not yet satisfactory especially in the presence of a compressed subarachnoid space.

However, tumors within the cord which markedly enhance with IV contrast injection such as astrocytomas and hemangioblastomas can be diagnosed (4, 18). A well-de-

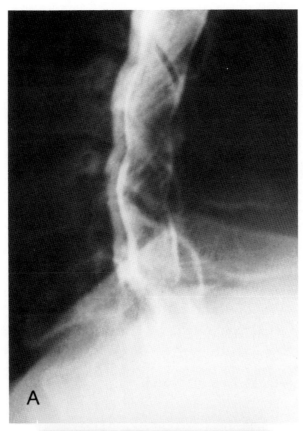

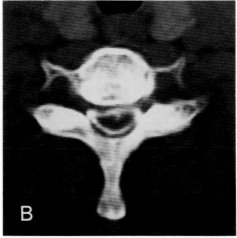

Figure 13.2. Posterolateral soft-disc protrusion at C6-C7. A 45-year-old female presented with persistent radicular pain radiating to the right hand, scapular pain, and numbness and weakness of the right hand. A. Cervical myelography on a lateral view shows an anterior defect with double density at C6-C7. B. Metrizamide CT at C6-C7 demonstrates a relatively small posterolateral disc with compression of the cord and roots. The anterior median raphe is also shifted.

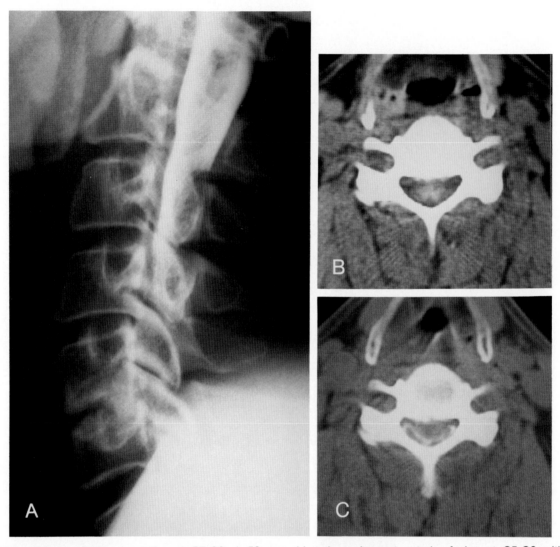

Figure 13.3. Midline soft-disc herniation at C5-C6. A 53-year-old male underwent anterior fusion at C5-C6 without any improvement. He was referred because of progressive gait disturbance over the past year. A. Cervical myelography via C1-C2 lateral puncture: A high-grade extradural block is noted from C4-C6. B. Plain CT at C5-C6 shows a large, high-density mass in the center of a slightly narrowed spinal canal. C. Metrizamide CT at C5-C6: The cord is compressed severely and becomes paper thin due to a large midline disc protrusion.

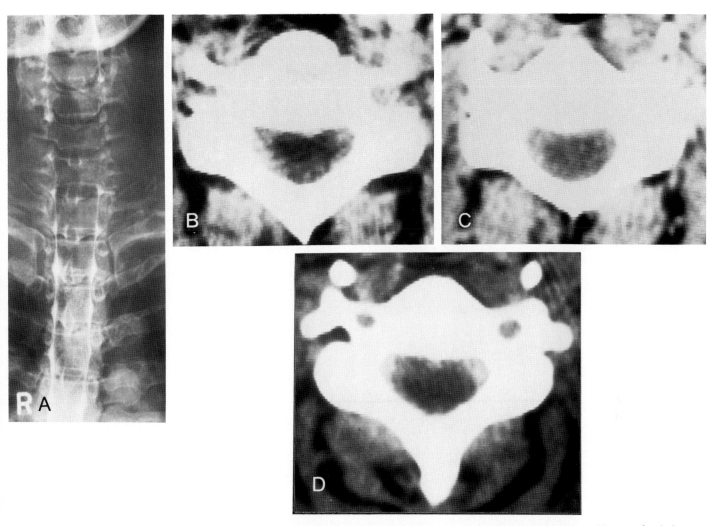

Figure 13.4. Intramedullary mixed glioma of the cervical cord. A 50-year-old female was admitted with 1-year history of pain in the neck and hands which recently had extended into the chest and shoulders. A. Myelography in anteroposterior view shows marked and diffuse swelling of the cord in the cervical and upper thoracic area. B. Plain CT at the C4 level suggests the presence of a low-density area in the anterior portion of the cord. C. Enhanced CT at the C4 level reveals that the cord has mixed densities with marginal enhancement. D. Metrizamide CT at almost the same level: The cord is swollen and hypodense and the subarachnoid space is narrowed.

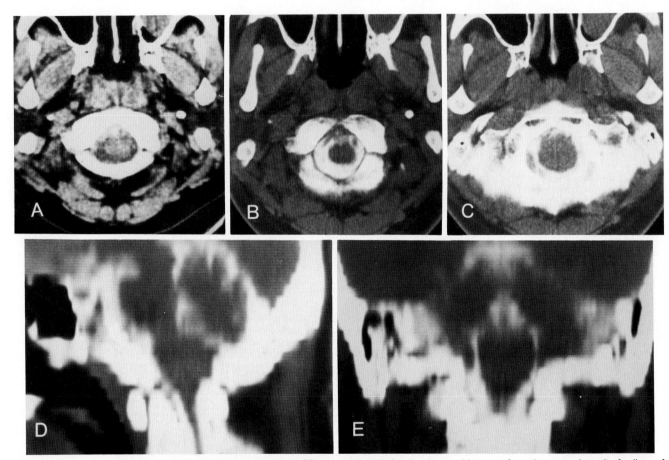

Figure 13.5. Astrocytoma of the medulla oblongata. A 26-year-old male had a 1-year history of vertigo, ataxic gait, feeling of tightness in the neck, and occasional difficulty in swallowing. A. Plain CT at the craniovertebral junction shows a lateral protrusion of the cord on the left. B. Metrizamide CT at this level confirms the presence of cord deformity on the left. C. Metrizamide CT at the foramen magnum reveals marked enlargement of the medulla oblongata. D. Metrizamide CT in sagittal reconstruction. E. Metrizamide CT in coronal reconstruction. The total configuration of the medullary mass is well-demonstrated. The 4th ventricle is elevated. At operation, a large intramedullary astrocytoma which originated in the medulla and extended to the inferior 4th ventricle through the obex was seen and partially removed.

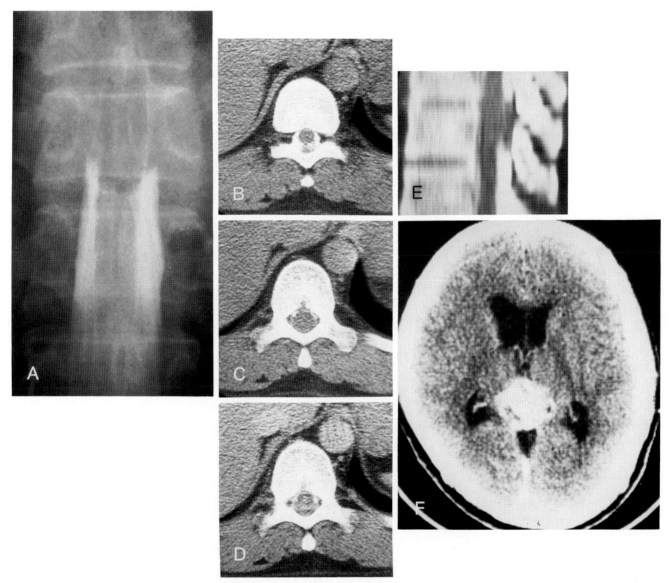

Figure 13.6. An intramedullary and extramedullary metastatic pineal body tumor at T11 in a 56-year-old male with a 3-month history of progressive numbness of the left leg, gait disturbance, and dysuria. A. Myelography via a lumbar puncture discloses an almost total block at T11. However, specific etiology of this block is not clear. B. Metrizamide CT at the inferior border of T11: The spinal cord is displaced anteriorly by the tumor, the lowest tip of which appears in a dilated subarachnoid space. C. Metrizamide CT at the superior border of T11: The tumor occupies the posterior half of the canal, flattening and anteriorly displacing the cord. D. Enhanced metrizamide CT at a slightly higher level: An irregularly enhanced tumor obviously invades the cord. E. Metrizamide CT in sagittal reconstruction shows the posteriorly located tumor and also slight swelling of the cord. F. Enhanced CT of the brain which was taken because of an amnestic episode after myelography clearly shows a large pineal body tumor.

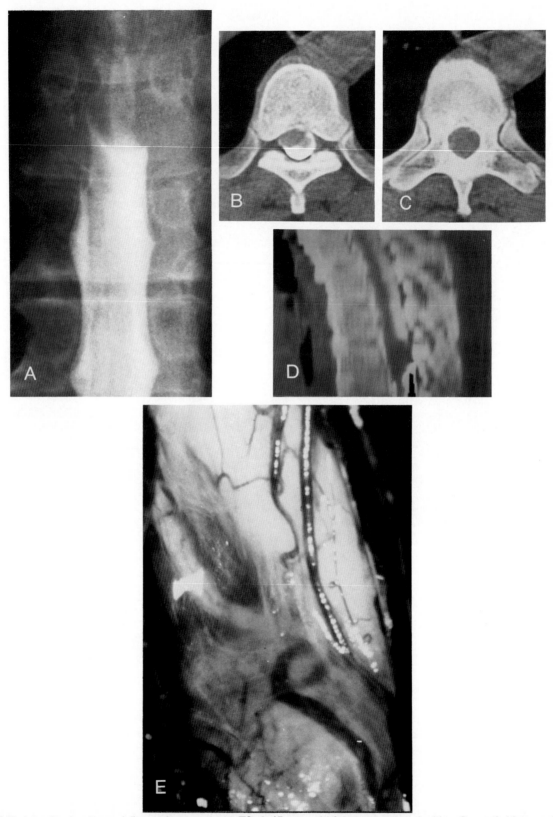

Figure 13.7. Intradural extramedullary schwannoma at T8. A 45-year-old farmer presented with a 5-month history of left flank pain and progressive numbness and weakness of the lower extremities of 3-weeks duration. A. Myelography via the lumbar route shows a complete block at T8 with a typical cupping appearance indicating an intradural extramedullary mass. B. Metrizamide CT at the T8-T9 level: The cord is displaced anteriorly and to the right. The lowest tip of the tumor is noted in the enlarged subarachnoid space. C. Metrizamide CT at T8: The compressed cord and the tumor are not definitely identified because of the high-grade block of the subarachnoid space. D. The sagittally reconstructed view discloses the upper and lower borders of the tumor. E. In a photograph through the operating microscope, a vascular extra-axial tumor apparently originates from a posterior root on the left.

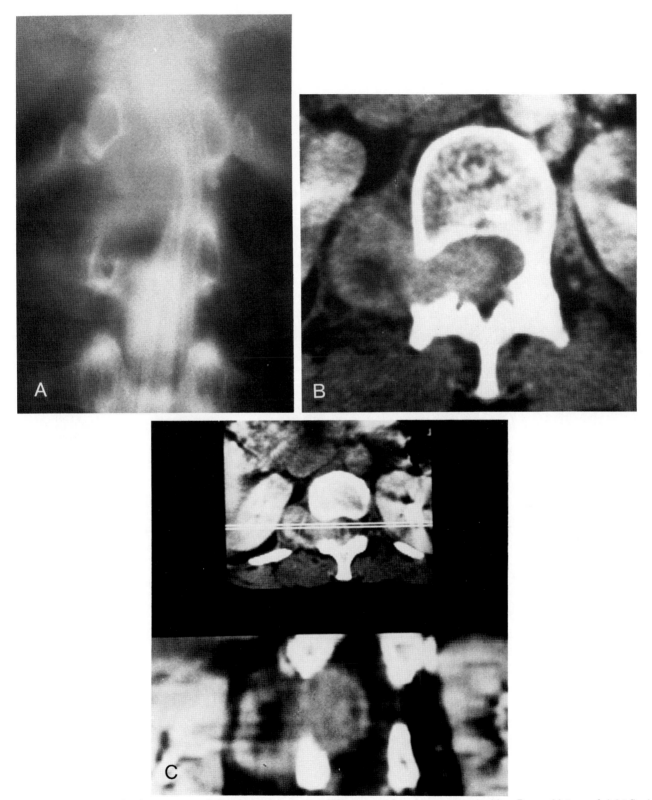

Figure 13.8. Dumbbell schwannoma of the T12 nerve root. A 36-year-old female presented with a 5-year history of right flank pain and a 1-month history of numbness of the right leg. Hypalgesia of the right T12 and L1 distribution was noted. A. Metrizamide myelography in an anteroposterior tomographic view: Clear-cut erosion of the pedicles of T12 and L1 was present on the right with marked displacement of the dural sac. B. Enhanced CT at the upper portion of L1 shows a typical appearance of a dumbbell schwannoma with intradural and paraspinal components. The pedicle is eroded on the right. C. A coronally reconstructed CT image corresponds well with the tomographic myelogram (A).

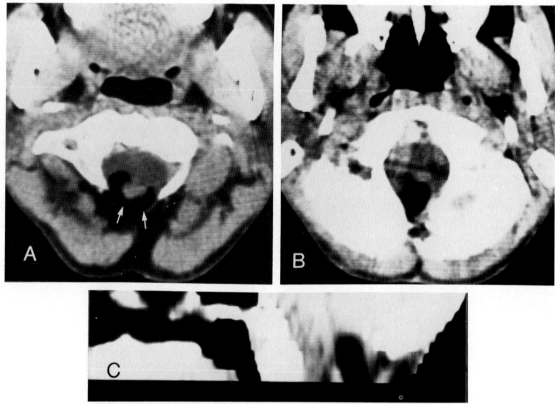

Figure 13.9. Intradural lipoma in the upper cervical region. A 36-year-old male who underwent an upper cervical laminectomy with partial removal of an intradural lipoma has had a full time job in spite of residual quadriparesis. A. Plain CT at the level of C1 shows a residual portion of the lipoma which encases two-thirds of the atrophic cord. B. Plain CT at the foramen magnum: The upper portion of the lipoma is located in the posterior portion of the foramen. C. Sagittal reconstruction reveals the upper extension of the tumor to be in the posterior fossa.

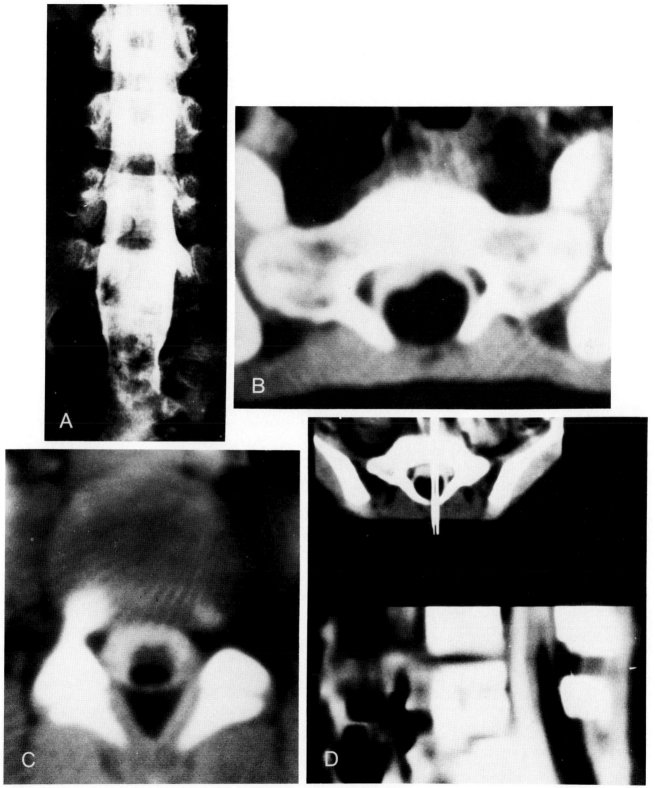

Figure 13.10. Sacral intradural lipoma and tethered cord. A 4-year-old male was noted to have a dimple 1 year ago and excision of a dermal sinus was performed. A. Lumbar myelography shows the presence of a tethered cord which connects to a mass in the sacral area. B. Metrizamide CT of the upper sacrum: There is a large lipoma in the enlarged canal which does not communicate with the subcutaneous fat tissue in spite of a spina bifida. C. Metrizamide CT at the L4-L5 space: The intradural lipoma is attached to the tethered cord and is separated clearly from the triangular epidural fat. D. In this sagittally reconstructed image, the superior extension of the lipoma into the tethered cord is visualized clearly.

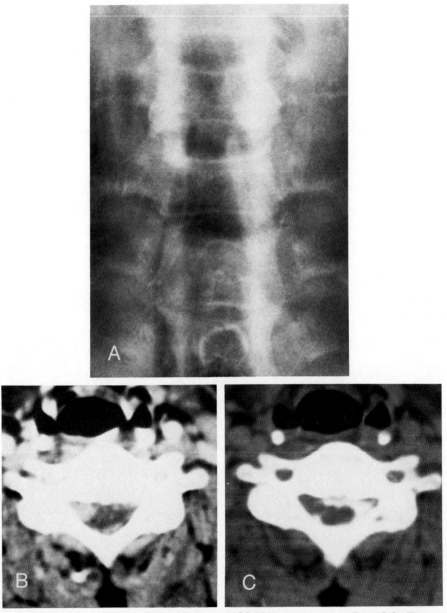

Figure 13.11. Subarachnoid seeding of the pineal body tumor at C5 (the same case as Fig. 13.6). The patient who underwent thoracic laminectomy with subtotal removal of intramedullary and extramedullary tumor and subsequently received radiotherapy to the head and the thoracic spine did well until 2 months ago when he developed radicular pain radiating to the right shoulder. A. Cervical myelography in an anteroposterior view shows a defect in right subarachnoid space. B. Enhanced CT with high-dose IV contrast injection at C5: There is an enhanced mass well-delineated in the right side of the canal in addition to other possible subarachnoid implants. C. Metrizamide CT at C5: An intradural extramedullary small mass is outlined clearly as well as a minimally deformed spinal cord.

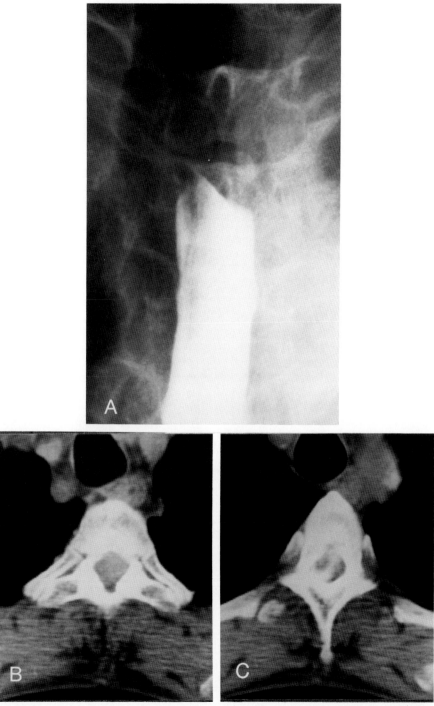

Figure 13.12. Epidural hemangioma at T3. A 73-year-old male was referred because of a 1-month history of back pain and progressive gait disturbance and frequency of urination. An incomplete Brown-Sequard phenomenon was noted. A. Thoracic myelography via a lumbar route shows a complete block at T3 with the cord being compressed and displaced to the right by an epidural mass. No evidence of bony destruction is present. B. Enhanced CT with IV contrast injection at T2 discloses a soft-tissue mass occupying two-thirds of the spinal canal on the left. C. Metrizamide CT at the superior aspect of T3: The lower portion of the epidural mass is present without bony erosion and the cord is compressed and shifted to the right.

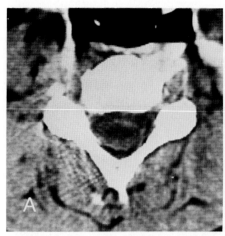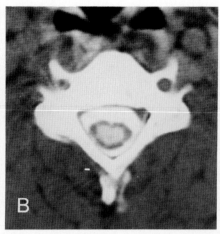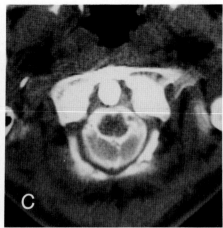

Figure 13.13. Syringomyelia with Arnold-Chiari malformation (type I). A 31-year-old male was admitted because of a 1-year history of progressive weakness and muscular atrophy of both hands and forearms. Sensory dissociation in the hands and hyperreflexia of the lower extremities also were noted. A. Plain CT at C4-C5: There is a low-density area in the center of the dilated cervical cord. B. Metrizamide CT taken 5 hours after the intrathecal injection of metrizamide: The syrinx is now filled with diluted metrizamide. The spinal canal and subarachnoid space also are enlarged significantly. C. Metrizamide CT at the craniovertebral junction shows downward displacement of the cerebellar tonsils.

fined cyst can also be seen (Fig. 13.4).

In our series, recognition of slight deformity of the cord at the C1 level on a plain CT actually led us to the diagnosis of astrocytoma of the medulla oblongata in a patient with a severe allergy to IV injection of iodine (Fig. 13.5). We found out that carefully performed intrathecal injection of metrizamide was less hazardous than IV contrast enhancement in a patient with an iodine allergy.

Another technique which we found useful was IV contrast enhancement combined with metrizamide CT. With this technique, the compressed cord and the narrow subarachnoid space were visualized along with an enhanced metastatic tumor invading the cord (Fig. 13.6).

INTRADURAL EXTRAMEDULLARY TUMOR

Schwannomas and meningiomas which are the most common intradural extramedullary tumors often demonstrate a characteristic CT picture, namely a dumbbell-type mass with bony erosion and a calcified intradural mass, respectively (2–5, 19).

On conventional myelography, a purely intradural extramedullary soft-tissue mass has a "cupped" appearance. It also appears this way on the transverse axial view of a metrizamide CT scan. The advantage of metrizamide CT over myelography is that in cases of myelographic block, it outlines the entire mass. It shows clearly, especially in sagittally reconstructed views, the superior and inferior extent of the tumor (Fig. 13.7).

In cases of dumbbell or hourglass schwannomas, an IV enhanced CT scan is the best study for outlining both the extradural and paraspinal components of these tumors and the associated pedicular and vertebral body destruction (Fig. 13.8). However, myelography or metrizamide CT is necessary for the demonstration of any intradural tumor involvement (2).

Schwannomas and meningiomas not infrequently originate at or extend to the foramen magnum, an area where

correct diagnosis is often difficult by conventional radiographic methods. The diagnosis, however, is facilitated greatly by metrizamide CT (4, 13, 20, 21).

The importance of CT in the diagnosis of an intradural lipoma has been well documented (2–5). Because the lipoma may originate in the extradural or intradural space or even in the subpial space (22) and often is associated with various congenital anomalies, metrizamide CT plays an important role in investigating the relationship between the lipoma and the cord which may be tethered down to the lower lumbar or even sacral area (23). Of great value is sagittal reconstruction which shows the longitudinal extension of the tumor (Figs. 13.9 and 13.10).

Seeding of intracranial tumors into the spinal subarachnoid space by way of cerebrospinal fluid is well known (22) and may occur in medulloblastoma, ependymoma, various gliomas, and in some pineal body tumors. Intraspinal implants can be visualized as soft-tissue masses on enhanced CT, whereas they can be identified as subarachnoid lesions by metrizamide CT (Fig. 13.11).

EPIDURAL TUMORS

The most frequent tumor of the spinal epidural space is a metastatic carcinoma. It often is accompanied by destruction of the vertebra.

CT is capable of demonstrating not only the details of bone destruction but also the exact extension of the soft-tissue mass into the spinal canal and into the paraspinal spaces (2–4).

With myelography, the differentiation between epidural and intradural extramedullary masses can be difficult. However with metrizamide CT, the diagnosis of an epidural mass is relatively easy to make because this study clearly demonstrates the separation of the dural sac from the neural arch. Figure 13.12, a benign epidural hemangioma, is a case in point.

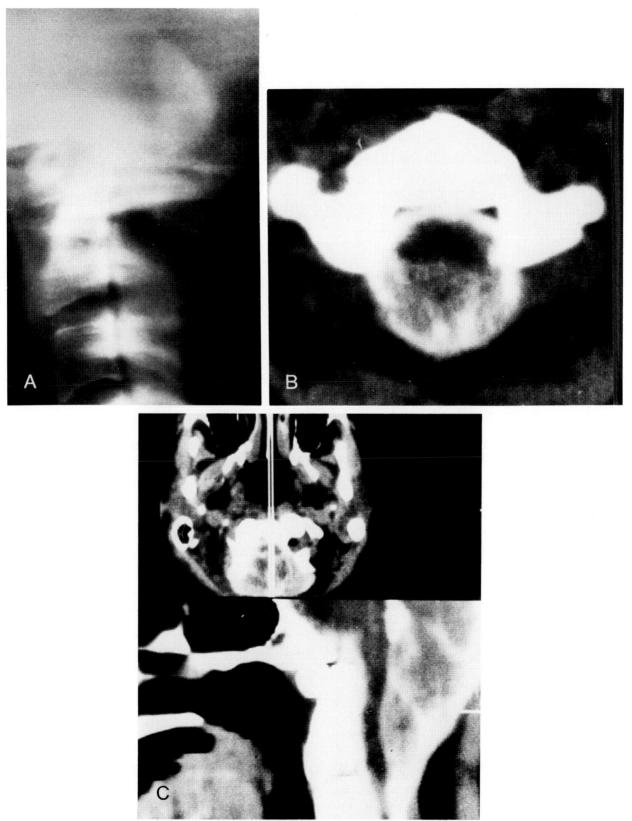

Figure 13.14. S/P decompression for an Arnold-Chiari malformation (type II). A 36-year-old female who had a suboccipital craniectomy and upper cervical laminectomy for Arnold-Chiari malformation was readmitted because of recent neurological deterioration. A. Metrizamide myeloencephalography with sagittal tomography shows downward displacement of a dilated 4th ventricle. B. Metrizamide CT at C2: The medulla remains compressed by herniated cerebellar tonsils in spite of the previous decompression. C. Metrizamide CT in sagittal reconstruction: Marked downward displacement of the cerebellar tonsils and vermis as well as the 4th ventricle and the medulla is clearly demonstrated.

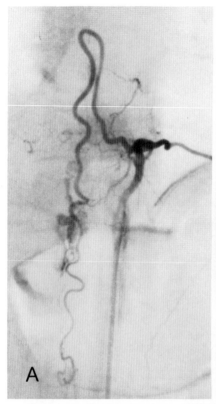 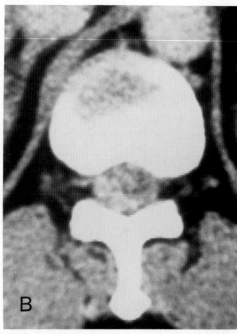 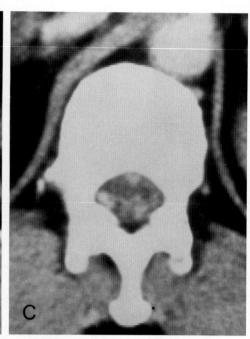

Figure 13.15. Arteriovenous malformation of the thoracolumbar cord. A 42-year-old patient with a several month history of progressive paraparesis. A. Selective spinal cord arteriography in a anterolateral view: The arteriovenous malformation was fed by the radicular artery of left T11. B. IV enhanced CT at T12-L1: Multiple densities which are markedly enhancing demonstrate that the AVM is in both an intramedullary and an extramedullary location. C. Enhanced CT at L1: AVM at this level appears to be mainly extramedullary.

SYRINGOMYELIA AND ARNOLD-CHIARI MALFORMATION

Previously, syringomyelia was evaluated by conventional contrast or air myelography, but not without some difficulty and risk. After the introduction of CT, there was great expectation that the diagnosis of syringomyelia would be simplified. However, initial whole body scanners were disappointing in regard to the complete delineation of a syrinx within the spinal cord and cerebellar tonsils (4, 24).

The advent of HRCT led to the more certain identification of a cystic cavity within a dilated cord. However, it did not resolve the difficulty on plain CT of identifying a cyst within a small cord, an occurrence not uncommon in syringomyelia (25).

With the use of intrathecal metrizamide during CT scanning, these diagnostic limitations were overcome. Metrizamide CT greatly increased diagnostic accuracy. It has now become the radiographic procedure of choice in evaluating syringomyelia (24–26).

Of a total of 64 cases of syringomyelia reported by Aubin et al. (25), the spinal cord appeared large on a metrizamide CT scan in 6, small in 29, and normal in 29, using the criteria established by Nordquist (27) at the C3-C4 level. Opacification of the syrinx cavity was seen in only 5 cases

(8%) on a scan 30 minutes after the injection of metrizamide. However, on a scan 6 hours after injection, the cavity was opacified in 59 of 64 (92%) cases (25).

Aubin et al. (25) also reported that there was a strong suggestion of transneural passage of metrizamide into the syrinx because the cavity was seen filled before the filling of the cisterna magna and the 4th ventricle. The possibility, however, of microscopic passage of metrizamide through the obex could not be eliminated.

As shown in Figure 13.13, metrizamide CT is probably the most reliable method of differentiating a syrinx from an intramedullary tumor with cyst formation.

The downward displacement of the tonsils and the medulla into the cervical canal also is outlined best by metrizamide CT (Fig. 13.14).

Axial and sagittally reconstructed scans demonstrate the Arnold-Chiari malformation to best advantage.

In Aubin's series, the Arnold-Chiari malformation was found in 48 of 64 (75%) cases, 47 being type I and one being a type II.

VASCULAR DISEASE

Arteriovenous malformations of the spinal cord can be diagnosed by myelography and selective angiography. However, angiography is an invasive and time-consuming procedure.

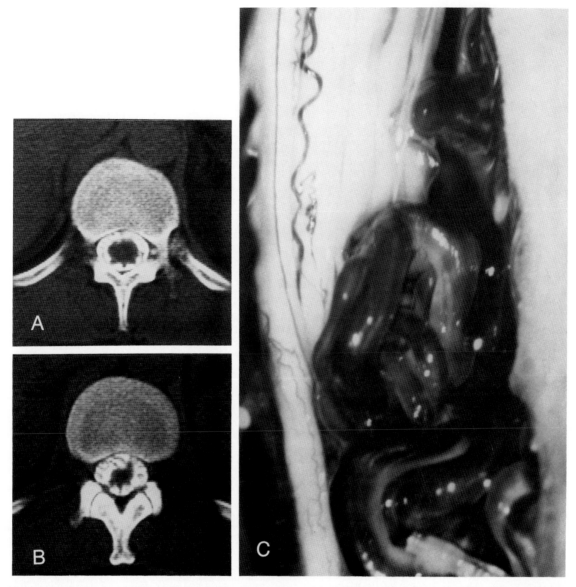

Figure 13.16. Arteriovenous malformation of the thoracolumbar cord and the cauda equina. A 40-year-old male with a 6-month history of back pain and numbness of the legs which were followed by gait disturbance and bladder and sphincter disturbance. Sensory level at T10, spastic paraparesis with absent ankle jerk and sacral anesthesia were found. Metrizamide myelography via C1-C2 lateral puncture vaguely showed abnormal vasculature in the cauda equina and a mass-like defect in the conus medullaris. A. Metrizamide CT at T11-T12: The spinal cord is enlarged and multiple defects due to the enlarged vessels are seen in the subarachnoid space. B. Metrizamide CT at T12-L1: The conus medullaris is deformed due to the abnormal vasculature. Selective spinal cord arteriography demonstrated an arteriovenous malformation in the cauda equina and the spinal cord which were fed by internal iliac arteries and the L4 lumbar arteries. C. Operative photograph through operating microscope: An extensive arteriovenous malformation was found and was totally removed.

With IV or intra-arterial contrast, CT can delineate abnormal intramedullary vessels (Fig. 13.15) (4, 29). With intrathecal metrizamide, CT can demonstrate vascular malformations in the subarachnoid sac as well as cord enlargement (Fig. 13.16).

Another vascular disorder which can be diagnosed easily by CT is massive hemorrhage in the spinal canal, whether occurring in the cord, in the subarachnoid sac, or in the subdural or epidural spaces. In cases of intra-spinal hemorrhage due to hemophilia where surgical treatment is not indicated, CT also can be used as a valuable follow-up procedure (Fig. 13.17).

CONCLUSIONS

There is no question that HRCT has improved visualization of intraspinal anatomy and pathology significantly. Carefully performed plain CT is capable of demonstrating

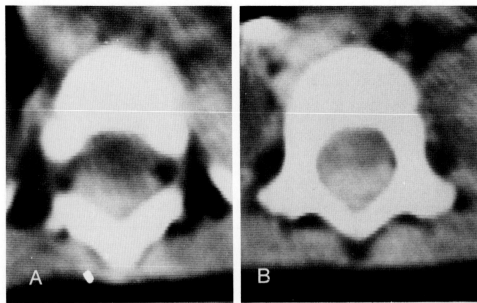

Figure 13.17. Intraspinal hemorrhage in hemophilia. An 8-month-old patient with known hemophilia was referred because of acute onset of paraplegia. A lumbar puncture showed grossly bloody cerebrospinal fluid. A. Plain CT at T12-L1. B. Plain CT at L1. There is a clearly demarcated area of high density in the posterior half of the canal which is compatible with a hematoma in the epidural space. Vague densities anteriorly suggest the presence of subarachnoid hemorrhage.

certain soft-tissue lesions such as cervical soft-disc herniations and cystic lesions of the cord. IV enhanced CT is capable of detecting certain vascular lesions such as arteriovenous malformations and vascular tumors.

Nevertheless, in order to visualize the spinal cord and the subarachnoid space clearly, it still is necessary to employ the intrathecal injection of metrizamide. Metrizamide CT enables us to evaluate the relationship of the lesion with the spinal cord directly. For this reason, metrizamide CT should be performed routinely after myelography.

Metrizamide CT is especially useful in the diagnosis of cervical central disc herniations which may be missed by myelography and in the detection (on a delayed scan) of syringomyelia.

References

1. Hammerschlag SB, Wolpert SM, Carter BL: Computed tomography of the spinal canal. *Radiology* 121:361–367, 1976.
2. Nakagawa H, Huang YP, Malis LI, et al: Computed tomography of intraspinal and paraspinal neoplasms. *J Comput Assist Tomogr* 1:377–390, 1977.
3. Aubin ML, Jardin C, Bar D, et al: Computerized tomography in 32 cases of intraspinal tumors. *J Neuroradiol* 6:81–92, 1979.
4. Nakagawa H, Malis LI, Huang YP: Computed tomography of soft tissue masses related to the spinal column. In: Post MJD: *Radiographic Evaluation of the Spine: Current Advances with Emphasis on Computed Tomography.* New York, Masson Publishing, 1980, pp. 320–352.
5. Isu T, Ito T, Iwasaki Y, et al: Computed tomography in the diagnosis of spinal cord tumor. *Neurol Med Chirurg* 20:833–844, 1980.
6. Post MJD: CT update: The impact of time, metrizamide, and high resolution on the diagnosis of spinal pathology. In: Post MJD: *Radiographic Evaluation of the Spine: Current Advances with Emphasis on Computed Tomography.* New York, Masson Publishing, 1980, pp. 259–294.
7. Haughton VM, Syvertsen A, Willims AL: Soft-tissue anatomy within the spinal canal as seen on computed tomography. *Radiology* 134:649–655, 1980.
8. Raskin SP: Demonstration of nerve roots on unenhanced computed tomographic scans. *J Comput Assist Tomogr* 5:281–284, 1981.
9. Taylor AJ, Haughton VM, Doust BD: CT imaging of the thoracic spinal cord without intrathecal contrast medium. *J Comput Assist Tomogr* 4:223–224, 1980.
10. Pullicino P, duBoulay GH, Kendall BE: Xenon enhancement for computed tomography of the spinal cord. *Neuroradiology* 18:63–66, 1979.
11. Coin CG, Coin JT: Contrast enhancement by xenon gas in computed tomography of the spinal cord and brain: preliminary observations. *J Comput Assist Tomogr* 4:217–221, 1980.
12. Di Chiro G, Schellinger D: Computed tomography of spinal cord after lumbar intrathecal introduction of metrizamide (Computer assisted myelography). *Radiology* 120:101–104, 1976.
13. Nakagawa H: CT diagnosis of the spinal disorders—Regional anatomy and pathology. 1. Craniovertebral junction and upper cervical spine. *Prog Comput Tomogr* (Eng. Abstr.) 3:5–12, 1981.
14. Nakagawa H: CT diagnosis of the spinal disorders—Regional anatomy and pathology. 2. Mid and lower cervical spine. *Prog Comput Tomogr* (Eng. Abstr.) 3:141–148, 1981.
15. Coin CG, Coin JT: Computed tomography of cervical disk disease: Technical considerations with representative case reports. *J Comput Assist Tomogr* 5:275–280, 1981.
16. Miyasaka K, Isu T, Iwasaki Y, et al. High resolution computed tomography in the diagnosis of cervical disc disease. *Neuroradiology* 24:253–257, 1983.
17. Nakagawa H, Okumura T, Sugiyama T, et al: Discrepancy between metrizamide CT and myelography in diagnosis of cervical disks. *AJNR* May/June 1983.
18. Handel S, Grossman R, Sarwar M: Computed tomography in the diagnosis of spinal cord astrocytoma. *J Comput Assist*

Tomogr 2:226–228, 1978.
19. Balériaux-Waha D, Terwinghe G, Jeanmart L: The value of computed tomography for the diagnosis of hourglass tumors of the spine. *Neuroradiology* 14:31–42, 1977.
20. Spallone A, Tanfani G, Vassilouthis J, et al: Benign extramedullary foramen magnum tumors: Diagnosis by computed tomography. *J Comput Assist Tomogr* 4:225–229, 1980.
21. Thijsen HOM, Keyser A, Horstink MWM, et al: Morphology of the cervical spinal cord on computed myelography. *Neuroradiology* 18:57–62, 1979.
22. Epstein BS: *The Spine, A Radiological Text and Atlas*, 4th Edition. Philadelphia, Lea and Febiger, 1976.
23. Resjö MI, Harwood-Nash DC, Fitz CR, et al: Computed tomographic metrizamide myelography in spinal dysraphism in infants and children. *J Comput Assist Tomogr* 2:549–558, 1978.
24. Forbes WSC, Ischerwood I: Computed tomography in syringomyelia and the associated Arnold-Chiari Type I malformation. *Neuroradiology* 15:73–78, 1978.
25. Aubin MC, Vignaud J, Jardin C, et al: Computed tomography in 75 clinical cases of syringomyelia. *AJNR* 2:199–204, 1981.
26. Bonafé A, Manelfe C, Espagno J, et al: Evaluation of syringomyelia with metrizamide computed tomographic myelography. *J Comput Assist Tomogr* 4:797–802, 1980.
27. Nordquist L: The sagittal diameter of the cord and subarachnoid space in different age groups. A roentgenographic postmortem study. *Acta Radiol (Stockh)* Suppl 227, 1964.
28. Di Chiro G, Doppman JL, Wener L: Computed tomography of spinal cord arteriovenous malformations. *Radiology* 123:351–354, 1977.
29. Nagashima C, Yamaguchi T, Tsuji R: Arteriovenous malformation of the cord: Computed tomography with intraarterial enhancement. *J Comput Assist Tomogr* 5:586–587, 1981.

SECTION III

Computed Tomography of the Pediatric Spine and of Congenital Abnormalities

CHAPTER FOURTEEN

Computed Tomography of the Pediatric Spine

HOLGER PETTERSSON, M.D., and DEREK C. HARWOOD-NASH, M.B., Ch.B., F.R.C.P.(C)

INTRODUCTION

During the first years after its introduction, CT in pediatric neuroradiology had its largest impact on the assessment of the skull and brain, just as in adult neuroradiology. The subsequent application of wide-aperture CT scanners provided the possibility to include also CT of the spine and spinal canal into the diagnostic arsenal, and a few years later, the diagnostic accuracy of the CT examinations was enhanced considerably due to the introduction of high-resolution technique. Concurrent with this development of the CT examination, metrizamide (Amipaque, Nyegaard & Co A/S, Oslo, Norway), a water-soluble cerebrospinal fluid (CSF) contrast medium, was introduced, primarily as a contrast medium designed for conventional myelography. The combination of CT and metrizamide has meant a minor revolution in the imaging of the spine and spinal canal in pediatric radiology, and spinal CT (SCT) and CT metrizamide myelography (CTMM) in children now occupies about 25% of the routine work load in pediatric neuroradiology. These examinations have improved our knowledge of the normal anatomy considerably as well as the pathology of the spine and its contents in children, and they consequently also have changed and improved the clinical management of the diseases in the areas of pediatric neurosurgery and neurology, orthopaedic surgery, and genitourinary surgery.

At the Hospital for Sick Children, Toronto, Canada, our initial CT experience was obtained from an Ohio Nuclear Delta 50 scanner (1–5). During the last 2½ years we have used a General Electric CT/T 8800, with a computer program providing high spatial resolution. The following chapter as well as the illustrations are based primarily on our experiences from this modern equipment.

Given the above-mentioned modern diagnostic tools, the following imaging modalities are now available in pediatric neuroradiology: Conventional radiography (plain films), conventional metrizamide myelography (MM), radionuclide bone scans, SCT and CTMM. In the following, we will give our experience concerning the technique, normal anatomy, and pathology concerning SCT and CTMM. SCT with or without enhancement with intravenous (IV) contrast medium injection, may give sufficient information in some cases, but often additional important information is provided if metrizamide is injected into the subarachnoid space and a CTMM is performed. For this reason, the findings at SCT and CTMM integrated will be described. The diagnostic accuracy of the CT examinations, as compared with conventional examinations then will be discussed, and ultimately, our protocols for the use of the available diagnostic modalities in different conditions will be given.

TECHNIQUE

Preparation and Positioning of the Patient

In infants and small children, the normal physiological state is disturbed easily by temperature loss, dehydration, or local pressure on the infant's body, and precautions must be taken against these risks. Thus, the CT room should be at the ambient hospital temperature. There is no need for starvation before the examination; on the contrary, a meal before the examination will act as a slight sedation. An IV drip infusion of saline, introduced before the examination, will prevent dehydration, and also will make IV contrast medium enhancement possible without disturbing the infant during the examination. Bundling of the neonates and small infants in a soft towel will protect and maintain some warmth. It also will minimize movements. A rubber blanket containing rubber tubes is then wrapped around the towel as described by Harwood-Nash and Fitz (5). Restraining bands across the wrapping stabilize the child on the table. Older children are secured only in a soft blanket. The supine position during the examination is most comfortable, and in this position the chest and abdominal movements during breathing are much less than in the prone position, providing less movement artifacts.

Sedation

If sedation is necessary, we use intramuscular Nembutal (pentobarbital) in a dose of 6 mg/kg body weight if the weight is 15 kg or less and 5 mg/kg body weight if the weight is more than 15 kg, to a maximum dose of 200 mg. A supplementary dose of 2 mg/kg body weight may be given 20 minutes after the initial injection. This sedation should be given at least 20 minutes before the procedure.

For SCT, sedation as described above seldom is demanded above the age of 3 or 4 years. For primary CTMM, in which the CT examination is performed immediately after the lumbar puncture and metrizamide injection, and in which no conventional metrizamide myelography has preceded the CT examination, general anesthesia is not necessary, and sedation as described usually is given up to an age of about 8 years. In secondary CTMM, in which a conventional metrizamide myelography precedes the CT examination, general anesthesia for the MM should be given to all children below the age of about 6, and to about 50% of the children between 6–12 years of age. This general anesthesia then is continued during the CTMM. In older children, a sedation as described above may be enough.

Metrizamide Injection

The technique of lumbar puncture and subarachnoid injection is the same as in conventional myelography, and will not be discussed here. In primary CTMM, small doses of metrizamide are sufficient. We use 1–7 ml, depending upon the age of the child, at a concentration of 170 mg iodine/ml, which is isotonic with the CSF. The patient is tilted and rolled after the metrizamide injection, to mix the contrast medium with the CSF, and after this the CT examination is performed. Too much metrizamide should be avoided, as large concentrations of iodine in the subarachnoid space will create an over-range in the image, with an obliteration of the small structures.

If secondary CTMM is performed, the dose of metrizamide given is that of the previously performed conventional MM (6, 7). We use between 2–12 ml metrizamide, with a concentration varying between 170–250 mg iodine/ml. As the adverse reactions to metrizamide are caused by effects on the central nervous system (CNS), the proper maximum amount given should be related to the child's age, and not to the body weight or size, as the size of the CNS is a function of the age (8). The optimal iodine concentration for the CT examination after a conventional metrizamide myelography is obtained during the first hours of the metrizamide injection, and an acceptable concentration often is maintained during the first 4 or 5 hours after the MM.

IV Contrast Medium Injection

IV contrast medium injection may be of value in the examination of, for instance, arteriovenous malformations or neoplasms. In these cases, we use Hypaque 60%, 3 ml/kg body weight, and most information is provided if CT

sections are performed both before and immediately after the contrast medium injection.

CT Technique

It is mandatory to get an exact identification of the anatomical level of the CT section. With modern CT equipment, this is obtained by a digital radiograph (ScoutView image, General Electric Medical Systems). Because the ScoutView image as well as the trans-sectional CT images are obtained by the same tube and detector systems, the ScoutView acts as a perfect localization system (9). Though the ScoutView still does not provide as high a spatial resolution as a conventional radiograph, it gives sufficient information to identify the anatomical areas to be scanned, and also provides information of the gross anatomy of the lesion to be examined (Fig. 14.1). On the ScoutView image, each section scanned may be marked by a computed superimposition of a cursor line (Fig. 14.2).

THE IMAGE

To enhance the spatial resolution and contrast discrimination, modern CT machines now provide a computer program giving target reconstruction of the raw data obtained during the scanning, as described in other chapters. This target reconstruction, combined with double-pass reconstruction for correlation of the bone hardening effect of the spine increases the spatial resolution and contrast discrimination considerably, and if possible, should be used in all examinations of the pediatric spine.

In older machines, in which no high resolution system is obtainable, the metrizamide as well as the surrounding bone with high attenuation values will cause over-range with "blooming" of the image on the screen. To diminish this, a wide window width and a high window level should be used. In this case, it also is valuable to reverse the color scale to black on white as structures with a low attenua-

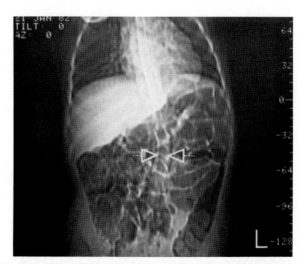

Figure 14.1. Digital radiograph of a 3-year-old girl. The anatomical landmarks are well outlined as is the scoliotic spine. Metrizamide has been injected in the subarachnoid space, and the widened low cord is visualized (*arrows*).

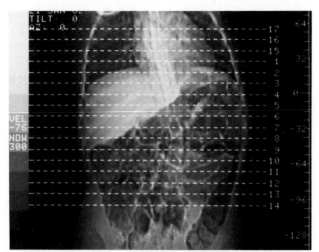

Figure 14.2. Digital radiograph—Cursor lines of same patient as in Figure 14.1. Cursor lines outline the levels of the CT sections.

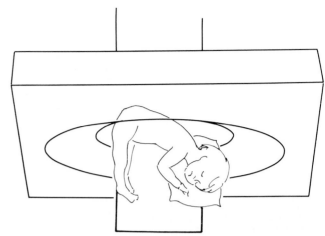

Figure 14.3. Direct coronal CT: Drawing of the position of the child, placed decubitus on the table with the long axis of the body parallel to the gantry. Reproduced by permission from: Pettersson H, Harwood-Nash DCF. *CT and Myelography of the Spine and Cord.* Berlin, Springer-Verlag, 1982.

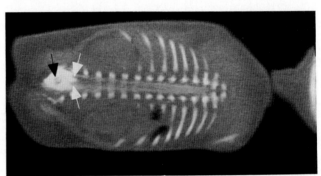

Figure 14.4. Direct coronal CT of a 10-day-old boy. Metrizamide has been injected in the thecal sac, outlining a low cord which is split in the lower lumbar region (*white arrows*). In the sacral region, the canal and thecal sac is widened, and there is a small lipoma (*black arrow*).

tion, for instance the cord and nerve roots, then will appear white. The unavoidable over-range on the screen then will make these structures apparently enlarged and more clearly visible.

RECONSTRUCTION TO OTHER PLANES AND DIRECT CORONAL SECTIONS

Performing transaxial CT, sections as perpendicular as possible to each part of the spine should be obtained, in order to assess the true size and form of the skeletal and intraspinal structures. To achieve this, the gantry may be angled, but this angling, at times, may be insufficient to overcome the lower lumbar lordosis or a severe kyphosis, for instance. In these instances, image reconstruction to planes angled to the initial sections may be obtained with the aid of the computer. In modern machines, the image may be reconstructed to any plane although the sagittal or coronal are the most often used. This technique has been described elsewhere in this book. However, the programs available for reconstruction to planes angled to the initial sections still do not give complete detailed information. A direct coronal section through the spine will provide much better spatial resolution than a coronal section reconstructed from transaxial scans (10), and we have found direct coronal sections of the pediatric spinal canal vary valuable (11). To obtain these direct coronal sections, the child is placed in the decubitus position across the examination table, the long axis of the spine being as parallel to the plane of the gantry as possible (Fig. 14.3). The head of the child often will be situated outside the CT table and may be supported by the radiologist's hands. Using the largest scanning circle and 10-mm thickness sections, we have obtained coronal images of the spinal canal with a considerably high accuracy (Fig. 14.4). However, this method is used best for small children up to the age of 5 years in most CT scanners because the size of the gantry hole is a limiting factor for older children. Direct coronal sections of the occipitocervical region and

the upper cervical vertebrae may be obtained from children of all ages if the patient is positioned supine with a pillow beneath the shoulders and the neck maximally extended, as described by Harwood-Nash and Fitz (5) (Fig. 14.5).

NORMAL ANATOMY

During growth the anatomy of the spine and its contents is subject to a dynamic change: not only the absolute size and shape of the vertebral bodies, the spinal canal and the dural sac and cord changes, but there is also a change in the relationship between the relative size of these different structures.

The Vertebral Column

In the small infant, the spine is straight from occiput to coccyx. When the infant begins to sit up and walk, the cervical and lumbar lordosis and the thoracic kyphosis

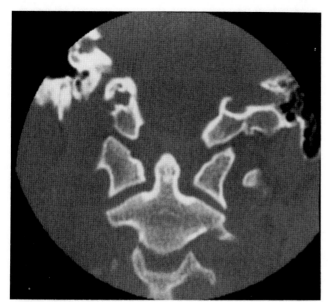

Figure 14.5. Direct coronal CT of a 13-year-old girl, upper cervical spine. The relationships between the occiput, the C1 and C2 vertebrae, including the odontoid, are well visualized.

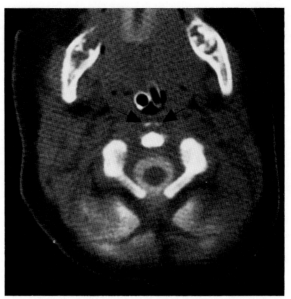

Figure 14.6. Normal cervical spine of an 8-month-old girl, C1. There are 2 small ossification centers of the C1 anterior arch (*arrows*). The neural arches are ossified from 2 C-shaped ossification centers, with small transverse processes. In the midline, there is 1 ossification center of the odontoid. Metrizamide has been injected into the subarachnoid space and the cervical cord is rounded and placed centrally in the thecal sac.

appear. This should be borne in mind when choosing the gantry angles, to get axial sections perpendicular to the spine.

At birth, there are usually 1 or possibly 2 ossification centers in each vertebral body. If there are 2 centers, they are divided by a sagittal or coronal cleft. The neural arch is ossified from 2 centers, 1 on each side (Fig. 14.6).

In the C1 vertebra, the anterior arch ossifies from 1–4 centers and there might be 1 small center posteriorly in the midline between the 2 ossification centers of the posterior arch.

The odontoid process normally contains two ossification centers, divided by a sagittal "cleft", symmetrically placed within the C1 arch, while the tip of the odontoid ossifies from 1 or 2 separate centers. The anatomy of the occipital condyles, and the relation between the occiput and the C1 and C2 vertebrae, often is demonstrated best in the coronal view (Fig. 14.5).

The pedicle-lamina complexes in the lower cervical vertebrae ossifies from 2 C-shaped ossification centers with very small transverse processes (Fig. 14.6). During the first year of life, the pedicles become thicker and the transverse processes become outlined by bone (Fig. 14.7). The transverse processes as well as the foramina transversaria are outlined completely by bone at the age of 3 (Fig. 14.12).

In the thoracic region, the pedicles are longer than the laminae (Fig. 14.8), whereas in the lumbar region, the pedicles are thick and of the same length as or shorter than the laminae (Fig. 14.9).

In the sacrum, the ossified parts of the pedicles and laminae are small in infancy and early childhood, and the sacroiliac joints are wide (Fig. 14.10). The heavy buttressing of these structures does not appear until about the age of 5.

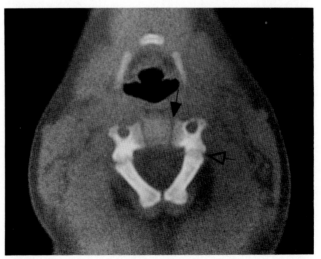

Figure 14.7. Normal cervical spine of a 1-year-old boy, C5. The transverse processes as well as the pedicles now are outlined by bone. The neurocentral synchondrosis (*black arrow*) as well as the interosseous cartilage (*open arrow*) still are open. Also, the posterior cartilaginous junction between the neural arches is open, and should not be mistaken for spina bifida.

The cartilaginous junctions between the above-described ossification centers disappear during the first years of life. The rare sagittal cleft in the vertebral bodies normally fuses before the age of 6 months. The junctions between the ossification centers of the anterior arch of the

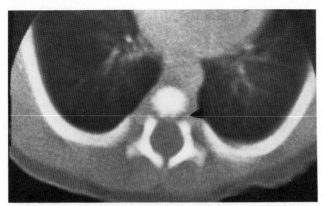

Figure 14.8. Normal thoracic spine of a 13-day-old girl, T7. In the thoracic region, the pedicles are longer than the laminae. The neurocentral synchondrosis is wide (*black arrow*).

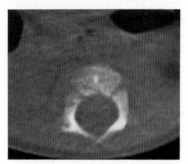

Figure 14.9. Normal lumbar spine of a 2-month-old boy. The pedicles are thick and of the same length as the laminae. The neurocentral synchondrosis is wide.

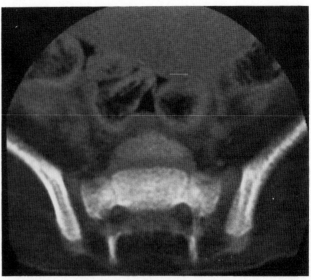

Figure 14.10. Normal sacroiliac joints of a 4-year-old boy. The sacroiliac joints are normally still wide. (There is a pronounced dysraphism, the neural arches of S1 vertebra being parallel.)

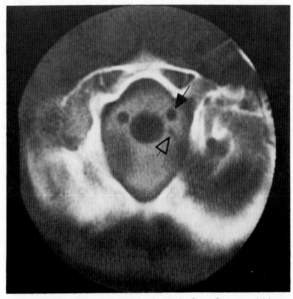

Figure 14.11. Normal cervical cord of an 8-year-old boy. At the foramen magnum, the cervical cord is round and centrally placed. The vertebral arteries (*black arrow*) are visualized as is one of the hypoglossal nerves (*open arrow*).

C1 vertebra disappears before the age of 3, as do the junctions between the ossification centers of the odontoid.

The neurocentral synchondrosis, positioned between the vertebral body and the neural arch, is wide in the infant (Fig. 14.8). It disappears at the age of 4, but often a thin area of increased density at the fusion site remains through childhood and early adolescence (Fig. 14.18).

The junction of the two halves of the spinal processes ossify during the first years of life, the latest to ossify being the junctions of C1 and L5, which usually have disappeared at the age of 5 years. These cartilaginous junctions should never be regarded as a spina bifida (Fig. 14.7).

The Spinal Canal

The absolute size of the spinal canal increases until the age of 16. Also, the size and shape of the canal relative to the size of the vertebral bodies changes with growth. Thus, in infants and small children, the transverse diameter of the canal is wider than that of the vertebral body in the whole spine (Fig. 14.8). From the ages of about 6–8 years, the transverse diameter of the cervical canal is about the same size as that of the cervical vertebral body (Fig. 14.12), whereas in the thoracic and lumbar area, the canal is smaller than the corresponding body (Fig. 14.13).

Also, the shape of the spinal canal changes with age: in infancy the cervical canal is oval with the large diameter oriented transversely, the thoracic canal is oval with the large diameter oriented sagittally, whereas the lumbar canal is shaped in the same way as the cervical. With increasing age, the shape of the canal becomes more triangulated, with the apex posteriorly.

The Contents of the Spinal Canal

As has been described above concerning the spinal column and canal, the shape and size of the dural sac and

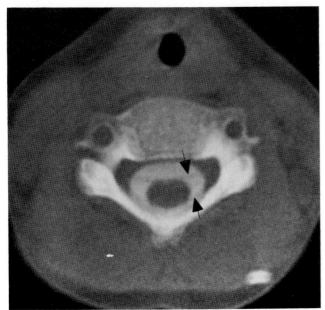

Figure 14.12. Normal cervical cord of an 8-year-old boy, C4. The dural sac and cord are oval with the large diameter oriented transversely. The roots are well visualized (*arrows*). The spinal canal is triangulated, and its transverse diameter is of the same size as the transverse diameter of the vertebral body.

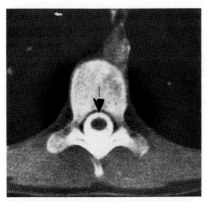

Figure 14.13. Normal thoracic cord of an 11-year-old boy, T6. In the upper thoracic region, the cord is placed anteriorly. The nerve roots and the anterior spinal artery (*arrow*) are visualized.

its contents also change during growth. However, at all ages, absolute symmetry from one side to the other is the rule throughout the canal.

SHAPE

At the foramen magnum and the C1–C2 level, the cord is round and placed centrally in the subarachnoid space. At this level, also, the vertebral arteries may be seen (Fig. 14.11). At the lower cervical level, the dural sac and the cord become oval with the large diameter oriented transversely (Fig. 14.12). During the first months of life, though, the subarachnoid space and the cord are more rounded

throughout the cervical region (Fig. 14.6).

At the cervicothoracic junction, the cord becomes relatively smaller and, at the T3 level, the dural sac is slightly oval with the large diameter in the sagittal plane, and the cord is now situated close to the anterior wall of the sac (Fig. 14.13). This is the only area in the canal in which the cord normally is placed anteriorly, and this is caused by the thoracic kyphosis.

At the T10–T11 level, where the cord widens to form the conus, it is placed centrally in the canal and subarachnoid space. Here the emerging anterior and posterior roots are large as are the anterior and posterior spinal arteries (Fig. 14.14). From this level on, the cord and roots have the same configuration regardless of age. At the L1–L2 level, the conus narrows forming the filum terminale, whereas the roots form the cauda equina (Fig. 14.15). Normally, the tip of the conus is at the level of L1–L2 at the age of 2 months, but to our experience it may be situated as low as at the L2–L3 disc space without any pathological significance, and at the age of 12 years, the

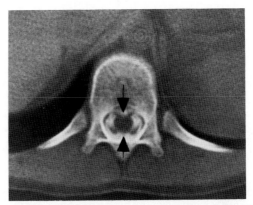

Figure 14.14. Normal conus of an 11-year-old boy, T12. At this level, the normal cord is thick, as are the emerging nerve roots. Note the anterior and posterior spinal arteries (*arrows*).

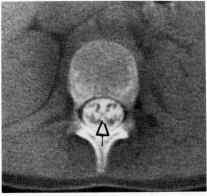

Figure 14.15. The tip of the conus of an 11-year-old boy, L2. This is the same patient as Figure 14.14. The tip of the conus has merged into the filum terminale (*arrow*). The nerve roots, collected in two pairs on each side of the filum will form the cauda equina.

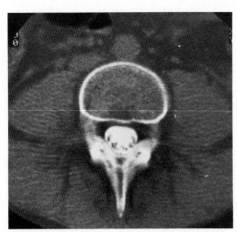

Figure 14.16. Normal cauda equina of a 16-year-old girl, L3. The roots are arranged in a crescentic shape, the sacral roots being situated medially to the lumbar. The filum terminale is still visible in the midline.

tip should be at or above the L2 level (12). Below the tip of the conus, the nerve roots and the filum terminale are situated in the posterior half of the dural sac in a crescentic or V-shaped form (Fig. 14.16), the sacral roots being situated medially to the lumbar roots.

SIZE AND ATTENUATION VALUES

The dimensions of structures as appearing in the CT images are influenced greatly by the window level whereas the window width is less important. Seibert et al. (13) recently showed that for measurements of the cord and roots the appropriate window level is the mean between the attenuation value for the metrizamide in the subarachnoid space and that of the cord. The measurements are performed most easily and accurately with a low window width (20 HU). In a recent investigation (10), we showed that the normal cord size according to age varies within a wide range at most spinal levels and age groups. Thus, the morphology of the cord rather than its size is the essential parameter in the evaluation of pathological conditions. However, the cord increases in size most rapidly during the first months of life, whereas this increase in size is much slower after the age of about 6 months. This probably is due to the rapid myelinization in the early infancy.

With the technical equipment available today, the dural sac and its contents at SCT appear as a homogeneous density within the spinal canal, except at the high cervical levels, where the cord may be seen within the subarachnoid space (14). The attenuation values of the cord before any contrast medium injection vary between 30–45 HU (5). After IV contrast medium injection as described earlier in this chapter, the attenuation values of the cord increase by about 10 HU. At the same time, there is an increase in the attenuation values of the epidural space. After metrizamide injection into the subarachnoid space, the attenuation value of the cord may increase with about 30 HU, caused by an absorption of metrizamide, probably in the Virchow-Robin spaces (5, 15).

PATHOLOGICAL CONDITIONS

Modern CT equipment with possibilities for high resolution and multiplanar reconstruction, has added dramatically to the diagnosing and understanding of the pathology of the spine and paraspinal structures in children. After introduction of metrizamide into the subarachnoid space also the anatomy of the intrathecal structures and their abnormalities may be studied in detail.

In the following, the pediatric pathological conditions will be described as appearing at SCT or CTMM. However, in most cases, the general geography of the spine must be considered initially, either by a digital radiograph, or a conventional examination. Also, conventional myelography and radionuclide bone scans still have application in many circumstances. Therefore, the appropriate place of the CT examination in the diagnostic protocols of different pediatric conditions will be discussed in the end of this chapter.

Congenital Anomalies

A major contribution of CT to the examination of the spine and its contents in pediatric praxis is within the area of congenital anomalies (10). Spinal dysraphism, including a vast variety of abnormalities of the skeleton, the thecal sac, and its contents, as well as surrounding structures, occupies an important part in the spectrum of congenital anomalies both from a clinical and a radiographic point of view. This spectrum also includes musculoskeletal disorders and dysplasias, as well as scoliosis.

DYSRAPHISM

The term "spinal dysraphism" denotes defective fusion of the neural tube (16). The abnormalities may involve the vertebral bodies, and/or the posterior neural arch. Thus, there may be hemivertebrae, cleft vertebrae, defect vertebral segmentation, spina bifida, or asymmetrical and widely spread neural arches. In the formation of the spinal cord, the dysraphism may be manifested as a thick filum terminale with tethering of the cord, or as myelomeningocele, diastematomyelia, or Chiari malformation. Overgrowth of tissue, sequestered during the fetal growth, may result in developmental mass lesions as dermoid, epidermoid, lipoma, or teratoma. A neuroenteric cyst is the result of persistance of the transient open passage in the embryo between the yolk sac and the notochordal canal.

The above-described anomalies may be occult, without any cutaneous abnormalities, or manifested by cutaneous abnormalities as a hairy patch or abnormal pigmentation, a vascular nevus, dermal sinus, lipoma, or an obvious meningocele or myelomeningocele.

The Tethered Cord Syndrome

The tethered cord or fixed conus syndrome is common in pediatric neuroradiology (10). In all cases, it is accompanied by some degree of vertebral dysraphism. Clinically, it may present as a pes cavus, as minor neurological changes in one or both legs, abnormal ankle jerks, or a straight back with minor bladder and bowel dysfunction.

At CTMM, the condition is detected easily (5, 10, 17). Normally, the tip of the conus is situated at or above the

L2–L3 level in infants and at or above the mid-L2 level at the age of 12 years. The tethered cord may appear as a thick filum terminale associated with a low situated normal conus (Fig. 14.17). The cord itself also may extend to lower levels, and a thin low cord may be differentiated from a thick filum by nerve roots emerging from the cord (Fig. 14.18). Lipomatous tissue often is attached to the thick filum and the low cord (Fig. 14.19).

Myelomeningocele

Distortion of the arachnoid membrane in dysraphism may involve only the meninges, and if this extends outside the spinal canal the condition is defined as a *meningocele*. If neural elements are involved in this extension, there is a *myelomeningocele*. A *lipomyelomeningocele* contains lipomatous tissue. Herniation of the meninges through the wall of the dural sac, but not through the wall of the spinal canal constitutes an *intraspinal meningocele*.

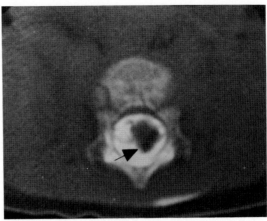

Figure 14.19. Low cord and lipomatous tissue of a 2-month-old boy, L3. There is a low cord, revealed by the emerging nerve roots. Lipomatous tissue is attached to cord (*arrow*).

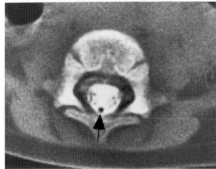

Figure 14.17. Thick filum terminale of a 1-year-old boy, L4. The diameter of the filum terminale is 3 mm which is abnormal (*arrow*). Although the filum is tethering the cord, the nerve roots in this case are arranged symmetrically.

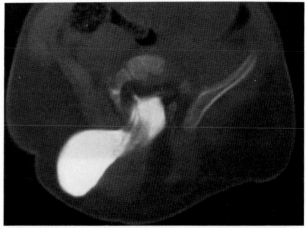

Figure 14.20. Myelomeningocele of a 6-month-old girl, S1. There is a pronounced dysraphism with widely open neural arches. Through this opening extends a large meningocele containing nerve roots.

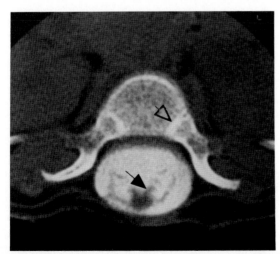

Figure 14.18. Low cord of a 3-year-old boy, L2. The low cord is identified by the emerging nerve roots (*black arrow*). There is a pronounced dysraphism, the posterior arches being widely spread apart and divergent. Note the normal increased density outlining the previous neurocentral synchondrosis (*open arrow*).

The different types of myelomeningoceles are revealed easily at the CTMM. In myelomeningocele, the neural elements may be seen entering the sac which may extend far posteriorly (Fig. 14.20). In pronounced dysraphic cases, the neural anatomy may be totally disorganized as a part of the grotesque spinal dysraphic abnormalities (Fig. 14.21).

Lipomatous tissue often is present in cases of myelomeningocele, and the fatty tissue may involve the cord, the intradural, extradural, intramuscular, and subcutaneous compartments. This lipomatous tissue should be differed from the discrete lipoma, i.e., occurring in the spinal canal may give specific neurological symptoms identical with those of other intraspinal mass lesions (see below).

Diastematomyelia

A split cord, situated in one dural sac or in separated subarachnoid spaces, may be divided by a bony, cartilag-

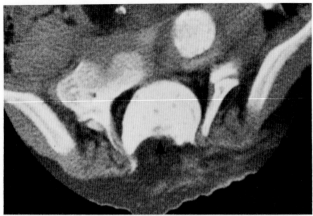

Figure 14.21. Pronounced dysraphic abnormalities of a 6-year-old boy, S1. There is a pronounced derangement of the S1 vertebra. The posterior arches are widely spread apart. The metrizamide-filled arachnoid space fills the spinal canal, and extends to the subcutaneous tissue dorsal to the vertebra. A neural placode (*arrow*) intrudes into the arachnoid space, and in this space there are nerve roots in a disorganized pattern.

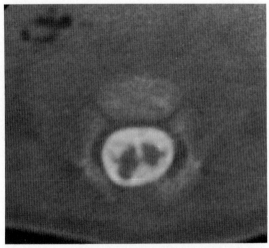

Figure 14.22. Split cord of a 1-month-old girl, L2. The two parts of the cord within one dural sac are separated partially and slightly asymmetrical. Nerve roots emerge from the lateral side of each part of the split cord.

inous, or fibrous spur, protruding into or through the sac. This condition previously was regarded as rare (18). However, the condition is revealed easily at SCT and CTMM (1, 19–22), and in a material of 110 children examined with CTMM because of dysraphism, we found diastematomyelia in 31 (28%) cases (10). A bony spur or bridge causing a split dural sac and cord is not as common as previously thought, and occurred in our material in only 10 (30%) cases. The remaining 70% had a split cord within a single dural sac, in accordance with the figures reported by Scotti et al. (22). The two parts of the cord may be separated totally or partially, these two parts being slightly

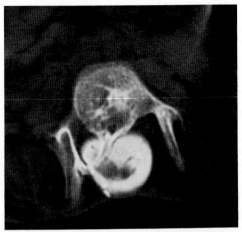

Figure 14.23. Diastematomyelia of an 8-year-old girl, L2. There is a pronounced dysraphism, the neural arches being spread widely apart. There is a bony spur, asymmetrically dividing the canal, and on each side of this spur there is a dural sac, containing a part of the cord.

asymmetrical (Fig. 14.22). At the CTMM, not only the parts of the cord but also the nerve roots emerging from the lateral sides of each part are visualized (Fig. 14.22). In all cases with a bony spur or bridge, commonly asymmetrical, there is a complete dural sac on each side of the division (Fig. 14.23). As is true for all other manifestations of dysraphism, diastematomyelia also often is accompanied by other abnormalities of the cord and meninges, for instance, myelomeningocele and syringohydromyelia.

Syringohydromyelia

The combined term syringohydromyelia denotes congenital dilatation of the central canal (hydromyelia) and/or cyst formation within the cord, separate from the central canal (syringomyelia). As these two conditions might be difficult to distinguish both clinically and radiologically, we prefer the combined term, as first proposed by Gardner in 1965 (23).

At the CT examination, the syringohydromyelia may appear as a wide cord in a large cystic canal. The partial collapse of the cord in the upright position, as described at air myelography (24), is seen seldom in CTMM (10). The contrast medium may enter the syringohydromyeliac sac by the 4th ventricle, given a patent obex (4, 25), but it also may migrate through the wall of the cavity (26). To detect this, a repeat CT scan should be performed about 5 hours after the contrast medium injection. At this later examination, the attenuation value of the fluid may arise with more than 100 HU.

In our opinion, if the syringohydromyelia does not collapse and if the obex is not open, the differentiation from a cystic neoplasm may be difficult or impossible with a CT examination, although others (14) have described detection of the cystic cavity in syringohydromyelia without metrizamide.

The syringohydromyelia also may appear as a flattened cord, and this was seen in 12 of our series of 23 cases (10).

The change in shape of the flattened cord between the supine and decubitus position is very slight, as the cord is fixed by the dentate ligaments and by the emerging nerve roots (Fig. 14.24). Also, the cavity of the flattened cord may be filled with contrast via an open obex (Fig. 14.25). In children, we have never seen a normal-sized, an atrophic, or small cord containing a syringohydromyeliac sac, as described in adults (14).

Syringohydromyelia often is accompanied by a Chiari malformation, and to assess this, the occipitocervical junction always should be scanned in cases of syringohydromyelia.

Neuroenteric Cyst

In anterior vertebral dysraphism, there rarely may be a persistence of the canal of Kovalevski between the yolk

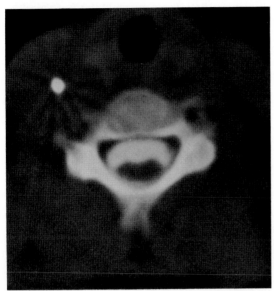

Figure 14.24. Syringohydromyelia of an 11-year-old boy, C5. This syringohydromyelia appears as a flattened cord. There is a slight indentation in the midline anteriorly.

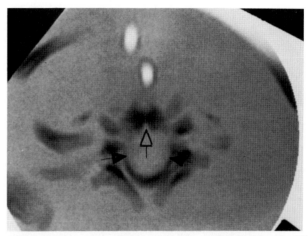

Figure 14.26. Neurenteric cyst of a 13-day-old girl, C7. There is a large cystic lesion occupying most of the cervical canal (*black arrows*). The canal of Kovalevsky is open (*open arrow*), and is in connection with the intraspinal cyst. The extraspinal portion, situated in the upper thoracic region, was removed surgically before the present examination.

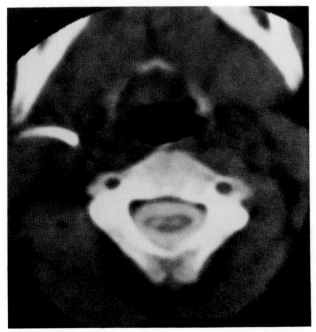

Figure 14.25. Syringohydromyelia shown in the same patient as in Figure 14.24, repeat CT 5 hours later. Metrizamide with high concentration fills the syringohydromyelic cavity.

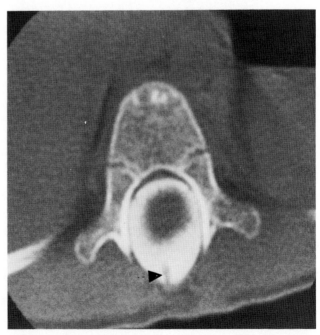

Figure 14.27. Dermoid of a 5-year-old girl, T12. There is an intramedullary mass lesion with attenuation value of minus 20 HU. The dermal sinus (*black arrow*) is pathognomonic for a dermoid or epidermoid.

sac and the notochordal canal. The presence of the intra-spinal part of the malformation, as well as the connection through the canal of Kovalevski and the enteric cyst is well visible at the CTMM (Fig. 14.26), and CT has proven to be of great value in the surgical approach to and successful treatment of this unusual abnormality (5).

Developmental Mass Lesions

Sequestration of normal tissue elements during fetal development and later overgrowth of these tissues result in developmental mass lesions. If the mass is derived from dermis and epithelium, a dermoid or epidermoid may appear, most often in the lumbar region (Fig. 14.27). A lipoma may be differed from the dermoid and epidermoid by the differing Hounsfield numbers: the attenuation value of the dermoid varies between +30 and −30 HU, the attenuation value of a lipoma is about −60 (Fig. 14.28). A teratoma, containing derivatives from mesoderm, ento-derm, and ectoderm often presents at a low age, and is one of the three mass lesions in pediatric neuroradiology that may involve the entire cord, the others being astro-cytoma and syringohydromyelia. An arachnoid cyst may be seen in dysraphism, but also may occur in neurofibro-matosis, or may be caused by arachnoiditis.

At CTMM, the exact localization of the mass lesions is obtained, and the attenuation values also will give a clue as to the type of the mass, but in many cases it may be difficult or impossible to differentiate between a dermoid, teratoma, and neoplastic mass lesion, as it also may be difficult to distinguish between a syringohydromyelia and cystic neoplastic mass lesion.

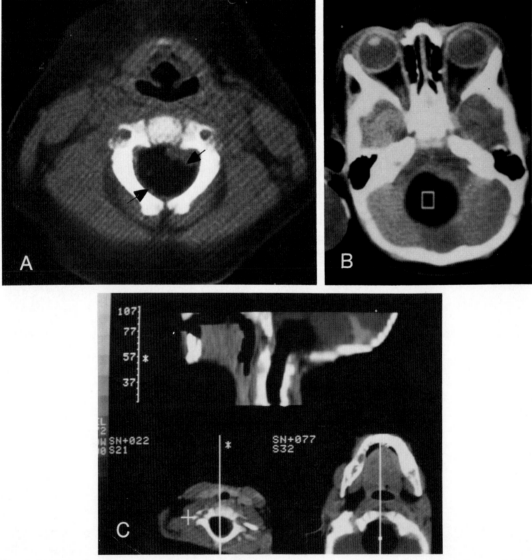

Figure 14.28.   A. Lipoma of a 7-month-old girl, C5. The spinal canal is occupied by a large mass lesion (*arrows*). The attenuation value is minus 90 HU, giving the diagnosis of a lipoma. B. The mass lesion extends up into the posterior fossa. C. Reformation in sagittal plane outlines the pronounced extension of the tumour.

Chiari Malformation

The Chiari malformation, being an abnormality of the lower brain stem and cerebellum, was earlier usually regarded to be associated with myelomeningocele (12). In conventional myelography, the primary radiological sign is tonsillar herniation, which might be difficult to distinguish from other masses in the craniocervical junction. The CTMM clearly outlines the cord and the herniated tonsils in Chiari malformation (Fig. 14.29), and the increased use of CT has revealed that Chiari malformation is combined more often with other manifestations of dysraphism than was previously supposed (10).

The Multifaceted Dysraphic State

The pathological entities occurring in dysraphism have

been discussed separately, but the dysraphic state to a varying degree involves tissues from ectoderm, entoderm, and mesoderm. Thus, in each case, there often is a spectrum of abnormalities not only in the structures derived from the cord, but there is often also skeletal abnormalities as deformed ribs, or there may be cardiopulmonary or gastrointestinal anomalies (12). All the changes are well suited for CT examination.

SCOLIOSIS

Scoliosis, be it idiopathic, secondary to neoplasia, infection, trauma or irradiation, or congenital as in dysraphism or skeletal dysplasias, may present considerable problems to the orthopaedic surgeon as far as corrective surgery is concerned. In all cases, it is necessary with a radiological evaluation of the skeletal anomalies, and in scoliosis with spinal dysraphism as well as in scoliosis with progressive neurological disturbances, also an extensive neuroradiological work-up is demanded (27). In these congenital scolioses, there might be dysraphic changes that must be considered before the orthopaedic treatment of the scoliosis, and in neurofibromatosis for instance, an intraspinal neurofibroma must be ruled out before surgical correction is performed. Also, other conditions responsible for a scoliosis must be ruled out, for instance, disc herniation, tumor, or infection.

The ScoutView at the CT examination gives information of the degree of scoliosis and from this, the gantry angles may be chosen. A series of transaxial sections through the scoliotic part of the spine gives information on the rotational deformities of the vertebral bodies, including the deformity of the spinal canal (Fig. 14.30), and if metrizamide has been introduced in the subarachnoid space, the asymmetrical position and rotation of the cord and roots also will be visualized (Figs. 14.30 and 14.31). The cord tries to take the shortest path through the curves, and, therefore, is situated in the concave part of each curve. In congenital scoliosis, for instance in dysraphism, most of the above-described changes within the dysraphic state

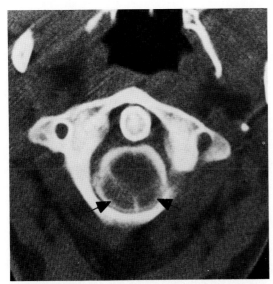

Figure 14.29.   Chiari malformation of a 17-year-old girl, C1. The cerebellar tonsils are herniated through the foramen magnum (*arrows*), displacing the medulla anteriorly.

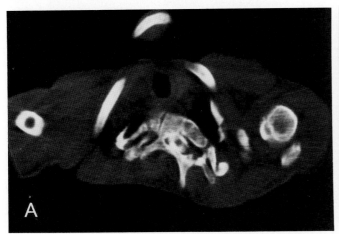 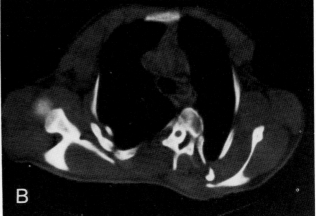

Figure 14.30. Scoliosis: A. At the level T1. B. At the level T5. The spinal anatomy is distorted, the thecal sac is placed asymmetrically in the distorted spinal canal. The dural sac as well as the cord are displaced to the concave side of the scoliotic curve.

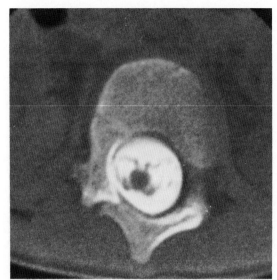

Figure 14.31. Scoliosis of a 3-year-old boy, L2. In mild scoliosis, there might be a deformation of the spinal canal and thecal sac. The cord is rotated slightly and placed asymmetrically in the sac.

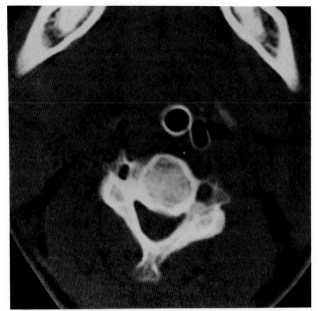

Figure 14.32. Achondroplasia of an 11-year-old girl, C3. The anatomy of the vertebral body is abnormal. The pedicles and the lamina are thickened, causing a narrowing of the spinal canal and intervertebral foramina.

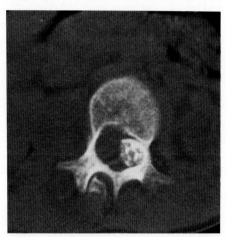

Figure 14.33. Neurofibromatosis of an 11-year-old girl, L2. There is a slight dysplasia of the vertebral body, and the spinal canal is widened asymmetrically. There is a large extradural tumour, that displaces and compresses the dural sac.

might be revealed concurrent with the scoliosis. The SCT or CTMM also will reveal the dysplastic changes, for instance in achondroplasia or neurofibromatosis, as well as the reason for a scoliosis secondary to, for instance, tumor, disc herniation, or trauma. These changes will be described later.

In a recent investigation (27), we found that in severe scoliosis, in cases of scoliosis combined with dysraphism, and in cases of scoliosis with localized neurological disturbances, CTMM added considerable information to the conventional MM and, in these cases, CTMM should be added to the MM or be the only examination.

MUSCULOSKELETAL DISORDERS AND DYSPLASIAS

SCT provides detailed information on the size and shape of the vertebrae and the spinal canal in musculoskeletal dysplasias. The spinal stenosis, for instance in achondroplasia or osteopetrosis, may involve the entire vertebral column and CTMM reveals not only the abnormal configuration of the abnormal bodies, it also shows the osseous stenosis as well as the impingement of the sac and cord caused by this stenosis (Fig. 14.32) (28). The gross changes of the spine, however, are shown best in conventional plain films. Acquired spinal stenosis, thoroughly studied at SCT in adults, is not common in children (5).

A widened spinal canal may be seen in dysraphism and in cases of space-occupying mass lesions within the spinal canal. We also have seen a slight widening and scalloping of the vertebral bodies in Marfan's disease, Ehlers-Danlos syndrome, and neurofibromatosis (10). The pathological changes in neurofibromatosis, a congenital neuroectodermal and mesenchymal dysplasia, are visualized remarkably well by SCT and CTMM. These examinations reveal the vertebral disorganization with kyphoscoliosis and posterior vertebral body scalloping, as well as dural ectasia

with herniation of the dura through widened intervertebral foramina. Also, the neurofibromas that might be extraspinal or extend into the extradural space are well visualized (Fig. 14.33) as are the single or multiple intradural neurofibromas without any extradural component (10, 29, 30).

Neoplasia

Primary neoplasms of the spine are rare in childhood. Their presence is easy to detect at the SCT, but the differentiation between, for instance, malignant lesions as

Ewing's sarcoma (Fig. 14.34), osteogenic sarcoma or rhab-domyosarcoma, and benign lesions such as giant cell tu-mor and hemangioma, may be difficult. All these tumors most often appear as multiple osteolytic areas, enhancing after IV contrast medium injection (5). These tumors most often are confined to the vertebral body, not impinging into the spinal canal. Osteoblastomas, often situated in the lamina or pedicles, seldom encroach upon the canal (Fig. 14.35), whereas aneurysmal bone cysts, occupying both the vertebral body and the neural arch may compress the neural structures (Fig. 14.36) (31, 32).

Paraspinal malignancies may spread to the intraspinal canal by direct intrusion, the most common tumors of this kind being retroperitoneal sarcomas and the neuroblas-toma-ganglioneuroma. This latter group of tumors, arising from the sympathetic chain is the most common malignant lesions in early childhood, with an annual incidence rate of about 8 per million (10). The CTMM will give informa-tion both of the extra- and the possible intraspinal part of the tumor and, in a recent examination, we found that primary CTMM is the method of choice in the examina-tion of these patients (33). Thus, the extension of the tumor in the abdomen, thorax, neck, or skull will be revealed, as will the extension of tumor from the paravertebral to the intraspinal space through the intervertebral foramina. It is very important to know preoperatively if there is an intraspinal extension because this will determine the sur-gical approach and/or the radiotherapy. The tumor growth within the spinal canal may displace the dural sac and cord slightly, or it may give an impingement on the dural sac, or in pronounced cases, there might be a com-

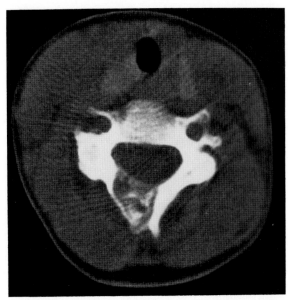

Figure 14.35. Osteoblastoma of a 16-year-old boy, C3. The tumor occupies part of the lamina and the spinous process, with very slight impingement upon the spinal canal.

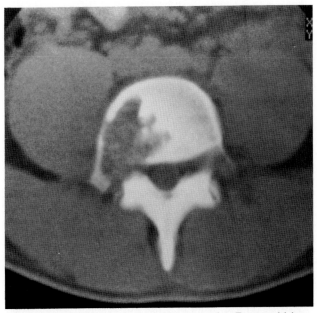

Figure 14.36. Aneurysmal bone cyst of a 7-year-old boy, L4. The tumor occupies part of the vertebral body and the dural arch impinging upon the spinal canal and the interver-tebral foramen.

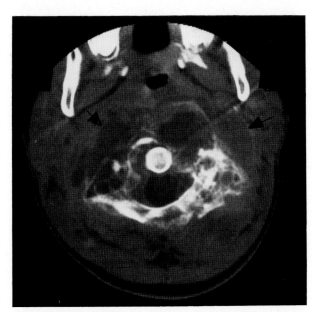

Figure 14.34. Malignant bone tumor of an 11-year-old boy, C1. The C1 vertebra is occupied by multiple osteolytic de-structions. The tumor has expanded the vertebra, and ex-tends far outside the vertebra into the soft tissues (*arrows*). Histological examination revealed a highly undifferentiated bone sarcomatous tumor.

plete block for the passage of contrast medium.

Primary neoplasms of neural origin, developing within the spinal canal are all rare, but astrocytoma, ependy-moma, and neurofibroma appear with an incidence of about 3 per million (10). The early clinical signs of these mass lesions are often subtle, and they may be large before they come to more sophisticated neuroradiological ex-aminations. On the CTMM, the astrocytoma may appear

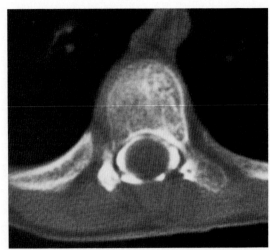

Figure 14.37. Astrocytoma of an 11-year-old boy, C5. The thoracic cord is enlarged irregularly by an intramedullary mass lesion. A laminectomy has been performed.

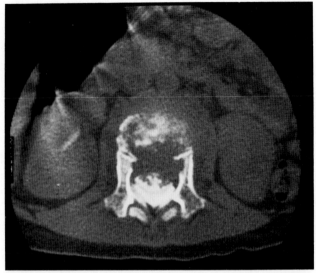

Figure 14.38. Histiocytosis X of a 3-year-old boy, L2. There is an osteolytic destruction occupying the vertebral body, with extension into the spinal canal. The dural sac is compressed significantly and displaced posteriorly.

cystic or solid, and the tumor may extend over several vertebral levels or even involve the whole cord (Fig. 14.37). Ependymoma, most often found in the lumbar region, appears as a smooth widening of the cord and the filum terminale. The neurofibroma, derived from the cells of Schwann in the nerve sheath, may appear as a solitary tumor, or multiple in neurofibromatosis as described earlier in this chapter.

It should be noted that although the existence and the extension of the tumor is revealed perfectly at the CT examinations, most of the tumors might be cystic and/or solid, and the differential diagnosis between, for instance, intramedullary astrocytoma, ependymoma, dermoid, teratoma, and syringohydromyelia with closed obex may be difficult or impossible.

Metastases to the vertebrae seldom are seen in children, but may appear in, for instance, rhabdomyosarcoma. These metastases often destroy the vertebral body, and extend both para- and intraspinally. Histiocytosis X, a generalized disease of the reticuloendothelial system, may occur as a localized osteolytic lesion in one vertebra with extension into the spinal canal (Fig. 14.38). The differentiation from both osteomyelitis and malignant lesions as Ewing's sarcoma may be difficult or impossible (10).

The secondary tumors within the spinal canal most often emanate from neoplasms elsewhere in the CNS (12). Intracranial medulloblastoma, ependymoma, astrocytoma, pineal neoplasms, and carcinoma of the choroid plexus are examples of primary tumors involved. The CTMM may reveal nodules around the nerve roots, and sheathing around the cord which then appears enlarged and irregular (Fig. 14.39) (3). Also, lymphoma and leukemia may spread to the intra- or extradural space, and may appear as multiple nodules along the cord and nerve roots (Fig. 14.40). This irregular enlargement of the nerve roots should be differentiated from the more smooth enlargement seen in the uncommon interstitial neuropathy known as Dejerine-Sotta's disease (12, 34).

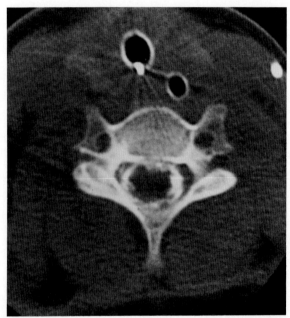

Figure 14.39. Metastatic pineal dysgerminoma of a 12-year-old girl, C4. The cervical cord is enlarged irregularly, caused by sheathing of the tumor around the cord.

IV contrast medium injection might be of value in paravertebral, vertebral, and intraspinal tumors (30, 33, 35), and there have been reports on considerable enhancement in cases of hemangioblastoma, hemangioma, and intraspinal arteriovenous malformations. This value of the IV contrast medium injection in CT examination probably will increase in the future, with increasing spatial resolution and contrast discrimination.

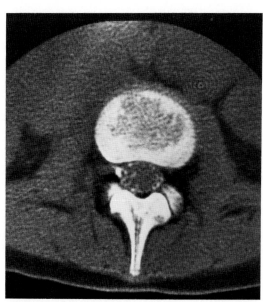

Figure 14.40. Intradural lymphoma of a 14-year-old girl, L3. There is a large amount of nodules of tumor tissue around the nerve roots in the cauda equina, giving the impression of a very large number of roots. The roots cannot be distinguished from the malignant tissue.

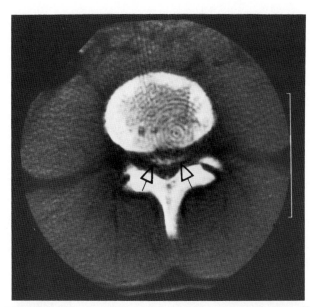

Figure 14.41. Avulsion of the posterior apophysis of a 15-year-old boy, L4. A part of the posterior apophysis (*arrows*) is avulsed from the vertebra, and posteriorly dislocated into the spinal canal.

Trauma, Infection and Inflammation

Severe trauma to the spine and infection and inflammation of the spinal column or content of the spinal cord is uncommon in children, but early and effective treatment in these cases may prevent serious irreparable damage, and the CT examinations have considerably improved the possibilities of an accurate diagnostic work-up (10).

After spinal trauma, standard radiographs of the spine give the best evaluation of the gross changes, although the CT examination demonstrates subtle fractures, as well as displacement of bony fragments and distortions of the canal (36–38). Not only the fractures, but also herniation of the intervertebral discs, spondylolysis, and spondylolisthesis (37) as well as avulsion of the vertebral apophyses (40, 41) (Fig. 14.41) are visualized clearly at SCT. CTMM adds information on the condition of the intraspinal contents, such as avulsion of nerve roots, intramedullary hematomas (42) and traumatic sequelae such as cord atrophy (Fig. 14.42).

Osteomyelitis of the vertebrae is well visualized at the CT examination, but may at times be difficult to differentiate from malignant neoplasms or histiocytosis X (Fig. 14.43). Transverse myelitis in our experience may appear as nonspecific swelling of the cord, but in many cases the cord as well may appear normal. Arachnoiditis, in a pediatric material most often caused by lumboperitoneal shunts, appears at the CTMM as a narrowing and irregularity of the lining subarachnoid sheath and the roots, over several vertebral levels (Fig. 14.44). The CTMM appearance of arachnoiditis may be similar to that of tumor seeding to the cord and roots, as well as to Déjérine-Sottas disease. The conditions may be differentiated by the fact that the tumor seeding appears in a normal-sized or ex-

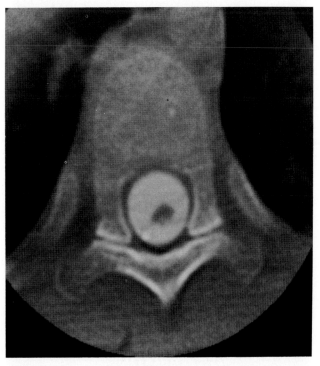

Figure 14.42. Cord atrophy of a 5-year-old girl, T12. As a sequelae of spinal trauma, the cord is atrophic and placed asymmetrically in the subarachnoid space.

panded subarachnoid space, whereas in arachnoiditis the dural sac is shrunken. In Déjérine-Sottas disease, the changes of the roots are more smooth and regular than in arachnoiditis and secondary malignancies (34).

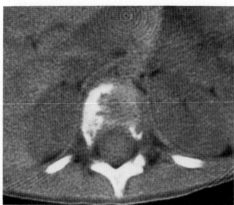

Figure 14.43. Osteomyelitis of a 4-year-old boy, T12. There is a pronounced osteomyelitic destruction of the vertebral body. This destruction may be difficult or impossible to distinguish from malignant destruction or histiocytosis X.

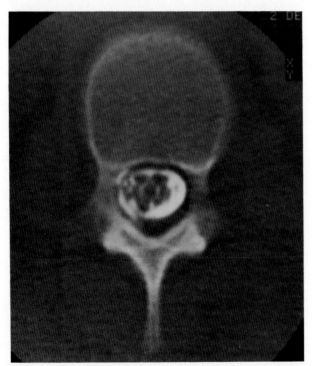

Figure 14.44. Arachnoiditis of a 12-year-old girl, L2. The dural sac is slightly asymmetrical. The nerve roots are disorganized and irregularly bunched.

THE DIAGNOSTIC ACCURACY OF CT EXAMINATIONS

The descriptions of normal anatomy and pathological conditions given above have demonstrated the high aesthetic quality and extensive anatomical detail with which normal and pathological structures are imaged with high-resolution CT. This good quality in imaging also means high diagnostic accuracy: in a recent review of 137 cases in which CT of the spine was performed, and in which the CT findings were controlled at operation or autopsy,

no false-negative diagnoses were seen (10). However, there were 5 false-positive diagnoses: 2 cases in which a neoplastic mass lesion was mistaken for a lipoma, and 3 cases in which CTMM suggested an intramedullary mass lesion, although no tumor was present at the surgical exploration. Thus, the greatest dubiety of the CT lies in the assessment of intramedullary mass lesions.

In another review of 100 consecutive cases in which both conventional metrizamide myelography and a subsequent secondary high-resolution CTMM was performed, we found CTMM to be superior in a considerable amount (31%) of the cases.

Of the 100 cases, 46 had dysraphic changes, and MM did not add any information to the CTMM in any of these. In 16 cases, however, CTMM added information concerning syringohydromyelia, diastematomyelia, lipoma, neuroenteric cysts, tethered cord, and Chiari malformation. In 18 cases of neoplasm, MM did not add any information to the CTMM, whereas CTMM added information in 8 cases, this time concerning the extension and composition of the tumor, as well as vertebral and paravertebral lesions. In 19 cases of trauma, CTMM added information in 4 cases, concerning vertebral fractures and cord compression. In 17 cases of musculoskeletal dysplasias, CTMM added information in 3 cases concerning spinal stenosis, cord atrophy, and 1 case of extraspinal neurofibromatosis. In none of the traumatic or dysplastic cases did MM add any information.

It should be stressed that the CTMM in these 100 cases was secondary and, thus, that the CT examination was guided by the preceding conventional MM. However, few, if any lesions would have been missed at repeat CTMM examination if the guidelines given in the protocols below had been followed. Thus, the diagnostic accuracy of the SCT and CTMM is very high, and the CT examination of the spine indeed adds considerable confidence to the diagnostic work-up of the spinal lesions in children.

DIAGNOSTIC IMAGING PROTOCOLS

As has been shown above, the images of the paravertebral, vertebral, and intraspinal structures obtained with modern CT equipment give detailed and profound information. However, as mentioned in the introduction, simpler means may give enough information for proper clinical management. Thus, in each individual patient, it is necessary to find the combination of diagnostic techniques that will give accurate information to as low a cost, risk, and discomfort for the patient as possible. The following protocols should be regarded as rough guide lines as to the use of plain film radiography, MM, radionuclide bone scanning, SCT, and CTMM (including reformation at any angle). Oil contrast media or air for myelography no longer are demanded, and conventional complex motion tomography is seldom requested.

The following protocols (Fig. 14.45), given for the most common situations in pediatric neuroradiology, never can be more than rough guidelines. The radiological findings made during the procedure, as well as the experience of

DIAGNOSTIC IMAGING PROTOCOLS

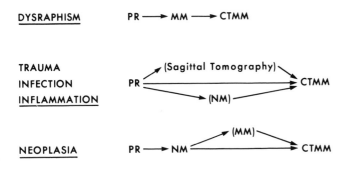

Figure 14.45. Diagnostic imaging protocols: PR = plain radiography, NM = nuclear bone scan, MM = metrizamide myelography, CTMM = CT metrizamide myelography.

the radiologist then may alter the course of the diagnostic events during the examination.

DYSRAPHISM

Plain radiographs give an overall survey of the skeletal changes, and conventional metrizamide myelography will provide a survey of the spinal canal lesions. If there is any doubt, no matter how minor, on the diagnosis on the conventional myelography, CT is demanded. The CT section then must cover the skeletal dysraphic changes, the conus, and, as mentioned above the cervico-occipital junction to rule out a Chiari malformation (Fig. 14.45).

NEOPLASTIC LESIONS

Plain radiographs give the morphology of the skeletal changes and radionuclide scan reveals the area or areas involved. Conventional metrizamide myelography is seldom necessary. The CTMM will give information on the paravertebral, vertebral, and intraspinal lesions and the CT sections should be performed over areas from which neurological disturbances emanate, as well as pathological areas detected at plain radiographs or radionuclide bone scan. In neuroblastoma and neurofibromatosis, intraspinal lesions may appear at a long distance from the paraspinal masses and, in these cases, a large area must be covered by the CT examination. If CSF-borne metastases are suspected, the whole canal must be covered. In these cases, we prefer low-dose CT for a survey, and if pathological changes in a specific area are found, this area might be examined also with scans using higher radiation dose, giving higher anatomical detail (10) (Fig. 14.45).

TRAUMA, INFECTION, AND INFLAMMATION

Plain radiographs and radionuclide bone scans give overall information. Conventional tomography in the sagittal plane may give additional information on fractures,

FUTURE PROTOCOLS

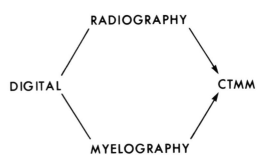

Figure 14.46. Future diagnostic protocols.

if high-detailed CT reconstruction is not available, otherwise, CT has replaced the complex motion tomography. Conventional myelography seldom is demanded. The levels of the CT sections should be guided by clinical findings, as well as findings on plain radiographs and radionuclide bone scans. In arachnoiditis, the whole spine must be covered, using a low-dose CT (Fig. 14.45).

MUSCULOSKELETAL DISORDERS AND DYSPLASIAS

Plain radiographs of the spine give overall information on the skeletal lesions, and conventional metrizamide myelography on the intraspinal changes. CTMM may add information of discrete areas from which clinical signs or symptoms emanate, or areas found at the MM (Fig. 14.45).

FUTURE PROTOCOLS

The information provided by high-resolution CT, combined with metrizamide myelography in the subarachnoid space is considerable. However, the technical quality of the CT equipment is improving steadily, and with only slightly better spatial resolution provided by the digital radiograph, this may replace the survey given by conventional MM. Subsequently, it also may replace the plain radiographs, and the diagnostic work-up will include only the digital radiograph and the CT examination after instillation of metrizamide in the subarachnoid space (Fig. 14.46). It also should be noted that although metrizamide is the only water-soluble CSF contrast medium available today, other water-soluble contrast media are in progress (43). Ultimately, after further increases in CT technology, it should be possible to perform direct imaging not only of the paravertebral and skeletal structures, but also of the cord and nerve roots, without any violation of the subarachnoid space caused by contrast medium injection.

References

1. Resjo IM, Harwood-Nash DC, Fitz CR, et al: Computed tomographic metrizamide myelography in spinal dysraphism in infants and children. *J Comput Assist Tomogr* 2:549–558, 1978.
2. Resjo IM, Harwood-Nash DC, Fitz CR, et al: Normal cord in infants and children examined with computed tomographic metrizamide myelography. *Radiology* 130:691–696, 1979.
3. Resjo IM, Harwood-Nash DC, Fitz CR, et al: CT Metrizamide

myelography for intraspinal and paraspinal neoplasms in infants and children. *AJR* 132:367–372, 1979.

4. Resjo IM, Harwood-Nash DC, Fitz CR, et al: Computed tomographic metrizamide myelography in syringohydromyelia. *Radiology* 131:405–407, 1979.

5. Harwood-Nash DC, Fitz CR. Computed tomography and the pediatric spine: computed tomographic metrizamide myelography in children. In: Post MJD: *Radiographic Evaluation of the Spine: Current Advances with Emphasis on Computed Tomography.* New York, Masson Publishing, 1980, pp. 4–33.

6. Fitz CR, Harwood-Nash DC, Barry JF, et al: Pediatric myelography with metrizamide. *Acta Radiol Suppl* 355:182–192, 1977.

7. Sortland O, Hovind K: Myelography with metrizamide in children. *Acta Radiol Suppl* 355:211–220, 1977.

8. Pettersson H, Fitz CR, Harwood-Nash DC, et al: Adverse effects to myelography with metrizamide in infants, children and adolescents. I. General and CNS effects. *Acta Radiol Diag* 23:323–329, 1982.

9. Blumenfeld SM: Physical principles of high resolution CT with the General Electric CT/T 8800. In: Post MJD: *Radiographic Evaluation of the Spine: Current Advances with Emphasis on Computed Tomography.* New York, Masson Publishing, 1980, pp. 295–307.

10. Pettersson H, Harwood-Nash DC. CT and myelography of the spine. Techniques, anatomy and pathology in children. Berlin, Springer-Verlag, 1982.

11. Kaiser MC, Pettersson H, Harwood-Nash DC, et al: Direct coronal CT of the spine in infants and children. *AJNR* 2:465–466, 1981.

12. Harwood-Nash DC, Fitz CR. *Neuroradiology in Infants and Children.* St. Louis, C. V. Mosby Co., 1976.

13. Seibert CE, Barnes JE, Dreisbach JN, et al: Accurate CT measurement of the spinal cord using metrizamide: physical factors. *AJNR* 2:75–78, 1981.

14. Ethier R, King DG, Melancon D, et al: Diagnosis of intra and extramedullary lesions by CT without contrast achieved through modifications applied to the EMI CT 5005 scanner. In: Post MJD: *Radiographic Evaluation of the Spine: Current Advances with Emphasis on Computed Tomography.* New York, Masson Publishing, 1980, pp. 377–397.

15. Isherwood I, Fawcitt RA, St. Clair Forbes W, et al: Computer tomography of the spinal canal using metrizamide. *Acta Radiol Suppl* 355:299–305, 1977.

16. Lichtenstein BW: "Spinal Dysraphism", spina bifida and myelodysplasia. *Arch Neurol Psychiatr* 44:792–810, 1940.

17. James HE, Oliff M: Computed tomography in spinal dysraphism. *J Comput Assist Tomogr* 1:391–397, 1977.

18. Dale AJD: Diastematomyelia. *Arch Neurol* 20:309–317, 1969.

19. Lohkampf F, Clausen C, Schumacher G: CT demonstration of pathologic changes of the spinal cord accompanying spina bifida and diastematomyelia. In: Kaufman HJ: *Progress in Pediatric Radiology.* Vol. 5:II. Basel, S. Karger, pp. 200–227, 1978.

20. Tadmor R, Davis KR, Roberson GH, et al: The diagnosis of diastematomyelia by computed tomography. *Surg Neurol* 8:434–436, 1977.

21. Wolpert SM, Scott RM, Carter BL: Computed tomography in spinal dysraphism. *Surg Neurol* 8:199–206, 1977.

22. Scotti G, Musgrave MA, Harwood-Nash DC, et al: Diastematomyelia in children: Metrizamide and CT metrizamide myelography. *AJNR* 1:403–410, 1980.

23. Gardner WJ: Hydrodynamic mechanism of syringomyelia: its relationship to myelocele. *J Neurol Neurosurg Psychiatr* 28:247–259, 1965.

24. Wickbom WI, Hanafee W: Soft tissue masses immediately below the foramen magnum. *Acta Radiol Diagnosis* 1:647–658, 1963.

25. Forbes WCS, Isherwood I. Computed tomography in syringomyelia and the associated Arnold-Chiari Type I malformation. *Neuroradiology* 15:73–78, 1978.

26. Aubin ML, Vignaud J, Jardin C, et al: Computed tomography in 75 clinical cases of syringomyelia. *AJNR* 2:199–204, 1981.

27. Pettersson H, Harwood-Nash DC, Fitz CR, et al: Metrizamide myelography (MM) and computed tomographic metrizamide myelography (CTMM) in scoliosis—a comparative study. *Radiology* 142:111–114, 1982.

28. Post MJD: Computed tomography of the spine: its values and limitations on a nonhigh resolution scanner. In: Post MJD: *Radiographic Evaluation of the Spine: Current Advances with Emphasis on Computed Tomography.* New York, Masson Publishing, 1980, pp. 186–258.

29. Hammerschlag SB, Wolpert SM, Carter BL. Computed tomography of the spinal cord. *Radiology* 121:361–367, 1976.

30. Nakagawa H, Huang YP, Malis LI, et al: Computed tomography of intraspinal and paraspinal neoplasms. *J Comput Assist Tomogr* 1:377–390, 1977.

31. Bonakdarpour A, Levy WM, Aegerter E: Primary and secondary aneurysmal bone cyst: a radiological study of 75 cases. *Radiology* 126:75–83, 1978.

32. McLeod RA, Dahlin DC, Beabout JW: The spectrum of osteoblastoma. *AJR* 126:321–325, 1976.

33. Armstrong E, Harwood-Nash DC, Fitz CR, et al: Computed tomography of the neuroblastoma-ganglioneuroma spectrum in children. *AJR* 139:571–576, 1982.

34. Rao CV, Fitz CR, Harwood-Nash DC: Dejerine-Sotta's syndrome in children. *AJR* 122:70–74, 1974.

35. Handel S, Grossman R, Sarwar M: Computed tomography in the diagnosis of spinal cord astrocytoma. *J Comput Assist Tomogr* 2:226–228, 1978.

36. Geehr RB, Rothman SL, Kier EL: The role of computed tomography in the evaluation of upper cervical spine pathology. *Comput Tomogr* 2:79–97, 1978.

37. Tadmor R, Davis KR, Roberson GH, et al: Computed tomographic evaluation of traumatic spinal injuries. *Radiology* 127:825–827, 1978.

38. Kershner MS, Goodman GA, Perlmutter GS: Computed tomography in the diagnosis of an atlas fracture. *AJR* 128:688–689, 1977.

39. Nakagawa H, Malis LI, Huang YP: Computed tomography of soft tissue masses related to the spinal column. In: Post MJD: *Radiographic Evaluation of the Spine: Current Advances with Emphasis on Computed Tomography.* New York, Masson Publishing 1980, pp. 320–352.

40. Handel SF, Twiford TW Jr, Reigel DH, et al: Posterior lumbar apophyseal fractures. *Radiology* 130:629–633, 1979.

41. Pettersson H, Harwood-Nash DC, Fitz CR, et al: The CT appearance of avulsion of the posterior vertebral apophysis: Case report. *Neuroradiology* 21:145–147, 1981.

42. Post MJD: CT update: the impact of time, metrizamide and high resolution on the diagnosis of spinal pathology. In: Post MJD: *Radiographic Evaluation of the Spine: Current Advances with Emphasis on Computed Tomography.* New York, Masson Publishing, 1980, pp. 259–294.

43. Lindren E (Ed): Iohexol. A non-ionic contrast medium. *Acta Radiol Suppl* (Stockh) 362, 1980.

CHAPTER FIFTEEN

Spinal Dysraphism

LARRY K. PAGE, M.D. and M. JUDITH DONOVAN POST, M.D.

INTRODUCTION

The term spinal dysraphism is used here to label a group of developmental anomalies that demand a separate nosological classification from spina bifida aperta (spina bifida cystica, meningocele, myelomeningocele, myeloschisis) (1–3). Spinal dysraphism (4–7) includes diplomyelia, diastematomyelia, dermal sinus tracts, dermoid cysts, neurenteric cysts, fibrous bands, and lipomas. In contrast to spina bifida aperta, these conditions are three or four times more common in females than males and ordinarily are not associated with the Arnold-Chiari malformation or hydrocephalus.

ETIOLOGY

Whereas myelomeningocele and myeloschisis can be explained as an arrest in embryological development, formation of the anomalies of spinal dysraphism is clearly of a different sort. Bremmer (8) offers the currently most acceptable etiological explanation: the neurenteric canal is a normal, but brief, communication between the yolk sac and amniotic cavity. It appears and regresses quickly, leaving the primitive knot (Hensen's node) as its only residual marker. The primitive knot lies at the tip of the coccyx, well below the levels of the anomalies under discussion here. Bremmer believes that the lesions of spinal dysraphism develop in association with an ectopic or accessory neurenteric canal, i.e., a dorsal intestinal fistula. Thus, if the ventral portion of an accessory neurenteric canal persists, duplication of the intestine results. If the midportion remains, a neurenteric cyst occurs. If the midportion is large, but disappears, medial pedicular processes that had formed hemivertebra may unite to produce the midline spur of diastematomyelia. If the terminal portion of the canal persists, even if fibrotic, the result may be an interaction with dermal elements to form a dermal sinus tract and/or cyst. Fibrous bands and lipomas similarly are induced.

CLINICAL ASPECTS

Spinal dysraphism often is associated with subcutaneous masses, skin dimples, sinus tract openings, cutaneous blood vessel malformations, and abnormal tufts of hair that are readily corrected by operation. However, the clinical importance of surgical repair lies with the potential for dermal sinus tracts to act as portals of entry for bacteria to produce meningitis, and for the deceptive tendency of the other lesions in this group toward a slowly progressive neurological deficit as expressed by spinal deformity, weakness, and/or deformity of the lower extremities and disturbances of bowel and bladder sphincters. These symptoms usually appear in childhood, but may begin for the first time in the late teens or rarely in the 3rd or 4th decades of life.

One or more bouts of bacterial meningitis may have occurred before the diagnosis of a dermal sinus tract. The sinus opening is invariably in or near the midline. It often is quite small but usually contains one or more coarse hairs. It may be possible to express a thin or purulent discharge from the sinus opening. Hemangiectatic discolorations of the adjacent skin are common with a number of these anomalies. Diastematomyelia often is associated with a large, luxuriant growth of hair in the overlying skin (Fig. 15.1).

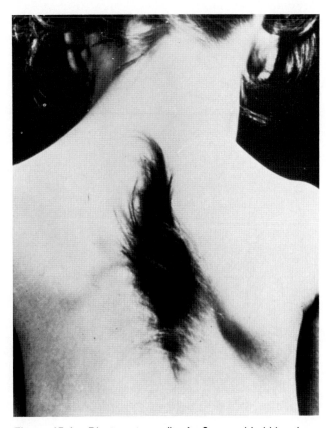

Figure 15.1. Diastematomyelia: An 8-year-old girl has luxuriant growth of hair overlying bony spur of dorsal spine.

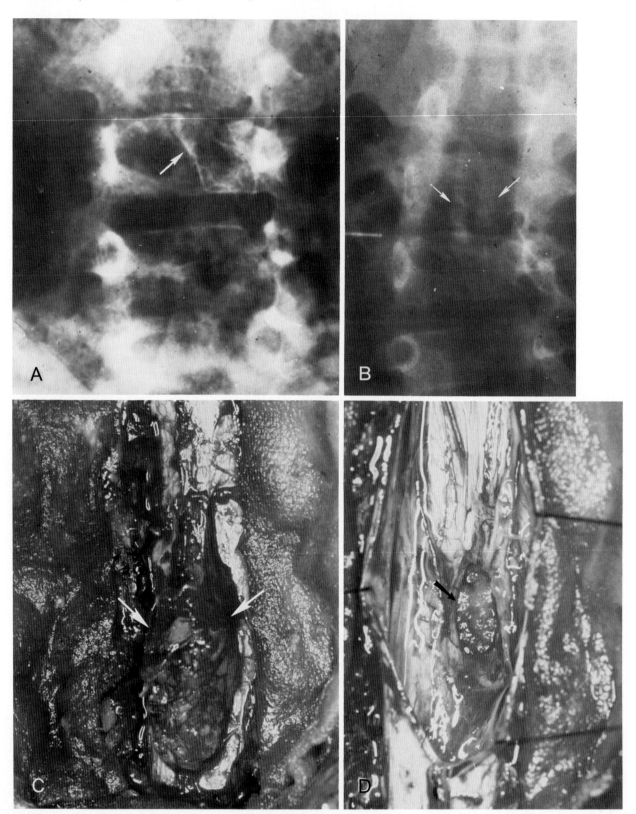

Figure 15.2. Diastematomyelia. A 10-year-old female has equinovarus deformity of the right foot and absence of right ankle jerk. Urinary incontinence had been present since birth. This child had complete bladder control by 48 hours after operation! A. Plain roentgenogram shows bony spicule at L4 (*white arrow*). B. Air myelogram reveals cleft between 2 halves of spinal cord (*white arrows*). C. Shows the laminectomy before the dura mater is opened. Note bony spur with associated cartilage and lipomatous tissue (*arrows*). It extends extradurally through cleft to join L4 body. D. Dura has been opened and transfixing spur removed along with its dural sleeve (*arrow*). Gelfoam is present in the depths of the cleft.

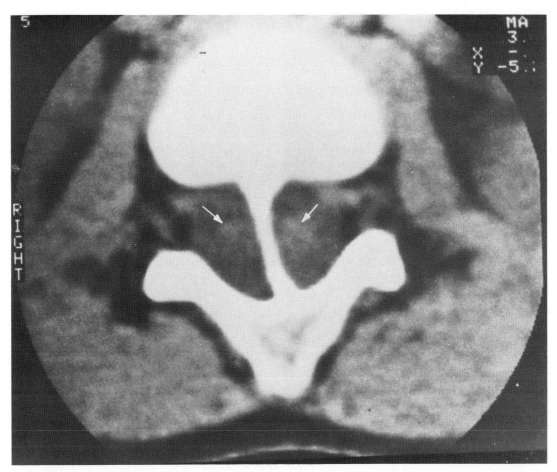

Figure 15.3.   A bony spur traversing the spinal canal is evident on this noncontrast high-resolution CT scan of the lumbar spine. Notice that the cord (*white arrows*) is split at the level of the spur. (Case courtesy of Dr. Victor Haughton and Dr. Alan Williams, Milwaukee County General Hospital, Milwaukee, Wisconsin.)

Tethered Cord

Dermoid cysts and neurenteric cysts can be expected to expand slowly and cause progressive signs and symptoms by a pressure mechanism similar to that of spinal cord tumors. However, lipomas ordinarily do not grow like neoplasms and should not be expected to cause progressive pressure on neural elements. Nor can this mechanism be evoked to explain the increasing deficits seen with diastematomyelia or fibrous bands. Rather, these lesions often are associated with a low-lying conus medullaris. Neurological deficit of the lower extremities and sphincters in association with a low-lying conus has been termed "tethered cord syndrome" and is seen most commonly in patients with intraspinal lipomas, diastematomyelia, and fibrous bands. It also occurs in patients with unoperated spina bifida aperta and occasionally may become manifest years after a repaired myelomeningocele or myeloschisis.

A tethered spinal cord must be assumed to be present when the conus medullaris is found to lie at abnormally low segments within the spinal canal. Although the tip of the conus lies at the caudal end of the spinal canal in early embryological life, axial growth of the vertebral column exceeds that of the central nervous system (5). Thus, the tip of the conus lies opposite the 4th lumbar vertebra halfway through gestation, near the lower border of L2 at birth and within the adult range at 2 months of age (9). Reimann and Anson (10) found the tip of the conus to be between the superior border of L1 and the inferior border of L2 94% of the time. The median position in their series was at the L1–2 interspace.

It is difficult to explain why most patients develop progressive symptoms months or years after all differential growth between spinal column and cord has ceased. Something more within the setting of failed rostral migration must occur over time to produce these late effects. Fitz and Harwood-Nash (11) suggest that the mechanism may be related to diminished mobility of the tethered cord during the normal flexion and extension of the spine that occur with the activities of daily living. This chronically intermittent stress presumably causes insufficiency of the vascular microcirculation within the spinal cord.

Symptoms and signs of tethered cord syndrome may present in adulthood (2, 12, 13), although most begin in infancy or childhood (7) and include kyphoscoliotic deformities of the spine. Bladder incontinence and weakness

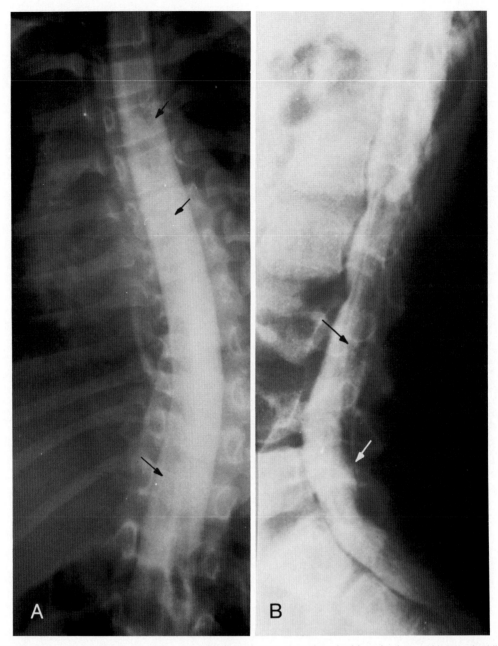

Figure 15.4.   Diastematomyelia without a bony or cartilaginous spur, associated with tethering and intraspinal lipoma. Scoliosis and widened lower thoracic and lumbar interpedicular distances in this child prompted a metrizimide myelogram (A) which revealed a single upper thoracic cord (*short black arrows*) which was split in the lower thoracic and lumbar canal (*long black arrow*). B. The split cord was low lying (*black arrow*) and tethered posteriorly at L4–5 (*white arrow*). The exact point of cord splitting was difficult to determine. However, CT scanning clearly demonstrated the levels at which the cord was single (C, and *short black arrow*, H) and split (D, and *long black arrows* H and I). Coronal reconstructions (H and I) showed the split cord to best advantage, demonstrating that the right cord was larger than the left. At the exact point of adhesion of conus and filum to posterior dura (*black arrow*, E), CT measurements revealed no lipomatous tissue (F) in the conus, but that a lipoma within the bifid spinous process of L4 extended inward to the point of cord tethering (G). The low lying split spinal cord (*black arrow*, J), its tethering at L4–5 level, and the adjacent lipoma within the spina bifida (*white arrow*, J) are especially well shown with sagittal reconstruction.

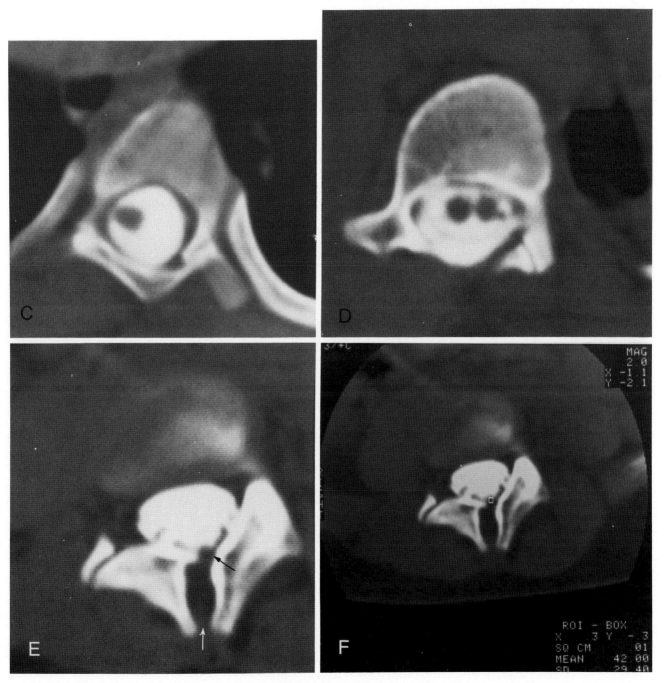

Figure 15.4.   C–F.

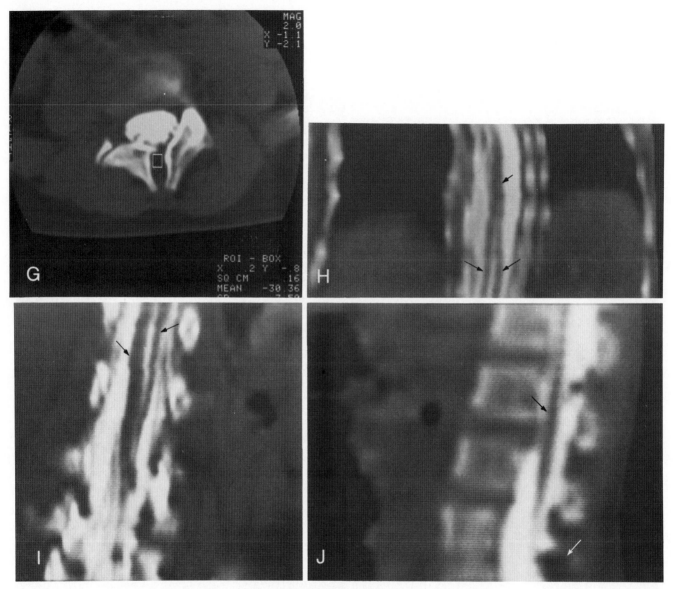

Figure 15.4.   G–J.

and numbness in one or both extremities often are seen. Equinovarus or other deformities of the feet with absent Achilles reflexes are common. There may be shortening or atrophy of the involved leg or foot. It is difficult to detect the progressive nature of the neurological deficits, especially in the pediatric age group. Many patients will have undergone one or more orthopaedic operations to correct deformities in their feet, legs, or spine before the abnormal neurological features of tethering are appreciated.

RADIOLOGICAL ASPECTS

Further evidence toward the diagnosis of spinal dysraphism is obtained through plain roentgenograms. Spina bifida, spinal deformities, hemivertebrae, diastemato-

myelic spurs, and widened interpedicular distances all may be seen. Pantopaque myelography was used in the past to confirm occult cases. This contrast material is so dense, however, that many of the subtle features of these anomalies are not demonstrated until the time of surgical exploration. Although air myelography was first popularized in 1939 by Lindgren (14) and further refined by Westberg (15) and by Scatliff et al. (16), it has not been used widely in this country. When properly carried out, however, air myelography is superior to Pantopaque as a myelographic agent for these conditions. More recently, metrizimide myelography, especially in combination with CT scanning (12, 17–20), has offered significantly better visualization of the often multiple features of spinal dysraphism. In addition, the more sensitive density discrimination afforded by CT has resulted in the identification

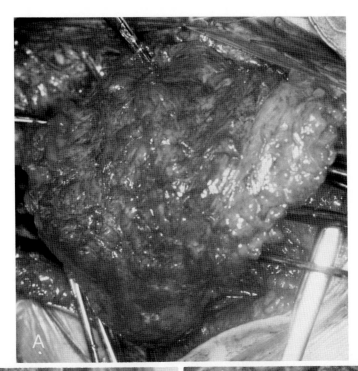

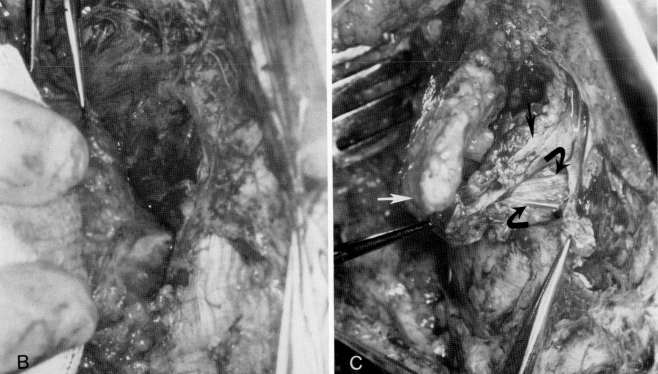

Figure 15.5.   Lipoma extending from subcutaneous level through spina bifida to cartilaginous junction with tethered myeloschisic conus medullaris. Subcutaneous lipoma (A) in lumbosacral area of 4-year-old boy that extends through the spinal bifida defect (B). After the lipoma has been removed (C), a large anomalous hemilamina (*white arrow*) can be seen, to which the tip of the conus is attached. The cartilaginous buffer (*straight black arrow*) between neural tissue and fat, and the rostrally slanting nerve roots are revealed (*curved arrows*).

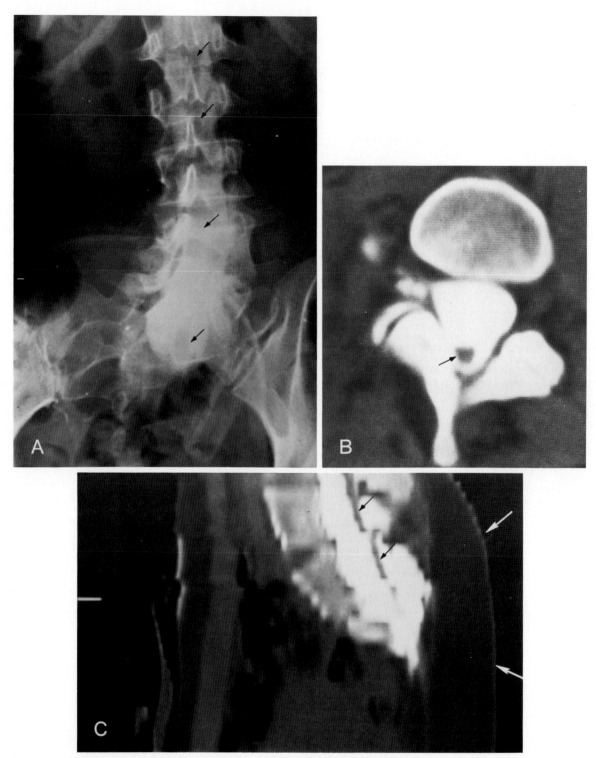

Figure 15.6. Lipoma extended from subcutaneous area of buttocks through spina bifida, attached to conus, and tethered it. The metrizamide myelogram (A) showed a low-lying cord (*arrows*) within a widened subarachnoid space in this 25-year-old woman. CT scan documented the position of the tethered cord in axial (*arrow*, B) and sagittally reconstructed (*black arrows*, C) views. This lipoma (*white arrow*, D) was attached through the spina bifida to the tethered conus (*black arrow*) within the sacrum. Absorption coefficients demonstrated that the tethered cord (F) was not infiltrated by lipomatous tissue (E).

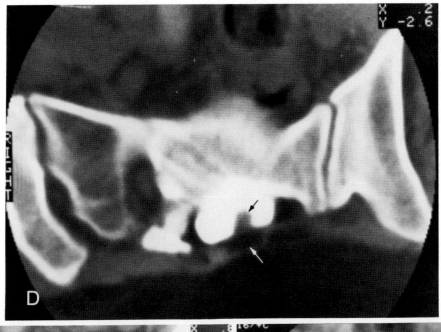

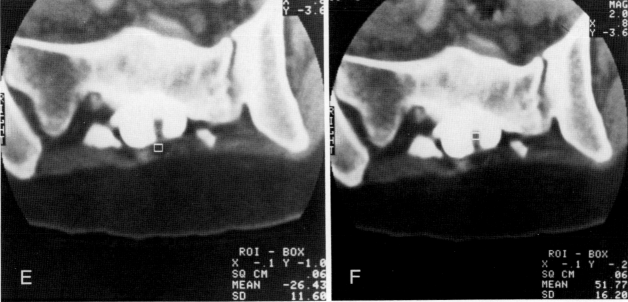

Figure 15.6.   D–F.

of extraspinal and intraspinal lipomas and in their clear-cut demarcation from an associated tethered cord.

Diplomyelia

Diplomyelia may be associated with extensive spina bifida and other skeletal deformities of the vertebra. In essence, however, it is a duplication of the spinal cord or a portion thereof. This is an extremely rare anomaly. It cannot be distinguished from diastematomyelia (cord split into 2 halves) with certainty except at postmortem, and has been described by Herrin and Edwards (21) as an attempt at twinning in which each duplicated segment contains 2 anterior horns, 2 posterior horns, and a central canal.

Cohen and Sledge (22) have questioned the existence of diplomyelia in most autopsied case reports. They point out that the presence of 2 anterior fissures does not distinguish diplomyelia from diastematomyelia because this may represent the rotation of each anterior horn around one branch of a bifid spinal artery. These authors believe that nerve roots exiting from the medial side of each duplication are a necessary feature of diplomyelia. The differentiation of this anomaly from diastematomyelia is further complicated by its association with duplications of

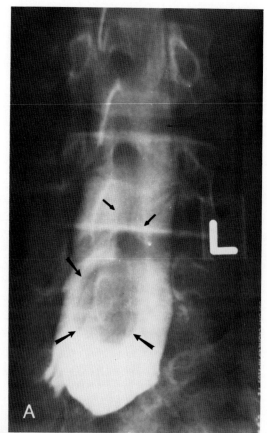

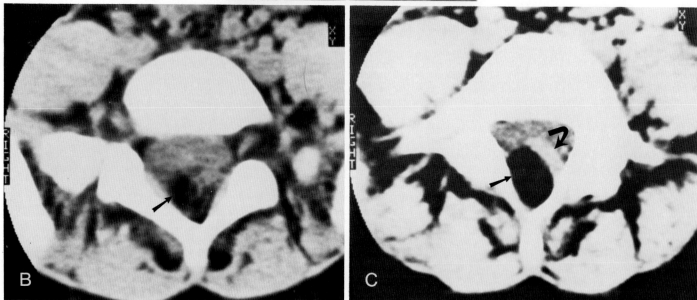

Figure 15.7. A metrizamide myelogram (A) showed a low-lying conus (*small arrows*) associated with a large smooth intradural mass (*large arrows*) and with a capacious subarachnoid sac. The plain high-resolution CT scan (B–F) offered valuable complementary as well as new diagnostic information. It demonstrated the exact position of the intradural mass (*arrow*, B and C), and showed its close proximity to the tethered conus (*curved arrow*, C). By absorption coefficients (D and E), it also revealed that the mass was a lipoma (measuring −49.12 EMI Units) and that it was not infiltrating the adjacent conus (which measured 17.47 EMI Units). It also documented the abnormal posterior position of the conus, (*arrow*, F).

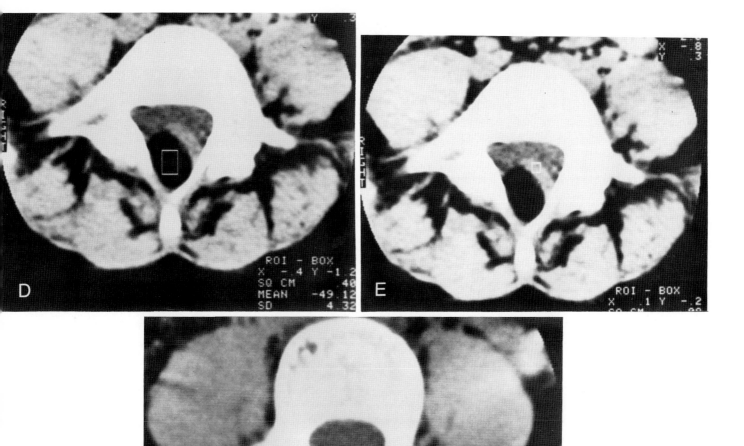

Figure 15.7.   D–F

the pia, arachnoid, and/or dura over varying portions of the involved segments, and by intervening bony or cartilaginous spurs. It is not clear whether tethering occurs in this condition and if so, whether it is amenable to operative correction. However, if a spur or tethered conus is found, the patient should be treated as though he has diastematomyelia. Because diplomyelia only can be distinguished by careful examination of the transected cord, James and Lassman (6) recommend that all such cases be termed diastematomyelia during life.

Diastematomyelia

Diastematomyelia is a congenital division of the spinal cord into 2 halves. It usually, although not invariably, is associated with a bony or cartilaginous spicule which extends posteriorly from the body of the vertebra to join an overlying lamina (Figs. 15.2 and 15.3). In the usual case (Fig. 15.2), the split in the spinal cord ends caudally at the level of the spur, extending several segments above it. Thus, the spur appears to split the neural tissue longitudinally due to the differential growth rates of the vertebral column and spinal cord. However, there is no such spicule within the split segment in some cases of diastematomyelia (Fig. 15.4). Rarely, the split cord may extend for several segments below the spicule as well as above it. Cohen and Sledge (22) reported a case of diastematomyelia in support of Bremer's theory (8) that this anomaly is due to the persistence of the midportion of an accessory neurenteric canal.

When diastematomyelia is discovered early in life, it should be repaired surgically (23). It is found occasionally in adults and if signs and symptoms are evident, operation should be carried out then as well. The spicule must be removed epidurally down flush to the posterior surface of the vertebral body. Its dural sheath should then be freed from adhesions to the 2 halves of the spinal cord and excised. The resulting anterior dural defect may be left open, but the posterior dural defect must be closed in water-tight fashion.

Lipoma

Lipomas are the most frequent variety of spinal dysraphism (Fig. 15.5–15.7). Although they occasionally are limited to the intradural compartment, these lesions usually are present at birth as subcutaneous collections of fat in the midline over the lumbosacral area and extend through a spina bifida defect to and usually through the dura, being attached to a myeloschisic plate, (Figs. 15.5 and 15.6). This particular lesion has been well described (24, 25) and sometimes is called "lipomyelomeningocele." Lipomatous collections of this sort are not neoplastic in nature and usually increase in size only relative to the general growth pattern of the patient. In some cases, however, the intraspinal portions of the lipoma appear to exert considerable mechanical pressure against nerve roots and/or the conus itself. Although nerve roots may travel through these lipomatous collections, this has been quite rare in the experience of the authors.

If the roots of the cauda equina are involved at all, they usually are adhered to the outer surface of the lipoma and can be dissected easily from it. These lesions should be removed except for the areas immediately adjacent to the central nervous system. This junctional zone between fat and conus is sometimes quite firm in consistency, may be cartilaginous (Fig. 15.5C) and is best *not* removed. However, the conus must be freed from the tethering effect of the lipoma during the course of the operative repair.

Dermal Sinus Tract

Congenital dermal sinuses commonly arise in the perineal or lower intergluteal area and extend into the anus or subcutaneous tissues of the buttocks. These are called pilonidal fistulas or sinuses. Those arising at or above the upper end of the intergluteal fold, especially if they are in the midline, may continue into the spinal canal and to or through the dural sac. Once through the dura, they continue in a cephalad direction (Fig. 15.8). There is a propensity to extend to the neural segment that corresponds to the dermatome of origin of the skin lesion, i.e., to the conus medullaris or above (1).

Because a dermal sinus tract that extends through the dura offers an excellent portal of entry for the production of bacterial meningitis, it should be excised whenever diagnosed. Every effort must be made to remove it in toto: beginning with an eliptical excision of the skin dimple

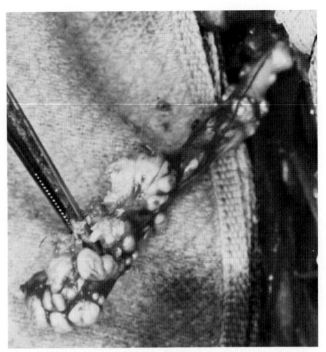

Figure 15.8. Dermal sinus tract with multiple dermoid cysts. This 6-year-old child had had multiple episodes of bacterial meningitis. The intradural portion of the sinus tract extended over several segments and was attached to the conus medullaris. Multiple laminectomies were required to effect its total excision. Note the numerous associated dermoid cysts along the course of the sinus.

and tracing the tract cephalad, via multiple laminectomies, if necessary, to its termination. If there have been previous bouts of meningitis, great patience with microsurgical technique may be required to free the lesion from the roots of the cauda equina and from the conus medullaris.

Dermoid Cyst

Although isolated dermoid cysts within the spinal cord can occur, they most often are associated with a dermal sinus tract. In this setting, one or several cysts may occur as local expansions of the sinus tract anywhere along its course from skin to spinal cord (Fig. 15.8). Bryant and Dayen (26) reported a case of a dermoid cyst that occurred after the repair of a thoracolumbar myelomeningocele. A dermoid cyst apparently developed after the neural plate had been replaced in the spinal canal, a small bit of dermis having been left on its surface. These cysts, as well as the sinus tracts of dermal origin, have a great propensity to recur so that every effort must be made toward complete excision.

Fibrous Band

Fibrous bands (6, 7) may tether the dorsal spinal cord or conus medullaris. They often run from the conus posteriorly and inferiorly to the dura (Fig. 15.9). However, lateral extension is not uncommon. Occasionally, they are

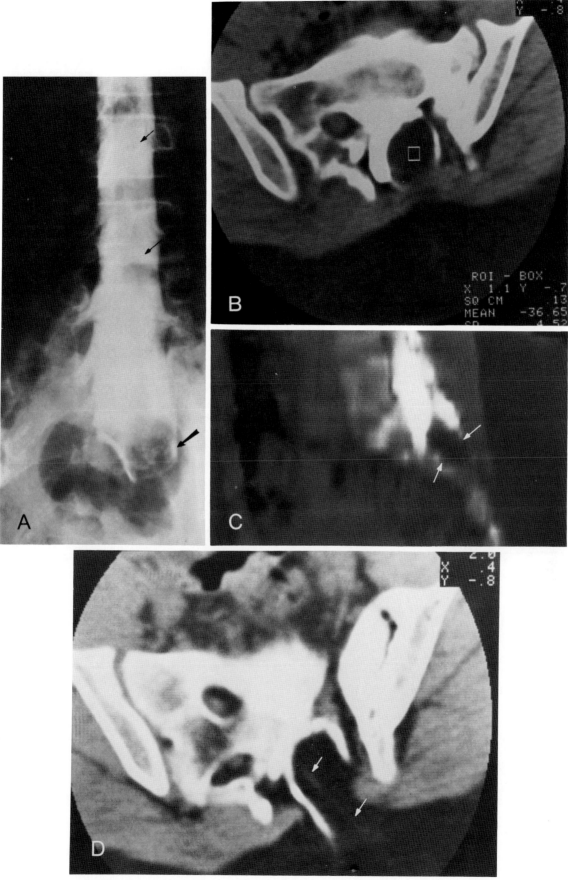

Figure 15.9. Lipoma and fibrous band extending from subcutaneous area into bifid sacral canal, tethering conus medullaris in a 9-year-old girl. A metrizimide myelogram demonstrates an abnormally low spinal cord (*small black arrows*, A) and a mass involving the caudal sac (*large black arrow*). CT scan in axial (B) and sagitally reconstructed views (C) shows the extent and position of the lipoma, −36.65 EMI Units, within the dysplastic sacrum. A fibrous band (*white arrows*, D) is attached to the conus and extends through the lipomatous tissue posterior to the sacrum.

found anteriorly. Bands may or may not continue through the dura, bone, and more superficial tissues to cause dimpling of the overlying skin. In some cases, the only explanation for the low-lying posteriorly displaced conus is a thickened filum terminale. Under such conditions, the filum may demonstrate excessive collagenous tissue, glia, or varying amounts of fat. It may be difficult grossly to distinguish the conus from the filum in these cases. Our practice is to section the filum 1.5–2 cm below the origin of the last spinal root.

Neurenteric Cyst

Neurenteric cysts are rare lesions that may be associated with intestinal duplication. Extension anteriorly from the spinal canal through a defect in a vertebral body is somewhat more frequent in the low cervical or upper thoracic level, although this may occur in the lumbosacral area as well. Bremer's explanation (8) of the development of these lesions and other types of spinal dysraphism has been discussed above. Theoretically, a complete accessory neurenteric sinus might be found, although persistence of only a segment along its course is the rule. Communication may exist through the vertebral column as either a fistula or a fibrous tract. Indeed, there may be only an isolated cyst inside the spinal canal with no anterior extension or bony defect. Intraspinal neurenteric cysts may be extradural, intradural extramedullary, or intramedullary in location. They cause symptoms either by expansive compression of neural tissue or by meningeal irritation. The picture of clinical meningitis may be seen, but bacterial cultures are usually negative. These lesions should be removed as completely as possible via laminectomy. If they extend anteriorly into the mediastinum or abdomen, another procedure in conjunction with thoracic or abdominal surgeons will be necessary.

Multiple Lesions

More than one type of spinal dysraphism is often present in the same patient. Thus, lipomas may be associated with fibrous bands (Fig. 15.9). Dermal sinus tracts frequently occur with dermoid cysts (Fig. 15.8). A fatty filum terminale may be present with other lipomata and a dermal sinus tract (Fig. 15.10). Chapman (27) has emphasized the importance of a thick filum in association with diastematomyelia. If complete neuroradiological studies are not carried out, the former may go unrecognized. Then, even though the diastematomyelic spur is removed satisfactorily, the cord remains tethered from below.

SUMMARY

Spinal dysraphism usually can be suspected clinically. Current practice should include formal neuroradiological evaluation using metrizimide myelography in combination with CT scanning. These anomalies are diagnosed ideally in infancy or early childhood when mechanical correction can be made of abnormal communications, tethering, or mass effects before the development of meningitis, progressive neurological deficit, or spinal deformity.

References

1. Matson DD: *Neurosurgery of Infants and Children*, 2nd Edition. Springfield, IL, Charles C Thomas, 1969.
2. Page LK, Berti AF: Myelomeningocele: Criteria for treatment and surgical management. *Contemp Neurosurg* 2:1–5, 1980.
3. Page LK, Welch FT: Neurosurgical care of the patient with spina bifida aperta. *J Fla Med Assoc* 63:892–894, 1976.
4. Anderson FM: Occult spinal dysraphism: a series of 73 cases. *Pediatrics* 55:826–835, 1975.
5. Ingraham FD: *Spina Bifida and Cranium Bifidum*. Cambridge, Harvard University Press, 1944.
6. James CCM, Lassman LP: *Spinal Dysraphism. Spinal Bifida Occulta*. London, Butterworths, 1972.
7. Till K: Spinal dysraphism: a study of congenital malformations of the lower back. *J Bone Joint Surg* 51B:415–422, 1969.
8. Bremer JL: Dorsal intestinal fistula; accessory neurenteric canal; diastematomyelia, A.M.A. *Arch Pathol* 54:132–138, 1952.
9. Barson AJ: Vertebral level of termination of spinal cord during normal and abnormal development. *J Anat* 106:489–497, 1969.

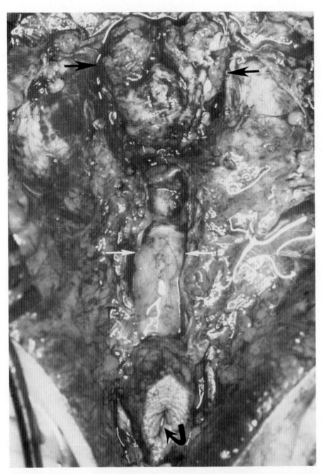

Figure 15.10.   Lipoma in a 3-year-old boy extended through spina bifida (*straight black arrows*) and attached to conus medullaris. Subcutaneous lipoma has been removed and the sacral canal unroofed to reveal a large fatty filum terminale (*white arrows*). Note the external opening of a dermal sinus tract which is attached to the filum (*curved arrow*).

10. Reimann AF, Anson BJ: Vetebral level of termination of the spinal sord with report of a case of sacral cord. *Anat Rec* 88:127–138, 1944.
11. Fitz CR, Harwood-Nash DC: The tethered conus. *Am J Roentgenol Radiat Ther Nuc Med* 125:515–523, 1975.
12. Kaplan JO: Quencer RM: The occult tethered conus syndrome in the adult. *Radiology* 137:387–391, 1981.
13. Yashon D, Beatty RA: Tethering of the conus medullaris within the sacrum. *J Neurol Neurosurg Psychiatr* 29:244–250, 1975.
14. Lindgren E: Myelography with air. *Acta Psychiatr Neurol* 14:385–388, 1939.
15. Westberg G: Gas myelography and percutaneous puncture in the diagnosis of spinal cord cysts. *Acta Radiol* Suppl 252, 1966.
16. Scatliff JH, Till K, Hoare RD: Incomplete, false and true diastematomyelia. *Radiology* 116:349–354, 1975.
17. Harwood-Nash DC, Fitz CR: Computed tomography and the pediatric spine: Computed tomographic metrizimide myelography in children. In: Post MJD: *Radiographic Evaluation of the Spine: Current Advances with Emphasis on Computed Tomography.* New York, Masson Publishing, 1980.
18. Kaiser MC, Pettersson H, Harwood-Nash DC, et al: Direct coronal CT of the spine in infants and children. *AJNR* 2:465–466, 1981.
19. Murtagh FR, Balis GA: Diagnosis of intradural sacral lipoma and tethered cord by computed tomography. *J Fla Med Assoc* 68:499–500, 1981.
20. Pettersson H, Harwood-Nash DC, Fitz CR, et al: Conventional metrizimide myelography (MM) and computed tomography metrizimide myelography (CTMM) in scoliosis. *Radiology* 142:111–114, 1982.
21. Herren RY, Edwards JE: Diplomyelia (Duplication of the spinal cord). *Arch Pathol* 30:1203–1214, 1940.
22. Cohen N, Sledge CB: Diastematomyelia: an embryological interpretation with report of a case. *Am J Dis Child* 100:257–263, 1960.
23. Kennedy PR: New data on diastematomyelia. *J Neurosurg* 51:355–361, 1979.
24. Bassett RC: The neurologic deficit associated with lipomas of the cauda equina. *Ann Surg* 131:109–116, 1950.
25. Emery JL, Lendon RG: Lipoma of the cauda equina and other fatty tumors related to neurospinal dysraphism. *Dev Med Child Neurol (Suppl)* 20:62–70, 1969.
26. Bryant H, Dayen AD: Spinal inclusion dermoid cyst in a patient with treated myelocystocele. *J Neurol Neurosurg Psychiatr* 30:182–184, 1967.
27. Chapman PH: Occult spinal dysraphic states. In: Schmidek HH, Sweet WH: *Current Techniques in Operative Neurosurgery.* New York, Grune and Stratton, 1977, pp. 265–277.

CHAPTER SIXTEEN

Syringomyelia and Arnold-Chiari Malformation

MARIE LOUISE AUBIN, M.D. and JACQUELINE VIGNAUD, M.D.

Syringomyelia represents an anatomical lesion: a cavity within the cord, involving several segments.

The cavity is completely or partly independent from the ependymal canal, thus, differentiating it from hydromyelia. The syringomyelic syndrome includes typical neurological syndromes.

Syringomyelia may be due to a congenital malformation; but may be of traumatic, tumoral, or infectious origin.

PATHOLOGICAL ANATOMY

The syringomyelic cavity lies in the central part of the cord, behind the ependymal canal. It mainly occupies the midpart of the central cord.

Superiorly, it often stops at C2 and inferiorly, it extends down to the thoracic or even lumbar part of the spinal cord.

Within the grey matter, the cavity extends into the posterior horns. Destruction of the anterior horns sometimes may occur. The cavity is covered by glial tissue, and not by ependyma.

Lesions of the medulla oblongata may lengthen the superior extent of the cavity. These lesions are referred to as syringobulbia. Anatomically, they are clefts which are in communication with the floor of the 4th ventricle.

The syringomyelic cavity involves the conducting pathways, thus, inducing degenerative lesions of the pyramidal pathways below the cavity, and the ascending lemniscal pathways above the cavity.

An Arnold-Chiari malformation often is associated with syringomyelia, including: a low position of the medulla oblongata and an ectopic low position of the tonsils which may extend down to the level of C2–C3. Theoretically, the 4th ventricle is in normal position in Chiari I malformation; whereas it is in low position in Chiari II malformation.

CLINICAL FINDINGS

When complete, the syringomyelic syndrome includes a dissociated sensory loss: loss of pain and temperature sense with preservation of touch and deep pressure in segments of the upper extremities.

Areflexia of the upper limbs is frequent. Paresis and amyotrophia of the arms is due to destruction of the neurons of the anterior horn.

Syringobulbia may cause nystagmus, 5th nerve pathology, and mixed nerve palsies as well as 12th nerve involvement.

Compression or destruction of the white matter by the cavity may induce a spastic paraplegia.

Clinical history and physical examination of the patient can give clues to the etiology of the lesion.

A long evolution of the disease, associated with cervical bony malformation, is in favor of a Chiari I malformation, which is by far the most frequent cause of syringomyelia (79% of our cases).

A rapid onset of the disease will favor a tumoral origin. The history of acute trauma will point to a traumatic etiology and the history of meningitis will favor the diagnosis of arachnoiditis.

PATHOGENESIS

Several theories (Fig. 16.1) have been proposed to explain the phenomenon of syringomyelia. According to Gardner and associates (1–3), failure of the foramina of the 4th ventricle to open at the 29th week of fetal life with continuing communication between the 4th ventricle and the central canal allows increased pressure within the ventricles to be transmitted to the central canal which then dilates. At the same time, the hydrocephalus causes inferior displacement of the cerebellum, thus, creating an Arnold-Chiari malformation. In such a case, the main abnormality is hydromyelia, which may be associated with a dissecting cyst within the cord thus called syringomyelia.

In the Williams theory (4), the resulting anatomical abnormality is approximately the same, except for the often observed lack of hydrocephalus. According to this theory, efforts such as the Valsalva maneuver produce increased venous pressure, which raises the cerebrospinal fluid (CSF) pressure within the ventricles, which in turn is transmitted to the central canal, whereas muscular efforts induce venous hypertension in the medullary veins and in the cavity.

Aboulker (5) believes that the Gardner et al. theory is only valid for children who have hydrocephalus, frequently associated with meningocele. According to Aboulker (5), the pathogenesis of the clinical syndrome of the adult is different: a cavity develops within the parenchyma of the cord without any relation to the central canal which, in adults, according to the pathologists mentioned by Aboulker, often is collapsed, closed, or absent. The abnormality is caused by stenosis at the level of the foramen magnum due to the Arnold-Chiari malformation, arachnoiditis, or tumors.

This theory is supported by canine experiments per-

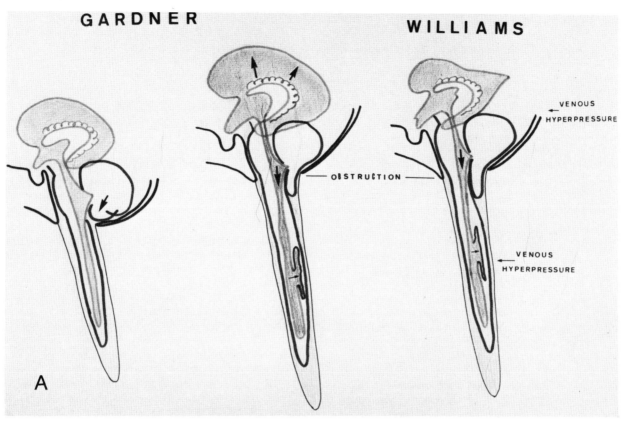

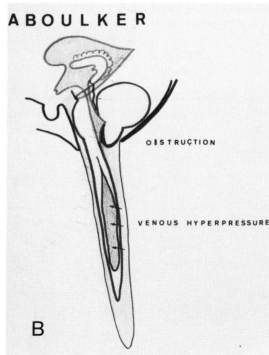

Figure 16.1.   In Gardner's theory, failure of the 4th ventricular foramina to open results in a persistent communication between the 4th ventricle and central canal. The resulting hydrocephalus causes increased pressure within the central canal and inferior displacement of the tonsils. In Williams' theory, intermittent venous hypertension results in increased CSF pressure which is transmitted to the persistent central canal. In Aboulker's theory, there is incomplete cistern obstruction, hydrocephalus, and high venous pressure with transmedullary passage of CSF creating a true syringomyelia cavity. (Reproduced with permission from *AJNR* 2:199–204, May/June 1981.)

formed by Sato et al. (6) that demonstrated that 30% of the CSF is produced in the spinal canal.

Due to the stenosis at the foramen magnum, the CSF finds its way with difficulty towards the intracranial areas of resorption. The pressure of the CSF within the spinal canal is higher than that of intracranial CSF, resulting in edema within the cord. The last stage of the edema is cavity formation; this mechanism is potentiated by increased venous pressure in the azygous system, which may be congenital or acquired.

According to Aboulker (5), the CSF filters through the parenchyma, or via a pathway along the posterior roots. Ball and Dayan (7) thought that it might be transmitted along the arteries. The cavity, which generally ends at the level C2, may sometimes dissect along the medulla oblongata to reach the 4th ventricle.

RADIOLOGICAL STUDIES

The aim of the radiological examination is to demonstrate the cavity; its exact location and extension; its relationship with surrounding structures, the ventricular system and subarachnoid spaces; and to try to find out its underlying etiology: an Arnold-Chiari malformation which is the more likely, and rule out a tumor.

Plain films of the spine have to be performed initially in anteroposterior (AP) and lateral projections. Conventional radiographs are, at the present time, more precise than the digital radiographs of CT. They may demonstrate abnormalities suspicious for an Arnold-Chiari malformation (Fig. 16.2A): a small posterior fossa; an enlarged foramen magnum with a convex posterior border; an enlarged diameter of the spinal canal which may be associated with scalloping of the posterior margins of the vertebrae (Fig. 16.3). Malformations of the vertebrae may also be seen: Klippel-Feil syndrome; basilar invagination; and spina bifida of the lumbar spine. Scoliosis very frequently is observed too.

However, the absence of cervical malformations does not exclude a Chiari I malformation.

Plain films sometimes may demonstrate a tumoral modification of the bone.

After plain films, the least invasive procedure is *plain CT* (i.e., without any kind of injection of contrast material).

It is performed in cases of suspected nontumoral syringomyelia. The cervical and thoracic levels should be examined, as well as the brain. Contiguous sections of 5–8 mm, should be obtained.

The cyst was visualized in 89% of our cases (67 of 75 cases). It appeared as a well-delineated area of low density (with an absorption coefficient equal to CSF) (Figs. 16.4A, B, and C).

The cysts which failed to show up on plain CT were those with a small collapsed cord. In such cases, they were demonstrated on the delayed metrizamide CT scan.

The top level of the cavity was C1–C2. The cervical cord was well delineated down to the level of C5–C6.

The lateral ventricles were dilatated in 17 cases of 75 (22%). Nine of these, in elderly patients with dilated sulci, were considered to be secondary to atrophy, so that only 11 cases (15%) had true hydrocephalus.

With plain CT, an Arnold-Chiari malformation may be suspected when no subarachnoid space is detectable at the level of the foramen magnum (Fig. 16.5).

This procedure which is a completely noninvasive technique is valuable in establishing the diagnosis of a cyst

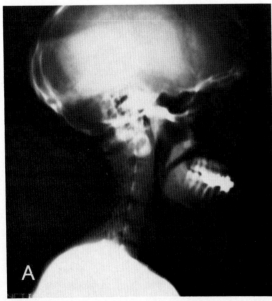
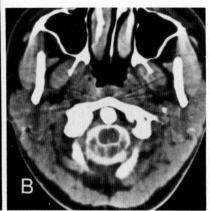

Figure 16.2. A. Cervical spine: lateral plain film demonstrates abnormalities suspicious for Chiari I malformation: small posterior fossa, basilar invagination, widening of the foramen magnum, and the AP diameter of the upper part of the cervical canal. B. In the same patient, Chiari I malformation is demonstrated after intrathecal metrizamide injection.

(89%) but it is unable to provide a complete anatomical description of the lesion.

When clinical findings suggest the possibility of a tumor, CT with intravenous injection should be performed. En-

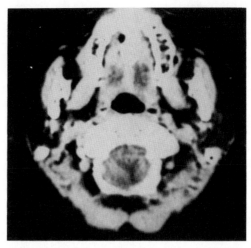

Figure 16.5. Plain CT scan with a slice through C1. Chiari I malformation. The tonsils are visible in low position posterior to the cervical cord.

hancement of the cord (in cases of intramedullary tumor) or of adjacent tissue in cases of extramedullary tumor may be demonstrated. (However, one must realize that isodense nonenhancing tumors may exist.)

For further information invasive procedures using intrathecal or intramedullary injection of contrast material must be performed.

Conventional techniques are: air or opaque myelogra-

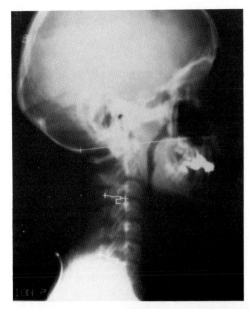

Figure 16.3. Cervical spine: lateral plain film shows enlargement of the AP diameter of the lower part of the cervical spine.

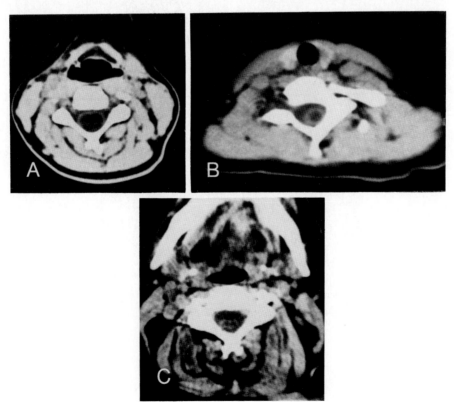

Figure 16.4. Plain CT scan. Syringomyelic cyst is visible. A. in a large cervical cord (C4); B. in a normal cord (C7); C. In a small cord (C3).

phy; cystic opacification by direct puncture into the cyst; CT metrizamide.

Air or opaque myelography may demonstrate indirectly the presence of a cyst by the fact that the cord enlarges or collapses depending on the position of the body; it may demonstrate an Arnold-Chiari malformation: small cisterna magna; low position of the tonsils, no filling of the 4th ventricle. However, the cyst is never spontaneously shown.

Since CT metrizamide may give all this information, and, in addition, demonstrate a cyst, we think that conventional myelographic procedures are of no particular diagnostic value.

Intracystic injection of contrast material via a direct intracystic puncture may be considered as a very invasive technique which must be employed when surgical shunting is to be performed and CT with sagittal reconstruction has failed to demonstrate the inferior portion of the cyst.

CT METRIZAMIDE

Intrathecal injection of metrizamide (7 ml of 170 mg/I/ml) is performed via lumbar puncture. The patient should be tilted head down for 1 minute prone, and for 1 minute supine in order to obtain a better view of the craniocervical junction.

IMMEDIATE CT METRIZAMIDE SCANS

With CT scans obtained shortly after myelography, the contrast medium generally fills the cisterns of the posterior fossa (in all but 1 case) and enters the ventricle [in 65 of 75 cases (86%)].

On these immediate scans, one has good visualization of the cord; in all cases, the opacified subarachnoid spaces are sharply delineated.

The cord. The AP diameter of the subarachnoid space and cord were measured and the ratio of these diameters were calculated. According to the criteria for normal cord measurements established by Nordquist (8) at the level C3–C4, we found 3 groups of measurements (Figs. 16.6A, B, and C): enlarged cords (10%), small cords (45%); and normal cords (45%). Opacification of the cavity in the first 30 minutes occurred in only 5 cases of the 64, suggesting a direct communication between the 4th ventricle or the posterior fossa and the cyst (Gardner's theory) (Fig. 16.7A

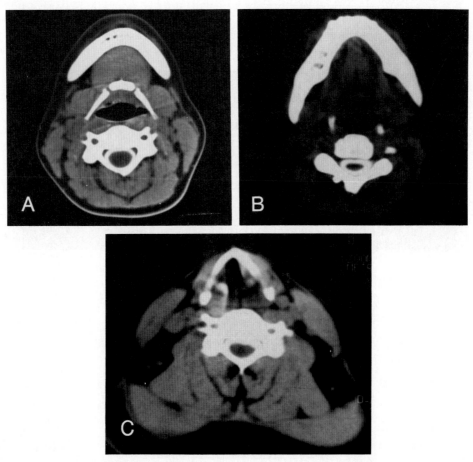

Figure 16.6.   Shape of the cervical cord after intrathecal metrizamide injection. A. enlarged cord (10%); B. small cord (45%); C. normal cord (45%).

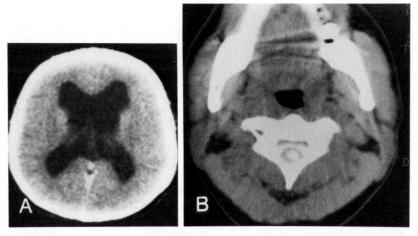

Figure 16.7.   Same patient: A. plain CT scan: hydrocephalus; B. cervical slice immediately after intrathecal metrizamide injection shows filling of the syringomyelic cavity (Gardner's theory).

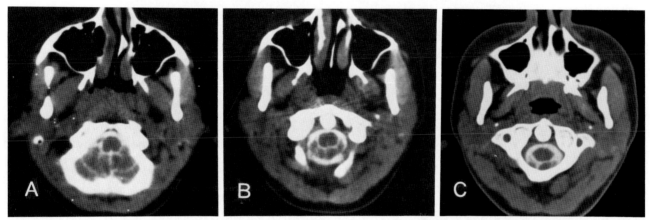

Figure 16.8.   A–C. Morphological aspects of Chiari I malformation, in axial projection, after intrathecal metrizamide injection.

and B). In the other 59 cases, the cavity was not opacified, and its natural low density could not be identified clearly due to the high concentration of metrizamide which necessitated wide window widths to visualize the cord. However, a density profile obtained in some of these cases demonstrated low-density variations suggesting a cyst. At the craniocervical junction, an Arnold-Chiari malformation was demonstrated in 48 cases (79%) (Figs. 16.8A, B, and C and 16.9A and B).

The 4th ventricle was in low position; and the tonsils clearly outlined by the contrast appearing as two filling defects, which may be asymmetrical on each side of the cord, or of the ectopic medulla oblongata.

The 4th ventricle was filled in 55 cases (86%).

DELAYED CT METRIZAMIDE SCANS

Delayed metrizamide CT scanning is performed 6–10 hours after intrathecal contrast injection. A central cavity was opacified in 59 of our 64 cases (Figs. 16.10 and 16.11). Amongst the 59 cases, 51 were demonstrated on plain CT. The 8 cases which failed to show up on plain CT had small cords. In these cases, the cord parenchyma was thin.

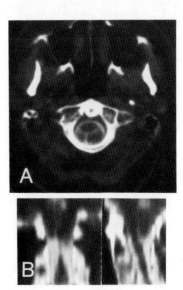

Figure 16.9.   A and B. Morphological aspects of Arnold-Chiari malformation after intrathecal metrizamide injection. A. Axial projection. B. Coronal and sagittal reconstruction.

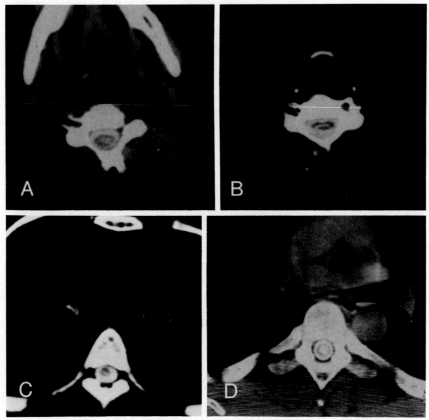

Figure 16.10. Syringomyelic cysts opacified by metrizamide 8 hours after intrathecal injection. A and B. Cervical cysts. C and D. Thoracic cysts.

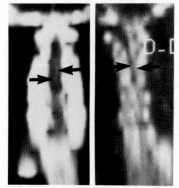

Figure 16.11. Coronal and sagittal reconstructions show the syringomyelic cyst (*arrows*) filled with metrizamide 8 hours after injection.

In 9 of the 59 cases, a posterolateral defect in the parenchyma was visualized clearly, on one (2 cases) or both sides (1 case) (Fig. 16.12A and B).

It should be mentioned that in 4 patients with hydrocephalus, the central cavity seen on the scan before metrizamide was not filled by metrizamide.

In some cases, delayed scans were obtained at 12, 24, and 48 hours after injection. The cavity remained opacified whereas the density of CSF and of the parenchyma decreased.

Changes in the densities of the CSF, cord, and cavity with time were recorded in 21 cases (Fig. 16.13A, B, and C). The mean densities of the CSF, cord, and cyst were plotted against time. The curves demonstrate that in all these cases, there is an increase in density of the parenchyma and a much greater increase in density of the cyst cavity. On the other hand, CSF density decreased with time, suggesting an active filling of the cavity with metrizamide. Delayed scans confirmed these findings. It recently was demonstrated that cysts due to a tumor associated with a syringomyelic syndrome were only demonstrated on very delayed CT scans (9).

DISCUSSION

CT is the safest technique for visualization of the syringomyelic cavity. Detection of the cavity is somewhat more accurate with CT metrizamide than with plain CT.

The diagnosis of an Arnold-Chiari malformation is straightforward and accurate with CT. In 48 of 59 cases who had an Arnold-Chiari malformation demonstrated by previous myelography, it was demonstrated as well by the metrizamide CT study. The ventricular system may be evaluated easily by CT and hydrocephalus demonstrated when present.

In order to determine the possible route of metrizamide penetration, particular attention was paid to the 59 patients who had a cavity opacified. In only 5 cases was a

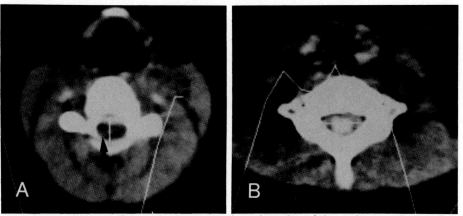

Figure 16.12. A. The metrizamide opacifies early the posterolateral portion of the syringomyelic cyst (*arrow*). B. In the same patient, 12 hours later, the syringomyelic cyst is completely filled by metrizamide.

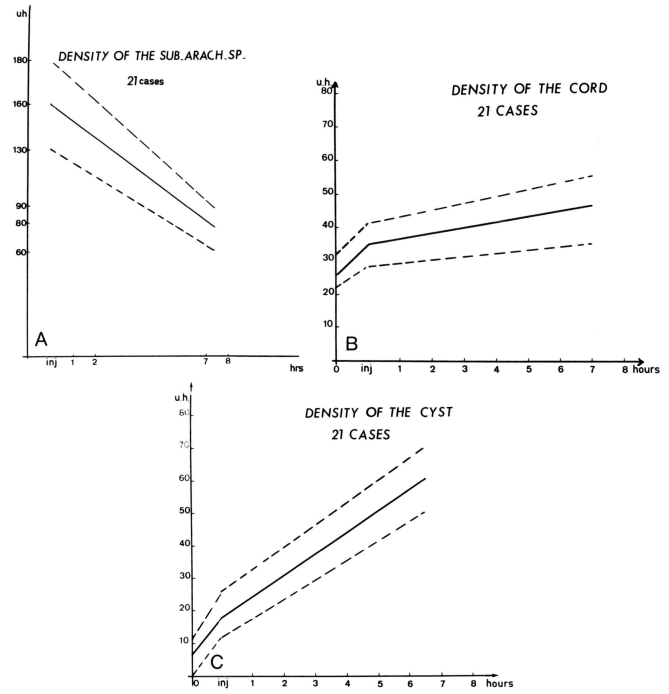

Figure 16.13. Relationship between the densities (HU) of the subarachnoid space (A), cord (B), and cyst (C) and time of examination in (hours). *Solid line* = mean; *dashed line* = 1 SD.

central canal demonstrated on the immediate CT metrizamide scan. This early filling of the cavity suggests that it fills from the region of the cisterna magna or 4th ventricle, through the obex of a patent central canal. In these cases, the 4th ventricle and the cisterna magna were opacified after tilting.

In 54 cases the filling was delayed. We cannot assess the exact time of the beginning of the filling because we did not obtain scans at frequent intervals and because of the potential error in the evaluation of the density measurements from the density profiles. However, the evidence for active filling of the cavity is convincing. It may be seen whether or not the 4th ventricle is filled. These observations strongly suggest transneural passage of metrizamide.

CONCLUSION

Plain CT and CT with metrizamide are the most accurate procedures for establishing the diagnosis of syringomyelia, for visualizing the cyst and an associated Arnold-Chiari malformation. However, these techniques may be complemented by a direct intracystic injection of contrast with conventional cystography when CT metrizamide fails to demonstrate the inferior part of the cyst, and surgical shunting of the cavity is to be performed.

In the future, the radiological protocol of syringomyelia may be completely modified by Nuclear Magnetic Resonance (NMR). A recent preliminary communication reported cases in which the cyst was spontaneously demonstrated by this technique.

REFERENCES

1. Gardner W: Hydrodynamic mechanism of syringomyelia: its relationship to myelocele. *J Neurol Neurosurg Psychiatr* 28:247–259, 1965.
2. Gardner W, Angel J: The mechanism of syringomyelia and its surgical correction. *Clin Neurosurg* 6:131–140, 1975.
3. Gardner W, Murry FML: Noncommunicating syringomyelia: a non existent entity. *Surg Neurol* 6:251–256, 1976.
4. Williams B: Pathogenesis of syringomyelia. *Lancet* 1:142–143, 1972.
5. Aboulker J: La syringomyélie et les liquides intra rachidiens. *Neurochirurgie* 25:suppl 1, 1979.
6. Sato O, Asai T, Amono Y, et al: Extraventricular origin of the cerebrospinal fluid: formation rate quantitatively measured in the spinal subarachnoid space of dogs. *J Neurosurg* 36:276–281, 1972.
7. Ball MJ, Dayan AD: Pathogenesis of syringomyelia. *Lancet* 2:799–801, 1972.
8. Nordquist L: The sagittal diameter of the spinal cord and subarachnoid space in different age groups. A roentgenographic postmortem study. *Acta Radiol* (Stockh) Suppl 227, 1964.
9. Kan S, Fox A, Vinuela F: Delayed CT metrizamide enhancement of syringomyelia secondary to tumor. XII Symposium Neuroradiologicum, Washington, D.C., 1982.
10. Aubin ML, Vignaud J, Bar D, et al: Apport de la scanographie à l'étude des syringomyélies. *Rev Neurol* (Paris) 136:271–277, 1980.
11. Aubin ML, Vignaud J, Jardin C, et al: Computed tomography in 75 clinical cases of syringomyelia. *AJNR* 2:199–204, 1981.
12. Bamberger-Bozo C: Malformation de Chiari II. Arnold Chiari de la littérature. *J Neuroradiol* 9:47–70, 1982.
13. Bonafe A, Ethier R, Melancon D, Belanger G, Peters T: High resolution computed tomography in cervical syringomyelia. *J Comput Assist Tomogr* 4:42–47, 1980.
14. Dubois PJ, Drayer BP, Osborne D, et al: Intramedullary penetrance of metrizamide in the dog spinal cord. Presented at the annual meeting of the American Society of Neuroradology, Toronto, Canada, May, 1979.
15. Ellertson AB: Syringomyelia and other cystic spinal cord lesions. *Acta Neurol Scand* 45:403–417, 1969.
16. Emde H, Piepgras U: Percutaneous injection of metrizamide into spinal cord cysts. X-ray, CT and reconstructed images in the preoperative diagnosis of syringomyelia. XII Symposium Neuroradiologicum Washington, D.C., 1982.
17. Escourolle R, Poirier J: Manuel élémentaire de neuropathologie. Paris, Masson Publishing, 1977.
18. Forbes W, Isherwood I: Computed tomography in syringomyelia and the associated Arnold Chiari I malformation. *Neuroradiology* 15:73–78, 1978.
19. Greenfield J: Neuropathology. Arnold, 1976.
20. Hiratsuka H, Fujinara K, Odaka K, et al: Modification of periventricular hypodensity in hydrocephalus with ventricular reflux in metrizamide CT cisternography. *J Comput Assist Tomogr* 3:204–208, 1979.
21. Lichtenstein BW: Syringomyelia-textbook of neuropathology. London, WB Saunders, 1949.
22. Naidich TP, Pudlowski RM, Naidich JB: Computed tomography signs of the Chiari II malformation. Part I—Skull and dural partitions. *Radiology* 134:65–71, 1980.
23. Naidich TP, Pudlowski RM, Naidich JB: Computed tomography signs of the Chiari II malformation. Part II—Midbrain and cerebellum. *Radiology* 134:391–398, 1980.
24. Naidich TP, Pudlowski RM, Naidich JB: Computed tomography signs of the Chiari II malformation. Part III—Ventricles and cisterns. *Radiology* 134:657–665, 1980.
25. Newman PK, Terenty TR, Fister JB: Some observations on the pathogenesis of syringomyelia. *J Neurol Neurosurg Psychiatr* 44:964–969, 1981.
26. Resjoe IM, Harwood-Nash DC, Fitz CR, et al: Computed tomographic metrizamide myelography in syringohydromyelia. *Radiology* 131:405–407, 1979.
27. Simmons J, Norman D, Newton T: Preoperative diagnosis of postinflammatory syringomyelia. XII Symposium Neuroradologicum, Washington, D.C., 1982.
28. Taylor J, Greenfield JC, Martin JP: Two cases of syringomyelia and syringobulbia. *Brain* 45:323–356, 1922.
29. Vignaud J, Aubin ML: Computed tomography in 25 cases of syringomyelia. Presented at the annual meeting of the American Society of Neuroradiology, Toronto, Canada, April, 1979.
30. West RJ, Williams B: Radiographic studies of the ventricles in syringomyelia. *Neuroradiology* 20:5–16, 1980.
31. Williams B, Timperley WR: Three cases of communicating syringomyelia secondary to mid brain gliomas. *J Neurol Neurosurg Psychiatr* 40:80–88, 1977.
32. Winkler SS, Sackett JF: Explanation of metrizamide brain penetration: a review. *J Comput Assist Tomogr* 4:191–193, 1980.

SECTION IV

Computed Tomography of the Adult Spine

A. DISC DISEASE
1. Diagnosis (Preoperative)

CHAPTER SEVENTEEN

Computed Tomographic Evaluation of Lumbar and Thoracic Degenerative Disc Disease

ALAN L. WILLIAMS, M.D. and VICTOR M. HAUGHTON, M.D.

INTRODUCTION

With the advent of high-resolution CT scanners which are able to differentiate the various soft-tissue structures within the vertebral canal, CT has become the primary neuroradiological modality for evaluating the spine in many institutions. In no area of spinal pathology has CT had greater impact than in degenerative disc disease, particularly herniated discs. Because of the relatively abundant epidural fat in the lumbar spine, CT scanning in this region has been more satisfactory than in thoracic or cervical. This chapter will emphasize CT scanning of lumbar disc disease, touching only briefly on disc herniation in the thoracic region.

TECHNIQUE

Patients are scanned in the supine position. They are instructed not to move or breathe while scans are obtained. After the patient is positioned by the technologist, a lateral localizer image is obtained, then levels and gantry tilt are selected using a computer program (Fig. 17.1) (1–3).

Angulation of the gantry makes possible CT slices in the plane of the disc. At L5-S1, slices precisely in the plane of the disc may be difficult to obtain as the normal lumbosacral angle approaches 30° and gantry tilt is limited to 15–20° in CT scanners currently available. However, in most cases, slight obliquity of CT sections at L5-S1 does not create a diagnostic problem because the posterior margin of the disc can still be visualized. A pillow placed beneath the patient's knees may reduce the lumbar lordosis, thus decreasing the lumbosacral angle. Similarly, a board elevating the patient's hips and legs will also decrease the difference between lumbosacral angle and max-

imal gantry tilt. Alternatively, a series of contiguous axial sections may be obtained at L5-S1 without gantry tilt. Using reformatting techniques, an image in the sagittal plane is obtained, followed by a reformatted axial image in the plane of the disc (Fig. 17.2) (4). In most cases, we prefer direct CT images at L5-S1 using maximal gantry tilt, even if images are not precisely in the plane of the disc, rather than reformatted scans because image resolution is higher and fewer slices are required to demonstrate the disc and adjacent tissues.

Either a 42-cm field of view (large-body calibration) with target reconstruction algorithm or a 25-cm field of view (infant calibration) may be used. Target reconstruction (ReView™), whereby a selected portion of a CT image is reconstructed on smaller pixels, theoretically increases the spatial resolution of various tissues (Fig. 17.4). In obese patients target reconstruction (soft-tissue algorithm) scans are superior to nontargeted images obtained with smaller calibrations.

In the lumbar region, where the normal height of the intervertebral disc is 5–8 mm (5), 5–7 axial sections are obtained routinely at each level of interest, one through the midplane of the disc and 2 or 3 contiguous slices on either side. Technical factors for routine lumbar spine scanning include 5-mm slice thickness, 500–600 MA, 120 KV, 3.3-millisecond pulse width code and 9.6-second scan speed. In the thoracic and cervical regions where the normal disc height is only 3–5 mm, and sometimes in narrowed lumbar discs, 1.5-mm thick slices are obtained (Fig. 17.3). When 1.5-mm slice thickness is selected, maximal techniques (600 MA) must be used to ensure optimal soft-tissue differentiation.

The vast majority of our patients with suspected disc disease have been studied by CT without a contrast me-

307

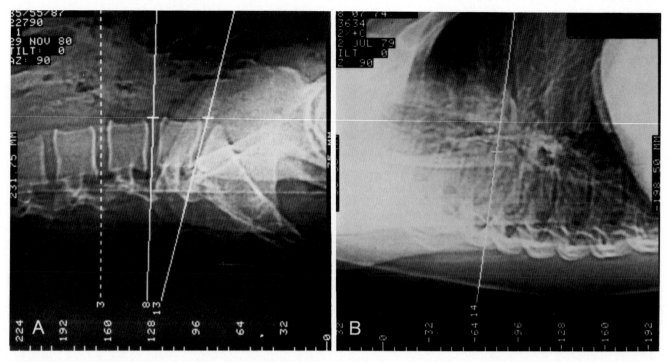

Figure 17.1. A lateral localizer image facilitates selection of levels of interest and gantry angulation. Cursor lines on lumbar (*A*) and thoracic (*B*) localizer images indicate the plane of section through intervertebral discs. [Reproduced with permission from Haughton and Williams (5).]

dium. Intravenous contrast, although able to enhance the epidural veins (2), has not provided useful diagnostic information in degenerative disc disease. Intrathecal metrizamide has been useful in at least two instances: 1) distinguishing a dilated nerve root sheath from a free disc fragment adjacent to the root sheath; and 2) demonstrating the dural sac and root sheaths in patients with extensive postoperative fibrosis.

NORMAL CT ANATOMY OF THE INTERVERTEBRAL DISC

The intervertebral disc is composed of a central nucleus pulposus, consisting of mucoid gelatinous material and thin fibrocartilaginous strands, surrounded by the anulus fibrosus, multiple layers of tough fibers which are collagenous at the periphery (Sharpey's fibers) and otherwise fibrocartilaginous (Fig. 17.5) (7, 8). Each anular layer contains nearly parallel, obliquely oriented fibers. The weakest fibers in the anulus are the thinner, more vertically oriented ones in the posterolateral portion. Because the anulus is thicker anteriorly than posteriorly, the nucleus pulposus is centered slightly posterior to the middle of the disc.

The superior and inferior surfaces of the fibrocartilaginous discs are covered by thin plates of hyaline cartilage. The end plate of hyaline cartilage is surrounded by a ring of bone, the ring apophysis, which fuses to the vertebral body in the second decade. Adjacent to the cartilaginous

disc end plate is a thin layer of cortical bone, the vertebral body endplate. The inner layers of the anulus fibrosus fuse with the cartilaginous end plate whereas the outer anular layers (Sharpey's fibers) insert into the vertebral ring apophysis.

In cross-section, the disc conforms to the adjacent vertebral bodies. Thus, the lumbar discs are oval in shape, the upper four with slight posterior midline concavity and L5-S1 with a nearly straight posterior margin (Fig. 17.6) (1). The thoracic discs are also characterized by concave posterior margins (Fig. 17.3) (5).

In CT images, the fibrocartilage of the nucleus and inner anulus appears homogeneous in density. The peripheral anular fibers, because of partial volume averaging of the ring apophysis or their greater collagen content, sometimes appear slightly more dense than the remainder of the disc. The dural sac, which appears slightly less dense than the disc in CT images, usually abuts the posterior margin of the disc in the thoracic and lumbar regions, exept at L5-S1 where the anterior epidural space is wide (Fig. 17.6). The posterior longitudinal ligament, which is attached to the anulus but not to the vertebral body, has a normal thickness of only 0.5–1.0 mm and, in most cases, cannot be distinguished from the anulus by CT. Because the attenuation values of the epidural fat are substantially less than those of the disc, the posterior margin of the disc can be demonstrated clearly by CT. The loss of epidural fat makes differentiation of the various intraspinal soft tissues difficult (Fig. 17.20).

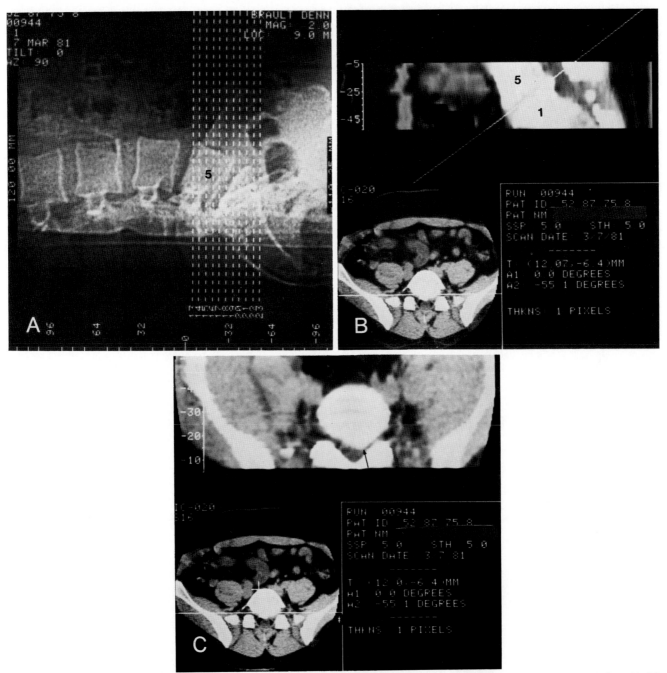

Figure 17.2. Reformatting of axial scans. A. A lateral localizer image demonstrates contiguous axial sections at L5-S1 with 0° gantry tilt. Following sagittal reformation which defines the L5-S1 disc space (B), an axial image in the plane of the disc is generated (C). A disc herniation (*arrow*) is demonstrated. [Reproduced with permission from Haughton and Williams (5).]

DEGENERATIVE DISC DISEASE

Pathophysiology

In the second decade of life the disc begins to degenerate (9). Gradual dessication of the nucleus pulposus results in decreasing turgor of the nucleus (10, 11) and elasticity of the anulus fibrosus. As a result, the disc becomes progressively less able to absorb and redistribute compressive forces. The anulus may develop tears which are concentric or, more commonly, radially oriented. These tears usually occur posteriorly or posterolaterally. Via such a radial tear nuclear material then may dissect through successive layers of the anulus to a position under the posterior longitudinal ligament (subligamentous herniation) or through it to lie within the epidural fat (extruded or free fragment). The nucleus becomes progressively more fi-

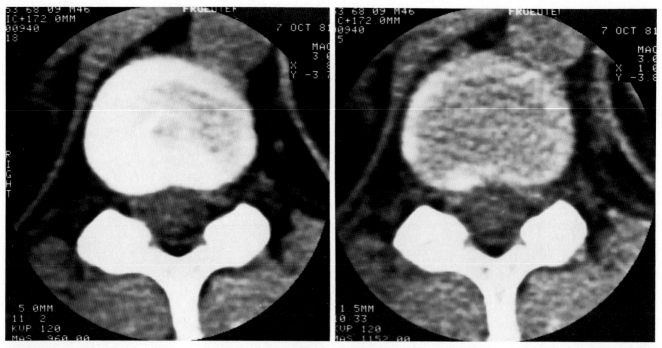

Figure 17.3. Effect of slice thickness on disc margins definition. Because of partial volume averaging of adjacent vertebral end plates, 5-mm thick slices (A) are less effective than 1.5-mm thick slices (B) for demonstrating the margins of normal thoracic and narrowed lumbar discs.

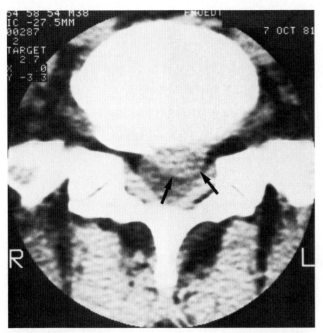

Figure 17.4. Target reconstruction. Using a computer program (ReView™) spatial resolution of an area of interest may be increased by reconstructing the data on smaller pixels. A target reconstructed image demonstrates a large midline disc herniation at L5–S1.

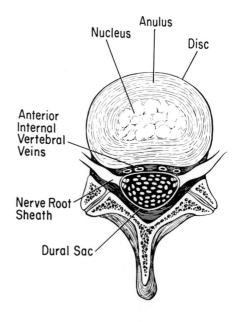

NORMAL

Figure 17.5. Artist's sketch of a normal lumbar disc showing the nucleus and anulus in axial projection.

brotic with advancing age and the likelihood of herniated nucleus pulposus diminishes. It becomes indistinguishable from the anulus by the 5th–7th decades.

Bulging Anulus

As the nucleus loses its turgor and the anulus its elasticity, the disc bulges outwardly beyond the vertebral body margins and the disc space decreases in height (Fig. 17.7). The CT diagnosis of a bulging but intact anulus is

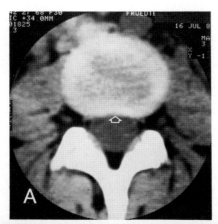

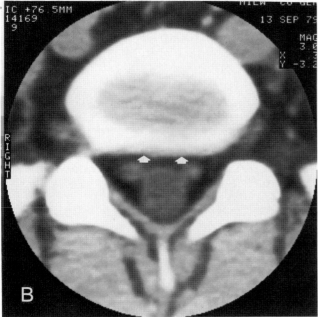

Figure 17.6. Normal lumbar discs. A. Lumbar discs exclusive of L5-S1 have a slight posterior midline concavity (*arrowhead*) of the disc margin and little anterior epidural fat. B. At L5-S1, the posterior disc margin is flat (*arrowheads*) and anterior epidural fat may be generous. [Reproduced with permission from Haughton and Williams (5).]

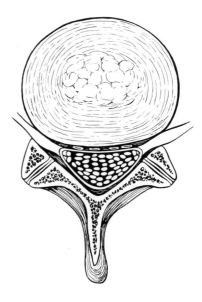

BULGING ANULUS

Figure 17.7. Artist's sketch of bulging anulus fibrosis. Note the convex posterior disc margin and flattening of the anterior dural sac.

based upon the identification in axial images of generalized extension of the disc margin beyond the vertebral end plates (12).

In the lumbar region, most bulging discs develop a convex posterior margin, however, in some cases the posterior margin retains its usual midline concavity, presumably because of buttressing by the posterior longitudinal ligament (Fig. 17.8) (12). Bulging discs usually appear symmetrical in CT images and somewhat asymmetrical in scoliosis (Fig. 17.8). Intradiscal gas (vacuum disc phenomenon) is demonstrated readily on CT scans when densities of −500 to −1000 HU are identified within the disc.

Bulging thoracic discs are less common than lumbar, but also may be identified on CT scans as generalized

extension of the disc beyond the vertebral body margins. The posterior disc margin may be convex or concave.

Herniated Nucleus Pulposus

In the lumbar region, herniation of nuclear material through a defect in the anulus most commonly occurs posterolaterally or posteriorly because the anulus is thinner posteriorly than anteriorly and the posterior longitudinal ligament is weaker than the anterior longitudinal ligament (Figs. 17.9–17.11) (5, 10, 13). When herniated nucleus lies beneath the posterior longitudinal ligament (subligamentous herniation), a smooth focal protrusion of the disc margin is identified on CT images (1, 3). When the herniation occurs within or lateral to the intervertebral foramen (lateral herniation), a myelogram may not demonstrate any deformity of the dural sac or root sheath. However, CT may identify such a lateral disc herniation readily (Fig. 17.12) (14).

When nuclear material passes through or around the posterior longitudinal ligament into the epidural space (free fragment) CT shows a different abnormality than in the subligamentous herniation (Fig. 17.13). In some cases the disc margin may not be deformed greatly despite the presence of an extruded fragment (Fig. 17.13). Once free in the epidural space extruded disc fragments may migrate in cephalad or caudad direction. Thus, CT sections adjacent to, as well as through, the disc space are mandatory if these fragments are to be identified (Fig. 17.14). If a free fragment lies adjacent to a root sheath, it may mimic a dilated root sheath (Fig. 17.15). A scan with intrathecal metrizamide may be necessary to distinguish such a free disc fragment from a dilated root sheath.

Calcification sometimes is observed with disc herniation

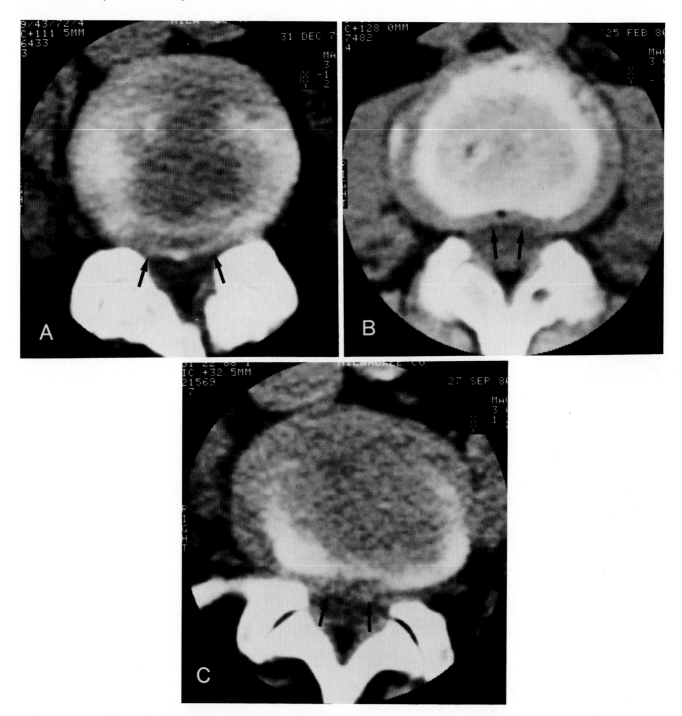

Figure 17.8. Bulging anulus fibrosis. In most cases of bulging anulus, the posterior disc margin becomes convex (*arrows*) (A), however the posterior midline concavity (*arrows*) may persist in some (B). [Reproduced with permission from Haughton and Williams (5).] Although most diffuse disc bulging is symmetrical, anular bulging may be slightly asymmetrical (C). Note the convex posterior disc margin (*arrows*).

in CT scans (Fig. 17.16). The presence of calcification is not diagnostically significant, as calcification within the nucleus pulposus or anulus fibrosis is commonly found in degenerated discs (10, 13).

Nuclear material may herniate through the cartilagi-

nous end plate of the disc and cortical end plate of the vertebral body, presumably through defects related to previously obliterated vascular channels (9, 13). Herniation of nuclear material into a vertebral body is referred to as a Schmorl's node. Commonly, sclerosis is identified at the margins of these intraosseous herniations. Schmorl's nodes are demonstrated readily on CT scans (Fig. 17.17). Osseous metastases treated with radiation or chemotherapy may develop a sclerotic margin, thus simulating a Schmorl's node on CT (Fig. 17.17) (5). A Schmorl's node should always be contiguous with the disc, whereas a metastatic deposit may be located more centrally within the vertebral body.

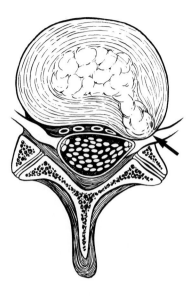

HERNIATED NUCLEUS

Figure 17.9. Artist's sketch of herniated nucleus pulposus. Note the focal protrusion of the disc margin (*arrow*) and nerve root compression secondary to herniated nuclear material.

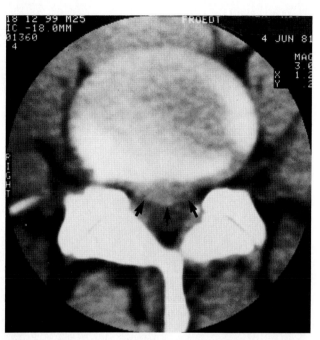

Figure 17.11. Central herniated disc: Focal protrusion of this L4–5 disc (*arrows*) deforms the dural sac.

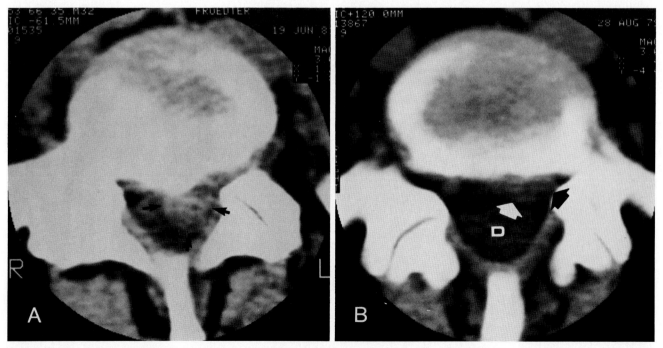

Figure 17.10. Posterolateral disc herniations. A. Marked focal protrusion of the disc (*arrows*) and compression of the dural sac are identified in another patient with an L5-S1 disc herniation. Note the absence of epidural fat on the left. B. There is focal protrusion of the L5-S1 disc (*arrowheads*) with displacement of anterior epidural fat and slight deformity of the dural sac (*D*). The left S1 root sheath is obscured.

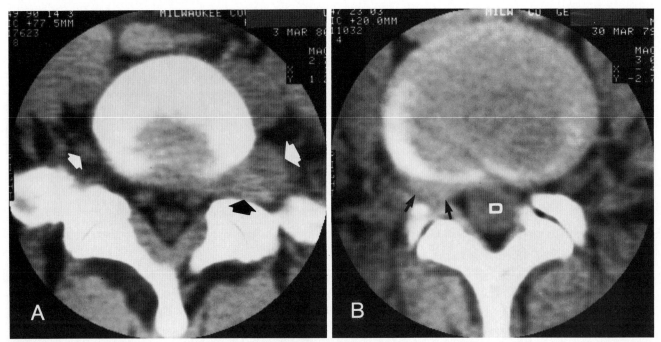

Figure 17.12. Lateral disc herniation: A. There is a large soft-tissue mass (*large arrowheads*) displacing fat within the left L5-S1 intervertebral foramen. The L5 nerve, seen on the contralateral side (*small arrowhead*), is obscured on the ipsilateral side. [Reproduced with permission from Haughton and Williams (5).] B. Focal protrusion (*arrows*) of the L4–5 disc is displacing fat within the right intervertebral foramen. Note that the dural sac (*D*) is not deformed.

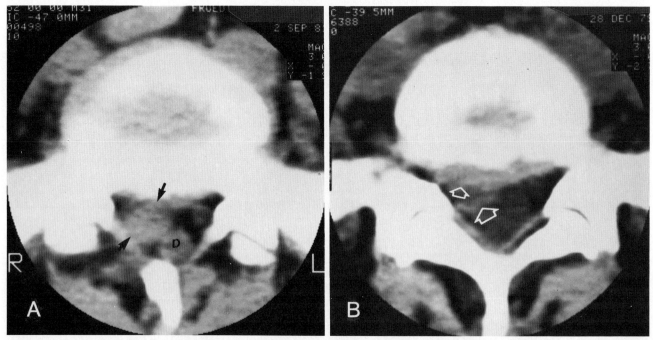

Figure 17.13. Herniated disc with free fragment: A. A soft-tissue mass (*arrows*) in the epidural space at the level of the L5-S1 disc obscures the S1 root sheath but does not deform the small dural sac (*D*). B. In addition to focal posterolateral protrusion of the L5-S1 disc (*small arrowhead*), a free disc fragment (*large arrowhead*) is identified within the epidural space in another patient. [Reproduced with permission from Haughton and Williams (5).]

Because the thoracic spine is a more rigid structure than the lumbar, degeneration of thoracic intervertebral discs progresses more slowly. Demonstration of thoracic disc herniations by CT depends in part upon the relative size of the subarachnoid and epidural spaces. A large subarachnoid space and correspondingly small epidural space should permit the demonstration of a herniated disc by CT without intrathecal contrast medium (Fig. 17.18).

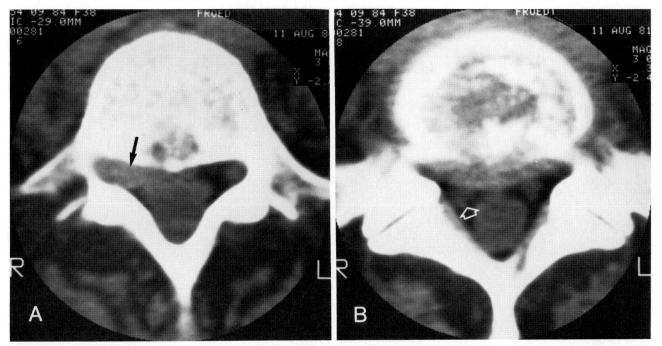

Figure 17.14.   Migration of free disc fragment: However, in a section (A) 10-mm craniad to the L5-S1 disc, a large disc fragment is identified in the right lateral recess (*arrowhead*). B. A CT image through the L5-S1 disc demonstrates only moderate symmetrical bulging of the posterior disc margin and minimal posterior displacement of the right S1 root sheath (*arrowhead*).

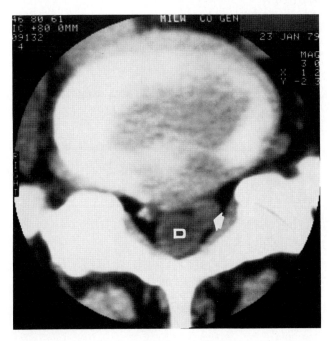

Figure 17.15.   Free disc fragment simulating dilated root sheath: In a patient with left S1 radiculopathy, an axial image through the L5-S1 disc demonstrates apparent enlargement of the left S1 root sheath (*arrowhead*) and focal midline protrusion of the disc. Note the absence of epidural fat between the root sheath and dural sac (*D*). At operation, a small disc fragment was identified between the dural sac and root sheath. [Reproduced with permission from Haughton and Williams (5).]

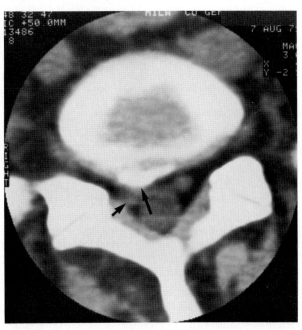

Figure 17.16.   Calcified lumbar disc herniation: Calcification is associated with this posterolateral herniated L5-S1 disc (*large arrow*). Note the posterior displacement of the right S1 root sheath (*small arrow*). [Reproduced with permission from Haughton and Williams (5).]

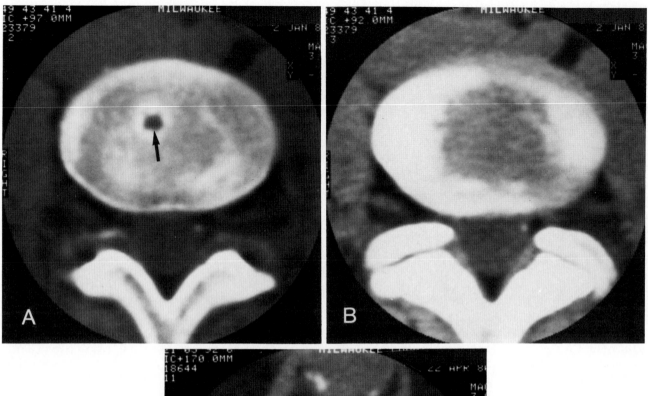

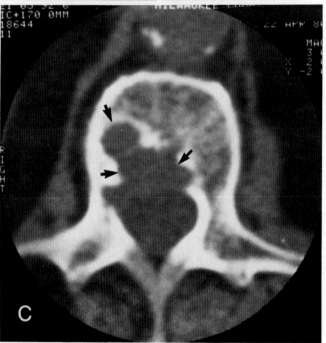

Figure 17.17. Schmorl's node: A. Protrusion of nuclear material thorugh the vertebral end plate has resulted in focal soft-tissue density (*arrow*), with a sclerotic margin, in the inferior portion of the L3 vertebral body. This osseous defect is just craniad to the L3–4 disc (B). C. Vertebral body metastasis (*arrows*) treated with radiation therapy or chemotherapy may develop sclerotic margins, thus, simulating a Schmorl's node in some cases. [Reproduced with permission from Haughton and Williams (5).]

Otherwise, a small amount of metrizamide (3–5 ml, 170 mg I/ml) will provide satisfactory opacification of the subarachnoid space, demonstration of the spinal cord and visualization of the herniated disc. Calcification commonly is associated with herniated discs in the thoracic region (5) and may appear as a dense epidural mass (Fig. 17.19).

PROCESSES SIMULATING HERNIATED NUCLEUS PULPOSUS ON CT

Because epidural fat is very important in differentiating soft tissues within the vertebral canal, any process which obliterates the fat makes accurate diagnosis more difficult. After laminectomy and discectomy, scar tissue replaces

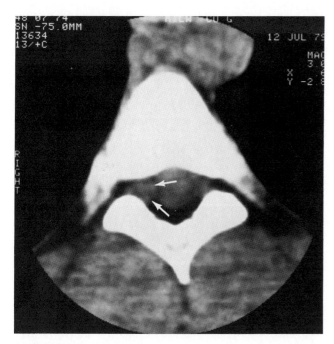

Figure 17.18. Thoracic disc herniation: A disc fragment (*arrows*) is identified in the right lateral epidural space. The lateral margin of the dural sac is deformed slightly. [Reproduced with permission from Haughton and Williams (5).]

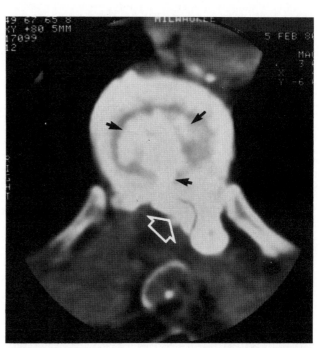

Figure 17.19. Calcified thoracic disc herniation: A calcified disc fragment (*large open arrowhead*) is identified within the anterior epidural space. Disc fragment calcification is contiguous with calcification within the disc (*small arrows*). The neural arch was removed at previous laminectomy. [Reproduced with permission from Haughton and Williams (5).]

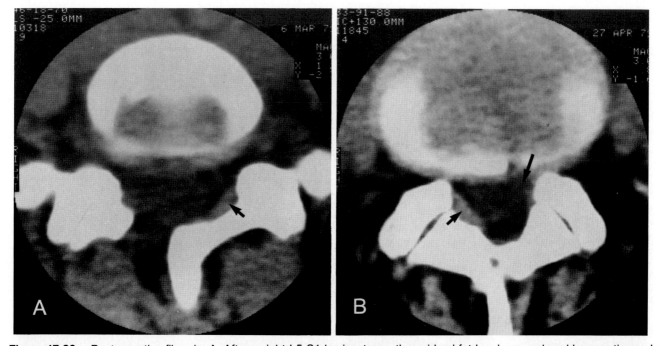

Figure 17.20. Postoperative fibrosis: A. After a right L5-S1 laminectomy, the epidural fat has been replaced by scar tissue. In addition, the ligamentum flavum, seen on the contralateral side (*arrow*), has been removed on the ispilateral side. B. In another patient with a previous left L4–5 laminectomy, scarring (*large arrow*) has obliterated the epidural fat. Note the absence of ligamentum flavum, seen on the contralateral side (*small arrow*), at the operative site.

epidural fat (Fig. 17.20) (1). Although the relative absorption coefficient of postsurgical fibrosis (35–70 HU) is usually slightly lower than disc (60–120 HU), there is suffi-

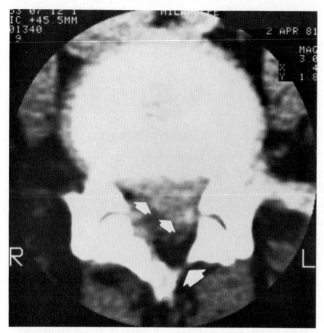

Figure 17.21.   Recurrent disc herniation at previously operated level: Herniated nuclear material (*small arrowheads*) contiguous with the L4–5 disc is compressing the dural sac. Note the laminectomy defect (*large arrowhead*). [Reproduced with permission from Haughton and Williams (5).]

cient overlap to invalidate tissue density as a definitive CT criterion. Thus, a residual or recurrent disc fragment may not be distinguishable from scar tissue by CT (Fig. 17.21). In our practice, the previously operated patient comprises 30–40% of lumbar spine CT scans. Patients in this group are particularly challenging to both the referring physician and the radiologist. Currently, the postoperative CT scan, like the myelogram, must be interpreted with caution.

Epidural fat may be replaced or displaced by neoplasms such as lymphoma (Fig. 17.22) or metastases, or by granulation tissue associated with infection (Fig. 17.23). Bony destruction or sclerosis are important CT findings when distinguishing tumor or infection from herniated disc. Spondylolisthesis may result in deformity of the posterior disc margin, simulating disc herniation (Fig. 17.24).

ACCURACY OF CT IN DISC HERNIATION

In the few clinical studies reported to date (15–20) CT has detected disc herniations as accurately or more accurately than myelography. The limitation of most comparative studies is the anatomical verification because surgical observations may not reliably distinguish all herniated and bulging discs. The sensitivity of CT (true positive rate) was 96% compared to 90–93% for myelography (16, 18) in 2 studies. False-negative diagnoses were caused by scanning the wrong level (16) or by diagnosing a bulging disc when the surgeon subsequently described a herniated one (18). Other potential causes of false-negative CT diagnoses include conus medullaris tumors or high lumbar disc herniations simulating an L4–5 or L5-S1 protrusion. The

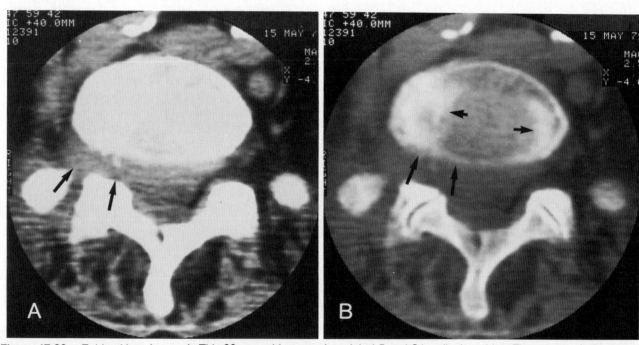

Figure 17.22.   Epidural lymphoma: A. This 60-year-old woman has right L5 and S1 radiculopathies. There is a soft-tissue mass within the right intervertebral foramen (*arrows*) obliterating the epidural fat. [Reproduced with permission from Haughton and Williams (5).] B. The same image viewed at a wide window for bone detail demonstrates poor definition of the posterior vertebral body cortex (*large arrows*) and focal sclerosis within the L5 vertebral body (*small arrows*).

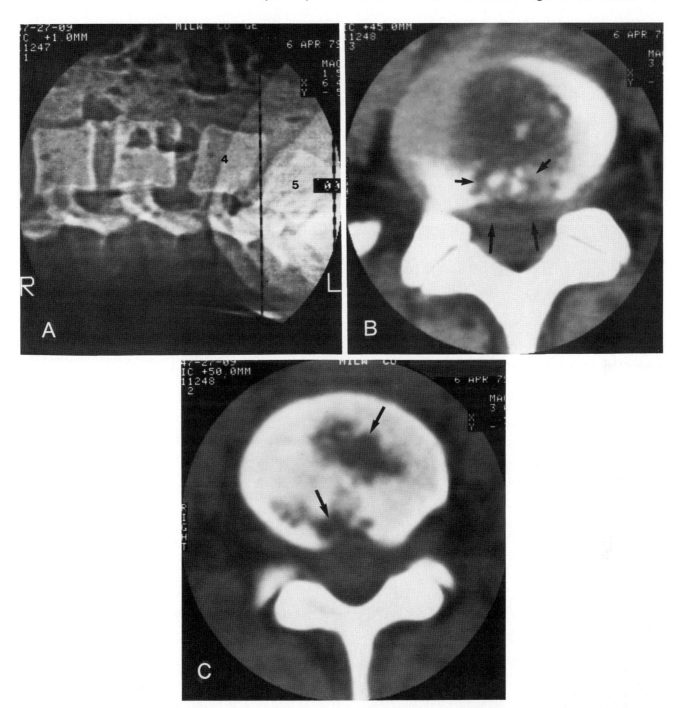

Figure 17.23. Granulation tissue simulating bulging disc: A. A lateral localizer image demonstrates poor definition of the vertebral endplates at L4–5 with minimal narrowing of the disc space in a patient with discitis. B. A section through the L4–5 disc demonstrates apparent bulging of the posterior disc margin (*large arrows*) with displacement of anterolateral epidural fat. However, focal lytic areas are identified within the vertebral endplate (*small arrows*). C. A contiguous image just craniad to the disc space demonstrates focal areas of bone destruction (*arrows*) within the L4 vertebral body. [Reproduced with permission from Haughton and Williams (5).]

CT detection of a herniation was more difficult when the epidural fat was replaced by scar or displaced by stenosis. False-negative myelograms were encountered in far lateral herniations and, in small caudal sacs, distant from the vertebrae (Fig. 17.25).

The specificity for CT also has exceeded that of myelography. When the interpretation was negative for herniated disc, or positive for another process, CT tended to be more reliable than myelography. Neoplasms, spondylolysis, discitis, and some other processes were detected more accu-

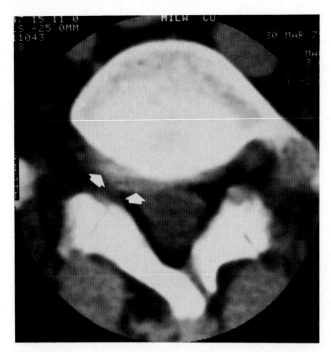

Figure 17.24. Disc herniation simulated by spondylolisthesis: Note the asymmetry of the posterior disc margin (*arrowheads*) secondary to grade I spondylolisthesis. [Reproduced with permission from Haughton and Williams (5).]

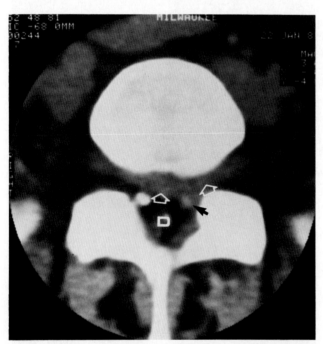

Figure 17.25. CT demonstration of herniated disc in a patient with a normal myelogram: This 28-year-old man had left sciatica. Iophendylate (Pantopaque) and metrizamide myelograms were negative for disc herniation. However, CT demonstrates focal protrusion of the disc (*open arrowheads*) with compression of the left S1 root sheath (*arrowheads*), consistent with herniated nucleus pulposus. Note the wide anterior epidural space and lack of dural sac (*D*) deformity despite the prominent disc protrusion.

rately by CT than myelography (18). The true-negative rate for CT was 92% in 1 study (16). False-positive diagnoses were due to scanning at the wrong level (16) or to interpreting osteophytes as calcified herniated discs (18). These interpretations, although technically false-positive diagnoses, accurately represented the pathological anatomy uncovered at surgery.

ROLE OF CT IN DISC DISEASE

Unlike CT of the head, spinal CT is not cost-effective as a screening modality. CT of the spine is most useful when specific clinical levels are designated for examination by the referring physician. When localization is possible clinically, as in patients with specific radiculopathy, CT is the most appropriate neuroradiological study. When localization is impossible or a large segment of the spine must be evaluated, myelography is the procedure of choice. Myelography also is preferred when levels some distance from one another, e.g., conus medullaris and L4–5 or L5-S1 disc, must be studied.

Because CT is more accurate than myelography in some processes, e.g., lateral disc herniation or wide epidural space (L5-S1), a negative myelogram does not obviate a CT scan. When a myelogram is positive, CT may provide further definition of the abnormality.

References

1. Williams AL, Haughton VM, Syvertsen A: CT diagnosis of herniated nucleus pulposus. *Radiology* 135:95–99, 1980.
2. Haughton VM, Syvertsen A, Williams AL: Soft tissue anatomy within the spinal canal as seen on CT. *Radiology* 134:649–656, 1980.
3. Carrera GF, Williams AL, Haughton VM: Computed tomography in sciatica. *Radiology* 137:433–437, 1980.
4. Glenn WV, Rhodes ML, Altschuler EM, et al: Multiplanar display computerized body tomography applications in the lumbar spine. *Spine* 4:202–352, 1979.
5. Haughton VM, Williams AL: *Computed Tomography of the Spine.* St. Louis, C.V. Mosby Company, 1982.
6. Shaffer KA, Haughton VM, Wilson CR: High resolution computed tomography of the temporal bone. *Radiology* 134:409–414, 1980.
7. Coventry MB, Ghormley RK, Kernohan JW: The intervertebral disc: Its microscopic anatomy and pathology. Part I. Anatomy, development and physiology. *J Bone Joint Surg* 27:105–112, 1945.
8. Parke WW, Schiff DCM: The applied anatomy of the intervertebral disc. *Orthop Clin North Am* 2:309–324, 1971.
9. Coventry MB, Ghormley RK, Kernohan JW: The intervertebral disc: Its microscopic anatomy and pathology. Part II. Changes in the intervertebral disc concomitant with age. *J Bone Joint Surg* 27:233–247, 1945.
10. Harris RI, MacNab I: Structural changes in the lumbar intervertebral discs. *J Bone Joint Surg* 36B:304–322, 1954.
11. Shapiro R: *Myelography* 3rd edition. Chicago, Year Book Medical Publishers Inc., 1975, pp. 357–360.
12. Williams AL, Haughton VM, Meyer GA, et al: CT appearance of bulging annulus. *Radiology* 142:403–408, 1982.
13. Coventry MG, Ghormley RK, Kernohan JW: The intervertebral disc: Its microscopic anatomy and pathology. Part III. Pathological changes in the intervertebral disc. *J Bone Joint Surg* 27:460–474, 1945.
14. Williams AL, Haughton VM, Daniels DL, et al: CT diagnosis of lateral lumbar disc herniation. *AJNR* 3:211–213, 1982.

15. Breun JF, Lin JP, George AE, et al: Pitfalls in the diagnosis of the lumbar spine in disk disease. Presentation at the 67th Scientific Assembly and Annual Meeting of the Radiological Society of North America. Chicago, November, 1981.
16. Gado MH, Chandra-Schur B, Patel J, et al: An integrated approach to the diagnosis of lumbar disc disease by computed tomography and myelography. Presentation at the 67th Scientific Assembly and Annual Meeting of the Radiological Society of North America. Chicago, November, 1981.
17. Glenn WV, Brown BM, Murphy RM, et al: Computed tomography and myelography in the evaluation of lumbar disc disease. Presentation at the 67th Scientific Assembly and Annual Meeting of the Radiological Society of North America.

Chicago, November, 1981.
18. Haughton VM, Eldevik OP, Magnaes B, et al: A prospective comparison of computed tomography and myelography in the diagnosis of herniated lumbar discs. *Radiology* 142:103–110, 1982.
19. Teplick JP, Peyster RG, Teplick SK, et al: Computed tomography and lumbar disc herniation. A prospective study. Presentation at the 67th Scientific Assembly and Annual Meeting of the Radiological Society of North America. Chicago, November, 1981.
20. Raskin SP, Keating JW: The relative accuracy of CT and myelography for lumbar disc disease. A collaborative study (100 cases). *AJNR* 3:215–221, 1982.

CHAPTER EIGHTEEN

Computed Tomography of the Spine: Correlation with Myelography

STEPHEN P. RASKIN, MD. and S. HENRY LaROCCA, M.D.

The patient with back pain often presents with ambiguous or contradictory subjective findings. To obtain objective information about the patient's disorder, the physician commonly will employ radiological methods. Most physicians consider myelography to be the most objective and informative test in evaluating the patient with back pain. Although myelography is not a perfect test, its strengths and limitations are well known, and most practitioners know when to rely on a myelographic diagnosis and when not to. This very extensive, albeit subjective, medical experience with myelography makes it the mainstay of diagnosis at this time.

If any new diagnostic procedure is to compete with myelography, it must undergo three levels of testing. It first must be proved as a technically practical procedure. Then it must be validated clinically by undergoing trials under controlled circumstances. After this "scientific" testing, the new procedure must stand the test of general usage, proving itself to each practitioner on a case-by-case basis.

CT of the spine is still a new modality, and its strengths and weaknesses have yet to be described fully. Early reports about CT have documented its ability to show spinal anatomy and pathology in isolated cases (1–8). Recent reports have compared larger series of CT examinations with myelography and surgery, although reports with clinical follow-up are still lacking (9, 10). Over the course of the next several years, we can expect reports which will deal with the failures of CT and the subtleties of its interpretation. Mature clinical judgment in the use and interpretation of CT will depend on this last phase of acceptance, as the rules of diagnosis and treatment become established and as we learn to recognize the exceptions to the rules.

IMAGING THE SPINAL SYSTEM

Myelography and CT produce radically different images of the spine. CT is a cross-sectional method which shows the dural and epidural spaces, the segmental nerves, the intervertebral discs, and the bony canal. Myelography, on the other hand, provides standard radiographic views of the subarachnoid space and its contents only.

The spinal system consists of a bony, cartilaginous, and fibrous skeleton which supports and protects nervous tissue. Sustaining these organs are vascular, neural, and synovial components. It is not unexpected that disorders of the lumbar spine may result from injury, degeneration, or derangement of many elements, and it is simplistic and

misleading to restrict our understanding of the lumbar spine to an abnormality of only one element, such as herniation of a nucleus pulposus.

Because myelography can depict only the subarachnoid space, there is a tendency to emphasize disease which causes an impression on this space. By and large, this approach is useful. Where the subarachnoid space does not encompass all the neural elements, however, myelography is recognized as being of limited value, and other studies such as epidural venography or epidurography have been necessary in the past.

CT has the advantage of portraying all the tissues and organs which compose the spinal system. Furthermore, it does this in a manner which maintains the exact anatomical relationships among these tissues. CT can show the neural components better than myelography can, because it depicts the segmental nerves all the way from the cauda equina to the paraspinous muscles. CT also can show the epidural space and the structural elements (bony, cartilaginous, synovial, fibrous, and muscular) which may be involved with disease processes.

Not only can pathology be identified in a wide range of tissues by CT, but when two or more pathological processes are active, the relative contribution of each to the patient's disease can be estimated, based on the CT findings. This aspect of CT is critical to the understanding of disorders of the lumbar spine, because disease of one component, e.g., anular bulging, commonly interact with disease of other elements, e.g., subluxation of the facet joints, to produce clinical findings. The interplay between disparate but mechanically coupled elements is so critical to an understanding of the spine, that emphasis on only one element cannot explain anything other than the most simple cases.

Myelography has had a profound effect on our conception of disorders of the spine. As we approach CT, therefore, it is useful as a learning device to compare it with myelography. This approach will have practical as well as didactic merit, because we can hope to derive preliminary guidelines for the choice of one or the other in clinical practice. This paper, therefore, compares these two modalities in case-by-case manner.

RECENT LITERATURE

Two recent studies have compared CT to myelography in large numbers of patients. The study by Haughton et al. (9) was a prospective, controlled study involving 107 patients who underwent myelography and CT. In this study, there was surgical follow-up in 52 patients. A comparable study has been published by one of us in which 108 examination pairs (CT-myelography) were analyzed in a retrospective, single-blind manner (10). There were 42 cases with surgical follow-up in this group.

In general, the results of these two studies were similar. Both groups found that CT was as effective as myelography in the diagnosis of lumbar disc disease. When discrepancies occurred, they usually were due to difficulties in distinguishing between herniated disc fragments and bulging of the anulus fibrosis. This same discrepancy was encountered in correlating both types of examination with the findings at surgery. It is likely that the significance of the bulging anulus will remain the center of controversy for some time.

Both groups of authors found the highest level of correlation in patients without prior surgery. We showed CT to be superior to myelography at the lumbosacral level, where the anterior epidural space is the widest. In patients without previous surgery in whom optimal technique was used (adequate photon flux, thin sections, and no contrast in the spinal canal) there were no false-negative CT examinations in one series and only one false-negative CT in the other. There were no false-positive CT examinations in either series, although we have encountered 2 cases in clinical practice.

ILLUSTRATIVE CASE 1: SIMPLE DISC HERNIATION

Figure 18.1 shows the classical CT and myelographic findings in a herniated nucleus pulposus. The CT section shows a capacious spinal canal with abundant epidural fat. The normal left S1 nerve root is seen surrounded by fat, which also extends posterior to the dural sac at the laminar junction point. The right anterolateral epidural fat is replaced, however, by a hyperdense (relative to the dural contents) soft-tissue structure. The posterior margin of the lumbosacral disc is asymmetrically protruding, and there is mass effect on the right S1 nerve. Our three criteria for a herniated disc fragment (disc protrusion, abnormal intraspinal fragment, and mass effect) are satisfied, and this diagnosis can be made with confidence.

The myelographic examination helps us to understand the CT findings better. The degree of mass effect being exerted on the dural sac is greater than one would estimate on casual inspection of the CT. The myelogram shows that the dural sac is compressed to the midline, and, on review of the CT, it is apparent that a thin low-attenuation interface can be recognized at the midline. This line would not have been noticed without knowledge of the myelogram; it probably represents the compressed right epidural fat remnant. It is possible that had greater radiographic technique (higher MAS) been used, this thin fat line would have been more apparent.

This very typical case shows that the same disease can look very different when studied by two radically different modalities. Even experienced observers are surprised sometimes at the differences between CT and myelography. The information content remains the same, however:

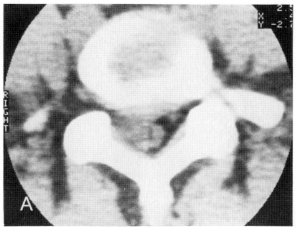
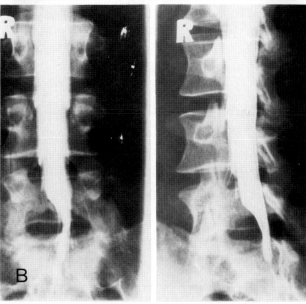

Figure 18.1. A. Axial CT section at L5-S1: There is an abnormal soft-tissue density inside the canal which is obliterating the right epidural fat. B. Metrizamide myelography: Frontal and oblique projections show an extradural defect. [Reproduced with permission from Raskin (8).]

this is an abnormal disc which almost certainly needs to be removed.

This case also highlights the dependence of the size of a myelographic defect on both the size of the disc fragment and on the size of the spinal canal. The fragment in Figure 18.1 would obliterate a smaller canal completely. CT demonstrates the geometry and size of the canal better than myelography. This information may aid the surgeon in planning the laminectomy and exploration preoperatively.

ILLUSTRATIVE CASE 2: DISC HERNIATION WITH MIGRATION

Figure 18.2 shows another case with the three major criteria of disc herniation (abnormal annular contour,

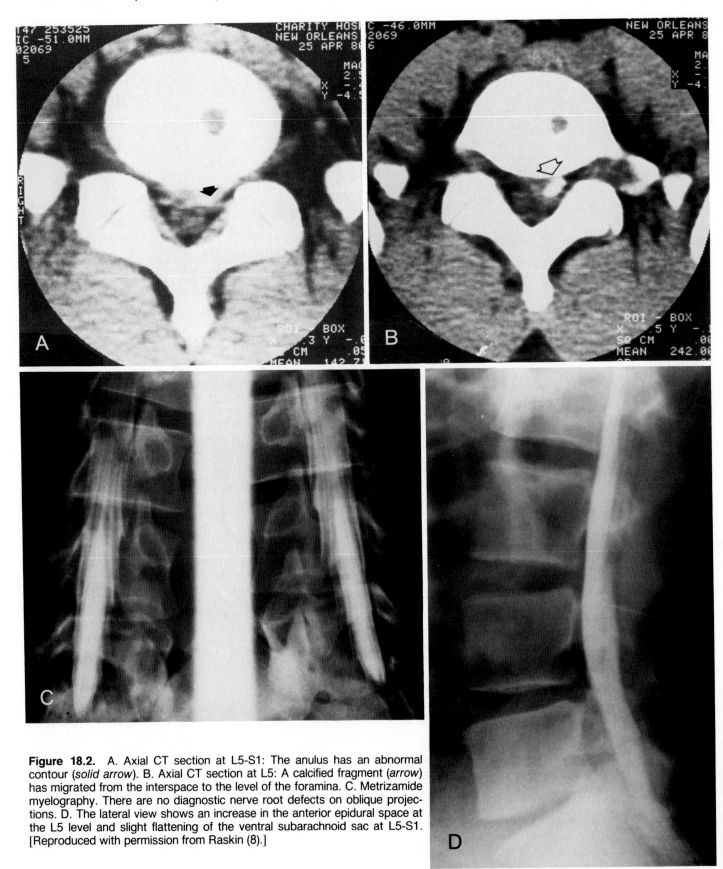

Figure 18.2. A. Axial CT section at L5-S1: The anulus has an abnormal contour (*solid arrow*). B. Axial CT section at L5: A calcified fragment (*arrow*) has migrated from the interspace to the level of the foramina. C. Metrizamide myelography. There are no diagnostic nerve root defects on oblique projections. D. The lateral view shows an increase in the anterior epidural space at the L5 level and slight flattening of the ventral subarachnoid sac at L5-S1. [Reproduced with permission from Raskin (8).]

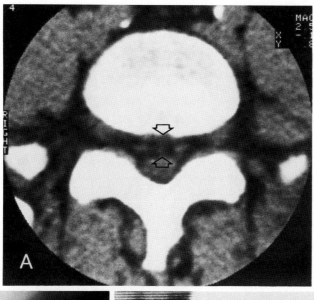

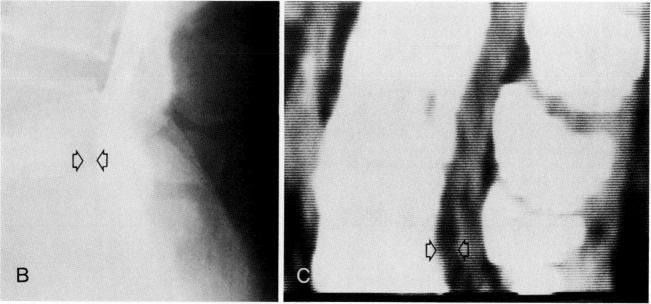

Figure 18.3.   A. Axial CT section at L5: The wide anterior epidural space (*arrows*) contains only fat and epidural vessels. B. Metrizamide myelography: A standing lateral view shows a wide space at this level (*arrows*). C. Reformatted sagittal CT image: There is a close correspondence between this view and the lateral myelogram. CT shows the contents of the epidural space, however. [Reproduced by permission from Raskin and Keating (10).]

abnormal intraspinal fragment, and mass effect). In this case, the abnormal intraspinal fragment is calcified. Furthermore, this small fragment has migrated up from the lumbosacral interspace, almost to the level of the L5 pedicle. Myelographic examination of the nerve roots shows no diagnostic defect. The myelographic examination does show a very wide and flat anterior epidural space at the L5 level and narrowing of the lumbosacral interspace.

It takes some sophistication and experience in order to interpret the wide anterior epidural space. Most experi-

enced myelographers would agree that this study is abnormal, although no one could predict from it the size or location of the fragment. CT, however, precisely locates the disc fragment. Even when the myelographic examination is as suspicious as in this case, CT still is more diagnostic because it shows the exact size, shape, and location of the lesion.

In our experience and that of others, migrating fragments are common (11). A migrated fragment which was not included in standard angled-gantry scanning of the lumbosacral disc space accounted for a false-negative CT examination in our series. It is for this reason that we routinely perform CT of the entire lower spine and do not focus on the disc spaces only.

ILLUSTRATIVE CASE 3: THE WIDE ANTERIOR EPIDURAL SPACE

Figure 18.3 shows another patient with a very large anterior epidural space at myelography. The myelographic diagnosis must be indeterminate at this level. CT shows the space to be normal. In our series, CT was superior to myelography at the lumbosacral level for this reason. Haughton et al. (9) did not publish their data in regard to the accuracy of CT at L5-S1 specifically, but in two of their cases (patients 29 and 44) CT was more diagnostic than myelography at this level.

Because CT is a tomographic study, it is possible to lose orientation if one relies on only one section. For this reason, it is imperative to identify the location of an abnormality by use of a planar image (preferably frontal and lateral) or of a reformatted sagittal image. In this case, despite the poor quality of the myelographic lateral, there is a remarkable correspondence between the myelographic lateral and the sagittal CT format. We consider the ability to perform multiplanar formatting to be an advantage of the "normal array" method of scanning (8).

Figure 18.4 shows another patient whose spinal canal is filled largely with epidural fat. The myelographic examination shows attenuation of the dural sac, which could be due to fibrosis, hemorrhage, tumor infiltration, or spinal stenosis. The CT is definitive, however, in excluding disease at this and other levels.

ILLUSTRATIVE CASE 4: THE ISODENSE FRAGMENT

The CT section in Figure 18.5 was photographed at narrow window settings to emphasize the soft-tissue contents of the spinal canal. The small spinal canal is occupied almost completely by a small, right-centered, high-attenuation structure. This is an "isodense" fragment which almost completely has filled the canal. In this case, the myelographic examination is unmistakably abnormal. We have found that these very large (relative to the spinal canal) fragments are the most difficult to appreciate on CT, unless the examiner personally examines the cases on the video console and manipulates the window and level controls.

The isodense disc in a small canal is another setting where normal array scanning and image reformatting can be of value. The patient whose CT is shown in Figure 18.6 underwent CT because of "dry taps" at two attempted myelographic examinations. Routine 5-mm sections were obtained and reformatted as shown in this figure. They show a small spinal canal and a large high-attenuation structure posterior to the L4-L5 space. In this setting, the spaces above and below this level act as the "normal controls" and allow one to diagnose a markedly bulging or herniated disc.

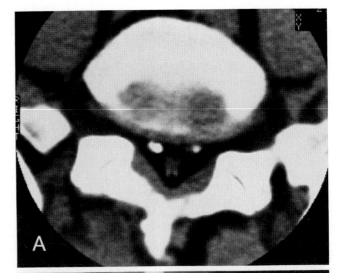

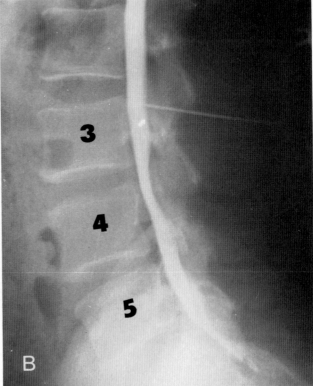

Figure 18.4. A. Axial CT section at L5-S1: The dural sac is thin but not compressed. B. Metrizamide myelography. The dural sac appears compressed at the L5-S1 level.

ILLUSTRATIVE CASE 5: THE BULGING DISC

The centrally bulging anulus (Fig. 18.7) is likely to become the most controversial subject in CT (12). Because CT is so sensitive to the contour of the anulus, it can detect slight bulges. Many clinicians consider anular bulging to be a normal phenomenon. The significance of an anular bulge may be assessed on reformatted images as shown in Figure 18.8.

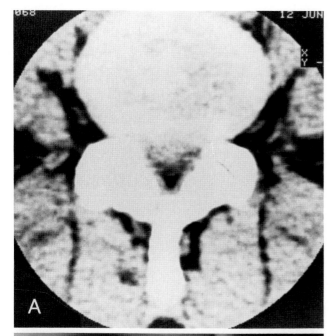

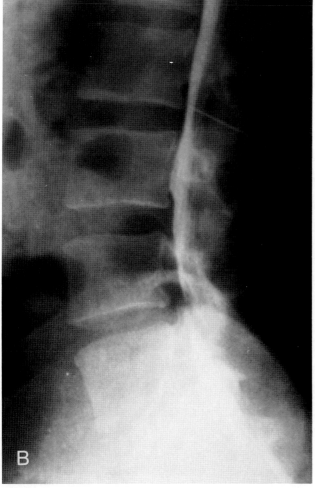

ILLUSTRATIVE CASE 6: FORAMINAL ENCROACHMENT

Myelography is unable to show disease except as it impinges on the subarachnoid space. CT maintains an advantage over myelography in locations such as the anterior epidural space and in the neural foramina. An example of this is shown in Figure 18.9. The patient shown here had had previous surgery which had failed to alleviate a right L5 radiculopathy. Multiple myelographic examinations had been interpreted as essentially unremarkable. The CT scan was performed in this difficult setting and provided a precise diagnosis.

CT shows a large lateral osteophyte occluding the outlet of the right L5 foramen. Reformatted views are very helpful in understanding the genesis of this osteophyte, which has arisen from the end plate of the S1 vertebral body and has probably developed as a response to bulging of the disc in this region. Figure 18.9 also provides comparison oblique reformatted displays of the normal left side. Although these can be displayed to correspond to the myelographic obliques, they contain much more information.

Oblique and off-center reformatted images have value in assessing other conditions. Figure 18.10 shows a patient with an L4 spondylolysis and spondylolisthesis. Two processes combine to markedly constrict the L4 nerve foramen. First is the forward and downward subluxation of L4 which reduces the cross-sectional area of the foramen. More important, perhaps, is the second component, stress on the L4-L5 anulus, which has produced anular bulging and calcification, much greater on the right than on the left. This reactive calcification further impinges on the already constricted foramen.

As indicated in the introduction to this chapter, an emphasis on the discs alone will result in an oversimplification of the disease processes active in the lumbar spine. Degeneration in the discs inevitably will lead to mechanical and reactive abnormalities elsewhere, especially in patients with small canals and no "spinal reserve." The spine must be considered as an intricate system of bone, cartilage, and nerve. Normal array scanning and extensive use of reformatting will prove invaluable in understanding a complex clinical problem such as this.

ILLUSTRATIVE CASE 7: NONDISCOGENIC DEFECTS

Extradural defects may often be seen at myelography which are not related to the discs. Figure 18.11 shows symmetrical defects at the disc space level, which usually are considered to be due to a large central protrusion of the disc with posterior displacement of contrast into the narrow posterior segment of the canal. The CT study, which was obtained prone after myelography, shows that the lateral defects are due to symmetrical encroachment

Figure 18.5. A. Axial CT section at L4-L5: The majority of the spinal canal is filled with high-attenuation material. B. Metrizamide myelography: There is a constriction of the contrast column at this level. [Reproduced by permission from Raskin (8).]

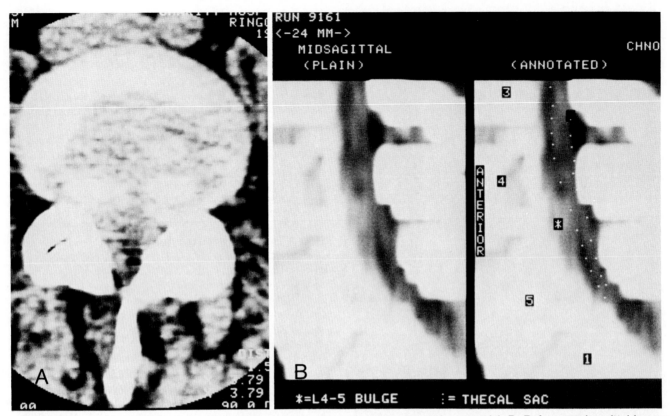

Figure 18.6. A. Axial CT section at L4-L5: The canal is filled with high-attenuation material. B. Reformatted sagittal image: The isodense fragment can be appreciated when the affected interspace is compared with other levels. A small spinal canal is apparent.

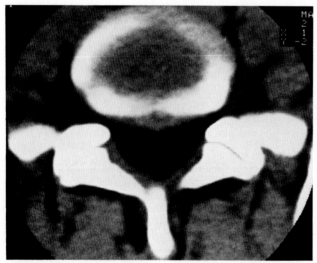

Figure 18.7. Axial CT image at L5-S1: The lumbosacral disc bulges symmetrically but does not compress the nerves or dural sac.

on the dural sac by osteophytes of the superior articular processes.

COMPARISON WITH OTHER MODALITIES

We have found CT to be superior to plain film tomog-

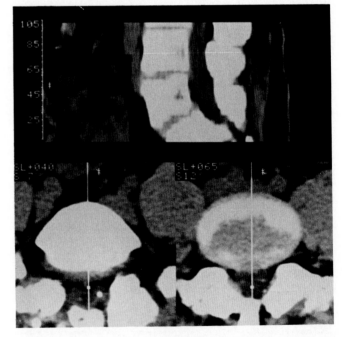

Figure 18.8. CT images with L5-S1 (S-7) and L4-L5 (S-12) referenced and sagittal reformatting shown above. The bulging lumbosacral anulus is outlined by epidural fat. There is no compression of the dural sac.

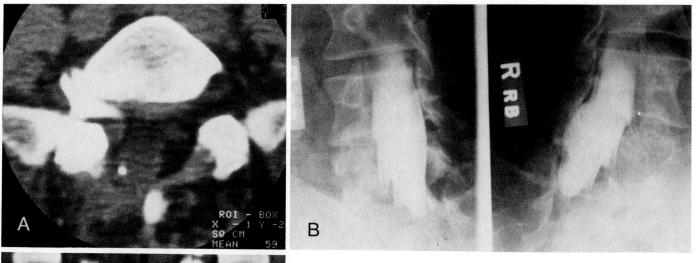

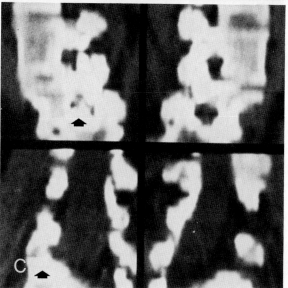

Figure 18.9. A. Axial CT section at L5: There is a large osteophyte in the right L5 foramen (subsequently proven at surgery). B. Pantopaque myelography: Only the proximal nerve segments are shown, and the distal foraminal disease is not revealed. (Incidentally noted is a postoperative pseudomeningocoele). C. Oblique reformatted CT images: Images obtained across and along the nerve roots at L5 show the foraminal occlusion (*arrows*).

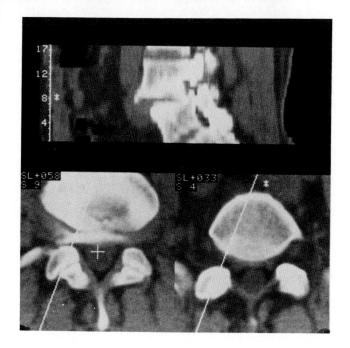

raphy in the evaluation of spinal fusions. The CT method is ideal because the digital information can be manipulated to demonstrate even the densest bone. Image reformatting is essential in relating a fusion to other elements of the spine. Another advantage of CT in this situation is the reduction in patient radiation because of the narrow collimation and the need to do only one series of tomographic sections.

Epidural venography is an indirect means of demonstrating the epidural space. It is a low-risk, invasive procedure, and it may be difficult to interpret due to marked variations in normal anatomy. It would be useful to correlate a large series of epidural venograms and relate the venous filling patterns to the capacity of the epidural spaces seen at CT (Fig. 18.12).

Figure 18.10. Axial and oblique reformatted view across the right L4 foramen. A spondylolysis has led to chronic stress on the L4-L5 annulus and subsequent calcification. Both the spondylolisthesis and the hypertrophic change in the anulus compromise the L4 foramina.

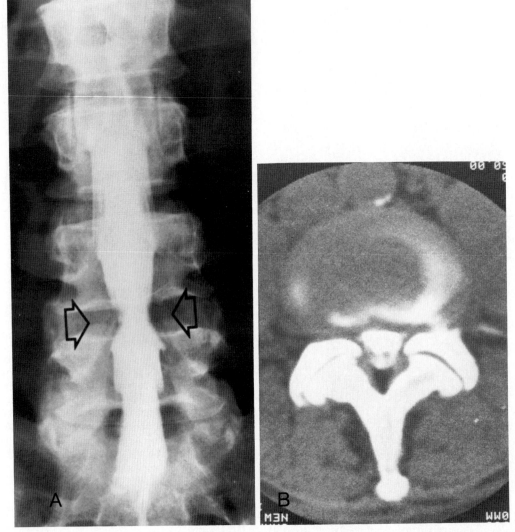

Figure 18.11.   A. Metrizamide myelography: Frontal view shows bilateral lateral constriction of the contrast column (*arrows*). This may be due to a large centrally bulging disc. B. Axial, prone CT section at L4-L5: The lateral constriction of the sac is due to osteophytes which originate on the L5 superior articular processes. [Reproduced by permission from Raskin (13).]

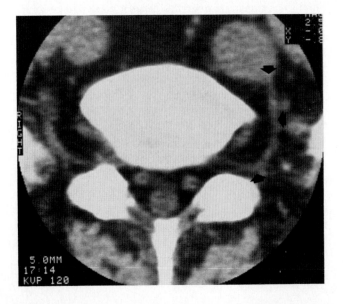

CT is incapable of demonstrating internal disc degeneration unless there is gas or calcification inside the disc space. Furthermore, CT is incapable of showing a tear in the anulus. The only method of directly assessing the disc for degeneration or an anular tear is discography. Discography is an invasive procedure which requires meticulous technique and careful interpretation. Nevertheless, we believe that in selected cases it can supplement CT.

Such a case is shown in Figure 18.13. This patient had a normal myelographic examination and a normal standard CT. Although the CT showed suspicious anular bulging and calcification at L5-S1 a volume-averaging artifact could not be excluded. The patient underwent lumbar discography because of strong clinical suspicion. The dis-

Figure 18.12.   Axial CT section at L5-S1: The course of the left ascending lumbar vein from the left common iliac vein to the epidural plexus is shown incidentally (*arrows*).

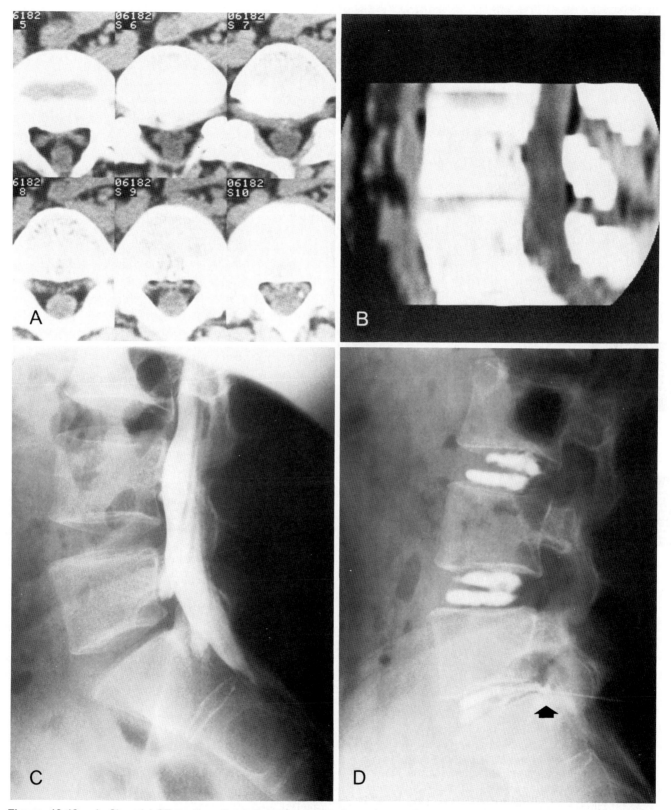

Figure 18.13. A. Six axial CT sections through the L5-S1 level are shown. The anulus bulges and may be partially calcified. B. Sagittal reformatted CT image: The bulging lumbosacral annulus may be due to volume averaging among the 5-mm sections. C. Metrizamide myelography: A lateral view shows a normal lumbosacral space. D. Lumbar discography. There is leakage of contrast posteriorly at L5-S1 (*arrow*). The other levels are normal.

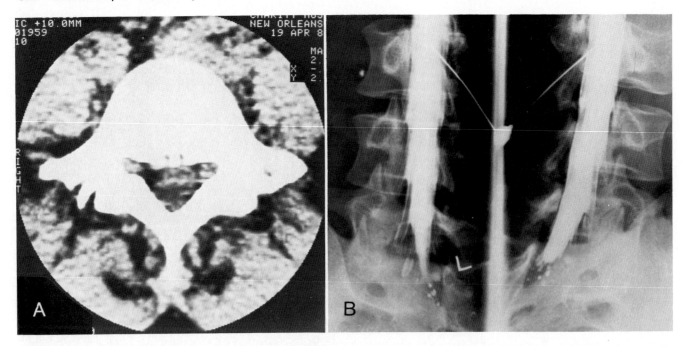

Figure 18.14. A. Axial CT image at L5: There is a hyperdense structure adjacent to the dural sac in the left epidural space. B. Metrizamide myelography: Oblique views show no nerve root defect. Subsequent surgery demonstrated no disc herniation, only dilated epidural veins.

cogram showed posterolateral leakage of contrast and was considered positive. At surgery, there was a large tear in the anulus which contained nuclear material. There was no disc herniation.

FALSELY POSITIVE CT

Figure 18.14 shows CT and myelographic findings in a patient who underwent surgery for a left S-1 radiculopathy. The CT was interpreted as suspicious for a herniated disc fragment because of asymmetry of the epidural spaces. At surgery, dilated epidural veins were found at this site; the disc was normal. On review of the CT, it was noted that the disc anulus was never shown to be abnormal and that there was no mass effect on the nerves or dural sac. Because of this case, we have learned to apply rigid criteria for the diagnosis of a herniated disc.

RISK/BENEFIT CONSIDERATIONS

CT and myelography are of comparable accuracy in the diagnosis of disorders of the lumbar spine. They are not of comparable ease and efficacy, however. Myelography is an invasive procedure, which requires introduction of contrast material into the subarachnoid space. Even with the use of water-soluble agents and small-gauge needles, it has a significant morbidity. It is common practice to perform myelography only on an inpatient basis. The usual admission for myelography only is of 2 days' length, even in the absence of headache or other postmyelographic complaints. Myelography, therefore, is an expensive and potentially dangerous procedure.

CT, on the other hand, is noninvasive and may be performed on an outpatient basis. The expense of a CT examination is more than offset by savings in unnecessary hospitalization and morbidity. CT, however, may result in more radiation exposure than myelography if a myelogram is restricted to only a few films. CT also requires patient cooperation. In addition, CT is limited in its ability to study the cervical spine at this time. For these reasons, it is unlikely that CT will supplant myelography completely. We have suggested, however, that CT become the initial radiological procedure after plain films in the evaluation of disorders of the lumbar spine (10).

CONCLUSIONS

1. CT is as accurate as myelography in the diagnosis of disorders of the lumbar spine.
2. CT is better tolerated than myelography. It is also less expensive than a myelogram if one takes into account the cost of hospitalization required for myelography.
3. CT may be unable to detect internally degenerated discs and anular tears which do not result in herniation of disc material.
4. False-positive CT diagnoses may result unless strict criteria for disc disease are applied.
5. More clinical experience will be necessary before the role of CT in the diagnosis of disc disease is known completely.

References

1. Di Chiro G, Axelbaum SP, Schellinger D, et al: Computerized axial tomography in syringomyelia. *N Engl J Med* 292:13–16, 1975.

2. Lee BCP, Kazam E, Newman AD: Computed tomography of the spine and spinal cord. *Radiology* 128:95–102, 1978.
3. Glenn WV, Rhodes ML, Altschuler EM, et al: Multiplanar display computerized body tomographic applications in the lumbar spine. *Spine* 4:282–352, 1979.
4. Meyer GA, Haughton VM, Williams AL: Diagnosis of herniated lumbar disc with computed tomography. *N Engl J Med* 301:1166–1167, 1979.
5. Naidich TP, King DG, Moran CJ, et al: Computed tomography of the lumbar thecal sac. *J Comput Assist Tomogr* 4:37–41, 1980.
6. Williams AL, Haughton VM, Syvertsen A: Computed tomography in the diagnosis of herniated nucleus pulposus. *Radiology* 135:95–99, 1980.
7. Federle MP, Moss AA, Margolin FR: Role of computed tomography in patients with "sciatica." *J Comput Assist Tomogr.* 4:335–341, 1980.

8. Raskin SP: Computed tomographic findings in lumbar disc disease. *Orthopedics* 5:419–431, 1981.
9. Haughton VM, Eldevik OP, Magnaes B, et al: A prospective comparison of computed tomography and myelography in the diagnosis of herniated lumbar disks. *Radiology* 142:103–110, 1982.
10. Raskin SP, Keating JW: Recognition of lumbar disk disease: a comparison of myelography and computed tomography. *AJNR* 3:215–221, 1982.
11. Thoen DD: The fallacy of gantry angling in CT evaluation of lumbar disc disease. International symposium and course on computed tomography, New Orleans, LA, April 14, 1981.
12. Williams AL, Haughton VM, Meyer GA, et al: Computed tomographic appearance of the bulging annulus. *Radiology* 142:403–408, 1982.
13. Raskin SP: Degenerative changes of the lumbar spine: Assessment by computed tomography. *Orthopedics* 4:186–195, 1981.

CHAPTER NINETEEN

Lumbar Disc Disease: Clinical and Computed Tomographic Evaluation

HAMILTON E. HOLMES, M.D. and RICHARD H. ROTHMAN, M.D. Ph.D.

INTRODUCTION

CT has become a valuable tool to the clinician who treats patients with lumbar degenerative disease and its clinical sequellae. In most centers where high-resolution CT (HRCT) is available, it has become or rapidly is becoming an integral radiographic study in the evaluation of sciatica in the virgin back. As new techniques for differentiating tissue density become available, HRCT also is becoming quite useful in the evaluation of the "failed back" (1, 2).

As radiologists and clinicians become more familiar with the diagnostic advantages of HRCT, this probably will become the next radiographic study ordered in the evaluation of lumbar disc disease after the plain lumbar films (2). More scientific data are needed, however, before definitively reaching this conclusion. Herkowitz et al. (3), in a prospective study, demonstrated that water-soluble myelography had 100% specificity and 97% sensitivity for surgically proven herniated lumbar discs and lumbar stenosis. In a prospective study involving 30 patients, comparing metrizamide myelography and epidural venography for evaluation of sciatica, the above figures for sensitivity and specificity were obtained for metrizamide myelography (3). If HRCT is to become the procedure of choice, these figures are the standard which must be approached. Haughton and associates (4) in a prospective study involving 107 patients, 52 of whom had operatively demonstrated pathology, found that HRCT and metrizamide myelography compared favorably. In the 52 patients with confirmed diagnoses surgically, 46 HRCT and 44 myelographic diagnoses agreed with the operative diagnosis. The patient selection included previously operated backs, possibly accounting for the high false-negative rate (4). More comparative data obviously are needed.

Perhaps the greatest value of HRCT in the future will be in providing a more precise initial preoperative anatomical diagnosis. The astute radiologist and clinician often can suspect lateral recess stenosis on the plain films and the metrizamide myelogram. If missed initially, the experienced spinal surgeon usually will detect this at surgery. However, HRCT usually will demonstrate lateral recess compromise quite well and would allow the surgeon to more precisely plan the operative procedure in advance (1, 2). The failure to recognize and treat lateral recess stenosis is probably a leading cause of failure in lumbar disc surgery in the properly selected patient (1). The resulting failed back syndrome patient remains one of our biggest medical and socioeconomic problems today.

HRCT may prove to be valuable in the evaluation of the failed back before further surgery. This patient has been perhaps the greatest diagnostic challenge in the past for both the radiologist and the spinal surgeon. With newer techniques for enhancement and with the continual development of new software, it is becoming easier to differentiate between scar tissue and recurrent disc herniation. Myelography has not been helpful in this regard in the past. If HRCT can provide this type of preoperative information accurately and consistently, improved patient selection will be possible. This should decrease the amount of unsuccessful back surgery performed, hopefully decreasing the enormous amount of pain, suffering, and financial burden presently seen with failed back surgery.

Lest we become overly enthusiastic with HRCT and its possibilities we must remember that in many places this test and its expert interpretation are not available. We, therefore, will discuss the more traditional methods of evaluating lumbar disc disease before discussing our use of HRCT in evaluation of our patients. We also will discuss the natural history of lumbar disc disease and its varied clinical presentations in order to correlate this disease with the CT findings. A thorough understanding of the natural history should be beneficial to both the radiologist and the clinician.

THE PATHOPHYSIOLOGY OF LUMBAR DISC DISEASE

An understanding of the progressive pathophysiology of lumbar degenerative disc disease allows the radiologist and the clinician to correlate clinical findings with radiographic findings better. A lack of clear understanding of the disturbed anatomy may give a confusing picture, often leading to misdiagnosis and improper treatment.

There are certain progressive biochemical changes which are associated with aging in the intervertebral disc of man. The etiological factors producing these events are not clear. Intensive research now is being conducted in this area. It is known that aging causes changes in the composition of the gelatinous nucleus pulposus with the end result being the loss of water. This causes the nucleus to act less like a gel, distributing forces on the disc unequally. The nucleus becomes less elastic and more fibrous and the disc is more subject to trauma from abnormal stresses. This process is progressive with increasing age. This process reaches its peak in the 4th and 5th decades at a time when the individual is still in a very active stage of life. This accounts for the high incidence of disc herniations seen in these age groups. A better understanding of the etiology and physiology of these changes in the nucleus hopefully will lead to a better understanding of the pathological process, and hopefully, eventually, to methods of blocking or at least slowing the degenerative process. A detailed description of this research is beyond the scope of this discussion.

Armstrong (5) and DePalma and Rothman (6) have recorded the pathological process clearly. Initially, the nucleus loses water and becomes more fibrous. The annulus becomes concurrently less elastic and begins to crack with stress. At this stage, the disc is extremely vulnerable and trauma may cause the nucleus to break through the anulus and the posterior longitudinal ligament. During the early stages of this process, which may take months or years, the individual experiences either no back pain or tolerable back pain. A rapid progression of these events may produce more severe back pain. Final protrusion of the disc usually leads to relief of back pain and produces leg pain. Most nuclear protrusions can be grouped into three categories: lateral protrusions, intraforaminal protrusions, and dorsal protrusions. Lateral protrusions are most common because the strong fibers of the posterior longitudinal ligament are not present laterally. Intraforaminal protrusions occur when nuclear material enters the spinal canal and migrates to the foramen. A midline protrusion may or may not break through the posterior longitudinal ligament. These produce the fairly classical picture of back pain, followed by sciatica in one leg or acute sciatica in one leg without back pain. We all are familiar with this clinical presentation.

These are some variations of the usual herniations which may produce a bizarre and confusing clinical picture. However, if one understands the nature of these lesions, the symptom complex becomes clear. These lesions are relatively infrequent and usually are encountered only a few times in one's career. An understanding of the nature of these lesions will make the clinical and radiological diagnosis more likely.

A massive disc protrusion, usually midline, may give sudden compression of the dural sac and cauda equina with the rapid onset of paraplegia and loss of sphincter control. Accurate diagnosis and immediate surgical treatment is essential in this instance.

Bilateral disc lesions may present as sciatica on both sides or as pain on first one side and then on the opposite side.

Disc herniations may occur at different levels because degenerative disc disease may affect any or all of the lumbar discs. Herniations may occur at several levels simultaneously or at separate times. Fortunately, when they occur simultaneously they are usually at contiguous discs and are on the same side.

In the final stages of degenerative disc disease, there is complete disintegration of the disc, followed by a reparative process which results in replacement of the disc by fibrous tissue that binds the vertebral bodies together. Nuclear extrusions may occur in this final stage but it is relatively rare. This final phase of degeneration results in a narrowed disc space with secondary changes in the vertebral bodies and the posterior articulations. The end plates of the vertebral bodies become sclerotic. Osteophytes frequently form along the rims of the vertebral bodies. Finally, with approximation of the vertebrae there is telescoping of the facet joints with eventual thickening of these structures. This usually leads to osteophytosis of the articular facets, narrowing the neural foramen and the subarticular gutter. Root irritation by foraminal or subarticular stenosis is frequently the end result of this process and usually requires surgical decompression.

A thorough understanding of this pathological process by the radiologist can be very helpful in his interpretation of the radiographic studies. He should suspect a disc protrusion as the primary culprit for sciatica in an individual under the age of 50 years. In the elderly individual, although a disc herniation must be ruled out, he should search much harder for foraminal or subarticular encroachment. A bulging disc in an elderly individual without definite nerve root compression would have much less significance than the same lesion in a younger individual. It is not unusual, however, to see mixed pathology with definite spinal stenosis and a superimposed disc hernia.

Some individuals progress to end-stage disease without having a disc protrusion or any significant back or leg pain. These individuals may have stable spines and minimal or no symptoms or signs.

Correlation of the pathological process with the clinical and radiographic findings can give a more reliable and accurate diagnosis and allow for more precise treatment of the patient.

CLINICAL FEATURES OF LUMBAR DISC DISEASE

The clinical presentation of lumbar disc disease may be highly variable. It has been said that the only truly constant feature of lumbar disc lesions is the great variability of signs and symptoms, not only from patient to patient, but in the same patient. A thorough knowledge of the different phases of the pathological process makes the findings easier to understand and correlate.

As in all other diseases, a careful history is important. A history of injury, whether acute or chronic, is elicited in many cases. However, there may be no history of injury or the injury may be minimal. Injury in a young adult causing a disc lesion is usually severe, whereas an injury in an older adult may be much less severe. This divergence can be explained on the basis of the pathological changes in the disc. In the young adult, with only minimal pathological changes, a violent injury will be required to cause retropulsion of the nucleus. In the older adult, degenerative changes have weakened the annulus to an extent that trivial trauma may cause a disc herniation. A true herniation of a completely normal disc is rare. It is believed, therefore, that in most cases an injury is the precipitating factor and not the actual causative factor in lumbar disc disease.

The pain pattern is important in determining the cause

of the pain. Sciatica secondary to nerve root compression usually improves with rest and generally resolves at night. Persistent night pain, be it axial or radicular, should be investigated aggressively. Night pain is not typical of lumbar degenerative disc disease but is more typical of tumors of the spine.

The soft-tissue components of a motor unit (a disc and its adjacent vertebra) usually are innervated by the sinuvertebral nerves and the posterior primary divisions of the lumbar nerve roots (7). These nerves contain sympathetic and sensory fibers. The sinuvertebral nerve originates near the spinal ganglion and through its branches innervates the peripheral layers of the anulus fibrosis of the disc above and below. Other branches innervate the dura, the vascular elements, the posterior longitudinal ligament, and the periosteum.

The posterior rami supply the skin and muscles of the lumbar region and, in addition, distribute sensory fibers to fasciae, ligaments, the periosteum, and the intervertebral joints.

The sinuvertebral nerve endings, when stimulated by noxious agents and events such as tearing of the posterior anulus and extrusion of disc material, not only evoke deep local pain but also produce reflex muscle spasm. The severity of this pain and spasm depends upon the intensity of the stimulus. If the stimulus is of great intensity, pain may radiate into the hip, the region of the sacroiliac joint, and the posterior aspect of the thigh. This type of radiating pain is diffuse and deep in nature and is localized poorly by the patient. This is often referred to as discogenic or nonradicular pain in contrast to the more specific pain of neurogenic origin caused by direct irritation of a nerve root (8).

Pain in the lumbar region alone, or associated with leg pain, is the result of stimuli applied to mesodermal structures of the spine or to the nerve roots. Based on the site of origin, pain can be classified as scleratogenous or dermatogenous pain.

The disruption of a disc and the subsequent deranged mechanics of the motor unit frequently are accompanied by deep, dull aching pain with wide radiation and poor localization. The pain radiates to structures of mesodermal origin (muscles, tendons, ligaments, and periosteum). These are structures innervated by nerve fibers from nerve roots of the same embryonic level as the affected disc. This deep pain is scleratogenous pain. This type of pain has no cutaneous distribution and is confined to deep structures connected to the skeleton. The area of radiation is called a sclerotome in contrast to a dermatome, which is a cutaneous area of pain radiation. Occasionally, severe stimulation of mesodermal tissues may cause the pain to be accompanied by a vasovagal response such as sweating, nausea, decrease in the blood pressure, or even collapse.

Dermatogenous or true radicular pain is superficial and localized to a specific cutaneous region. This pain follows direct irritation of nerve roots. Each nerve root has its specific dermatome. There are two types of dermatogenous pain, fast and slow. Dermatogenous pain is typically sharp, lancinating, and well-delineated. This pain can be evoked by minimal pressure on a nerve root (9). Any form of pressure, tension, or traction can produce radicular pain and the extension of pain along a dermatome will depend on the intensity of the stimulus. Severe pressure on a nerve root may cause loss of function with disappearance of pain and the development of motor or sensory deficits.

It was noted previously that degenerative disc disease frequently progresses to its end stage without ever presenting with significant sciatica. It is sciatica, however, which is most amenable to precise diagnosis and surgical treatment. For our discussion, therefore, we are most interested in the characteristics of sciatica.

The disc levels most affected in degenerative disease in the lumbar spine are the L5-S1 and the L4-L5 discs. L3-L4 lesions are not common but are perhaps more frequent than previously recognized. L1-L2 and L2-L3 lesions are rare and are more prone to occur in young adults subjected to violent flexion of the spine. Table 19.1 shows the salient features of the major nerve roots usually involved. The nerve roots most involved in a herniated nucleus pulposus and in bony encroachment syndromes (spinal stenosis) are the L4 (L3-L4 disc), L5 (L4-L5 disc) and S1 (L5-S1 disc) levels. Once a nerve root is involved, its functional deficits tend to be more enduring than the low back symptoms. Pain in the sciatic distribution is usually the initial presenting complaint. By the time neural changes occur, the process is far advanced and, in some cases, irreversible.

Cauda equina syndrome, although rare, deserves mention here because of its frequent catastrophic consequences. This lesion must be diagnosed and treated sur-

Table 19.1.
Clinical Features of Lumbar Root Syndromes

	Pain and Numbness	Weakness	Atrophy	Reflexes
L4	Posterolateral aspect of thigh, across patella, along anteromedial aspect of leg	Extension of knee	Quadriceps muscle	Decrease of patellar reflex
L5	Anteromedial aspect of leg and foot	Dorsiflexion of foot and great toe	Anterior tibial muscle	No change
S1	Posterolateral aspect of leg	Plantar flexion of foot and great toe	Calf	Decrease or absence of ankle jerk

Table 19.2.
Clinical Features of Cauda Equina Syndrome

Pain	Numbness	Weakness	Atrophy	Paralysis
Backs of thighs and legs	Buttocks, backs of legs, soles of feet	Paralysis of legs and feet	Calves	Bladder and bowel

Table 19.3.
Signs of Nerve Root Compression

1. Neurological deficit
2. Positive tension sign (sciatic stretch)
3. Positive radiographic contrast study (myelogram, epidural venogram) or HRCT that corresponds to the neurological deficit

gically immediately. The lesion is usually a massive midline disc extrusion at the L3-L4, L4-L5, or L5-S1 disc levels. A period of even a few hours of massive unrelieved cauda compression may cause irreversible sphincter changes. The salient clinical features of this lesion are shown in Table 19.2.

EVALUATION OF LUMBAR DISC DISEASE

In the treatment of lumbar disc disease we continue to believe that the precision and accuracy of the spinal surgeon's decision-making is more important than his technical excellence in the operating room. The goal of the surgeon should be to return the patient with lumbar disc disease as promptly as possible to a normal functional existence. In an effort to help surgeons improve their decision-making capacities, a systematic approach to the evaluation and treatment of patients incapacitated with lumbar disc disease was devised (10). This approach has withstood the test of time, and with minor variations, continues to be used in our evaluation of lumbar disc disease. From this, an algorithm for the radiographic evaluation of lumbar disc disease was extracted (11). We have found this plan valuable for solving a particular problem in a finite number of steps.

We continue to begin our radiographic evaluation of lumbar disc disease with anteroposterior, lateral, and oblique plain lumbar films. Patients with low back pain resistant to the usual nonoperative measures of treatment receive further evaluation. A Technetium bone scan is performed to rule out tumor, infection, and inflammatory disease of the spine.

Linear or complex motion tomography may be helpful in questionable bone lesions. CT body scanning may be helpful in demonstrating pathology adjacent to the spine such as retroperitoneal neoplasm which may present as low back pain. CT scans also may help to delineate the extent of tumor or infection in the spine and in the paraspinal soft tissues. Evaluation of these areas by CT may be especially helpful if surgery is contemplated.

Recent advances in CT have been of great help in the diagnosis of neural compression. With continued improvements in the software, this diagnostic modality may well

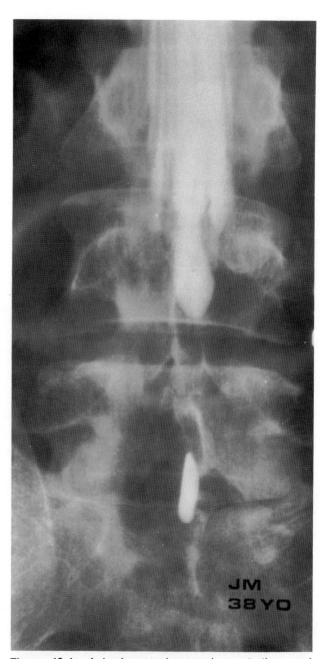

Figure 19.1. A lumbar myelogram demonstrating arachnoiditis at the L4-L5 level. This patient had a previous myelogram and lumbar disc surgery 10 years earlier with excellent relief of pain. Nine years later, he developed recurrent sciatica.

become the standard by which all other modalities are compared.

In the evaluation of sciatica, we obtain standard lumbar

films as the initial diagnostic test. If these are not remarkable and if there are no rapidly progressive neurological findings, the patient is started on a nonoperative treatment regimen of rest, exercises, anti-inflammatory medication, and mild analgesics. This may take up to 6 weeks occasionally. After 6 weeks of such treatment without significant improvement, further evaluation is required. At this point, the primary decision is differentiation between mechanical and nonmechanical sciatica. In mechanical sciatica, there is definite compression of a spinal nerve or the cauda equina. These individuals are amenable and respond quite well to surgical decompression. On the other hand, persons whose sciatica is not mechanical (i.e., inflammatory) are not candidates for surgery. Should they undergo a surgical procedure they most certainly would be therapeutic failures. It becomes evident, therefore, that a precise diagnosis is imperative before proceeding with surgery.

It should be evident, but we nonetheless emphasize, that radiographic data will have pertinence only as they correlate with the clinical findings. We believe that a patient should not undergo decompressive laminectomy unless he has at least two of the three key signs of nerve root compression (Table 19.3). The patient, therefore, must be evaluated clinically and should have either a neurolog-

ical deficit or positive tension sign before further radiographic studies are ordered. Positive radiographic data without the correlative clinical findings would not be adequate substantiation for a surgical procedure.

In the evaluation of the patient with mechanical sciatica, we still rely primarily on the metrizamide myelogram. As mentioned before, this test has a very high specificity and sensitivity in the evaluation of nerve root compression (3). This test will continue to be valuable because many practitioners do not have HRCT or its expert interpretation readily available. We also are concerned about the over-reading of HRCT scans by inexperienced radiologists and clinicians. We have seen patients operated upon for benign central disc bulges, without relief of their sciatic symptoms. It is of no consequence that a disc bulges abnormally. The germane issue is whether or not that abnormal disc entraps a nerve root. We must learn to "think nerve root." Unless we can demonstrate nerve root compression in our radiographic study, be it from a soft disc, bony encroachment, or both, that study must be viewed as inconclusive. We do believe, however, that HRCT has a future in the evaluation of nerve root compression, as will be discussed later.

We rarely use epidural venography at the present time. With the advent of metrizamide myelography and HRCT

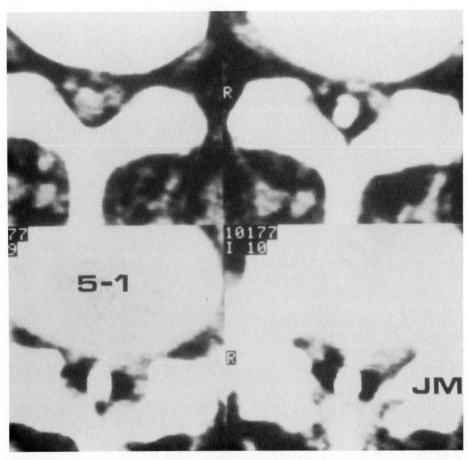

Figure 19.2. A HRCT scan of the same patient shown in Figure 19.1. The scan demonstrates a recurrent L5-S1 disc herniation.

this test retains little usefulness.

We currently are assessing the relative accuracy of HRCT versus metrizamide myelography in our institutions. We are obtaining metrizamide myelography and a HRCT scan preoperatively on our patients with mechanical sciatica and correlating these findings with the operative findings. If HRCT proves to be comparable in specificity and sensitivity to metrizamide myleography in our hands, then it will probably become our test of choice. Heithoff (2) has noted a specificity and sensitivity of 98% in 290 patients diagnosed as having a herniated disc by HRCT. Two of the very definite advantages of HRCT compared to metrizamide myelography are less cost (myelography requires hospitalization) and its noninvasive nature.

HRCT is especially useful in those cases when myelography is less than adequate. In arachnoiditis, myelography often is of no benefit to the radiologist or the clinician. HRCT in this instance may provide the evidence needed for a definitive diagnosis of mechanical root compression. Figure 19.1 represents the myelogram of a 38-year-old male who had an L4-L5 disc removed 10 years previously. He was readmitted with acute sciatica on the same side with a positive straight-leg raising test and absent Achilles reflex. The myelogram showed marked arachnoiditis at the L4-L5 level with no significant amount of contrast below. The clinical diagnosis of recurrent disc hernia could not be confirmed. A HRCT scan (Fig. 19.2) was performed revealing an L5-S1 disc herniation on the involved side. The scan in this instance helped to confirm the clinical impression and allowed for more precise preoperative planning.

Although most radiologists, who are experienced with HRCT, believe it now to be the procedure of choice in evaluating mechanical sciatica in the virgin back, the possibility of its usefulness in the failed back syndrome excites clinicians more. Many failed backs occur because of the failure to recognize lateral recess or foraminal stenosis at the time of disc surgery by the inexperienced spinal surgeon. HRCT can detect these areas of stenosis reliably, hopefully decreasing this common cause of the failed back.

HRCT eventually may be of most value to the spinal surgeon in the evaluation of the failed back syndrome before further surgery. With the use of intravenous contrast enhancement and with the evolution of new software with the "blink mode", we now are able to differentiate better between tissue densities. An important step in the surgical management of the failed back would be the differentiation of neural compression secondary to fibrosis and neural compression secondary to a recurrent or new disc herniation. This should increase the success rate in the multiply-operated back markedly by allowing more precise preoperative planning.

With further clinical experience and further technological advances, HRCT rapidly is becoming the procedure of choice in the evaluation of sciatica. It is also a valuable addition to our diagnostic armamentarium for the evaluation of resistant low back pain.

References

1. Burton CV: Conservative management of low back pain. *Postgrad Med* 70:168–183, 1981.
2. Heithoff KB: High-resolution computed tomography of the lumbar spine. *Postgrad Med* 70:193–213, 1981.
3. Herkowitz HN, Wiesel SW, Booth RE, et al: Metrizamide myelography and epidural venography. Their role in the diagnosis of lumbar disc herniation and spinal stenosis. *Spine* 7:55–63, 1982.
4. Haughton VM, Eldevik OP, Magnoes B, et al: A prospective comparison of computed tomography and myelography in the diagnosis of herniated lumbar disks. *Radiology* 142:103–110, 1982.
5. Armstrong JR: *Lumbar Disc Lesions.* Baltimore, Williams & Wilkins, 1965.
6. DePalma AF, Rothman RH: *The Intervertebral Disc.* Philadelphia, WB Saunders, 1970.
7. Roofe PG: Innervation of annulus fibrosus and posterior longitudinal ligament. *Arch Pathol* 27: 201–211, 1939.
8. Cloward RB: The clinical significance of the sinuvertebral nerve of the cervical spine in relation to the cervical disc syndrome *J Neurol Neurosurg Psychiatr* 23:321–6, 1960.
9. Smyth MJ, Wright V: Sciatica and the intervertebral disc. An experimental study. *J Bone Joint Surg* 40-A:1401–1418, 1958.
10. Holmes HE, Rothman RH: The pennsylvania plan: An algorithm for the management of lumbar degenerative disc disease. Instructional course lectures. *AAOS* 28:193–200, 1979.
11. Holmes HE, Rothman RH, Meyer JD: An algorithm for the radiographic evaluation of low back pain. In Post MJD: *Radiographic Evaluation of the Spine: Current Advances with Emphasis on Computed Tomography.* Chap. 33. New York, Masson Publishing, 1980.
12. Pederson HE, Blunck CFV, Gardner E: The anatomy of the lumbosacral posterior rami and meningeal branches of spinal nerves (sinu-vertebral nerves). *J Bone Joint Surg* 38-A:377–391, 1956

CHAPTER TWENTY

The Computed Tomographic Differential Diagnosis of Disc Disease

JOHN R. MANI, M.D.

High-resolution CT (HRCT) scanning has become indispensable in the diagnosis of spine disease. This computerized x-ray tool is accurate, functionally simplistic, and accepted by the medical community (1–4). Spine CT has completely restructured the diagnostic protocol applied to the back patient. Today's schematic, however, is under continuous modification as experience widens and CT metrizamide myelography (CTMM) gains greater acceptance. The present protocol includes the following:

1. Complete history and clinical examination
2. Routine spine films/tomograms
3. Routine HRCT scan
4. Myelogram
5. CTMM
6. CT guided-needle biopsy

The sequence of applicability of these diagnostic modes depends primarily upon the individual skill of the diagnostician and the clinical presentation. However, all patients should have a detailed history and physical examination at the outset. The anatomical area of clinical interest dictates the type of study and sequence. For example, the cervical spine may be evaluated satisfactorily by routine films and a CTMM. The anatomical area is compact and disc disease usually is found between the C3–4 and C7-T1 levels. A myelogram is not always indicated although it may be comforting. A routine plain CT scan will demonstrate the "hard" (calcified) cervical disc but may not detect the less dense "soft" disc herniation (5).

The thoracic spine, the longest anatomic segment, is optimally screened by routine films followed by a myelogram. If needed, an immediate CTMM may be performed if metrizamide had been used. An appropriate delay may be necessary for dilutional purposes. If Pantopaque had been the contrast agent used, its removal can be followed by the introduction of dilute metrizamide for immediate CT myelography (4).

Lumbar spine disease can be assessed accurately by routine spine films, routine CT scan (2, 6) and, if necessary, a myelogram and/or CTMM (3).

CT guided needle biopsy (7) may be utilized to differentiate a lesion with an unusual presentation, unusual location, or if a neoplasm or abscess is suspected.

Disc herniations are grouped into two distinct presentations:

A. Central (posterior)
B. Lateral

Central discs are posterior herniations of nuclear material into the spinal canal. Impingement against the thecal sac or upon emerging nerve roots may be demonstrated by CT (2, 6, 8). Impression on a myelographic contrast column may be seen if adjacency exists.

Lateral discs herniate into the lateral spinal recess, the intervertebral foramen, or rarely, may herniate extraspinally in a very lateral location (2). These lateral presenting discs often are identified only by spine CT.

The most common surgical lesion of the spine is the herniated disc (3). Regardless of location, surgically correctable disc disease requires nerve root entrapment. Occasionally, however, disc "imitators" are uncovered (6). These may be either surgical or histological surprises.

The expanding impact of HRCT scanning and/or CTMM, thrusts the radiologist into a prominent role in dealing with patients suspected of spine disease and their referring physicians. Often, it is the radiologist who recommends which diagnostic study to use, in what manner, and the sequence. The accuracy of CT in spine disease provides the radiologist with the unusual opportunity of frequently identifying the type of lesion and its exact anatomical location (6).

A thorough knowledge of the possible disc "mimickers" aids the radiologist in his broadening role. Wider experience and awareness may increase CT's diagnostic sensitivity but specificity actually may diminish. This phenomenon parallels the recent advent of cranial CT.

Dissimilar spine lesions, i.e., degenerative facets, discs, tumors, infections, etc., may have identical clinical presentations (2, 6). Clinical and historical data may not be available. The CT scan may be the only information upon which the radiologist must base a vital clinical diagnosis.

The differential diagnoses listed below are not necessarily in order of occurrence. This list is incomplete and will lengthen continuously. Examples have been included from both HRCT and HRCT metrizamide myelograms.

THE CT DIFFERENTIAL DIAGNOSIS OF DISC DISEASE

Central Presentation

1. Posterior Disc Herniation
2. Postoperative Scarring
3. Post-Traumatic Disc
4. Pseudodisc of Spondylolisthesis

5. Prominent Epidural Veins
6. Metastatic Neoplasm
7. Spinal Dysraphism
8. Primary Spine Neoplasm
9. Ossified Posterior Longitudinal Ligament
10. Infection
11. Epidural Hemorrhage
12. Postpuncture Spinal Fluid Leak

A-1: POSTERIOR DISC HERNIATION

The most common surgical lesion of the spine is the *posterior disc herniation* (7). A posterior rounded mass, based on the anulus, is the usual appearance (2) (Fig. 20.1) and represents 95% of all disc herniations. Calcification is common (9). Effacement of epidural fat between the herniation and the thecal sac is a strong diagnostic feature (2). Displacement and/or impression of the thecal sac and nerve roots are the significant CT findings of disc herniation. A disc fragment may burst free through the anulus and present as an untethered *free fragment* which may migrate superiorly, inferiorly, or present as a contralateral lesion. Rarely, the disc herniation may penetrate into the thecal sac and present as an *intradural free fragment*.

Central discs are more common in the thoracic and lumbar regions (9). Lateral discs are slightly more prevalent in the cervical area. Surgically amenable disc disease is defined narrowly as nerve root impingement. A diminutive spinal canal in the thoracic and cervical areas permits small disc protrusions to impinge on nerve roots (*radiculopathy*) or on the cord itself (*myelopathy*) (Fig. 20.2) (10). This relative spinal stenosis is in contrast to the lumbar region where, normally, a capacious spinal canal

is found (10). Here, the spinal canal may accommodate a large disc herniation without symptoms.

Sagittal reconstructions may be helpful in the differential diagnosis of central presenting lesions. Normal discs and herniations have identical CT measurements: 75–130 HU, whereas other lesions may have different values (2). CTMM is usually unnecessary to diagnose central lumbar discs (Fig. 20.3), but it is critical for the study of thoracic and cervical discs (Fig. 20.4).

A-2: POSTOPERATIVE SCARRING

The failed back surgery syndrome is defined as unsatisfactory results following back surgery, and has an incidence of 25% (11). The known causes are recurrent disc herniation, lateral spinal stenosis, central spinal stenosis, lumbar adhesive arachnoiditis, epidural scarring, and direct nerve injury syndromes (11–13). Lateral spinal stenosis is thought to be responsible for more than 50% of the "*failed backs*" (11–14). HRCT and CTMM permits the radiologist to evaluate these patients for any of the above factors.

Epidural scarring, however, provides an interpretive challenge. All spine surgery patients develop *epidural fibrosis* to some degree. Surgical exploration of the epidural space requires evacuation of epidural fat which is the normal inherent CT contrast agent. Following surgery fibroblasts, originating from the traumatized overlying paraspinal muscles, migrate into the vacant epidural space and create epidural scarring (13). The resultant fibrosis may obliterate the anatomical planes sufficiently within the spinal canal to prevent the exclusion of concomitant disc herniation (15–16). Resorting to CTMM may surmount the epidural scarring impediment (Fig. 20.5). Un-

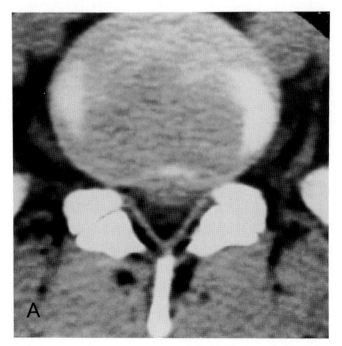
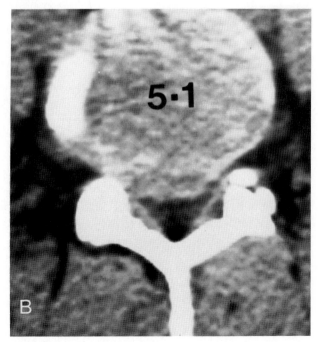

Figure 20.1. A and B. Typical posterior disc herniations.

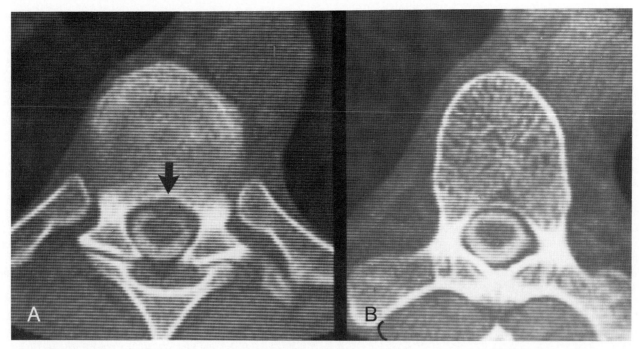

Figure 20.2.   A. CTMM. Small symptomatic thoracic disc (*arrow*). B. Normal thoracic CTMM, same patient.

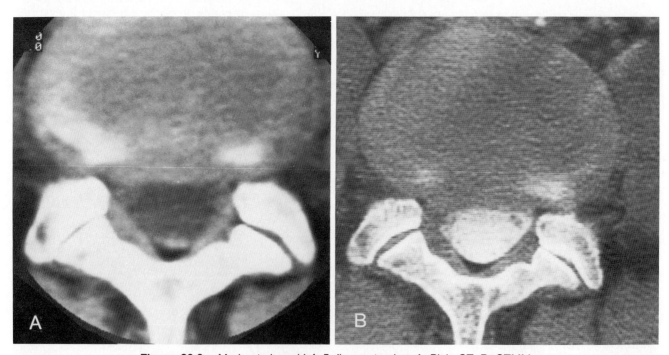

Figure 20.3.   Moderate broad L4–5 disc protrusion. A. Plain CT. B. CTMM.

fortunately, extensive scar retraction may occur, deforming or retracting the thecal sac sufficiently to simulate a herniated disc or other mass lesion (Figs. 20.6 and 20.7).

The attenuation values of epidural scarring vary from 35–75 HU with an average of 40–50 HU. Disc *attenuation* values are generally 75–130 HU (usually 30–50 HU more than epidural scarring). These relative values may be of aid in forming a CT impression on a failed back patient with scarring.

Recently, a Swiss group reported on pre- and postiodine contrast-enhanced CT scanning of the failed back (16). This report indicated 100% correlation in 36 failed backs.

Epidural scarring demonstrated contrast enhancement whereas recurrent discs did not. All cases were reoperated for surgical verification.

Occasionally, postoperative rods or grafts may impinge

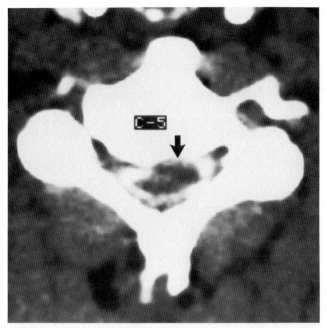

Figure 20.4. CTMM demonstrating left central C5–6 "soft" disc (arrow).

into the spinal canal, displacing the thecal sac and imitating a disc (Fig. 20.8).

A-3: POST-TRAUMATIC DISC HERNIATION

Spinal trauma is increasing due to smaller, lightweight vehicles, increased use of motorcycles, and expanding recreational facilities. The main thrust of post-traumatic spinal CT is the evaluation and delineation of acute spinal stenosis (17–19). The determination of neural injury (spinal cord and/or nerve root compression) and the instability of bony fragments can be displayed best with CT. The accurate assessment of spinal trauma is critical to proper patient management and often dictates therapeutic management (17).

CT scanning can be performed easily on the injured whether in tongs, traction, or with paralyses (19). After plain films, CT and CTMM have become the diagnostic procedures of choice.

Comminuted fractures with posterior displacement of fragments into the spinal canal can impinge upon the spinal cord or emerging nerve roots (18, 20, 21). Associated *traumatic disc herniation* also may be present (Fig. 20.9) (19). Careful scrutiny of adjacent CT scans is necessary to differentiate epidural hematoma from the partial volume effects of bone fragments (Fig. 20.10) (17).

The CT appearance of post-traumatic posterior disc herniation may be identical to degenerative discs, since both have trauma as an indirect or direct cause. The post-traumatic etiology is recognized by concomitant bony injury (Fig. 20.11). Image reconstructions may have greater injury assessment capabilities than axial scans.

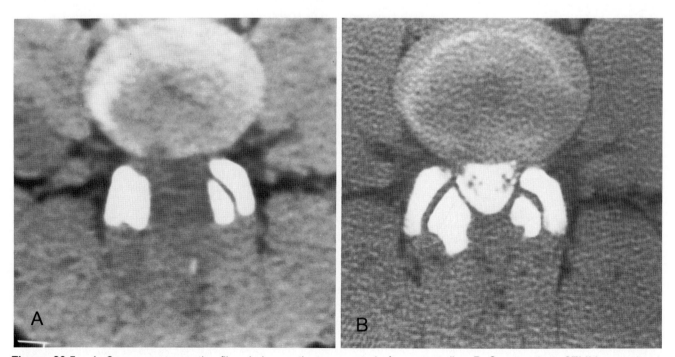

Figure 20.5. A. Severe postoperative fibrosis in a patient suspected of recurrent disc. B. Same patient, CTMM, same level: normal disc; mild arachnoid scarring with "clumped" nerve roots.

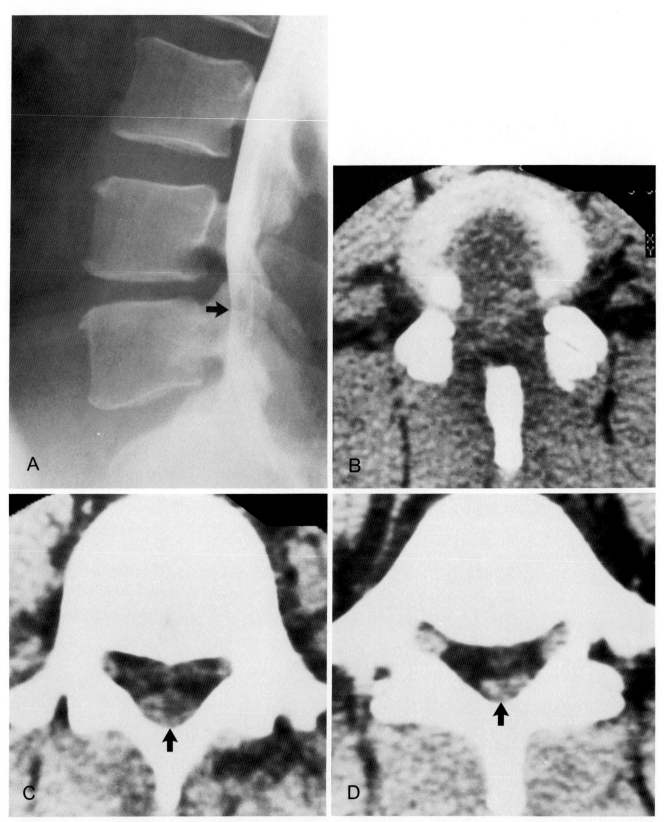

Figure 20.6. A. Postoperative myelogram in patient with recurrent back pain. Thecal sac displaced posteriorly at L4–5 suspicious for recurrent disc (*arrow*). B. L4–5 routine CT scan demonstrating severe postoperative scarring. Disc margins obscured. C. Upper L5 CT scan revealing thecal sac posteriorly displaced (*arrow*). D. Mid L5 CT scan. Same finding: posterior position of thecal sac. Surgery: No disc. Thecal sac retracted by scar tissue.

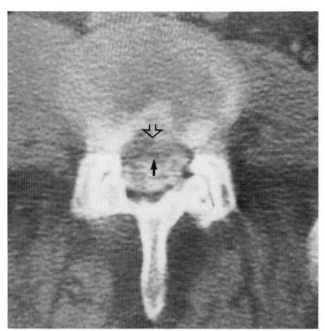

Figure 20.7. CTMM of postoperative patient with back pain. Space between arrows interpreted as probable disc. Surgery: Epidural fibrosis, no disc recurrence.

A-4: SPONDYLOLISTHESIS

Spondylolistheses are divided into two types: 1) Degenerative: occurring mainly at L4–5 after disc degeneration, and 2) Isthmic Defects: acquired stress fractures of the pars interarticularis, usually of L5 (22–24). The statistics of this spinal abnormality are impressive: spondylolysis, the pars defect alone, occurs in 7.6% of the U.S population (50% in Eskimos); spondylolisthesis in 3.5%. Back pain is present in 50% of patients with spondylolysis and will occur in 100%, at some time, in those with spondylolisthesis (25).

Spondylolysis may be missed at spine CT as the bony defect occupies the same plane as the CT slice and the pars area is below the disc level. In addition, if attention is concentrated to soft-tissue detail, the osseous lesion may be missed. One safeguard is to duplicate the CT images of the facet scans in both soft-tissue and bone settings. Plain spine films and image reconstruction are more reliable for evaluation in spondylolysis alone.

Spondylolisthesis also provides some difficulty during CT analysis. The vertebral displacement takes place at the disc level. A CT scan centered exactly at that level will frequently demonstrate a "*pseudodisc*" defect (Figs. 20.12 and 20.13). This is a scanning artifact due to a "partial volume" error. Each vertebral plate contributes to some degree to the CT slice thickness. The malalignment is perceived as "disclike" in appearance. Close inspection reveals no effacement of the thin epidural fat plane between the thecal sac and the pseudodisc (Fig. 20.12A). Spinal stenosis and foraminal narrowing also may exist in the presence of spondylolisthesis.

A-5: PROMINENT EPIDURAL VEINS

The vertebral epidural venous system is composed of 2 thick lateral venous bands extending vertically from the base of the skull to the sacrum (26). In the center of each vertebral body exists a flat, horizontal venous plexus (Fig. 20.14) that connects the lateral venous bands and anastamoses with the basivertebral vein that drains the vertebral body. Each venous band is composed of a medial and a lateral *epidural vein*. This entire venous system lies in the anterior limits of the spinal canal situated between the thecal sac and the posterior vertebral body wall (26–29).

The epidural space anterior to the thecal sac has enormous size variation. When this space is generous, the thecal sac may lie quite posterior in the spinal canal and raise the suspicion of displacement by a mass lesion such as a posterior disc herniation (Figs. 20.15–20.17). When confronted with this finding on CT, isolate and analyze the scans of the adjacent discs. If the disc/thecal sac interfaces are of normal appearance at the disc levels, the wide epidural space and prominent epidural veins are probably normal variants. Other causes of posteriorly displaced thecal sac can be ruled out by judicious use of image reconstructions, CT measurements, myelography, and CTMM.

Enhancement of epidural veins may be seen during CTMM.

A-6: METASTATIC NEOPLASM

Extension of tumor to the central nervous system is found in 20% of cancer patients, with *epidural metastases* noted in 5%. Intraspinal metastases are virtually all epidural and rarely extend through the dura to invade the cord directly. Back pain, indistinguishable from disc disease, is the earliest manifestation (30, 31). Later developing myelopathy and radiculopathy indicate spinal cord and nerve root compression caused by growing neoplastic masses (Figs. 20.18 and 20.19).

Early detection of these metastases is of particular concern as the onset of spinal cord compression may be abrupt, progressive, and irreversible. Despite myelography, at the initial sign of myelopathy and followed by aggressive surgical decompression, 50% of such patients will incur irreversible loss of ambulation.

Existence of vertebral osseous lesions portends epidural metastases as the dispersion of tumor is usually by direct extension rather than hematogeneous (Figs. 20.20–20.22). Intraspinal extension through spinal foramina occurs in 15% of epidural metastases with resultant radiculopathy. Virtually any tumor may metastasize to the epidural space, but 50% are due to lung and breast carcinoma. Solid tumors, sarcoma and carcinoma, account for 90% of epidural metastases whereas hematological tumors, myeloma and lymphoma, make up the balance.

CT is effective in evaluating cancer patients for all forms of spine involvement because soft tissues, bone, and neural elements may be visualized. The epidural space is identified readily by utilizing the abundant epidural fat as an inherent contrast medium, or by instilling metrizamide (32). The objective is to define threatening epidural

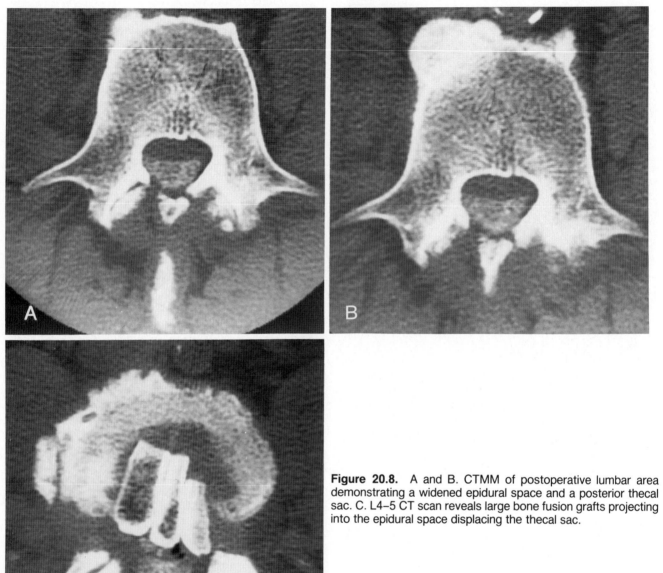

Figure 20.8. A and B. CTMM of postoperative lumbar area demonstrating a widened epidural space and a posterior thecal sac. C. L4–5 CT scan reveals large bone fusion grafts projecting into the epidural space displacing the thecal sac.

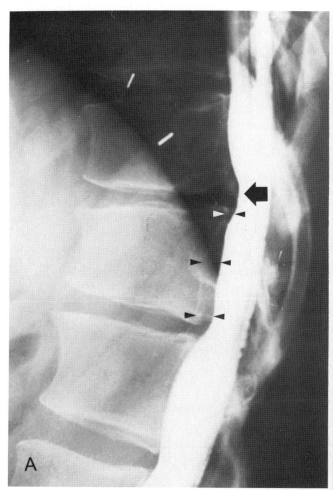

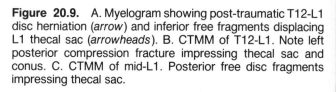

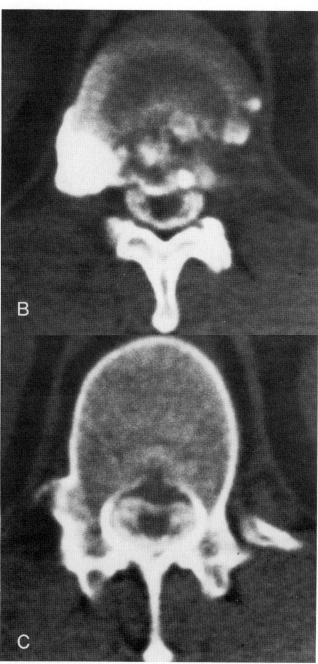

Figure 20.9.   A. Myelogram showing post-traumatic T12-L1 disc herniation (*arrow*) and inferior free fragments displacing L1 thecal sac (*arrowheads*). B. CTMM of T12-L1. Note left posterior compression fracture impressing thecal sac and conus. C. CTMM of mid-L1. Posterior free disc fragments impressing thecal sac.

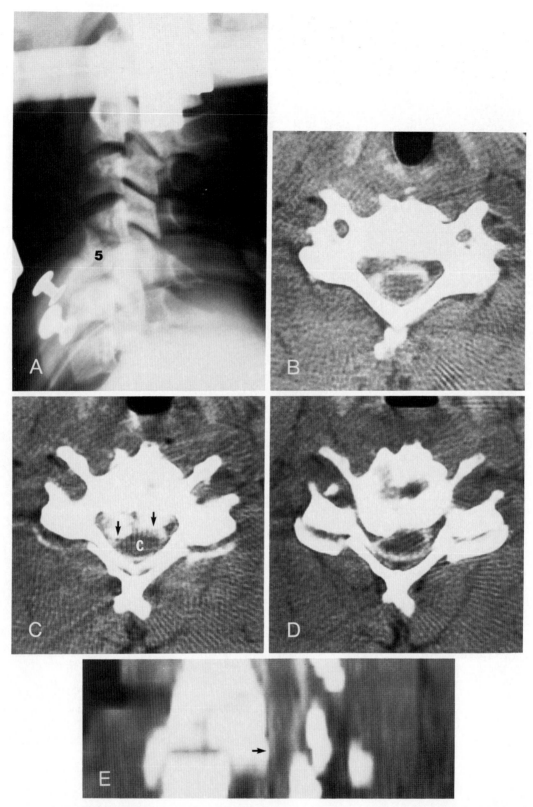

Figure 20.10. A. Quadraplegic patient with comminuted fracture of C5. B. CTMM scan of C6 revealing slight posterior displacement of thecal sac and ? defect of right lateral recess. C. CTMM of upper C6. Comminuted bone fragments (*arrows*) displaced into the spinal canal and compressing cord (C). Partial volume effect of these fragments mimic epidural hemorrhage. D. CTMM of C5–6 confirms fracture/dislocation causing acute spinal stenosis. E. Sagittal reformation displays comminuted fracture/dislocation of C5 with posterior displaced bone fragments (*arrow*).

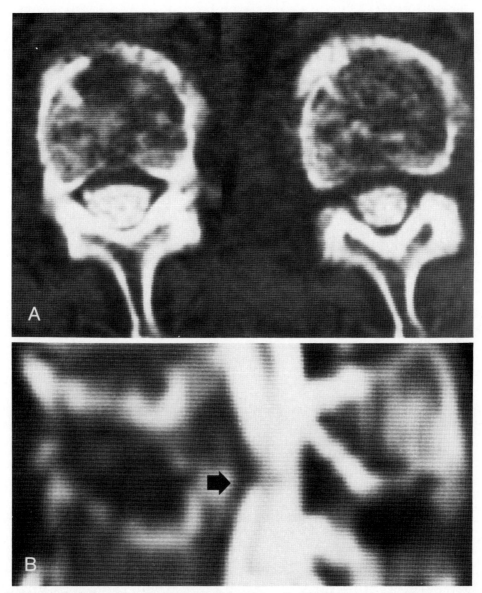

Figure 20.11. A. CTMM of L2. Posterior displacement of thecal sac. B. CTMM of L2–3 reveals same thecal sac displacement with widened anterior epidural space. C. Sagittal reformation of CTMM reveals compression fracture of L2 and L3 with bony fragments displacing thecal sac (*arrow*). At surgery, bone fragments and extruded disc were found and removed.

metastases before irreversible spinal blockage occurs.

A rare form of CNS metastasis is *leptomeningeal infiltration*. This sheetlike infiltration of the pia-arachnoid produces bizarre myelographic patterns which mimic severe arachnoid scarring. This entity is not a form of epidural metastasis, but the CT myelographic appearance may be similar and confusing. Leptomeningeal infiltration most often is seen with systemic lymphoma (33).

A-7: SPINAL DYSRAPHISM

Dysraphic spine indicates congenital anomalies arising from abnormal development of neural, mesodermal, and cutaneous elements in the embryo (34). CTMM is the study of choice in analyzing the various components of this complex syndrome (35). The vast array of data displayed by CTMM in these patients is, at times, overwhelming. Listed below are the various abnormalities which may be found in spinal dysraphism (34–38):

Vertebral bony abnormalities:

scoliosis
spina bifida
mal segmentation
split vertebra
fusions
scalloped posterior vertebrae

wide spinal canal
sacral agenesis
diastematomyelia
  fibrous
  fibrocartilage
  bony

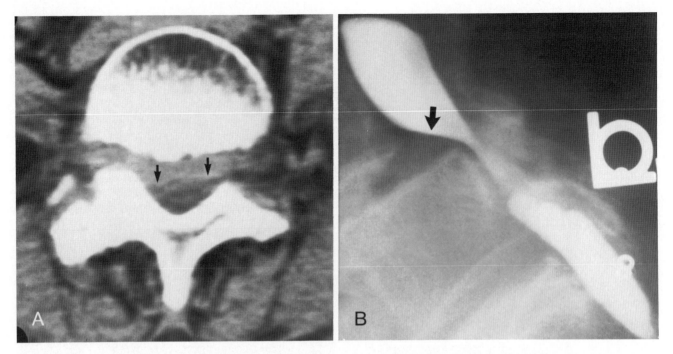

Figure 20.12. A. CT scan at L4–5 in a patient with degenerative spondylolisthesis. Apparent broad disc noted (*arrows*) is a "pseudodisc." B. Lateral myelogram reveals forward slip of L4 but not posterior disc (*arrow*).

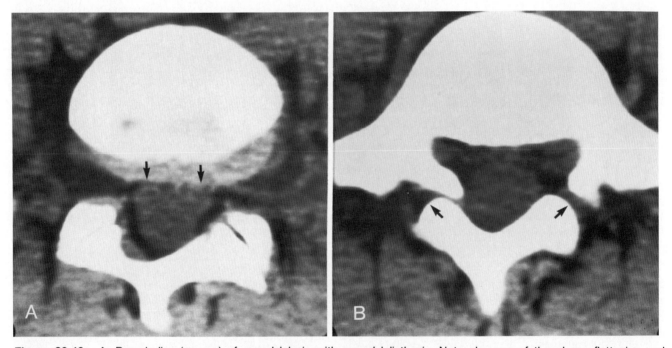

Figure 20.13. A. Pseudodisc (*arrows*) of spondylolysis with spondylolisthesis. Note absence of thecal sac flattening and presence of thin epidural fat plane between pseudodisc and thecal sac. B. Bilateral spondylolysis defects (*arrows*).

Neural abnormalities:
tethered cord
widened filum
low-lying conus
capacious thecal sac
split cord/split thecal sac

meningocoele, posterior/
    sacral
myelomeningocoele
Chiari malformation
arachnoid bands
cord-dural adhesions

Soft-tissue abnormalities:
lipoma, simple/complex
angioma
epidermoid
dermoid

teratoma
hamartoma
neurenteric cyst
paravertebral cyst

A tethered cord indicates longitudinal traction producing some form of neural deterioration. The actual "tethering" may be due to numerous causes (36):

thickened filum   diastematomyelia
lipoma   conus-dural adhesions
lipomeningocoele   myelomeningocoele
fibrous adhesions   myelomeningocoele/re-
pair/adhesion

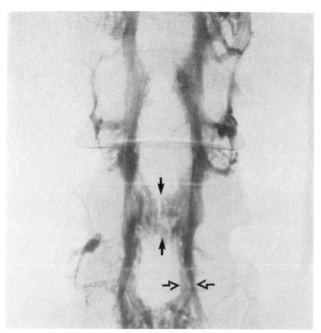

Figure 20.14. Lumbar epidural venogram. Horizontal epidural venous plexus (*solid arrows*) interconnecting the lateral epidural veins (*open arrows*).

Cord tethering is the result of conus fixation in the lumbar region. Normal growth then creates cord traction and stretching. The thoracic spinal cord, in response to tension, migrates anteriorly and flattens against the inner curve of the thoracic kyphosis. CT or CTMM of this abnormal cord position and contour will display a filling defect which may be mistaken for a mass or disc (Fig. 20.23). Image reconstructions will aid in obtaining an anatomical overview. Spinal puncture must be performed with caution in these patients due to the possible presence of a low conus and Chiari malformation.

The presence of intraspinal lipomata in dysraphic spines may create anatomical distortion sufficient to mimic posterior disc herniation (Figs. 20.24 and 20.25).

A-8: PRIMARY SPINE NEOPLASM

Intraspinal tumors may originate from any vertebral component: vascular, meninges, cord, nerve sheaths, embryonal rests, epidural fat, or bone (39). CT, when coupled with myelography to detect multiple lesions, contributes great accuracy to the radiological survey (40).

Because CT inherently produces exquisite anatomical detail, many primary spine tumors may be identified correctly. The lipoma with its low CT numbers is labeled easily (Fig. 20.26). *Meningiomas* often contain fine calcifications which readily are noted by CT (41). *Paget's disease of bone* and vertebral *hemangioma* display coarse bony trabeculations, which, although differing, are characteristic (42). A *neurilemmoma*, usually presenting as an extradural foraminal mass, has CT numbers in the 60–65 HU range (thecal sac: 15–30 HU), and may enhance with iodine to still higher number (43). The neural tumors,

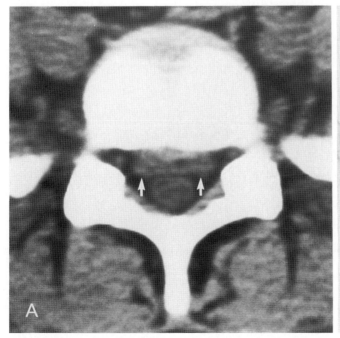 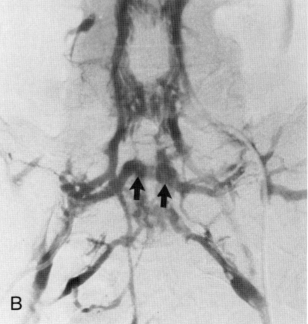

Figure 20.15. A. Large epidural mass anterior to thecal sac, mimics a disc (*arrow*). B. Lumbar epidural venogram. CT mass caused by anomalous horizontal vein at L5-S1 level (*arrows*).

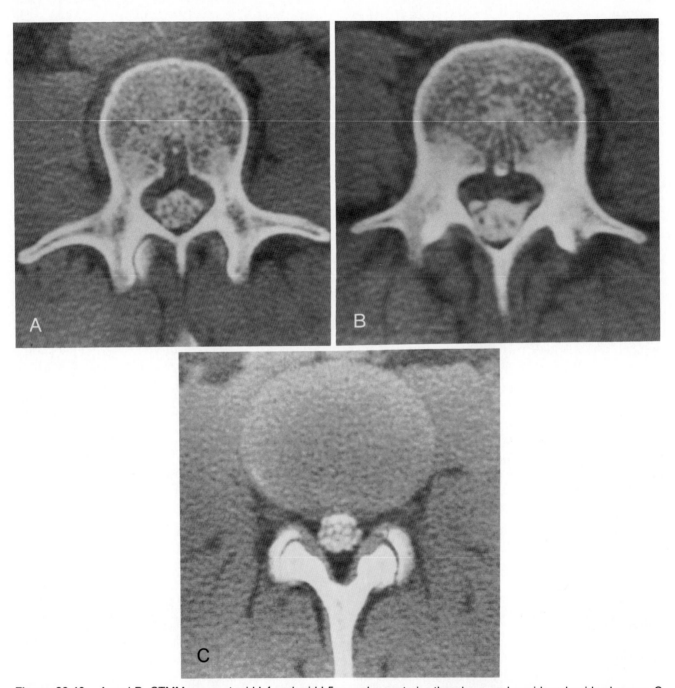

Figure 20.16.   A and B. CTMM scans at mid-L4 and mid-L5 reveal a posterior thecal sac and a widened epidural space. C. CTMM at L4–5 disc level reveals mild canal narrowing but no disc herniation. Findings on A and B are due to normal variation and prominent epidural veins.

ependymomas and *astrocytomas*, may display a widened cord or obstruct at myelography (44).

Osseous tumors are identified by bony distortion and destruction (Fig. 20.27). *Osteoid osteoma* exhibits focal bony sclerosis or a dense nidus centered within a round lucent defect. *Osteochondromas* produce large, rounded, irregular, sclerotic bony overgrowths, exterior to or within

the spinal canal (45). Vascular tumors may present with irregular contrast enhancement patterns due to entangled vascular channels. Finally, a dilated central canal, within the cord and noted on delayed CTMM scans, indicates a *syrinx* which may be associated with an obstructing tumor.

Historically, a spine tumor will mimic a disc in its

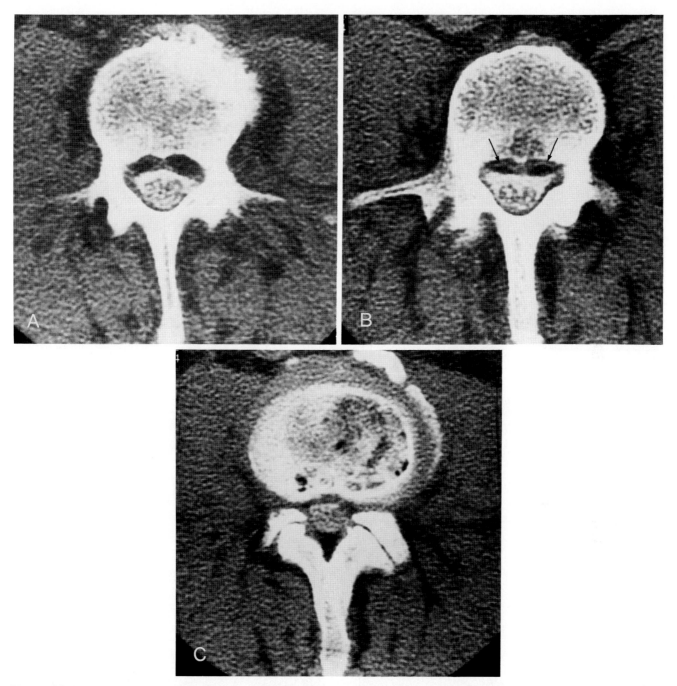

Figure 20.17.   A. Mid-L3 CTMM displaying widened epidural space. B. Mid-L 4 CTMM revealing a widened epidural space containing metrizamide enhanced epidural venous plexus (*arrows*). C. L3–4 CTMM. Mild spinal stenosis. Degenerative nonprotruding disc. Widened epidural spaces at L3 and L4 are normal variants and prominent veins.

clinical presentation (39). This mimicry extends to CT appearance as well (Fig. 20.28). Puzzling cases may require *CT guided-needle aspiration* or open biopsy (46).

CT permits the radiologist to scrutinize and evaluate lesions as to whether solid or cystic (CT numbers), vascular or avascular (contrast enhancement), and infiltrative or sharply marginated.

A-9: OSSIFIED POSTERIOR LONGITUDINAL LIGAMENT

The *posterior longitudinal ligament* is a fibrous reinforcing band attached to the posterior borders of the vertebrae and discs. It extends from the clivus to the coccyx (47, 48). Ossification of this ligament (OPLL) occurs as part of the

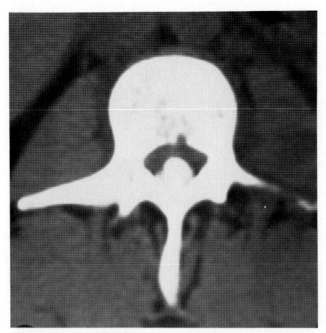

Figure 20.18. Epidural metastatic choriocarcinoma shown on CTMM of L2 producing widened epidural space.

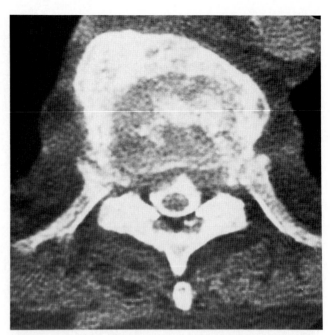

Figure 20.20. Metastatic carcinoma of prostate involving T8–9. CTMM. Bone destruction and epidural metastases impressing thecal sac.

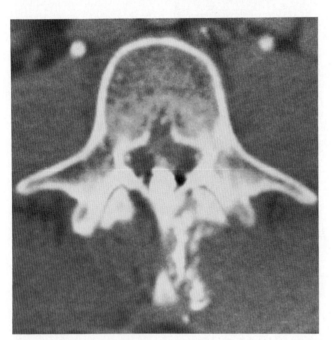

Figure 20.19. Metastatic chemodectoma of L4. CTMM reveals thecal sac displaced posteriorly and severely compressed by epidural metastases.

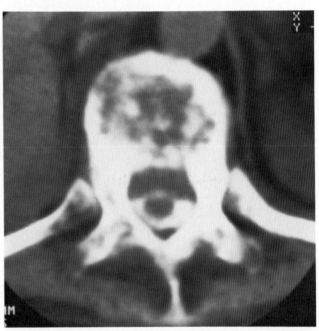

Figure 20.21. Metastatic breast carcinoma of L1. CTMM exhibits epidural metastasis plus vertebral and rib lesions.

aging process. Excessive ossification of PLL, with varying degrees of spinal stenosis, was first described by the Japanese in 1960 (47–51). Subsequently, OPLL has been found to occur in 1–3% of Orientals and 0.2% of Caucasians (48–50).

OPLL is found throughout the spine but is most prevalent in the cervical area (47–52). Ten percent of patients with cervical OPLL also will manifest similar changes in the lumbar and thoracic regions. Skip areas are common. Ono (47) suggests that OPLL merges with disseminated idiopathic spinal hyperostosis (DISH) whose bony changes are similar. The pathogenesis of OPLL is poorly understood.

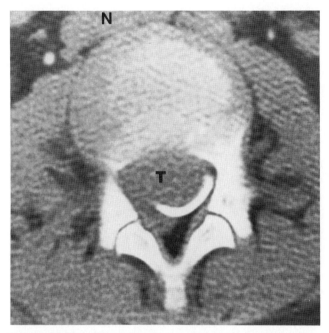

Figure 20.22. Epidural and paraspinal lymphoma. Large epidural tumor mass (*T*) flattening thecal sac on CTMM. Note retroperitoneal nodal involvement (*N*).

The spinal canal may be diminished by OPLL by more than 50% (48). The resultant spinal stenosis clinically mimics disc disease, tumor, spondylosis, and myelitis. Typically, large calcified masses are found projecting into the spinal canal from the posterior vertebral borders (Fig. 20.29). These osseous projections may appear identical to degenerative spurs or calcified discs on CT scanning (Fig. 20.29D) (48–52). Radiculopathy and myelopathy are common findings in OPLL. Neural injury is enhanced as the cord has less space or cushion to adjust to violent forces.

CT affords optimal spinal cross-sectional anatomy and easily displays OPLL. An assessment of CT disc disease must include OPLL in the differential diagnosis.

A-10: SPINE INFECTION

Spine infection has been depicted previously as diagnostically difficult (53–56). Today, CT is capable of displaying all of the subtle characteristics of inflammatory spine disease (57, 58). These include: discitis, osteomyelitis, epidural abscess, paravertebral abscess, and psoas abscess (59–61). Merging acute and chronic patterns are found. Causal agents include both pyogenic and granulomatous organisms.

The clinical onset may be abrupt, gradual, or insidious and indistinguishable from lumbar disc disease (56). The lumbar area is the most frequent location. Pathogenesis includes hematogenous metastasis and direct extension. The initial radiological findings include disc narrowing and epidural mass (56). Bone destruction is a later event and the development of spinal cord compression or cauda

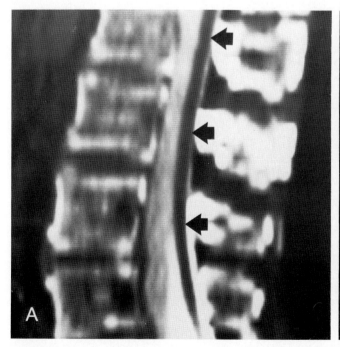
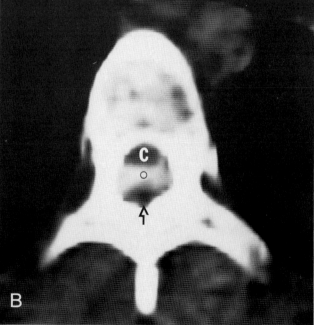

Figure 20.23.   A. Lumbar CTMM sagittal reformation demonstrating spinal cord tethered to posterior dural walls (*arrows*). B. Resulting growth traction causes cord (*C*) to migrate anteriorly, in this midthoracic CTMM, and mimic a disc. 0 = metrizamide filled thecal sac; *arrow* = epidural fat.

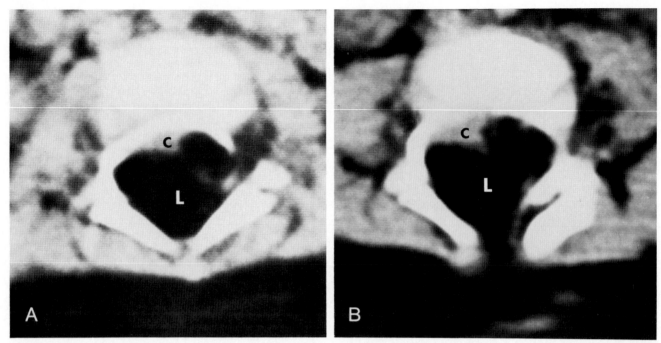

Figure 20.24.   Spinal dysraphism deformity imitating a disc. A. L3 CT scan reveals capacious spinal canal with diminutive thecal sac (C) displaced against vertebral body mimicking disc. Large epidural lipoma (L). B. L4 CT scan reveals spina bifida with lipoma (L) continuous with subcutaneous fat. Deformed thecal sac (C) fixed to posterior vertebral surface.

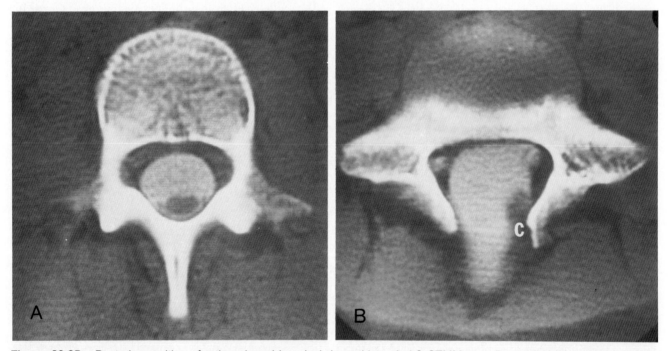

Figure 20.25.   Posterior position of tethered cord in spinal dysraphism. A. L3 CTMM revealing typical large thecal sac and capacious spinal canal. Note posterior low lying tethered cord. B. L5 CTMM demonstrating myelomeningocoele. Deformed tethered cord (C) is flattened against left wall of thecal sac.

equina syndrome is an ominous finding. Arrest of this process may occur in any stage if proper treatment is instituted (53). Previously, this disease complex was typified by delayed discovery. The advent of CT, CTMM, and

CT guided biopsy now provides early diagnosis, sometimes in the *cellulitis* stage, before the development of a true pus bearing *abscess*. Frequently, the primary source of infection may not be found (56). Originating sources include

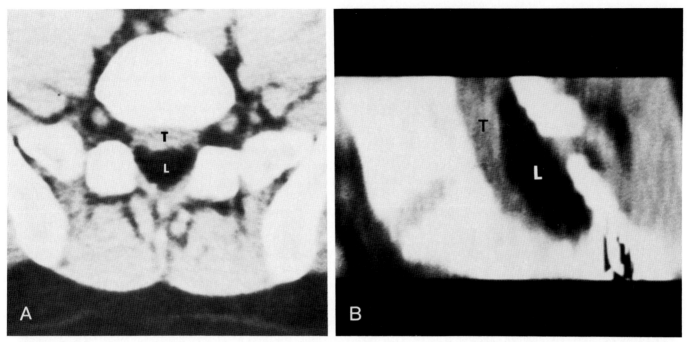

Figure 20.26. Primary intraspinal lipoma. A. L5-S1 CT scan reveals a low-density posterior intraspinal lipoma (*L*). Thecal sac is deformed, displaced anteriorly, and mimics a disc. B. Sagittal reconstruction displays relationship of lipoma (*L*) to thecal sac (*T*).

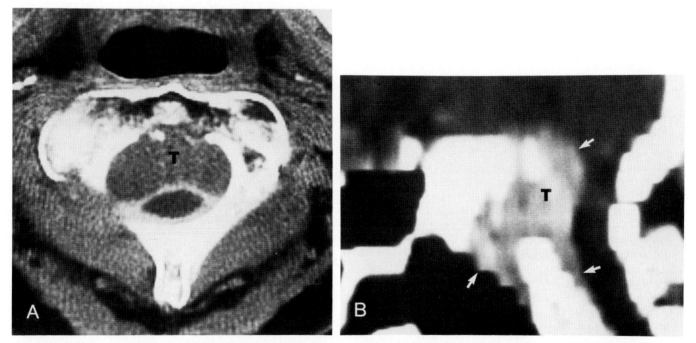

Figure 20.27. Clivus chordoma extending into upper cervical spine. A. C2 CTMM revealing tumor mass (*T*) displacing thecal sac and cord posteriorly. B. Lateral reformation of plain CT disclosing destructive clivus chordoma (*T*) extending into posterior fossa, hypopharynx, and upper cervical spinal canal (*arrows*).

the respiratory system, gastrointestinal tract, genitourinary system, and skin.

If the inflammatory spine process involves the epidural space anterior to the thecal sac, the CT findings may mimic posterior disc herniation (58), especially at CT myelography (Figs. 20.30–20.32). The availability of detailed clinical data and close communication with the referring physicians is critical in these diagnostic problem

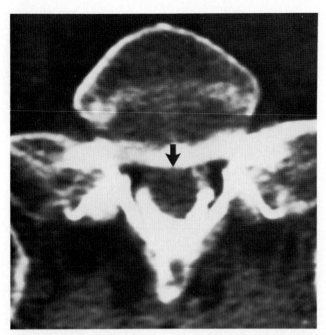

Figure 20.28. Primary hemangioblastoma (*arrow*) of S1 mimicking a disc on CTMM.

cases. Open aspiration or closed-needle biopsy may be needed for confirmation.

A-11: EPIDURAL HEMATOMA

Intraspinal hematoma may form in the epidural, subdural, and subarachnoid spaces, or in the spinal cord itself (62, 63). These collections of blood may be isolated to one compartment or involve all of them and the cord. Hematoma limited to the epidural space is the most common type. Fortunately, intraspinal bleeding is rare. Clinically, the onset is one of sudden severe back pain. Rapidly progressive myelopathy follows and the prognosis is poor (64). The most common locus is the thoracic area, followed by the cervical region; whereas the lumbar area is the least affected site (65).

Epidural hematomas develop from trauma, neoplasm, pregnancy, infection, arteriovenous malformations, venous angiomas, or epidural varicosities. Some are spontaneous whereas others follow lumbar puncture, spine surgery, spinal anesthesia, or anticoagulant therapy. The usual patient is elderly, hypertensive, and on anticoagulants (65).

This catastrophic uncommon event presents two imperatives: immediate diagnosis and surgical decompression (66). Cognizance of this entity coupled with careful CT analysis should provide adequate protection against diagnostic error. The CT characteristics of epidural hematoma may mimic a disc (65). The usual epidural hematoma is dorsal, may involve the ligamentum flavum, and if studied in the fresh state, will be seen as an area of increased density (Fig. 20.33).

A more common form of intraspinal hemorrhage is ligamentum flavum/epidural hematoma. This topic is discussed in Section B-8, and represents degenerative facet joint disease expressed in intraspinal abnormalities (100).

A-12: POSTLUMBAR PUNCTURE SPINAL FLUID LEAK

CT scanning may follow metrizamide myelography immediately if contrast dilution is permitted. This may be accomplished by 1) delaying CT scanning for 4 hours, or 2) placing the patient erect for a few moments and removing a volume of spinal fluid/contrast equal to the volume introduced and immediately scanning the patient. Both methods achieve the desired effect, that is, to dilute the metrizamide sufficiently to allow CT display of cord and nerve root detail. Delay is the method most often used as it permits needle removal for ease in fluroscopy and filming. Delay, however, also may allow spinal fluid to extravasate from the punctured dura and accumulate in the epidural space. Spinal fluid egress is enhanced by use of larger bore needles, multiple attempts, and by placing the patient in upright positions (67–69). *Spinal fluid leak* following metrizamide myelography will contain contrast material. CT scanning, under these circumstances, may be perplexing. If sufficient contrast/fluid collects anterior to the thecal sac a herniated disc may be simulated. Fortunately, this is a rare occurrence.

However, such a case came to our attention. A 32-year-old male underwent lumbar metrizamide myelography at a nearby hospital that did not possess a CT unit. The study was normal (Fig. 20.34A) but a disc was suspected and the patient was transported to our center for CT scanning four hours later. He volunteered that he had sat upright the entire interval to avoid metrizamide spill into his head. Initial CT scans show a vague density (CT measurement: 190 HU) anterior to the thecal sac, which is displaced posteriorly, at mid-L4, L4–5, and mid-L5 levels (Fig. 20.34B–D). An L4–5 central disc and *prominent epidural veins* were the considerations. However, the lateral myelogram film clearly demonstrates the thecal sac hugging the posterior spinal borders four hours earlier. A prone scan (Fig. 20.34F) suggests disc still more. Sagittal reconstruction (Fig. 20.34E) certifies wide separation of thecal sac from the spine—a marked change from the earlier lateral myelogram film. A prone cross-table lateral plain film confirms fluid anterior to the thecal sac, from L2–L5 (Fig. 20.34G), consistent with spinal fluid extravasation.

THE CT DIFFERENTIAL DIAGNOSIS OF DISC DISEASE
Lateral Presentations

1. Lateral Disc Herniation
2. Postoperative Epidural Scarring
3. Metastatic Spine Neoplasm
4. Conjoined Nerve Root
5. Arachnoid Scarring
6. Primary Spine Neoplasm
7. Infection
8. Ligamentum Flavum/Epidural Hemorrhage
9. Spinal AVM
10. Nerve Root Avulsion

B-1: LATERAL DISC HERNIATION

Lateral herniations of nucleus pulposus may occur into the lateral spinal recess, foramen, or far lateral in an actual extraspinal location (70). A well-controlled series of 1523 patients with low back and/or sciatic pain underwent CT and disclosed 274 herniated discs (18%), of which 14 (5%) were lateral disc herniations (71). These relatively rare disc presentations perplex the traditional back clinician because the myelogram is frequently normal. Spine CT is remarkably accurate in assessing the lateral discs, due to its ability to display both soft-tissue and osseous detail (72). *Lateral disc herniations* are most often found at the L4–5 level, decreasing at L3–4 and L2–3. They are rare at L5-S1—probably due to limited lateral bending at this level, which is thought to be the etiology (70). An analysis of the lateral recess syndrome must include a search for a possible lateral disc herniation (73).

CT can be of great aid to the surgeon in extreme lateral disc protrusions. The surgical approach may be quite different from the usual laminotomy most often used. The approach may be extraspinal or may require facet removal (70, 71, 73).

The differential diagnosis of the lateral disc includes *conjoined nerve root*, primary intraspinal tumor, especially neurolemmoma, free disc fragment, and metastasis. The use of historical data, CTMM, myelography, and CT attenuation values should differentiate all lesions but the neoplasms. Surgery or CT-guided biopsy may be required (Figs. 20.35–20.39).

B-2: POSTOPERATIVE LATERAL EPIDURAL SCARRING

Epidural fibrosis or scarring is the nemesis of the disc surgeon (74). Postoperative scarring results from fibroblasts laying down collagen resulting in dense fibrous tissue binding together the thecal sac, nerve roots, and the paraspinous muscles (11–13). Excessive epidural fibrosis replacing epidural fat significantly diminishes the diagnostic accuracy of spine CT. The use of CTMM, "stacked" scans, and image reconstruction is beneficial in determining disc versus scar (Figs. 20.40–20.44).

A disc may be reapproached surgically with reasonable expectation of favorable results. However, Benoist et al. (14) reported surgical dissection of epidural fibrosis and decompression of nerve roots in 38 patients, without discs, with recovery from radicular pain in only 13 cases. Typically, these "scar formers" will redevelop epidural fibrosis postoperatively (74).

The main differential diagnosis facing the radiologists in these postoperative *failed backs* is disc versus scar. This topic is discussed in detail in Section A-2: Posterior Postoperative Scarring.

Hopefully, the use of *free fat grafts* (13, 14) will eliminate or markedly diminish the development of epidural scarring. This procedure involves dissecting a large segment of subcutaneous fat from the operative site and wedging this fatty tissue into the laminotomy defect against the dura and closing conventionally. This free-fat graft will gain blood supply, survive, and, most importantly, retard or prevent epidural fibrosis (Fig. 20.45) (13, 14, 74).

B-3: LATERAL METASTATIC SPINE NEOPLASMS

The 20% incidence of neural complication in cancer patients is increasing (30). This fact is not indicative of medical failure so much as it is a tribute to extended survival times. Epidural metastases represent 25% of these neural complications. Although any tumor may metastasize to the epidural space, 50% of these lesions are due to carcinoma of the lung and breast (30).

Epidural metastases have a predilection for the lateral spinal recess and the spinal foramen. Their CT presentation is often most difficult to differentiate from lateral discs and isolated lateral *epidural scarring* (Figs. 20.46–20.52). A known primary tumor history or known metastasis should arouse suspicion. However, cancer patients may have disc disease as well. Perplexing cases may require CT guided-needle biopsy (75).

If bone destruction is present (Figs. 20.47 and 20.49), the differential tilts away from disc and toward infection, primary spine tumor, or metastasis. The history, clinical course, and CT guided biopsy all may be needed to determine the diagnostic probabilities. Infiltrating paraspinous muscle involvement often is noted in lung metastases (Figs. 20.46 and 20.51). Enlarged retroperitoneal nodes suggest lymphoma. Additional peripheral CT findings such as adrenal masses, paravertebral masses, and sacral or pelvic destructive lesions may also be present.

B-4: CONJOINED NERVE ROOT

Spine CT has stimulated renewed interest in the *conjoined nerve root* anomaly because it is easily seen at CT and it is frequently confused for a disc or mass.

Simply defined, a conjoined nerve root is two nerve roots arising from the same point of the thecal sac, sharing a large common dural nerve sheath, and finally separating and exiting through their respective foramina (Fig. 20.53) (77). Conjoined nerve root is the most common nerve root anomaly, occurs most often at the L5-S1 level, and has an incidence of 1.3% (78–81).

The CT image of a conjoined nerve root resembles a "teardrop" (Figs. 20.54 and 20.55) and mimics a lateral disc herniation, a free fragment, or a mass. CT measurements of this anomaly may be misleading. If the CT slice measured contains more dura than nerve root the CT numbers will be similar to thecal sac: 10–20 HU. But, if the CT scan contains nerve root and ganglion the CT numbers will be high, 65–80 HU, and approach disc values.

The diagnosis of conjoined nerve root is established easily by CTMM. The dural sac and the large nerve root sheath housing four nerve roots will be readily exposed (Fig. 20.56). Placing the patient prone, momentarily, before scanning will promote contrast filling of the nerve root sheaths.

The surgical literature claims the presence of conjoined nerve root presents an increased hazard at surgery (77–79). Wider bony resection and great care is recommended. The mere presence of conjoined nerve root offers no

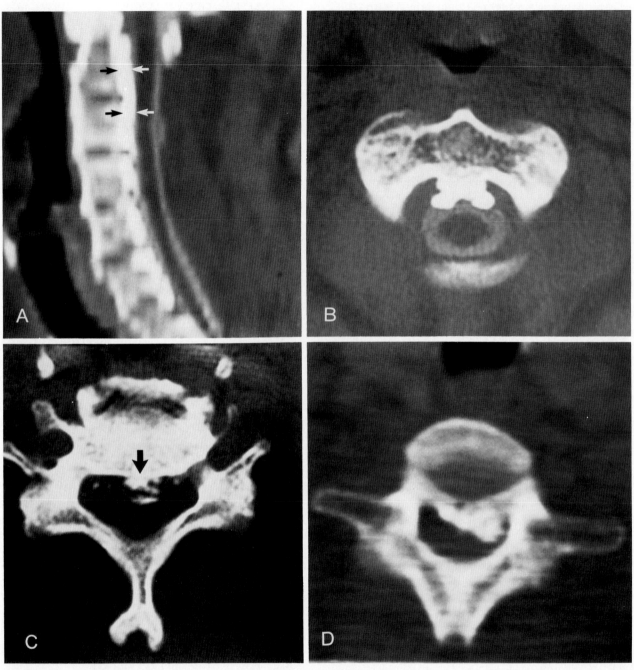

Figure 20.29. Ossified posterior longitudinal ligament (OPLL). A. Cervical sagittal CTMM reformation. OPLL seen as marked ossification of posterior vertebral borders (*arrows*). Note total bilateral decompressive cervical laminectomy. B. Large bilobed upper cervical ossification impressing thecal sac and producing spinal stenosis (CTMM). C. Midcervical irregular ossification (*arrow*). D. Huge C7 ossified mass. Mimics "hard" disc. E. Postoperative CTMM revealing a large degenerative posterior longitudinal ligament with peripheral ossification (*arrows*). F. Tiny L4 OPLL.

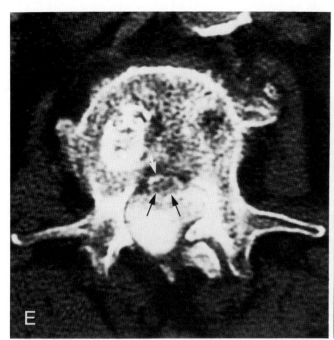

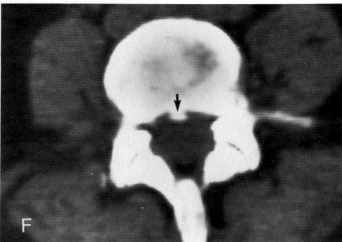

Figure 20.29. E and F.

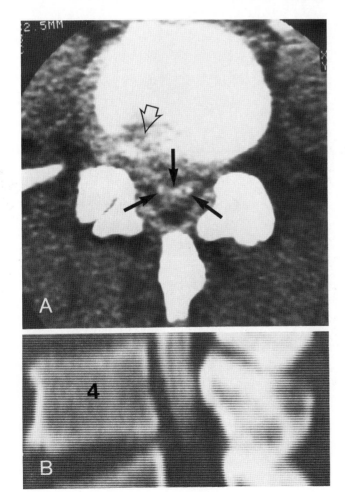

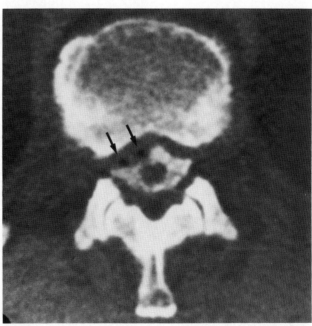

Figure 20.31. Acute epidural abscess in an 80-year-old male with fever and back pain. CTMM revealed anterior epidural mass at T12. Note gas collections (*arrows*). Abscess confirmed at surgery.

Figure 20.30. Pyogenic epidural abscess. A. CTMM demonstrates an irregular compressed thecal sac at L4–5 (*arrows*). Irregular bone destruction (*open arrow*). B. Sagittal reformation reveals circumferential abrupt termination of contrast column at L4–5. Surgery: Pyogenic epidural abscess surrounding thecal sac.

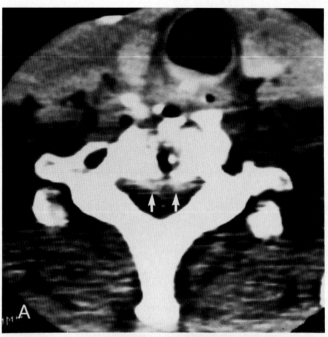

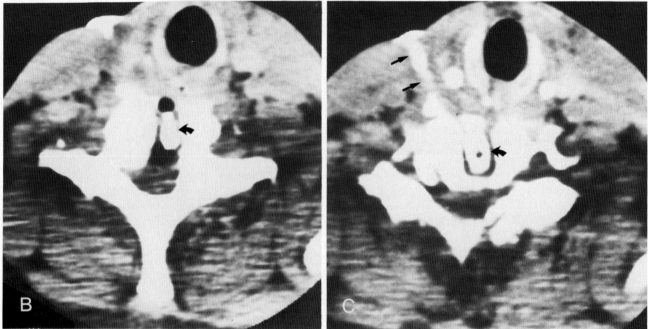

Figure 20.32. Chronic cervical epidural abscess. A. A 23-year-old quadraplegic, 1 year post C4–5 anterior cervical fusion. CT scan of C5 shows epidural abscess (*arrows*). Note lucency of midcentrum and prevertebral gas collections indicating infected graft (patient has draining skin wound). B. C5, 10 mm superior. Unfused bone graft (sequestrum) seen surrounded with gas (*arrow*). C. C4–5 scan. Unfused sequestrum noted (*curved arrow*). Metrizamide injected via skin wound outlines fistulous tract (*arrows*).

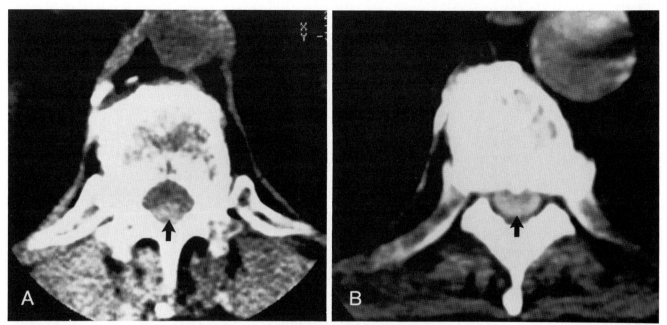

Figure 20.33. Epidural hematoma. A. Epidural hemorrhage (*arrow*) simulates disc disease. (The posterior density is fresh blood.) B. Subarachnoid hemorrhage (*arrow*). [Reproduced with permission from Post et al. (65).]

increased incidence for spontaneous injury. However, because the anomalous nerve roots present a bulky mass they are more susceptible to entrapment by disc herniation and compression by degenerative changes in the lateral recess (79).

B-5: ARACHNOID SCARRING

The arachnoid membrane reacts to the slightest trauma by producing an inflammatory reaction (82). A fibrin exudate forms, covering the nerve roots and arachnoid, which subsequently fuse together as the inflammation resolves (83). Resulting fibrinous bands attract fibrocytes which lay down collagen to convert the bands into adhesions.

The term *adhesive arachnoiditis* represents the end stage repair of arachnoidal inflammation (83). The major etiological agents are Pantopaque myelography and back surgery (83–90). Other causes include hemorrhage, trauma, infection, disc herniation, spinal stenosis, and thoratrast (85). The Pantopaque/arachnoid scarring link is so notorious that its use in Scandinavia is restricted and, in Sweden, forbidden by law (90). The presence of blood potentiates the inflammatory effects of Pantopaque. Fortunately, metrizamide, in normal concentrations, does not produce arachnoiditis and can be used in the presence of a bloody tap (91).

Arachnoiditis has no uniform accepted definition. Yet, many radiographic reports contain "arachnoiditis" in their conclusions. Some of the abnormal changes noted are dural, some arachnoidal, yet neither may be symptomatic. The patient may suffer from indiscriminate use of the term as the referring physician may be reluctant to impose

still another investigatory or surgical trauma on an existing inflammatory process.

Some clinicians reserve the term arachnoiditis for patients with radiological changes plus clinical findings of intractable pain, multiple nerve root involvement, and incontinence (84). Other clinicians deny this syndrome unless chills and fever are recorded as part of the clinical picture.

CTMM affords unparalleled visualization of the cauda equina. Spectral arachnoid adhesions are seen, some minor, other alarming. The uncertainty is: which are symptomatic? One alternative is the use of the term "arachnoid scarring" until the clinical obfuscation clears.

Proliferating postoperative *epidural scarring* may infiltrate the dura and secondarily cause arachnoid adhesions. Neither epidural scarring nor *arachnoid scarring* have effective remedies. Microscopic lysis of lumbar epidural, dural, or arachnoid adhesions has failed. There is no method to prevent the reaccumulation of scar tissue and the return of symptoms (86). The use of *free fat grafts* seems promising in preventing postoperative intraspinal scarring.

The CT display of arachnoid scarring ranges from minor *nerve root clumping* (Figs. 20.57 and 20.58) to massive agglutination of the entire cauda equina into an irregular neural mass (Figs. 20.59–20.61). The disposition of these neural masses within the dura dictates whether they mimic intradural tumors, "drop" metastases, posterior or lateral disc herniations, or epidural deforming fibrosis. If symmetric diffuse dura-arachnoid scarring occurs the *cauda equina* nerve roots may fuse into the wall of the thecal sac, presenting an *"empty" caudal sac* at CTMM

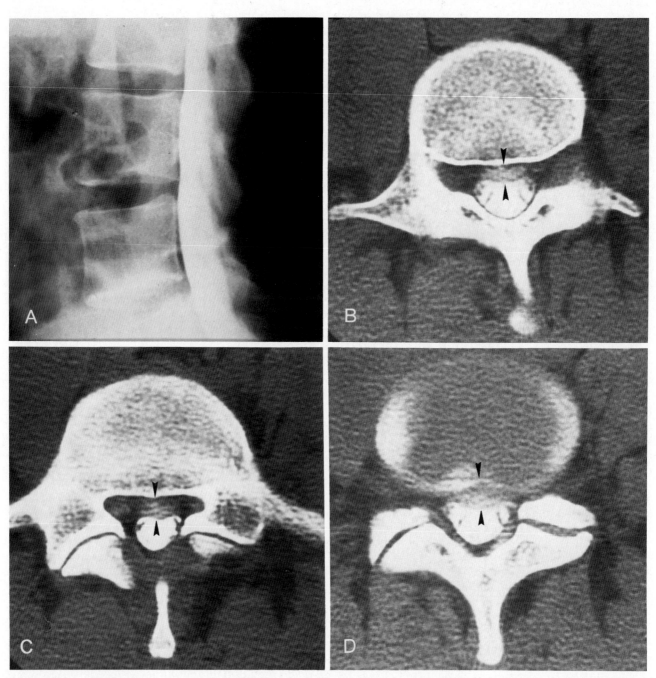

Figure 20.34.   Postlumbar puncture spinal fluid leak. A. A 32-year-old male with back pain. Normal metrizamide myelogram. Note close proximity of thecal sac to posterior vertebral bodies. B and C. CTMM scans of mid-L4 and mid-L5, 4 hours later, reveal thecal sac displaced posteriorly by vague density (*arrowheads*). D. CTMM scan of L4–5: same finding. Appears disclike but incompatible with myelographic film 4 hours earlier. E. Sagittal reformation confirms posterior thecal sac displacement (*arrows*). F. L4–5 CTMM prone scan: Posterior displacement of thecal sac is even greater and wider. CT measurement of this area (*between arrowheads*) is 190 HU. Etiology: leaking spinal fluid containing dilute metrizamide and pooling anterior to thecal sac. G. Prone cross-table lateral film, 5½ hours post myelogram, reveals the separation of thecal sac from entire vertebral border (*arrows*) confirming spinal fluid leak.

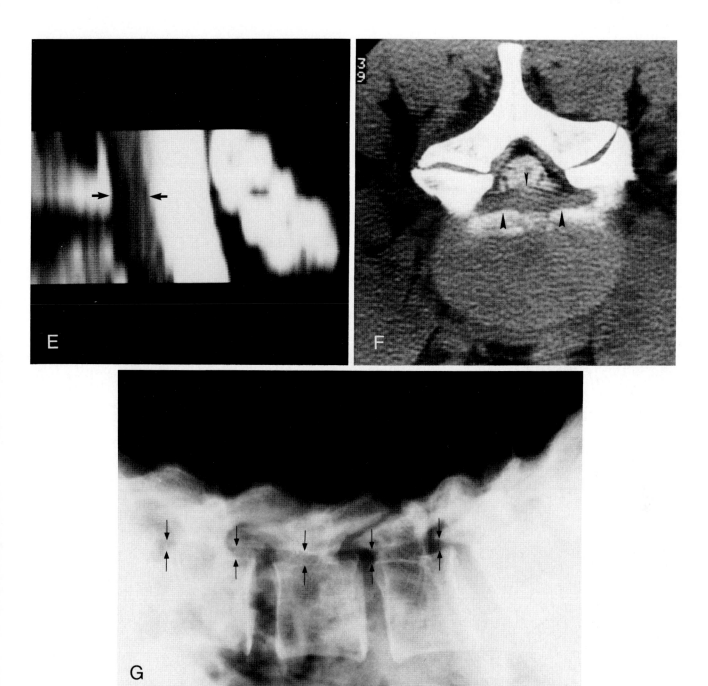

Figure 20.34.   E–G.

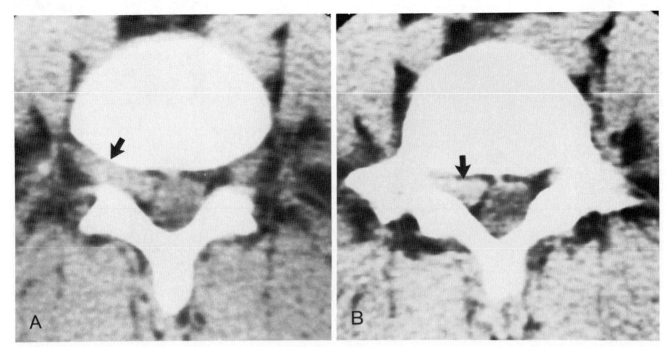

Figure 20.35. Right lateral disc herniation with inferior free fragment. A. Disc herniation (*arrow*) fills right lateral recess, right foramen, and extends extraspinally. L4–5 level. B. L5 scan 10 mm inferior. Inferior "free fragment" (*arrow*) noted, filling right lateral recess and compressing thecal sac.

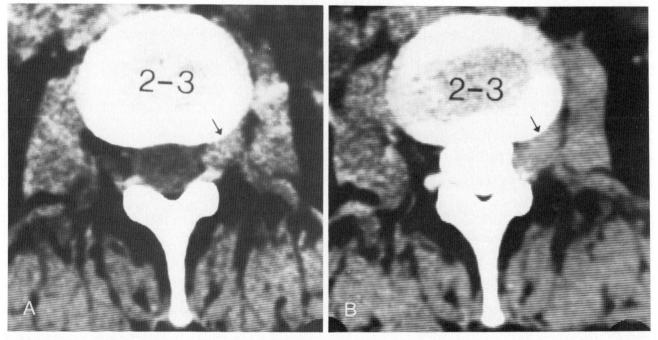

Figure 20.36. Left lateral disc herniation. A. Plain CT revealing left lateral L2–3 foraminal disc (*arrow*). B. Diagnosis doubted. CTMM 6 months later: Left foraminal disc still larger and compressing thecal sac (*arrow*). Surgery: disc.

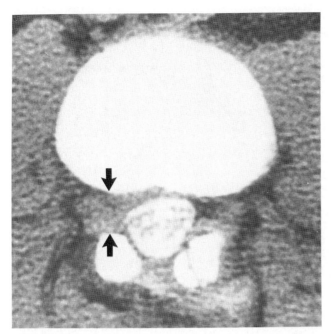

Figure 20.37. Failed back; CTMM: Right lateral L4–5 disc (*arrows*). Note total laminectomy and severe epidural scarring. Surgery: confirmed and removed disc.

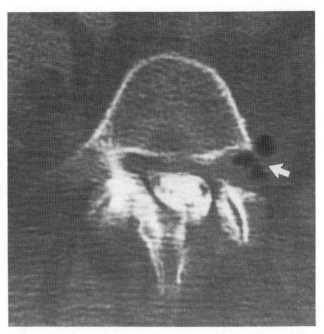

Figure 20.39. Left lateral L5-S1 disc. CTMM demonstrating a very lateral disc herniation with gas (*arrow*) in the herniation. Note blunting of left thecal sac. Previous left laminotomy

formation of an *arachnoid cyst* or the development of a *syrinx* (Fig. 20.64).

B-6: PRIMARY SPINE NEOPLASM

CTMM, coupled with newer computer software, allows exceptional evaluation of spinal and paraspinal tumors (93). CT imaging can define the location, extension, *calcification*, bony involvement, and composition of neoplasms readily. Depending upon cellular type, total surgical extirpation of spinal tumors is frequently the only hope for cure. The surgeon can identify, in easily accepted visual detail, the surgical landmarks he needs to plan his approach (40, 94, 95).

Neurilemmomas and *meningiomas* comprise the bulk of the extramedullary, intradural, and extradural tumors (41). Virtually all are benign and rarely undergo malignant degeneration. The neurilemmomas occur, evenly distributed, throughout the spine. Meningiomas are found mainly in the thoracic region, often calcify, and rarely ossify. An enlarged foramen is the hallmark of the neurilemmoma, whereas the meningiomas almost never produce bony abnormalities in the spine (43, 96).

Paraspinal and intraspinal tumors have easy access to the *lateral spinal recess*. These tumors frequently imitate lateral discs in CT appearance (Figs. 20.65–20.73) and clinical presentation. CT guided-needle biopsy may be necessary for adequate differential diagnosis.

B-7: SPINE INFECTION

The epidural space is continuous with the *retroperitoneal* and *paraspinal* spaces through the conduit of the vertebral foramina and wicks of adipose tissue. Thus,

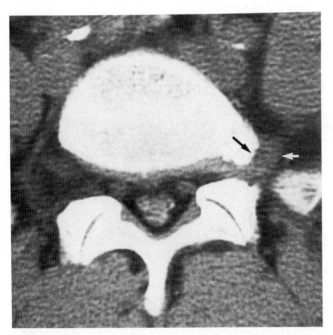

Figure 20.38. Left lateral extraspinal disc herniation. A combined hard and soft disc herniation is noted in an extreme left lateral L5-S1 extraspinal location (*arrows*).

(Fig. 20.62). The most spectacular example of this phenomenon is *ankylosing spondylitis* in which *dural ectasia* and the *cauda equina syndrome* (Fig. 20.63) also may be found (92). Finally, arachnoid scarring may be manifest by the

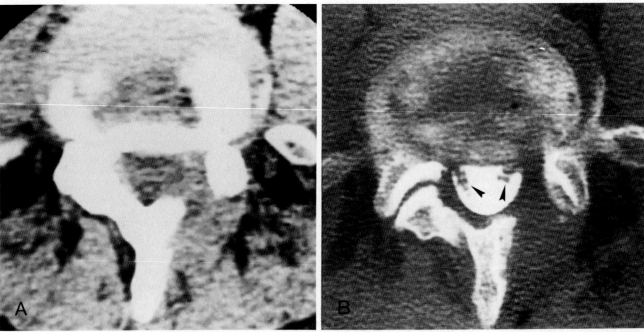

Figure 20.40. Postoperative scarring. A. Severe left lateral L4–5 epidural scarring. B. CTMM: no disc. Note arachnoid scarring with "clumped" nerve roots (*arrowheads*).

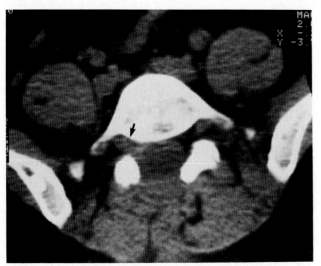

Figure 20.41. Postoperative right epidural scarring at L5-S1 (*arrow*).

inflammatory processes quite remote from the epidural space may extend intraspinally (97). The source of the infection may be by hematogenous route or by direct extension (61).

Granulation tissue located in the lateral recess may mimic a lateral disc or present in the foramen as a neurilemmoma imitator. A needle biopsy often is required for differentiation (Figs. 20.74–20.76) (46).

Epidural abscesses, predictably, will be on the increase because this area has received much recent attention and now is explored more often.

B-8: LIGAMENTUM FLAVUM/EPIDURAL HEMORRHAGE

The *ligamentum flavum* is composed of elastic connective tissue which is yellow in hue, hence its name: *yellow ligament* (98). This structure covers the lower one-half of each lamina and attaches to the superior lip of the lamina below. Thus, the upper one-half of each lamina has no ligamentum flavum. This ligament extends laterally to form the capsule of the spinal facet joint (99).

Degenerative disc narrowing creates abnormal stress on the zygapophyseal joints. In response, these joints develop irregularity, narrowing, subluxation, vacuum change, spurring and fusion. Such alterations are common, familiar, and easily demonstrated on plain films and CT. What cannot be seen are the intrafacet phenomena of articular cartilage degeneration, joint effusion, capsular swelling, capsular rupture, and attendant hemorrhage into the joint capsule (ligamentum flavum), and the epidural space (100). These *capsular ruptures* typically occur at the junction of the joint capsule and the ligamentum flavum. This is well known to physicians who perform facet injections. *Epidural hemorrhage* and swelling may lead to impingement of the thecal sac or nerve roots leading to myelopathy or radiculopathy.

The scenario depicted above is not uncommon and many ligamenta flava surgical specimens contain *synovial fragments* or *synovial cysts*. Postsurgical and histological reports include statements such as: "degenerative ligamentum flavum with hemorrhage", "hemorrhagic fibroma of ligamentum flavum", or "ligamentum flavum hemorrhage with synovial cyst" (100).

The clinical presentation may be identical to a disc

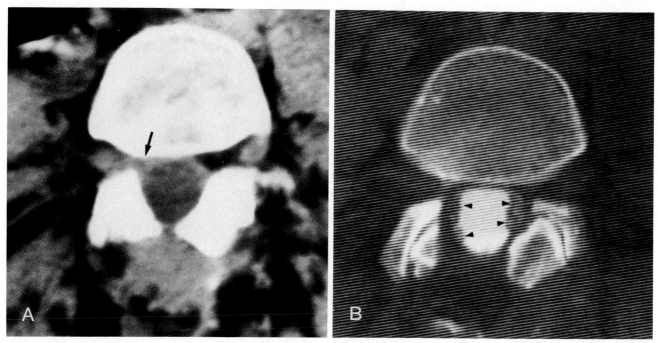

Figure 20.42.   A. Epidural fibrosis at L4–5 (*arrow*). History of five back surgeries. B. CTMM of L4–5. No disc. Severe arachnoid scarring with nerve roots (*arrowheads*) fused to walls of "empty" thecal sac.

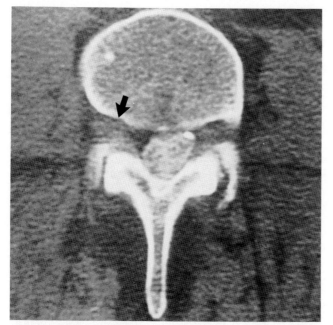

Figure 20.43.   CTMM of failed back at L4–5 reveals vague mass (*arrow*) with amputation of right thecal sac. Impression: right lateral disc. Surgery: epidural fibrosis, no disc.

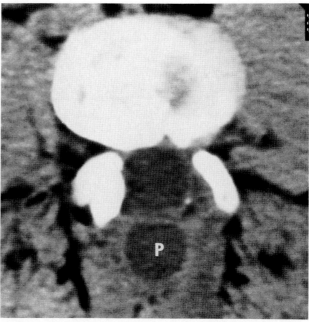

Figure 20.44.   Postoperative scarring and pseudomeningocoele (*P*). Back pain was due to a dural rent and spinal fluid leak into the paraspinal muscles. Reoperated and corrected.

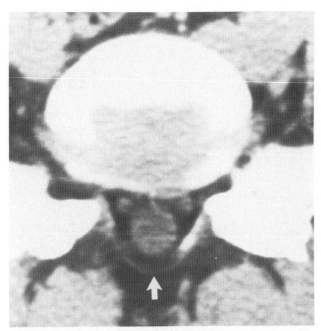

Figure 20.45. L5-S1 postoperative free fat graft changes. Note the absence of epidural fibrosis. Thecal sac is clearly seen. A "pseudomembrane" (*arrow*) has formed over the fat graft.

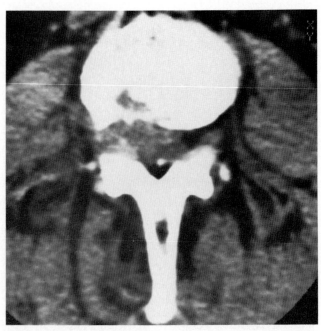

Figure 20.47. Metastatic carcinoma of lung. Mimics right lateral disc but note bony destruction.

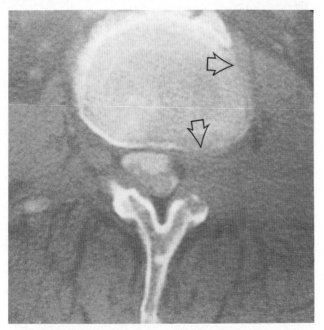

Figure 20.46. Metastatic carcinoma of lung (*arrows*).

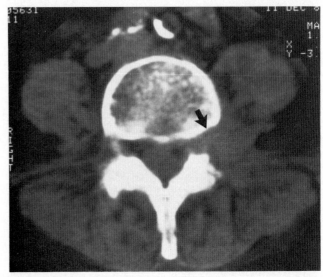

Figure 20.48. Metastatic oat cell carcinoma of lung (*arrow*). Disc mimic.

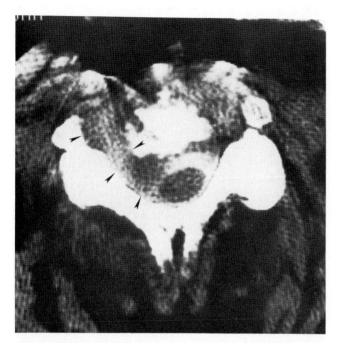

Figure 20.49. Metastatic renal cell carcinoma to C2 (*arrowheads*). Note bony destruction.

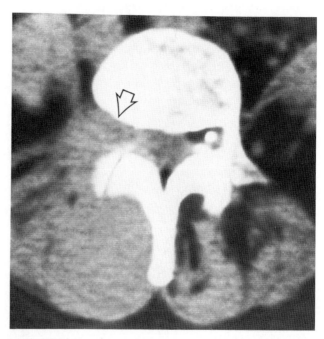

Figure 20.51. Metastatic carcinoma of lung (*arrow*). Disc mimic. Massive extension into right paraspinous muscles.

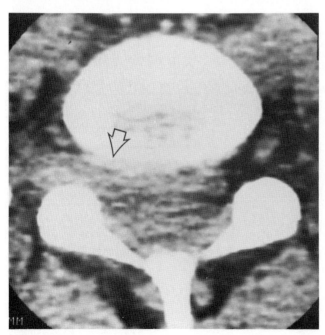

Figure 20.50. Metastatic choriocarcinoma (*arrow*). Disc mimic.

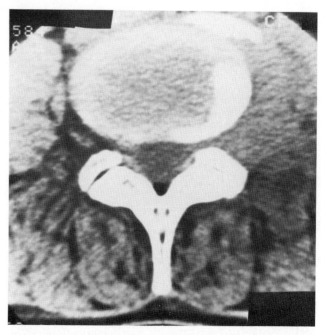

Figure 20.52. Metastatic carcinoma of nasopharynx. Note large left extraspinal mass that fills the left lateral recess and foramen (*arrows*).

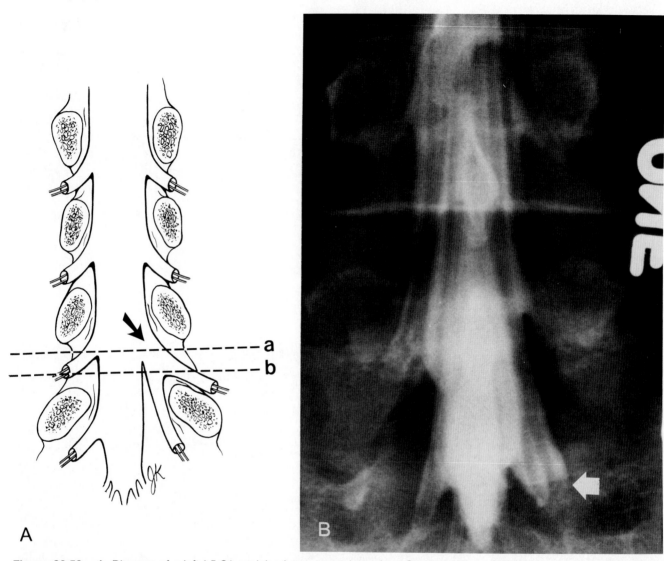

Figure 20.53. A. Diagram of a left L5-S1 conjoined nerve root (*arrow*). *a*. Corresponds to CTMM scan of Figure 20.56A. *b*. Corresponds to CTMM scan of Figure 20.56B. B. Myelogram of a left L5-S1 conjoined nerve root (*arrow*). (Note a second conjoined nerve root at the right L4–5 level.)

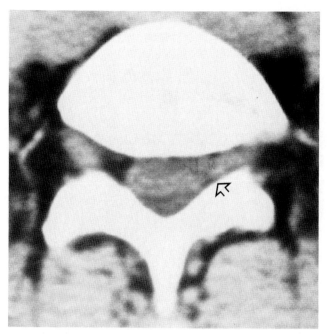

Figure 20.54. Plain CT of L4–5 left conjoined nerve root (*arrow*). Note "tear drop" shape.

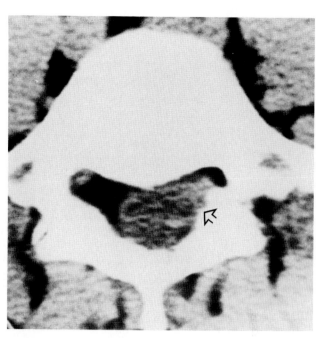

Figure 20.55. Conjoined nerve root of left L5-S1 (*arrow*).

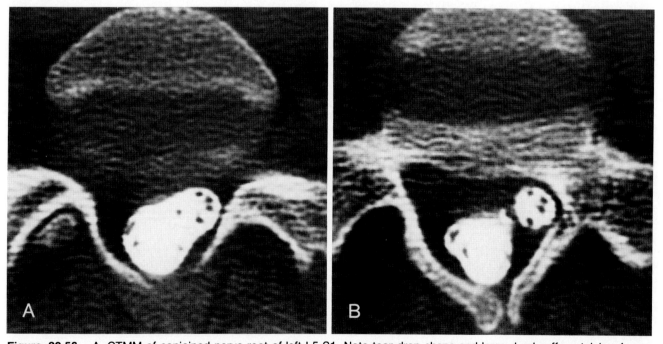

Figure 20.56. A. CTMM of conjoined nerve root of left L5-S1. Note tear drop shape and large dural cuff containing 4 nerve roots. (This CT scan corresponds to line "*a*" in Figure 20.53A.) B. CTMM 5 mm inferior. Conjoined nerve root has separated from thecal sac and still contains four nerve roots. (This CT scan corresponds to line "*b*" in Figure 20.53B.)

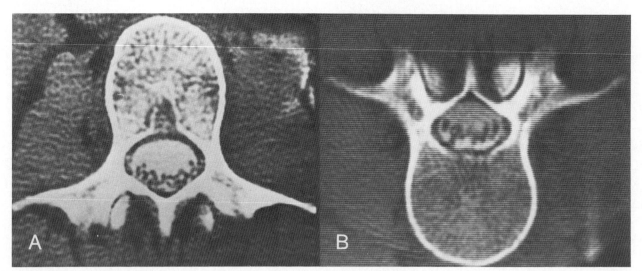

Figure 20.57.   A. Normal CTMM of cauda equina. Nerve roots lying in a relaxed arc in dependent portion of thecal sac. B. Same patient, prone CTMM. Nerve roots settle to a new dependent position.

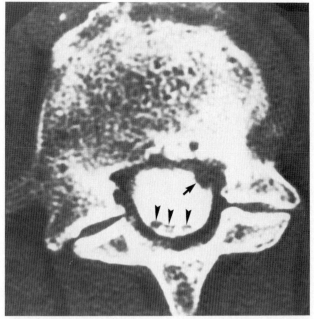

Figure 20.58.   Mild arachnoid scarring. Nerve roots fused to dura (*arrow*) mimic disc. Minor nerve root clumping (*arrowheads*).

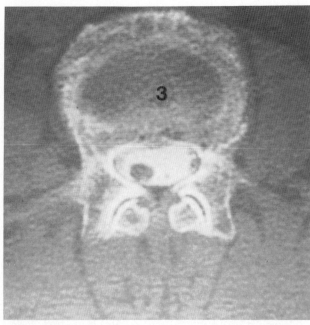

Figure 20.59.   Severe arachnoid scarring. Clumping of nerve roots simulate intradural masses.

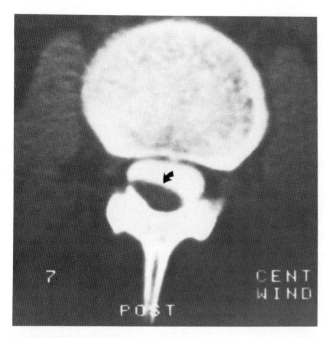

Figure 20.60. Severe arachnoid scarring. Entire cauda equina fused into neural mass (*arrow*).

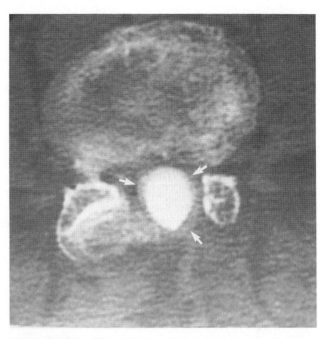

Figure 20.62. "Empty" thecal sac appearance of severe arachnoid scarring. The nerve roots are adherent to the dural wall (*white arrows*).

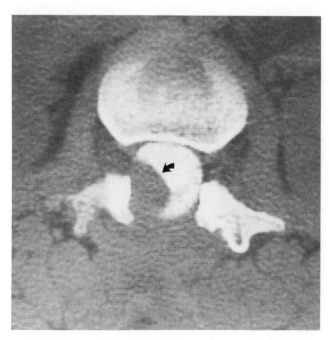

Figure 20.61. Severe arachnoid scarring mimicking a mass or lateral disc (*arrow*).

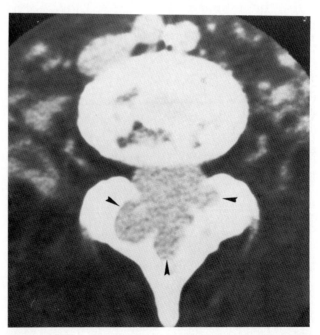

Figure 20.63. Severe dural ectasia in ankylosing spondylitis (*arrowheads*). CTMM revealing an empty thecal sac due to severe adhesive arachnoid scarring caused by chronic spondylitic inflammation. Nerve roots fused to dural margins and obliterated.

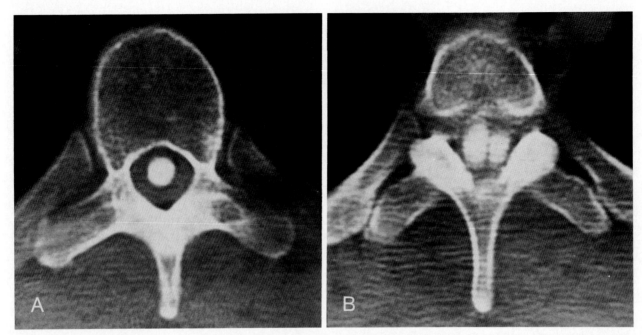

Figure 20.64. A. Thoracic syrinx created by severe obstructing arachnoid scarring. CTMM at 4 hours demonstrating a dilated central canal containing metrizamide. B. Same syrinx, lower level, revealing septation. CTMM at 4 hours. Cause: obstructing arachnoid scarring.

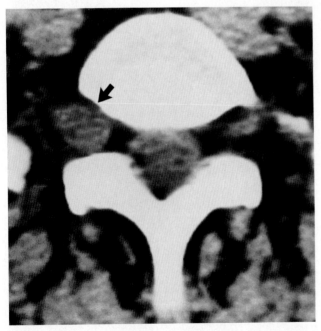

Figure 20.65. L4–5 neurilemmoma (*arrow*). Mimics disc, mass, focal abscess, meningocoele, etc.

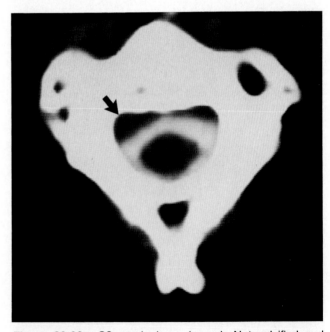

Figure 20.66. C2 meningioma (*arrow*). Not calcified and mimics soft disc.

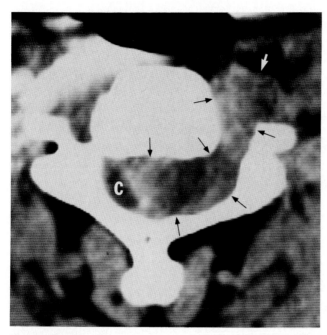

Figure 20.67. Chondrosarcoma (*arrows*). Spinal cord (*C*) markedly displaced to the right.

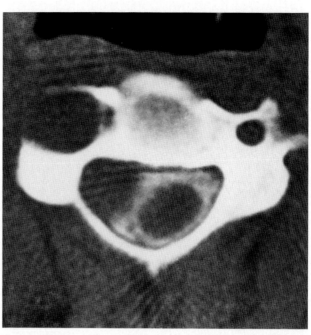

Figure 20.69. C5 neurilemmoma. CTMM simulates a right lateral soft disc. Note enlarged right foramen transversarium.

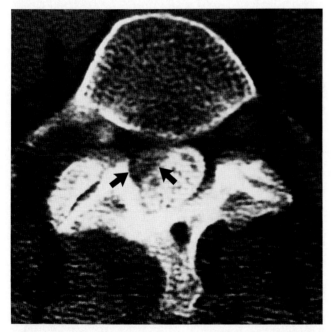

Figure 20.68. Intradural ependymoma of cauda equina (*arrows*) imitates a disc.

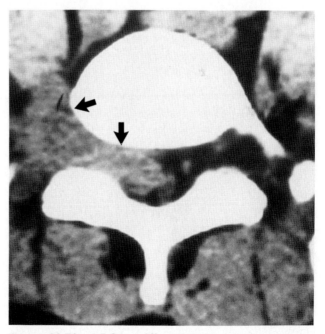

Figure 20.70. L5-S1 undifferentiated mesenchymal tumor (*arrows*). Disc mimic.

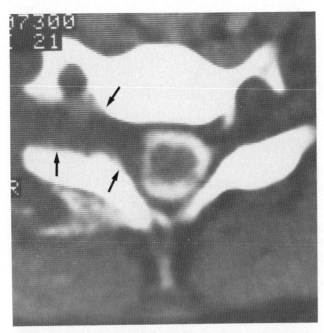

Figure 20.71. Cervical aneurysmal bone cyst (*arrows*). Contrast column compressed. Bone destruction (*lower arrows*) suggests tumor. CTMM.

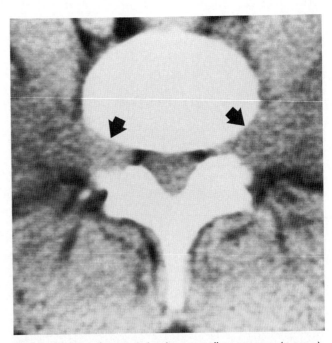

Figure 20.73. Bilateral lumbar neurilemmomas (*arrows*). Masses extending from foramina into the psoas muscles.

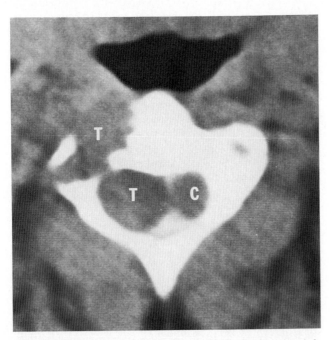

Figure 20.72. C4 chordoma (*T*). Cord (*C*) displaced to left. Note bone erosion and destruction. CTMM.

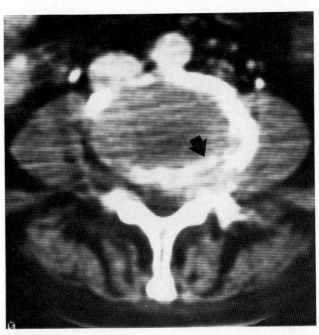

Figure 20.74. Left lateral disc space infection. L4–5 CT scan reveals a left lateral recess mass (*arrow*) simulating a disc. Bone destruction is typical of inflammatory origin.

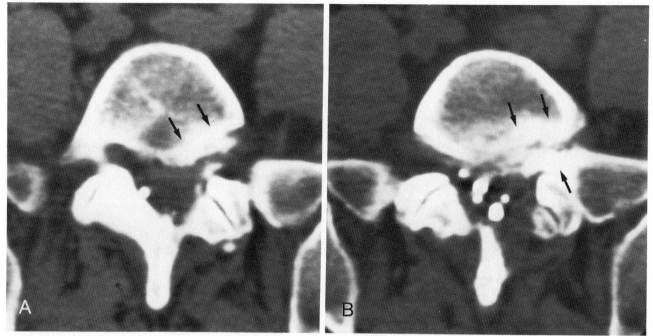

Figure 20.75.   A. Postoperative left lateral recess chronic asceptic discitis (*arrows*). Note reactive bone changes. B. CT scan 5 mm inferior. Reactive bone changes of "discitis" are more marked (*arrows*).

herniation. The patients are generally in the older age groups. Routine CT may not show a small hemorrhage unless scanned in the fresh state. These small hematomatas frequently are passed off erroneously as degenerative calcifications. The usual CT appearance is a vague area of increased density extending toward the lateral recess and the theca (Fig. 20.77) and may mimic a disc with very similar CT attenuation readings. A distended synovial cyst with hemorrhagic walls will be seen as a thin cyst-like density (Figs. 20.78–20.80) and simulates calcification.

If the clinical presentation can be tolerated, these traumatic events will subside and the CT may clear. Alarming clinical findings, myelographic changes, or the unique CT display may initiate immediate surgical exploration. The facet joint in question may demonstrate development of *vacuum phenomenon* on follow-up CT scanning (100).

B-9: SPINAL ARTERIOVENOUS MALFORMATION

Spinal arteriovenous communications are of two types: congenital and acquired. The congenital ones are *arteriovenous malformations* (AVM), whereas the acquired ones are *arteriovenous communications* (101). Previously, selected arteriography was considered the definitive diagnostic procedure for vascular mapping of spinal arteriovenous malformations. However, both selective and nonselective arteriograms may have serious sequellae (102, 103). *Digital subtraction angiography* coupled with *dynamic CT* scanning with *bolus technique*, offers a safer alternative (104).

The vascular architecture of spinal AVM may be bizarre with ipsilateral and contralateral communications involv-

ing both intraspinal and extraspinal vessels (101). Unusual vessels may be demonstrated, due to *arterialization of veins*. The intraspinal lesions generally are located on the dorsal or lateral aspects of the cord.

The spinal AVM is a rare lesion, often benign, occurring equally in both sexes, in all age groups, and presenting with a myriad of symptoms. These include: *bruit, cord ischemia* (steal?), spontaneous hemorrhage, and cardiac failure in children (101). These lesions rarely calcify and may enlarge the *foramina transversaria*.

Myelographic obstruction can create *serpentine nerve roots* often mistaken for dilated vessels. *Epidural varicosities* can simulate herniated discs (104, 105) at myelography, CT, or CTMM (Figs. 20.81 and 20.82).

B-10: NERVE ROOT AVULSION

Avulsion of a cervical nerve root is not uncommon and most frequently follows trauma to the shoulder. This neural injury represents intraspinal separation of a nerve root from the cord. A cuff of dura-arachnoid usually is torn from the thecal sac as well. Stump retraction and shrinkage creates a cavity which fills up with spinal fluid, forming a *traumatic meningocoele* (106–109). This cavity also may be termed a *pseudomeningocoele*. With time this sac, bathed in spinal fluid becomes lined with a smooth proliferating membrane, which may obliterate the cavity. Thus, although immediate myelography may demonstrate extraspinal extravasation of contrast material, a delayed myelogram or CT myelogram may not. Rarely, the nerve roots may be torn but the tougher dura-arachnoid remains intact (109).

The usual nerve roots involved are C5, 6, 7, 8, and T1.

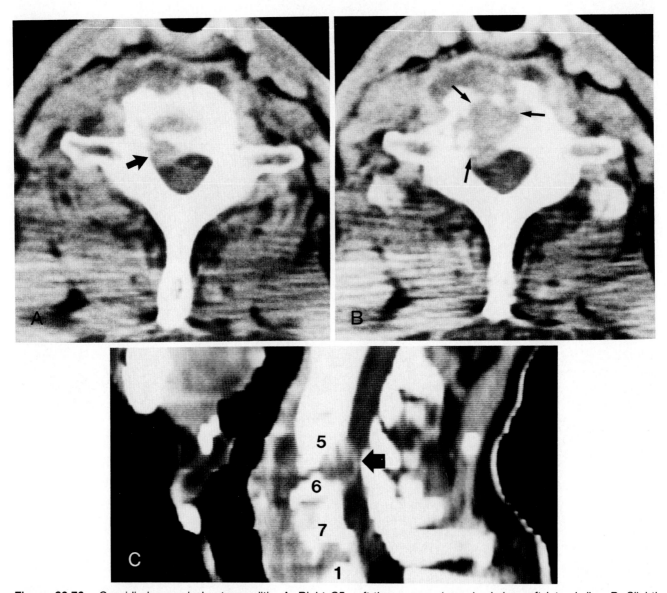

Figure 20.76. Coccidiodes cervical osteomyelitis. A. Right C5 soft-tissue mass (*arrow*) mimics soft lateral disc. B. Slightly lower scan reveals marked bone destruction (*arrows*). C. Sagittal reformation demonstrates Coccidioides disc space infection at C5–6 with epidural extension (*arrow*). C7-T1 also involved.

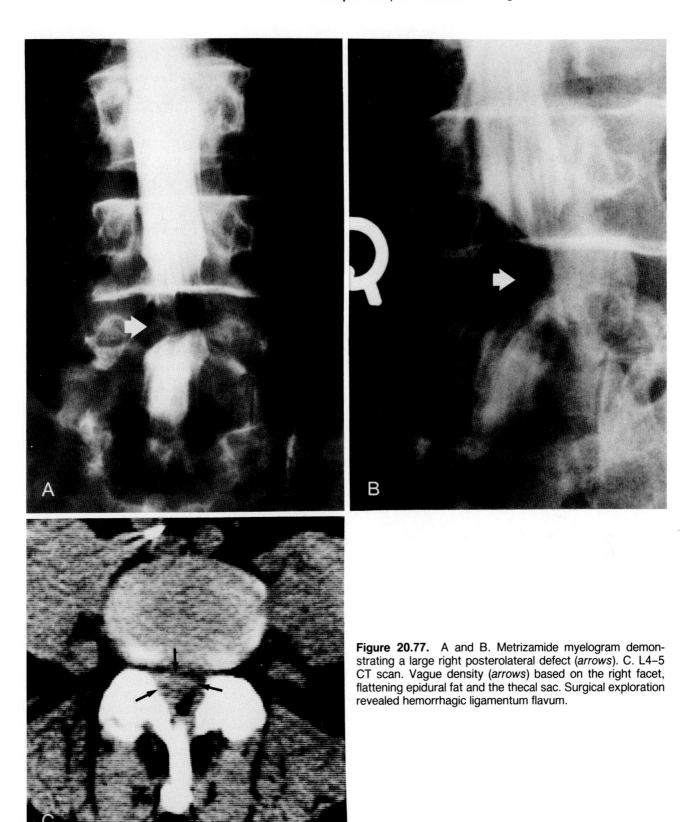

Figure 20.77. A and B. Metrizamide myelogram demonstrating a large right posterolateral defect (*arrows*). C. L4–5 CT scan. Vague density (*arrows*) based on the right facet, flattening epidural fat and the thecal sac. Surgical exploration revealed hemorrhagic ligamentum flavum.

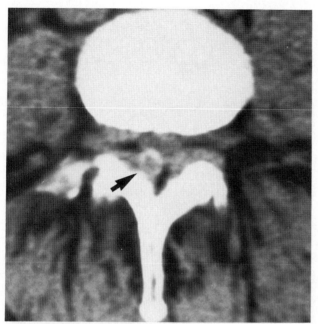

Figure 20.78. A 75-year-old male with severe sudden back pain. Hemorrhagic distended synovial cyst (*arrow*).

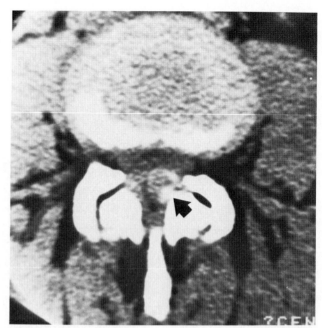

Figure 20.80. Distended synovial cyst with hemorrhagic areas within (*arrow*). Thickened ligamentum flavum with synovial and hemorrhagic components found at surgery.

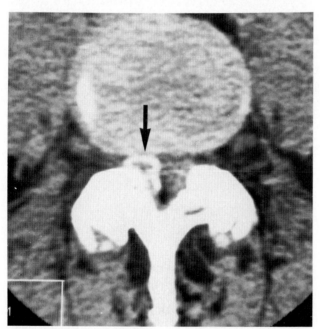

Figure 20.79. Hemorrhagic and distended synovial cyst (*arrow*) interpreted on CT scan as calcified ligamentum flavum. Surgery revealed degenerative ligamentum flavum with old hemorrhage; no calcifications found.

If T1 is torn, a *Horner's syndrome* may result due to involvement of sympathetic fibers to the stellate ganglion (108).

Treatment consists of expectant delay for approximately 6 months to permit spontaneous healing to occur. Periph-

eral nerve tears may respond to surgery. Central avulsions have no remedy.

CTMM or routine myelography can demonstrate patent pseudomeningocoeles with equal facility. Sealed tears and torn roots with intact dura-arachnoid are suggested by clinical deficits and normal diagnostic studies.

Spinal nerve roots are invested with a venous plexus (26). *Nerve root avulsions* produce *epidural hematomatas* of varying proportions. These hemorrhages may organize, fibrose, and persist as a mass lesion to indent or displace the thecal sac. Under these circumstances, a traumatic or degenerative disc herniation is simulated (Figs. 20.83 and 20.84).

Elongated normal cervical root pouches and lateral *intraspinal meningocoeles*, occasionally associated with neurofibromatosis, may mimic root avulsion (107). The clinical history and clinical levels may aid in this differentiation.

CONCLUSION

CT scanning of the spine has reorganized the approach to back disease completely. The ability to evaluate simultaneously and accurately the osseous, soft tissue, and neural elements of the vertebral column is an unprecedented advance. CTMM affords a still further detailed inspection of the cord, nerve roots, and spinal canal. Simultaneously, this study has been converted into a well-accepted outpatient procedure.

Paradoxically, many lesions displace the spinal cord, thecal sac, and nerve roots. Virtually all spinal masses may mimic or imitate the ubiquitous herniated disc. Fur-

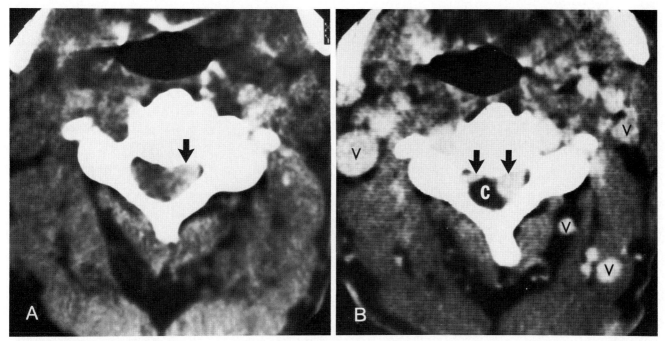

Figure 20.81. A. Cervical CT scan revealing a vague density (*arrow*) consistent with soft disc. B. After intravenous contrast, enhancement of enlarged intraspinal varices noted (*arrows*). This venous engorgement displaces the cord (*C*) to the right. Note enlarged extraspinal veins (*V*). An AVM was located in the extraspinal soft tissue (not shown).

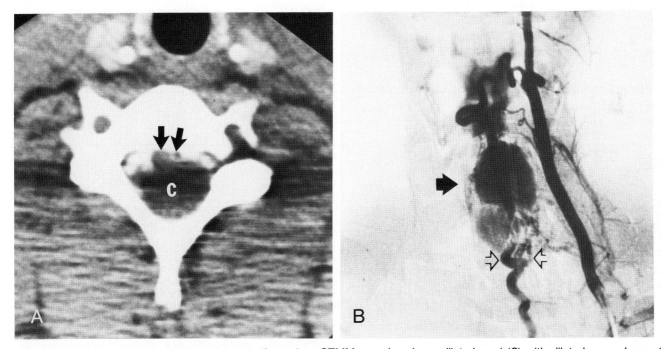

Figure 20.82. A. Intraspinal arteriovenous malformation. CTMM reveals a large dilated cord (*C*) with dilated, nonenhanced venous varices (*arrows*). B. Selected left vertebral angiogram demonstrates the intraspinal arteriovenous malformation (*arrow*). Note inferior dilated draining veins (*open arrows*).

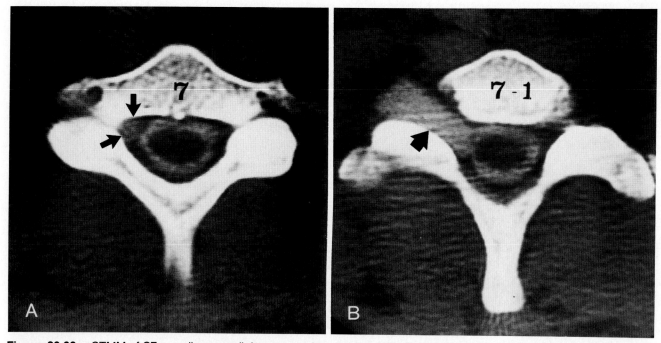

Figure 20.83. CTMM of C7 revealing a small dense mass (*arrows*) indenting the thecal sac. B. CTMM of C7-T1 reveals a large traumatic pseudomeningocoele (*arrow*) filled with metrizamide. At surgery, the right lateral defect of A was found to be an organized hematoma.

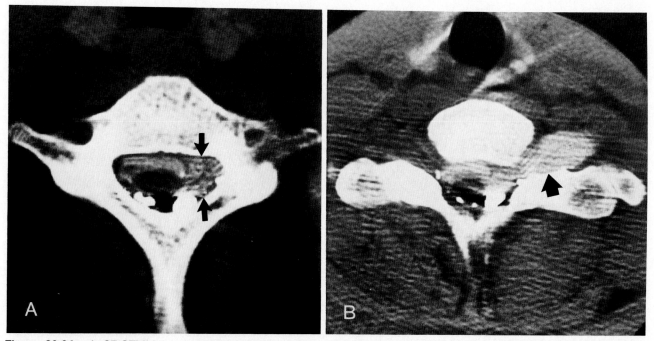

Figure 20.84. A. C7 CTMM demonstrating a left lateral dense mass (*arrows*) consistent with metrizamide enhancing organized hematoma. The thecal sac and cord are shifted to the right. B. C7-T1 CTMM. A large left traumatic pseudomeningocoele is noted (*arrow*). Surgery confirmed the hematoma and pseudomeningocoele.

ther CT exposure to the subtle, unusual, and rare lesion will, predictably, increase our sensitivity but possibly at the expense of specificity.

The judicious application of clinical and historical data, CTMM, CT attenuation measurement, image reformation, and CT guided-needle biopsy will ensure high levels of sensitivity and specificity.

A giant step forward in radiological diagnosis has been achieved.

References

1. Guillermo FC, Williams AL, et al: Computed tomography in sciatica. *Radiology* 137:433–437, 1980.
2. Heithoff KB: High-resolution computed tomography of the lumbar spine. *Postgrad Med* 70:193–228, 1981.
3. Raskin SP, Keating JW: Recognition of lumbar disk disease. *AJNR* 3:215–221, 1982.
4. Kieffer SA, Sherry RG, et al: Bulging lumbar intervetebral disk. *AJNR* 3:51–58, 1982.
5. Coin GC, Coin JT: Computed tomography of cervical disk disease. *J Comput Assist Tomogr* 5:275–280, 1981.
6. Williams AL, Haughton VM, et al: Computed tomography in the diagnosis of herniated nucleus pulposus. *Radiology* 135:95–99, 1980.
7. Adapon BD, Legada BD Jr, et al: CT-guided closed biopsy of the spine. *J Comput Assist Tomogr* 5:73–78, 1981.
8. Williams AL, Haughton VM, et al: Computed tomographic appearance of the bulging annulus. *Radiology* 142:403–408, 1982.
9. Hochman MS, Constantino P, et al: Calcified herniated thoracic disc diagnosed by computerized tomography. *J Neurosurg* 52:722–723, 1980.
10. Varughese G, Quartey GRC: Familial lumbar spinal stenosis with acute disc herniations. *J Neurosurg* 51:234–236, 1979.
11. Burton CV, Kirkaldy-Willis WH, et al: Causes of failure of surgery on the lumbar spine. *Clin Orthop Rel Res* 157:191–199, 1981.
12. Jacobs RR, McClain O, et al: Control of postlaminectomy scar formation. *Spine* 5:223–229, 1980.
13. Yong-Hing K, Reilly J, et al: Prevention of nerve root adhesions after laminectomy. *Spine* 5:59–64, 1980.
14. Benoist M, Ficat C, et al: Postoperative lumbar epiduro-arachnoiditis. *Spine* 5:432–436, 1980.
15. Meyer JD, Latchaw RE, et al: Computed tomography and myelography of the postoperative lumbar spine. *AJNR* 3:223–228, 1982.
16. Schubiger O, Valavanis A: CT differentiation between recurrent disc herniation and postoperative scar formation. *Neuroradiology* 22:251–254, 1982.
17. Faerber EN, Wolpert SM, et al: Computed tomography of spinal fractures. *J Comput Assist Tomogr* 3:657–661, 1979.
18. Coin GC, Pennink M, et al: Diving-type injury of the cervical spine. *J Comput Assist Tomogr* 3:362–372, 1979.
19. Brant-Zawadzki M, Jeffrey RB Jr, et al: High resolution CT of thoracolumbar fractures. *AJNR* 3:69–74, 1982.
20. Colley DP, Dunsker SB: Traumatic narrowing of the dorsolumbar spinal canal demonstrated by computer tomography. *Radiology* 129:95–98, 1978.
21. Hasue M, Kikuchi S, et al: Posttraumatic spinal stenosis of the lumbar spine. *Spine* 5:259–263, 1980.
22. Kestler OC: Spondylolysis and spondylolisthesis. Updated review. *NY State J Med* 79:700–708, 1979.
23. Taddonio RF Jr, McLachlan JE, et al: Consultation Corner. *Orthopedics* 1:233–235, 1978.
24. Privett JTJ, Middlemiss JH: Multiple lower lumbar spondylolyses. *Br J Radiol* 48:866–869, 1975.
25. Magora A, Schwartz A: Relation between low back pain and x-ray changes. *Scand J Rehab Med* 12:47–52, 1980.
26. Theron J, Monet J: *Spinal Phlebography.* Berlin, Springer-Verlag, 1978.
27. Dorwart RH, DeGroot J, et al: Computed tomography of the lumbosacral spine. University of California Printing Department, San Francisco, CA, May 1982.
28. Haughton VM, Syvertsen A, et al: Soft-tissue anatomy within the spinal canal as seen on computed tomography. *Radiology* 134:649–655, 1980.
29. Theron J, Houtteville JP, et al: Lumbar phlebography by catheterization of the lateral sacral and ascending lumbar veins with abdominal compression. *Neuroradiology* 11:175–182, 1976.
30. Rodichok LD, Harper GR, et al: Early diagnosis of spinal epidural metastases. *Am J Med* 70:1181–1187, 1981.
31. Federle MP, Moss AA, et al: Role of computed tomography in patients with "sciatica". *J Comput Assist Tomogr* 4:335–341, 1980.
32. Dorwart RH, Wara WM, et al: Complete myelographic evaluation of spinal metastases from medulloblastoma. *Radiology* 139:403–408, 1981.
33. Kim KS, Ho SU, et al: Spinal leptomeningeal infiltration by systemic cancer. *AJNR* 3:233–237, 1982.
34. James HE, Oliff M: Computed tomography in spinal dysraphism. *J Comput Assist Tomogr* 1:391–397, 1977.
35. Scotti G, Musgrave MA, et al: Diastematomyelia in children. *AJNR* 1:403–410, 1980.
36. Pang D, Wilberger JE, Jr: Tethered cord syndrome in adults. *J Neurosurg* 57:32–47, 1982.
37. Resjo IM, Harwood-Nash DC, et al: Computed tomographic metrizamide myelography in spinal dysraphism in infants and children. *J Comput Assist Tomogr* 2:549–558, 1978.
38. Arredondo F, Haughton VM, et al: The computed tomographic appearance of the spinal cord in diastematomyelia. *Radiology* 136:685–688, 1980.
39. Traub SP: Mass lesions in the spinal canal. *Sem Roentgenol* 7:240–258, 1972.
40. Nakagawa H, Huang YP, et al: Computed tomography of intraspinal and paraspinal neoplasms. *J Comput Assist Tomogr* 1:377–390, 1977.
41. Puljic S, Schechter MM: Multiple spinal canal meningiomas. *AJNR* 1:325–327, 1980.
42. Hammerschlag SB, Wolpert SM, et al: Computed tomography of the spinal canal. *Radiology* 121:361–367, 1976.
43. Yang WC, Zappulla R, et al: Neurolemmoma in lumbar intervertebral foramen. *J Comput Assist Tomogr* 5:904–906, 1981.
44. Handel S, Grossman R, et al: Computed tomography in the diagnosis of spinal cord astrocytoma. *J Comput Assist Tomogr* 2:226–228, 1978.
45. Spallone A, di Lorenzo N, et al: Spinal osteochondroma diagnosed by computed tomography. *Acta Neurochirurg* 58:105–114, 1981.
46. Quencer RM: Needle aspiration of intramedullary and intradural extramedullary masses of the spinal canal. *Radiology* 134:115–126, 1980.
47. Ono M, Russell WJ, et al: Ossification of the thoracic posterior longitudinal ligament in a fixed population. *Radiology* 143:469–474, 1982.
48. Murakami J, Russell WJ, et al: Computed tomography of posterior longitudinal ligament ossification. *J Comput Assist Tomogr* 6:41–50, 1982.
49. Yamamoto I, Kageyama N, et al: Computed tomography in ossification of the posterior longitudinal ligament in the cervical spine. *Surg Neurol* 12:414–418, 1979.
50. Hirabayashi K, Miyakawa J, et al: Operative results and postoperative progression of ossification among patients with ossification of cervical posterior longitudinal ligament. *Spine* 6:354–364, 1981.
51. Hyman RA, Merten CW, et al: Computed tomography in ossification of the posterior longitudinal spinal ligament. *Neuroradiology* 13:227–228, 1977.

52. Miyasaka K, Kaneda K, et al: Ossification of spinal ligaments causing thoracic radiculomyelopathy. *Radiology* 143:463–468, 1982.
53. Onofrio BM: Intervertebral discitis. *Clin Neurosurg* 27:481–515, 1980.
54. Postacchini F, Montanaro A: Tuberculosis epidural granuloma simulating a herniated lumbar disk. *Clin Orthop Rel Res* 148:182–185, 1980.
55. Buruma OJS, Craane J, et al: Vertebral osteomyleitis and epidural abcess due to mucormycosis. *Clin Neurol Neurosurg* 81:39–44, 1979.
56. Ettinger WJ Jr, Arnett FC Jr, et al: Intervertebral disc space infection. *John Hopkins Med J* 141:23–27, 1977.
57. Haughton VM, Eldevik OP, et al: A prospective comparison of computed tomography and myelography in the diagnosis of herniated lumbar disks. *Radiology* 142:103–110, 1982.
58. Williams AL, Haughton VM, et al: Computed tomography in the diagnosis of herniated nucleus pulposus. *Radiology* 135:95–99, 1980.
59. David CV, Balasubramaniam P: Acute osteomyelitis of the spine with paraplegia. *Aust NZ J Surg* 51:544–545, 1981.
60. Braithwaite PA, Lees RF: Vertebral hydatid disease. *Radiology* 140:763–766, 1981.
61. Russell NA, Heughan C: Pyogenic psoas abscess secondary to infection of the lumbar disc space. *Surg Neurol* 13:224–226, 1980.
62. Rengachary SS, Murphy D: Subarachnoid hematoma following lumbar puncture causing compression of the cauda equina. *J Neurosurg* 41:252–254, 1974.
63. Nagashima C, Yamaguchi T, et al: Clinical images. *J Comput Assist Tomogr* 5:586–587, 1981.
64. Kirkpatrick D, Goodman SJ: Combined subarachnoid and subdural spinal hematoma following spinal puncture. *Surg Neurol* 3:109–111, 1975.
65. Post MJD, Seminer DS, et al: CT diagnosis of spinal epidural hematoma. *AJNR* 3:190–192, 1982.
66. Pear BL: Spinal epidural hematoma. *AJR* 115:155–164, 1972.
67. Colletti PM, Siegel ME: Posttraumatic lumbar cerebrospinal fluid leak. *Clin Nuclear Med* 6:403–404, 1981.
68. Gass H, Goldstein AS, et al: Chronic postmyelogram headache isotopic demonstration of dural leak and surgical cure. *Arch Neurol* 25:168, 1971.
69. Silverman ED, Davis WB, et al: Spinal cerebrospinal fluid leak demonstrated by retrograde myeloscintigraphy. *Clin Nuclear Med* 6:27–29, 1981.
70. Postacchini F, Montanaro A: Extreme lateral herniations of lumbar disks. *Clin Orthop Rel Res* 138:222–226, 1979.
71. Williams AL, Haughton VM, et al: CT recognition of lateral lumbar disk herniation. *AJNR* 3:211–213, 1982.
72. Risius B, Modic MT, et al: Sector computed tomographic spine scanning in the diagnosis of lumbar nerve root entrapment. *Radiology* 143:109–114, 1982.
73. Ciric I, Mikhael MA, et al: The lateral recess syndrome. *J Neurosurg* 53:433–443, 1980.
74. Dohn DF: Complications of lumbar disc surgery. In: Hardy RW (Ed): *Seminars in Neurological Surgery; Lumbar Disc Disease*; Raven Press, New York, 1982, pp. 165–176.
75. Adapon BD, Legada BD, et al: CT-guided closed biopsy of the spine. *J Comput Assist Tomogr* 5:73–78, 1981.
76. Damgaard-Pederson K: Neuroblastoma follow-up by computed tomography. *J Comput Assist Tomogr* 3:274–275, 1979.
77. White JG III, et al: Surgical treatment of 63 cases of conjoined nerve roots. *J Neurosurg* 56:114–118, 1982.
78. Bouchard JM, Copty M, et al: Preoperative diagnosis of conjoined roots anomaly with herniated lumbar disks. *Surg Neurol* 10:229–231, 1978.
79. Epstein JA, Carras R, et al: Conjoined lumbosacral nerve roots. *J Neurosurg* 55:585–589, 1981.
80. Fox AJ, et al: Myelographic cervical nerve root deformities. *Radiology* 116:355–361, 1975.
81. Nathan H, et al: Multiple meningeal diverticula and cyst associated with duplications of the sheaths of spinal nerve posterior roots. *J Neurosurg* 47:68–72, 1977.
82. Benner B, Ehni G: Spinal arachnoiditis. *Spine* 3:40–44, 1978.
83. Quiles M, Marchisello PJ, et al: Lumbar adhesive arachnoiditis. *Spine* 3:45–50, 1978.
84. Brodsky AE: Cauda equina arachnoiditis. *Spine* 3:51–60, 1978.
85. Little JR, Bryerton B: Chronic lumbar arachnoiditis. In: Hardy RW (Ed): *Seminars in Neurological Surgery; Lumbar Disc Disease*. Raven Press, New York, 1982, pp. 277–286.
86. Johnson JDH, Matheny JB: Microscopic lysis of lumbar adhesive arachnoiditis. *Spine* 3:36–39, 1978.
87. Burton CV: Lumbosacral arachnoiditis. *Spine* 3:24–30, 1978.
88. Nainkin L: Arachnoiditis ossificans. *Spine* 3:83–86, 1978.
89. Auld AW: Chronic spinal arachnoiditis. *Spine* 3:88–94, 1978.
90. Skalpe IO: Adhesive arachnoiditis following lumbar myelography. *Spine* 3:61–64, 1978.
91. Haughton VM, Ho KC: Effect of blood on arachnoiditis from aqueous myelographic contrast media. *AJNR* 3:373–374, 1982.
92. Kramer LD, Krouth GJ: Computerized tomography. *Arch Neurol* 35:116–118, 1978.
93. Armstrong EA, Harwood-Nash DCF, et al: CT of neuroblastomas and ganglioneuromas in children. *AJNR* 3:401–406, 1982.
94. Schwimer SR, Bassett LW, et al: Giant cell tumor of the cervicothoracic spine. *AJR* 136:63–67, 1981.
95. Kamano S, Amano K, et al: The contributions of computed tomography in the choice of an anterolateral approach, for treating cervical dumb-bell tumors. *Neurochirurgia* 23:121–125, 1980.
96. Baleriaux-Waha D, Terwinghe G, et al: The value of computed tomography for the diagnosis of hourglass tumors of the spine. *Neuroradiology* 14:31–32, 1977.
97. Bullock R: Unusual presentation of pyogenic spinal epidural abscess. *SA Med J* 9:723–724, 1982.
98. Beamer YB, et al: Hypertrophied ligamentum flavum. *Arch Surg* 106:289–292, 1973.
99. Ramani PS, Perry RH, et al: Role of ligamentum flavum in the symptomatology of prolapsed lumbar invertebral discs. *J Neurol Neurosurg Psychiatr* 38:550–557, 1975.
100. Mani JR: (unpublished data).
101. Lawson TL, Newton TH: Congenital cervical arteriovenous malformations. *Radiology* 97:565–570, 1970.
102. Di Chiro G, Rieth KG, et al: Digital subtraction angiography and dynamic computed tomography in the evaluation of arteriovenous malformations and hemangioblastomas of the spinal cord. *J Comput Assist Tomogr* 6:655–670, 1982.
103. Di Chiro G, Wener L: Angiography of the spinal cord. *J Neurosurg* 39:1–29, 1973.
104. Di Chiro G, Doppman JL, et al: Computed tomography of spinal cord arteriovenous malformations. *Radiology* 123:351–354, 1977.
105. Cohen I: Extradural varix simulating herniated nucleus pulposus. *J Mt Sinai Hosp* 8:136, 1941.
106. Epstein BS: Low back pain associated with varices of epidural veins simulating herniation of nucleus pulposus. *AJR* 57:736, 1947.
107. Varley WJ: The importance of cervical myelography in cervical and upper thoracic nerve root avulsion. *Radiology* 76:376–380, 1961.
108. Epstein BS: *The Spine, A Radiological Text Book and Atlas*. 4th ed., Lea and Febiger, Philadelphia, 1976, pp. 578–582.
109. Shapiro R: *Myelography*. 2nd ed., Year Book Publishers, Chicago, 1978, pp. 195–198.
110. Jaeger R, Whiteley WH: Avulsion of the brachial plexus. *JAMA* 153:644, 1953.

CHAPTER TWENTY-ONE

Computed Tomography of Cervical Disc Disease (Herniation and Degeneration)

C. GENE COIN, M.D.

Computed tomography (CT), which has revolutionized the diagnosis of intracranial disease in less than a decade, also has made substantial progress in spinal diagnosis in the last few years (1). CT is rapidly becoming the preferred method for diagnosis of lumbar disc herniation (1–9). The ability of CT to demonstrate very small cervical disc herniations has been shown in laboratory animals (10) as well as in humans (11, 12). This capability is further documented here along with a discussion of the clinical syndromes associated with this condition. Precise anatomical determination of the herniation site, size of herniation, and capacity of the vertebral canal, uniquely available by CT, are critical factors affecting proper medical or surgical treatment of these syndromes.

DISCUSSION

Cervical disc disease affects the lives of a major portion of the world's population. This illness may be characterized by a gradual onset of symptoms spanning the adult life or can occur as a single event without warning or may follow acute injury. The symptoms might be slight and intermittent or disabling and progressive. Significant herniation may be so small that it is undetectable or so large that diagnosis is obvious. Below are typical clinical examples of cervical disc disease.

Cervical Disc Disease—"A Scenario"

Patient 1. A 17-year-old male football player suffers a minor injury during a scrimmage. There is acute neck pain, muscle spasm, and mild "tingling" in the right shoulder and arm. Symptoms gradually subside over the next few days without any neurological deficit.

Patient 2. A 28-year-old male engineer wakes one morning with a painful "crick" in his neck accompanied by muscle spasm and "tingling" sensation down his right arm. He sees the family physician who prescribes analgesics and physiotherapy. Pain varies in severity during the next few weeks. The patient is referred to a neurosurgeon. A myelogram confirms the clinical diagnosis of a C6–7 disc herniation. The patient then follows a program of conservative treatment.

Patient 3. A 45-year-old consultant has mild symptoms of neck stiffness and pain and complains of "popping" in the neck, headaches, and soreness in his shoulders made worse by tension. During the next 10 years, he has several episodes of severe neck pain and muscle spasm. An orthopaedist prescribes muscle relaxants, physiotherapy, and cervical traction. This treatment gives reasonable relief.

Patient 4. A 65-year-old retiree suffers from bouts with "arthritis" of the neck over a period of years. Initially

minimal neurological findings become disastrous and disabling with progressive quadriparesis. Extensive surgical decompression of the cervical cord is required.

These cases illustrate typical phases of cervical disc disease. In fact, these might represent the history of just 1 patient with this disease at various stages. Medical or surgical management varies according to the phase of the illness observed at any given time. Initially, the young man injured on the football field and seen by the team physician would be treated for acute muscle and ligament injury. This period of acute illness frequently is followed by a relatively long quiescent period lasting years. The only complaint might be occasional neck pain and stiffness. During this time, the lower cervical intervertebral discs would be undergoing a complex biochemical alteration. A degenerative process dehydrates the nucleus pulposus causing loss of elasticity and impairs the ability to transmit shock and stress evenly to the anulus and other support structures of the disc. This increase in mechanical stress accompanied by biochemical change eventually causes structural weakness of the anulus. Clefts and fissures appear. Calcification and alteration of the collagen content of the nucleus occur. Small fragments of nuclear material may herniate slightly causing a localized inflammatory reaction.

The next major event may be acute rupture of a substantial fragment of the now abnormal nucleus pulposus into the surrounding tissues. Symptoms and neurological sequelae at this point depend upon the location of the herniation and relationship to the spinal cord, nerve roots, and associated vascular structures. Severity of the clinical findings are influenced considerably by adequacy of the spinal canal and mobility of the spine and cord. The neurologist and neurosurgeon seeing the patient diagnose acute herniation of the disc. Management at this time depends upon severity of clinical findings, response to conservative treatment, the medical condition of the patient, as well as the training and experience of the physician.

The next stages of this disease most frequently are characterized by periods of exacerbation and remission. There is continued physical and biochemical derangement of the nucleus pulposus and anulus of the discs accompanied by fissures and by deterioration and fragmentation of the nucleus with small herniations of nuclear and anular material (13). Vascular granulation tissue may intrude into the defects (14). Inflammatory changes in the adjacent tissue result in calcification and marginal hypertrophic bony spurs (15). Etiology of disc degeneration, although not completely understood, is most frequently associated with trauma and aging (13, 16–18). In degeneration, the biochemical changes result in dehydration of the nucleus and alteration in its shock absorbing ability (19–22). Resultant abnormal stresses are transmitted to the annulus, facet joints, and joints of Luschka. These joints also deteriorate producing hypertrophic degenerative changes of varying degrees. Symptoms and neurological findings formerly produced by disc herniation are replaced by a symptom complex influenced by arthritic changes and marginal spurring affecting nerve roots and spinal cord in addition to symptoms produced by new herniations. Volume of both intradiscal material and herniated cartilage gradually is reduced by autogenous proteolytic enzymes (23). Partial fusion of adjacent vertebral bodies may occur as a result of hypertrophic bridging and degeneration of facet joints. Former symptoms may change or disappear as a result of these processes. Different cervical discs may be at various stages of herniation and degeneration simultaneously. This results in a puzzling complexity of symptoms and findings.

At the time of death, the cervical spinal cord may be ridged by several degenerated and protruding discs with their accompanying marginal hypertrophic changes. The spinal canal will be compromised further by marginal spurring from the uncovertebral joints of Luschka and by thickening of the ligamenta flava. Intervertebral foraminae may be narrowed by disc space collapse and hypertrophic changes. Vertebral arteries sometime afflicted by coexisting arteriosclerosis are narrowed further or even occluded by the adjacent degenerative process.

Gross changes generally increase in severity from C3–4 to C6–7. Disc degenerative disease will be most severe at C6–7 and C5–6 but, not infrequently, also will be present at C4–5 and less commonly at C3–4. The gross appearance of the intervertebral disc at C2–3 may be remarkably normal with only minimal degenerative changes. The disc at C7–T1 may also be nearly normal in appearance. All discs show microscopic evidence of degeneration and biochemical abnormality (20). Differentiation between anulus and nucleus is less marked or nonexistent. Calcification of the nucleus pulposus frequently seen radiographically in the degenerated disc (24, 25) is seen much more frequently by CT. The anulus fibrosus, anterior and posterior longitudinal ligaments, and ligamentum flavum may be calcified (26) (Case 9). Disc volume is reduced. Air frequently is present in the disc (27). Gas also may be seen in the facet joints. Final pathological diagnosis is "cervical spondylosis."

TECHNIQUE

The patient is examined in the supine position. A digital radiographic ScoutView* performed by the CT scanner is first obtained in the lateral projection (Fig. 21.4). This

---

* Manufactured by General Electric Co. Studies are performed with a GE CT/T 8800 whole body scanner.

digital radiograph then serves as the basis for correct positioning of the CT slices which are obtained in the axial plane through the disc spaces approximately parallel to the vertebral body horizontal plates at the level of each disc space to be examined. Precise positioning of thin sections in the disc space is required for accurate diagnosis. Three contiguous slices 1.5-mm thick usually are needed for each disc examined. The remainder of the study of the cervical spine is completed by contiguous thick sections (5-mm or 10-mm each).

No injections of either intravenous or intraspinal contrast material are utilized for the diagnosis of disc herniations. Epidural fat and spinal fluid with absorption values in the range of −100 and +10 HU, respectively (scale ± 1000), provide excellent contrast with disc herniations which are usually in the range of +100 HU.

Present technique is to examine all disc spaces from C2–3 to C7–T1. (There is no disc space at C1–2.) Cervical traction and shoulder traction are usually utilized to immobilize the patient and to reduce artifacts from the shoulders in the lower cervical region. Shoulder artifacts are most troublesome at the level of the C7-T1 disc; however, rarely do they prevent a diagnostic study and, in general, are less troublesome technically than in lateral radiography of the cervical-thoracic junction during myelography. Patient motion will degrade the CT image substantially. Accurate examination may not be possible in an uncooperative patient; but unsatisfactory studies for this reason are uncommon because the complete study is done in the supine position without changing position of the patient. Optimum quality of disc spaces on the present scanner is obtained with a 10-second exposure. Preferably, respiration is suspended during examination of disc spaces although results in this area are almost as good if quiet respiration is maintained throughout the examination. Faster scanners capable of acquiring the same amount of data in 2 seconds or less are now available which will make the technique faster and easier. After data are acquired, the CT image is reconstructed for optimal contrast and then also is reconstructed for maximum spatial resolution. Electronic images are used for critical diagnostic interpretation. Accurate measurements of canal diameter and shape are obtained from sections that are perpendicular to the long axis of the vertebral canal. Size and density of herniations are measured by region-of-interest (ROI) programs of the computer display. These measurements provide an objective basis for diagnosis and also are useful in evaluation of treatment results.

Providing information not otherwise obtainable except by surgery or autopsy, CT is useful in the study of degenerative disease and disc herniation, giving insight into age and chronicity of herniation—a basis used by the author for classification of this disease.

Classification of Cervical Disc Herniation

Considerable variation in terminology is found in the literature dealing with cervical disc herniation. A simple form of classification of these herniations is listed below:

I. Acute herniation of the normal intervertebral disc.

II. "Bulging" disc.
III. Acute herniation of the degenerated disc.
IV. Chronic herniation of the degenerated disc.
V. Cervical spondylosis.

TYPE I. ACUTE HERNIATION OF THE NORMAL INTERVERTEBRAL DISC

This is the least frequent herniation. This classification may be reserved for herniations caused by a severe injury. Nearly all occur in young patients. The normal intervertebral disc rarely ruptures. When present acute herniation of the normal disc is associated with severe neck injury and usually is overshadowed by other evidence of bone and soft-tissue injury. Real incidence of herniation in these cases is unknown because myelography, previously required for diagnosis, is not indicated routinely in these cases of acute severe neck injury. Even when indicated, myelography may be difficult to accomplish in the severely injured patient and, therefore, often not done. In some of these cases, the evidence for herniation of the normal disc is conclusive, i.e., demonstration of herniation immediately after diving injury (28), vehicular accident (15), or other severe neck injury in young patients. In these cases, radiographs of the cervical spine show absence of hypertrophic changes. CT demonstrates that herniation is only disc material without evidence of calcification or "vacuum" intervertebral disc. Acute herniation of the normal disc may occur in severe flexion or extension injuries of the cervical spine. Severe vertical compression injuries with "burst" fractures are accompanied by herniation of the nucleus into the vertebral body through the inferior end plate (29). When herniation does not occur immediately, such injuries may initiate premature degeneration of the disc resulting in herniation at a later date.

TYPE II. BULGING DISC

This term means the protrusion of a bulging anulus and is a sign of disc degeneration. The distinction between bulging lumbar disc and herniation beyond the anulus may be shown by CT (7). The cervical herniations are similar but smaller in size. A bulging disc will present as a simple increase in convexity of the anulus protruding midline of the anterior margin of the vertebral canal (Fig. 21.5a). A relative barrier to posterolateral disc protrusion is provided by the uncinate processes and joints of Luschka (15). Calcification or air may be present in the nucleus or anulus indicating degeneration of the disc. Macroscopic and microscopic examination may show radiating ruptures, fissures, and small herniations of degenerated nucleus into the anulus, but there is no herniation beyond the anulus by definition in this classification.

The CT appearance is that of a "bulge" no more than 2 mm beyond the normal confines of the disc; larger lesions usually indicate herniation of nuclear material through the anulus. By conventional myelography, Type II lesions rarely are visible. Discography may be positive due to tears in the anulus but also may be negative if the bulging anulus is intact. These small lesions are of little immediate clinical importance because the symptoms, if any, are minor unless accompanied by spinal stenosis. Their importance lies in the potential for future protrusion.

Degeneration and weakness of the anulus make the disc "ripe" for rupture. These "discs at risk" represent a vast reservoir of potential disasters ready to befall an unsuspecting population.

TYPE III. ACUTE HERNIATION OF THE DEGENERATED DISC

This is a sequel to Type II lesions. Degenerated nuclear material is herniated acutely through a weakened anulus.

Herniation may occur in patients who present no history of trauma (awakening in the morning and becoming progressively more symptomatic) or in cases with an obvious injury to the neck. Hypertrophic spurs, an indicator of prior herniation and chronicity, are generally not present in these or Type II cases although several types of herniations are often present at different levels in the same patient. Calcification may or may not be visibly present in the herniation by CT. Absorption values will be generally higher than in the normal disc, however, these values are variable. Surgeons frequently refer to this type as a "soft" herniation.

TYPE IV. CHRONIC HERNIATION OF THE DEGENERATED DISC

In this condition, the soft herniation has been transformed into a "hard" herniation accompanied by calcification of ligaments and marginal hypertrophic changes. In time, components of the herniation may be absorbed partially or almost completely; on the other hand, they may be converted to hard nodules of bone firmly attached to the underlying vertebral body. This type herniation is an essential precursor to the next class, "cervical spondylosis."

TYPE V. CERVICAL SPONDYLOSIS

This term is subject to variability in definition. Some authorities consider that chronic degenerative disease of the cervical disc and cervical spondylosis are synonyms whereas others also include osteitis deformans, degenerative arthritis, and hypertrophic arthritis (30).

A practical definition of spondylosis is the anatomical condition of narrow spinal canal produced by chronic degeneration and herniation of one or more cervical intervertebral discs with hypertrophic changes. This condition usually is accompanied by degenerative changes in the facet joints, joints of Luschka, and spinal ligaments—particularly the anterior and posterior longitudinal ligaments and the ligamenta flava. Degeneration and chronic herniation of cervical discs at one or more levels is always present in this condition, however, spondylosis may be present without clinical evidence of myelopathy.

The separation between these various classifications is not always distinct. Various types may occur in the same patient. Classification is much less important than the effect on the canal—particularly whether or not cord and nerve roots are compromised.

TOTAL CERVICAL HERNIATIONS SHOWN BY CT ■ vs □ MYELOGRAPHY

KEY

■ BLACK — Herniations shown by CT

□ WHITE (Open bar) — Herniations shown by Myelography

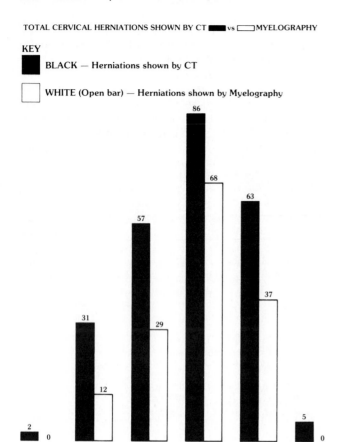

Table 21.1.

ETIOLOGY AND INCIDENCE

Degeneration of the Disc

Degeneration of the intervertebral disc is the most important precursor to herniation of all types except Type I (acute herniation of the normal intervertebral disc). Because degenerated discs are seen with great frequency in the aged, it might be assumed that aging is the cause of degeneration; however, this is still unproven. High incidence should not be confused with normalcy. Association does not imply cause. The etiology of disc degeneration remains an intriguing question only partially answered.

Complete review of incidence and the biochemical and structural changes that occur in this process will not be undertaken here. Informative sources on this subject, which are themselves extensively referenced, are listed here (12, 14, 15, 17, 19–22, 24, 30–34). Degeneration of the nucleus may begin in the 2nd or 3rd decade. This involves a complex process with alteration of the collagen content and water retaining ability of the nucleus. Similarly, biochemical and structural changes occur in the anulus. Small cracks and fissures form in these structures. Chondrification of the disc occurs with loss of distinction between annulus and nucleus. Calcification frequently appears within the nucleus. Small ruptures of nuclear material into the fissures and into the anulus and uncovertebral joints may appear. There is a loss of disc volume and bulging of the anulus. Weakness of the anulus permits rupture.

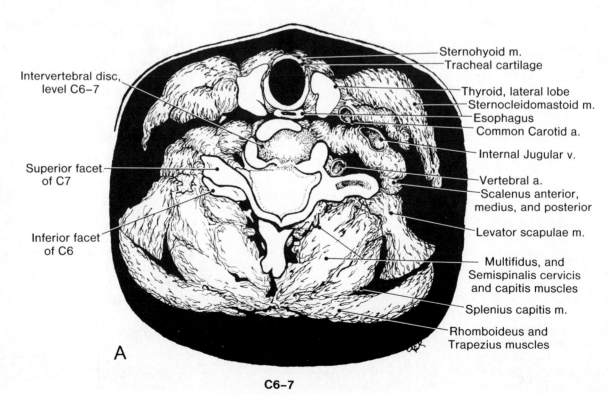

C6–7

Figure 21.1. A. Schematic illustration of normal C6–7 level.

TRAUMA AS AN INSTIGATOR OF DISC DEGENERATION AND HERNIATION

It previously was noted that the normal disc rarely herniates. On the other hand, herniation of the abnormal degenerated disc is common.

History of a specific traumatic event will be obtained in 10–30% of cases (35). It is reasonable to assume that trauma, even though mild, may play a part in the actual event when a degenerated nucleus pulposus herniates through a weakened or fissured anulus fibrosus to produce symptoms. The importance of trauma in the etiology of degenerative disc disease has been emphasized by multiple reports since 1886 (36). Hohl (37) suggested that there was an increased incidence of disc degeneration in individuals who suffered a severe extension injury of the spine. McNabb (38) noted the frequency of continued neck pain after extension-type acceleration injuries of the spine. Jackson (15) implicated trauma in 90% of cervical spine disorders.

Premature degeneration of cervical discs after trauma may be documented by CT (Case 6). Although there are other factors in degeneration of these discs, trauma is one of the major causes.

Autopsy evidence may indicate degenerative changes at all levels (20), but radiographic and clinical studies indicate a predilection for the lower cervical discs. C6–7, C5–6, and C4–5 discs are most frequently abnormal with C3–4 and C7-T1 being uncommonly affected and C2–3 being rarely affected. This distribution is documented in the author's series studied by CT (Table 21.1). Myelographic and CT distribution of cervical disc herniation indicate a similar distribution of herniation. In this series, CT is shown to be more sensitive for this diagnosis. Of 468 cervical CT studies performed, 144 also had myelograms. Two hundred forty-four herniations were shown by CT scans, and 146 herniations were shown by myelograms. CT and myelographic diagnoses were identical in 122 of these herniations. Only 25 herniations were demonstrated by myelography that were not diagnosed by CT. CT showed 127 herniations that were not demonstrated by myelography. Many small herniations shown by CT were not thought to be of immediate surgical significance. On the other hand, some of these small lesions were judged to be responsible for significant symptoms or neurological findings even though not seen by myelography. *Fifty-three patients had surgical exploration. At operation, the CT findings were confirmed in 47 cases and the myelographic findings in 45 cases.*

This series does not yet warrant a definitive statement regarding the relative clinical efficacy of each technique, but the series does support the impression that CT is capable of more accurate anatomical diagnosis of cervical disc herniation than radiographic myelography.

The distribution of disc disease in the cervical spine is

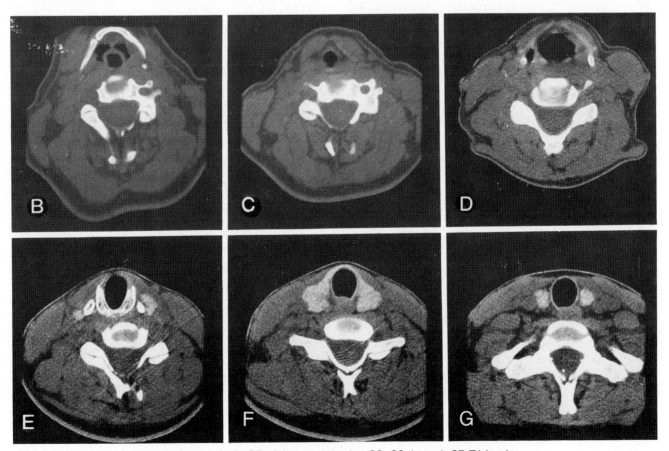

Figure 21.1.   B–G. CT of the normal spine C2–C3 through C7-T1 levels.

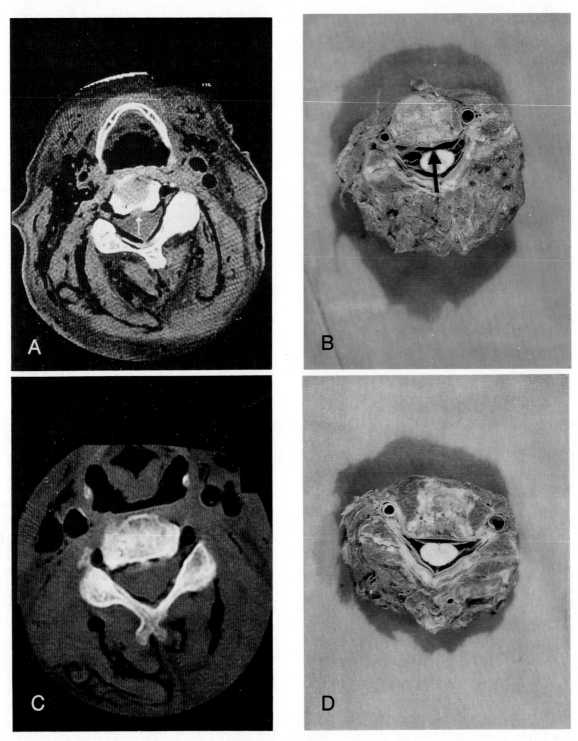

Figure 21.2.

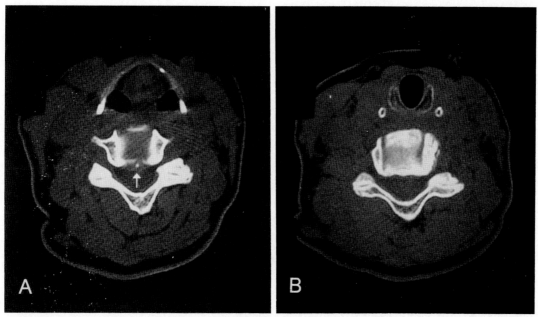

Figure 21.3.

similar in all types and has obvious implications regarding physical stress, mobility, and susceptibility to trauma. Similar incidence related to age and location of degenerative disc disease has been shown in the lower lumbar discs (14).

The use of this technique (CT diagnosis of cervical disc herniation) is reported here with representative cases. For comparison, a series of normal CT scans at the disc levels from C2–3 through C7-T1 (Fig. 21.1B–G), precede the abnormal cases. An artist's illustration of the C6–7 level (Fig. 21.1A) accompanies the CT spine images for anatomical correlation.

CASE 1. SMALL DISC HERNIATION AT C3–4, POSTMORTEM ANATOMICAL STUDY

A very small central herniation of a degenerated disc at C3–4 is shown by postmortem CT scan (Fig. 21.2A). Anatomical dissection confirms the CT findings (Fig. 21.2B). A degenerated disc without herniation is shown for comparison (Fig. 21.2C and D). The herniation measures only 2.7 mm in diameter. Herniations of this size are not likely to be clinically significant in the presence of an adequate spinal canal; however, the CT capability to demonstrate even these small herniations is evident. A small punctate nidus of calcification within the herniation is an interesting finding in this study and has been frequently observed in the author's clinical cases (Fig. 21.3A). Larger calcifications are also frequently noted on CT (Figs. 21.5B). Calcifications within cartilaginous herniations are seen much more frequently on CT than by standard radiography. Calcification within the intervertebral disc first described by Luschka in 1858 (25) and present in up to 71% of all spines in Schmorl's Institute (24) increasing in frequency with age is an indicator of degeneration of the disc.

CASE 2. SMALL C4–5 DISC HERNIATION

A 52-year-old female developed severe posterior cervical pain radiating into both arms after a recent minor neck injury. Radiographs of the cervical spine were unremarkable. Neurological examination was essentially normal. CT demonstrates a small central disc herniation containing a calcific nidus at C4–5 (Fig. 21.3A, *arrow*). The anteroposterior (AP) diameter of the spinal canal is reduced measuring 8 mm at this level. Note the similarity between this herniation and the postmortem study (Fig. 21.2A). The CT appearance of a nonherniated degenerated C5–6 disc in this patient is shown for comparison (Fig. 21.3B). The spinal canal is relatively narrow, measuring 9 mm in midsagittal AP diameter. Moderate degenerative changes involve the facet joints contributing to narrowing of the intervertebral canal at this level.

CASE 3. TYPE III HERNIATION AT C6–7

A 59-year-old man presented with neck pain, weakness of the right arm and right leg, dyspraxia and numbness of the left leg, and numbness of the left side of the body. CT demonstrates a small soft disc herniation at C6–7 level (Fig. 21.4A). Digital radiograph shows precise positioning of CT slice (Fig. 21.4B). A radiographic myelogram (Fig. 21.4C, D, E) was normal failing to demonstrate the C6–7 herniation readily shown by CT; however, the lateral view was of limited technical quality in the lower cervical region due to inability to clear the C6–7 disc space from the shoulders (a common radiographic problem in shortnecked individuals). This problem is much less troublesome in the axial image provided by CT.

CASE 4. C5–6 DISC HERNIATION WITH SPINAL STENOSIS, TYPE V

A 44-year-old male presented with neck pain radiating down both arms to the elbow of 3 years' duration. Recently, the pain became more severe and was accompanied by a tingling sensation in the right arm. Pantopaque myelogram shows a partial block with slight apparent widening of the spinal cord image centered at C5–6 junction (Fig. 21.5A). CT scan demonstrates a calcified disc herniation at C5–6 with significant stenosis of the spinal

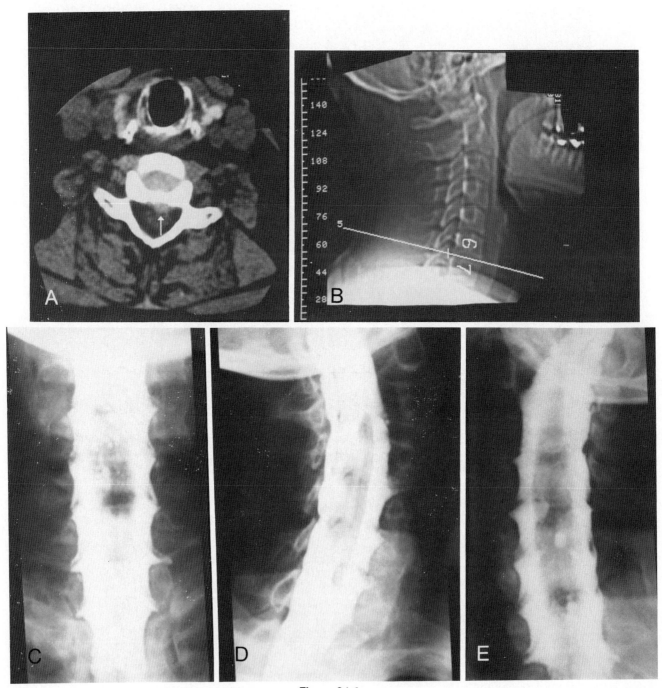

Figure 21.4.

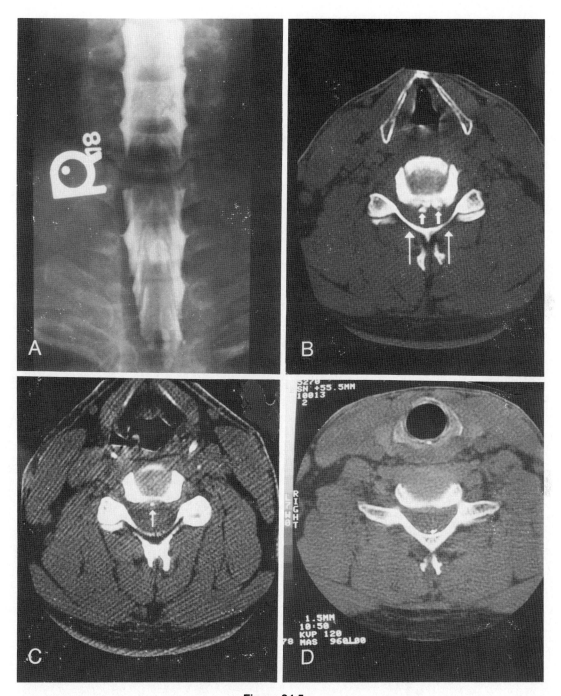

Figure 21.5.

canal (Fig. 21.5B, *short arrows*). The laminae were also thinned at this level (Fig. 21.5B, *long arrows*), probably an indicator of chronic pressure phenomenon. An incidental small central disc herniation at C4–5 also is shown by CT (Fig. 21.5C, *arrow*), but is not visible on the myelogram. A normal disc in this patient at C6–7 is shown for comparison (Fig. 21.5D).

CASE 5. MULTIPLE DISC HERNIATIONS

A 41-year-old male physician complained of neck pain of 5 years' duration. In addition to neck pain, there was radiation of pain into the left shoulder and into the 4th and 5th fingers of the left hand. A cervical myelogram 2 years ago was normal. CT reveals multiple abnormalities of the cervical discs. CT at C3–4 shows a normal disc (Fig. 21.6A). A Type II bulging disc is present at C4–5 (Fig. 21.6B, *arrow*). Herniation at C5–6 contains punctate calcification (Fig. 21.6C, *arrow*). Herniation at C6–7 has adjacent osteophytes intruding into the canal (Fig. 21.6D, *arrow*).

Decompressive laminectomies were performed at C4, C5, and C6. After a complicated postoperative course,

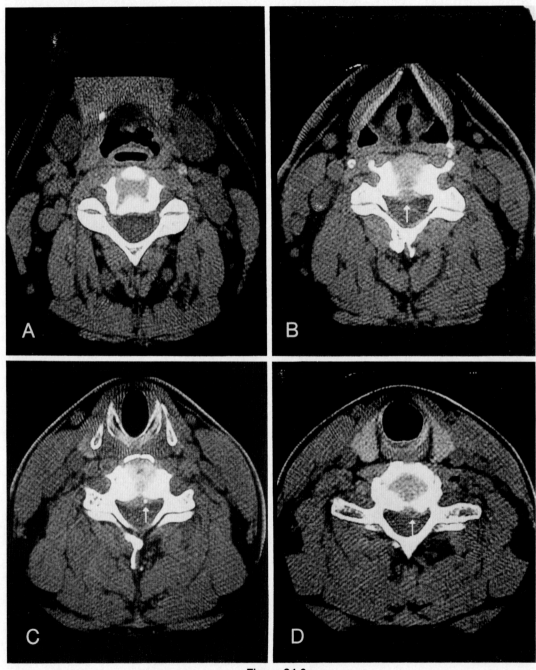

Figure 21.6.

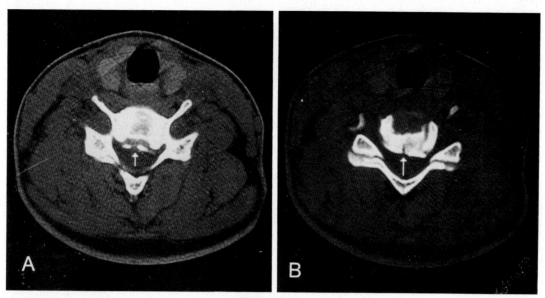

Figure 21.7.

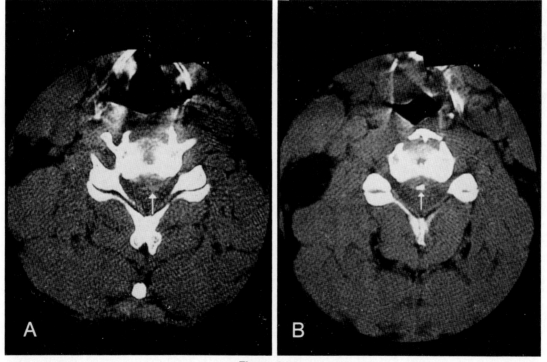

Figure 21.8.

there has been overall improvement. At present, there is only dull neck pain aggravated by neck flexion and normal use of a microscope. Ulnar radiation of pain is no longer present. There is now radial radiation of mild pain into the left arm and left hand. Neurological examination is unremarkable.

CASE 6. TRAUMATIC DISC RUPTURE IN A DIVING INJURY

A 17-year-old girl became quadriparetic immediately after a dive into shallow water 1 year ago. Spastic quadriplegia was present except for movement of both arms from shoulder to wrists. Pin prick and light touch sensation were present to T-6 level and spotty sensation was present over the thumbs. Repeated cervical spine X-rays were negative for fracture.

CT demonstrated both disc herniation and fracture at C5–6: A calcified barlike herniation at C5–6 (Fig. 21.7A, *arrow*), and comminuted fracture of C6 body (Fig. 21.7B, *arrow*).

This case documents the sensitivity of CT in demonstration of obscure cervical fracture and traumatic disc herniation similar to previous experience with this technique (28).

CASE 7. C4–5 AND C5–6 DISC HERNIATIONS

A 60-year-old male farmer (weight, 270 pounds) became immediately quadriparetic after being knocked down by a hog. Cervical spine X-rays showed evidence of degenerative changes. A myelogram attempt was unsuccessful. CT demonstrated a large, soft-disc herniation at C5–6 with prominent cartilaginous intrusion into the spinal canal (Fig. 21.8A, *arrow*). A significant herniation was also present at C4–5 level (Fig. 21.8B). This herniation was partially calcified (*arrow*).

CASE 8. DISC HERNIATIONS AT C4–5 AND C5–6

This is the case of a 56-year-old male laborer with chronic neck and shoulder pain, reduced tendon reflexes in both upper extremities, and decreased sensation in the thumb and index finger of the right hand. CT sections demonstrate a small central cartilaginous herniation at C4–5 (Fig. 21.9A) and a calcified herniation at C5–6 (Fig. 21.9B) accompanied by marginal degenerative changes.

CASE 9. DEGENERATIVE DISC DISEASE AND CALCIFIED LIGAMENTUM FLAVUM

A very active, trim 79-year-old female has chronic neck and shoulder pain of at least 10 years' duration. A degenerated bulging disc is present at C3–4 level (Fig. 21.10A). Calcified ligamentum flavum is also seen at this level (*arrow*). C6–7 disc is degenerated (Fig. 21.10B) and a small calcific density intrudes into the epidural space (*arrow*). C4–5 disc appears normal at this level (Fig. 21.10C).

CASE 10. CERVICAL SPONDYLOSIS, TYPE V

A 60-year-old female complains of neck pain and left shoulder pain with radiation down the left arm and numbness in the left hand of 1 year's duration. CT at C3–4 reveals a soft herniation bulging into the vertebral canal (Fig. 21.11A, *arrow*). At C4–5, there is a hard calcified central herniation (Fig. 21.11B, *arrow*). C5–6 disc is degenerated with a moderate calcified herniation into the vertebral canal producing significant stenosis (Fig. 21.11C, *arrows*). Below C5–6 level, a dense nodule extends several millimeters caudad to the level of the disc space apparently representing a free disc fragment that has become ossified (Fig. 21.11D, *arrow*). C6–7 level shows a moderate calcified disc herniation (Fig. 21.11E, *arrow*).

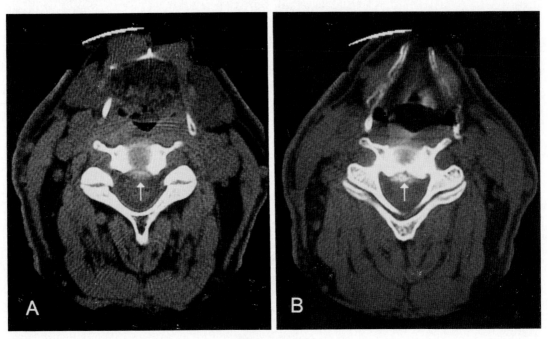

Figure 21.9.

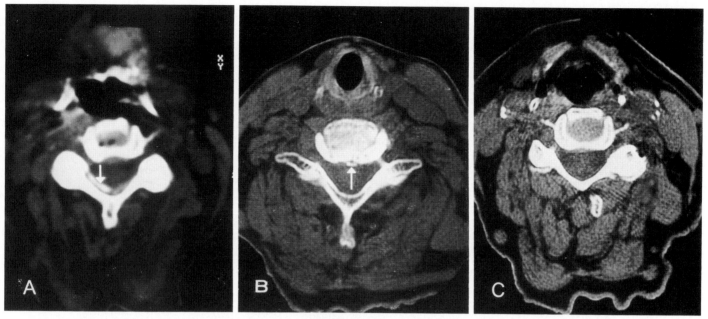

Figure 21.10.

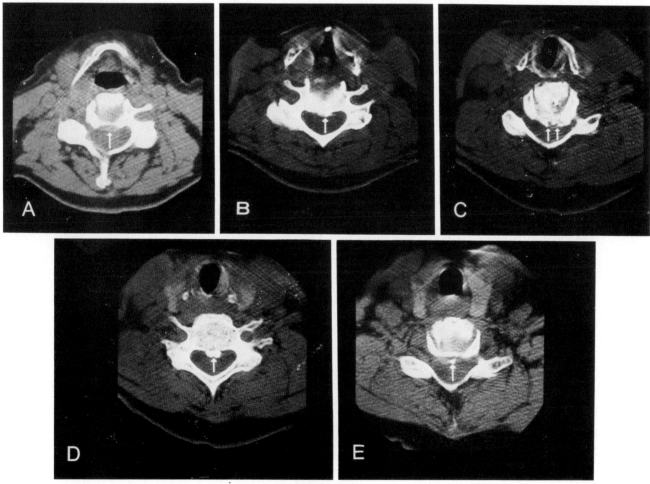

Figure 21.11.

CASE 11. C5–6 AND C6–7 HERNIATION WITH CERVICAL SPONDYLOSIS

A 45-year-old female has had neck and lower back pain intermittently over the last 20 years. The pain has become increasingly severe in the last 5–6 years. CT scan shows disc herniations at C5–6 (Fig. 21.12A, *arrow*) and C6–7 (Fig. 21.12B, *arrow*). Myelogram performed two days after the CT scan confirmed a disc protrusion at C6–7 (Fig. 21.12C and D, *arrow*). Degenerative changes are seen at C5–6; however, the herniation shown by CT is not clearly visible on the myelogram.

CASE 12. POST-TRAUMATIC DISC HERNIATION, C5–6, TYPE I

A 25-year-old male is quadraparetic after an auto accident 2 years ago. The car he was driving rolled, and the convertible roof collapsed, compressing his head and neck. He had been regaining movement gradually in all extremities until a recent fall from a wheelchair resulted in deterioration of neurological status. CT shows a slightly depressed fracture of C5 lamina and stellate fracture of C5 body (Fig. 21.13A, *arrows*). There is also herniation of the C5–6 disc (Fig. 21.13B, *thin arrows*) and calcification in

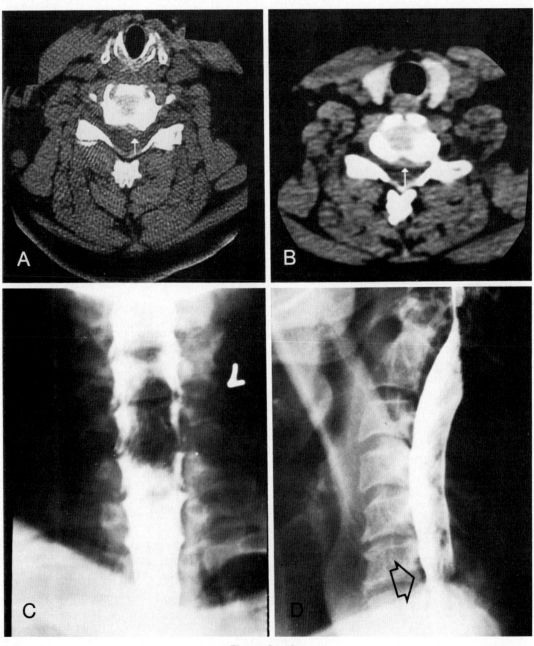

Figure 21.12.

the region of the anterior longitudinal ligament and anulus (Fig. 21.13B, *thick arrow*).

CASE 13. SCHMORL'S NODE AND DISC HERNIATION AFTER COMPRESSION INJURY

A 35-year-old female was seen 2 years after an auto accident. She ran over a large metal pipe and violently struck her head against the roof of the car. Since the accident she has suffered chronic neck pain, shoulder pain, severe headaches, fatigue, and emotional disturbances. X-rays of the cervical spine (Fig. 21.14A) are unremarkable except for slight narrowing of the C5–6 disc

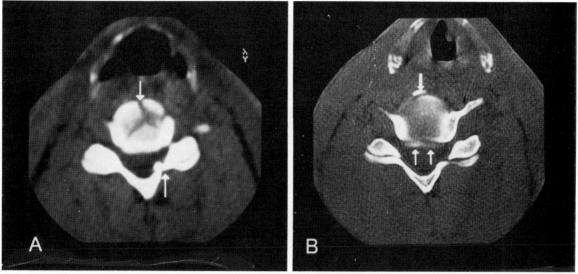

Figure 21.13.

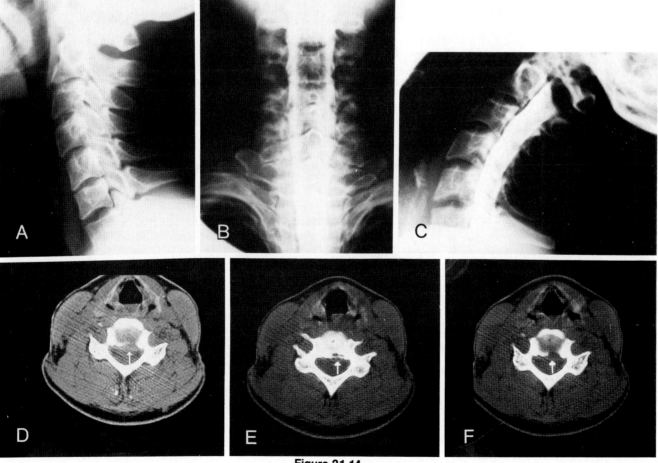

Figure 21.14.

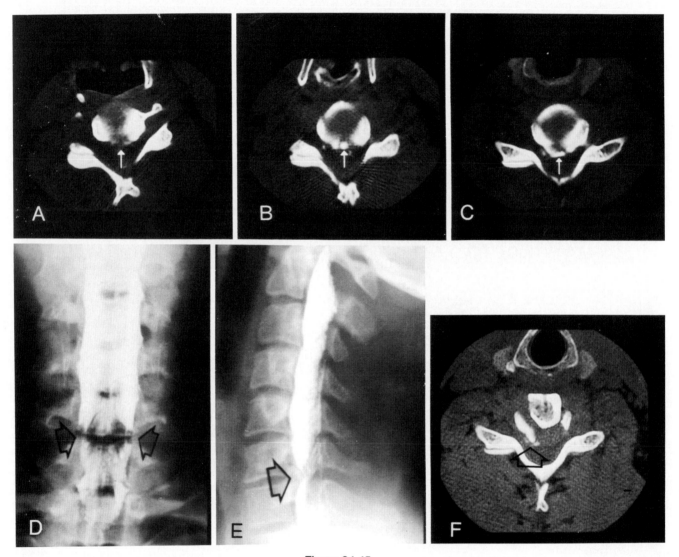

Figure 21.15.

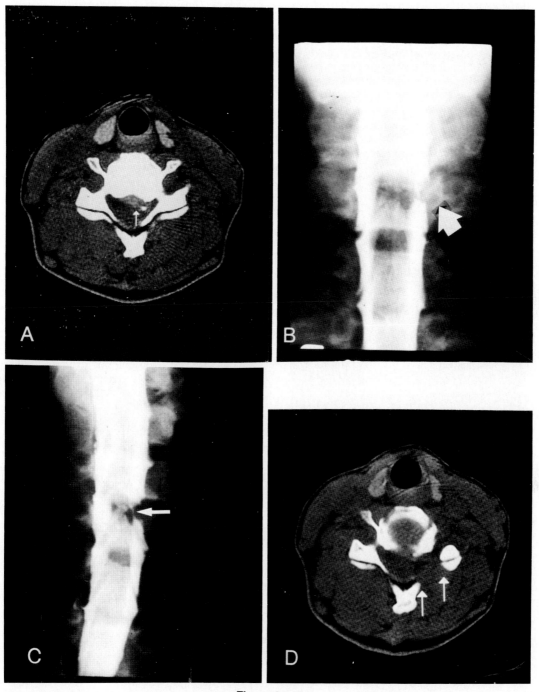

Figure 21.16.

space. Myelography (Fig. 21.14B and C) is inconclusive. CT demonstrates a soft herniation of the C5–6 disc (Fig. 21.14D, *arrow*). A small Schmorl's node is also shown in the superior horizontal surface of C6 body (Fig. 21.14E and F *arrows*).

CASE 14. MULTIPLE HERNIATIONS

A 39-year-old male has had stiffness of the neck and numbness of the index and middle fingers of the left hand of only 1 month's duration. There is no history of trauma. CT demonstrates three-level disease with different stages of disc herniation at these levels: C4–5, Type II bulging

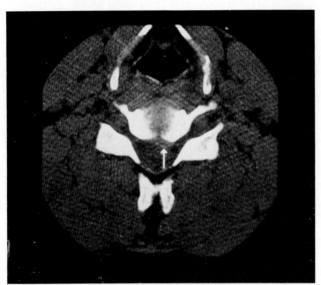

Figure 21.17.

disc (Fig. 21.15A, *arrow*); C5–6, Type IV chronic calcified herniation (Fig. 21.15B, *arrow*); C6–7, Type V spondylosis (Fig. 21.15C). Myelogram demonstrates the C6–7 herniation (Fig. 21.15D and E, *arrowheads*); however, the C4–5 protrusion is not visible and C5–6 defect is only questionable. Surgical decompression was accomplished by means of anterior discectomy and interbody fusion. Postoperative CT at C6–7 shows interbody fusion is in good position (Fig. 21.15F). Canal has been decompressed anteriorly. Residual degenerated disc fragments and spur on the right were significant postoperative findings not identifiable by other methods (Fig. 21.15F, *arrowhead*).

CASE 15. C5–6 HARD DISC HERNIATION

A 39-year-old female has left arm pain radiating to all fingers of the left hand since lifting a heavy bag of manure 9 years ago. On examination, weakness and diminished tendon reflexes in the left arm and hand are present. CT scan shows a partially calcified disc herniation at C5–6 (Fig. 21.16A, *arrow*). Myelogram performed after the CT scan shows a lateral extradural defect at the same level with obliteration of the nerve root sleeve on the left (Fig. 21.16B and C, *arrows*). Laminectomy and partial discectomy were performed with clinical improvement. CT scan 6 months later shows laminectomy defect (Fig. 21.16D, *arrows*). The C5–6 intervertebral foramen on the left has been decompressed. Herniation is reduced.

CASE 16. C5–6 TYPE III HERNIATION

A 38-year-old male laborer in heavy industry was injured while "twisting" a heavy piece of metal 4 weeks before examination. He complains of left shoulder pain along with pain and numbness in his left hand. There is a history of previous lumbosacral disc herniation. CT shows a small soft (Type III) C5–6 herniation (Fig. 21.17, *arrow*).

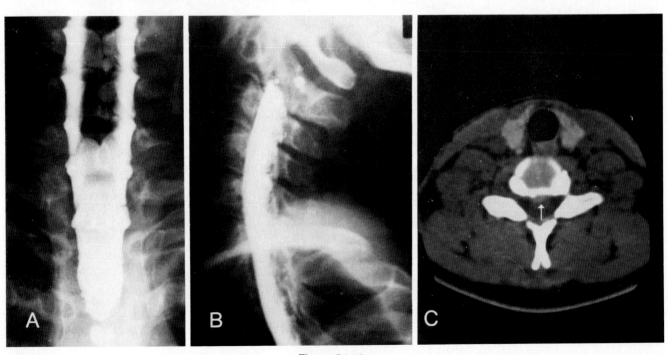

Figure 21.18.

CASE 17. C6–7 TYPE III HERNIATION

A 28-year-old female was injured in an industrial accident 3 years ago. She has had persistent pain in the right shoulder and lower cervical region with pain radiating down the right arm. Myelogram is unremarkable (Fig. 21.18A and B). CT shows a small cartilaginous herniation at C6–7 (Fig. 21.18C, *arrow*).

SUMMARY

CT provides an accurate, noninvasive means for anatomical evaluation of cervical disc disease. This method has considerable promise for aiding in the medical management, surgical treatment, and postoperative follow-up of cervical disc problems.

References

1. Gonzalez ER: CT beats myelography for lumbar spine diagnosis. Medical News. *JAMA* 246:2112–2113, 1981.
2. Coin CG, Chan YS, Keranen V, et al: Computer assisted myelography in disk disease. *J Comput Assist Tomogr* 1:398–404, 1977.
3. Glenn WV Jr, Rhodes ML, Altschuler EM, et al: Multiplanar display computerized body tomography applications in the lumbar spine. *Spine* 4:282–352, 1979.
4. Meyer GA, Haughton VM, Williams AL: Diagnosis of herniated lumbar disk with computed tomography. *N Engl J Med* 301:1106–1107, 1979.
5. Post MJD: CT update: The impact of time, metrizamide, and high resolution on the diagnosis of spinal pathology. In: Post MJD: *Radiographic Evaluation of the Spine: Current Advances with Emphasis on Computed Tomography.* New York, Masson Publishing, 1980, pp. 259–294.
6. Glenn WV Jr, Rhodes ML, Altschuler EM: Multiplanar computerized tomography of lumbar disc abnormalities: The proponent's viewpoint. In: Post MJD: *Radiographic Evaluation of the Spine: Current Advances with Emphasis on Computed Tomography.* New York, Masson Publishing, 1980, pp. 108–138.
7. Williams AL, Haughton VM, Syvertsen A: Computed tomography in the diagnosis of herniated nucleus pulposus. *Radiology* 135:95–99, 1980.
8. Coin CG: Computed tomography of the spine. In: Post MJD: *Radiographic Evaluation of the Spine: Current Advances with Emphasis on Computed Tomography.* New York, Masson Publishing, 1980, pp. 391–412.
9. Haughton VM, Eldevic PO, Magnaes B, et al: A prospective comparison of computed tomography and myelography in the diagnosis of herniated lumbar disks. *Radiology* 142:103–110, 1982.
10. Coin CG, Coin JT, Garrett JK: Computed Tomography of Canine Disc Herniation with CT Controlled Chemonucleolysis by Collagenase Injection. Exhibit. Radiological Society of North America, Chicago IL, November 15–20, 1981.
11. Coin CG, Coin JT: Technical note. Computed tomography of cervical disk disease. Technical considerations with representative case reports. *J Comput Assist Tomogr* 5:275–280, 1981.
12. Coin CG, Herman GT, Coin JT: Computed tomography of the spine: Techniques and procedures. *Comput Radiol* 6:69–74, 1982.
13. Schmorl G, Junghanns H: *The Human Spine in Health and Disease*, translated and edited by Wilk SP, Goin LS. Grune and Stratton, New York and London, 1957.
14. Hirsch C, Schajowicz F: Studies on structural changes in the lumbar annulus fibrosus. *Acta Orthop* 22:184–231, 1953.
15. Jackson R: The mechanism of cervical nerve root irritation (Chap. 3) and Etiology (Chap. 4). In: *The Cervical Syndrome, Fourth Edition.* Springfield IL, Charles C Thomas, 1978.
16. Brain WR: Cervical spondylosis. In: Beeson PB, McDermott W: *Cecil-Loeb Textbook of Medicine.* WB Saunders, Philadelphia and London, 1963, pp 1705.
17. Simeone FA, Rothman RH: Cervical disc disease. Chap. 7. In Rothman RH, Simeone FA: *The Spine.* Philadelphia, WB Saunders, 1974, pp 387–433.
18. Harner RN, Wienir MA: Differential diagnosis of spinal disorders. Chap 3, In: Rothman RH, Simeone FA: *The Spine.* Philadelphia, WB Saunders, 1974, pp 53–68.
19. Brain WR, Wilkenson M: *Cervical Spondylosis.* WB Saunders, Philadelphia, 1967, pp 232.
20. DePalma A, Rothman R: *The Intervertebral Disc.* Philadelphia, WB Saunders Co., 1970.
21. Rothman RH: Pathophysiology of disc degeneration. *Clin Neurosurg* 20:174–182, 1973.
22. Naylor A: Intervertebral disc prolapse and degeneration. *Spine* 1:108–114, 1976.
23. Coin CG, Coin JG, Garrett JK: Experimental computed tomography controlled discolysis. In: Post MJD: *Computed Tomography of the Spine.* Chap. 27. Baltimore, Williams & Wilkins, 1984.
24. Schmorl G, Junghanns H: *The Human Spine in Health and Disease.* First American Edition. Translated and edited by SG Wilk, SG Louell. Grune & Stratton, New York, London, 1932, pp 166, 172–173.
25. Luschka H: Die halbgelenke des menschlichen Korpers, Berlin, 1858.
26. Kubota M, Baba I, Sumida T: Myelopathy due to ossification of the ligamentum flavum of the cervical spine, a report of two cases. *Spine* 6:553–559, 1981.
27. Marr JT: Gas in intervertebral discs. *Am J Roentgenol Rad Ther, Nucl Med* Vol. 70:804–809, 1953.
28. Coin CG, Pennink M, Ahmad WD, et al: Diving-type injury of the cervical spine: Contribution of computed tomography to management. *J Comput Assist Tomogr* 3:362–372, 1979.
29. Harris JH: In: Harris JH Jr: *The Radiology of Acute Cervical Spine Trauma.* Williams & Wilkins Co, Baltimore, 1978, pp 47–48, 59, 80–81, 83.
30. Dunsker SB: Cervical spondylotic myelopathy. In: Dunsker SB: *Cervical Spondylosis.* Raven Press, New York 1980, pp 104, 126–127, 131–132.
31. Smith BH: *Cervical Spondylosis and Its Neurological Complications.* Charles C Thomas, Springfield IL, 1968, pp 23–24, 105, 160.
32. Friberg S, Hirsch C: Anatomical and clinical studies on lumbar disc degeneration. *Acta Orthop* 19:222–237, 1950.
33. Coventry MB, Chormley RK, Kernohan JW: The intervertebral disc: Its microscopic anatomy and pathology. *J Bone Joint Surg* 27:105–112, 1945.
34. Brown MD: The pathophysiology of the intervertebral disc. Anatomical, physiological and biochemical considerations. PhD Thesis, Jefferson Medical College, Philadelphia, 1969.
35. McLaurin RL: Diagnosis and Course of Cervical Radiculopathy. In: Dunsker SB: *Cervical Spondylosis*, page 104, Raven Press, New York 1981.
36. Jeffreys E: *Disorders of the Cervical Spine.* Butterworths & Co., Ltd., London, 1980, pp 82–104.
37. Hohl M: Injuries of the neck in automobile accidents. *J Bone Joint Surg* 56A:1675–1682, 1974.
38. McNabb I: Acceleration extension injuries of the cervical spine. In: Rothman RH, Simeone FA: *The Spine.* WB Saunders, Philadelphia, 1975, pp 515–528.

A. DISC DISEASE
2. Diagnosis (Postoperative)

CHAPTER TWENTY-TWO

The Postoperative Lumbar Spine

J. GEORGE TEPLICK, M.D., STEVEN K. TEPLICK, M.D., and MARVIN E. HASKIN, M.D.

INTRODUCTION

A significant percentage of patients who have had prior lumbar surgery for herniated disc, or for conditions like spondylolisthesis or stenosis develop low back pain and radiculopathy months or years after surgery. These postoperative symptoms may be different from the preoperative pain and radiation, but more often they are strikingly similar.

Once the physician (usually the orthopaedic surgeon or neurosurgeon) has determined that the new and persistent symptoms are not due to some form of musculoskeletal strain, other possible causes must be considered, especially those related to the prior spinal surgery. These possibilities will include extradural scarring, recurrent disc herniation, postoperative bone overgrowth with stenosis, facet subluxation, and postoperative arachnoiditis (1).

In such cases, radiographs of the spine generally add little information, showing the usual postoperative bone findings. The myelogram frequently will show a defect at the operative site, but its significance is uncertain. Infrequently, there will be findings of arachnoiditis on the myelogram, sometimes confined to the operated interspace, but often involving the sac also well above or below the operated interspace.

As experience with high-resolution CT scanning of the lumbar spine has increased, it is becoming apparent that this noninvasive modality can give considerably more information about the postoperative spine than any other current imaging modality. In our experience with approximately 600 CT scans of the postoperative lumbar spine, *metrizamide* was virtually never used except in an occasional special case. We do not believe that a *metrizamide* CT is ordinarily more valuable than a plain CT for evaluating the postoperative spine.

THE LAMINECTOMY AND LAMINOTOMY

In order to identify an extradural soft-tissue density on the CT scan as possible scar or fibrosis, the lesion must be at the level and site of the laminectomy. Ordinarily, the exact site of the prior surgery will be recognized when a laminectomy is done since there will be absence of bone. However, in many cases where a laminectomy was done with removal of little or no bone, the recognition becomes important because sometimes the operative record of the exact interspace of the surgery can be confusing, especially where there has been a sacralized lumbar body or a lumbarized sacral segment. Another possible cause of error may be a failure of the referring physician to know actually when or what level laminectomy had been performed in the past because operative records may not be available.

The laminectomy bone defect usually is recognized very easily in most cases (Fig. 22.1). However, after a laminotomy, particularly a minilaminotomy where almost no bone has been removed, the only definite way to identify the site of the laminectomy is by the absence of some or most of the ligamentum flavum (Fig. 22.2). Because some portion of the ligamentum flavum must be resected in every case where the canal is to be explored surgically, the absence of a portion of the ligamentum flavum clearly indicates the site of the previous surgery, even when the newer microtechniques are employed.

THE UNCOMPLICATED POSTOPERATIVE LUMBAR CANAL

In the absence of extradural scarring or fibrosis or postoperative bony overgrowth, the spinal canal appears quite similar to the preoperative canal in the normal patient. The thecal sac is central in position and is surrounded by epidural fat, especially anterolaterally and posteriorly. If extensive laminectomies have been performed, fibrotic replacement of the posterior epidural fat may appear to "touch" the posterior thecal sac. The ligamentum flavum, of course, will be missing on the side of the laminectomy (Fig. 22.3). Frequently in the soft tissues immediately behind the laminectomy site, the fatty tissue will be replaced by fibrous tissue (Fig. 22.3), a finding readily rec-

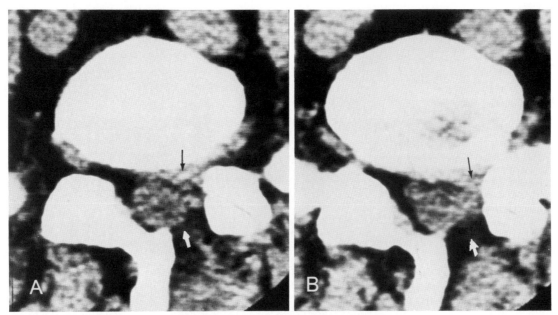

Figure 22.1. A and B. Classical CT appearance of laminectomy; discectomy scar: Successive slices show the absence of the left lamina and of the ligamentum flavum, a characteristic finding of a laminectomy. There is complete absence of fibrosis or scarring at the laminectomy site, and the posterior canal epidural fat (*white arrows*) is intact.

The triangular soft-tissue density (*black arrows*), from its CT appearance could be either a scar or a recurrent herniated disc. At surgery, it proved to be a scar.

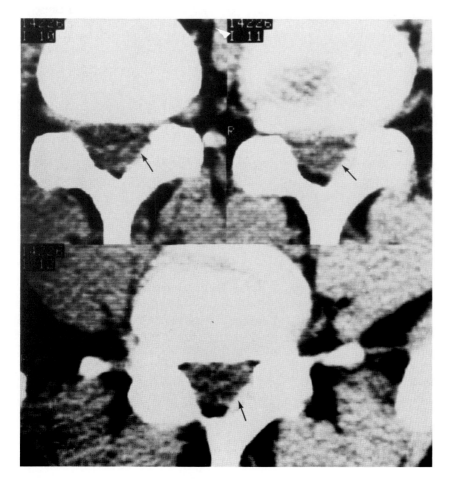

Figure 22.2. Identification of site of minilaminectomy (laminotomy): On 3 successive slices, the ligamentum flavum is seen on the left side (*black arrows*), but not on the right. This absence of one ligamentum flavum is virtually pathognomonic of laminectomy, even though clear-cut resection of the lamina cannot be identified on the scans, as illustrated above.

When very little bone is removed, the procedure is more accurately a laminotomy, in which the ligamentum flavum is removed in part, but very little of the bony lamina is resected.

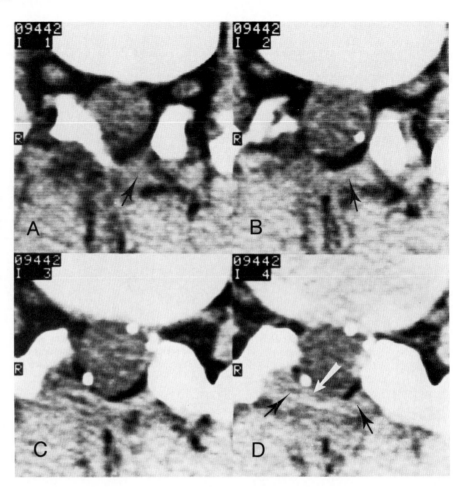

Figure 22.3. Bilateral laminectomies without significant scarring: Four successive CT sections (A–D) at L4–5 disclose extensive bilateral laminectomies with complete absence of the bony laminas. Both ligamentum flavum have been removed. Droplets of old Pantopaque are seen within the sac.

Note that the thecal sac is still entirely surrounded by epidural fat, and soft-tissue fibrosis has not replaced any of the fat in the canal.

A band of fibrosis (*black arrows*) has replaced the lamina and the fibro-fatty tissue behind the canal. The fibrosis appears to barely touch the thecal sac at one point (slice D, *white arrow*).

The irregularity and decreased volume of the posterior facets is seen when the laminectomy is extensive and portions of the facets have been resected.

ognized on the CT. With extensive bilateral laminectomies, the thecal sac may be located slightly more posteriorly than usual (Fig. 22.4), certainly a desired result when spinal stenosis is the underlying problem.

With an extensive laminectomy, portions of the posterior articular facet, which merges with the lamina, will be removed. In surgery on a stenotic canal or foramen, often the medial aspects of both the anterior and posterior articular facets are resected. The spinous process generally is removed when extensive bilateral laminectomies are performed.

EXTRADURAL SCARS OR FIBROSIS

The terms "scar" and "fibrosis" will be used interchangeably in our forthcoming discussions.

Orthopaedic surgeons and neurosurgeons frequently have encountered extradural scars in the lumbar canal during reoperation (2–6). In one series of postoperative myelograms, defects at the site of surgery were found in 38% (5), due, in most cases, to extradural scars and less frequently due to recurrent herniated discs.

In approximately 600 patients in our group who had had previous laminectomy and usually discectomy, extradural scarring of some degree was noted in approximately 75% and sizeable scars were found in about 40%.

The extradural scar appears as a soft-tissue density in the spinal canal, virtually always of greater CT density than the thecal sac.

The scar or fibrosis always is found on the side of the surgery and apparently a scar or fibrotic area can develop in 1 of 3 surgical sites: 1) in the posterior portion of the canal at the site of the laminectomy and flavum excision; 2) in the anterior canal at the site of the discectomy, most often in a recess, although it can occur centrally, particularly if a large central disc has been removed; 3) in the lateral wall of the canal at the site of a facetectomy.

Frequently, the scar is a combination of 2 or 3 of the primary scars.

The Posterior Laminectomy Scar

This area of fibrosis may be limited to the laminectomy site (Fig. 22.4), or may be incorporated into the postsurgical fibrotic changes which often replace the fibro-fatty muscular tissue behind the lamina (Figs. 22.3 and 22.6). The anterior portion of the laminectomy fibrosis may not extend into the canal and then the thecal sac will be seen completely separate from the scar (Fig. 22.3). This type of fibrosis, which does not compromise the canal, is probably of no clinical significance.

Not infrequently, however, the laminectomy scar extends into the canal and seems to merge with the posterior

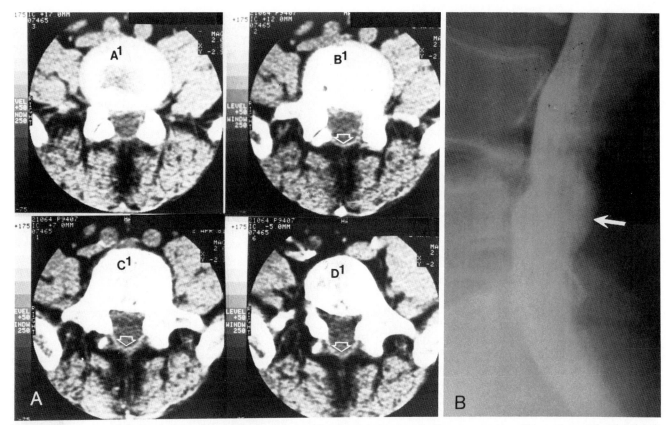

Figure 22.4. A and B. Posterior bulge of the thecal sac after laminectomies: A. Four successive CT sections (A¹, B¹, C¹, D¹) at L4–5 show the progressive posterior bulging of the thecal sac (*white open arrows*). Note the extremely thin line of fibrosis at the laminectomy site, with preservation of the fibro-fatty tissue behind it. B. The posterior bulge of the sac is well seen on the lateral myelogram (*arrow*).

portion of the sac (Figs. 22.5 and 22.6). Less often, the thecal sac is retracted by an adherent laminectomy scar (Fig. 22.7).

The Lateral Wall Scar

This is seen less frequently than the others in our group of postoperative patients. Most often, it is seen at the site of the facetectomy (Fig. 22.8), which is often done for the relief of canal or neural foraminal stenosis. This lateral fibrosis may encroach upon the wall of the dural sac (Figs. 22.8 and 22.9) or may retract the sac (Fig. 22.10), but more often, barely touches or is totally separate from the sac (Figs. 22.11 and 22.12). The lateral wall scar often merges with a discectomy and/or laminectomy scar, producing larger scar masses.

The Discectomy Scar

After discectomy, some degree of scarring or fibrosis in the anterior canal or recess is seen in most cases. The scar may vary from a small thin fibrous-like strand or a small soft-tissue density in the recess, replacing some of the epidural fat (Figs. 22.13 and 22.16) to a large mass resembling a herniated nucleus pulposus. The classical small discectomy scar appears as a replacement of recess fat by a soft-tissue density which tends to conform to the curve

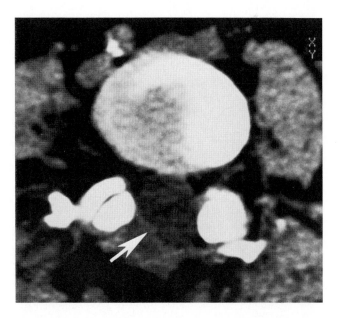

Figure 22.5. Laminectomy scar; sac encroachment: The trapezoid shaped laminectomy scar on the right is encroaching on the right posterior aspect (*arrow*) of the thecal sac.

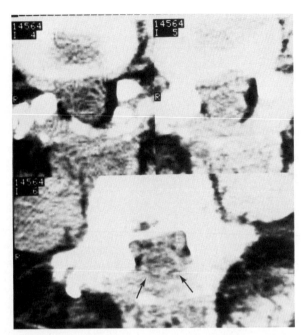

Figure 22.6. Laminectomy scar; sac encroachment: Sequential CT scans show that the fibrosis at the laminectomy site is merging with the bilateral posterior aspects (*arrows*) of the thecal sac.

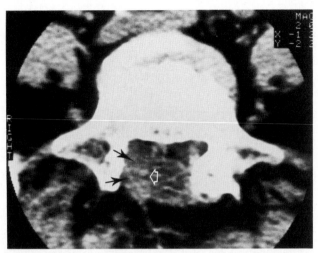

Figure 22.8. Lateral canal scar: Fibrous tissue (*black arrows*) has replaced the resected portions of the right facets, which were removed as part of a foraminotomy. The sharp medial border of the canal scar (*open white arrow*) is apparently in contact with the right side of the thecal sac.

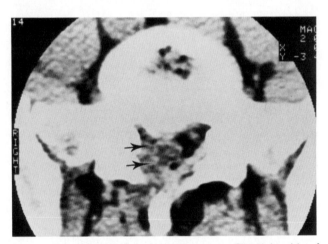

Figure 22.9. Canal scar; thickened dura: The right side of the canal is filled with soft-tissue scar (*arrows*) which appears attached to the right side of the thecal sac.

Note the thickened wall of the sac, possibly an indicator of dural thickening and this could be part of focal arachnoiditis.

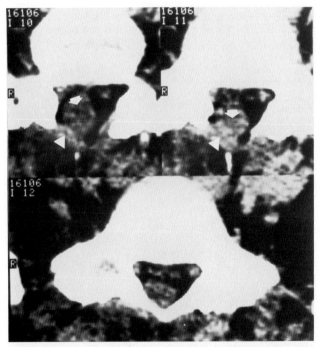

Figure 22.7. Small laminectomy scar; retraction of sac: The small right laminectomy scar (*arrowheads*) has become fixed to the thecal sac (*short arrows*) and has retracted the sac to the right.

Significant retraction of the thecal sac conceivably may put the emerging roots on stretch and cause symptoms on the side opposite the scar.

of the sac, without any apparent deformity of the sac (Figs. 22.14 and 22.15). A very important clinical consideration is the distinction of a discectomy scar from a recurrent herniated nucleus pulposus (HNP). This will be considered in more detailed discussion in a following section.

Combined Scars

Extensive scarring or fibrosis in the canal results usually from combined scars which apparently arose from two or more of the primary sites; for example, a combined unilateral discectomy and lateral wall scar. These larger scars may surround one side of the thecal sac (Figs. 22.12 and 22.17). When a laminectomy scar is also present and

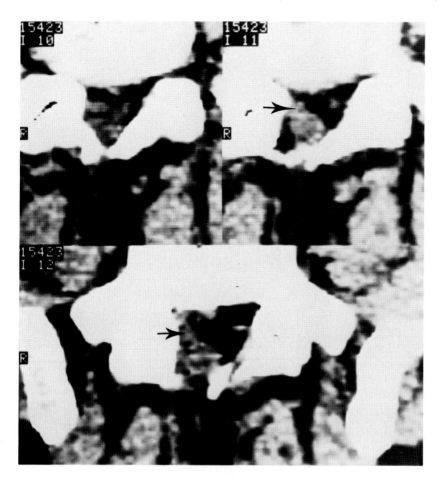

Figure 22.10. Small scar in canal wall with retraction of sac: The right facetectomy and foraminotomy have resulted in a relatively small scar (*arrows*), but this scar has retracted the thecal sac to the right.

merges with the above, over one-half of the sac may appear surrounded by scar (Fig. 22.18). Bilateral surgery can result in complete replacement of epidural fat by fibrosis and the sac will appear then as a relatively rounded lucent area completely encircled by denser fibrotic tissue (Fig. 22.19).

Clinical Significance of Extradural Scarring

The relationship between extradural scars and recurrent symptoms is extremely difficult to evaluate. In well over one-half of the patients examined because of late postoperative recurrence of symptoms, sizeable scarring was present on the side of the recurrent radiculopathy. However, in many patients with similar symptoms, there was no evidence of significant extradural scarring and, in fact, in many of these there was no CT evidence of any postoperative complications such as recurrent HNP, bony stenosis or facet disease, or myelographic evidence of arachnoiditis.

In many cases, the scar apparently is compromising the ipsilateral nerve root and occasionally even the dural sac, both from the CT appearance and the clinical findings. However, surgical scar excision and freeing of the nerve root is rarely undertaken, because clinical relief too often is followed by second recurrence of symptoms due to new and often greater scar formation (Fig. 22.20). This was true in 2 of 5 patients whose scar was removed surgically.

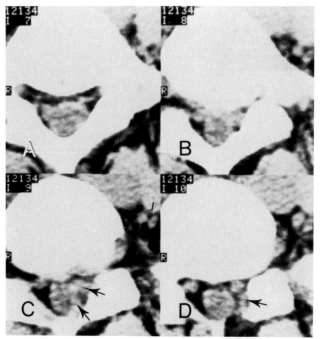

Figure 22.11. Lateral canal scar: At B and C, the scar (*arrows*) appears to be overlying the left side of the thecal sac. However, in D, 4 mm below, the scar (*arrow*) is clearly separate from the sac.

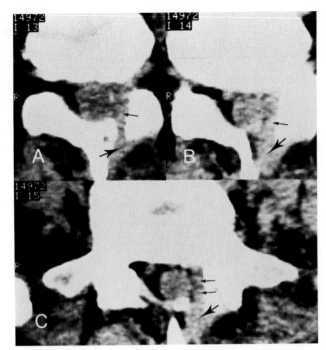

Figure 22.12. Combined foraminectomy (facetectomy) and laminectomy scars: The left lateral canal scar (*small black arrows*) is continuous with the laminectomy scar (*large black arrows*). At A, the scar merges with the left side of the thecal sac; at B and C, a distinct plane of separation is seen between the sac and scar.

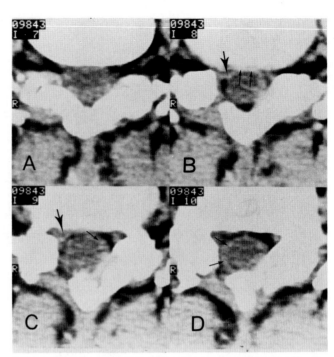

Figure 22.14. Classical discectomy scar: The density replacing the epidural fat in B and C (*large arrows*) conforms to the curve of the adjacent thecal sac and does not press upon or deform the sac.

Note the thickening of portions of the wall of the thecal sac (*small arrows*).

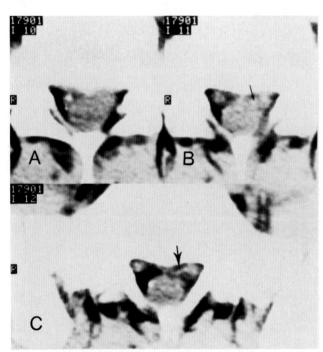

Figure 22.13. Minimal discectomy scar: At section B, the small density (*arrow*) medial to the left nerve root is probably a small scar. The left root has somewhat fuzzy borders, probably from minimal scarring.

At C, 4 mm below B, the scar takes the form of a linear strand (*arrow*) extending from the anterior sac to the left nerve root.

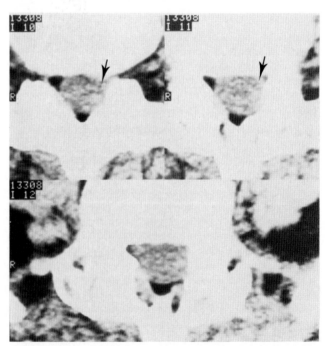

Figure 22.15. Classical discectomy scar: The left recess epidural fat has been replaced by soft tissue (*arrows*), which lies adjacent to the thecal sac without pressure or compromise of the sac. The classical discectomy scar is sufficiently characteristic to allow distinction from a recurrent herniated disc.

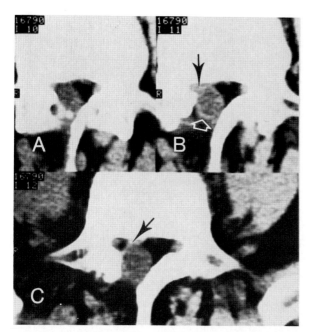

Figure 22.16. Discectomy scar; retraction of sac: At A, the sac is obviously pulled over to the right side. At B, a classical discectomy scar (*black arrow*) is apparent. At C, the scar has become a linear strand (*arrow*) extending from the superior facet to the posterior vertebral body. All these changes are virtually pathognomonic of scar! Note the thickened sac wall on the right (*open white arrow*).

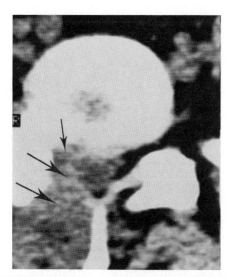

Figure 22.17. Combined discectomy and laminectomy scar: The discectomy scar (*small arrow*) in the right recess is almost continuous with the laminectomy scar (*larger arrows*). This combined scar is encroaching on the right side of the thecal sac.

Indeed, the operation is generally undertaken in hope of finding a recurrent herniated disc rather than a symptomatic extradural scar! In one reported series of 34 reoperated cases (6), 20 had extradural scars only, 10 had

recurrent HNP only, and 4 had both scars above and below the interspace and a recurrent HNP at the interspace.

The clinical effects and significance of scars which are limited to the lateral canal wall or laminectomy site, or

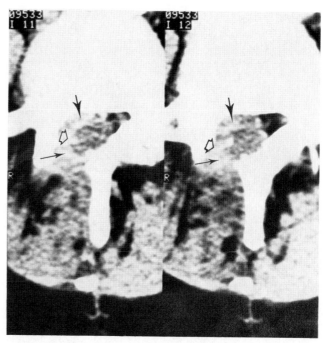

Figure 22.18. Combined laminectomy, foraminotomy, and discectomy scar: At L4–5, the right-sided laminectomy scar (*small black arrows*), the foraminotomy (facetectomy) scar (*open arrows*), and the discectomy scar (*large black arrows*) have become one confluent scar which is encroaching on the entire right half of the sac. Droplets of residual Pantopaque are present in the sac. Surgery was performed subsequently to free the entrapped right L5 root from the scars.

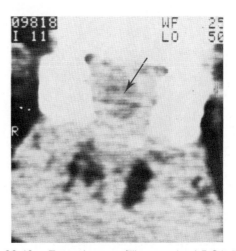

Figure 22.19. Extensive scar filling canal at L5-S1: Bilateral laminectomies and discectomies were performed 5 months previously, but symptoms gradually returned. The thecal sac appears as a rounded lucency (*arrow*) completely surrounded by denser scar tissue.

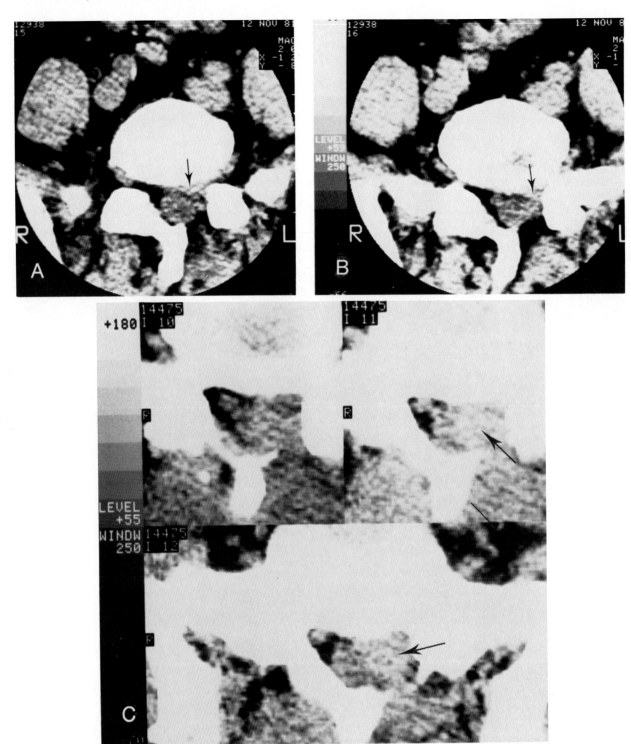

Figure 22.20. Recurrent symptomatic scar after surgical removal of discectomy scar: A and B. Two slices of L5-S1 show a soft-tissue density in the left recess (*arrows*). This was considered more likely to be scar than recurrent HNP. However, the possibility of a recurrent HNP was clinically considered because of the severe radiating pain and, therefore, surgery was done. Only an extradural scar was found and this was removed and the nerve root freed. C. Three months after surgery, the symptoms recurred and were more severe than before the scar surgery. Three consecutive CT slices at L5-S1 reveal a large scar (*arrows*) which is filling almost the entire left half of the canal, with obliteration of the left side of the sac and of the left recess.

both, is uncertain even when this scar will encroach and perhaps deform the lateral or posterior portion of the thecal sac or retract the thecal sac. This type of scar often will cause posterolateral deformations on the myelogram. Apparently some extradural scars extend to the dura and seem to be associated with dural thickening focally. This will be discussed under arachnoiditis.

The Recurrent Disc Herniation (HNP) versus The Discectomy Scar

The clinician, faced with the discectomy patient who has a recurrence of pain and radiculopathy, often quite similar to the preoperative symptoms, usually entertains the possibility of a recurrent HNP or a postoperative spinal stenosis. More recently, consideration is being given to symptomatic discectomy scars. The distinction between a recurrent HNP and a large discectomy scar becomes very important, because surgical excision may be indicated for a recurrent HNP, whereas an excision of an extradural scar is too often unrewarding (Fig. 22.20) and may even eventuate a more disabled patient (3).

Myelography can sometimes suggest the distinction. Cronquist (6) believed that deformation on the postoperative myelogram limited or most marked at the intervertebral level indicates a recurrent herniated disc, but if the deformation extended significantly above or below the excised disc level, an extradural scar was present. Irstam and Rosencrantz (5) however, did not believe that this myelographic distinction was valid, especially because focal adhesive arachnoiditis can produce myelographic changes that simulate recurrent disc herniation or extradural scar. However, the arachnoiditis myelographic picture has no definite extradural counterpart on CT and does not enter into the CT differential diagnosis. Arach-noiditis and the CT scars will be discussed in a later section.

The discectomy scar frequently will have features on the CT scans which can distinguish it from a recurrent herniated disc. The following CT characteristics are much more typical of scar than of recurrent HNP (see Table 22.1):

1. Retraction of thecal sac toward the soft-tissue lesion (Fig. 22.16).
2. Discectomy scar often will contour itself around the thecal sac (Figs. 22.14 and 22.15). This latter type scar will more often than not be associated with a negative myelogram.
3. Linear strandlike densities will occur frequently in scars and not in HNP (Figs. 22.13 and 22.16).
4. The bulk of the scar is often above or below the disc interspace (Fig. 22.21) in contrast to the recurrent HNP. This deformation, above or below the interspace, is also a myelographic criteria for extradural scarring; however, only larger scars will be apparent on the myelogram.
5. The anterior border of the discectomy scar may sometimes not appear to be a direct extension from the intervertebral anulus in contrast to a disc herniation.
6. The discectomy scar will enhance appreciably after intravenous contrast, whereas a herniated disc will not enhance significantly (Fig. 22.22) (8).

The recurrent HNP has a CT appearance which is quite similar to the ordinary HNP seen in the nonoperated patient. Thus, it may press upon the thecal sac, and does not conform to the shape of the sac. The posterior border of a recurrent HNP is generally sharp and discrete. It may displace a nerve root posteriorly. The bulk of the soft tissue of a HNP is at the interspace level and appears to be a continuation of the anulus, although a large HNP

Table 22.1.

CT Characteristics	Discectomy Scar	Recurrent Disc Herniation
Shape contour	From strands to mass, often irregular, but can be regular. Often contours around thecal sac	Masslike density. Does not follow sac contours
Location	Frequently extends well above or below the interspace. Largest portion may not be at interspace	Usually limited to interspace. (Rarely, fragment may migrate above or below)
Relation to thecal sac	Often retracts the sac. Often conforms to contour of sac. Rarely compresses sac	Never causes sac retraction. May compress or deform sac
Associated scars	May be solitary, or continuous with canal wall scar	Very infrequently associated with sizeable scarring. If associated, usually appears somewhat denser than adjacent scar
Free border into canal	Either sharp or indistinct	Free border usually sharp and distinct
Anterior (vertebral body) border	May not appear to be direct extension of anulus	Usually appears to be direct extension of anulus
Intravenous contrast enhancement	Shows marked enhancement	Little or no enhancement

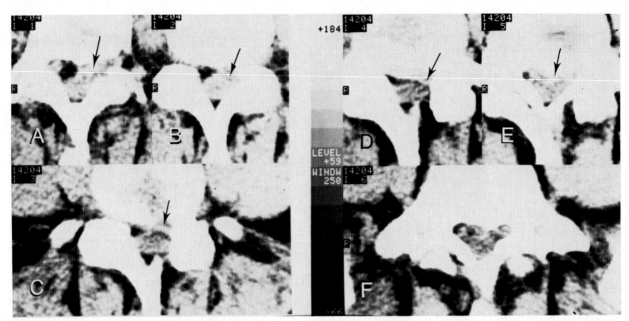

Figure 22.21. Recurrent HNP versus scar: About 1 year after a left discectomy at L4–5, the patient began experiencing recurrent left radiculopathy. The CT scan at L4–5 shows that a soft-tissue density (*arrows*) is in the left recess, not only at the interspace level (C and D) but also well above the interspace (A and B) and a bit below it (E and F). Although the posterior border of the density appears sharp at C and D, note how it appears to maintain the contour of the sac. In addition, the density appears more bulky and more irregular on the most cranial section A. This was considered to be a scar from the above-mentioned CT criteria. Myelogram showed a defect at L4–5, suspicious of a recurrent HNP. At surgery, only scar and no disc herniation was found.

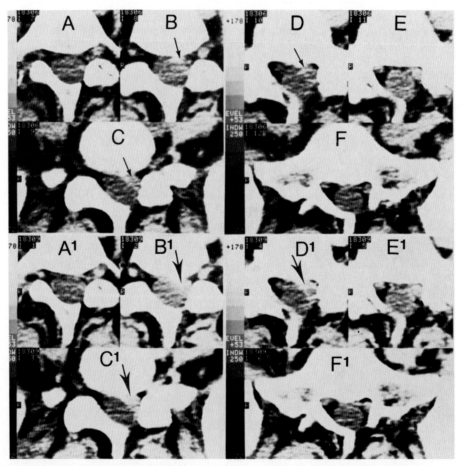

Figure 22.22. Scar versus recurrent disc; enhancement distinction: A, B, C, D, E, and F are successive slices of L5-S1 made before enhancement. The soft-tissue density (*small arrows*) in B, C, and D, extending across the left upper border of the thecal sac had a CT appearance more characteristic of a scar, but recurrent HNP could not be entirely excluded, particularly because the lesion was largest at the interspace and had rather sharp borders. A¹, B¹, C¹, D¹, E¹, and F¹ are corresponding sections made after rapid infusion of 150 cc of conray. Marked enhancement of the density is seen at B¹, C¹, and D¹ (*large black arrows*), indicating that the lesion is a scar and not a HNP.

may also extend above or below the interspace. The HNP does not enhance after intravenous contrast.

Table 1 lists the distinguishing figures of discectomy scar and recurrent HNP.

The majority of discectomy scars can be identified fairly accurately on the CT scans. Features such as retraction of the thecal sac, linear stranding, contours that follow the curve of the sac and the continuity and merging with canal scars, and their major location above or below the interspace generally will allow confident assessment of the lesion as scar. This type of lesion will usually not be mistaken for a recurrent herniated disc on CT. If myelography is performed, more often than not the deformation of the contrast column at the interspace, which is thought to be characteristic of HNP, is not seen.

However, when the CT reveals a sharply demarcated density which is quite similar to a HNP, it is virtually impossible to make a CT distinction between a HNP and a sharply marginated scar. In such cases, enhancement techniques after rapid intravenous contrast (8) might allow distinction because the scars will enhance markedly whereas a herniated disc will enhance little or not at all (Fig. 22.22). In the cases of recurrent HNP proven by surgery (Figs. 22.23 and 22.24) the myelograms were positive, showing a deformation at the interspace level. Our current impression is that a recurrent HNP cannot be distinguished unequivocally from a masslike scar by CT appearance alone (Figs. 22.1, 22.25, and 22.26) but, an enhancement study may prove more conclusive. On the other hand, a typical scar with its characteristic CT appearances can be distinguished from a recurrent HNP (see Table 1) and enhancement studies are not needed. It should be emphasized that an extradural scar which is identified readily as such on the CT, is a far more frequent occurrence in our experience than either a recurrent herniated disc or a scar which closely resembles the latter.

Our experience with intravenous contrast enhancement has been limited to about 30 patients. In only 3 of these was a recurrent disc herniation diagnosis made after the enhancement study; one of these has been surgically verified. The remaining patients were considered to have enhancing scars and no recurrent herniation. Three of these have been reoperated; in 2, only scar tissue was found; in 1, a disc fragment was found anterior to a thick scar.

We find the enhancement study very encouraging, and hope it will become more widely used and more fully evaluated.

When the CT findings are indecisive, the clinical history may prove helpful. If recurrent symptoms have appeared as early as a month or as late as a year or so after the discectomy and continue to worsen, the possibility of a scar etiology is high, although, of course, a recurrent herniated disc is by no means ruled out. However, if symptoms recur several years or more after the surgery, then an anterior soft-tissue mass on the CT is much more likely to be a recurrent herniated disc.

The distinction between an extradural discectomy scar and a recurrent HNP is important for treatment planning.

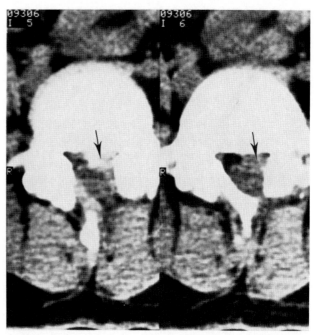

Figure 22.23. Recurrent HNP: Sections from an L5-S1 scan of a patient who had a left discectomy 2 years previously and now has recurrence of left radiculopathy, reveals a partially calcified density (*arrows*) in the anterior left canal. On CT, this had the appearance of a calcified herniated disc. This was found at surgery.

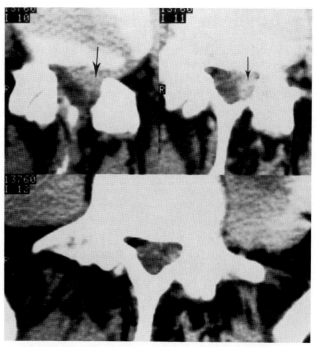

Figure 22.24. Recurrent HNP—L4–5: Eight years after a left discectomy, this patient developed left sciatica. Scans at L4–5 show a large, soft-tissue mass (*large arrow*) projecting from the left side of the anulus and extending considerably posteriorly (*small arrow*). This proved to be a large recurrent HNP.

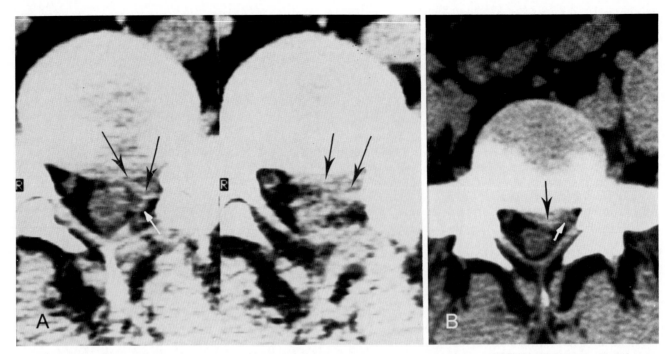

Figure 22.25. Recurrent HNP or scar?? A. Preoperative scan reveals a left-sided HNP at L5-S1 (*black arrows*); the left nerve root (*white arrow*) is displaced posteriorly. B. Pain recurred 6 months after the discectomy. Scan shows a soft-tissue mass (*black arrow*) at the interspace, impinging on a left root (*white arrow*), but not on the sac. While the CT appearance is fairly typical of a HNP, a sharply marginated scar can produce an identical CT appearance. Enhancement studies probably would clarify the problem because a herniated disc would not enhance significantly.

When only a scar is found at surgery, the ultimate clinical result is often poor because new and sometimes extensive extradural scarring and symptoms may develop later (Figs. 22.20 and 22.27). The surgeon, therefore, is reluctant to operate if an extradural discectomy scar is the expected finding. On the other hand, removal of a recurrent HNP is much more likely to provide a long-term satisfactory clinical result.

THE POSTOPERATIVE EXTRADURAL HEMATOMA

In 13 patients who had undergone discectomy, CT studies of the postoperative site were made from 4–14 days after surgery. In 2, the scans were done because of unexpected and unexplained postoperative radicular pain; in the other 11, the early postoperative scans were investigational to determine the appearance of the canal after successful surgery.

In 11 of the 13, extradural soft-tissue densities were seen at the operative site. Although none of these cases were reoperated and, therefore, positive identification of these extradural densities was not obtained, it seems reasonably certain that they represented postoperative hematomas (Figs. 22.28–22.32). In only 2 patients was there virtually no evidence of postoperative hematoma; 1 of these did have microsurgery. However, in another case of microsurgery, the hematoma was quite sizeable. Although this series is small and limited, it suggests that the majority of patients develop hematoma at the discectomy site. To

date, 4 of these patients have been re-examined by CT 2 months or later after surgery, to determine the fate of these hematomas. In every case, the extradural soft-tissue shadow has persisted with minimal changes (Figs. 22.31 and 22.32). This finding suggests that the hematoma has become an extradural scar or fibrosis. Corroboration of hematoma converting to an extradural scar would require, of course, a much larger series, which we hope to obtain. This conversion is not entirely unexpected; Cronquist in 1959 (6) believed that extradural scars were frequently the result of organization of a postoperative extradural hematoma.

If hematoma changing into scar proves to be true in most or even many cases, and because extradural scarring does seem to be a possible cause of postoperative recurrent low back pain and radiculopathy, it would seem that minimizing the postoperative hematoma might minimize the incidence and extent of extradural scarring. Certainly this could be verified by a large series of both immediate and late postoperative CT scans. Hopefully, with the rapid proliferation of high-resolution scanners, such series will be forthcoming from various centers within the next few years.

THE POSTLAMINECTOMY PSEUDOMENINGOCELE (PLP)

This rare complication apparently results from an inadvertent tear of the dura during spinal canal surgery. The cerebrospinal fluid extravasates posteriorly and forms

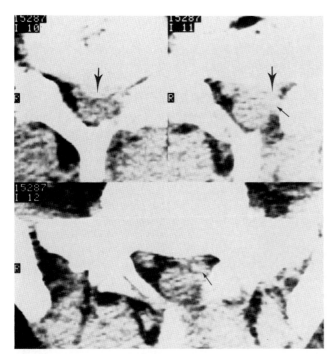

Figure 22.26. Scar or recurrent HNP? After a successful left discectomy at L5-S1 6 years ago, this 45-year-old woman developed a left radiculopathy. Sections from the current scan at L5-S1 show a soft-tissue mass (*large arrows*) at the level of the intervertebral space, pressing on the sac and displacing the somewhat enlarged left nerve root (*small arrow*). The CT findings are characteristic of a recurrent disc herniation, but surgery has not been performed. An intravenous contrast enhancement study was not done. Occasionally, even a characteristic lesion like this one can turn out to be a solid masslike scar rather than a disc herniation.

a rounded collection of low CT density (Figs. 22.33 and 22.34) behind the laminectomy at or very near midline. The appearance is quite characteristic on the CT.

Although most of these collections are extravasations or leaks of cerebrospinal fluid which develop a fibrous capsule, in some cases, apparently a superficial dural tear will allow herniation of the intact arachnoid, which gradually enlarges. This becomes an arachnoid-lined true meningocele, but apparently this type is much less common.

Because the PLP frequently loses its communication with the dural sac after the tear heals, it is not surprising that the myelogram often will fail to demonstrate the presence of the PLP. This was true in several of our cases. Obviously, CT of the operative site is the most accurate modality for uncovering a PLP. This has been an unexpected CT finding in 9 of our 10 cases. The earliest PLP encountered was 1 month postoperatively (Fig. 22.33); the latest was seen 6 years postoperatively (Fig. 22.34).

Clinically, a PLP may be totally asymptomatic or may cause a localized backache. This is more likely to occur if the PLP is still connected to the dural sac; coughing or sneezing may then cause ballooning of the PLP and local pain. If a root is trapped or herniates partially into the PLP tract, severe radiculopathy can occur. Some neurosur-

geons believe that a PLP should be suspected if symptoms recur shortly after surgery, particularly if the surgeon has manipulated the thecal sac. A PLP, which is due to a dural tear and extravasation posteriorly, should not be confused

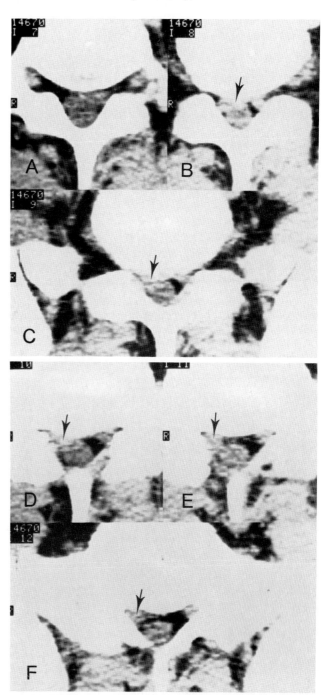

Figure 22.27. Recurrent scarring after scar excision: This 34-year-old man had a right discectomy at L5-S1. Because of recurrent symptoms, surgery was done 1½ years ago. No HNP was found, but a sizeable scar was removed. Recently, the right radiculopathy recurred. The CT scan at L5-S1 (A to E) shows a sizeable scar has reformed (*arrows*), extending from about 5 mm above the interspace (B), to about 12–14 mm (F) below the interspace.

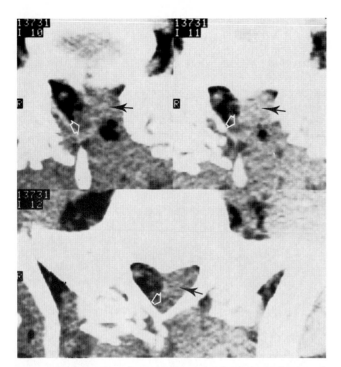

Figure 22.28. Postdiscectomy extradural hematoma: A scan at L5-S1 made 8 days postoperatively shows the large, soft-tissue density (*black arrows*) filling the left canal, extending from the posterior vertebral area to the small thecal sac (*white open arrows*). The epidural fat in the left recess is not entirely obliterated.

with posterior displacement of the thecal sac that may occur after bilateral laminectomy (Figs. 22.3 and 22.35). Unfortunately, this displacement of the sac has also been called pseudomeningocele in the literature.

POSTOPERATIVE STENOSIS

Bony overgrowth or spur formation of a facet or vertebral body sometimes can be secondary to the resection and traumatic irritation of these bony structures during spinal surgery. If the spur or bony overgrowth compromises the canal or a neural foramen, clinical symptoms may occur (Figs. 22.36 and 22.37). However, recurrent symptoms in the postdiscectomy patient are due far more often to extradural scar or recurrent disc herniation than to postoperative spinal stenosis. Before the information gained from spinal CT, the principal causes of recurrent symptoms were thought to be either spinal stenosis or a recurrent HNP.

ARACHNOIDITIS

Chronic adhesive arachnoiditis of the lower spine is a myelographic diagnosis. The majority of cases, by far, are found in patients who have had previous spine surgery (2–7). The name arachnoiditis is a misnomer, because, histologically, all layers of the meninges are involved and invariably the dura is quite thickened.

Although arachnoiditis can be one of the causes of postoperative symptoms (2), no distinct clinical symptom

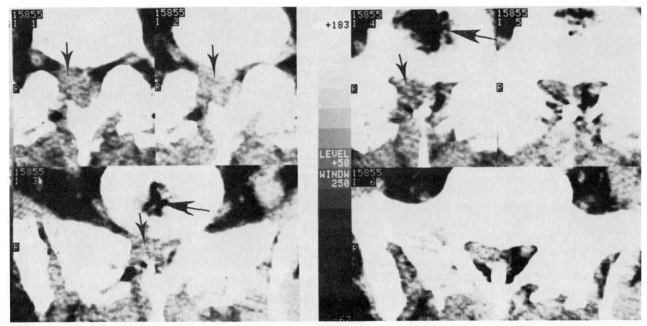

Figure 22.29. Postoperative hematoma and vacuum disc: A scan of L5-S1 made 8 days after right discectomy reveals a sizeable hematoma (*smaller arrows*). Note that a considerable portion of the hematoma is well above the actual interspace, a finding consistent with the fact that extradural scars are frequently most marked above or below the interspace, in contradistinction to a recurrent HNP. A vacuum disc (*large arrows*) has developed; this was not present on the preoperative scan. Postdiscectomy development of a vacuum disc frequently is encountered.

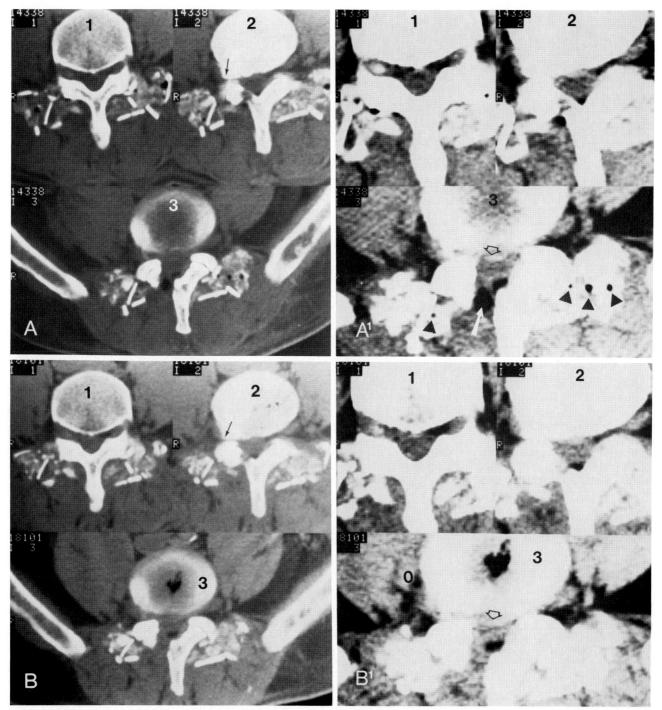

Figure 22.30.   Early and late postoperative changes: A and A¹ are both three successive cuts of an L4–5 scan made 8 days after a right discectomy and posterior fusion. A is the bone window, while A¹ is the soft-tissue window. Similarly, B and B¹ are the equivalent sections made 6 months after surgery. These were done because of recurrent right radiculopathy. The patient was a 41-year-old man. A number of interesting and significant points are illustrated:

1. A vacuum disc, not present immediatley after surgery (B3) developed on the later scan (B¹3).
2. A fairly severe right foraminal stenosis due to a spur (*small black arrows*) was overlooked at surgery, and possibly is responsible for some of the current symptoms.
3. The discectomy hematoma in A¹ (*open black arrows*) has become a scar of the same shape and size (3B¹) (*open arrow*).
4. The bone chips behind and lateral to the lamina remain more or less discrete and unchanged in 6 months, and have not yet fused or become attached to the laminas or spinous process.
5. The air bubbles in the fusion operative sites (*black arrowheads in A¹*) have been introduced by the recent surgery and gradually disappear.
6. The piece of fat (or gelfoam) (*white arrow, A¹*) has been replaced by fibrosis (section 3 in B¹).

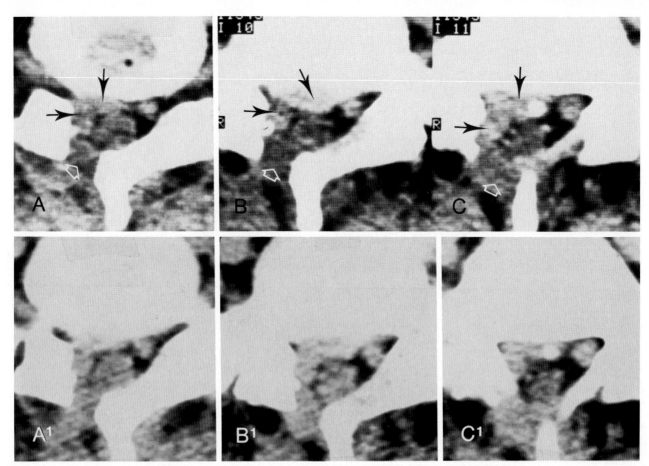

Figure 22.31. Hematoma changing into scar: Because of recurrence of pain a few days after discectomy, CT scans (A, B, C) were made 2 weeks after the surgery. The extensive extradural soft-tissue densities (*arrows*) undoubtedly represent hematomas at the discectomy and facetectomy sites. Repeat scans 2 months later (A¹, B¹, C¹) show that the hematomas have contracted slightly in size and become slightly more dense, indicative, we believe, of contracting scars. The patient was symptom free at this time. Note that the soft tissue at the laminectomy site (*white open arrows*) changed from low density (edema?) at 2 weeks to higher density (fibrosis) in 2 months.

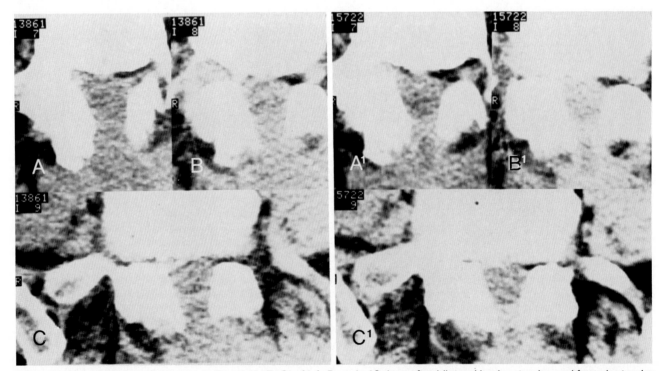

Figure 22.32. Hematoma into scar: A. Scans (A, B, C) of L4–5 made 10 days after bilateral laminectomies and foraminotomies, show the canal almost entirely filled with densities surrounding the more lucent thecal sac. These are presumably hematomas. B. Repeat scans (A¹, B¹, C¹) of the same area made 3 months after surgery, show an identical appearance suggesting that the hematomas have now become fibrosis.

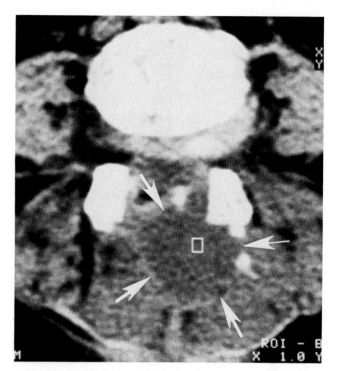

Figure 22.33. Postlaminectomy pseudomeningocele: CT made 1 month after bilateral facetectomies reveals a 2-cm low-density rounded mass (*arrows*) behind the laminectomies. The appearance is characteristic of a pseudomeningocele.

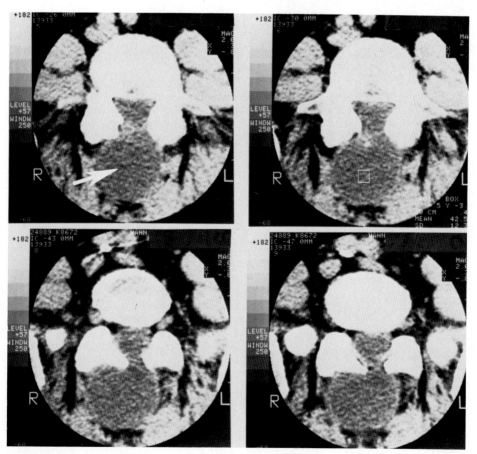

Figure 22.34. Postlaminectomy pseudomeningocele: A low-density rounded area (*arrow*) just behind the laminectomy at L4–5, is the typical CT picture of a pseudomeningocele. The bilateral laminectomy was performed 6 years previously. The fluid collection was 3 cm wide and 4 cm deep. Its relationship to the current bilateral leg pain is uncertain.

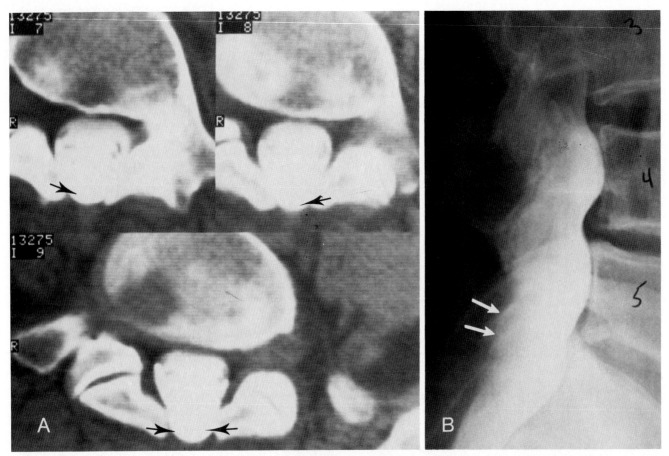

Figure 22.35. Posterior "herniation" after bilateral laminectomy: A. The posterior portion of the metrizamide-filled thecal sac (*arrows*) is protruding posteriorly through the bilateral laminectomy site at L5-S1. This posterior herniation has produced a pear-shaped thecal sac. B. On myelography, the posterior bulge of the column at L5-S1 (*arrows*) is characteristic. This herniation also has been termed pseudomeningocele, but it is unrelated to the PLP.

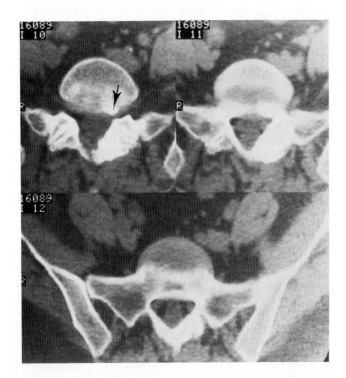

Figure 22.36. Postdiscectomy spur and foraminal stenosis: The spur at the discectomy site (*arrow*) is seriously compromising the left neural foramen. Some irregularity of bone of the posterior vertebral body at the discectomy site is a not uncommon finding on postoperative CT scans.

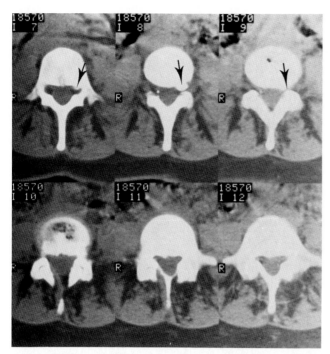

Figure 22.37. Postdiscectomy foraminal stenosis: About 6 years after a left laminectomy and discectomy at L4–5, an increasing left radiculopathy developed. CT scans revealed a large bony spur (*arrows*) at the discectomy site; the left neural foramen is seriously compromised by the spur.

complex is associated with the myelographic diagnosis of arachnoiditis (3). In the relatively few cases of arachnoiditis which were reoperated (2, 3, 5), there was always some epidural scarring around the sac associated with thickened dura. These findings were always at the previous operative site; the proliferative dural changes were also mostly on the side of the discectomy but might extend well above and below the operated interspace. The mechanism of the development of postoperative chronic adhesive arachnoiditis is still somewhat of a mystery.

On CT, thickening of the dural sac is occasionally seen in the postoperative patient (Figs. 22.9, 22.14, 22.16, 22.43, and 22.44). This thickening also was seen in a myelographic proven case of arachnoiditis. In our enhancement studies performed to distinguish scar from recurrent HNP, we have noted distinct enhancement of a thickened wall of the sac in many of these (Figs. 22.32 and 22.33). It seems likely that this represents thickened dura and probably arachnoid which somehow are related to the surgery and are most prominent on the side of surgery. Perhaps this dural thickening of the sac may be the CT manifestation of postoperative arachnoiditis.

Probably considerable information on arachnoiditis could be obtained if postoperative myelograms and intravenous enhanced CT studies could be performed on a series of both symptomatic and asymptomatic postoperative patients. Nevertheless, our current experience suggests that a thickened dural sac can be seen with or without contrast enhancement and often may occur in the

postdiscectomy patient. This thickening may encircle the sac uniformly or may be segmental and nonuniform. When segmental, the thickening occurs most often on the side of the laminectomy. We can postulate that if the dural thickening compromises the arachnoid space, even focally, some degree of arachnoiditis may be seen on the myelogram. Dural sac thickening on the postoperative CT scans without metrizamide cannot indicate accurately the presence or severity of arachnoiditis. This still remains an exclusive myelographic diagnosis.

MISCELLANEOUS POSTOPERATIVE CT FINDINGS

Fusion

The CT appearance of early and late posterior fusion by bone chips (Figs. 22.30 and 22.38) is characteristic and easily recognized. It is curious that the degree of fusion seen on CT many years after surgery can vary from almost none, as evidenced by persistence of the multiple discrete bone fragments, to solid bony bridging.

An interesting CT appearance is the bone fragments within the disc and partially into the adjacent bodies (Figs. 22.39 and 22.40). These are bone chips inserted within the disc and adjacent edges of the vertebra to promote interbody fusion. This type of anterior bone fusion apparently is performed infrequently.

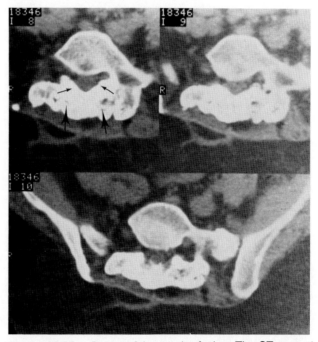

Figure 22.38. Successful posterior fusion: The CT scan at L5-S1 shows the mass of solid bone (*large arrows*) posterior to the intact lamina (*small arrows*), fused to the facets and lamina. The spinous process has been resected. The new bone extends more laterally than the facet. This type of total fusion across midline is performed when the lamina are intact. If a sizeable laminectomy is done, the bone chips are more laterally placed away from the midline.

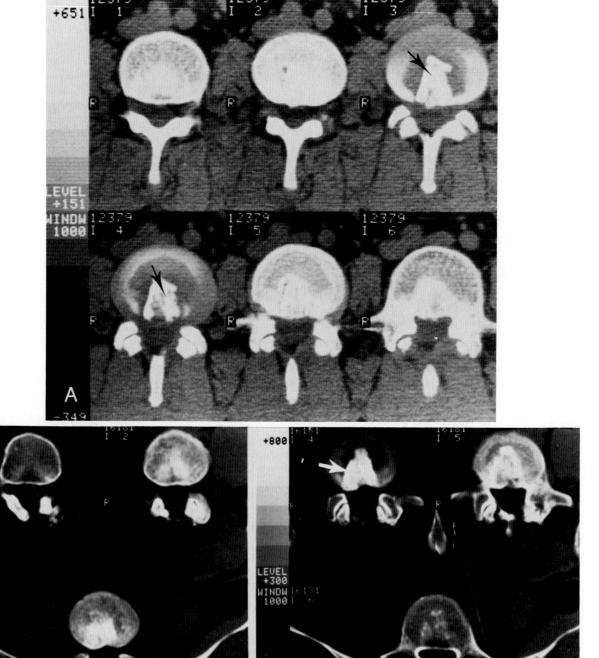

Figure 22.39. Interbody fusion—2 cases: Scans of L4–5 of 2 patients show the bone chips (*arrows*) which had been inserted into the posterior intervertebral space. Large bilateral laminectomies are present on both patients. Interbody fusions currently are performed rarely and CT recognition of this characteristic appearance will avoid any considerations of other bone pathology.

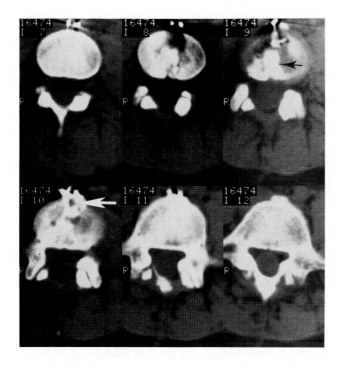

Figure 22.40. More extensive interbody fusion: CT scans of L4–5 show that pieces of bone have been inserted in both the posterior (*black arrows*) and in the anterior (*white arrow*) intervertebral spaces.

The Postoperative (Vacuum) Disc

In a number of patients who had a preoperative lumbar CT for comparison, a postoperative CT disclosed that a vacuum disc had developed shortly after the discectomy (Figs. 22.29 and 22.30). This apparently results from surgical extraction of degenerated disc material through the defect of the anulus fibrosis. This leads to a "hole" in the anulus where the degenerated or fragmented nucleus pulposis had been; the vacuum quickly fills with gas.

Air in the Thecal Sac

A unique complication occurred when the dura was torn accidentally and repaired during a discectomy. The patient developed unexpected low back pain very shortly after surgery. A CT scan 4 days postoperatively (Fig. 22.41A) showed an air-distended thecal sac. The patient was allowed to stand and move and his symptoms became less severe within a few days. A CT scan 6 days later, (10 days postoperatively) (Fig. 22.41B), showed that there was considerably less air and distention of the sac. It is interesting that as the sac distention subsided, the soft-tissue hematomas became visible. Incidentally, this patient also developed a vacuum disc postoperatively.

Postoperative Facet Disturbances

Facet subluxations have been encountered in a few patients. The subluxation is usually on the same side as the laminectomy and sometimes is associated with a facetectomy done to correct foraminal stenosis. However, the mechanism of the focal apophyseal joint subluxation is not clear in many cases.

One interesting example was severe recurrent radiculopathy after an apparent successful discectomy. The CT (Fig. 22.42) disclosed small recess scar and a mild bony excrescence from the vertebral body into the neural foramen and a dislocated anterior facet pushing into the foramen. At surgery, the left L5 root was found trapped between the scar, the bony overgrowth from the vertebral body, and the subluxed facet. Freeing the nerve has provided prolonged relief.

CONCLUSIONS

High-resolution CT of the postoperative spine in the symptomatic patient offers a great deal of information. The location and size of extradural scars, the recurrent HNP, postoperative bony stenosis, postoperative facet abnormalities, and iatrogenic pseudomeningoceles all are revealed considerably more accurately on CT than on myelography. The degree of extradural hematoma formation can be assessed readily on early postoperative scans. Postoperative arachnoiditis still remains a myelographic diagnosis.

Perhaps, when high-resolution CT studies will eventually be performed on *asymptomatic* postoperative patients, the clinical significance of the postoperative CT changes will be assessed more accurately.

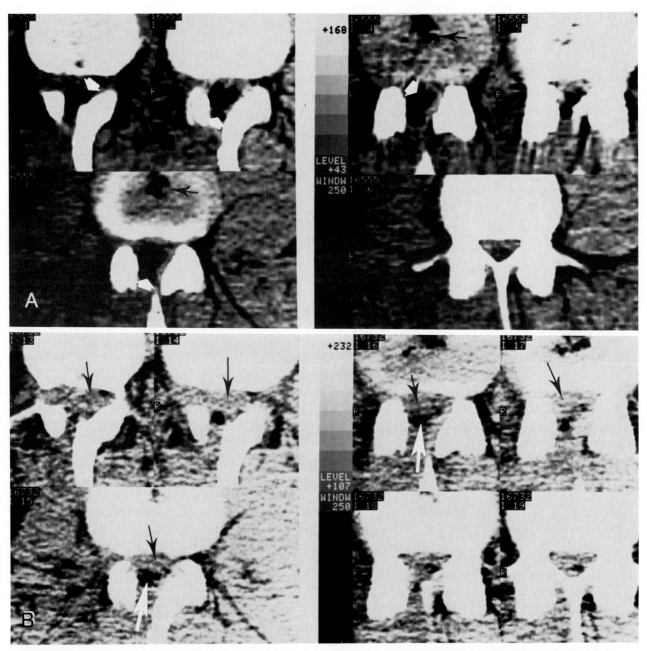

Figure 22.41. Postoperative complications; air in the thecal sac: A. CT scans of L4–5 were made 4 days after a right discectomy because of severe back pain. The surgeon had inadvertently opened the thecal sac but the tear was repaired. The thecal sac is distended with air (*white arrows*). Note the vacuum disc (*black arrows*) which was a postoperative development. B. Six days later, the CT scans shown considerably less gas and less distention (*white arrows*). The soft-tissue hematomas (*black arrows*) are now much more apparent. Clinically the patient, who had been allowed to stand and walk, was considerably improved. It is difficult to understand why air which entered the sac, undoubtedly from the inadvertent tear, should remain within the sac at the site of the tear unless one postulates that there was exudate within the sac which attached itself to the air bubbles.

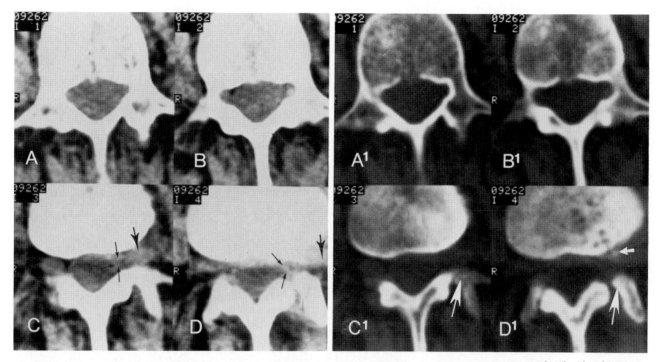

Figure 22.42.   Late postdiscectomy radiculopathy (facet subluxation): The successive scans of L4–5 (A¹, B¹, C¹, D¹) are seen in the soft-tissue window in A and in the bone window in B. This woman had recurrence of left radiculopathy 5 years after a successful left discectomy at L4–5. The following abnormalities are apparent on the scans:

1. A small discectomy scar adjacent to the sac (*small black arrows* in A—slices C¹ and D¹).
2. An enlarged nerve root on the left (*large black arrows* in A—scans C¹ and D¹).
3. A subluxed superior facet (*large white arrow*, B—scans C¹ and D¹).
4. A bony spur (*small white arrow*) extending from the body into the neural foramen.

The myelogram (Pantopaque) showed a large defect on the left at L4–5 interpreted as a recurrent HNP. At surgery, the swollen left root was found entrapped between the scar, the subluxed facet, and the bony spur. No recurrent HNP was found. The postoperative CT scan is generally more informative than the postoperative myelogram.

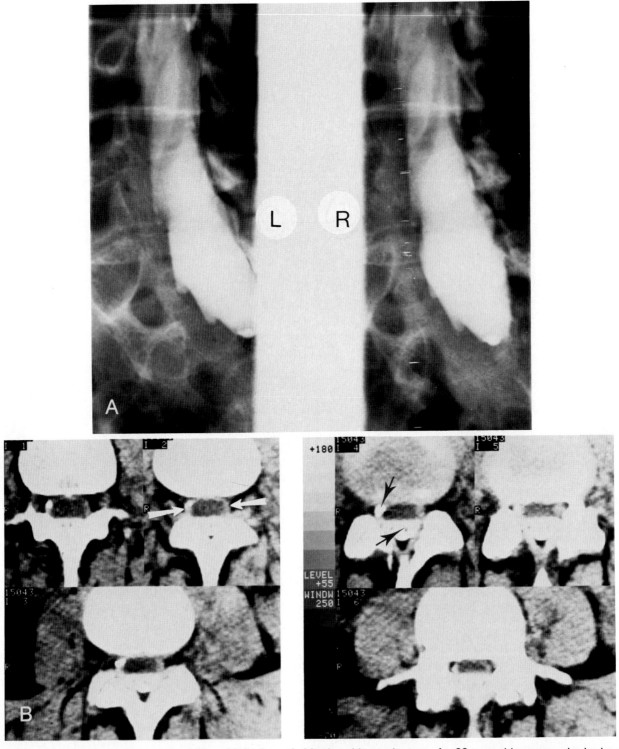

Figure 22.43. Postoperative arachnoiditis—CT findings: A. Metrizamide myelogram of a 32-year-old woman who had a right laminectomy at L5-S1, shows the typical changes of arachnoiditis; blunted nerve roots and thickening of the intradural nerve roots in the L3 to L5 area. B. A CT scan at L4–5 made shortly after the myelogram shows layered metrizamide (*black arrow*) in the sac and in a proximal nerve sleeve (*black arrow*). The wall of the sac is markedly thickened in all the sections (*white arrows*) which probably represents the marked thickening of the dura and the arachnoid. A thickened wall of the sac seen on CT probably represents thickened meninges, but the effect of this on nerve sleeves and roots cannot be assessed by CT. Only myelography can evaluate the extent and severity of arachnoiditis.

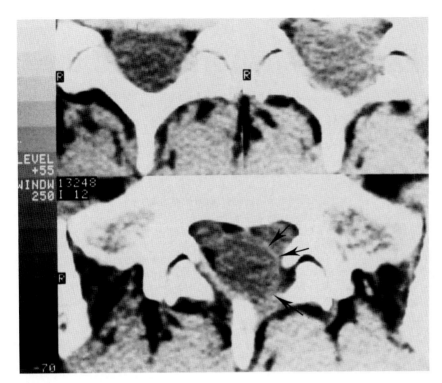

Figure 22.44. Postoperative arachnoiditis?? A CT scan of L5-S1 made 10 months after a left discectomy at L5-S1 reveals thickening of the left wall of the sac (*arrows*). This thickening of the wall has been seen not infrequently in postoperative scans, and is almost always more marked on the side of the previous laminectomy and discectomy (see Figs. 22.9, 22.14, and 22.16). It is more often apparent after enhancement studies.

References

1. Winkleman NW, Gotten N, Scheibert D: Localized adhesive spinal arachnoiditis. *Trans Am Neurol Assoc* 78:15–18, 1953.
2. Smolik EA, Nash FP: Lumbar spinal arachnoiditis: A complication of the intervertebral disc operation. *Ann Surg* 133:490–495, 1951.
3. Jørgensen J, Hansen PH, Steenskuv V, et al: A clinical and radiological study of chronic lower arachnoiditis. *Neuroradiology* 9:133–144, 1975.
4. Irstam L, Sundström R, Sigstedt B: Lumbar myelography and adhesive arachnoiditis. *Acta Radiol (Diag)* 15:356–366, 1974.
5. Irstam L, Rosencrantz M: Water soluble media and adhesive arachnoiditis. *Acta Radiol (Diag)* 15:1–15, 1974.
6. Cronquist S: The postoperative myelogram. *Acta Radiol* 52:45–51, 1959.
7. Quencer RM, Tenner M, Rothman L: The postoperative myelogram. *Radiology* 123:667–679, 1977.
8. Schubiger O, Valavanis A: CT differentiation between recurrent disc herniation and postoperative scar formation: The value of contrast enhancement. *Neuroradiology* 22:251–254, 1980.

CHAPTER TWENTY-THREE

Computed Tomographic Myelography of the Postoperative Spine

JOHN D. MEYER, M.D.

INTRODUCTION

Radiological examination of the lumbar spine after operation may be very difficult. The problem arises because alterations produced by previous myelography and operation are not only confusing themselves, but often superimposed upon developmental variation, degenerative changes, and the problems arising from acute and chronic disc disease (1–8). Myelography alone, particularly Pantopaque, may cause confusing chronic alterations. Dural-arachnoid scarring patterns may produce a broad range of deformity from minimal root sleeve defects to a complete block. Spinal stenosis, which may be developmental, acquired, or both, is difficult to study properly without axial tomography, either computed or not. Complex degenerative changes make matters more difficult. The recognition of the herniated disc, either recurrent or newly herniated, therefore, becomes most difficult in a postoperative spine. In particular, differentiation of disc from scar has been a problem.

Earlier reports have demonstrated the usefulness of CT examination of the spine with and without metrizamide in various conditions (9–27). CT scanning also should be of use, therefore, in evaluating the postoperative spine. Because of the complex alterations present, it was assumed that maximum available information would be most useful; therefore, CT scanning after metrizamide myelography was utilized. No comprehensive review of the postoperative metrizamide myelogram was available, nonetheless it was assumed that although more details would be available with metrizamide, metrizamide, per se, would not solve the diagnostic dilemma. Pending additional data, it also was assumed that plain CT scanning alone might not provide sufficient data. However, future developments and additional data might make metrizamide usage unnecessary.

MATERIALS AND METHODS

Clinical

Currently, there are 78 adult men and women of average age 45, all of whom had had at least one previous myelogram and lumbar operation, usually a laminectomy for herniated disc. Many patients had had multiple operations and myelograms. Backache, sciatica, or both persisted or recurred in all patients studied, and all had had a failure of conservative therapy before a decision to restudy the spine.

Technique

All patients were studied by metrizamide myelography, followed by a lumbar spine scan on the General Electric 8800 Scanner. Metrizamide at 190 mg/cc concentration in a volume of 10–12 cc was utilized. Filming was obtained immediately in the semierect position, generally without flexion or extension views. Delayed filming was not performed. All CT scans were performed within 4 hours, usually 1 hour, with the patient supine and the legs straight. Most were scanned at L5-S1 and L4-5, with about one-half at L3-4. Five-mm thick adjacent sections were obtained from approximately pedicle to pedicle through the disc space. Thin sections of 1.5 mm or overlapping 5-mm sections were not obtained due to time constraints. Gantry angle was chosen by localizer as the closest angle parallel to the disc at the respective levels. No attempt was made to correct for lordosis by changing the patient's position. Scans were performed at 120 kVp, 600 MA. Routine image display at 2X magnification was utilized. No reformatting or sagittal/coronal reconstruction was used. A window-width of 500 was generally used, with window levels of approximately 80–120.

CT Diagnostic Criteria

Observed abnormalities were classified by the dominant pathological alteration. These categories were herniated disc, scarring patterns, central stenosis, lateral stenosis, indeterminate, and normal.

HERNIATED DISC

Figures 23.1–23.3: Disc material was considered to be herniated if a smooth and rounded or roughly-rounded mass of the same relative density as disc material was found in relation to the disc and in continuity with it. Actual measurement of CT number was not performed since it was found that the relative density was the important criterion. Herniated disc material was always of disc density.

SCARRING PATTERNS

Figures 23.4–23.8: These changes were represented by replacement of epidural tissues by denser tissue, but without any significant focal mass effect, in general. The normal epidural fat was replaced. The density of this tissue, which was not measured consistently, was found to be of the same relative density as herniated disc material. A tendency was observed for scar tissue to be relatively radiolucent, but this was not found consistently. It also was noted that some disc material was of lesser density than the majority of disc, either herniated or not herniated. Scar tissue usually did not relate solely to the disc space alone, but was found removed from the disc space as well. A tendency to be related to epidural spaces between the disc spaces was observed. In contrast, herniated disc material related primarily to the disc space. Scars tended to produce angular or irregular and roughened tissue alteration, not a smooth and rounded focal mass like the herniated disc produced. Even though myelograms revealed extensive root sleeve and thecal sac distortions, a lack of focal mass effect was noted with scarring patterns. In only one instance (Fig. 23.5) was a scar noted to have mass effect visible on both myelogram and CT scan.

STENOSIS

Figures 23.9 and 23.10: Central canal stenosis (28–35) (Fig. 23.10) may result from either developmental narrowing or acquired narrowing of the canal. The developmental type may demonstrate short pedicles, thick laminae, and facet joints, with sagittal canal narrowing. Degenerative changes also may produce central canal narrowing, secondary to thickened laminae and facet joint degenerative changes. These findings may be superimposed, especially in the patient with a relatively small canal and concomitant change. Lateral canal stenosis (36–39) (Fig. 23.9) may result from peripheral narrowing of the spinal canal, lateral recess, or root exit zone. This may be caused by spurs, thickened superior articular facet, and other developmental and degenerative alteration.

INDETERMINATE

Figure 23.11: In this small group, the canal was surrounded by dense tissue with no visualization of epidural fat or root sleeves. The canal was well seen, however, but was somewhat narrow and distorted. No distinguishing characteristics, however, with respect to other diagnostic categories were noted. There was an element of "fibrous" stenosis seen in this group. The bony canal appeared to be normal in the patients examined. It is possible that findings generally represent scarring only, but this has not been confirmed concretely at this point. Surprisingly, the number of indeterminate scans was quite small, considering the large number of markedly altered myelograms.

NORMAL

Figure 23.6: In the absence of any of the above criteria, essentially, the CT scan findings were considered normal at the level in question.

RESULTS

Myelography

All myelograms were abnormal at least at one level, usually the level in question. At L3–4, the myelogram was usually normal. The defects ranged from small root sleeve pressure alterations, such as splaying or widening, to a complete subarachnoid block. Very often, unfilled root sleeves were noted bilaterally, at L5-S1 and L4–5, accompanied by minor extradural pressure defects on the contrast column. Herniated discs tended to produce focal and relatively smooth defects, but the sign itself was not specific enough for discs to be reliable, unless the defect was very prominent and very focally related to the disc space. This presentation, per se, was not extremely common. Both herniated discs and scarring produced single unfilled root sleeves, but none of the defects otherwise had any consistent specificity: root sleeves tended to be visualized with the same degree of alteration in any of the conditions. Root sleeves that were unfilled or poorly filled at myelography were seen better on CT, a tendency which enabled metrizamide CT to be more helpful than either myelography or plain CT alone.

CT Scanning

There are three tables in which data are organized by CT diagnosis at the interspace levels indicated. Table 23.1 presents data for patients not reoperated upon for various reasons, such as confusing clinical findings, poor operative risk, or failure to demonstrate convincingly an operable lesion consistent with clinical findings. In Table 23.2, a similar organization is displayed. This group included levels scanned in all the patients that were reoperated upon. Not all levels were operated upon, just the principal levels, and these data are displayed in Table 23.3, which includes the diagnosis and the operative findings in 24 patients reoperated upon. Table 23.4 summarizes all data. The main difference between Tables 23.1 and 23.2, the reoperated and nonreoperated groups, was the presence of herniated disc, which when discovered by CT, usually was operated upon. A few patients that had recurrent or new herniated discs were not operated upon, however. There were 6 of these. An unexpected finding was the large number of normal levels identified, even though myelograms demonstrated extensive abnormality. This finding alone, abnormal myelogram with normal CT, indicates the value of CT scanning after metrizamide myelography. As noted above, the number of indeterminate scans was rather small, another surprising finding, considering the range of abnormal myelographic findings.

Spinal stenosis remains an important consideration, and one that needs to be stressed. CT affords a much easier route of recognition of stenosis than previous methods. Stenosis reported herein does not include the postoperative variety noted after fusion, because no patient with this condition was identified. Similarly, no patient with Paget's disease, achondroplasia, or other acquired bone disease was found. Stenosis referred to the congenital or developmental type commonly with superimposed degenerative change. Undoubtedly, lateral stenosis commonly has combined developmental alterations and superimposed degenerative change. A review of 227 patients needing operations for symptoms of disc syndrome found a significant number of patients having stenosing conditions, either alone or with combination with herniated disc (40). This attests to the frequency of stenosing conditions.

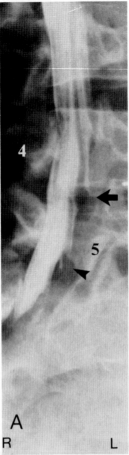

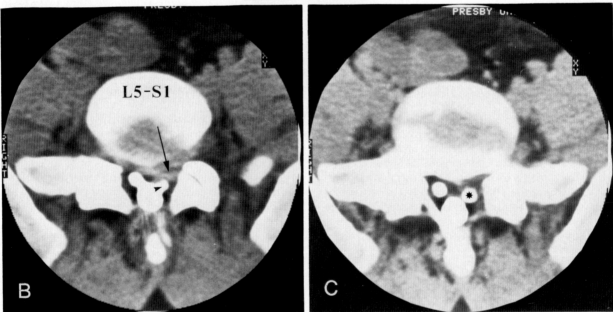

Figure 23.1. New Herniated Disc at L5-S1 and Disc Protrusion Without Herniation Accompanied by Some Scarring at L4–5, Operatively Proved: In A, the myelogram, the S1 root sleeve is incompletely filled (*arrowhead*). One level above at L4–5 (*arrow*), the root sleeve apparently is widened, although this partly is due to incomplete filling of the sleeve, as noted in other views. In B, a section through the disc level at L5-S1, a roughly-rounded focal mass of disc density is seen projecting posterolaterally (*arrow*), and also displaces the root sleeve posteriorly (*arrowhead*). C taken just inferior demonstrates that the focal mass is related essentially to the disc space and is not as prominent as in the section above. The root sleeve is better filled (*star*) and is not quite as posteriorly displaced. This tendency to be filled better is commonly observed at CT compared to myelography alone. D, E, and F, were obtained at L4–5, the level of previous operation. In D, the anterior epidural space and root sleeve is essentially symmetric. Arrow indicates no focal mass of disc density. Slightly below, in E, the *arrow* indicates a nonfilled root sleeve, but no mass effect is observed. Similarly, slightly below in F, the *white arrow* indicates again nonfilling of the root sleeve on the left. The *black arrow* indicates fairly good filling of the root sleeve on the right side. These findings at L4–5 were due to scar tissue and "disc bulge" but no recurrent herniation was found at operation. Some scar tissue prevented the root sleeve from filling properly.

434

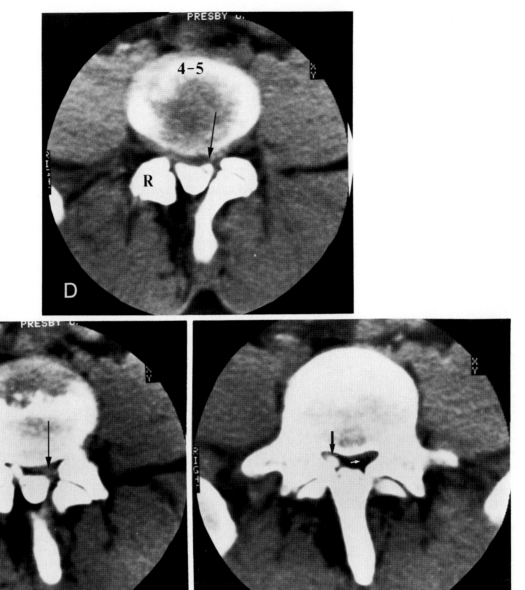

Figure 23.1. D–F.

DISCUSSION AND CONCLUSIONS

From the good correlation of operative findings with suspected diagnosis at the principal level, as noted in Table 23.3, herniated discs, either recurrent or new, can be differentiated from scarring patterns and from other pathological changes by metrizamide CT myelography. If one adheres fairly strictly to the criteria for definition of herniated disc, then results are good. These criteria, as described above, should include focal mass related to the disc space. All cases of herniated disc, operatively proved, demonstrated a focal mass effect at the disc space, while only 1 patient with a scar presented with focal mass effect. It may be in the future that measurement of the actual

density of scar and disc material may be of some use. It seems at this point that there is a tendency for scar tissue to be more radiolucent than herniated disc, however, the reliability of numbers does not seem adequate. This is due partly to the various densities observed within disc material itself, ranging from relatively lucent to the more commonly observed denser tissues, and also because of various densities of scar tissue per se. Complex anatomical changes observed in the lumbar spine, especially in the postoperative state, make measurement more difficult. Morphological criteria, as described herein, seem to be more important in distinguishing scar and herniated disc. It also should be noted that a single unfilled root sleeve, seen either myelographically or on CT scanning, might be

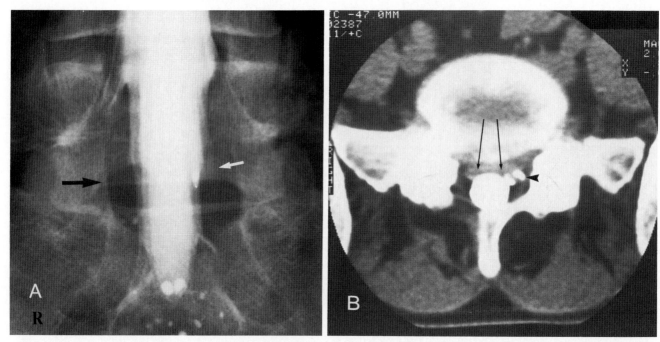

Figure 23.2. Recurrent Herniated Disc, Operatively Proved: In the myelogram, A, the right S1 root sleeve is not filled (*black arrow*). The left S1 root sleeve (*white arrow*) is widened somewhat and poorly filled. No other distortion or displacement is noted. This is L5-S1, the level of previous operation. A CT scan obtained at the level of the *black arrow* on the myelographic film demonstrates a curvilinear mass of disc density projecting posteriorly (*black arrows*). The left S1 root sleeve appears somewhat widened, but is better filled (*arrowhead*). The right S1 root sleeve does not fill. This was a surgically confirmed recurrent herniated disc.

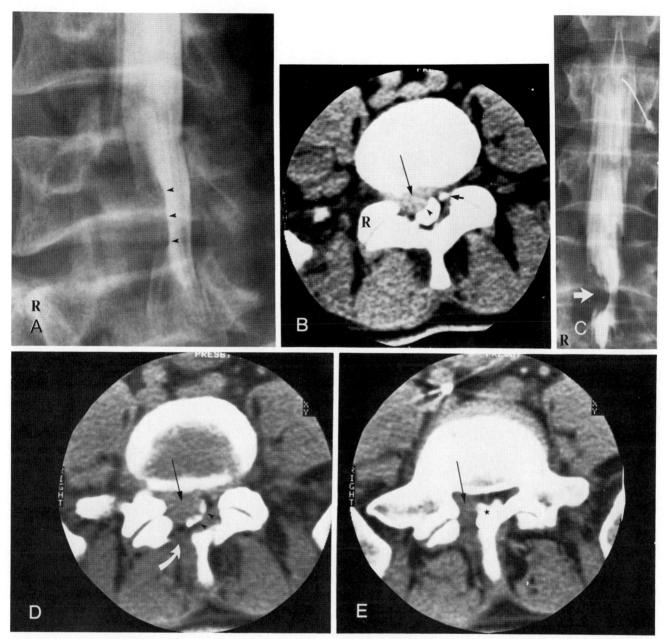

Figure 23.3.   Two Large Recurrent Herniated Discs in the Same Patient—Same Level, Different Times, Operatively Proved: In A, the first postoperative myelogram, a prominent right-sided extradural defect was noted with posterior and slight medial displacement of the contrast (*arrowheads*) at the level of previous operation. CT scan at that time, B, demonstrated a prominent focal mass of disc density on the right side (*arrow*), indenting the contrast column (*arrowhead*). The right L5 root sleeve did not fill, but the left (*small arrow*) did. At operation, this was a recurrent herniated disc. In C, a myelogram was obtained a year later after presentation with similar symptoms. An extradural defect of very large size is noted at L4–5 once again (*white arrow*). In D, CT scan through the L4–5 level demonstrates once again a very prominent focal mass of disc density projecting posterolaterally (*arrow*). The contrast column is markedly distorted and displaced (*arrowheads*). The site of previous laminectomy (*white arrow*) is well demonstrated. A section slightly below at E demonstrates still the mass produced by herniated disc (*arrow*), but it is not as prominent as seen in the section above, which is at the disc space. The thecal sac and root sleeve are distorted and displaced toward the left (*star*).

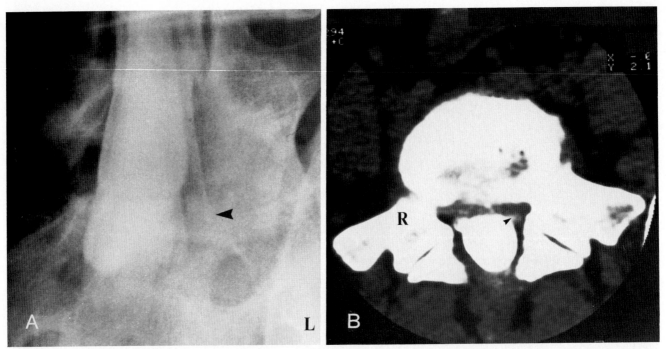

Figure 23.4. Scarring Pattern, Not Operatively Proved: In the myelogram, the S1 root sleeve at the level of previous operation is filled incompletely and appears to be widened slightly (*arrowhead*) and the thecal sac may demonstrate a slight extradural defect as well. However, the CT scan, although showing that the S1 root sleeve is filled incompletely and flattened slightly (*arrowhead*), fails to demonstrate any material of disc density in the epidural space. Also the thecal sac and root sleeve are not displaced. No evidence of disc herniation is identified.

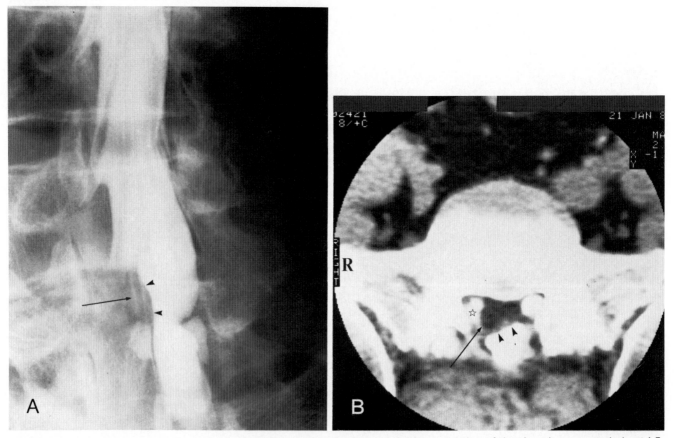

Figure 23.5. Scarring Pattern, Operatively Proved: In the myelogram, A, the lower portion of the thecal sac posteriorly at L5 and L5-S1 demonstrates prominent distortion, secondary to scarring. However, there is an extradural defect on the contrast column (*arrowheads*) accompanied by some distortion and displacement of the S1 root sleeve (*arrow*). This is the site of previous operation. The CT scan obtained at the top of S1 level demonstrates the posteromedial distortion and displacement of the contrast column in the thecal sac (*arrowheads*). This distortion seems to be caused by a *lucent* extradural defect which has some mass effect (*arrow*). There is also distortion of the S1 root sleeve (*star*). At operation, the findings were due to scarring with no evidence of recurrent herniated disc.

438

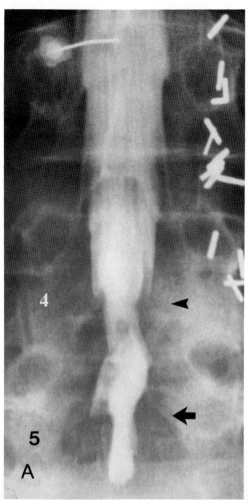

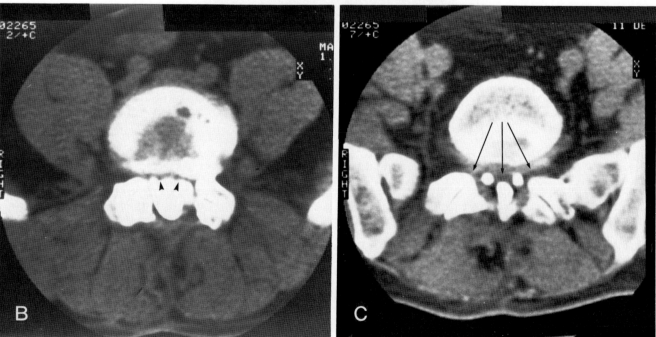

Figure 23.6. Minor Scarring at L4–5 and Normal CT at L5-S1, Not Operatively Proved: In the myelogram, irregular constriction of the contrast column is noted from the lower half of L4 caudally. Previous operations were at L4–5 and L5-S1. The contrast does not appear to pass below the midportion of L5. Root sleeves are poorly filled. In B, a section obtained at the level of the *arrowhead*, the contrast column and root sleeves appear to be filled fairly well with little distortion of the epidural space (*arrowheads*). There is no evidence of herniated disc. The next section obtained at the level of the arrow on the myelogram film demonstrates good filling of the root sleeves, although the myelogram fails to show them well filled. The *arrows* indicate the posterior aspect of the disc. No evidence of herniation observed. The thecal sac also is filled somewhat better on the CT myelogram than conventional myelogram alone. Some of the distortion of the thecal sac appears to be due to possible primary scarring process, and not to displacement extrinsically.

439

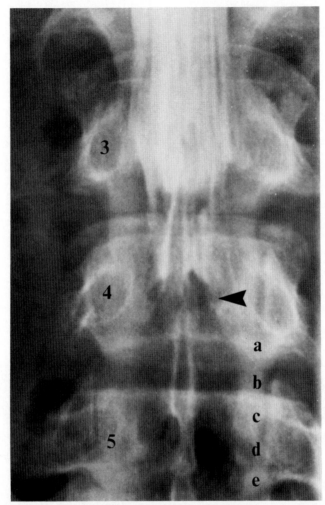

Figure 23.7. Extensive Scarring Pattern, Proved at Operation: The myelogram demonstrates a block to caudal flow of contrast at the midportion of L4 (*arrowhead*). Previous operation was at L4–5. No distinguishing characteristics at all can be identified below the level of block. The letters a-e indicate the levels of the scans obtained in A-E. In A, the anterior and anterolateral epidural space contains somewhat irregular densities which are associated with some distortion of the thecal sac (*arrowhead*). This distortion appears to continue caudally as noted in B-E. In B, *small white arrows* indicate anterior distortion of the thecal sac, which is nonspecific in that section. The distortion continues and in C, there is marked distortion of the thecal sac, with only a small portion of the subarachnoid space filling with contrast (*star*). Continuing caudally, marked distortion is still noted and a continuous irregular band to the level of the next disc. This is not the pattern noted with herniated disc since there is no focal mass of disc density, and the distorting tissues are not related only to the disc space, but continue extensively above and below. No disc was found at operation, only scar tissue.

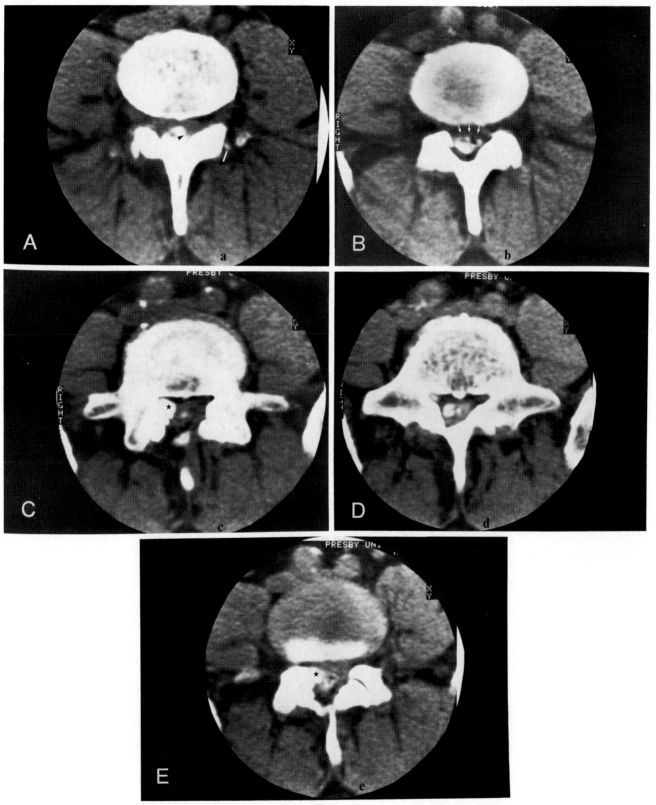

Figure 23.7. A–E.

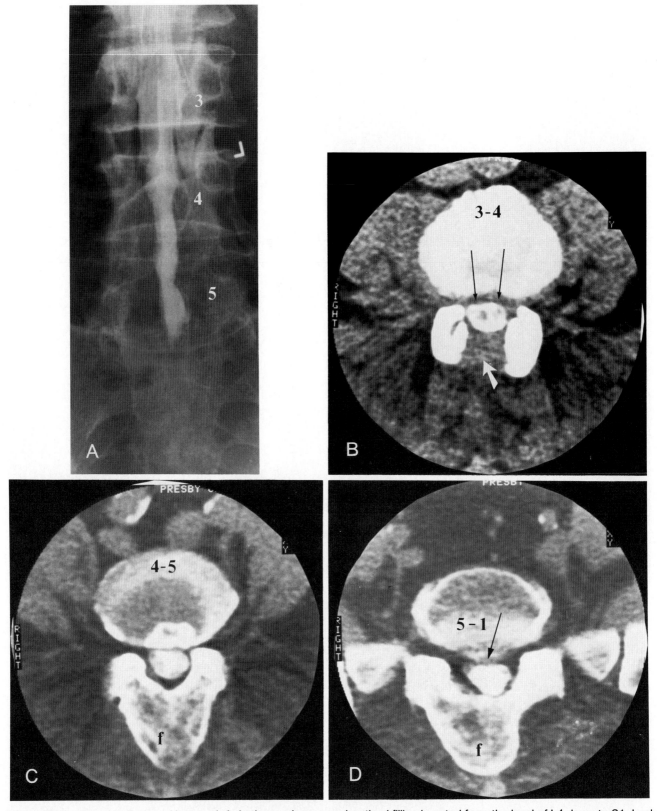

Figure 23.8. Scarring Pattern, Unproved: A. In the myelogram, suboptimal filling is noted from the level of L4 down to S1. Lack of symmetry is noted with very poor root sleeve filling and irregular distortion. Evidence of previous laminectomy at L3–4, L4–5, and L5-S1 is noted. Fusion at L4–5 and L5-S1 was also performed. In B, a section obtained at L3–4, the anterior epidural space is essentially intact (*black arrows*) with no evidence of herniation or any significant scarring deformity. The site of previous laminectomy is noted (*white arrow*). Caudally, at L4–5 in C, fusion bone is noted posteriorly (*f*). The anterior epidural space, although somewhat thin, is normal with no distortion or displacement of the contrast material. In D, at L5-S1, the posterior portion of the edge of the vertebral body projects slightly into the anterior epidural space (*arrow*) without any associated significant distortion of the contrast column.

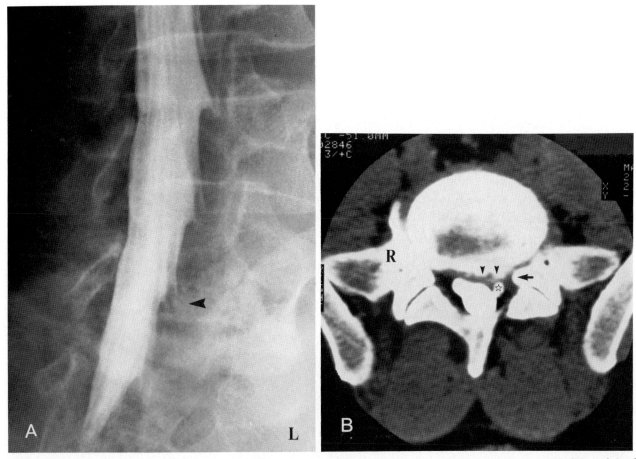

Figure 23.9.   Lateral Recess Stenosis, Operatively Proved: In A, the myelogram, the *arrowhead* indicates poor filling of the S1 root sleeve. Some sclerosis is observed in the facet joint. Previous operation occurred at this level. CT scan, however, much better shows that the root sleeve (*star*) is displaced somewhat posteriorly by a combination of roughening and thickening of the posterior portion of the vertebral body (*arrowheads*) and by medial projection of a portion of the superior articular process (*arrow*). No disc material was found at operation.

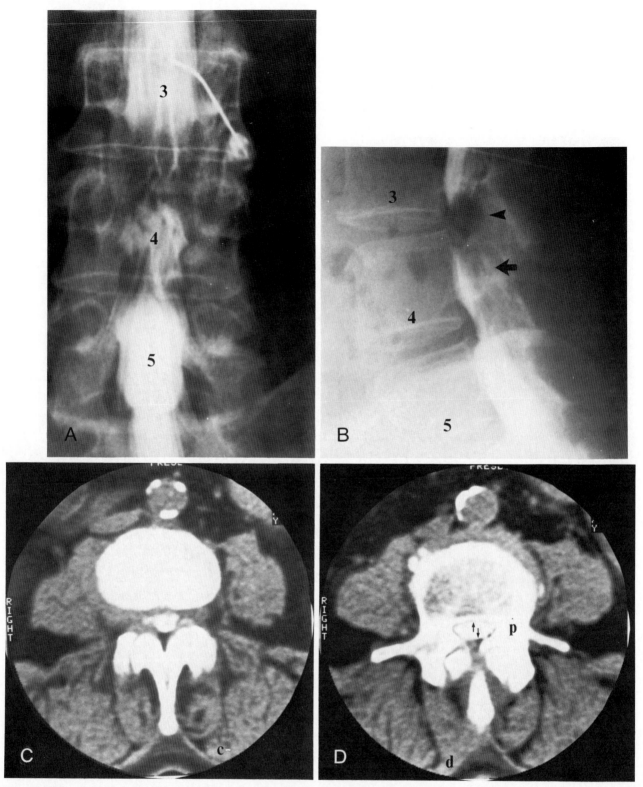

Figure 23.10.   Central Spinal Stenosis, Operatively Proved: A and B are anteroposterior and lateral myelographic films. At the site of previous operation, L5, the spinal canal is normal with good filling of the root sleeves. CT at this level was unremarkable. At L3–4, there is slight anterolisthesis with a very prominent constriction of the subarachnoid space with diminution in the rate of caudal flow. C was obtained at the level of the *arrowhead*, D at the level of the *arrow*. Redundant nerve roots are noted within the subarachnoid space. Constriction at L4–5 was not as marked as that at L3–4. In C, the laminae and facet joints are relatively thick. The subarachnoid space is reduced in diameter. No evidence of a herniation is identified. In D, the pedicles are short and there is reduction in the anteroposterior diameter of the spinal canal (*arrows*). This is the typical developmental stenotic pattern.

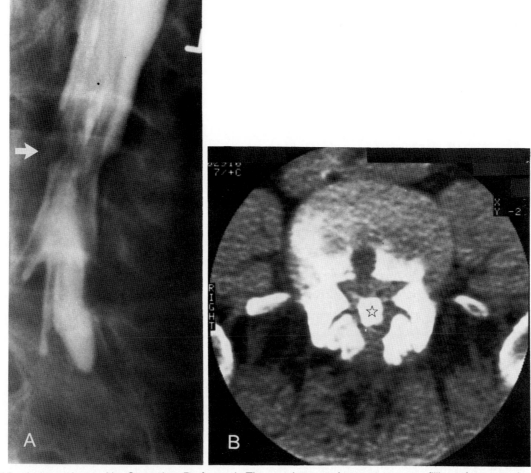

Figure 23.11. Indeterminate, No Operation Performed: The myelogram demonstrates nonfilling of a root sleeve, L5, and generalized narrowing at the level of previous operation, L4–5, and the proximal portion of L5. CT scan, which was obtained at the level of the *arrowhead*, demonstrates that the thecal sac (*star*) is surrounded by dense tissue, but no specific characteristics are present to distinguish disc or scar. It may be that this represents all scarring, but more data are needed to confirm the appearance.

Table 23.1.
CT Findings: No Reoperation Group—54 Patients

Diagnosis	L5-S1	L4–5	L3–4
Recurrent disc herniation	3	1	0
New disc herniation	0	2	0
Scar	13	15	10
Central stenosis	0	5	3
Lateral stenosis	3	2	0
Normal	28	26	29
Indeterminate	2	3	1

Table 23.3.
Operative Findings at Principal Level—24 Patients

Diagnosis	Number	Findings
Recurrent herniated disc	9	9
New herniated disc	4	4
Scar	4	4
Stenosis	8	8
Normal	2	2

Table 23.2.
CT Findings: Reoperated Group—24 Patients

Diagnosis	L5-S1	L4–5	L3–4
Recurrent disc herniation	7	2	0
New disc herniation	2	1	1
Scar	3	4	3
Central stenosis	1	3	2
Lateral stenosis	2	1	0
Normal	9	9	9
Indeterminate	0	2	0

Table 23.4.
CT Findings: All Patients—78 Patients

Diagnosis	L5-S1	L4–5	L3–4
Recurrent disc herniation	10	4	0
New disc herniation	2	3	1
Scar	15	19	13
Central stenosis	1	3	5
Lateral stenosis	5	3	0
Normal	37	35	38
Indeterminate	2	5	1

due to herniated disc or scar, but more likely herniated disc if mass effect is present. Although it is true also that a herniated disc may be present with very little mass effect, or perhaps none, no patient operated upon presented radiographically in this manner. Patients were chosen for operation not simply on the basis of radiographic findings but on clinical findings. It seems that maximum available anatomical data are necessary to study the postoperative spine. Therefore, utilization of metrizamide provides the maximum amount of data available. Good visualization of root sleeves at CT scanning was observed, even though myelograms showed nonfilling of the same sleeve. This probably is due to the tendency for metrizamide to slowly pass an area of partial obstruction and the great sensitivity of CT scanning. Without metrizamide present in the root sleeves, their location is not always apparent, even with high-resolution overlapping sections of the lumbar spine. An important finding noted as well by this technique was the large number of normal levels identified by CT scanning in patients whose myelograms were abnormal. This again is believed to be due to the better visualization of root sleeves by CT scanning and the fact that the scanning is performed at least an hour after the contrast material has been placed in the subarachnoid space. It has been observed that simply obtaining a delayed myelographic film after placement of contrast material demonstrates better filling of root sleeves at myelography. The identification of normal CT levels is a very useful addition and further reduces the possibility of reoperation that might produce a poor result.

The number of indeterminate scans was relatively small. This pattern of density surrounding the thecal sac is an unusual finding at CT scanning because most patients demonstrated filling of the root sleeves. It might be that this is a diffuse scarring pattern which is rather symmetrical in appearance. Luckily, the number of indeterminate scans was relatively small which, therefore, allowed for accurate classification in most patients and in most levels scanned.

References

1. Mosley I: The oil myelogram after operation for lumbar disc lesions. *Clin Radiol* 38:267–276, 1977.
2. Burton C: Lumbo-sacral arachnoiditis. *Spine* 3:24–30, 1978.
3. Castan P, Bourbotte G, Herail J, et al: Follow-up and postoperative radiculography, a radiological analysis of 640 patients. *J Neuroradiol* 4:49–93, 1977.
4. Picard L, Roland J, Blanchot P, et al: Scarring of the theca and the nerve roots as seen at radiculography. *J Neuroradiol* 4:29–48, 1977.
5. Benoist M, Ficat C, Baraf P, et al: Post-operative lumbar epiduroarachnoiditis, diagnostic and therapeutic aspects. *Spine* 5:432–436, 1980.
6. Benner B, Ehni G: Spinal arachnoiditis, the post-operative variety in particular. *Spine* 3:40–44, 1978.
7. Quiles M, Marchisello P, Tsairis P: Lumbar adhesive arachnoiditis, etiologic and pathologic aspects. *Spine* 3:45–50, 1978.
8. Brodsky A: Cauda equina arachnoiditis, a correlative, clinical, and roentgenologic study. *Spine* 3:51–60, 1978.
9. Ullrich C, Binet E, Sanecki M, et al: Quantitative assessment of the lumbar spinal canal by computed tomography. *Radiology* 134:137–143, 1980.
10. Di Chiro G, Schellinger D: Computed tomography of spinal cord after lumbar intrathecal introduction of metrizamide (computer-assisted myelography). *Radiology* 120:101–104, 1976.
11. Lee B, Kazam E, Newman A: Computed tomography of the spine and spinal cord. *Radiology* 128:95–102, 1978.
12. Hammerschlag S, Wolpert S, Carter B: Computer tomography of the spinal canal. *Radiology* 121:361–367, 1976.
13. Scotti L, Marasco J, Pittman T, et al: Computed tomography of the spinal canal and cord. *Comput Tomogr* 1:229–234, 1977.
14. Federle M, Moss A, Margolin F: Role of computed tomography in patients with "sciatica." *J Comput Assist Tomogr* 4:335–341, 1980.
15. Roub L, Drayer B: Spinal computed tomography: limitations and applications. *AJR* 133:267–273, 1979.
16. Burton C: Computed tomographic scanning and the lumbar spine, Part 1: Economic and historic review. *Spine* 4:353–355, 1979.
17. Burton C, Heithoff K, Kirkaldy-Willis W, Ray C: Computed tomographic scanning and the lumbar spine, Part 2: Clinical considerations. *Spine* 4:356–368, 1979.
18. Verbiest H: The significance and principals of computerized axial tomography in idiopathic developmental stenosis of the bony lumbar vertebral canal. *Spine* 4:369–378, 1979.
19. Livingston P, Grayson E: Computed tomography in the diagnosis of herniated discs in the lumbar spine. In: Post MJD: *Radiographic Evaluation of the Spine: Current Advances with Emphasis on Computed Tomography*, Masson Publishing USA Inc., New York, 1980, pp. 308–319.
20. Post M: CT update: The impact of time, metrizamide, and high resolution on the diagnosis of spinal pathology. In Post MJD: *Radiographic Evaluation of the Spine: Current Advances with Emphasis on Computed Tomography*, Masson Publishing USA Inc., New York, 1980, pp. 259–294.
21. Baleriaux-Waha D, Soeur M, Stadnik T, et al: CT of the adult spine with metrizamide. In Post MJD: *Radiographic Evaluation of the Spine: Current Advances with Emphasis on Computed Tomography*, Masson Publishing USA Inc., New York, 1980, pp. 353–365.
22. Coin CH, Ying-Sek C, Keranen V, et al: Computed assisted myelography in disc disease. *J Comput Assist Tomogr* 1:398–404, 1977.
23. Arii H, Takahashi M, Tamakawa Y, et al: Metrizamide spinal computed tomography following myelography. *Comput Tomogr* 4:117–125, 1980.
24. Naidich T, King D, Moran C, Sagel S: Computed tomography of the lumbar thecal sac. *J Comput Assist Tomogr* 4:37–41, 1980.
25. Haughton V, Syvertsen A, Williams A: Soft-tissue anatomy within the spinal canal as seen on computed tomography. *Radiology* 134:649–655, 1980.
26. Williams A, Haughton V, Syvertsen A: Computed tomography in the diagnosis of herniated nucleus pulposus. *Radiology* 135:95–99, 1980.
27. Carrera G, Williams A, Haughton V: Computed tomography in sciatica. *Radiology* 137:433–437, 1980.
28. Lee C, Hansen H, Weiss A: Developmental lumbar spinal stenosis, pathology and surgical treatment. *Spine* 3:246–255, 1978.
29. Kirkaldy-Willis W, Wedge J, Yon-Hing K, et al: Pathology and pathogenesis of lumbar spondylosis and stenosis. *Spine* 3:319–328, 1978.
30. Kirkaldy-Willis W, Hill R: A more precise diagnosis for low-back pain. *Spine* 4:102–109, 1979.
31. Roberson G, Llewellyn H, Taveras J: The narrow lumbar spinal canal syndrome. *Radiology* 107:89–97, 1973.
32. Yamada H, Ohya M, Okada T, et al: Intermittent cauda equina compression due to narrow spinal canal. *J Neurosurg* 37:83–88, 1972.

33. Wedge J, Kinnard P, Foley R, et al: The management of spinal stenosis. *Orthop Rev* 6:89–93, 1977.
34. Verbiest H: Fallacies of the present definition, nomenclature, and classification of the stenoses of the lumbar vertebral canal. *Spine* 1:217–225, 1976.
35. Verbiest H: Results of surgical treatment of idiopathic developmental stenosis of the lumbar vertebral canal, a review of 27 years' experience. *J Bone Joint Surg* 59:181–188, 1977.
36. Mikhael M, Ciric I, Tarkington J, et al: Neuroradiological evaluation of lateral recess syndrome. *Radiology* 140:97–107, 1981.
37. Epstein J, Epstein B, Rosenthal A, et al: Sciatica caused by nerve root entrapment in the lateral recess: the superior facet syndrome. *J Neurosurg* 36:584–589, 1972.
38. Ciric I, Mikhael M, Tarkington J, et al: The lateral recess syndrome, a variant of spinal stenosis. *J Neurosurg* 53:433–443, 1980.
39. Epstein J, Epstein B, Lavine L, et al: Lumbar nerve root compression at the intervertebral foramina caused by arthritis of the posterior facets. *J Neurosurg* 39:362–369, 1973.
40. Paine K, Haung P: Lumbar disc syndrome. *J Neurosurg* 37:75–82, 1972.

CHAPTER TWENTY-FOUR

The Computed Tomographic Appearance of the Lumbar Spine Following Disc Surgery: An Analysis of Findings in Asymptomatic Volunteers

IRA F. BRAUN, M.D., JOSEPH P. LIN, M.D., VALLO BENJAMIN, M.D., and IRVIN I. KRICHEFF, M.D.*

A most difficult diagnostic problem from both the clinical and radiographic standpoint occurs in the evaluation of patients who present with recurrent symptoms after surgery for disc disease. Whereas postoperative arachnoiditis, disc herniation at a remote level, infection, acquired spinal stenosis, cyst and meningocele formation and mechanical instability may cause or contribute to the patient's symptom complex, the most commonly encountered causes are recurrent herniation at the operative level and postoperative scarring (1).

It is well known that myelographic differentiation between postoperative scarring and recurrent disc herniation is at best difficult and considered by many impossible (2–10). The anatomical site of deformity of the contrast column produced by scar and recurrent disc herniation are usually the same (3). Myelographic examinations of 5 asymptomatic postoperative patients reported by Lindblom (11) and Knutsson (2) were reported as "normal", whereas 4 symptom-free postoperative patients examined by Soule et al. (12) had "slight but definite distortions of the canal at the level of former protrusions." In another series, 22 of 38 patients presenting with recurrent pain in the postoperative period had myelograms which the authors considered normal (13). In addition, the finding of nerve root sheath obliteration, a reliable sign for disc herniation in the preoperative myelogram, especially with water-soluble contrast material, has limited significance in the postoperative study. This finding has been observed sufficiently frequently in patients without recurrent herniation to be of little, if any, diagnostic value (9).

The advent of high-resolution CT coupled with a localizing digital radiographic scout imaging system has been shown to be an effective, noninvasive means of evaluating preoperative patients with suspected lumbar disc disease (14). This diagnostic modality also is being used extensively in the evaluation of the symptomatic postoperative patient. In an attempt to provide a "baseline" for the evaluation of the changes seen on CT in the symptomatic

patient after surgery for lumbar disc disease, we have scanned a series of asymptomatic patients at various intervals, ranging from 4 weeks to 7 months after surgery. The CT appearance of physiological postoperative healing with subsequent scar formation then was analyzed. Seven patients had surgery without the use of fat allograft whereas 2 patients had fat allografts in an attempt to decrease postoperative scar formation. All surgery was performed by the same neurosurgeon (MVB).

DESCRIPTION OF SURGICAL TECHNIQUE

The surgical procedure performed on all volunteers included in this report was the same (Figs 24.1 and 24.2). It consisted of a hemilaminotomy of the inferior and superior one-half of the lamina at the involved interspace. One-half of the ligamentum flavum was removed in its entirety. The medial one-third to one-half of the superior and inferior facets of the operated interspace is removed, flush with the radical removal of the nucleus pulposus. Gelfoam pads are left covering the opening of the anulus, nerve root, and the dorsal aspect of the dural theca.

RADIOGRAPHIC TECHNIQUE

All volunteers were scanned using the General Electric CT/T 8800 high-resolution scanner equipped with a digital radiographic scout imaging system (ScoutView) which was used to identify scanning planes. A scanning slice thickness of 5 mm was used to decrease partial volume effects from thicker cuts. Technical factors included a kVp of 120, mAs of 760, pixel size of 0.75 mm, and scan time per slice of 10 seconds.

Only the level of surgery was studied. Four to five slices were obtained routinely; 2–3 scans through the surgically violated disc space, one slice approximately 5 mm below the disc space through the superior aspect of the subjacent vertebral body, and an additional slice approximately 5 mm above the disc space through the intervertebral foramen of the superjacent vertebral body. All scans were obtained parallel to the disc space and its adjacent vertebral body endplates (15). Reformatting was done as necessary in order to obtain slices parallel to the disc space

* The authors wish to thank Linda Michaels, Jill Tepper, Lydia Logozo, Kate Marshall, and Francine Hollowell for their valuable assistance in the preparation of this chapter.

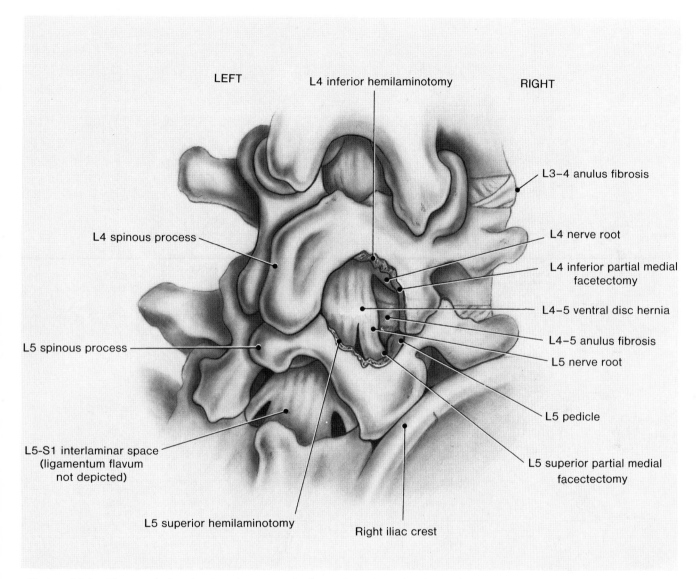

LEFT

L4 inferior hemilaminotomy

RIGHT

L3–4 anulus fibrosis

L4 spinous process

L4 nerve root

L4 inferior partial medial facetectomy

L4–5 ventral disc hernia

L4–5 anulus fibrosis

L5 spinous process

L5 nerve root

L5 pedicle

L5-S1 interlaminar space (ligamentum flavum not depicted)

L5 superior partial medial facetectomy

L5 superior hemilaminotomy

Right iliac crest

Figure 24.1. The surgical procedure for removal of a unilateral paramedian soft-disc hernia is done through a unilateral subperiosteal dissection of paravertebral muscles. Figure 24.1 illustrates the extent of inferior L4 and superior L5 hemilaminotomy. This bony exposure affords complete removal of the interlaminar portion of the ligamentum flavum. Medially, the ligament is removed close to the interspinous ligament. Laterally, the medial one-third of both facets in normal size canals, and one-half in stenotic canals, are removed, including the portion of the ligamentum flavum covering the neural foramen.

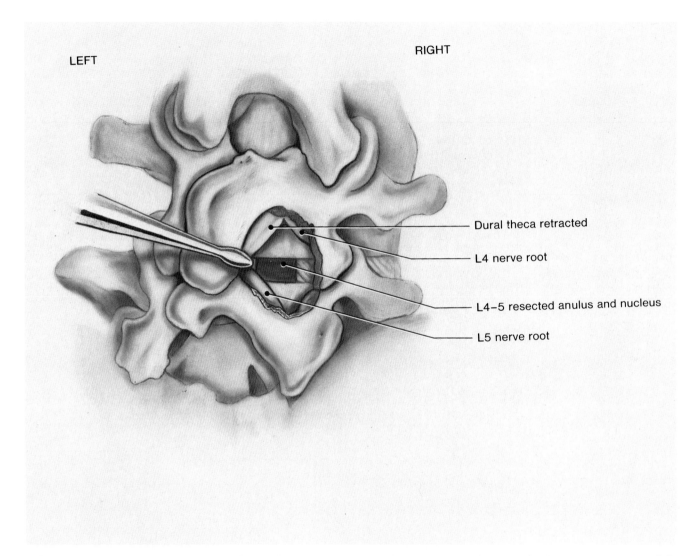

LEFT

RIGHT

———— Dural theca retracted

———— L4 nerve root

———— L4–5 resected anulus and nucleus

———— L5 nerve root

Figure 24.2. After thorough bipolarization and section of adjacent epidural venous plexus, the dural sac is retracted medially. A rectangular opening is made in the posterior aspect of the anulus, flush with the vertebral end plates. The contents of the nucleus is removed radically with angled currettes and pituitary forceps.

in patients whose L5-S1 interspace required gantry angulation greater than the tilting capability of the scanner (15°).

All scans were done with the patient in a supine position without attempts at bolstering the lower lumbar spine. Because we have noted no significant intravenous contrast enhancement of intraspinal structures in a large group of symptomatic postoperative patients, and for ethical reasons, intravenous contrast material was not administered to these asymptomatic volunteers. Several patients had preoperative CT as part of their initial evaluation.

RESULTS

Several features were seen consistently in this group of asymptomatic volunteers in whom fat allografts were not used, and are listed in Table 24.1. The CT studies of 4 of the 7 volunteers revealed an eccentric vacuum phenomenon (Figs. 24.3–24.6), which was seen in patients scanned as early as 5 weeks and as late as 7 months postoperatively. One volunteer studied 5 weeks into the postoperative period had gas within the spinal canal (Fig. 24.6B and C) in addition to a vacuum phenomenon at the disc space.

All volunteers without fat grafts with a nonstenotic canal (4 of 7) displayed retraction of the dural tube toward the side of surgery (Figs. 24.3 and 24.5). Of 7 patients, 6 displayed accumulation of relative hyperdense intraspinal tissue on the side of surgery which blended anteriorly with the disc, coursed around the lateral aspect of the dural tube, and extended posteriorly to the laminotomy defect (Figs. 24.3–24.5 and 24.7). Associated findings included effacement of normal epidural fat, a finding again appreciated in all volunteers with a nonstenotic canal (Figs. 24.3–24.5 and 24.7), loss of distinction of the nerve root ipsilateral to the surgical side (Figs. 24.3 and 24.5), and extension of relatively hyperdense soft tissue into the neural foramina seen in both cases in which a foraminal disc had been removed previously (Figs. 24.4 and 24.5).

Relatively poor definition of intraspinal contents was appreciated in those asymptomatic volunteers with a stenotic spinal canal. In addition, all cases in which a preoperative study was available, displayed a decrease in height of the surgically violated disc space as seen on the preliminary digital postoperative scout radiograph (Figs. 24.3E and F).

The CT scans of the 2 asymptomatic volunteers who received fat allografts are shown in Figures 24.8 and 24.9

and reveal no significant differences in appearance. A lucent area was seen within the epidural scar on 1 patient (Fig. 24.8) which presumably represents persistent fat. No difference in the amount or quality of fibrous tissue was observed, however, in this admittedly limited series of volunteers with fat allografts when compared to studies on patients without fat grafts.

DISCUSSION

In our routine clinical practice, only those postoperative patients with clinical complaints and symptomatology are referred for radiographic study. The CT appearance of the postoperative disc space in these symptomatic patients consistently includes vacuum changes, increased density obliterating nerve root and dural tube landmarks on the side of surgery, effacement of epidural fat, and retraction of the dural tube. Although our series of asymptomatic volunteers is admittedly small in number, every one of these asymptomatic postoperative patients had several or all findings commonly seen in the majority of symptomatic postoperative patients.

A vacuum phenomenon was seen consistently in our group of asymptomatic volunteers. The vacuum phenomenon commonly seen in the lumbar spine in patients without a history of previous surgery is thought to be due to liberation of gas, usually nitrogen, into fissures within the degenerated disc material (16). A vacuum formation also may be seen when the disc is injured (17) secondary to either metabolic disease which interferes with nutrition of the disc or to simple mechanical trauma such as occurs during disc removal. The gas in the region of the disc shortly after surgery probably represents sequelae of the recent surgical manipulation, whereas that seen 6 or 7 months after surgery is a reflection of postoperative disc degeneration and disc space collapse, a normal postsurgical phenomenon.

Dural tube retraction toward the side of surgery is consistent with postoperative healing and scar formation with subsequent cicatrization and adhesions of the thecal sac. Whereas we would expect to see this change in all patients as a result of normal physiological healing, the only asymptomatic volunteers in whom this change was not demonstrated on CT were those with a relatively stenotic canal. The paucity of visualized epidural fat on CT in the stenotic canal precludes this dural tube retraction from being seen.

The accumulation of a band of relatively hyperdense soft tissue on the side of surgery coursing from the disc margin around the lateral aspect of the dural tube and extending to the laminotomy defect is seen in all asymptomatic volunteers, both with and without fat allografts, with a canal capacious enough to demonstrate intraspinal contents. This CT manifestation is the result of postoperative healing and fibrosis. Indeed, this accumulation of fibrous tissue extended laterally through the neural foramina simulating recurrent lateral herniation in those asymptomatic volunteers operated on for a laterally herniated disc (Figs. 24.4 and 24.5). Effacement of epidural fat

Table 24.1.
CT Features of the Asymptomatic Postoperative Spine

Eccentric vacuum phenomenon
Gas within spinal canal
Dural tube retraction toward surgical side (in nonstenotic canal)
Intra- and extraspinal tissue accumulation
Effacement of epidural fat
Loss of distinction of ipsilateral nerve root
Decrease in height of surgically violated disc space

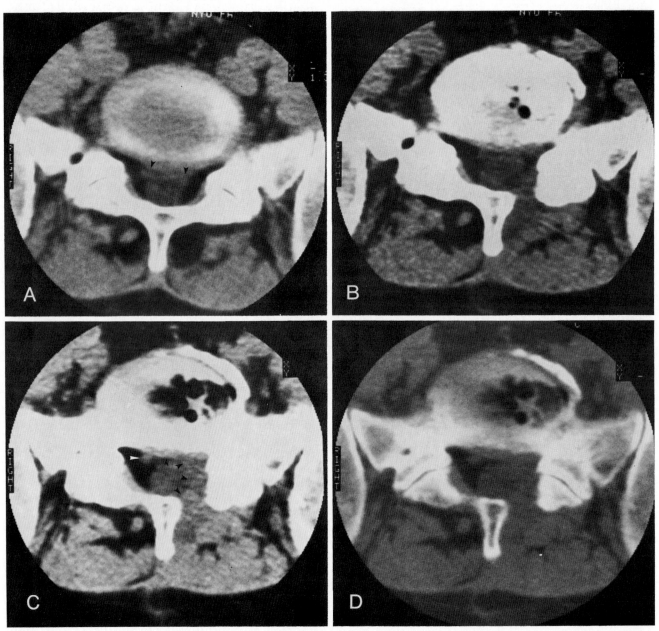

Figure 24.3.   A. Preoperative CT image through the L5-S1 interspace demonstrating a large centrally herniated disc (*arrowheads*) compressing the anterior aspect of the dural tube in this patient with a capacious spinal canal. Symmetric areas of epidural fat are noted bilaterally on either side of the dural tube. A moderate amount of facet joint hypertrophy is appreciated as well. B, C, and D. Postoperative scans obtained 5 months after surgery from the same patient who is now symptom-free. Slice B is obtained at the same level as the preoperative slice in A, whereas slices C and D demonstrate a contiguous area. Slice C is imaged using a soft-tissue window, whereas slice D is the same slice imaged at a bone window. An eccentric vacuum phenomenon is appreciated. A band of relatively hyperdense soft tissue courses from the disc margin anteriorly, around and abutting the lateral aspect of the dural tube and extending posteriorly to the laminotomy defect (*arrowheads*) (seen best in C). Effacement and distortion of ipsilateral paraspinal musculature is noted. Minimal retraction of the dural tube toward the surgical side associated with effacement of the ipsilateral nerve root is appreciated. The contralateral nerve root is well seen in C (*white arrowhead*). E and F. Digital scout radiographs, obtained from the pre- and postoperative studies (E and F, respectively). Despite the change in magnification a decrease in the height of the L5-S1 disc space is clearly seen. A vacuum phenomenon is also appreciated on postoperative digital radiograph (*arrowheads*).

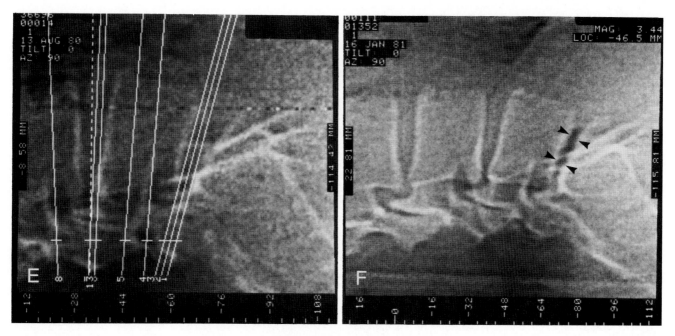

Figure 24.3. E and F.

and loss of distinction and displacement of nerve roots occurred in several of the volunteers secondary to healing and scar formation.

Early in our experience with CT scanning of the lumbar spine in symptomatic postoperative patients, scans were done both pre- and postintravenous contrast administration. In our experience, intravenous contrast enhancement was of no value in differential diagnosis and indeed no significant changes other than some enhancement of epidural venous structures could be seen when comparing pre- and postcontrast images. For this reason and for ethical considerations, contrast was not administered to our group of asymptomatic volunteers.

In an attempt to distinguish recurrent disc herniation from fibrosis we have measured the range of attenuation coefficients for known herniated disc material and have compared these values to those obtained by measuring areas of postoperative fibrosis in asymptomatic volunteers. No distinguishing ranges of attenuation coefficients were noted in our analysis. Indeed, even if differing measurements were obtained, their usefulness would be doubtful. The spine is a particularly difficult area for computer reconstruction because of the close proximity of adjacent bone. The beam hardening effect along with scatter from adjacent bone affect those detectors not directly imaging bone and make absolute and relative measurements in this area notoriously unreliable. Small attenuation differences on the order of 20 HU, may be seen with millimeter placement changes of the cursor. Furthermore, it is not infrequent for patient anatomy to extend beyond the scan field further invalidating attenuation coeffcents.

All of these findings seen in our group of asymptomatic postoperative volunteers have been seen in a large majority of symptomatic patients. Whereas scarring and subsequent nerve root retraction and effacement commonly are implicated as a cause for recurring symptoms in the postoperative period, this finding was seen in all asymptomatic patients with a canal capacious enough for visualization of intraspinal contents and was indistinguishable from that seen in symptomatic patients. Hasso (18) has seen contralateral displacement of the dural tube due to a recurrent herniated disc, but we have not yet observed this finding. We, therefore, agree with Williams et al. (14), Carrera et al. (19), and Haughton et al. (20) that the CT differentiation of symptomatic scarring versus asymptomatic fibrosis secondary to physiological healing and its differentiation from recurrent disc herniation is extremely difficult to make. Similarly, the finding of a vacuum in the postoperative period seen in both groups of patients, provides no diagnostic information.

The CT appearance of the postoperative lumbar spine both in asymptomatic volunteers and in symptomatic patients will depend necessarily, to a great extent, on the type of surgery performed. In the majority of cases, 2 basic surgical procedures are in use for the treatment of herniated lumbar discs. The simplest, least radical technique is an interlaminar approach without laminotomy and facetectomy with limited removal of disc fragments. The more radical approach, and the one used in our institution (described in detail in a preceding section), consists of a hemilaminotomy with partial medial facetectomy and radical disc removal. The former method of treatment

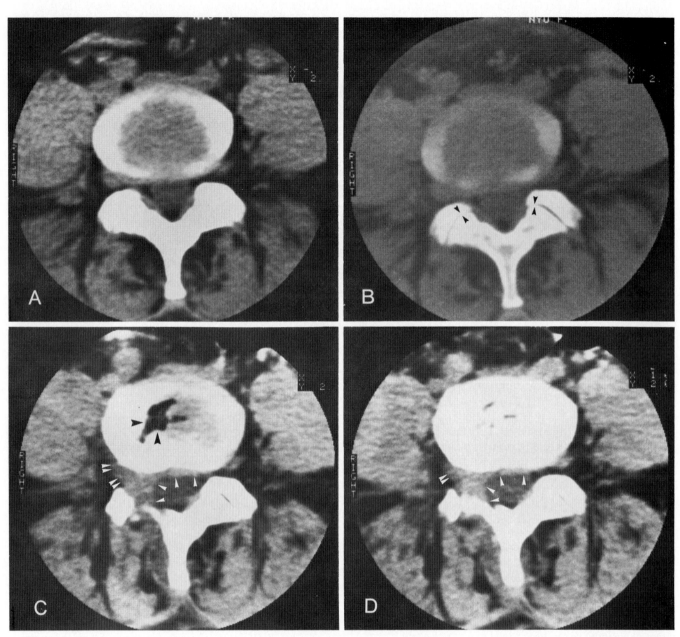

Figure 24.4.   A and B. Preoperative slices through the L4–5 disc space in a patient with severe right L4 radiculopathy, imaged at soft-tissue and bone windows, respectively. A soft-tissue mass, representing surgically verified herniated disc material extends from the posterolateral disc margin on the right extending through the intervertebral foramen. Little, if any distortion of the dural tube is appreciated. A negative lumbar myelogram (not pictured) confirmed this finding. Mild to moderate facet joint hypertrophy and narrowing is seen in the bone-window image (B) (*arrowheads*). C and D. Contiguous slices imaged at a soft-tissue window obtained 5 months postoperatively in this patient who is now asymptomatic. An eccentric vacuum phenomenon is again noted (*large arrowheads*). A band of relatively hyperdense soft tissue extends from the disc margin anteriorly, around the right lateral aspect of the dural tube, courses through the right intervertebral foramen and abuts on the postoperative bony defect (*white arrowheads*). The soft tissue within the foramen (*double arrowheads*) should not be misconstrued as recurrent foraminal disc herniation. Postoperative changes in the right paraspinal musculature are noted.

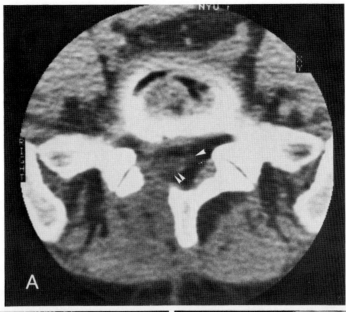

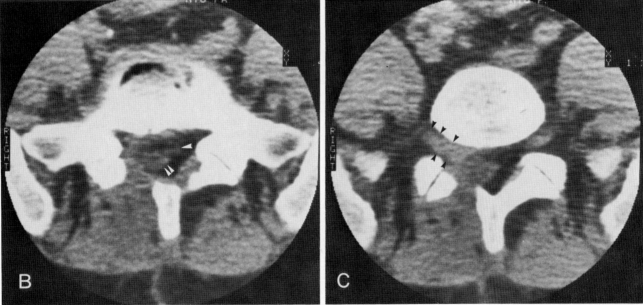

Figure 24.5. A and B. Postoperative contiguous CT images through the L5-S1 interspace in this patient who has been asymptomatic 5 months since surgery. A vacuum phenomenon again is appreciated. Marked retraction of the dural tube to the right is noted (*double arrowhead*) in this capacious canal associated with a band of soft tissue extending from the disc margin coursing around the right lateral aspect of the dural tube to the laminotomy defect. The nerve root is well seen on the left (*single arrowhead*) whereas the ipsilateral root is effaced. Degenerative productive changes of the facet joints are appreciated. Postoperative distortion of ipsilateral right paraspinal musculature is visualized. C. Postoperative image through the L5-S1 intervertebral foramen demonstrating the band of relatively hyperdense soft tissue noted in A and B, extending laterally through the foramen at this level (*arrowheads*) simulating a recurrent foraminal herniation.

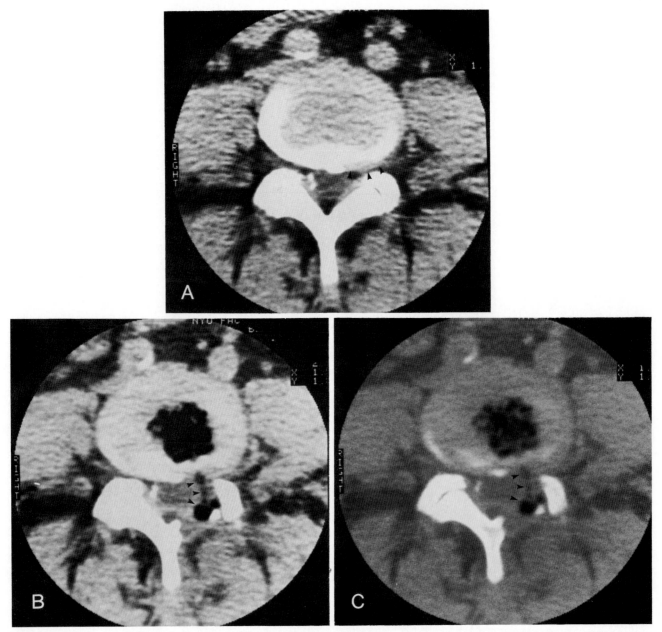

Figure 24.6.   A. Preoperative axial image through the L4–5 disc space in this patient with a 6-month history of low back pain radiating to the left lower extremity. A small left lateral herniation (*arrowheads*) is seen which was confirmed at surgery. A relatively narrow spinal canal and moderate facet joint hypertrophy are appreciated. Residual myelographic contrast material is seen on the right. B and C. Postoperative images through the L4–5 disc space obtained 4 weeks after surgery in this now symptom-free patient. The slice is imaged using soft-tissue (B) and bone (C) technique. An eccentric vacuum phenomenon is appreciated. Intraspinal gas (*arrowheads*) extends from the left posterolateral disc margin around the left lateral aspect of the dural tube and terminates at the bony laminotomy defect. The intraspinal gas appears almost continuous with the disc vacuum (seen best in C).

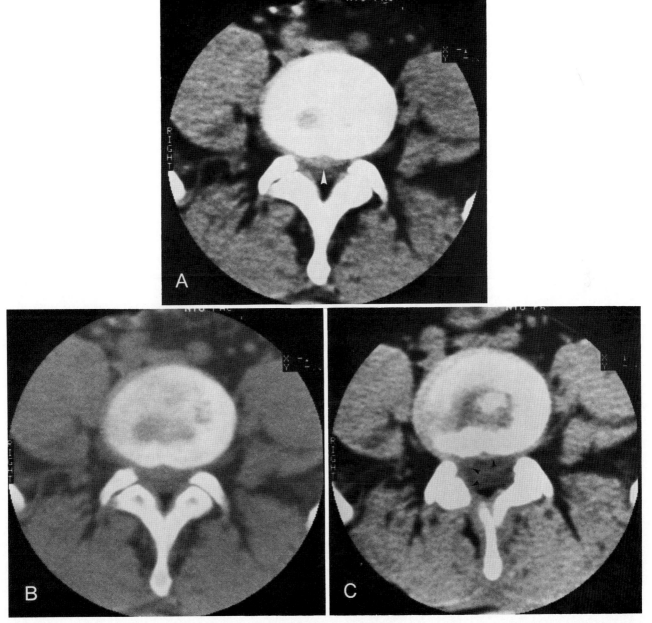

Figure 24.7. A and B. Preoperative images taken contiguous to the L4–5 disc space using soft-tissue (A) and bone (B) techniques in this patient with a 20-year history of low back pain radiating to both lower extremities. A central disc herniation is seen. C. Postoperative images obtained through the L4–5 region in this patient who is asymptomatic 5 months after surgery. A band of soft tissue abuts the right posterolateral aspect of the disc and courses around the lateral aspect of the dural tube (*arrowheads*). Visualization of dural tube retraction is precluded by the narrow canal.

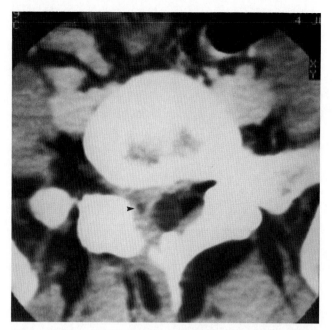

Figure 24.8. Axial image through the region of the L5-S1 disc space in a patient asymptomatic 10 months since surgery. A fat allograft was placed around the nerve root intraoperatively in an attempt to decrease scar formation. Findings similar to those seen in the previous patients are again noted. A lucency, however, is appreciated (*arrowhead*) within the fibrous tissue which probably represents residual fat.

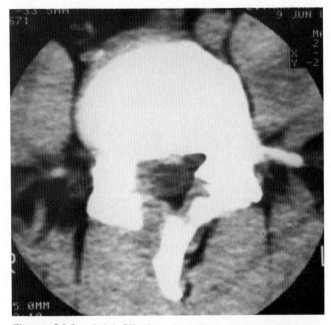

Figure 24.9. Axial CT slice through a region contiguous with the L4–5 disc space in this patient asymptomatic 6 months since surgery. This patient also had the benefit of a fat graft. No lucencies in the fibrous tissue are seen either in this slice or in contiguous sections.

involves sectioning of the ligamentum flavum with disc fragment removal and preservation of epidural fat, whereas the latter involves removal of bone, ligamentum flavum, as well as epidural fat. The use of fat allografts placed around nerve roots in an attempt to decrease scar formation is also widely popular. No significant difference in the CT appearance of scar formation was encountered, however, comparing those volunteers with and without benefit of this procedure. Our series of patients with fat allografts is rather limited, however, and this is the subject of future investigation.

In view of the changes seen in asymptomatic patients secondary to physiological healing and fibrosis, herniated nuclear material superimposed on these findings may be difficult and, at times, impossible to discern. Partial volume effect from adjacent bone and fibrous material would require a relatively large mass of herniated nuclear material to make itself evident. CT myelography with metrizamide may provide a means for this differentiation by allowing visualization of subtle changes in the course of the dural tube caused by herniated disc material.

References

1. Quencer RM, Murtagh FR, Post MJD, et al: Post-operative bony stenosis of the lumbar spinal canal: Evaluation of 164 symptomatic patients with axial radiography. *AJR* 131:1059–1064, 1978.
2. Knutsson F: The myelogram following operation for herniated disc. *Acta Radiol* 32:60–65, 1949.
3. Cronquist S: The postoperative myelogram. *Acta Radiol* 52:45–51, 1959.
4. Maltby GL, Prendergrass, RL: Pantopaque myelography: Diagnostic errors and review of cases. *Radiology* 47:35–46, 1946.
5. Leader SA, Russel JJ: The value of Pantopaque myelography in the diagnosis of herniation of the nucleus pulposus in the lumbosacral spine. *AJR* 69:231–241, 1953.
6. Borelli FJ, Maglione AA: The importance of myelography in spinal pathology: Analytic study of 150 cases. *AJR* 76:273–289, 1956.
7. Wright FW, Sanders RC, Steel WM, O'Connor BT: Some observations in the value and techniques of myelography in lumbar disc lesions. *Clin Radiol* 22:33–43, 1971.
8. Shapiro R: *Myelography*, 3rd Ed. Year Book Medical Publishers, Chicago, 1975, p. 203.
9. Moseley I: The oil myelogram after operation for lumbar disc lesions. *Clin Radiol* 28:267–276, 1977.
10. Sackett JF, Strother CM (Eds): *New Techniques in Myelography*, Harper & Row Publishers, Hagerstown, 1979, p. 84.
11. Lindblom K: Lumbar myelography by abrodil. *Acta Radiol* 27:1–7, 1949.
12. Soule AB, Gross SW, Irving JG: Myelography by the use of Pantopaque in the diagnosis of herniations of the intervertebral discs. *AJR* 53:319–340, 1945.
13. Silver MI, Field FA, Silver CM, Simon SD: The post-operative lumbar myelogram. *Radiology* 72:344–347, 1959.
14. Williams AL, Haughton VM, Syvertsen A: Computed tomography in the diagnosis of herniated nucleus pulposus. *Radiology* 135:95–99, 1980.
15. Braun IF, Lin JP, George AE, et al: Pitfalls in the computed tomographic evaluation of the lumbar spine in disc disease. Presented at the Sixty-Seventh Scientific Assembly and Annual Meeting of the Radiological Society of North America, Chicago, IL, November, 1981.
16. Ford LT, Gilula LA, Murphy WA, et al: Analysis of gas in

vacuum lumbar disc. *AJR* 128:1056–1057, 1977.

17. Resnick D, Niwayama G, Guerra J Jr, Vint V, Usselman J: spinal vacuum phenomena: Anatomical study and review. *Radiology* 139:341–348, 1981.

18. Hasso AN: Commenting on presentation #265. The CT appearance of the lumbar spine in the asymptomatic patient after disc surgery. Braun IF, Lin JP, Benjamin MV, et al: Sixty-Seventh Scientific Assembly and Annual Meeting of the Radiological Society of North America, Chicago, IL, November, 1981.

19. Carrera GF, Williams AK, Haughton VM: Computed tomography in sciatica. *Radiology* 137:433–437, 1980.

20. Haughton VM, Elderik OP, Magnaes B, Amondsen P: Prospective comparison of computed tomography and myelography in the diagnosis of herniated lumbar discs. *Radiology* 142:103–110, 1982.

A. DISC DISEASE
3. Discolysis

CHAPTER TWENTY-FIVE

Computed Tomography Before and After Chemonucleolysis

JOHN A. McCULLOCH, M.D., F.R.C.S.(C)

INTRODUCTION

Since 1963, the concept of chemically removing herniated nuclear material in the lumbar spine without open surgery has followed a controversial and checkered course. It is still not universally accepted as a method of treatment for sciatica due to a herniated lumbar nucleus pulposus and a number of world government regulatory agencies, including the United States, have just approved its general use. However, many countries are using chymopapain (Discase)* for chemically removing nuclear material and it is the author's opinion that evidence, including further double-blind trials, is weighing in favor of chemonucleolysis as a clinical tool.

However, two problems remain unsolved, namely, reconstitution of the disc space after chemonucleolysis (Fig. 25.1) and the occasional persistence of the CT scan defect after chemonucleolysis in spite of a good result. It is this latter problem that will be addressed in this chapter.

ACTION OF CHYMOPAPAIN

Briefly, chymopapain, a plant protein, is a proteolytic enzyme that interferes with or breaks the mucopolysaccharide protein core bond of the proteoglycan of nucleus pulposus (1). This impairs nuclear ability to retain water and, thus, decompresses, through volume alteration, the mass of nucleus both normal in position and herniated (herniated nucleus pulposus, HNP).

TYPES OF DISC HERNIATION

Chemonucleolysis has been limited to the lumbar spine (2). The clinically significant lumbar disc migrations in the adult population are represented in Figure 25.2. Mye-

_____
* Discase = Chymopapain, Baxter Laboratories

lography will demonstrate abnormal canal migration of disc material (Fig. 25.3) but it is more common that the characteristics of the myelographic defect, in most cases, will not allow for separation of protrusions, extrusions, and sequestrations.

One of the many criticisms of chemonucleolysis is that it will not dissolve sequestered disc material for two reasons. Firstly, chymopapain when injected into the central nuclear region of the disc space cannot reach a free fragment of disc material in the spinal canal. Secondly, if, by chance, the injected chymopapain leaks out of the nuclear region through a rent in the anulus, to come in contact with a predominately collagenous, sequestered mass of nucleus that has lost a substantial portion of its proteoglycan content, dissolution cannot occur. At this moment, the only reliable available demonstration of a sequestered disc is operative exposure of the disc space (segment) but CT scanning, in its increasingly refined way may be of assistance (Fig. 25.4).

PATIENT SELECTION FOR CHEMONUCLEOLYSIS

As the last step in conservative treatment for sciatica due to a HNP, chemonucleolysis should be reserved for those patients in whom a surgeon could confidently expect a good result from laminectomy discectomy. Chemonucleolysis is only used for lumbar disc herniations. It is of no use in patients with symptoms due to degenerative disc disease or spinal stenosis. The criteria for sciatica due to a herniated intervertebral disc are outlined in Table 25.1.

THE ROLE OF CT IN THE DIAGNOSIS OF HNP

There is no doubt, in the author's opinion, that CT scanning will play an increasing role in the diagnosis of a herniated lumbar nucleus pulposus. As dosimetry, tech-

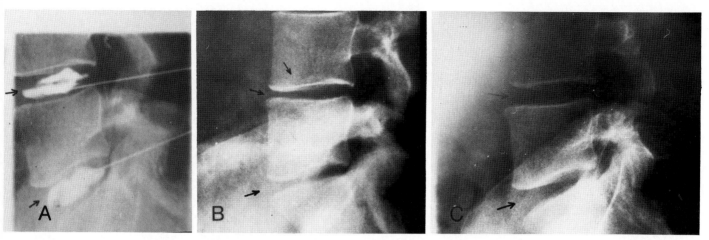

Figure 25.1. L4-L5 and L5-S1 disc space (A) before chemonucleolysis (at the time of discography), (B) 2 months after chemonucleolysis and (C) 3 years after chemonucleolysis. After narrowing of both disc spaces at 2 months, the disc spaces have reconstituted to normal height at 3 years. (Courtesy of Leon Wiltse, M.D.)

DISC HERNIATIONS

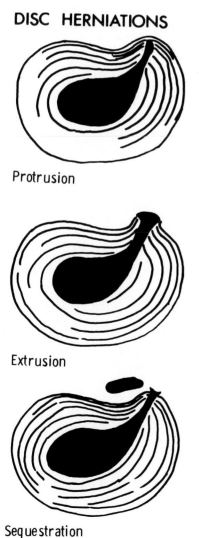

Protrusion

Extrusion

Sequestration

nique, and software improve, so myelography and venography ultimately will play a subordinate role.

Two words of caution:

1. Noninvasive CT scanning is simple and safe and with its increasing use will occur the increasing incidence of false-positive scans and the resulting unnecessary surgery. The CT scan is only valuable when interpreted in light of the clinical presentation and will assume an increasingly valuable role if the clinician closely correlates his surgical findings in a team approach with the reporting radiologist.

2. It is easy to limit CT examination to the last two mobile levels (L4–L5, L5–S1) and miss a disc at another level (Fig. 25.5).

THE ROLE OF CT IN THE DIAGNOSIS OF A MIDLINE DISC HERNIATION

Midline HNP—A Concept

The patient with a classic disc herniation is outlined in Table 25.1. The patient with a *central* disc herniation with cauda equina compression, including bladder and bowel involvement, is also classic in its presentation and, fortunately, is a rare clinical event. Chemonucleolysis should not be used in this surgical emergency. Between these two classic presentations lies a group of patients with a midline disc herniation. In the past, these patients were grouped with all the other patients with "lumbago" and treatment prescribed accordingly.

Figure 25.2. The three degrees of clinically significant displacement of nuclear material beyond the normal confines of the anulus. Note the gradation of anular disruption (protrusion, incomplete; extrusion and sequestration, complete) and nuclear mass continuity (protrusion and extrusion, continuous; and sequestration, free fragment in spinal canal).

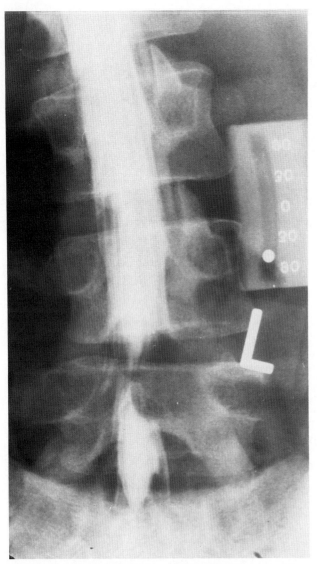

Figure 25.3. Water-soluble myelography showing a large HNP L4-L5 left, with a significant portion of the defect away from the disc space. The patient had a sequestered disc at surgery.

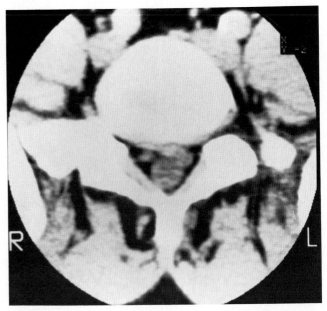

Figure 25.4. CT scan L5-S1 showing HNP midline and left. Notice the apparent separation between the disc fragment and the posterior limits of the vertebral body/disc space, possibly indicating a sequestered disc. However, the patient has an excellent response to chemonucleolysis.

Table 25.1.
Criteria for Diagnosis of HNP Causing Sciatica. Patients with 4 or 5 Criteria probably have a HNP, Patients with 3 Criteria possibly have a HNP, Patients with less than 3 Criteria do not likely have a HNP as the Cause of their Sciatica

1. Leg (and buttock) pain is the dominant symptom when compared with midline back pain, affecting 1 leg only and following a typical sciatic nerve distribution.
2. Paresthesiae are localized to a dermatomal distribution.
3. Straight leg raising is reduced by 50% of normal (when compared to the opposite normal side) and/or pain crosses over to the symptomatic leg when the unaffected straight leg is elevated and/or pain radiates proximally or distally with digital pressure on the tibial nerve in the popliteal fossa.
4. Two of 4 neurological signs are present (wasting, motor weakness, diminished sensory appreciation, or diminution of reflex activity).
5. Investigation in the form of myelography, venography, or CT scanning is positive.

CT scanning is helping to identify these patients with a midline disc herniation who present with intermittent episodes of acute back and bilateral leg pain, often with bilateral neurological symptoms but frequently yielding no neurological signs. Bilateral reduction in straight leg raising is an essential component of the clinical diagnosis. Unequivocal evidence of a midline HNP may come in the positive Bowstring test (back pain on pressure directed over the tibial nerve in the popliteal fossa). The plain radiographs are often normal and myelography may reveal a defect that is indistinguishable from a mild anular bulge of no clinical significance, or show nothing at all (especially at S1) (Fig. 25.6). CT scanning is helpful in delineating this clinical condition but the author would caution that this diagnosis and its CT scan support is an area of lumbar spinal practice that can be overcalled and lead to unnecessary and unwise invasive surgical procedures, especially in the litigation conscious, compensation patient where nonorganic features can cloud the assessment of the less astute clinician who, in turn, relies on a sensitive false-positive CT scan on which to act.

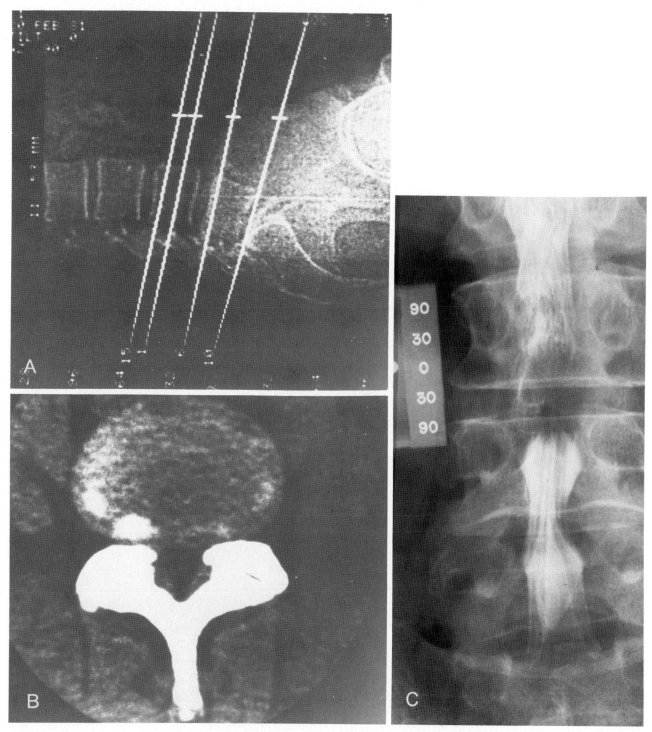

Figure 25.5.   A. Localizer film accompanying patient sent for chemonucleolysis. B. CT scan L4-L5 which was negative (L5-S1 was also negative). C. Subsequent myelogram showing defect at L3-L4.

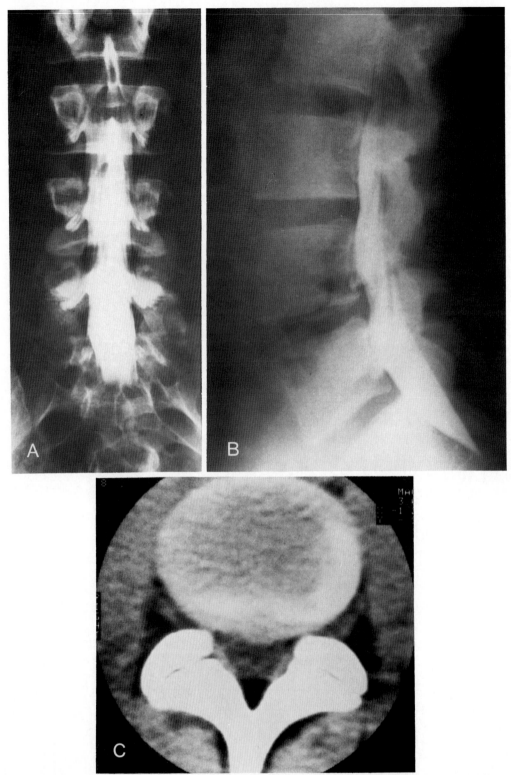

Figure 25.6. A. Anteroposterior myelogram that is essentially normal. B. Lateral myelogram showing midline defect at L4-L5 that might be interpreted as a clinically insignificant anular bulge. C. CT scan showing HNP L4-L5. NOTE: This concept is even more important at L5-S1 where lateral myelogram shows even less (or no) defect.

TECHNIQUE OF CHEMONUCLEOLYSIS

Chemonucleolysis is done after lateral insertion of a needle in the nuclear space of the offending disc segment (3). Needle placement must be between the medial borders of the pedicles and in the center of the disc space on lateral x-ray. This author uses noncontrast discometry rather than discography to assess the integrity of the disc (4) before injecting 2 cc (4000 units or 8 mg) of chymopapain into the disc space. Injection usually is done at one disc level only but there are a few, infrequent, exceptions to this statement.

POSTINJECTION COURSE

The patients have variable amounts of back pain after the procedure, ranging from the infrequent patient with severe back spasms to the infrequent patient with minimal or no back pain. Most patients like the support of a corset for the first 2–4 weeks after injection to help control their discomfort.

Most patients who are going to obtain a good result will notice alteration (sometimes total relief) of leg pain immediately. Some will notice gradual reduction in leg symptoms up to 1 month after injection, but any patients with significant leg pain persisting beyond a month are considered failures and operative intervention is recommended.

RESULTS

Numerous reports (5–7) in the literature describe a 60–90% success rate with chemonucleolysis. It is the author's opinion that, if the procedure is confined to patients as described in Table 25.1, approximately 80% will be relieved of symptoms. The remaining 20% will have operative diagnoses such as sequestered disc, lateral recess stenosis, and minor disc protrusions and/or adhesions. There is no detrimental effect of chymopapain leaking into the extradural space at the time of injection. The author has operated on approximately 125 patients after chemonucleolysis and has noticed no adverse effects, such as excessive scarring.

COMPLICATIONS

The most serious complication to injection of the plant protein chymopapain is anaphylaxis (incidence ½%). The reaction is manifested by profound cardiovascular collapse with little or no respiratory distress. Treatment is quick intravenous infusion of (a) epinephrine, (b) steroids, (c) antihistamines, (d) large volume of fluids. To date, 4 deaths have occurred, in other centers, as a result of anaphylaxis after administration of chymopapain. All 4 patients were under general anesthesia which only served to complicate the treatment of anaphylaxis. The procedure should be done under local anesthetic with minimal neuroleptic augmentation so that an anaphylactic reaction can be more readily handled. Other less severe reactions include angioneurotic edema, hives, and a chemical discitis, each with no long-term consequences.

DISCUSSION

CT scanning is assuming an increasingly important role in the diagnosis of a HNP. It localizes HNP material better than myelography by demonstrating defects laterally and lying in the foramen (Fig. 25.7). It characterizes nuclear material, easily demonstrating calcified nuclear material (Fig. 25.8). There is a real possibility, that with further refinements, it will demonstrate the sequestered disc clearly. Like everything new and dramatic in medicine,

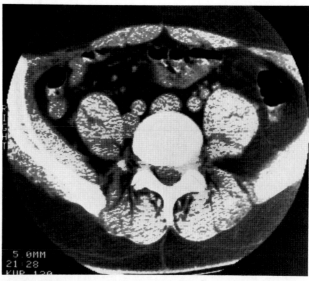

Figure 25.7.   CT scan showing HNP in left foramen at L5-S1. The myelogram was normal.

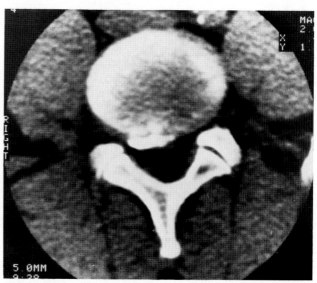

Figure 25.8.   CT scan showing calcified HNP—a contraindication to chemonucleolysis.

there is a possibility that the CT scanner will be overused and overinterpreted in making invasive surgical decisions. However, as the clinician and radiologist gain experience as a team, the pendulum will swing to CT scanning being used as the "gold standard" instead of myelography to

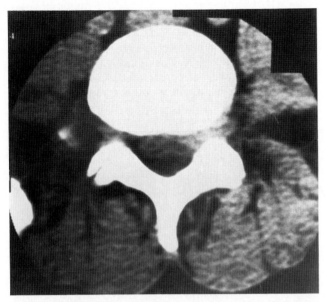

Figure 25.9. CT scan of patient in Figure 25.7, 3 months postchemonucleolysis with persistant foraminal defect. The patient has an excellent result.

support the clinician's decision to remove (chemically or surgically) offending herniated disc material.

On occasion, CT scan defects do persist on CT scanning (Figs. 25.9–25.11) after chemonucleolysis. We have demonstrated persistent defects on myelography after chemonucleolysis but we have also demonstrated their disappearance (8). The author cannot give an incidence for persisting CT defects for two reasons. The constraints of Canadian Government funded medical care are such that very limited time is available on our single GE 8800 unit which is serving a number of hospitals. Policy does not allow the establishment of privately controlled units outside of our public hospital systems. Secondly, the author sees patients from widely spread areas of the Americas and, although attempted, it has been logistically and financially impossible to establish an incidence. But there is no doubt, that CT scan defects do persist after successful and unsuccessful chemonucleolysis.

The first question to be asked, when faced with a healthy postchymopapain patient, relieved of sciatica, yet demonstrating a persistent defect on CT scan, is whether the defect originally shown was, in fact, a disc herniation.

Many studies, correlating clinical, investigational, and surgical findings, have been published (9, 10) to support the fact that CT scan defect is indeed a HNP. In addition, the author has satisfied himself, through numerous combined studies (Fig. 25.12) that the defect seen before and after chemonucleolysis is herniated nuclear material.

The persistent defect on postinjection CT scan is com-

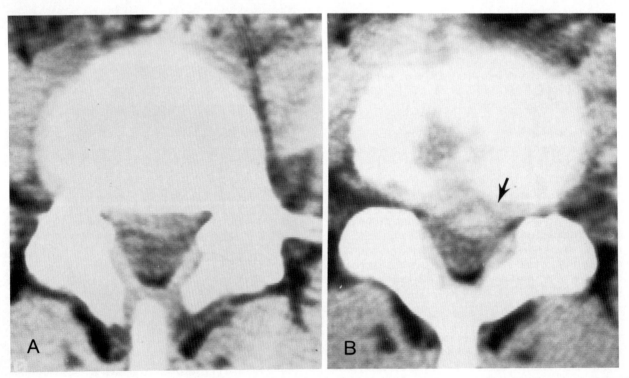

Figure 25.10. A. CT scan young woman with HNP L4-L5. B. CT scan 1 month postinjection showing persistence of the disc herniation, (*arrow*). The patient has an excellent response.

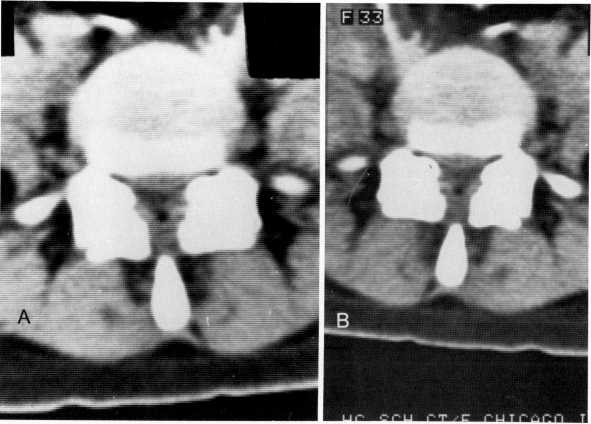

Figure 25.11.   A. CT scan showing midline HNP L5-S1. B. CT scan 3 months postinjection showing persistent midline defect. The patient has a good result.

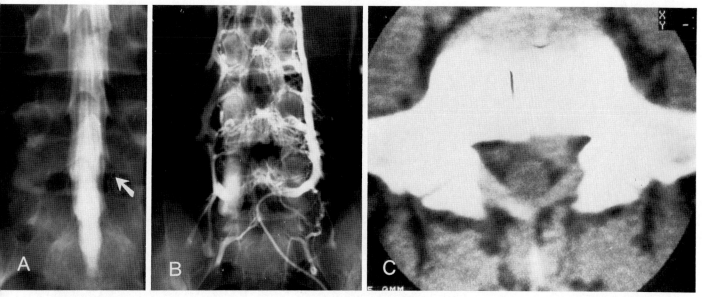

Figure 25.12.   A. Anteroposterior myelogram showing root cut off (S1) at L5-S1 left. B. Venogram. C. CT scan.

patible with a good result to chemonucleolysis when one appreciates the cause of sciatica pain when nuclear material herniates into the spinal canal. Three local mechanisms of pain production ensue:

a. The mass of nuclear material (collagen, proteoglycan, and water) presses on the nerve root. It is this mass that constitutes the CT scan defect.

b. Within the mass, distention occurs through the binding of water and proteoglycan. Chymopapain breaks this chemical bond and the resulting hydrolysis of the mass

converts the pressure on the nerve from that of a distended nuclear fragment (hard "golf ball") to an undistended nuclear fragment (soft "cotton ball"). Thus, the remaining mass of nucleus is merely collagenous but still appears on the CT scan. Over months or years, this collagenous mass will gradually disappear (Fig. 25.13). The optimal time for observing this disappearance on CT scan is at least beyond 2 months in most cases and may even be up to 1 year postinjection.

c. Finally, the distended herniated nuclear fragment sets up an inflammatory reaction around the nerve root

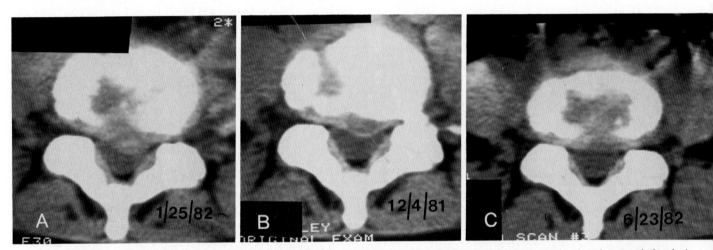

Figure 25.13.   A. CT scan showing large left L4-L5 HNP. B. CT scan 7 weeks postchemonucleolysis showing persisting but smaller defect. C. CT scan 6 months postchemonucleolysis showing shrinking defect. Patient is a young woman who had an immediate excellent result which she maintains to date.

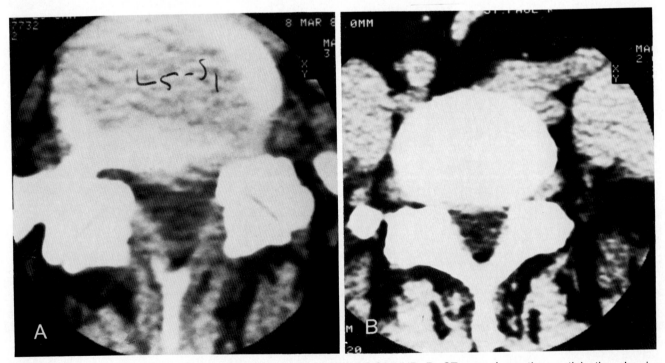

Figure 25.14.   A. CT scan preinjection showing midline and left L5-S1 HNP. B. CT scan 4 months postinjection showing reduction of defect. The procedures (CT scan and chemonucleolysis) were done on an outpatient basis.

to contribute to the pain of sciatica. Somehow, chymopapain neutralizes this chemically mediated pain reaction which explains the often observed dramatic relief of sciatica within minutes of injection of chymopapain. (Obviously this does not bear on the continuing defect appearance on postinjection CT).

OP CHEMONUCLEOLYSIS

The author performs chemonucleolysis on an increasing number of patients using outpatient hospital facilities to relieve pressure on costly hospital beds. Similarly, CT scanning, in replacing myelography, will reduce demands on hospital facilities. The combination of the two outpa-

tient procedures has allowed for the treatment of many patients suffering with sciatica without introducing foreign material (metrizamide) into the subarachnoid space and without hospital admission. Nothing foreign enters the patient's spinal canal and the patient does not see a hospital bed overnight (Fig. 25.14). This will reduce the incidence of a number of complications that arise in the investigation and treatment of sciatica due to a HNP.

To date, chemonucleolysis has been limited to those patients who have the clinical presentation of a herniated nucleus pulposus. Twenty percent will fail to respond to the procedure for various reasons, the most common being an extruded or sequestered disc. With improving CT scan-

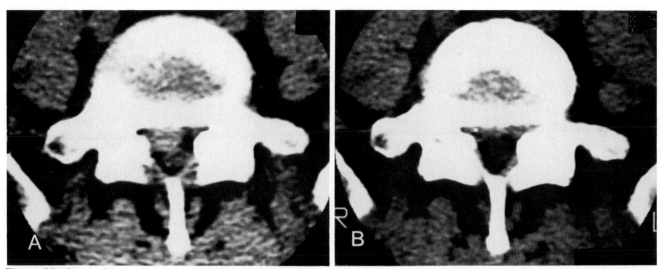

Figure 25.15. A. CT scan showing large HNP L5-S1 right. B. CT scan 2 months postinjection showing disappearance of HNP.

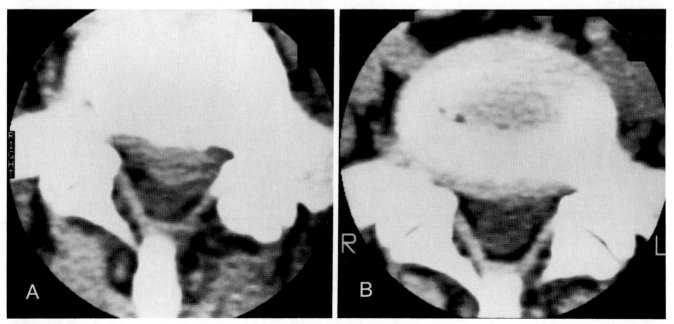

Figure 25.16. A. CT scan showing large midline and left HNP. B. CT scan 2 months postchemonucleolysis showing defect largely resolved.

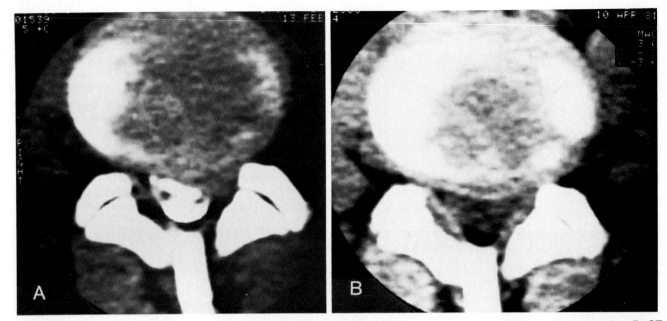

Figure 25.17. A. Augmented CT scan showing HNP L4-L5 midline and left. Addition of metrizamide emphasizes lesion. B. CT scan 2 months postinjection showing resolution of HNP. With improved CT scan technique, it will be less necessary to augment with contrast material.

ning dosimetry, technique, and software, it is likely a sequestered disc will be demonstrated and the patient will be saved the fruitless step of chemonucleolysis. The present state of the art of CT scanning demonstrates calcified disc herniations (Fig. 25.8) that will not respond to chemonucleolysis. CT scanning also will demonstrate lateral foraminal disc herniations (Fig. 25.7) and, with further experience, we will be able to decide which of these lateral foraminal herniations is sequestered and will not respond to chemonucleolysis.

In summary, noninvasive CT scanning is allowing for increasing confidence in diagnosis of herniated nuclear material. The persistence of a CT scan defect after chemonucleolysis in the presence of a good result helps us to understand further the multifaceted cause of the pain of sciatica. CT scans showing disappearance of the HNP fragment (Figs. 25.15–25.17) verify the clinical efficacy of chemonucleolysis. With further refinements, it is anticipated that CT scanning will allow for the more accurate depictment of the character of a disc herniation and save some patients the unnecessary and fruitless step of chemonucleolysis.

References

1. Garvin PJ, Jennings RB, Stern IJ: Enzymatic digestion of the nucleus pulposus: A review of experimental studies with chymopapain. *Orthop Clin North Am* 8:27–35, 1977.
2. Smith L: Chemonucleolysis. *Clin Orthop* 67:72–80, 1969.
3. McCulloch JA, Waddell G: Lateral lumbar discography. *Br J Radiol* 51:498–502, 1978.
4. McCulloch JA, Ferguson JM: Outpatient chemonucleolysis. *Spine* 6:606–609, 1981.
5. McCulloch JA: Chemonucleolysis: Experience with 2000 cases. *Clin Orthop* 146:128–135, 1980.
6. Smith L, Brown JE: Treatment of lumbar intervertebral disc lesions by direct injection of chymopapain. *J Bone Joint Surg* 49B:502–519, 1967.
7. Parkinson D, Shields C: Treatment of protruded lumbar intervertebral discs with chymopapain (Discase). *J Neurosurg* 39:203–208, 1973.
8. Macnab I, et al: Chemonucleolysis. *Can J Surg* 14:280–209, 1971.
9. Burton CV, Heithoff KB, Kirkaldy Willis W, et al: Computed tomographic scanning and the lumbar spine, Part II: Clinical considerations. *Spine* 4:356–368, 1979.
10. Glenn WV, Rhodes ML, Altschuler EM, et al: Multiplanar display computerized body tomography applications in the lumbar spine. *Spine* 4:282–352, 1979.

CHAPTER TWENTY-SIX

Computed Tomography of Canine Disc Herniation: A Potential Diagnostic Model for the Evaluation of Disc Disease and Discolysis in Humans

C. GENE COIN, M.D., J. THADDEUS COIN, Ph.D., and J. K. GARRETT, D.V.M.

INTRODUCTION

Canine disc herniation, like the human counterpart, is a serious and common problem in veterinary medicine. Chondrodystrophoid breeds such as dachshunds, Pekingese, cocker spaniels, poodles, and beagles most commonly are affected; however, all breeds may suffer from this ailment. Among the nonchondrodystrophoid, German shepherds and Labrador retrievers predominate. The discs at T12–13 and T13-L1 in the thoracic lumbar region and at C2–3 and C3–4 in the cervical region most frequently herniate; however, any level may be affected. This subject is well-covered and extensively referenced by Hoerlein (1).

Clinical manifestations occur earlier in life and are more severe in the chondrodystrophic breeds. Similar findings are observed in human achondroplasia. Accompanying narrow spinal canal is an important contributing factor in this condition. Like the human counterpart, symptoms and neurological findings in canine disc herniation vary greatly, ranging from asymptomatic incidental occurrence to quadriplegia and death. Remissions and exacerbations of symptoms are common in canines and man, making objective evaluation of treatment extremely difficult. Neurological manifestations are due to the location and extent of spinal cord and nerve injury which may be the result of direct trauma or secondary to interference with the blood supply.

Roentgen studies include radiography, discography, venography, and myelography. Plain film abnormality may include narrowing of disc spaces, apparent narrowing of intervertebral foraminae, and calcification of the intervertebral disc (1). Unlike the human counterpart, multiple disc calcifications frequently are visible on plain films. These changes are helpful indicators of the presence of disc disease; however, as in man, the plain film studies are not highly accurate indicators of specific location and extent of herniation except when a calcified mass in the spinal canal is visualized. This viewpoint (nonspecificity of plain film studies) is supported by radiographic anatomical studies (Figs. 26.1 and 26.2) and by the CT evidence presented here. Myelography, a technically difficult procedure in dogs (as in achondroplastic humans), has been

required for determination and precise localization of canine disc herniation.

CT is the only accurate noninvasive method for the visualization of cartilaginous disc herniation in humans and is capable of showing very small herniations in man (2–8). We have applied this method of diagnosis (CT) to canine disc disease and demonstrate similar capability. We report here our technique with postmortem anatomical studies and representative clinical cases. Similarities in the CT appearance of canine and human disc disease are also shown. These similarities suggest that CT of canine disc herniation can serve as a model for the evaluation of discolysis in humans. This aspect of our study will be addressed further in the next chapter.

METHODS

CT was performed utilizing either the General Electric CT/T 8800 equipped with ScoutView or the Elscint 905 whole body scanner. Postmortem studies were done on recently euthanized dogs or dissected specimens including spinal cord, spine, and adjacent muscles. These studies included detailed radiography by plain films, multiple thin-section high-resolution CT, and anatomical dissection of the spine and intervertebral discs. Anatomical, radiographic, and CT findings are compared. Clinical cases were performed utilizing general anesthesia. Typical technical factors for CT were:

GE CT/T 8800—
   120 kVp
   600 MAs
   1.5-mm slice thickness
   9.6-second scan time
Elscint 905—
   138 kVp
   646 MAs
   5-mm slice thickness
   17-second scan time

POSTMORTEM STUDIES

Case 1. An 8-year-old German Shepherd Mixture

This animal had developed sudden quadriplegia. Euthanasia was performed. Radiographs of the live dog (not illustrated) were normal except for calcification of the C4–5 disc. Postmortem radiographs of the dissected neck specimen were obtained by using detail screens (Fig. 26.1A). On these studies, additional faint calcification also could be seen in other disc spaces. Extensive thin-section CT of the entire neck specimen was performed, then the intervertebral discs were dissected. These studies were compared. A high degree of correlation between CT and the anatomical sections was noted (Fig. 26.1). There was little specific correlation between plain film study and location of a large disc herniation found at C3–4 and a very small herniation found at C5–6. CT, on the other hand, readily demonstrated these herniations and correctly predicted the absence of herniation at other levels (Fig. 26.1B-E).

Case 2. A 3-year-old Miniature Poodle

Postmortem CT, radiographic, and gross anatomical studies were performed on a 3-year-old miniature poodle (Fig. 26.2). This dog had posterior paraparesis for 2 weeks' duration. Detailed screen radiographs showed extensive degenerative changes including calcifications of intervertebral discs and narrowing of disc spaces. These changes were most prominent in the lower thoracic and upper lumbar region (Fig. 26.2A); however, radiographic abnormalities were present in every disc level from D6 through L7. Multiple thin section (1.5 mm) CTs were obtained through all disc spaces. Anatomical dissection of disc spaces was performed. Small (2–4 mm) herniations were found at D13-L1 and L2–3. CT correctly displayed the only

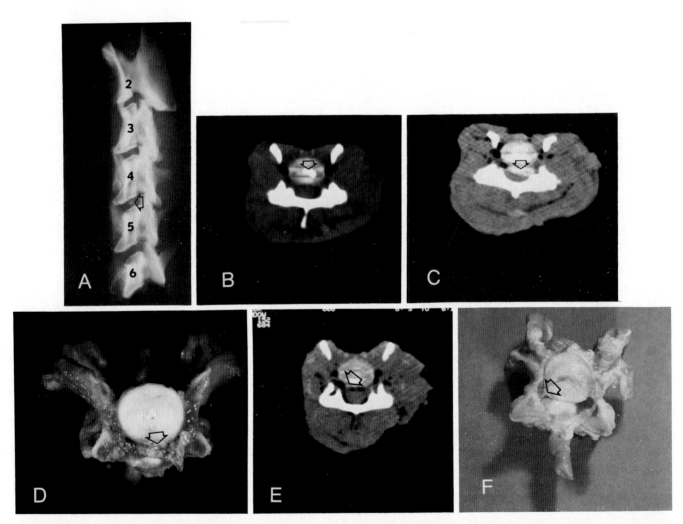

Figure 26.1. Postmortem radiographic and CT study of excised German shepherd cervical spine with anatomical comparison: A. Radiograph of excised neck (C2-C6) reveals a prominent calcification at C4–5 (*arrow*). B. CT slice at C4–5 confirms calcification (*arrow*) within the intervertebral disc. The disc is otherwise normal with no evidence of herniation into spinal canal. C. CT slice at the level of C3–4 reveals large calcified herniated disc severely compromising the canal (*arrow*). D. Specimen at the C3–4 level confirms the CT findings of a large herniation (*arrow*). Spinal cord was necrotic at this level. E. CT of C5–6 reveals a very small lateral herniation of disc anulus (*arrow*) without significant herniation into the canal. F. Specimen at C5–6 disc confirms CT findings (*arrow*). Herniation measures 2 mm in diameter.

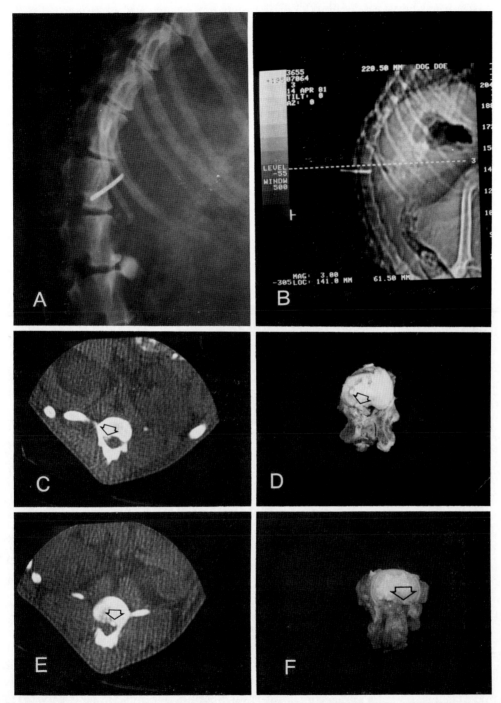

Figure 26.2. Postmortem radiographic, CT, and anatomical study of miniature poodle's thoracic-lumbar spine: A. Lateral radiograph. Extensive disc calcification and degenerative changes are shown. Radiodense marker needle is at the level of L1. B. Digital radiograph (General Electric Co., ScoutView) is used to position CT slice. C. 1.5-mm thick CT section at level of D13-L1 disc space. A small, partially calcified disc herniation (*arrow*) is present. D. Dissection of spine at the D13-L1 disc level confirms presence of herniated disc material (*arrow*). E. CT slice demonstrates calcified herniation at L2–3 (*arrow*). F. Specimen at L2–3 confirms the CT findings (*arrow*).

two herniations found and correctly predicted absence of other herniations. Plain film radiographs correctly showed abnormalities including narrow disc space at the level of herniations; however, plain film radiographs also demonstrated abnormalities at multiple levels where herniation was not found. Small, calcified disc herniations were shown on CT of D13-L1 (Fig. 26.2C) and L2–3 (Fig. 26.2E). These findings were correlated on dissected specimen (Fig. 26.2D and F).

CLINICAL STUDIES

During the past 4 years, we have studied clinical cases of canine disc herniation by radiography and by CT. Similarities of disc disease in man and dog have been previously reported (1, 9). Major differences between canine and human disc disease appear to be related to caudal continuation of the canine spinal cord (to about Lumbar 6–7), relatively small spinal canal, and compressed time frame of the evolution and history of the disease in dogs. All of these features favor canine disc disease as a suitable animal model of the human ailment. We note a striking similarity in the CT appearance of disc herniation in dog and man. The only major difference we have noted is the apparent frequency of roentgenographically visible calcifications in discs of dogs. This may be related to the compressed time frame and is deserving of further investigation.

Intervertebral disc calcification in humans [first reported by Luschka in 1858 (10) and not reported radiographically until 1921 (11)] increases steadily with advancing age (12). Disc calcifications both in the anulus and in the nucleus frequently are visualized by CT when they cannot be seen on standard radiographs. Similarities in appearance of human and canine herniations are displayed here (Figs. 26.3–26.5), along with representative clinical cases of canine disc herniation shown by CT.

Case 3. Normal Intervertebral Disc

The CT appearance of a normal canine intervertebral disc is shown in comparison to a freshly dissected canine disc and CT of a normal human intervertebral disc (Fig. 26.3).

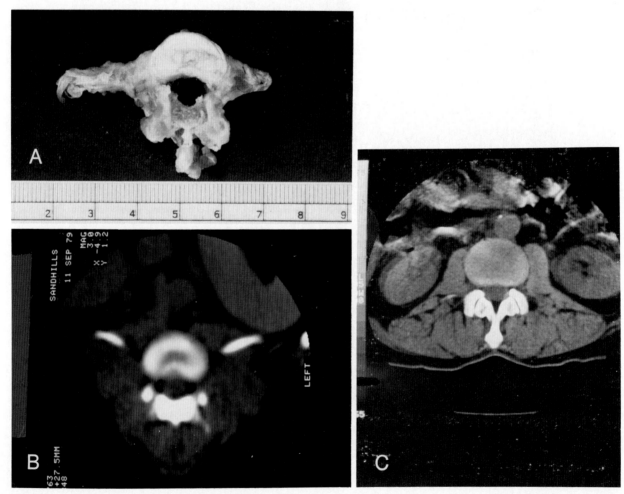

Figure 26.3.   Normal intervertebral disc: A. Fresh specimen of an essentially normal canine intervertebral disc. B. CT of a normal canine disc. C. CT of a normal human disc.

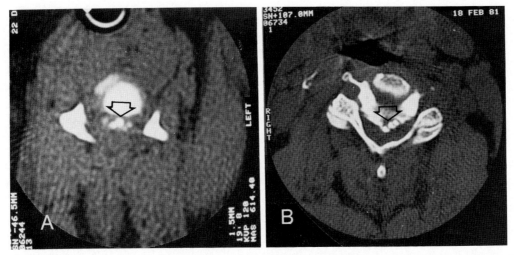

Figure 26.4.   Cervical disc herniation: A. Large canine disc herniation at C5–6 (*arrow*). B. Human disc herniation at C3–4 (*arrow*).

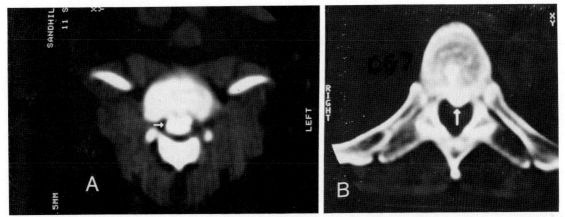

Figure 26.5.   Thoracic-lumbar disc herniation: A. Canine herniation at L2–3. A large calcified herniation (*arrow*) occupies much of the spinal canal. B. A small calcified midline herniation is present in the lower thoracic spine (*white arrow*) of a 62-year-old man. Level is D6–7.

Case 4. Cervical Disc Herniation

A 9-year-old male dachshund presented with evidence of severe neck pain accompanied by muscle spasm and quadriparesis. CT of the neck demonstrated a large calcified disc herniation with significant intrusion into the spinal canal at C5–6 disc space (Fig. 26.4A). Note the striking similarity in comparison to a 54-year-old male human presenting with severe neck pain and bilateral "tingling" sensation in both upper extremities immediately after a serious automobile accident. A calcified disc herniation at C3–4 level is shown by CT (Fig. 26.4B).

Case 5. Calcified Thoracic-Lumbar Disc Herniation

A 5-year-old beagle-corgi mixture had well-documented episodes of paralysis of posterior extremities occurring intermittently over 4 months' duration. A large calcified disc herniation at L2–3 is well shown by CT (Fig. 26.5A).

A very similar human thoracic herniation also is shown for comparison (Fig. 26.5B).

Case 6. Lumbar Disc Herniation

A 3-year-old female cocker spaniel suffered from posterior paralysis of 1 week's duration. Paralysis was sudden in occurence without prior symptoms. A large cartilaginous herniation of L2–3 disc was demonstrated by CT (Fig. 26.6A). This case was unusual in our series in that calcification usually was visible in these herniations. It is pertinent to note that we are referring to calcification in the range of Hounsfield numbers greater than 100. Many of these herniations were not visibly calcified on standard radiographs which are inherently much less sensitive in contrast resolution. A human cartilaginous disc herniation at L5–S1 is shown in a 25-year-old male who experienced low back pain with radiation into the right leg after a parachuting accident (Fig. 26.6B).

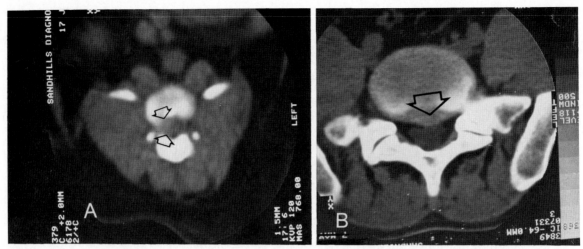

Figure 26.6. Lumber disc herniation: A. Canine herniation at L2–3 (*arrows*) is cartilaginous. B. Human disc herniation (*arrow*) at L5-S1 is also of cartilage density.

SUMMARY

We report here the noninvasive diagnosis of canine disc herniation by CT. CT is capable of demonstrating very small disc herniations in dogs as in man.

Anatomical documentation supported by postmortem studies is provided. Similarities between human and dog disc herniations are noted. Spontaneously occurring canine disc herniation studied by CT may provide a suitable diagnostic model for the evaluation of human disc disease and discolysis.

CONCLUSION

1. Plain film radiography provides high sensitivity with low specificity for the diagnosis of disc disease. This is identical to our human experience.

2. CT provides a highly accurate noninvasive means for diagnosis of canine disc herniation.

3. Many similarities between canine and human herniation are apparent.

4. Spontaneously occurring canine disc herniation studied by CT may provide a suitable diagnostic model of human disc herniation and discolysis.

References
1. Hoerlein BF: Intervertebral disks. Chap 14. In: *Canine Neurology Diagnosis and Treatment*. 3rd Ed. W. B. Saunders, Philadelphia, 1978, pp. 470–555.
2. Coin CG, Chan YS, Keranen V, et al: Computer assisted myelography in disk disease. *J Comput Assist Tomogr* 1, 1977.
3. Coin CG, Coin JT: Computed tomography of cervical disk disease: Technical considerations with representative case reports. *J Comput Assist Tomogr* 5:275–280, 1981.
4. Di Chiro G, Schellinger D: Computed tomography of spinal cord after lumbar intrathecal introduction of metrizamide (computer assisted myelography). *Radiology* 120:101–104, 1976.
5. Glenn WV Jr, Rhodes ML, Altschuler EM, et al: Multiplanar display computerized body tomography application in the lumbar spine. *Spine* 4, 1979.
6. Meyer GA, Haughton VM, Williams AL: Diagnosis of herniated lumbar disk with computed tomography. *NZ J Med* 301:1166–1167, 1979.
7. Post MJD: CT update: The impact of time, metrizamide, and high resolution in the diagnosis of spinal pathology. Chap. 8. In: Post MJD: *Radiographic Evaluation of the Spine: Current Advances with Emphasis on Computed Tomography*. New York, Masson Publishing, 1980, pp. 259–294.
8. Williams AL, Haughton VM, Syvertsen A: Computed tomography in the diagnosis of herniated nucleus pulposus. *Radiology* 135:95–99, 1980.
9. Riser WH: Posterior paralysis associated wtih intervertebral disc protrusion in the dog. *North Am Vet* 27:633, 1946.
10. Luschka H: Die Halbgelenke des menschlichen. Korpers, Berlin, 1858.
11. Calva UU, Galland M: Sur une affection particuliere de la colonne vertebrale simulant de mal de Pott. *J Radiol* 21, 1921.
12. Schmorl G, Junghanns H: *The Human Spine in Health and Disease*. First American edition. Translated and edited by SP Wilk, LS Goin. New York and London, Grune and Stratton, 1932, p. 166.

CHAPTER TWENTY-SEVEN

Experimental Computed Tomographic-Controlled Discolysis

C. GENE COIN, M.D., J. THADDEUS COIN, Ph.D., and J. K. GARRETT, D.V.M.

Enzymatic dissolution is a promising method of treatment for disc herniation in man and dogs (1–22). Clinical results, although encouraging, are controversial. Rational evaluation of these treatment results is hampered by the lack of an objective, noninvasive method to determine the drug's effect on disc herniation. The purpose of this study is to establish a method for objective evaluation of enzymatic dissolution of disc herniation in animals with a view to developing this technique for human use.

Although myelography is a relatively safe and useful method for diagnosis of disc herniation, it is not suitable for this study. Intraspinal injection of any other drug would introduce an unfavorable bias into the study for evaluation of enzymatic discolysis. Modern thin-section CT, on the other hand, offers an accurate method for diagnosis of disc herniation without need for spinal tap or introduction of foreign material into the spinal canal. Present equipment provides slice position of fractional millimeter accuracy. Slice thickness is down to 1.5 mm. Contrast resolution is such that cartilage may be differentiated readily from epidural fat, dura, and spinal fluid.

Absorption values showing the relative density of the herniation may be measured accurately and comparison made before and after treatment. The ability of CT to demonstrate even very small disc herniations in dogs has been shown previously (4).

This study utilizes CT for the diagnosis of paralyzing canine disc herniation, for control of injection of highly purified collagenase (Advance Biofactures Corporation, Lynbrook, NY), and for objective analysis of discolysis. These cases show objective CT evidence that collagenase is effective in producing substantial lysis of canine disc herniations. The nonherniated component of these discs is reduced, and calcification is reduced both within the confines of the disc and herniation into the spinal canal. While clinical results were not a major objective of this investigation, it is interesting to note that recovery from paralysis occurred in 10 of the 13 dogs treated. Techniques, results, and representative cases are reported here.

TECHNIQUE

CT is utilized to confirm specific location and extent of clinically suspected disc herniation in symptomatic dogs. Under general anesthesia, axial thin-section CT of the suspected disc spaces is performed. After diagnosis of herniation, treatment is performed utilizing CT stereotaxy. An outer 22-g needle is positioned in the lateral margin of the affected disc. An inner 28-g needle is then inserted into the intervertebral disc. Fifty microliters of collagenase solution (Advance Biofactures—300 units) is injected into the disc. Additional scans of the affected disc verify the injection site.

Lateral spine radiographs and follow-up CT scans are obtained for the duration of the study (in this study—1 year). Digital radiographic positioning and general anesthesia ensure precise positioning of the follow-up sections in the previously treated disc spaces. Postmortem study is performed in selected studies (Fig. 27.5).

COLLAGENASE

The enzyme used for the intradiscal injection is collagenase, a proteolytic enzyme with a high degree of substrate specificity. Collagenase catalyzed peptide bond cleavage occurs at amino acid sequences found in few proteins other than collagen (23, 24). Mammalian collagenases expressed into the interstitial space by osteoclasts and fibroblasts are instrumental in bone remodeling and connective tissue regulation, respectively (25). Bacteria secrete collagenases presumably as part of the infectious offense. Mammalian collagenases cleave collagen into relatively large fragments ¼–¾ of the original size whereas the bacterial enzymes produce smaller fragments (23, 25). Otherwise they may be considered functionally identical. Bacterial collagenase from *Clostridium histolyticum* has been isolated (23), highly purified (24), and produced commercially (Advance Biofactures Corporation, Lynbrook, NY) for a variety of pharmaceutical uses including lysis of the intervertebral disc.

The collagenase molecule [molecular weight = 81,000 (25)] is much smaller than the collagen fiber which it attacks. Triple helix collagen units (molecular weight = 300,000) aggregate in a regular fashion to form fibers of undetermined length (25). The matrix of collagen fibers allows ample space for other structural components and infiltration of interstitial fluid [e.g., hyaline cartilage contains 75% of its fresh weight in fluid contained in a collagen matrix which is 40% of its dry weight (26)]. Relatively tiny collagenase molecules can diffuse easily through the interstitial fluid and attack at a multitude of sites on the collagen fiber matrix. Similarly collagen fragments produced by enzymatic hydrolysis may readily diffuse away.

A hypothetical mode of therapeutic collagenase lysis of the nucleus pulposus of the intervertebral disc follows:

1. Injected collagenase solution first displaces its vol-

ume in interstitial fluid contained in the nucleus pulposus;

2. Collagenase molecules diffuse throughout the interstitium producing countless molecular lesions in the collagen matrix until the enzyme is inactivated by endogenous proteases or diluted and removed to the circulation;

3. Collagen fragments diffuse away as do other components which were supported by the previously intact matrix.

The high degree of substrate specificity of collagenase precludes a large range of toxic effects due to general protein destruction. Inadvertent extradiscal injection or leakage of collagenase would produce only interstitial damage. A similar misplacement of a general protease is likely to produce more serious cellular as well as interstitial destruction.

CASE REPORTS

Case 1. Plain Film Changes after Collagenase Treatment

A 7-year-old male dachshund with posterior paralysis secondary to T12–13 disc herniation was treated with an intranuclear injection of 300 units of collagenase. Plain films before and 21 days after treatment show that both calcification and volume within the disc are reduced (Fig. 27.1 A–C). This dog experienced clinical recovery within 3 days after treatment and had remained well for 6 months when he suffered another paralyzing herniation—this time at L3–4 level (Fig. 27.1D). The L3–4 disc then was treated by intranuclear injection of 300 units of collagenase. There was recovery from posterior paralysis in 4 days. Narrowing of disc space and disappearance of calcification is noted on plain films made 6 weeks after treatment (Fig. 27.1E).

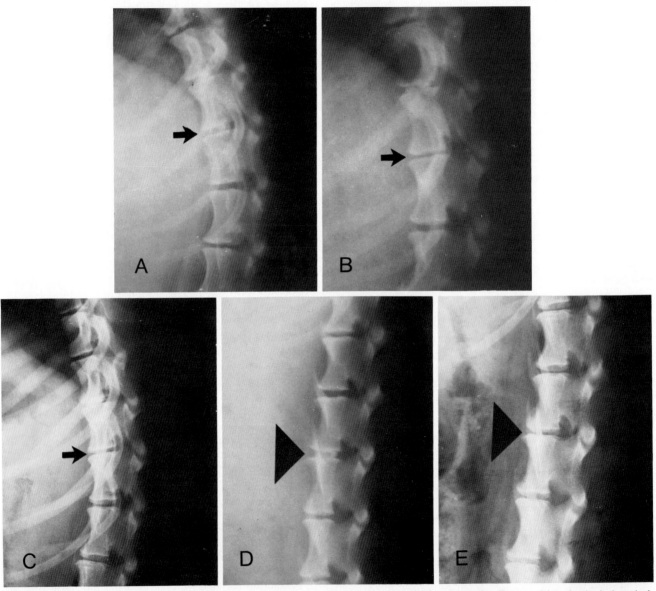

Figure 27.1. Case 1. Plain film changes after collagenase treatment: Lateral radiographs of a 7-year-old male dachshund. A. Precollagenase radiograph reveals calcified T12–13 intervertebral disc (*arrow*). B. T12–13 is narrowed with no visible calcification (*arrow*) on postcollagenase radiographs 21 days after treatment and (C) 1 year after treatment. D. L3–4 before collagenase treatment. Disc is calcified. E. Six weeks later, calcification is no longer visible. The disc space is narrowed.

Case 2. CT-Controlled Treatment of T13–L1 Disc Herniation in a 5-year-old Dachshund

This 5-year-old male dachshund had paresis of pelvic limbs for 9 weeks with muscle atrophy. CT scan of the T13–L1 disc level revealed a large calcified disc herniation obstructing more than one-half of the canal (Fig. 27.2A). Collagenase (300 units) were injected into the disc during the same scan session (Fig. 27.2B). Clinical improvement occurred in less than 1 week. The animal completely recovered from posterior paresis and was essentially normal at 6 months post-treatment. Follow-up CT at 3 months post-treatment showed prominent reduction in the herniation; even the calcification has been reduced (Fig. 27.2C).

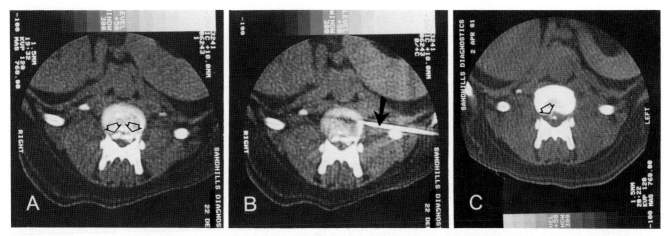

Figure 27.2. Case 2. Collagenase injection and follow-up CT of T13-L1 in a 5-year-old dachshund: A. Large, calcified disc herniation (*arrows*) is shown on 1.5-mm CT slice at T13-L1. B. Needle (*arrow*) is in place for collagenase injection. C. CT follow-up 3 months postcollagenase treatment shows herniation substantially reduced in size and reduction of calcification (*arrow*).

Case 3. Treatment of L2–3 Herniation in a 3-year-old Female Cocker Spaniel

Rapid onset of posterior paresis without prior symptoms occurred 1 week before treatment. CT of the L2–3 disc level reveals a large cartilaginous herniation (confirmed by repeat sections) occupying about one-half of the canal (Fig. 27.3A). This herniation was not significantly calcified. The disc was injected with 300 units of collagenase by CT-controlled stereotaxis (Fig. 27.3B). One week post-treatment there was clinical recovery with ability to walk and run. CT follow-up at 16 days post-treatment shows reduction in the herniation with a small amount of residual material in the canal (Fig. 27.3C). This animal remains clinically well at 6 months after treatment.

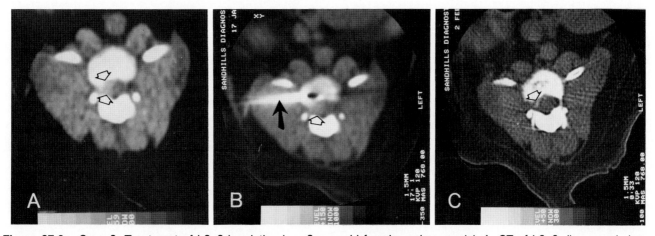

Figure 27.3. Case 3. Treatment of L2–3 herniation in a 3-year-old female cocker spaniel: A. CT of L2–3 disc reveals large cartilaginous herniation (*arrows*). B. Needle is in place (*solid arrow*) immediately postcollagenase injection. *Open arrow* shows herniation. C. Follow-up CT 16 days postcollagenase treatment shows marked reduction in herniation (*arrow*).

Case 4. Collagenase Treatment of Cervical Disc Herniation in a 9-year-old Male Dachshund

Severe neck pain was accompanied by quadriparesis. CT scan of the C5–6 level demonstrates a calcified disc herniation (Fig. 27.4A). Collagenase, 300 units, was injected at that time (Fig. 27.4B). The dog improved with

relief of pain and returned to normal walking. A relapse of pain at about 2 months post-injection was treated successfully by conservative management. CT follow-up study at 3 months shows that disc material in the canal at C5–6 was reduced in size; extent of calcification was also reduced (Fig. 27.4C). This animal was clinically normal at 8 months post-treatment.

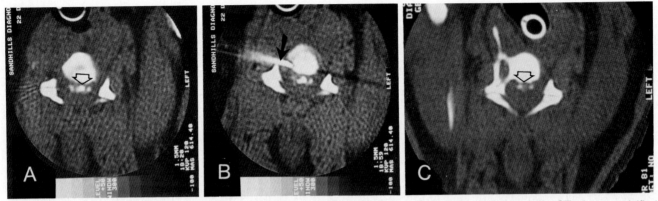

Figure 27.4. Case 4. Collagenase injection and follow-up CT of C5–6 in a 9-year-old dachshund: A. CT shows calcified herniated disc at C5–6 (*arrow*). B. Needle is in place (*arrow*) for collagenase injection. C. Three-month follow-up CT reveals significant reduction in herniation. Calcified material in the canal also has been reduced.

Case 5. Multiple Disc Herniations in a 10-year-old Dachshund

This dog first developed symptoms of hypersensitivity and pain followed by progressive posterior paralysis which began 1 week before treatment. CT scan of T13-L1 disc demonstrated a large, partially calcified herniation occupying at least ¾ of the canal at this level (Fig. 27.5A). Collagenase was injected into the T13-L1 disc (Fig. 27.5B). Follow-up CT of T13-L1, 16 days later showed prominent

reduction of herniated disc material (Fig. 27.5C). This animal was still paraplegic at the time of the 16-day follow-up study; there was dense paralysis of the hind extremities. Additional small disc herniations at L1–2 and L2–3 each were treated by CT-controlled intradiscal injection of 300 units of collagenase. Paraplegia remained unchanged. Euthanasia was performed 60 days after original treatment. CT and gross anatomical findings are shown in Figure 27.5.

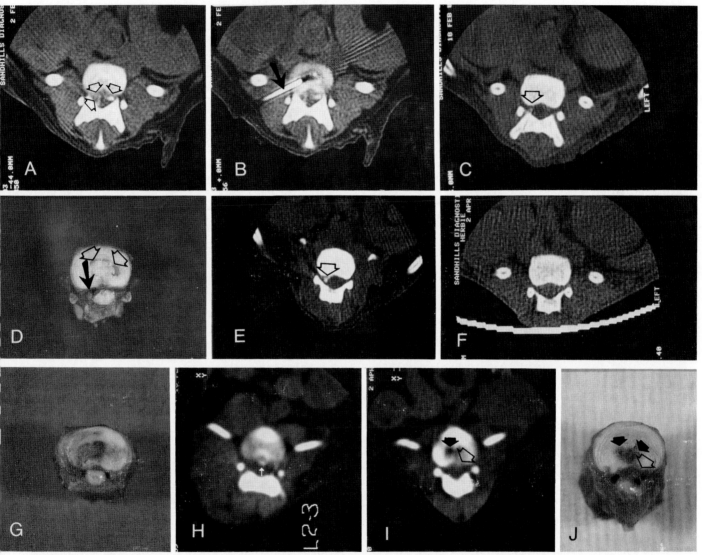

Figure 27.5. Case 5. Collagenase injection and postmortem correlation in a 10-year-old male dachshund: A. CT at T13-L1. A very large, partially calcified herniation (*arrows*) severely compromises the spinal canal. B. Needle is in place (*arrow*) immediately postcollagenase injection. C. Follow-up CT 16 days postcollagenase injection reveals only a small residual lateral herniation (*arrow*) in the spinal canal. D. Dissected specimen of the T13-L1 disc. There is excellent correlation with the antemortem CT scan. There has been lysis of the nucleus (*open arrows*). Small lateral herniation remains (*arrow*). The cord was soft and necrotic at this level. E. Antemortem CT scan at L1–2. A partially calcified lateral herniation is present (*arrow*). F. Postmortem CT scan of L1–2 6 weeks after intranuclear treatment with collagenase. Herniation is no longer visible. G. L1–2 disc, dissected frozen specimen. There is excellent correlation with the CT findings postmortem. H. Pre-mortem CT at L2–3. A central partially calcified disc herniation intrudes significantly into the territory of the spinal cord (*arrow*). I. L2–3 postmortem CT scan 6 weeks after collagenase treatment. Calcification is diminished (*open arrow*). Significant central nucleolysis with "vacuum" intervertebral disc is present (*arrow*). J. L2–3 anatomical specimen showing correlation with the CT scan. Central nucleolysis has occurred (*open arrow*). There is necrosis of the cord at this level due to herniation.

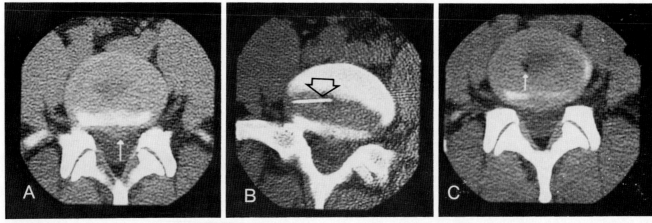

Figure 27.6. Case 6. CT-controlled discolysis, human technique: A. Paracentral herniation at L4–5 (*arrow*). B. CT scan at L4–5 shows needle in good position before collagenase injection (*open arrow*). C. Air in disc (*arrow*) confirms injection site.

RESULTS

Nineteen discs were injected with collagenase in 13 dogs suffering from paralyzing disc herniations. In these cases diagnosis, treatment, and follow-up studies were performed utilizing precisely controlled thin-section high-resolution CT under general anesthesia. Three of these treated discs in 1 dog were also studied by postmortem CT and autopsy examination. All injected discs showed loss of volume on follow-up radiographs. Calcifications within the discs and in herniations diminished or disappeared. CT demonstrated reduction in herniation and reduced absorption values both within the nucleus and in the herniations in all cases studied. There was good correlation between CT and autopsy findings.

Ten of the 13 dogs treated promptly recovered from paralysis (within 2 weeks of treatment) and have remained well up to 1 year afterwards. Two dogs remained paralyzed. In both of these, there was CT evidence that substantial lysis of both the nucleus and herniation had occurred. One dog was lost to follow-up and is presumed to be unimproved.

HUMAN CT-CONTROLLED DISCOLYSIS

The canine technique described has been modified for human use. After the CT diagnosis of lumbar disc herniation, CT-controlled discolysis is performed utilizing 600 units of collagenase (Case 6, Fig. 27.6). CT then is utilized for the objective evaluation of discolysis results (Case 7, Fig. 27.7).

Case 6. L4–5 Disc Herniation in a 34-year-old Male Human*

This man was injured in an industrial accident 6 months before the study. Immediately after an attempt to restrict the fall of a gasoline pump, the patient suffered from severe low back pain with extreme pain radiating down his left leg. During the following 6 months of conservative management, he was unable to resume work due to persistent low back and leg pain. Radicular symptoms were referred to the L5 root on the left. Valsalva maneuver caused back and leg pain. Sensory examination revealed diminished sensation over the distribution of the 5th nerve root on the left. Deep tendon reflexes were normal. Straight leg raising was positive at 30° on the left, and greater than 60° on the right. There was slight weakness of eversion of the left foot and moderate dorsiflexion weakness. CT demonstrated the presence of a central and paracentral 5-mm disc herniation at L4–5 on the left side. Under CT control, intradiscal injection of collagenase was performed at the L4–5 level (Fig. 27.6).

Case 7. Human Disc Herniation at L4–5†

A 39-year-old male physician presented with a history of low back pain of 14 months' duration. In the past 3 months, the pain had become progressively more severe with radiation into the right buttock, down the posterior aspect of the right thigh, and posterior lateral aspect of the calf. Straight leg raising on the right was positive at 20° and 50° on the left. Slight toe extension and anterior tibial weakness was present on the right as well as hyperesthesia in the distribution of L5 nerve root. Symptoms did not respond to conservative management.

This patient was a participant in phase 2 of the Food and Drug Administration-approved evaluation of the effect of intradiscal collagenase on herniated intervertebral discs. Because of previous protocol requirements radiographic myelography (Fig. 27.7A) was performed, also showing herniation of L4–5 disc. The L4–5 disc was injected with 600 units collagenase (Nucleolysin, Advance Biofactures Corporation, Lynbrook NY).

The patient's symptoms increased in severity and dorsiflexor weakness increased for approximately 10 days after injection. Progressive improvement began thereafter.

---

* This case illustrates the human technique of CT-controlled discolysis.

---

† Figure 27.7 Clinical case courtesy of John W. Bromley, M.D. This case shows the ability of CT to provide objective evidence of discolysis.

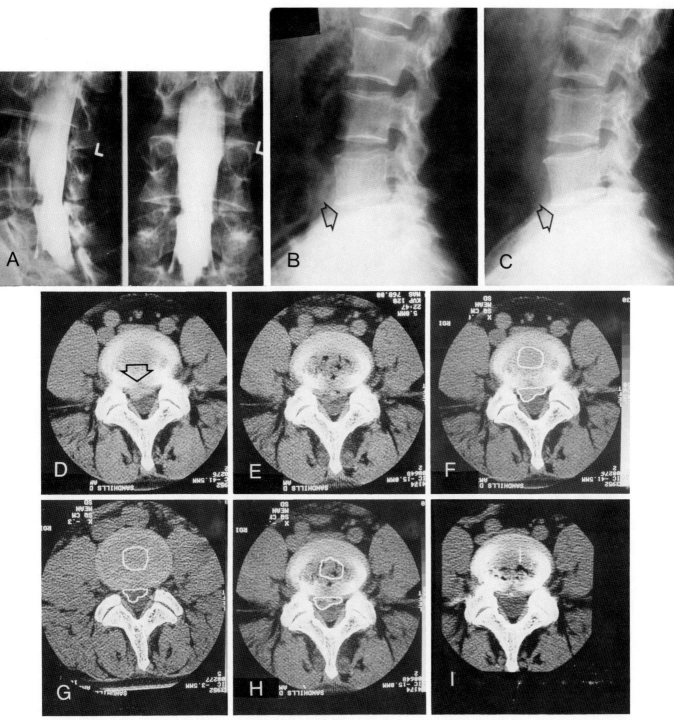

Figure 27.7. Case 7. L4–5 disc herniation in a 39-year-old male before and after collagenase treatment: A. Radiographic myelogram. There is an extradural defect at L4–5 on the right characteristic of disc herniation. B. Lateral radiograph before treatment. The L4–5 disc is normal. C. Lateral radiograph 4 weeks later. The L4–5 disc space is narrowed. D. CT at L4–5. A large cartilaginous herniation is present (*arrow*). E. Same level CT 4 weeks later. There is obvious evidence of discolysis. F. Density studies before treatment. Mean value in the disc 100 HU and 96 in the herniation. G. Control study. Normal (L3–4) disc. Mean value in the disc 100 HU and in a comparable portion of the spinal canal 30 HU. H. Density studies of L4–5 4 weeks after treatment. Mean value in the disc is 40 HU, and 48 HU in the region of the herniation. I. CT scan at 10-months postinjection shows no residual herniation. Gas is shown in the disc (*arrow*).

The patient returned to work at 3½ weeks. At 6 weeks, appreciable recovery in dorsiflexor power was noted as well as marked relief of preinjection back and leg pain.

Radiographic and CT studies were performed before, 1 month, and 10 months after injection of the L4–5 disc. The 1-month follow-up study shows conclusive evidence of lysis of cartilage both within the disc and of the herniation into the spinal canal (Fig. 27.7E). The L4–5 disc space became narrowed on plain x-rays (Fig. 27.7B and C). The herniation obviously was diminished in size and density on the CT images. Absorption values within the disc and in the herniation diminished significantly averaging about 40 HU less than the pretreatment studies.

CT scan at 10 months postinjection showed no residual herniation (Fig. 27.7I).

CONCLUSIONS

1. CT and plain lateral radiographs of the spine provide an accurate objective means for evaluation of lysis of the intervertebral disc nucleus and for evaluation of lysis of disc herniation in the dog.

2. Spontaneously occurring canine disc herniation is a promising model of the human disease and may provide a valuable adjunct for the evaluation of human treatment, particularly in enzymatic discolysis.

3. Collagenase is effective in the lysis of both the disc and the herniation in canine disc herniation. Early human results also are encouraging.

References

1. Bromley JW, Hirst JW, Osman M, et al: Collagenase. An experimental study of intervertebral disc dissolution. *Spine* 5:126–132, 1980.
2. Brown MD: Chemonucleolysis with Discase, techniques, results, case reports. *Spine* 1:115–120, 1976.
3. Brown MD, Daroff RB: The double-blind study comparing Discase to placebo: An editorial comment. *Spine* 2:233–236, 1977.
4. Coin CG, Coin JT, Garrett JK: Canine disc herniation, diagnosis by computed tomography. Exhibit at the Annual Scientific Meeting of RSNA, Chicago, IL, November 15–21, 1981; and Exhibit at the American Veterinary Medical Association meeting, Salt Lake City, UT, July 1982
5. Garvin PJ: Toxicity of collagenase: The relation to enzyme therapy of disc herniation. *Clin Orthop Relat Res* 101:186–291, 1974.
6. Gomez JG, Patino RM, Fonnegrap J: Lumbar discolysis with collagenase. *Neurolog Columbia* 355:362, 1979.
7. Nordby EJ, Brown MD: Present status of chymopapain and chemonucleolysis. *Clin Orthop Relat Res* 129:79–83, 1977.
8. Onofrio BM: Injection of chymopapain into intervertebral discs. *J Neurosurg* 42:384–388, 1975.
9. Popovic J, Tabor L, Cerk M: Nucleolysis by papain in intervertebral disc herniation. *Rheumatizam (Zagreb)* 22:16–20, 1975.
10. Ravichandran G, Mulholland RC: Chymopapain chemonucleolysis a preliminary report. *Spine* 5:380–384, 1980.
11. Schwetschenau RR, Ramirez A, Johnston J, et al: Double-blind evaluation of intradiscal chymopapain for herniated lumbar discs: Early results. *J Neurosurg* 45:622–627, 1976.
12. Smith L: Enzyme dissolution of the nucleus pulposus in humans. *JAMA* 187:137–140, 1964.
13. Smith L, Brown JE: Treatment of lumbar intervertebral disc lesions by direct injections of chymopapain. *J Bone Joint Surg* 49B:502–519, 1967.
14. Smith L, Garvin PJ, Gesler RM, et al: Enzyme dissolution of the nucleus pulposus. *Nature* 1981:1311–1312, 1963.
15. Stern EW, Coulson WF: Effects of collagenase upon the intervertebral disc in monkeys. *J Neurosurg* 44:32–44, 1976.
16. Stern IJ, Smith L: Dissolution by chymopapain in vitro tissue from normal or prolapsed intervertebral discs. *Clin Orthop Relat Res* 50:269–277, 1967.
17. Sussman BJ: Inadequacies and hazards of chymopapain injection as treatment for lumbar intervertebral disc disease. *J Neurosurg* 42:389–396, 1975.
18. Sussman BJ: Intervertebral discolysis with collagenase. *J Nat Med Assoc* 60:184–187, 1968.
19. Sussman BJ, Bromley JW, Gomez J: Injection of collagenase in the treatment of herniated lumbar disc. *JAMA* 245:730–732, 1981.
20. Sussman BJ, Mann M: Experimental intervertebral discolysis with collagenase. *J Neurosurg* 31:628–635, 1969.
21. Widdowson WL: Effects of chymopapain in the IV disc of the dog. *J Am Vet Med Assoc* 150:608, 1967.
22. Wiltse LL, Widell EH, Hausen AY: Chymopapain chemonucleolysis in lumbar disc disease. *JAMA* 231:474–479, 1975.
23. Mandl I, Zipper H, Ferguson LT: *Clostridium histolyticum* collagenase: Its purification and properties. *Arch Biochem Biophys* 74:465–475, 1958.
24. Lwebuga-Mukasa JS, Harper E, Taylor P: Collagenase enzymes for *Clostridium*: Characterization of individual enzymes. *Biochemistry* 15:4736–4741, 1976.
25. Goldberg B, Rabinovitch M: Connective tissue. In Weiss L, Greep RO: *Histology*. McGraw-Hill, New York, 1977, pp. 145–178.
26. Belanger LF: The skeletal tissues. In: Weiss L, Greep RO: *Histology*. McGraw-Hill, New York, 1977, pp. 145–178.

CHAPTER TWENTY-EIGHT

Computed Tomography of the Lumbar Facet Joints

GUILLERMO F. CARRERA, M.D.

INTRODUCTION

The lumbar facet joints are a well-recognized source of low back and radiating leg pain which can be confused with sciatica due to herniated disc (1–6). CT with high-resolution techniques can clearly demonstrate not only the soft-tissue structures of the spinal canal, but also can provide clear images of the lumbar facet joints (7–10). Pathological processes such as narrowing of the facet joint, subchondral sclerosis, articular erosions and subchondral cysts, osteophytes, and juxtaarticular calcification are evaluated much more easily using CT than conventional radiographic techniques (7, 8). The combination of high-resolution CT and intra-articular lumbar facet block form an effective method for diagnosis and evaluation of lumbar facet arthropathy in the patient with low back and leg pain (11–13).

CT TECHNIQUE

Numerous imaging protocols have been proposed for properly evaluating the neural arches and lumbar facet joints (8, 10, 14). There is uniform agreement that adequate CT studies should include contiguous or overlapping images through the lumbar facet joints and pars interarticularis. High-resolution techniques such as small field-of-view calibration or target-reconstruction algorithms should be used to minimize pixel size and improve spatial resolution.

The protocol in general use at the Medical College of Wisconsin was established for the General Electric CT/T 8800 scannner with a tilting gantry and large patient aperture. The patients were studied in the supine position, and a lateral localizer (ScoutView) image of the lumbar spine is obtained before transaxial study. A computer program is used to select appropriate gantry angles and table positions for transaxial CT images in, and adjacent to the plane of the intervertebral disc (Fig. 28.1). Contig-

uous 5-mm slices are obtained at each intervertebral level, 1 in the plane of the disc and 2 or 3 on either side. Using a 10-second scan time, 5-mm slice thickness, 25-cm field-of-view, 120 kV and 960–1152 mA provides contrast resolution of less than 0.5%, spatial resolution of 0.75 mm and a radiation dose of 4–6 Rads to the skin per examination. A wide window width (1000–4000 HU) and window level of 250–350 HU are optimal for studying the bony anatomy of the neural arch.

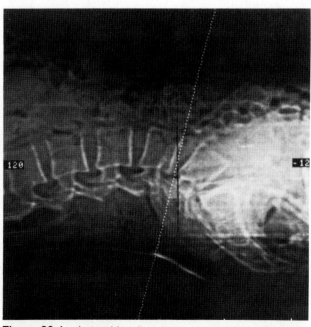

Figure 28.1. Lateral localizer image (computed radiograph) shows the level and gantry tilt used to obtain a transaxial image at mid-L4–5 disc level. This cut also passes through the L4–5 facet joints. [Reproduced with permission from Carrera et al (7).]

CLINICAL SIGNIFICANCE AND PATHOPHYSIOLOGY OF LUMBAR FACET SYNDROME

Numerous investigators have recognized that the lumbar facet joint can be a source of low back and sciatic pain which is similar to, or indistinguishable from the pain syndrome caused by herniated disc (1–5). The clinical differentiation of compressive neuropathy from referred pain due to lumbar facet arthropathy rests on several distinctions (4, 13). The pain of lumbar facet arthropathy clinically radiates to a myofascial sclerotomal rather than a cutaneous dermatomal distribution. The classical findings of motor weakness and reflex abnormalities found in herniated disc frequently are absent in lumbar facet syndrome. Despite these theoretic differences, however, the distinction between lumbar facet arthropathy and compressive neuropathy due to herniated disc remains frequently confusing and is one of the major challenges in diagnostic medicine today.

Some of the similarities in the pain syndromes of herniated disc and lumbar facet arthropathy can be understood by studying the anatomy and innervation of the lumbar facet joints (6, 15–17). The lumbar facets are paired, diarthrodial articulations between the superior articular facet of a lumbar segment and the inferior articular facet from the segment above. The joint surfaces are curved, and the plane of the joint surface is oriented between the sagittal and coronal plane (Fig. 28.2). The normal lumbar lordosis causes the plane of the lowest facet joints to tilt with respect to the coronal plane.

The lumbar facet capsule is formed in part, particularly anteriorly, by ligamentous structures including the ligamentum flavum. The lumbar facet capsule itself is spacious, and contains large fat pads in superior and inferior capsular recesses. The synovial membrane and underlying fat pad form prominent, richly vascularized and innervated villi which extend between the articulating cartilages in normal individuals (15).

The lumbar facet capsules as well as the underlying bony structures receive innervation from recurrent branches of the posterior primary ramus. A medial branch supplies the facet joint at its own level, and a lateral branch from each posterior primary ramus sends sensory innervation not only to the facet joint at its own level, but also to the joint one segment below (Fig. 28.3).

Because the sensory innervation of the lumbar facet joints is derived from an overlapping distribution of spinal nerve segments, pain originating in the facet joints may be referred along the distribution of the sclerotomes supplied by the spinal nerves in an overlapping pattern.

CT OF LUMBAR FACET ARTHROPATHY

The CT appearance of normal lumbar facet joints varies somewhat, depending on the width of the articular carti-

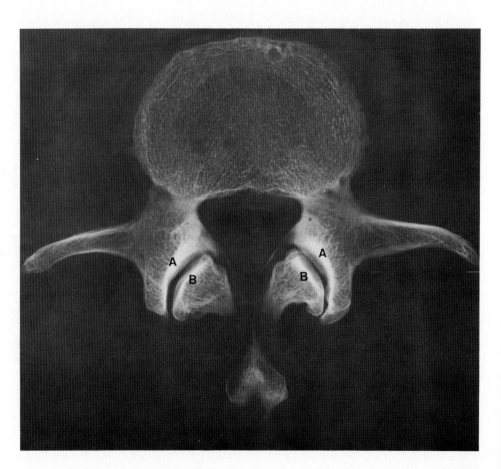

Figure 28.2. Specimen radiograph of a transaxial slice through the L4–5 lumbar facet joints. These joints are curved toward the midline. A. superior articular facet (L5); B. inferior articular facet (L4). [Reproduced with permission from Carrera (11).]

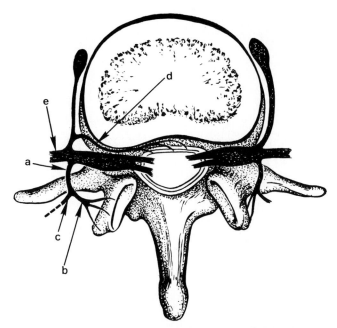

Figure 28.3. Diagrammatic representation of the sensory innervation of the lumbar facet joints and posterior anulus fibrosis. Pain fibers from the posterior primary ramus (a) and the sinuvertebral nerve (d) can refer pain to the distribution of the spinal nerve (e). a: posterior primary ramus, b: lateral branch supplying facet joints, c: medial branch descends to supply facet joint below, as well as sending small branches to the joint at the same level, d: sinuvertebral nerve which supplies pain fibers to the anulus fibrosis, e: spinal nerve.

lage (measured by computer program in normal volunteers as 2.5–4.0 mm), and the curvature of the joint. Normally the subchondral bone is uniform, with a sharp corticomedullary demarcation. The articular surfaces should be parallel (Fig. 28.4).

The most frequent CT findings in lumbar facet arthropathy are hypertrophy of one of the articular processes and osteophyte formation at the margins of the facet joints. The superior articular facet is the most common structure to hypertrophy in an abnormal joint, and is seen as an enlarged articular process which can deform the spinal canal or lateral recess (Fig. 28.5). Osteophytes appear on CT images just as they appear on conventional films, a uniformly dense bony excrescence which originates at the articular margin (Fig. 28.6).

Subchondral abnormalities characteristic of degenerative arthritis are important in the diagnosis of facet arthropathy by CT as they are in the diagnosis of degenerative arthritis on plain films. Subchondral sclerosis, cartilage narrowing, and erosions are important signs of degenerative abnormality of the lumbar facet joints (Figs. 28.6 and 28.7).

Juxta-articular calcification which can be identified in the joint capsule as well as in the ligamentum flavum is present with a surprisingly high frequency in patients with lumbar facet arthropathy (Fig. 28.8). These calcifications are found in patients who have no disorder of calcium metabolism or crystal deposition, and presumably represent a degenerative calcification which is better visualized using CT (with its high contrast sensitivity) than with plain films in the radicular skeleton.

In a series of 963 patients studied at the Milwaukee Regional Medical Center with CT scanning for low back pain or sciatica, 176 patients (18%) were identified with herniated disc, but 414 patients (43%) were identified with abnormal lumbar facet joints (Table 28.1). Little overlap was found in these populations.

CT scanning is a sensitive and accurate technique for demonstrating anatomical abnormality and lumbar facet arthropathy, but the presence of significant anatomical alteration in the lumbar facet joints in patients without back pain is well recognized (4, 5, 15). Because of this phenomenon, a more specific examination should be applied to patients suspected of having symptoms from abnormal lumbar facet joints as demonstrated by CT.

LUMBAR FACET INJECTION

Mooney and Robertson (13) used fluoroscopically guided intra-articular stimulation of the lumbar facet capsule, as well as intra-articular lumbar facet block in studying the pain pattern of lumbar facet syndrome as well as the potential role of steroid injection in treating patients with facet syndrome. Of a series of 110 patients studied with intra-articular lumbar facet block at the Milwaukee Regional Medical Center, 47 were examined with CT scanning before facet block (Table 28.2).

Following intra-articular placement of a 3½-inch, 22-gauge needle and facet arthrography, the lumbar facet joint is injected with a mixture of 15 mg of Depo-Methylprednisolone acetate suspension and 3 ml of 1% lidocaine solution in order to assess both the results of local anesthesia of the capsular innervation and the long-term effects of intra-articular corticosteroid administration (Figs. 28.9 and 28.10) (11, 18). Immediate relief of pain after anesthetic injection into the lumbar facet joint is considered diagnostically positive for facet syndrome, because such pain relief presumably results from anesthesia of the capsular and synovial nerves supplying a lumbar facet joint. Of the 39 patients with CT evidence for lumbar facet arthropathy who received facet block, 28 responded diagnostically to intra-articular local anesthetic injection, thus, confirming symptomatic lumbar facet arthropathy (Table 28.2).

Long-term relief after injection of intra-articular corticosteroids was found in 11 of these patients. This phenomenon presumably results from retraction of the adipose villi which can become traumatized by an abnormal lumbar facet joint (15). Patients who do not respond to intra-articular anesthesia and corticosteroid suspension presumably have pain either originating in structures other than the lumbar facet joints, or are experiencing the chronic bone pain of osteoarthritis which is not originating in a capsular sensory nerve supply.

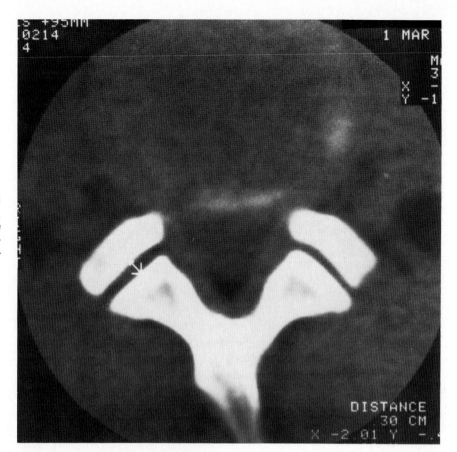

Figure 28.4. CT image through normal L4–5 facet joints shows sharply defined, intact, parallel articular surfaces. The spinal canal is undistorted by hypertrophic changes. [Reproduced with permission from Carrera et al. (7).]

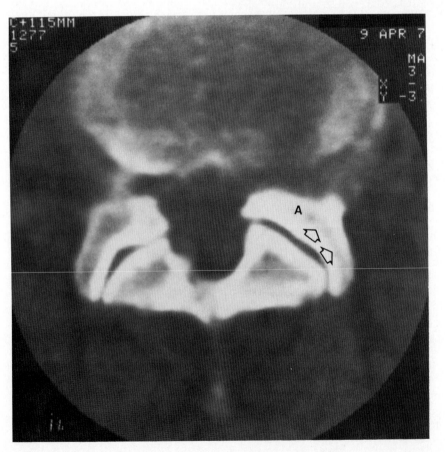

Figure 28.5. Hypertrophy of the left superior articular facet of L5 (A) causes distortion of the spinal canal. Corticomedullary discrimination is preserved (*arrows*). [Reproduced with permission from Carrera et al. (7).]

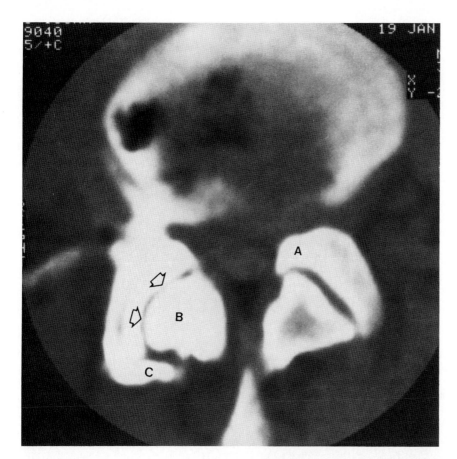

Figure 28.6. CT image through the L5-S1 facet joints shows asymmetric arthropathy. The left joint is normal except for a large anterior osteophyte (A) from the articular margin of the superior facet. The right joint is extensively diseased, with severe joint narrowing (*arrows*) and sclerosis of the inferior facet of L5 (B). A posterior osteophyte projects from the superior facet of S1 on the right (C). [Reproduced with permission from Carrera et al. (7).]

Figure 28.7. CT image through the L5-S1 facets of a postlaminectomy patient shows severe sclerosis and subchondral erosions (*arrows*) on the right. [Reproduced with permission from Carrera et al. (7).]

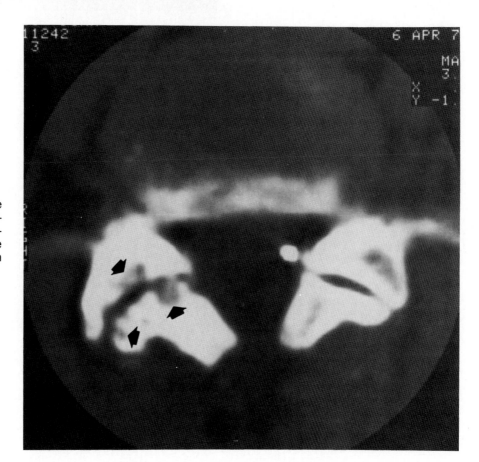

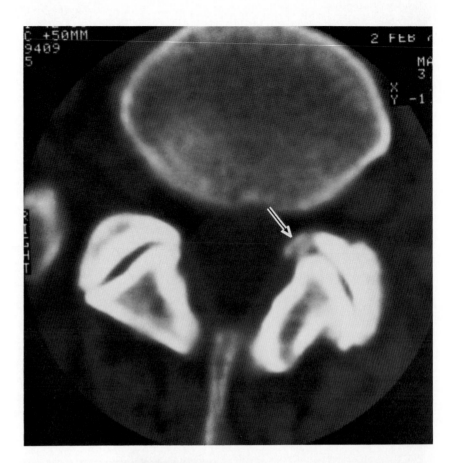

Figure 28.8. CT image through the L5-S1 facet joints shows a bilaminar juxta-articular calcification on the left. The anterior calcification (*arrow*) is the ligamentum flavum, the posterior is the joint capsule. [Reproduced with permission from Carrera et al. (7).]

Table 28.1.
CT Findings in 963 Patients Studied for Low Back Pain/Sciatica

Total number of patients	963
Lumbar facet arthropathy	414 (43%)
Herniated disc	176 (18%)

Table 28.2.
CT/Facet Block Correlation in 47 Patients

	Facet Block	
	Positive	Negative
CT		
Positive	28	11
Negative	1*	7

* This patient had well-documented abnormal psychological testing and was involved in compensation litigation. He reported 1 day of relief after facet block, then return of his full symptom complex.

SUMMARY

The complex anatomy and pathophysiology of the lumbar facet joints makes clinical and conventional radiographic study of lumbar facet syndrome difficult. Precise anatomical delineation of degenerative and arthritic changes in the lumbar facet joints now can be accom-

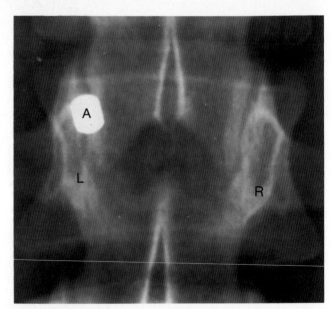

Figure 28.9. Fluoroscopic spot film obtained with the patient prone shows the hub of a 3½-inch needle (A) which has been inserted vertically into the left L4–5 facet joints.

plished using high-resolution CT. Facet joints with significant anatomical abnormalities are at risk for causing trauma to richly innervated adipose villi which extend

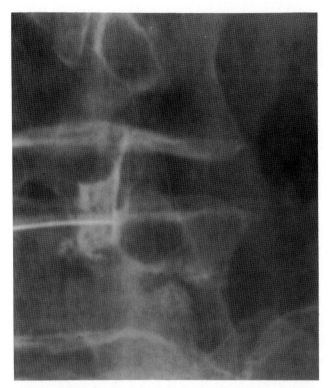

Figure 28.10. Fluoroscopic spot film after injection of 0.5 ml Reno-M-60^R into the right L4–5 facet joint. This technique assures intra-articular position of the needle tip before facet block. [Reproduced with permission from Carrera (11).]

into the facet articulation. Some patients, however, may have extensive abnormalities anatomically demonstrable by CT but have pain originating in other sources. For this reason, definition of a patient population at risk for facet syndrome by means of CT is an important first step in the diagnosis of low back pain in these patients. After the CT demonstration of facet arthropathy, selective intra-articular lumbar facet block can provide a safe and reliable means for establishing the diagnosis of facet syndrome. Patients with facet syndrome who do not respond with long-term relief to intra-articular steroid injection remain a difficult clinical problem. Numerous possibilities for treating these patients, ranging from medication to aggressive surgery must be considered after the initial step of accurate diagnosis (3, 4, 13, 19).

References

1. Badgley CE: Articular facets in relation to low back pain and sciatic-radiation. *J Bone Joint Surg* 23:481–496, 1941.
2. Brown HA: Enlargement of the ligamentum flavum—a cause of low back pain with sciatic radiation. *J Bone Joint Surg* 20:325, 1938.
3. Ghormley RK: Low back pain with special reference to the articular facets, with presentation of an operative procedure. *JAMA* 101:1773–1777, 1933.
4. Inman VT, Saunders JBDM: The clinico-anatomical aspects of the lumbosacral region. *Radiology* 38:669–678, 1942.
5. Oppenheimer A: Diseases of the apophyseal (intervertebral) articulations. *J Bone Joint Surg* 20:285–313, 1938.
6. Pedersen HE, Blunck CFJ, Gardener E: Anatomy of lumbosacral posterior rami and meningeal branches of spinal nerves (sinu-vertebral nerves) with experimental study of their function. *J Bone Joint Surg* 38A:377–391, 1956.
7. Carrera GF, Haughton VM, Syvertsen A, et al: Computed tomography of the lumbar facet joints. *Radiology* 134:145, 1980.
8. Carrera GF, Williams AL, Haughton VM: Computed tomography in sciatica. *Radiology* 137:433, 1980.
9. Lee BCV, Kazam E, Newman AD: Computed tomography of the spine and spinal cord. *Radiology* 128:95, 1978.
10. Williams AL, Haughton VM, Syvertsen A: Computed tomography in the diagnosis of herniated nucleus pulposus. *Radiology* 135:95, 1980.
11. Carrera GF: Lumbar facet joint injection: Low back pain and sciatic (I) and (II). *Radiology* 137:661–667, 1980.
12. Carrera GF: Lumbar facet arthrography and injection in low back pain. *Wisc Med J* (Symposium on Low Back Pain) 78:35–37, 1979.
13. Mooney V, Robertson J: The facet syndrome. *Clin Orthop Relat Res* 115:149–156, 1976.
14. Genant HK: Computed tomography of the lumbar spine: Technical considerations. In Genant KH, Chafety H, Helms CA: *Computed Tomography of the Lumbar Spine.* Univ. of Calif. Press, 1982, pp. 23–52.
15. Hadley LA: Anatomico-roentgenographic studies of the posterior spinal articulations. *AJR* 86:270–276, 1961.
16. Lewin T, Moffett B, Viidik A: Morphology of the lumbar synovial intervertebral joints. *Acta Morphol Neurol Scand* 4:299–319, 1962.
17. Stillwell DL Jr: Nerve supply of vertebral column and its associated structures in the monkey. *Anat Res* 125:139–169, 1956.
18. Ghelman B, Doherty JH: Demonstration of spondylolysis by arthrography of the apophyseal joint. *AJR* 130:986–987, 1978.
19. Williams PC, Yglesias L: Lumbosacral facetectomy for post-fusion persistent sciatica. *J Bone Joint Surg* 15:579–590, 1933.

CHAPTER TWENTY-NINE

Computed Tomographic Guided Anesthesia and Steroid Injection in the Facet Syndrome

F. REED MURTAGH, M.D.

Local anesthesia and steroid injection of facet joint complexes as a diagnostic maneuver and as a treatment for facet syndrome is well established (1–4). The facet complexes were first recognized by Ghormley (5) as a possible site of origin of pain in specific syndromes since 1933. Since then the facet complex has been ignored largely by the medical community in favor of herniated disc or spondylolisthesis, with most research and treatment directed toward these entities. However, with the ready availability of imaging in the axial plane which has come with the advent of CT, the role of facet disease in the overall picture of low back pain has been amplified (4). Indeed, other authors (5, 7) have suggested that in addition to pain related to the facet joints, pain which has its origin in the myofacial regions of the posterior compartment of the back such as the joint capsules, ligaments, and muscles of the multifidous group and others might be considered causative in the overall picture of "posterior compartment pain syndrome." For the most part, however, facet disease continues to be the focus of attention in these syndromes.

Pain originating in the facet complexes may have a characteristic clinical presentation with the patient complaining of difficulty maintaining one position such as sitting for long periods of time and pain increased with certain positions of the back such as reaching and stretching and leaning to one side or the other. In addition, people who are suffering from the facet syndrome very often have direct tenderness to digital palpation over the affected facets in the deep areas of the back.

A needle placed in the facet joint from the dorsal aspect can be used to deliver xylocaine into the synovial-lined joint capsule and if pain is originating in this complex the patient usually experiences immediate relief. This serves as a diagnostic maneuver isolating the pain by attributing it to this portion of the anatomy. If the xylocaine is then followed with steroids (such as betamethasone preparation), then the patient may be expected to achieve extended relief. The needle placement can be performed under fluoroscopic guidance; however, with the advent of CT, the image produced in the axial plane is ideally suited to the placement of a needle tip directly into the dorsal aspect of the facet joint (Fig. 29.1). This is especially true in cases where there is a great deal of osteophytic overgrowth of the facet joints in which case the dorsal opening into the facet joint may come to lie very medially and actually may be sheltered from the dorsal aspect by a large osteophytic spur arising from the inferior facet at that level and extending into the deep muscles of the back.

At our institution, we studied 38 patients who met the criteria noted above with respect to the clinical presentation of possible facet syndrome. All patients had had plain lumbar spine films, CT scan, and myelography before the attempted facet injection and results varied from completely negative studies to frankly herniated discs. In the cases with herniated discs, there was some component of the patient's pain syndrome which suggested that the pain might be due to the facet compartment rather than to the clearly herniated disc seen on the studies. The 38 patients underwent 140 separate injections into the facet joints of the lumbar spine. All of these patients were selected because of point tenderness and it is interesting that all of the patients using this selection technique in our group had a positive response to facet injection; that is, they had immediate and complete relief of pain after the injection of xylocaine. In some cases, more than one facet complex needed to be injected; in several cases an injection in one joint which was tender tended to unmask another joint which was also tender which was then injected. Other cases had multiple areas of tenderness initially which were obliterated completely by injection into a single joint. These probably represented patients who had recruitment phenomena of pain due to extensive neural connections of the lumbar spine.

The xylocaine injected was usually in the amount of 1–1.5 cc of 2% xylocaine which was always sufficient to produce the results we were seeking. In each case when pain was obliterated and the diagnosis made by injection, the patient was then injected through the same needle with 1–1.5 cc of betamethasone in the preparation Celestone. We then attained follow-up on these patients using established criteria in which long-term relief was defined as relief lasting more than 3 months. It was found that more than 62% of these patients with 140 injections produced long-term relief (87 injections).

Good evidence exists that the facet joint can be a source of pain (1–14). The facet joint is primarily a diarthrodial joint with synovial lining and, therefore, predisposed to degenerative changes and osteophyte formation with overgrowth of bone. If osteophytosis takes place in the side facing the spinal canal the syndromes of lateral recess encroachment or canal stenosis may result. Severe degenerative changes in any joint may themselves be a source of pain since synovium is richly innervated tissue and degenerative changes in the bone directly affect the synovial lining. The synovial lining of the joint capsule of the facet is supplied by a dorsal primary ramus nerve which arises near the dorsal root ganglion of the sensory

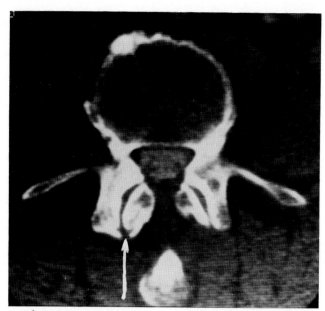

Figure 29.1. CT slice of the lumbar spine with isotonic metrizamide in the thecal sac. The facet joint on the patient's right is much more osteophytic and overgrown than that on the left. A *white line* indicates the angle one must take to enter this joint. Angling the tip more laterally from a more medial approach could also help.

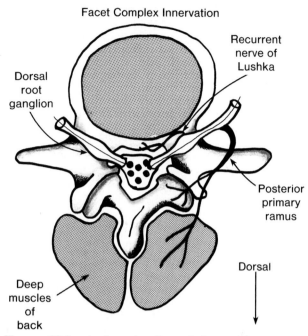

Facet Complex Innervation

Figure 29.2. A line drawing of facet joint anatomy demonstrates an idealized course of the posterior primary ramus branch of the dorsal root.

nerve of the adjacent vertebral body (Fig. 29.2). These dorsal primary rami are known sometimes to supply adjacent facet joints at the level of their emergence. Dorsal primary rami are not known to innervate a contralateral facet joint.

Injection of facet joints with xylocaine was performed originally as a diagnostic procedure before attempts to sever the dorsal primary ramus by direct knife insertion (6). Knife insertion tended to create complications such as large hematomas and has since proven to be anatomically unsound. Radiofrequency lysis efforts with concurrent denudation of the joint capsule and percutaneous approach was shown to produce good results and came into vogue in the late 1960s (7, 8). While preparing patients to have a radiofrequency lysis of the joint capsule, several authors found that direct injections of steroids into the facet joint, much in the same manner that a painful knee or shoulder joint is injected, often produced long-term relief which could not be explained adequately other than on the basis of improvement of inflammatory change of the synovium by contact with steroids. It is, therefore, believed that after a specific diagnosis of pain arising in the facet joint is obtained after xylocaine injection, a trial of steroid injection into the joint is warranted on the well-established grounds that it may relieve the inflammatory changes in the joint and allow the joint to return to normal physiological status. The patient must have a concurrent program of exercise to help the joint return to anatomic normalcy as well.

Destouet et al. (1) in 1981 injected 50 patients all of whom were unselected as to direct tenderness and

achieved a 60% long-term relief, using the same definition of long-term relief that we used (over 3 months). Carrera and associates (2–4) in 1980 injected 20 unselected patients, 13 of whom had short-term relief and 6 had long-term relief described as being over 6 months. Other authors (12–14) have obtained similar results. Criteria varied in these series, some of the patients had pain on straight leg raising as well as other neurologica symptoms which were thought to be relieved possibly by the xylocaine and steroid injections.

In none of the case series is there any mention of selecting the patients with reference to direct tenderness of the lumbar spine to direct our attention to which joints need injection. The usefulness of facet injection in positive straight leg raising has been attributed to the fact that inflammation from the facet complexes sometimes can spread through the myofacial areas and involve several localized nearby nerve roots, perhaps through recruiting phenomena. This, in turn, may cause positive straight leg raising or irritation of the sciatic nerve.

It is believed that the most important physical factor on examination in selecting the patients for possible facet injections is the presence of tenderness in the dorsal compartment of the lumbar spine. This is reflected in our finding that every 1 of our 38 patients when injected in the 140 sites had immediate relief of pain. It should be noted, however, that the long-term pain relief remains the same (62%) as other authors have experienced not using direct tenderness as a selection technique. Early in our trial, 5 patients who did not have direct tenderness localized in the spine but had diffuse low back pain were injected in facet joints which appeared to be somewhat degenerative. These patients did not have relief of pain and so were not included in our study and support our feeling that patients without direct tenderness in the spine would not benefit from this technique. This raises another interesting finding in that the appearance of the facet joints under fluoroscopy or CT did not necessarily correlate with the fact that the specific joint was a cause of pain. Many joints which appeared extensively osteophytic and degenerative were not tender and many joints which looked perfectly normal were tender and did benefit from the facet injection. It appears at this time that the state of degenerative disease in a facet complex does not necessarily correlate with the facet syndrome although 93% (120/130) of the painful facet complexes did have some degenerative osteoarthric changes on CT.

Follow-up in our series was from 3 weeks to 11 months total. As noted, 62% of the injections performed provided relief over 3 months. Several patients who had reinjections reported that they received initial relief from the xylocaine injection which lasted only a few weeks. Other patients who had reinjections had complete relief in their original pain site only to have delayed "unmasking" of pain in other sites nearby after several weeks. At least 1 patient has had three separate injections at the same areas of pain; each time the injection gave relief for 3–4 months but then recurred. One must begin to question what the long-term effects of steroids in a facet joint are and whether the repeated injection of steroid should be contraindicated on the grounds that it might cause some degenerative changes of its own in the synovium and associated bony structures. Once a diagnosis of facet syndrome is made, possible surgical approaches might include fusion across that joint or permanent radiofrequency lysis of the nerve endings.

References

1. Destouet JM, Gilula LA, Murphy WA, et al: Lumbar facet injection indications, technique, and pathological correlation. *Radiology* 145:321–325, 1982.
2. Carrera GF: Lumbar facet joint injection in low back pain and sciatica: Technique. *Radiology* 137:661–664, 1980.
3. Carrera GF: Lumbar facet joint injection in low back pain and sciatica: Preliminary results. *Radiology* 137:665–667, 1980.
4. Carrera GF, Williams FA, Haughton VM: Computed tomography in sciatica. *Radiology* 137:433–437, 1980.
5. Mooney V, Robertson J: The facet syndrome. *Clin Orthop Relat Res* 115:149–156, 1976.
6. Shealy CN: Facet denervation in the management of back and sciatic pain. *Clin Orthop Relat Res* 115:157–164, 1976.
7. King JS, Lagger R: Sciatica viewed as a referred pain syndrome. *Surg Neurol* 5:46–50, 1982.
8. Ogsbury JS, Simon RH, Lehman RA: Facet denervation in the treatment of low back syndrome. *Pain* 3:257–763, 1977.
9. Mehta N, Sluijter ME: The treatment of chronic back pain—a preliminary survey of radiofrequency denervation of the posterior vertebral joints. *Anesthesia* 34:768–775, 1979.
10. Pantabi MM, Goel VK, Takata K: Physiologic strains in the lumbar spinal ligaments. *Spine* 7:192–203, 1982.
11. Dory MA: Arthrography of the lumber facet joints. *Radiology* 140:23–27, 1981.
12. Maldague B, Mathurin P, Malohem J: Facet joint arthrography in lumbar spondylosis. *Radiology* 140:29–36, 1981.
13. Epstein BS: *The Spine: a Radiographic Text and Atlas.* 4th ed. Lee and Febiger, Philadelphia, 1976, pp. 417–418.
14. Grieve GP: *Common Vertebrae Joint Problems.* Churchill, Livingstone, New York, 1981, pp. 82–124.

CHAPTER THIRTY

The Orientation and Shape of the Lower Lumbar Facet Joints: A Computed Tomographic Study of Their Variation in 100 Patients with Low Back Pain and a Discussion of Their Possible Clinical Implications

JAN P. J. van SCHAIK, M.D., HENK VERBIEST, M.D., Ph.D., and FRANS D. J. van SCHAIK, M.A.*

INTRODUCTION

The facet joints are parts of the spinal motion segments. The term spinal motion segment is the Anglo-American translation of the German and Latin expressions: Bewegungssegment, or segmentum mobilitatis, introduced by Junghanns to indicate the unit of mobility of the spine (1). In his definition, the Bewegungssegment is formed by all connections between two bony vertebrae: disc, ligaments, joint capsules, and spinal muscles. Therefore, in Junghanns' view, the Bewegungssegment consists of both a purely mechanical portion whose functions are determined only by the physical properties of its constituents, and a physiological or dynamic portion: the muscles. Regarding the latter, Junghanns' definition is vague. It is, indeed, no easy matter to identify the muscles of the Bewegungssegment, because there are spinal muscles bridging more than one Bewegungssegment, muscles which have their origin on the processes of the spine and their insertion on other bones of the skeleton, and muscles having their origin and insertion on other than the vertebral bones, but producing spinal movements indirectly. Only the intertransversarii and interspinales muscles are limited to one motion segment, but their part is of minor importance in the functional integration of muscular activity in spinal movement.

For the reasons mentioned above, it seems preferable to limit the definition of the motion segment to the mechanical part of Junghanns' Bewegungssegment. The motion segment usually is not considered a joint itself, though it represents the union between two bones. It is stated, instead, that it contains three joints, the amphiarthrosis between the vertebral bodies, and two posterior diarthrodial or facet joints. Yet these joints are connected between

each other by the quasirigid bony structures, so that the motion in each of the three joints is track-bound (2). This implies that the instantaneous axis of rotation of the posterior joints is extra-articular, localized, with healthy motion segments, in the vicinity of, or inside the intervertebral disc.

White and Panjabi (3) call the motion segment the functional spinal unit which is the smallest segment of the spine that exhibits biomechanical characteristics similar to those of the entire spine. It is generally accepted that the motion segments have six degrees of freedom of motion. The term degree of freedom of motion was introduced by Steindler for describing joint function. Therefore, the use of this term for the movements in the motion segment implies a sort of recognition of its joint like function as a whole. The six degrees of freedom of motion of the motion segments are three rotations around and three translations along the three axes of the coordinate system. Having six degrees of freedom of motion means having the maximal possibility of joint movement. Therefore, the motion segment can be defined as a so-called universal joint. The movements in the motion segment are described relative to the subjacent vertebra.

It is in studies limited to the kinematics of the single motion segments in health and disease that attention is focussed on the function of its three track-bound joints. The ranges of motion in the motion segments greatly depend on the differences in orientation and shape of the facet joints in the various areas of the spinal column.

The only purely rotatory movement in the motion segment is flexion/extension. Each of the other rotatory movements is combined with motion about a second axis. These combined motions are indicated by the word "coupling." Of all ranges of motions, the rotatory are the most precisely known. They are expressed in degrees. As this study is limited to the facet joints L4-L5 and L5-S1, the data about the ranges of rotation at these levels, published by White and Panjabi (3) and Farfan (4) are:

* The authors want to thank Ingrid Janssen, Utrecht University Hospital, for preparing the graphs, and Mr. F. J. van Waert, medical photographer of the Pediatric University Hospital, for the photographic work.

	Flexion/ extension		Lateral bend (side to side)	Rotation (around longitudinal axis)
L4-L5	17°(3)	22°(4)	6°(3)	2°(3)
L5-S1	20°(3)	18°(4)	3°(3)	5°(3)

This simplified introduction to the biomechanics of the motion segments forms the background of our CT studies of the lower lumbar facet joints. They are aimed at an evaluation of the possible contribution of this diagnostic aid to the understanding of normal and pathological biomechanics of the lower lumbar spine. This initial publication deals with the following two topics:

The Orientation and Shape of the Lower Lumbar Facet Joints in the Axial Plane

Studies published so far on the orientation of the facet joints were based on findings on plain PA and oblique radiographs of the spine, in cadaver studies or during operation (Fig. 30.1). CT provides a superior means of visualizing the orientation and shape of the facet joints (5), and may provide references for mechanical studies on rotation of the lower lumbar motion segments around the longitudinal (Y−) axis. To this purpose, standard methods of measuring orientation and shape of the facet joints are described.

Asymmetry of the Facet Joints

This phenomenon occurs rather frequently, in 25% of Farfan's series of the three lower lumbar interspaces, and in 32% of Brailsford's cases (6, 7). Farfan stated that people with backache show a significantly higher incidence of facet asymmetry. In his experience, there was also a high degree of correlation between the side of sciatica and disc protrusion with the side with the most oblique facet. The validity of this statement has been checked in our series.

The data obtained so far in 100 patients suffering from low back problems were fed into a computer and the results are presented in the form of statistical judgments.

SELECTION OF PATIENTS

This study is not representative from an epidemiological point of view as it is not a sampling of ordinary human variation. For obvious reasons, CT scanning has not been performed in asymptomatic individuals. It is, instead, a collection of 100 patients suffering from backache and/or sciatica. This collection does not include:

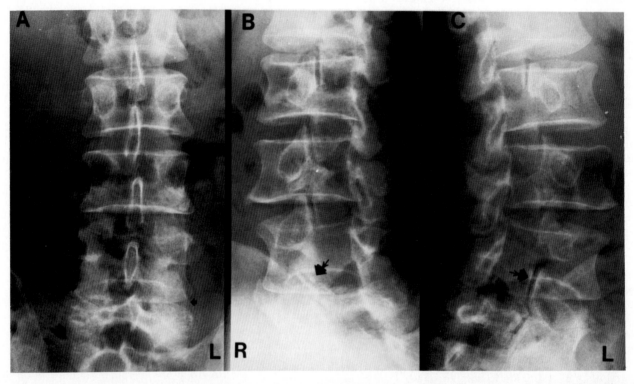

Figure 30.1. Information on orientation and shape of facet joints that can be obtained by means of plain radiographs. A. Anteroposterior view shows right-sided articulation between the tip of the transverse process of L5 and the adjacent sacrum and iliac bone. Spondylolysis is suggested in C. The AP view shows no evidence of asymmetric angulation of the facet joints of L4-L5 (*arrows*), as is demonstrated on the CT scan of the same patient (Fig. 30.5A). The oblique views B and C show the difficulty usually encountered in obtaining perfectly symmetric oblique views. There is asymmetry between the slope of the right (B) and left (C) facet joints of L4-L5 (*arrows*). The joint space is cut tangentially in C, but not in B, which may depend partly upon the difference in the incidence of the central ray. Yet it is obvious that the oblique views, apart from problems in symmetric positioning of the patient, do not allow an estimation of the angulation of the facet joints in the axial plane, and therefore, exclude any possibility of quantification.

1. Patients who previously had been treated by means of a posterior approach to the lumbar spine because of the possibility of surgically induced changes of the facet joints.

2. Asymmetric CT scans because of malposition of the patient, or abnormal curvature of his spine.

3. Patients presenting with asymmetric neural arches because of unequal length of the pedicles, although they may be subject to later studies.

4. Patients presenting with pronounced arthritic deformities of the facet joints.

EQUIPMENT

Two high-resolution general purpose CT scanners were used, the Philips Tomoscan 300 and 310. Field-of-view (FOV) was 160 (=160 × 160 mm²), in some of the patients enlarged by zoom reconstruction to 120. Slice thickness was 3 mm, and table incrementation 4.5 mm, so the intervals between the sections were 1.5 mm. The scan plane was chosen perpendicular to the longitudinal (Y−) axis of the spinal canal by means of the scanogram (lateral localizer view). The resulting sections are shown in Figure 30.2.

METHODS OF MEASUREMENT

The symmetry of the axial sections was ascertained in the sections through the transverse processes and pedicles of the vertebrae above and below the transarticular section. The transarticular sections through the middle portions of the facet joints were chosen for measurement because they visualized most clearly the orientation and

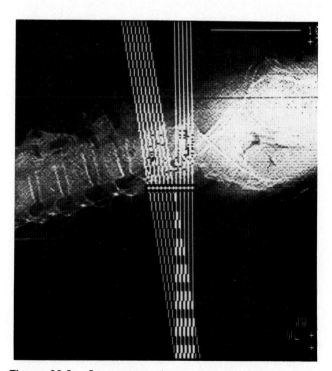

Figure 30.2. Scanogram shows the angulation of the planes of CT sections at the L4-L5 and L5-S1 levels.

shape of these joints. Anteriorly, the transarticular sections passed through the disc space or through the area of the upper end plate of the vertebral body below (Fig. 30.3A). For more accurate measurement, the CT images were magnified and printed in the reversed mode (Fig. 30.3B). All CT images were printed at a window level of 200 HU and a window width of 1000 HU. A comparative study of orientation and shape of the facet joints requires the use of uniform reference lines.

Definitions

1. The *orientation* of the facet joints in the axial plane has been defined by the angle between the following two lines: line f.l. (facet line) connects the anteromedial and posterolateral margin of the superior articular facet. This means that the orientation of the superior facet is measured, rather than that of the facet joint as a whole. Line c.i.l. (central interfacet line) is drawn between the central points of the right and left f.l. lines. The orientation is, in this paper, expressed in degrees of angulation between the lines f.l. and c.i.l. on the right and left sides, respectively (Fig. 30.3B).

The question of whether line c.i.l. parallels the frontal plane through the vertebrae cannot be answered exactly. The great variation in shape and the frequent occurrence of minor or more significant asymmetries of the vertebral bodies impede the placement of constant reference points needed for the exact determination of the frontal plane through these bodies. For this reason, such frontal planes were not used for measuring the degree of orientation of the superior facets, since the line c.i.l. allows more accurate comparative measurement. Yet we got, with the exclusion of CT scans mentioned in the section on patient selection, the visual impression that line c.i.l. paralleled more or less the posterior border of the corresponding vertebral bodies.

2. For measuring the *shape* of the facets in the axial plane it was not practical to quantify the entire curvature. Instead we used as a first step a curvation index, which gives some expression of the shape. For determining the curvation index, a line was drawn from the point of maximal curvature of the facet perpendicular to line f.l. This line is called c.d. (curvation depth) (Fig. 30.3C).

The curvation index is $\frac{c.d.}{f.l.} \times 100$.

It should be noted that the point of maximal curvature does not always coincide with the center of the facet surface.

An iconography of examples of variation in angulation and curvation, as well as of symmetry and asymmetry of the facet joints as visualized by means of CT is presented in Figures 30.4–30.7.

Measurements of angulation (orientation) and curvation index (shape) were made at the levels L4-L5 and L5-S1 in all patients. The resulting data were analyzed statistically. Correlations between the measured parameters were calculated with the Spearman rank-order correlation test; the linear regressions were calculated by the least-squares method. Statistical significance in differences of measure-

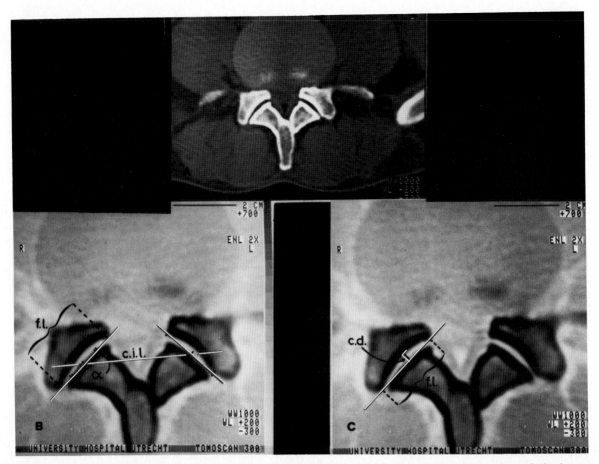

Figure 30.3. A. CT section through the middle portion of the facet joints L4-L5. The section passes through the intervertebral disc anteriorly. B. Same section, magnified and printed in the reversed mode. The angulation (orientation) α of the superior facet of L5 in the axial plane is determined by the angle between the lines *f.l.* and *c.i.l.* (see text). C. Same section. Lines *c.d.* and *f.l.* are used for determination of curvation index (see text).

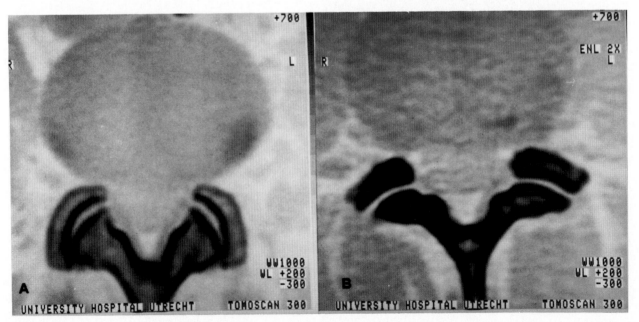

Figure 30.4. A and B. Symmetric angulation of the facet joints of L4-L5. The orientation of the facet joints in A is close to the sagittal plane, and in B close to the frontal plane.

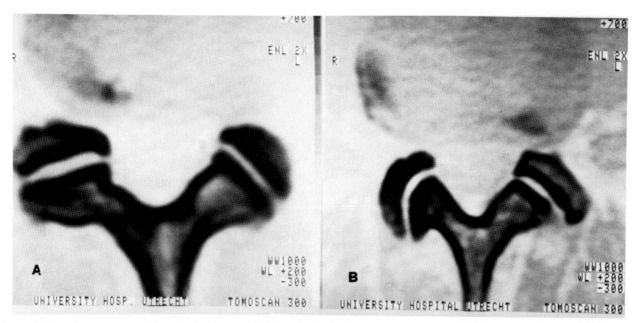

Figure 30.5. Asymmetry of the facet joints of L4-L5. A. Right facet joint oriented close to the frontal plane, left facet intermediate between frontal and sagittal plane (same patient as in Fig. 30.1). B. Right facet oriented close to the sagittal plane, left facet intermediate orientation.

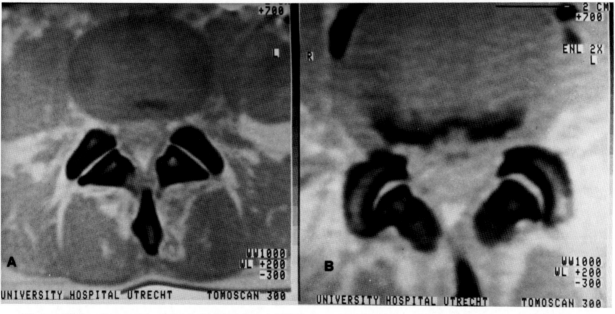

Figure 30.6. Symmetric shape of facet joints L4-L5 in A and B. Curvation almost absent in A, and marked in B.

ments was calculated by the Student's *t*-test.

The term orientation of the facets was replaced by angulation, expressed in degrees of the angles between the lines f.l. and c.i.l. as described above.

RESULTS

The values of angulation and curvation index of the superior articular facets L5 and S1 are shown in Table 30.1. The correlation coefficients between the various parameters are shown in Table 30.2.

Superior Articular Facets L5

ANGULATION

The angulation of the superior articular facet L5 (mean ± SD) is 39.1° ± 9.8° on the left side and 42.9° ± 9.5° on the right side. The frequency distributions are shown in Figure 30.8. The range of observed values are 19–71° on

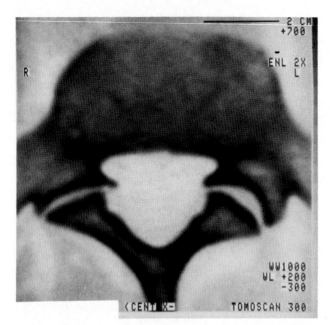

Figure 30.7. Asymmetric curvation of the superior facets of S1. Note the small osteophyte at the anteromedial edge of the right superior facet.

Table 30.1.
Angulation and Curvation Index of the Lower Lumbar Facet Joints[a]

	Angulation (mean ± SD)[b]	Curvation index (mean ± SD)[c]
Left sup. art. facet L5	39.1° ± 9.8°	15.4 ± 6.4
Right sup. art. facet L5	42.9° ± 9.5°	16.8 ± 6.2
Difference between left and right sup. art. facet L5	−3.8° ± 8.3° p ≤ 0.001	−1.4 ± 6.2 p ≤ 0.01
Left sup. art. facet S1	34.3° ± 9.2°	11.9 ± 6.4
Right sup. art. facet S1	36.4° ± 8.9°	12.1 ± 5.9
Difference between left and right sup. art. facet S1	−2.1° ± 7.8° p ≤ 0.001	−0.1 ± 5.9 NS
Difference between left sup. art. facets L5 and S1	4.8° ± 10.3° p ≤ 0.001	3.5 ± 8.1 p ≤ 0.001
Difference between right sup. art. facets L5 and S1	6.5° ± 9.9° p ≤ 0.001	4.8 ± 8.5 p ≤ 0.001

[a] Abbreviations used: SD = standard deviation; p = significance of the differences (paired Student's t-test); NS = not significant.
[b] Negative values in the middle column (angulation) indicate that the right facet is more sagittally oriented than the left.
[c] Negative values in the right column (curvation index) indicate that the right facet is more curved than the left.

the left and 15–72° on the right.

A striking feature is the significant difference in the mean values of angulation between left and right side of −3.8° ± 8.3° (p ≤ 0.001), the minus sign before the mean value signifying a greater occurrence of a sagittal orientation with the right facet L5 than with the left facet L5. The number of patients with a more sagittally oriented right or left facet were 68 and 28, respectively. The frequency distribution of the differences is shown in Figure 30.9. Maximal values are −28° and +25°, which means a marked asymmetry of the facet joints in these cases. Again, the minus sign indicates a more sagittal orientation of the right facet. Examples of marked asymmetry are shown in Figure 30.5.

Another interesting point is the correlation of angulations between left and right superior facets in each of the patients. These values are plotted in Figure 30.10, showing a significant positive correlation (r = 0.60, p ≤ 0.001). The extreme values in the diagram relate to the patients with a marked asymmetry.

CURVATION INDEX

The mean curvation indices of the superior facets L5 are 15.4 ± 6.4 on the left and 16.8 ± 6.2 on the right. The ranges of observed values of the curvation indices are 5–35 and 1–33, respectively. The frequency distributions are shown in Figure 30.11. The mean difference between left and right side is −1.4 ± 6.2 (p ≤ 0.01), the minus sign before the mean value signifying that the right facet is generally more curved than the left. The range of observed differences is −17 through +16. The correlation coefficient between left and right curvation indices is 0.50, being highly significant (p ≤ 0.001).

CORRELATIONS BETWEEN ANGULATION AND CURVATION INDEX

An interesting positive correlation was found between the angulation and the curvation index. The correlation coefficient is 0.57 on the left side (see plot diagram in Fig. 30.12), and 0.46 on the right side (no plot diagram given because this provides no important additional information). Both correlations are significant (p ≤ 0.001). The practical conclusion is that, in general, it can be stated that the greater the facet angle is, the more curved its joint surface. The higher mean curvation index of the right facets corresponds with their greater mean angulation.

Superior Articular Facets S1

ANGULATION

The angulation of the superior articular facets S1 (mean ± SD) is 34.3° ± 9.2° on the left side and 36.4° ± 8.9° on the right side. The frequency distributions are shown in Figure 30.13. The ranges of observed values are 10–60° on the left and 15–57° on the right.

Although less pronounced than at the level L5 there is also a significant difference in the mean values of angulation between left and right side, namely −2.1° ± 7.8° (p ≤ 0.001). As in angulation of superior articular facets L5, these values show that a sagittal orientation occurred

Table 30.2.
Some of the Correlation Coefficients between the Various Parameters[a]

Parameters	Correlation r	Significance p≤
Superior facets L5:		
left an—right an	0.60	0.001
left an—left ci	0.57	0.001
right an—right ci	0.46	0.001
left ci—right ci	0.50	0.001
Superior facets S1:		
left an—right an	0.58	0.001
left an—left ci	0.37	0.001
right an—right ci	0.43	0.001
left ci—right ci	0.49	0.001
Correlations between L5 and S1:		
left an L5—left an S1	0.39	0.001
right an L5—right an S1	0.40	0.001
left ci L5–left ci S1	0.26	0.005
right ci L5—right ci S1	0.05	0.304 (NS)

[a] Abbreviations used: r = correlation coefficient according to Spearman; p = significance; an = angulation; ci = curvation index; NS = not significant.

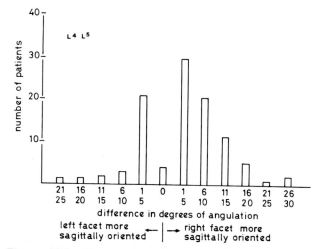

Figure 30.9.   Frequency distribution of the differences between left and right superior articular facet angulation L5. Patients with a more sagittally oriented left facet L5 are presented on the left side of the histogram, patients with a more sagittally oriented right facet L5 on the right. In the text, the latter group is indicated with a minus sign. Compare to Figure 30.14.

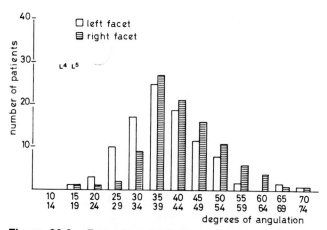

Figure 30.8.   Frequency distribution of degrees of angulation of the left and right superior articular facet L5. Compare to Figure 30.13.

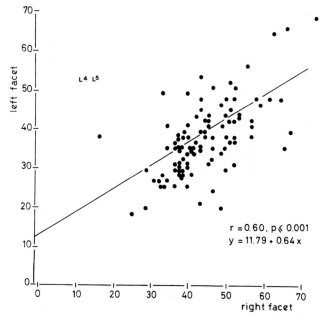

Figure 30.10.   Correlation between the degrees of angulation of the left and right superior articular facets L5. Compare to Figure 30.15.

more frequently with the right facet than with the left facet. The numbers of patients with a more sagittally oriented left or right facet were 37 and 54, respectively. The frequency distribution of the differences is shown in Figure 30.14. Maximal values are −23° and +20° (the significance of the minus sign is already discussed).

The correlation of angulations between left and right superior facets in each of the patients is presented in Figure 30.15, showing a significant positive correlation (r = 0.58, p ≤ 0.001).

CURVATION INDEX

The mean curvation indices of the superior facets S1 are 11.9 ± 6.4 on the left and 12.1 ± 5.9 on the right. The ranges of observed values of the curvation indices are 0–

29 and 0–25, respectively. The frequency distributions are shown in Figure 30.16.

No significant mean difference is found between left and right side. The range of observed differences is −15 through +15.

The correlation coefficient between left and right curvation indices is 0.49, which is significant (p ≤ 0.001) (no plot diagram given).

CORRELATIONS BETWEEN ANGULATION AND
CURVATION INDEX

The correlation coefficients between facet angulation
and curvature index are 0.37 on the left and 0.43 on the
right, both being significant (p ≤ 0.001). Although at L5-
S1 there is also a positive correlation between angulation
and curvature index, there is the remarkable finding that
the small but significant difference in angulation between
left and right side is not associated with a significant
difference in curvature index between left and right side
at this level. This fact needs further investigation.

Correlations between Superior Articular Facets L5 and S1

On both the left and right side the S1 facet is in the
mean more frontally oriented than the L5 facet, the differences being 4.8° ± 10.3° and 6.5° ± 9.9°, left and right,
respectively. Also, the mean curvature index at the S1
level is less on both sides than at the L5 level, the differences being 3.5 ± 8.1 and 4.8 ± 8.5, left and right. The
practical conclusion is that the S1 facets are generally
more frontally oriented, and have a less curved joint
surface than the L5 facets.

Correlation between Facet Asymmetry and Side of Unilateral Disc Protrusion

Of the 100 patients, 46 had a total number of 51 unilateral disc protrusions. Farfan stressed the high degree of
asymmetry of the facet joints in cases of sciatica and/or
disc protrusion (4, p. 161), namely, in 74% of 97 patients.
In our 100 patients examined at the levels L4-L5 and L5-
S1, 53% of the 200 levels showed no asymmetry, or asymmetry was less than 6° (see Table 30.3).

Farfan also stressed the high degree of correlation between the side of unilateral disc protrusion with the side
of the more oblique facet. This statement was based on
the findings in 51 cases of unilateral disc protrusion. This

relatively small number of cases is exactly the same as in
our series.

Table 30.4 shows no significant differences in localization of the disc protrusion with respect to a more sagittally
or frontally oriented facet joint with symmetry, or asymmetry of these facet joints of less than 11°. This holds for
37 (72%) of the 51 protrusions. With higher degrees of
asymmetry there was a greater incidence of localization
of a unilateral disc protrusion L4-L5 on the side of the
facet which was more frontally oriented (6 of 8 cases) than
on the side of the more sagittally oriented facet (2 of 8
cases). Unilateral disc protrusion L5-S1 did not show any
relation with respect to the orientation of the facet.

Our findings differ from Farfan's as to the frequency of
high degrees of asymmetry of the facet joints and give
some support to his view regarding correlation between

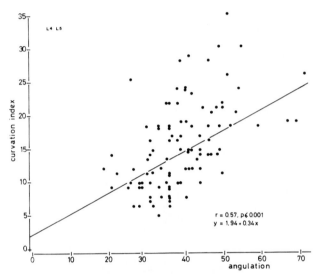

Figure 30.12. Correlation between the degrees of angulation and the curvature index of the left superior articular facet
L5.

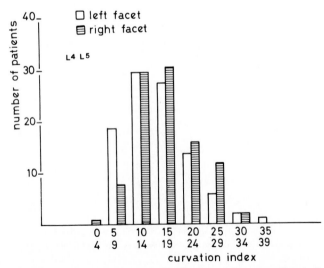

Figure 30.11. Frequency distribution of the curvature indices of left and right superior articular facet L5. Compare to
Figure 30.16.

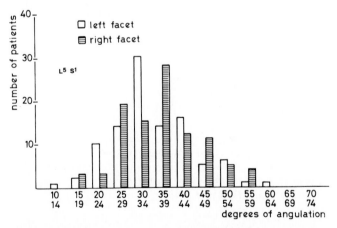

Figure 30.13. Frequency distribution of degrees of angulation of the left and right superior articular facet S1. Compare
to Figure 30.8.

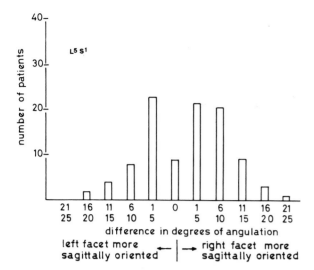

Figure 30.14. Frequency distribution of the differences between left and right superior articular facet angulation S1. As in Figure 30.9, patients with a more sagittally oriented left facet are presented on the left side of the histogram, and patients with a more sagittally oriented right facet on the right. In the text, the latter group is indicated with a minus sign.

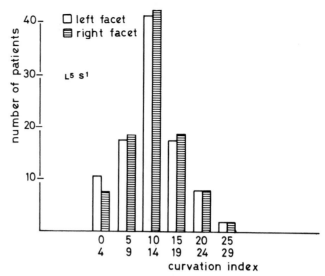

Figure 30.16. Frequency distribution of the curvation indices of left and right superior articular facet S1. Compare to Figure 30.11.

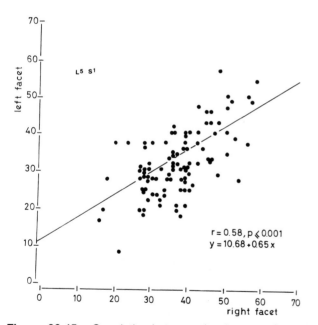

Figure 30.15. Correlation between the degrees of angulation of the left and right superior articular facets S1. Compare to Figure 30.10.

Table 30.3.
Frequency Distribution of Degrees of Asymmetry of the Facet Joints in Presence and Absence of Unilateral Disc Protrusion

Difference in degrees of angulation	Unilateral disc protrusion at L4-L5 and L5-S1 (51 levels)[a]	Absence of unilateral disc protrusion at L4-L5 and L5-S1 (149 levels)[a]
None (symmetric)	n = 4 (8%)	n = 9 (6%)
1–5°	n = 24 (47%)	n = 69 (46%)
6–10°	n = 9 (18%)	n = 43 (29%)
11–15°	n = 8 (16%)	n = 18 (12%)
16–20°	n = 3 (6%)	n = 8 (5%)
21–25°	n = 2 (4%)	n = 1 (1%)
26–30°	n = 1 (2%)	n = 1 (1%)
Totals	n = 51 (101%)[b]	n = 149 (100%)

[a] n = number of disc levels.
[b] The percentages do not always total 100% due to rounding error.

localization of the unilateral disc protrusion and the side of the more oblique facet (in our terminology, the more frontally oriented facet) in a small number of unilateral protrusions L4-L5 in the presence of asymmetry of more than 10°.

In addition, we want to stress that the distribution of degrees of asymmetry in our 51 unilateral disc protrusions and in the 149 disc levels without a unilateral protrusion presented in Table 30.3 does not show impressive differ-

ences. Asymmetry greater than 10° is found in 28% of unilateral disc protrusions and in 19% of the levels without unilateral protrusions. Gross asymmetry, therefore, is not frequent in both groups. The values mentioned above show, however, that in the group of unilateral disc protrusions the occurrence of asymmetry more than 10° is relatively higher than in the group without unilateral disc protrusions.

DISCUSSION AND CONCLUSIONS

According to Farfan (4) the mean value of the facet angle for the L4-L5 joint is 43°, and for the L5-S1 joint approximately 52°. The mean values found in our series are slightly lower for the left facet L4-L5, and about the same as in Farfan's series for the right facet (39.1° ± 9.8° and

Table 30.4.
Unilateral Disc Protrusion and Symmetric or Asymmetric Facet Angulation

Asymmetric angulation	Disc protrusion on side of facet closer to sagittal plane[a,b]	Disc protrusion on side of facet closer to frontal plane[a,b]	
1–5°	n = 12 (6; 6)	n = 12 (5; 7)	
6–10°	n = 4 (2; 2)	n = 5 (3; 2)	
11–15°	n = 3 (1; 2)	n = 5 (3; 2)	
16–20°	n = 1 (1; 0)	n = 2 (1; 1)	
21–25°	n = 1 (0; 1)	n = 1 (1; 0)	
26–30°	n = 0	n = 1 (1; 0)	
Totals	n = 21 (10; 11)	n = 26 (14; 12)	n = 47 (24; 23)
Symmetric angulation			n = 4 (3; 1)
Total number of protrusions			n = 51 (27; 24)

[a] n = number of protrusions
[b] In parentheses: first number applies to the level L4-L5, second number to the level L5-S1

42.9° ± 9.5° for left and right side, respectively). The reference system used by Farfan for measuring angulation is, however, different from ours. The statistically significant difference between left and right side of −3.8° ± 8.3°, the right facet generally being more sagittally oriented, is striking. We have not found any explanation of this fact. Statistical correlation and causal relationships are different matters. Concerning the curvation of the joint surfaces, a significant difference in curvation index has been found between left and right side at the L4-L5 level (15.4 ± 6.4 and 16.8 ± 6.2, respectively, with a difference of −1.4 ± 6.2, the right facet generally being more curved). Furthermore, we found a significant positive correlation between angulation and curvation of the joints: the more sagittally oriented, the more curved their surfaces. The generally more curved surface of the right facet corresponds to its more sagittal orientation.

At the level L5-S1 the mean values of the angulation on left and right side were 34.3° ± 9.2° and 36.4° ± 8.9°, respectively. There was a significant difference between the values for left and right side of −2.1° ± 7.8°. The curvation indices were 11.9 ± 6.4 and 12.1 ± 5.9, without significant difference.

Comparing the L5-S1 facets with the L4-L5 facets the more frontal orientation of the L5-S1 facets is clear, as is the lesser curvation of the joint surfaces at this level. The less curved joint surfaces of the L5-S1 level as compared to the L4-L5 level corresponds with the more frontal orientation of the L5-S1 joints.

The greater range of axial rotation at the L5-S1 level as compared to the L4-L5 level, found by the authors quoted in the introduction, may be explained by the more frontal orientation and the lower curvation index of the facets at this level.

The clinical significance of our findings of asymmetry of the facet joints is not clear yet. In the majority of our cases no gross asymmetry was found; no asymmetry in

6.5%, asymmetry less than 6° in 53%, asymmetry less than 11° in 79% of the disc levels.

As stated before, these findings were acquired from patients with low back problems, and are not representative of normal human variance. Therefore, it is not possible to evaluate exactly the importance of minor degrees of asymmetry, though it seems probable that minor asymmetries are natural phenomena.

Regarding the relation between the development of disc protrusions and asymmetry of the facet joints this study was limited to unilateral protrusions. No relation was found between type of asymmetry and side of disc protrusion at the level L5-S1. At the level L4-L5 there was no correlation between the side of unilateral disc protrusions and the type of asymmetry of the facets with asymmetries less than 11°. With greater degrees of asymmetry the localization of the unilateral disc protrusions was slightly more frequent on the side of the more frontally oriented facet. These findings show that great asymmetry of the facets may be of influence on the development of disc protrusion but that asymmetry is not the principle determinant.

This report is a first step in the evaluation of the properties of the various structures of the neural arch as visualized by CT, and their possible pathological, morphological, and functional consequences.

SUMMARY

Facet joint orientation and curvation in the lower lumbar spine in the axial plane were studied by CT in a hundred patients with low back pain and/or sciatica. The orientation of the facet joints was defined in terms of degrees of angulation between two reference lines. These reference lines were drawn between points which are constant in all vertebrae, thus allowing comparative measurements. At the L4-L5 level, the degree of angulation was found to be 39.1° ± 9.8° and 42.9° ± 9.5° (mean ± SD) for left and right side, respectively. There was a statistically significant difference of −3.8° ± 8.3° (p ≤ 0.001), the right being more frequently sagittally oriented than the left.

A parameter for curvation (shape) is proposed, and is called the curvation index. This curvation index was determined by two lines which equally allowed comparative measurements. The degree of curvation had a positive correlation with facet joint angulation: a more sagittal orientation of the joint was in general associated with a greater curvation of its surface.

At the level L5-S1, the angulation was found to be 34.3° ± 9.2° and 36.4° ± 8.9° for left and right side, respectively, with a statistically significant difference of −2.1° ± 7.8°. Here, also, a positive correlation existed between angulation and curvation. The joint surfaces L5-S1 are generally flatter than at the L4-L5 level, corresponding to their more frontal orientation. No relation was found between asymmetry of facet joints and side of localization of unilateral disc protrusions, with the exception of gross asymmetry at the L4-L5 level.

References

1. Junghanns H: *Die gesunde und die kranke Wirbelsäule in Röntgenbild und Klinik.* 5th Ed. G. Thieme Verlag, Stuttgart, 1968.
2. Steindler A: *Kinesiology of the Human Body.* 4th printing. Charles C Thomas, Springfield, 1973.
3. White AA, Panjabi MM: *Clinical Biomechanics of the Spine.* J. B. Lippincott Co., Philadelphia, 1978.
4. Farfan HF: *Mechanical Disorders of the Low Back.* Lea and Febiger, Philadelphia, 1973.
5. Carrera GF, Haughton VM, Syvertsen A, et al: Computed tomography of the lumbar facet joints. *Radiology* 134:145–148, 1980.
6. Farfan HF, Sullivan JD: The relation of facet orientation to intervertebral disc failure. *Can J Surg* 10:179–185, 1967.
7. Brailsford JF (cited by Farfan): Deformities of the lumbosacral region of the spine. *Br J Surg* 16:562, 1929.

CHAPTER THIRTY-ONE

High-Resolution Computed Tomography and Stenosis: An Evaluation of the Causes and Cures of the Failed Back Surgery Syndrome

KENNETH B. HEITHOFF, M.D.

INTRODUCTION

The failed back surgery syndrome (FBSS) is not, unfortunately, an uncommon sequela of back surgery. Of the approximately 200,000 patients having lumbar spine surgery each year, an estimated 25–40% have persistent or recurrent symptoms (1, 2). Before the use of high-resolution computed tomography (HRCT), accurate diagnosis of FBSS was difficult because the syndrome represents a spectrum of organic disease processes. Diagnosis in some patients was complicated further by the possibility of financial gain and by learned chronic pain behavior (3). HRCT has enhanced the physician's understanding of the various physiological entities involved in FBSS and their contribution to the individual patient's problem.

The recent advent of HRCT provides the diagnostician with far more specific and precise anatomical information regarding soft-tissue and bony nerve root impingement syndromes than was previously available. This has led to more accurate preoperative diagnoses and a much clearer understanding by the roentgenologist and surgeon of the scope and extent of the pathological condition to be encountered at surgery. Consequently, we have noted both a decrease in the incidence of FBSS in our patients operated for the first time, and an increased salvage rate among those patients operated on for surgically correctable causes of FBSS (4). Although HRCT has become the diagnostic procedure of choice in the evaluation of lumbar disc disease (5), it is through the clear, detailed depiction of bony nerve root impingement syndromes that HRCT has contributed most to the successful treatment of the FBSS patient.

We have found that the most frequent and significant lesion involved in FBSS is lateral spinal stenosis. Recurrent disc herniation, central spinal stenosis, lumbosacral adhesive arachnoiditis, epidural fibrosis, and other direct nerve root impingement syndromes play less important roles. The previous literature indicates that recurrent herniated nucleus pulposus (HNP) was the most common cause of the FBSS (6, 7). In our experience, however, unrecognized lateral spinal stenosis is a considerably more common cause of FBSS, representing between 53–58% of the cases evaluated at Sister Kenny Institute of Minneapolis and the University of Saskatoon (8).

Crock (8) has described two postsurgical failure patterns: outright failure, and failure after initial temporary relief.

Outright failure usually is related to inappropriate surgery performed because of a faulty preoperative diagnosis. Kirkaldy-Willis et al. at the University of Saskatoon (9), found that 56% of the patients diagnosed as having a herniated disc had concomitant lateral spinal stenosis, or lateral spinal stenosis alone, as the cause of FBSS upon reoperation. Current data at our institution, consisting of a 2-year review of HRCT scanning of the lumbar spine in 500 patients with FBSS, demonstrated lateral spinal stenosis in 53% of the cases.

Spinal stenosis is a heterogeneous group of abnormalities producing neural entrapment or compression. Before HRCT, no satisfactory means of preoperatively identifying spinal stenosis was available. This explains why lateral spinal stenosis has only now been recognized as an increasingly common cause of FBSS. In our experience, unrecognized lateral spinal stenosis with nerve root impingement is the most common cause of outright failure with persistent or recurrent symptoms after the performance of simple laminectomy and discectomy.

Myelography has proved unreliable in diagnosing lateral stenosis. This is particularly true of iophendylate because of limited filling of the nerve root sheaths, but is also true with metrizamide myelography. Myelography inherently is limited to providing information regarding lesions of the central spinal canal.

HRCT now can diagnose lateral stenosis readily as a cause of FBSS in the postoperative patient, and as a potential cause of this syndrome if recognized before the first surgical procedure. When studying postoperative patients, one cannot predict whether the stenosis was present before the surgical procedure or acquired thereafter. However, statistics are now available to indicate the high probability that, in most cases, stenosis antedated surgery and was responsible for the FBSS. In these cases, the patient was unrelieved of his symptoms after surgical procedures (Fig. 31.1).

This chapter will describe the use of HRCT in the following areas: evaluation of lateral spinal stenosis, differentiation between stenosis of the lateral intervertebral nerve root canal (lateral stenosis) and subarticular recess stenosis, evaluation of the postoperative patient with fibrosis and herniated disc, the prevention of the postoperative fibrosis by use of large-volume free-fat grafts, and use of HRCT in the selection of the proper patient for chymopapain.

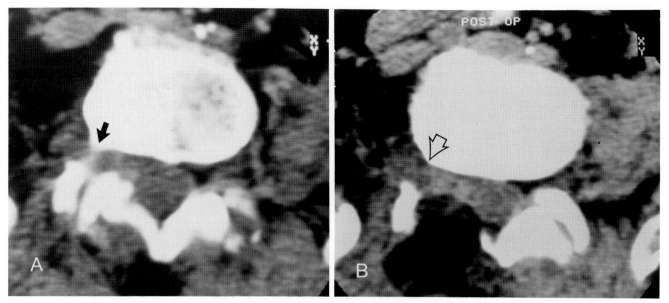

Figure 31.1. Pre- and postoperative HRCT scan of a failed back surgery patient with previous hemilaminotomy and partial facetectomy for L4–5 lateral spinal stenosis. A. Note partial surgical resection of the lamina and postsurgical distortion of the right L5-S1 zygoapophyseal joint as well as residual stenosis of the right L4–5 nerve root canal (*arrow*). B. Postoperative CT scan showing a hemilaminectomy and a subtotal facetectomy resulting in surgical decompression of the right L5-S1 nerve root canal (*arrow*). Also, note the large free-fat graft which has been placed and the absence of postoperative fibrosis.

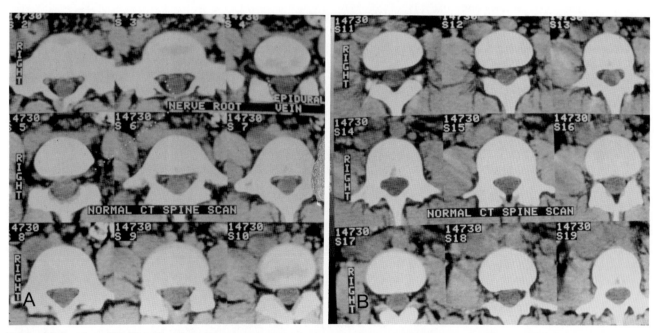

Figure 31.2. A and B. Note that the spine consists of a series of intraosseous segments with a complete bony envelope of the central spinal canal (S6–9, S13–15, and S19) and interosseous segments with an incomplete bony canal (S4, S5, S10–12, S16–18). The nerve roots and epidural veins are outlined by low density epidural fat and well visualized.

NORMAL ANATOMY AND ANATOMICAL VARIANTS

The spine consists of a series of intraosseous and interosseous segments (Fig. 31.2). The epidural space within the interosseous segments of the lumbar spine is occupied by fat, which provides a low-density envelopment of the thecal sac and nerve roots. This fat surrounds the lumbosacral nerve roots as they emerge from the thecal sac, course within the subarticular and lateral recesses, and traverse the intervertebral nerve root canal to enter the retroperitoneum (Fig. 31.3).

Figure 31.3. Normal appearance and course of the lumbosacral nerve roots, ganglia, and nerves. A. Note the symmetry and clear definition of the L5 and S1 nerve roots as they lie within the central spinal canal (*small arrows*), and as they traverse the nerve root canals (*large arrows*). B. Coronal reconstructed image obtained from the axial scans reveals the normal course and position of the nerve root ganglia and nerves. Note that the ganglia lies within the cephalic portion of the nerve root canal immediately beneath the pedicle and that the nerve courses inferiorly and laterally from the ganglia (*curved arrow*).

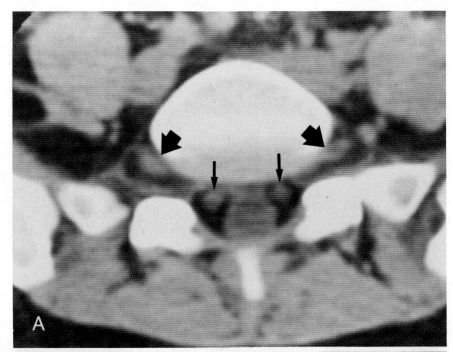

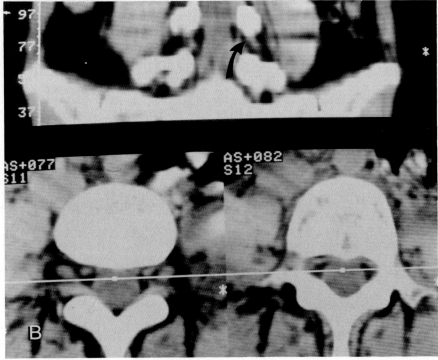

Normal measurements of the lumbar spine, including the central spinal canal and intervertebral nerve root canals, are available elsewhere in the literature, and will not be discussed here (11–13). However, these are artificial designations and direct visualization of the normal bony canal, the soft tissue within these canals, as well as the direct and indirect effects of their pathological correlates,

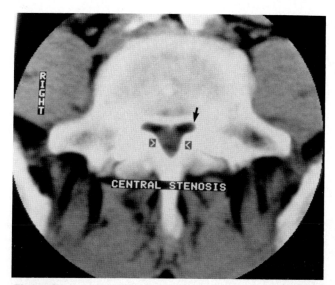

Figure 31.4. Axial CT scan reveals a small central spinal canal with diminished anteroposterior (AP), interfacet, and interpediculate measurements. Note the trefoil configuration of the spine. Although small, the lateral recesses are rounded in configuration and the L5 nerve roots which lie within the recesses are not compressed (*arrow*).

has made measurements largely superfluous. HRCT permits the evaluation of the thecal sac, nerve roots, and epidural fat in relation to the surrounding bony structures and allows comparison of the relative size of the neural elements with their respective bony nerve root canals.

Patients with congenitally diminished measurements of the central spinal canal often have diminished measurements of the intervertebral nerve root canals as well (Fig. 31.4). These patients often do not experience difficulty until they develop superimposed degenerative changes in the disc and posterior elements. Because the size of the canal already is diminished, a relatively minor superimposed degenerative narrowing is likely to produce critical stenosis and symptomatology.

It is our experience that a trefoil configuration of the lumbar spine (which is relatively common at L5) does not, in and of itself, cause nerve root entrapment. These lateral extensions of the central canal are rounded in configuration and are adequate for the size of the nerve roots coursing within them (Fig. 31.5A). However, this configuration may have a predisposition to the development of acquired subarticular recess stenosis when associated with degenerative hypertrophy of the superior articular process, degenerative bulging of the disc anulus, or posterolateral protrusion of an osteophyte. Any combination of these events may produce additional narrowing and nerve root compression (Fig. 31.5B).

The nerve roots and nerve root sheaths are normally symmetrical in their level of origin from the thecal sac, the course that they follow within the central canal and nerve root canals, and their size and configuration. Diffuse enlargement of the nerve root nerve root sheath complex in the absence of systemic disease often is due to sym-

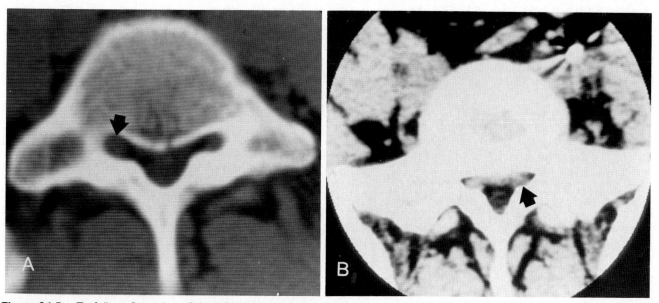

Figure 31.5. Trefoil configuration of the L5 lumbar vertebrae. A. Despite the marked trefoil configuration, the lateral recesses are rounded in configuration and are adequate for the size of the L5 nerve roots which lie contained within them (*arrow*). B. Trefoil configuration of the S1 vertebral body with superimposed pathological disc protrusion which is producing compression of the S1 nerve roots within the lateral recesses; left more than right (*arrow*).

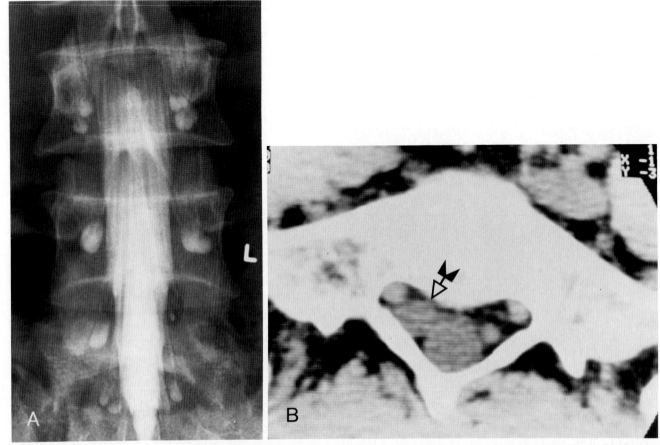

Figure 31.6. Enlargement of the nerve root-nerve root sheath complex due to dilatation of the nerve root sheaths. A. Myelogram demonstrating that an apparent nerve root enlargement seen on CT can be merely due to symmetrical bilateral dilatation of the nerve root sheaths. B. Asymmetric enlargement of the right S2 nerve root sheath, (*arrow*), in a different patient than illustrated in A. Note that the attenuation values of the enlarged nerve root sheath are similar to those of the thecal sac and less than that of the S1 nerve root ganglia.

metrical enlargement of the nerve root sheaths (Fig. 31.6A). Asymmetric imaging of the patient due to faulty positioning and/or roto scoliosis may produce asymmetry on a single image, but the cause of the asymmetry is made obvious by observation of adjacent images. When not due to patient tilt or scoliosis, the asymmetry may be due to asymmetrical enlargement of a nerve root sleeve (Fig. 31.6B). Asymmetry of the nerve root sheaths of the S1 nerve roots is not uncommon.

Conjoined nerve roots (most commonly L5-S1) are an important cause of nerve root asymmetry (Fig. 31.7). Failure to recognize a conjoined nerve root in patients with an underlying herniated disc may lead to operative damage of the conjoined nerve root, resulting in poor surgical results (16).

LATERAL SPINAL STENOSIS

The pathogenesis of degenerative disease of the lumbar spine is discussed in detail in another chapter in this book (Kirkaldy-Willis, Heithoff et al.).

For the purpose of this treatise, the following shall suffice: Repeated rotational strains produce simultaneous degeneration of the lumbar disc and posterior zygoapophyseal joints (Z-A) joints. Degenerative changes in the posterior joints consist of ligamentous laxity, cartilage destruction, and secondary subperiosteal bone deposition resulting in spondylosis and osteophyte formation. Pathological disc protrusion also may occur. It is these concomitant degenerative changes in the disc and facets which result in subarticular and lateral stenosis, which accompany pathologic disc disease (Fig. 31.8).

The most common cause of bony nerve root entrapment is lateral spinal stenosis produced by compression of the exiting nerve root within the nerve root canal by the superior articular process (SAP), i.e., the L4 nerve root within the L4-5 nerve root canal (Fig. 31.9). In addition to the hypertrophic enlargement of the SAP due to subperiosteal bone deposition, associated loss of disc height is often present, causing diminution in the superior-inferior dimension of the nerve root canal. This causes the SAP to under-ride the pedicle above (Fig. 31.10). This same mech-

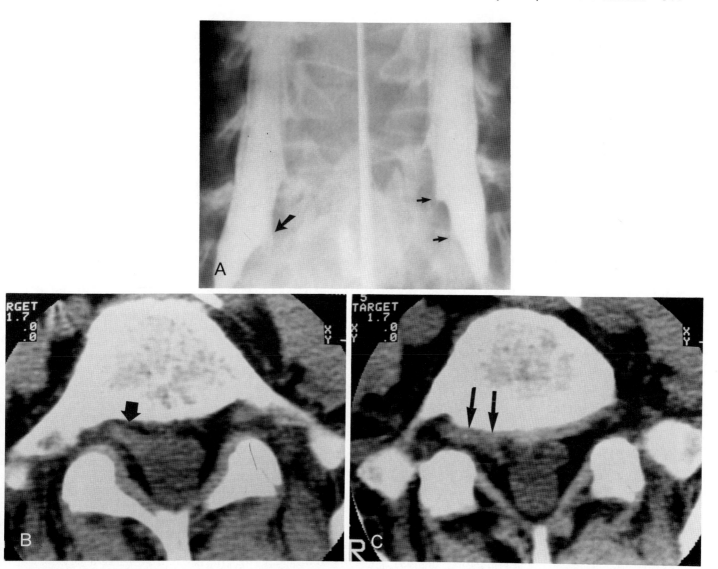

Figure 31.7. Conjoined nerve roots. A. Myelogram showing a conjoined left S1-S2 nerve root (*arrow*). Note that the conjoined nerve root emanates from the thecal sac approximately midway between the normal right-sided S1 and S2 nerve roots (*small arrows*). B. CT scan showing a conjoined L5-S1 nerve root. Note the lateral course of the conjoined nerve root from the thecal sac because of its more distal take-off (*arrow*). Note the higher density of the conjoined nerve root mass as opposed to the thecal sac. C. The increased density of the nerve root mass as it parallels the L5-S1 disc simulates asymmetric protrusion of the disc which may result in a false diagnosis of disc herniation (*arrows*). There is no separate origin of the S1 nerve root and it arises from the conjoined nerve root mass just medial to the pedicle of S1. In some cases, the S1 nerve root is very tightly opposed to the pedicle and appears splayed around it as it enters the subarticular recess of S1.

anism is responsible for nerve root entrapment in degenerative spondylolisthesis and retrolisthesis. Lateral spinal stenosis is not uncommon in retrospondylolisthesis (Fig. 31.11); whereas in degenerative spondylolisthesis (pseudospondylolisthesis) central and subarticular stenosis are common and bony lateral stenosis is unusual (Fig. 31.12).

Hypertrophy and superior subluxation of the SAP produces a CT image showing the nerve root ganglia to be compressed tightly between the SAP dorsally, the vertebral body ventrally, and the pedicle superiorly. The normal fat within the nerve root canal is replaced and the

compressed ganglia occupies the entire narrowed canal. The ganglia is flattened in appearance rather than having its normal rounded configuration (Fig. 31.13). The compressed nerve root often is pathologically enlarged. Swelling of the nerve root may occur both proximal and distal to the impingement, and when present, is a highly accurate direct sign of significant bony stenosis (Fig. 31.14). In addition to enlargement, there is often a loss of the sharp delineation of the nerve root border. This is due either to edema of the nerve root and adjacent tissue, or to venous engorgement on the surface of the nerve root sheath (Fig.

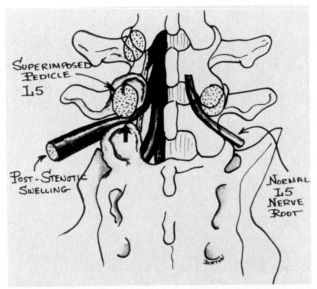

Figure 31.8. Line drawing demonstrating lateral spinal stenosis with compression of the left L5 nerve root secondary to hypertrophic overgrowth of the SAP of S1 (reader's left). There is compression of the nerve root between the pedicle of L5 and the SAP of S1 (*arrow*). Note the poststenotic swelling of the L5 nerve root and nerve. A normal configuration is demonstrated on the right. (Copyright: Dr. Charles V. Burton, Director, Institute for Low Back Care, Minneapolis, MN.)

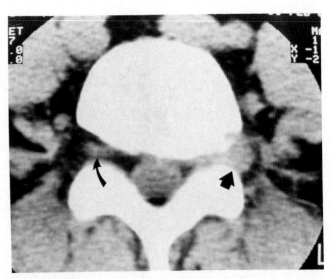

Figure 31.9. Lateral spinal stenosis at L4–5 on the left demonstrating narrowing of the nerve root canal caused primarily by a large posterolateral calcified osteophyte. Note marked swelling of the left L4 nerve root when compared to the right (*arrow*). The swelling of the nerve root, as well as the encroachment on the canal by the osteophyte, completely replaces the normal epidural fat within the nerve root canal and causes loss of definition of the nerve root which is seen on the normal right side (*curved arrow*).

31.15).

The spinal nerve root ganglia lies within the very cephalad aspect of the intervertebral nerve root canal, immediately below the pedicle and approximately 1–1.5 cm cephalad to the intervertebral disc at that level. Therefore, simple lateral bulging of the disc anulus without cephalad herniation is not a cause of lateral nerve root impingement (Fig. 31.16A). However, at the lumbosacral junction, the course of the nerve root is more directly caudal and, therefore, it lies in close proximity to the L5-S1 disc and may be trapped between the disc and the transverse process of L5 and/or sacral ala (Fig. 31.16B).

In the evaluation of patients for lateral nerve root entrapment, one must always carefully observe the appearance of the nerve root relative to the bony abnormalities. Hypertrophic overgrowth of the facets (Fig. 31.17) does not automatically translate to nerve root compression and one must carefully observe the serial images to determine the course of the nerve root with respect to the bony pathology noted. Although severe bony hypertrophic changes may be present, the nerve root may pass adjacent to the hypertrophic facets without being trapped. Similarly, even though the nerve root canal is narrowed with respect to its companion on the opposite side and is smaller than normal, if the nerve root passing through that narrowed canal is also small, and there is adequate remaining space for the nerve root, stenosis is not present (Fig. 31.18). Because of this variability and because of our ability to image the nerve roots directly, we do not use absolute

measurements as a guideline for stenosis, but rather, consider the size of the canal and the nerve root in each individual anatomical situation. Narrowing of the bony nerve root canal in conjunction with pathological swelling of the nerve root is virtually pathognomonic of significant stenosis.

When axial images are questionable for stenosis and no definite nerve root swelling is identified, reformatted sagittal images through the nerve root canals are very useful (Fig. 31.18). It is rare that reformatted images detect abnormalities unsuspected from axial images. We utilize routine sagittal image reformatting. Five images are obtained; 2 through each L5-S1 intervertebral nerve root canal, and a single midsagittal image through the central spinal canal. This is performed by the technician using the GE Arrange program. These are screening images. If stenosis is detected it is confirmed by the radiologist at the independent console at the time of interpretation. Specific planes are selected in the sagittal, coronal, and off-axis planes in an attempt to answer a specific diagnostic question. No attempt to completely reformat the entire spine is made.

Discectomy may produce postoperative lateral spinal stenosis due to reduction of disc height. Prophylactic foraminotomies are now being performed by our surgeons who have been forewarned of this eventuality by HRCT depiction of preoperatively narrowed nerve root canals. HRCT scans have demonstrated conversion of narrowed intervertebral nerve root canals (which preoperatively are not producing significant nerve root impingement) to sig-

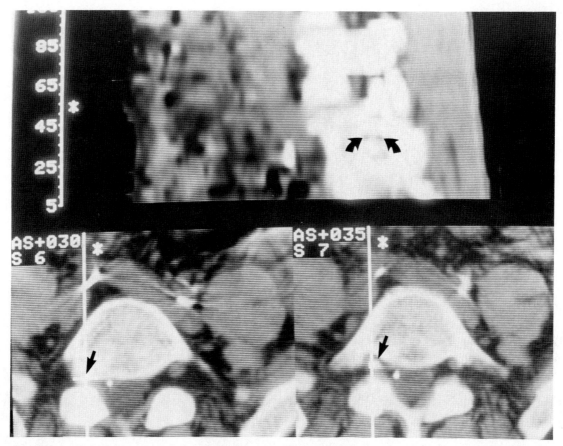

Figure 31.10. Severe lateral spinal stenosis at L5-S1 on the right showing marked compression of the right L5 nerve root between a calcified osteophyte which projects into the inferior aspect of the nerve root canal and compresses the exiting L5 nerve root against the pedicle of L5 (*arrows*).

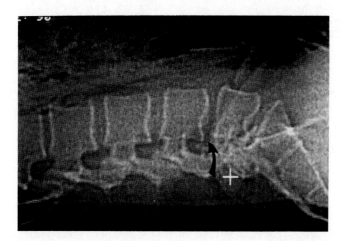

Figure 31.11. Retrospondylolisthesis: Lateral computed radiograph shows the posterior displacement of L4 on L5. Note the narrowing of the AP dimension between the posterior aspect of the vertebral body of L4 and the SAP of L5. This narrowing of the AP dimension of the nerve root canal is responsible for the not uncommon association of lateral spinal stenosis. Associated loss of disc height produces constriction of the superior-inferior dimension of the nerve root canal and allows compression of the nerve root ganglia between the SAP of L5 and the pedicle of L4.

nificant bony stenosis postoperatively (Fig. 31.19). Therefore, to prevent FBSS due to unrecognized lateral stenosis, it is strongly recommended that all patients undergoing surgery for degenerative lumbar disease have HRCT of the lumbar spine including reformatted images.

Postoperative lateral stenosis after spinal fusion may result from fusion overgrowth into the intervertebral nerve root canal (Fig. 36.20), or be due to a displaced bone plug in patients with posterior interbody fusions (Fig. 31.21A). These bony impingements on the nerve roots are identified easily by axial HRCT. Because of the lordotic curvature of the spine at the lumbosacral junction, axial images may seem to show posterior displacement of a normally situated plug, however, sagittal reformatted images show that the bony plug does not protrude beyond the posterior aspects of the L5 and S1 vertebral bodies (Fig. 31.21B).

Sagittal reformatted images are recommended strongly as an adjunct to axial images in all postoperative cases with spinal fusion. In addition to assisting in the evaluation of possible stenosis, sagittal reformatted images are invaluable in the evaluation of the solidity of fusion itself and the exclusion of pseudarthrosis and fusion failure, which are relatively common, occurring in 9–26% of cases (Fig. 31.22), (2, 14, 15).

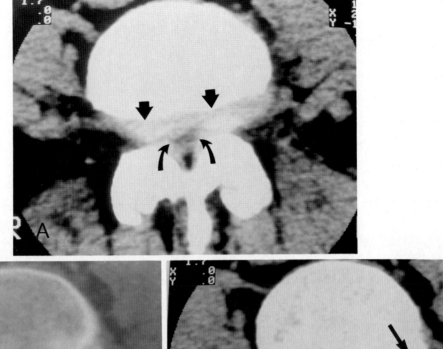

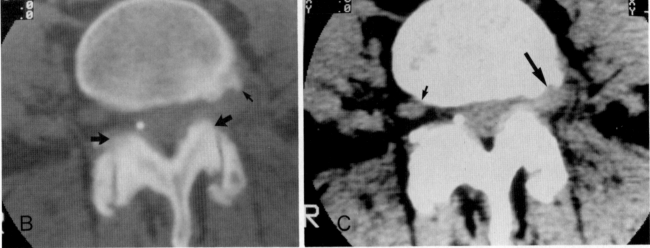

Figure 31.12.   Degenerative spondylolisthesis. A. Axial CT scan demonstrating anterior subluxation of the vertebral body of L4. This produces the prominent imaging of the disc dorsal to the L4 vertebral body (*arrows*). The anterior subluxation of the lamina and inferior facets of L4 produces both severe central stenosis and bilateral subarticular stenosis (*curved arrows*). B. L4–5 nerve root canals of the same patient with a wide window setting for bone detail demonstrates the anterior subluxation of the lamina and inferior facets of L4 which is greater on the left than the right (*large arrows*). There is also an associated large posterolateral osteophyte arising from the vertebral body of L4 which produces lateral spinal stenosis on the left (*small arrow*). C. Narrow, soft-tissue window setting of the same image as B demonstrates the pathological enlargement and loss of definition of the exiting L4 nerve root due to postimpingement swelling and edema (*arrow*), as compared to the normal contralateral L4 nerve root (*small arrow*).

Differentiation Between Lateral and Subarticular Recess Stenosis

Lateral spinal stenosis (nerve root impingement within the intervertebral nerve root canal) causes entrapment of the exiting nerve root; subarticular recess stenosis produces entrapment of the nerve root which is crossing the intervertebral disc within the lateral aspect of the central spinal canal and exits at the level below (Fig. 31.23). The use of the adjective "lateral" in stenoses of both the nerve root canal as well as subarticular regions has led to considerable confusion of the terms in the radiological as well

as the neurosurgical and orthopaedic literature. We propose "subarticular recess" as the preferred term for that proximal portion of the lateral recess which underlies the medial portion of the SAP.

A subarticular recess is only present in the pathological spine. It is defined as that portion of the anterolateral aspect of the central spinal canal whose cephalic margin is the intervertebral disc and the caudal margin is the superior aspect of the pedicle of the vertebra immediately below that disc. Stenosis of the subarticular recess may be caused by pathological bulging of the intervertebral disc (Fig. 31.24A), medial hypertrophy of the base of the supe-

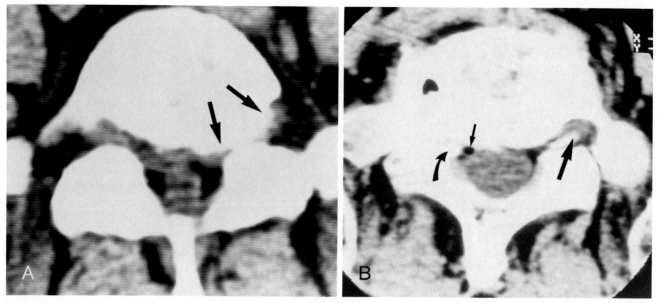

Figure 31.13. Lateral spinal stenosis with compression of the exiting nerve root ganglia. A. A large broad-based posterolateral osteophyte arising from the L5-S1 disc margin virtually occludes the L5-S1 nerve root canal (*arrows*) with compression and displacement of the L5 nerve root ganglia. B. Lateral spinal stenosis at L5-S1 on the left due to an osteophytic spur which impinges on the posterior aspect of the L5 nerve root ganglia within the proximal aspect of the L5-S1 nerve root canal (*large arrow*). Note also on the right considerable hypertrophic overgrowth of the medial aspect of the SAP of S1 (*curved arrow*) as well as gas within the epidural space due to a degenerated disc protrusion (*small arrow*).

rior articular process (Fig. 31.24B), or a combination of the two (Fig. 31.24C). The distal portion of the lateral recess which is medial to the pedicle and within the intraosseous segments of the central spinal canal is rarely involved in the stenosis (Fig. 31.24D).

These two entities can be distinguished easily by considering the nerve roots involved. Lateral stenosis of the intervertebral nerve root canal produces impingement of the exiting nerve root, whereas subarticular recess stenosis at the same level produces entrapment of the nerve root which is crossing the intervertebral disc to exit the foramen at the next level below (Fig. 31.25). A trefoil spine is a normal variant; however, it may contribute to subarticular recess stenosis when superimposed disc protrusion or hypertrophy of the superior articular process is present (Fig. 31.26). Subarticular nerve root entrapment occurs most commonly at the L4-5 level and somewhat less frequently at the L5-S1 level. Subarticular recess stenosis is commonly present in degenerative spondylolisthesis. Anterior subluxation of the inferior articular facets of the cephalad vertebra (most commonly L4) results in subarticular compression of the extradural nerve roots which traverse that disc space and exit the next intervertebral nerve root canal i.e., the L5 nerve root is compressed by subarticular stenosis at L4–5 proximal to its entering the L5–S1 nerve root canal (Fig. 31.27).

At the L5-S1 level, epidural fat outlining the S1 nerve roots is abundant. Therefore, subarticular impingement of the S1 nerve roots is identified easily. However, within the L4-5 subarticular recess, there is often no fat outlining

the L5 nerve root and direct visualization of nerve root impingement is not possible. One then must diagnose subarticular impingement based on the anatomical narrowing of the subarticular recess itself. In questionable cases, metrizamide-enhanced HRCT is diagnostic (Fig. 31.28).

Reports in the radiographic, neurosurgical, and orthopaedic literature often have not distinguished between lateral stenosis and subarticular impingement. Operative reports are often vague and merely speak of nerve roots compressed by "bony overgrowth" without specifically naming the processes involved. Lack of distinction or understanding between subarticular recess stenosis and stenosis of the intervertebral nerve root canal (lateral stenosis) in operative summaries promulgates the confusion. Thus, it is often difficult to obtain operative confirmation of the accuracy of CT in the diagnosis and differentiation of these two entities.. Often, no specific terminology is utilized and a general description of bone removal to "free up tight nerve roots" is all that is given. The term "foraminotomy" is used to describe relief of both subarticular and lateral stenosis. For example, a patient recently studied by HRCT and found to have subarticular recess stenosis at the L4–5 level was described on the operative report as having had a foraminotomy to free up the L5 nerve root at the L4–5 level. Obviously, a foraminotomy at the L4–5 level would have addressed lateral stenosis of the intervertebral nerve root canal and the exiting L4 nerve root. However, postoperative CT scanning showed that the patient actually had the appropriate me-

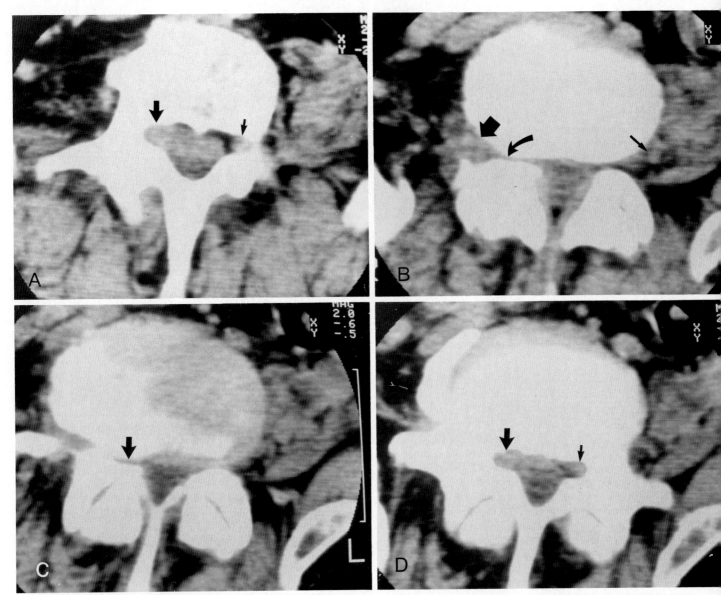

Figure 31.14.   Lateral spinal stenosis with swelling and edema of the involved nerve roots. A. Pathological enlargement of the right L4 nerve root just proximal to its entering a stenotic right L4–5 nerve root canal (*arrow*). Note normal L4 nerve root on left (*small arrow*). B. Marked enlargement of the right L4 nerve root as it emerges from the very stenotic right L4–5 nerve root canal (*arrow*). The stenosis is due almost entirely to marked overgrowth of the right L5 SAP (*curved arrow*). Note the normal left L4 nerve root and nerve (*small arrow*). C. Marked medial hypertrophy of the SAP of S1 in the same patient producing marked constriction of the subarticular recess (*arrow*). There is marked flattening of the right L5 nerve root and obliteration of its outline. D. Adjacent axial CT scan obtained 5 mm distal to C. Note the swelling of the right L5 nerve root as it emerges from the constricted subarticular recess (*arrow*). Compare with the normal left L5 nerve root (*small arrow*).

dial facectomy of the SAP of L5 for relief of the subarticular impingement of the L4 nerve root (Fig. 31.29).

Unfortunately, this lack of specificity between subarticular and lateral stenosis is the rule rather than the exception, and speaks strongly for the necessity of a standard nomenclature.

Stenosis of the subarticular recess produces myelographic abnormalities consisting of flattening of the nerve

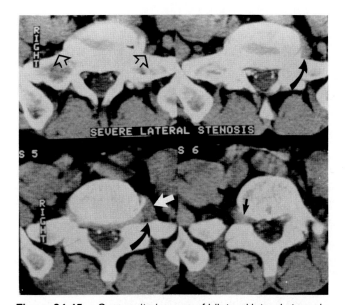

Figure 31.15. Composite images of bilateral lateral stenosis at L5-S1. Note the flattening of the right L5 nerve root ganglia (S6, *small arrow*). On the left, there is swelling of the left L5 nerve root proximal to the constricted canal. Marked edema surrounding the left L5 nerve produces obliteration of the margin of the L5 nerve distal to the nerve root canal (*curved arrows*). The swelling is contained laterally by the iliolumbar ligament which is responsible for the triangular appearance of this soft-tissue density (*white arrow*). Also, note the considerable enlargement of the edematous left L5 nerve when compared to the right (*upper left, arrowheads*).

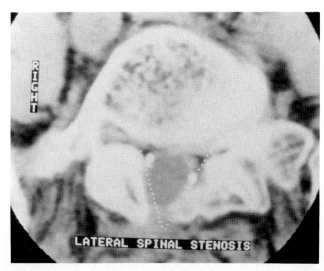

Figure 31.17. Marked spondylosis of the L5-S1 nerve root canal, more marked on the left. Marked hypertrophy of the facets of L5-S1 is seen.

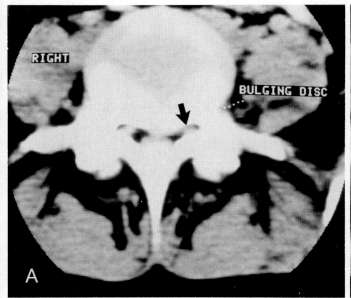
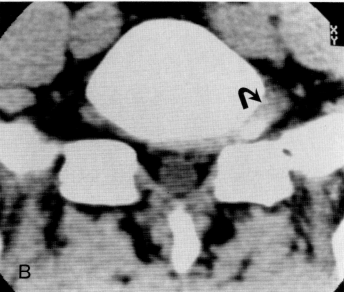

Figure 31.16. Bulging disc anulus as a cause of nerve root impingement: A. Centrally bulging disc at the L4–5 level. Because the disc is at the inferior aspect of the nerve root canal, no impingement of the exiting L4 nerve root occurs. However, bulging of the disc anulus narrows the subarticular recess and may produce subarticular recess impingement of the L5 nerve root at the L4–5 level (*arrow*). B. Lateral spinal stenosis at L5-S1 on the left. Note the edema of the exiting L5 nerve root (*arrow*) secondary to impingement by a laterally bulging calcified L5-S1 disc anulus. The more caudal course of the L5 nerve root causes it to lie adjacent the L5-S1 disc which may result in entrapment by lateral bulging of the disc anulus. This does not occur at more proximal levels of the lumbar spine.

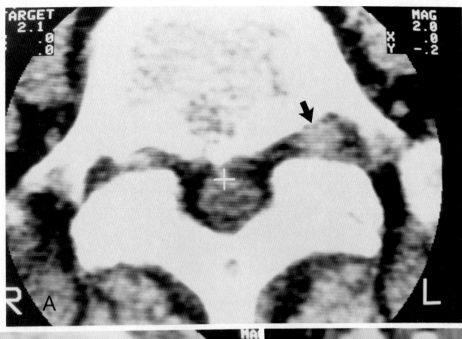

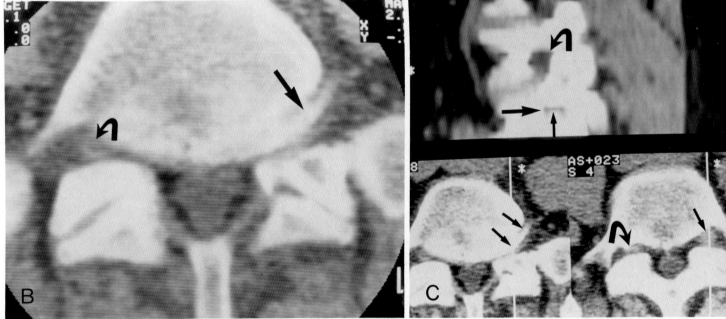

Figure 31.18.   Axial and reformatted sagittal images of constriction of the superior-inferior dimension of the L5 nerve root canal. A. Axial image (see also S4 in C) in a patient with left L5 radiculopathy shows a normal AP dimension of the left L5-S1 nerve root canal, but an enlarged left L5 nerve root ganglia (*arrow*). On the right, the scan passes through the very superior aspect of the right L5-S1 nerve root canal and simulates pathological narrowing of that nerve root canal. The adjacent, more caudal image showed a normal nerve root canal (B). B. The 5-mm axial scan obtained immediately caudal to A shows a large osteophytic ridge projecting into the left L5-S1 nerve root canal. The L5 nerve root ganglia is poorly imaged because of its superior displacement and compression by this large osteophyte arising from the superior and posterior aspect of the S1 vertebral body (*arrow*). Note also the normal-appearing right L5-S1 nerve root canal and right L5 nerve root ganglia (*curved arrow*). (Same image as S3 in C.) C. Sagittal reformatted image obtained through the mid aspect of the left L5 nerve root ganglia demonstrates marked constriction of the superior-inferior dimension of the nerve root canal resulting in the flattening of the left L5 nerve root ganglia (*arrows*). Note also the normal size of the L4–5 nerve root canal (*curved arrow*).

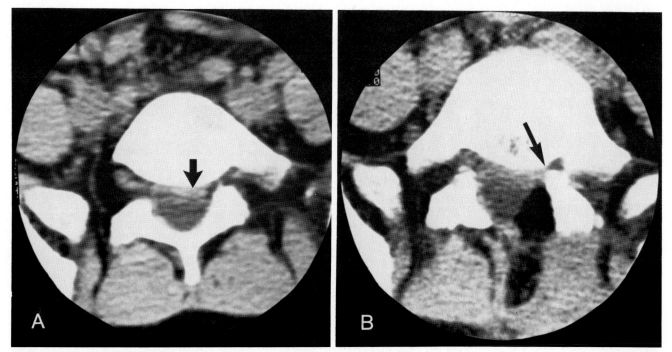

Figure 31.19.   Lateral stenosis after disectomy: A. Preoperative CT scan showing small left L5-S1 herniated disc (*arrow*). Note the narrowing of the left L5-S1 nerve root canal when compared to the right. However, no stenosis is present. B. Postoperative CT scan of the same patient after discectomy. The patient had been well for a period of time after surgery, but then developed gradual worsening with recurrent left leg pain. Note the compression of the left intervertebral nerve root canal by the SAP of S1 (*arrow*).

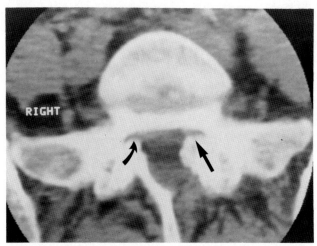

Figure 31.20.   Postoperative CT scan showing a left-sided hemilaminectomy and the inferior margin of a dorsolateral fusion. Bony overgrowth of the inferior margin of the fusion is extending into the central canal and causing marked compression of the S1 nerve root within the subarticular recess (*arrow*). An osteophyte arising from the SAP of S1 on the right is also causing constriction of the right subarticular recess and impingement on the right S1 nerve root (*curved arrow*).

root and nerve root sheath beneath the medial aspect of the base of the superior articular process. Filling of the nerve root sheath beyond occurs in mild cases, whereas complete amputation of the nerve root sheath occurs in

more severe cases (Fig. 31.30). The myelographic defects produced by subarticular impingement are often misinterpreted as herniated discs by the roentgenologist unfamiliar with subarticular stenosis. The differentiation between disc herniation and subarticular impingement is made easily with HRCT. It is the simplest, most accurate and economical means of establishing the correct diagnosis.

Dynamic Stenosis

Dynamic lateral stenosis occurs in patients with ligamentous laxity in whom rotatory motion of the spine causes anterior and superior subluxation of the SAP. This results in impingement on the nerve root either within the subarticular gutter or, more commonly, the intervertebral nerve root canal (Fig. 31.31). To demonstrate this lesion with HRCT, rotation-extension HRCT views of the lumbar spine are obtained after a routine flexion study. If weight loading of the spine is added to the rotation-extension views, it is our experience that this lesion is demonstrated more easily (Fig. 31.32). Extension-weight loading views have also successfully demonstrated dynamic pathological bulging of the disc anulus, producing subarticular nerve root impingement (Fig. 31.33).

Lytic Spondylolisthesis

Stenosis of the nerve root canals with impingement of the exiting nerve roots can occur in patients with spondylolysis and spondylolisthesis. This is most common at L5-S1. If the disc height is normal or mildly decreased in height, nerve root entrapment is unusual (Fig. 31.34).

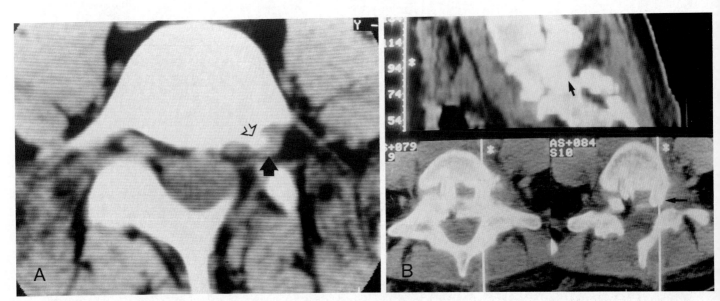

Figure 31.21. A. Posterior interbody fusion with posterolateral displacement of a bone plug into the intervertebral nerve root canal (*arrowhead*). The bone plug is impinging on the anterior aspect of the left L4 nerve root ganglia as it emerges from the canal (*arrow*). B. Axial and sagittal reformatted images through bone plugs of a posterior interbody fusion demonstrate no abnormal posterior displacement of the bone plugs on the sagittal reformatted images (*small arrow*) despite apparent encroachment on the intervertebral nerve root canal on the left on the axial images (*arrows*). The accentuated lumbar curvature is responsible for the apparent posterior displacement on the axial images.

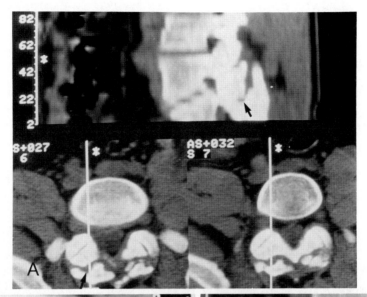

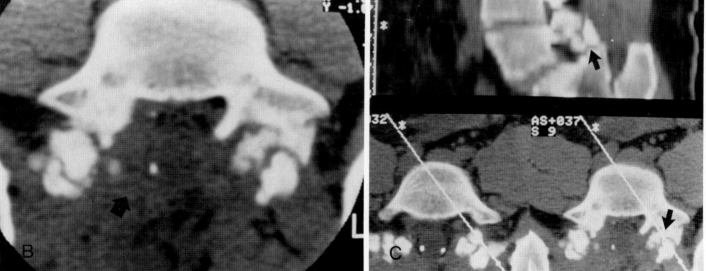

Figure 31.22.   A. Sagittal reformatted imaging of a failed L5-S1 dorsal fusion. Note the normal unfused appearance of the L5-S1 zygoapophyseal joints and the lack of fusion of the dorsally situated fusion bone with the inferior facet of L5 (*arrows*). B. Decompressive laminectomy and attempted lateral fusion at L5-S1. Note the lack of fat-grafting and marked postoperative epidural fibrosis (*arrow*) which completely envelopes the thecal sac and S1 nerve roots. The axial image is inadequate to determine the adequacy of the fusion. C. Off-axis reconstructed image of the L5-S1 fusion shows failure of fusion with a pseudarthrosis of the attempted L5-S1 fusion on the left (*arrow*).

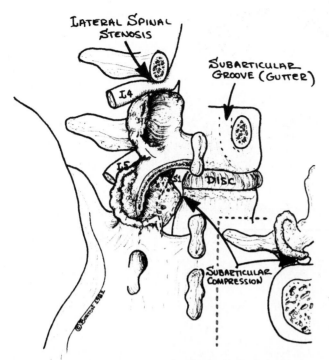

Figure 31.23. Line drawing: lateral and subarticular stenosis: L4–5 lateral spinal stenosis and L5-S1 subarticular stenosis as a sequelae to lumbar spondylosis. Marked overgrowth as well as superior subluxation of the SAP of L5 traps the exiting L4 nerve root by compressing it against the pedicle of L4, whereas, medial hypertrophy of the base of the SAP of S1 causes flattening and compression of the S1 nerve root immediately below the level of the L5-S1 disc. This is shown as broadening on the AP view and compression of the nerve root in the AP dimension on the cutout. Note on the AP view that the subarticular recess lies between the inferior aspect of the disc and the superior and medial aspect of the pedicle. The more caudal portion of the lateral recess which lies medial to the pedicle and caudal to the base of the SAP is not involved in this process. (Copyright: Dr. Charles V. Burton, Director, Institute for Low Back Care, Minneapolis, MN.)

However, degenerative loss of disc height in association with spondylolytic spondylolisthesis and overgrowth of the pars often is associated with entrapment of the L5 nerve root at the L5-S1 level. This stenosis of the bony nerve root canal is predominantly in the superior-inferior dimension (Fig. 31.35). The anteroposterior dimension of the nerve root canal may be normal on the axial images. Significant impingement may produce apparent enlargement of the L5 nerve root ganglia. However, the nerve root itself as it passes through the narrowed distorted nerve root canal, is often poorly visualized on axial images because of partial volume imaging of the pedicle and pars proximally and the intervertebral disc and vertebral body distally. In fact, whenever the course of a lumbar nerve root is tangential to the plane of the axial scan, we have found that sagittal and off-axis reformatted images which are perpendicular to the course of the nerve root have been extremely helpful in assessing whether a bony nar-

rowing or impingement was causing compression of that nerve root (Fig. 31.36).

Lateral Herniated Discs

Lateral herniated discs which protrude into the intervertebral nerve root canal but not into the central spinal canal are an infrequent, but important cause of FBSS. Because of their location, these lateral (foraminal) herniations may produce very subtle or no abnormality on the myelogram and may be inapparent at surgery when a simple hemilaminecotomy is performed.

Lateral herniated discs are identified easily on HRCT as high-density, soft-tissue masses which fill the intervertebral nerve root canal and obliterate visualization of the nerve root ganglia (Fig. 31.37). Lateral herniated discs, in our experience, occur more commonly at L3–4 than L4–5. Therefore, our routine examination extends from S1 to the midpedicle of L3. Lateral herniated discs at L5-S1 are rare (Fig. 31.38). We have studied patients with up to 8 years of undiagnosed back pain and sciatica with lateral herniated discs at L3–4. Previous diagnostic studies and exploratory surgery had been unable to detect any lesions. Because of the involvement of the L3 nerve root in these patients, there may be neither loss of knee jerk or ankle jerk, and these patients not uncommonly have severe pain (and insignificant) neurological deficit.

POSTOPERATIVE CT

The HRCT appearance of the spine is changed considerably by surgery. Bony alterations consisting of laminectomies, hemilaminectomies and laminotomies, partial and total facetectomies, as well as interbody and dorsolateral fusions may be present (Fig. 31.39). Postoperative epidural fibrosis is an invariable accompaniment of lumbar spine surgery unless fat grafting is utilized (Fig. 31.40).

Epidural fibrosis replaces the normal epidural fat as it extends into the central canal and onto the thecal sac (Fig. 31.41A). In severe cases, it extends into the anterior aspect of the canal and envelopes the nerve roots (Fig. 31.41B). This perineural fibrosis causes apparent enlargement of the nerve root, and in some cases, a solid sheet of fibrosis envelopes both the thecal sac and the nerve roots (Fig. 31.41C). There is correlation between the extent of the surgical procedure and the amount of fibrosis. Posterior interbody fusions associated with complete laminectomies, in our experience, produce the most severe fibrotic reactions.

When present, postoperative epidural fibrosis causes the nerve roots, epidural veins, and ligamentum flavum as well as dura to become indistinguishable. When the fibrosis extends anteriorly to interface with the disc, the sharp definition of the posterior margin of the disc is lost, making diagnosis of recurrent disc protrusion more difficult. Because the margin of the disc is obscured by the epidural fibrosis and fibrosis is indistinguishable from the nerve root sheath, the usual HRCT findings of disc herniation present in a previously unoperated patient are lost (Fig. 31.42).

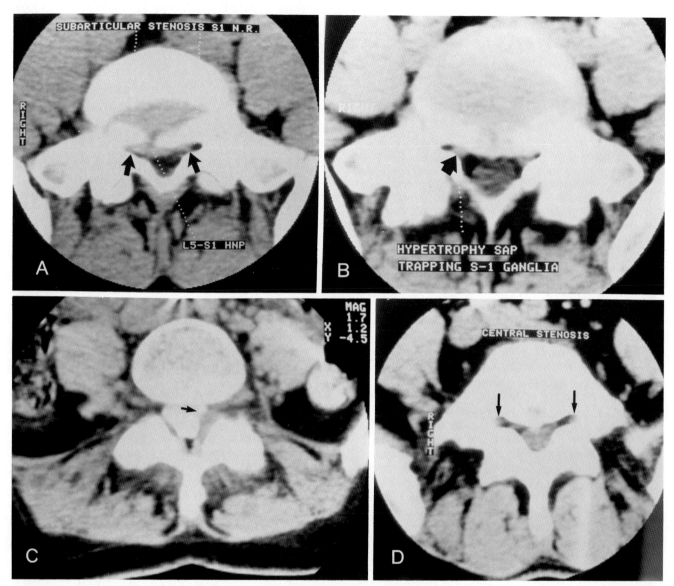

Figure 31.24. Subarticular recess stenosis; A. Bilateral subarticular stenosis at L5-S1 caused by pathological bulging of the L5-S1 disc anulus. This is more prominent on the right than the left. Note the marked flattening of both S1 nerve roots (*arrows*). B. Moderate subarticular recess stenosis at L5-S1 with flattening of the right S1 nerve root ganglia by medial hypertrophy of the SAP of S1 (*arrow*). C. Metrizamide-enhanced CT scan at L4–5 showing encroachment on the subarticular recess by marked thickening of the ligamentum flavum on the left. Note the encroachment on the dorsal aspect of the left L5 nerve root sheath (*arrow*). D. Lateral recess of the central spinal canal which lies distal to the subarticular recess and medial to the pedicle is usually not stenotic despite a marked trefoil configuration. Ordinarily the lateral recesses are rounded in configuration and large enough for the nerve root coursing through this recess (*arrows*), and because this is within the intraosseous segment of the spine, impingement by neither disc nor SAP is possible.

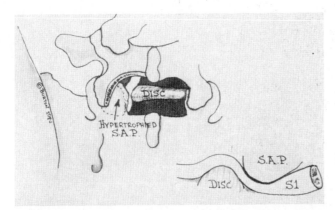

Figure 31.25. Line Drawing: Subarticular Stenosis: Subarticular recess stenosis due both to disc protrusion and hypertrophy of the medial aspect of the SAP produces a roller-coaster effect in which the nerve root coursing through the stenotic subarticular recess follows a roller-coaster course over the disc and beneath the hypertrophied SAP. The nerve root gets "guillotined" between these two impinging processes. It is the nerve root crossing the disc which is entrapped, not the nerve root exiting the foramen at that level. (Copyright: Dr. Charles V. Burton, Director, Institute for Low Back Care, Minneapolis, MN).

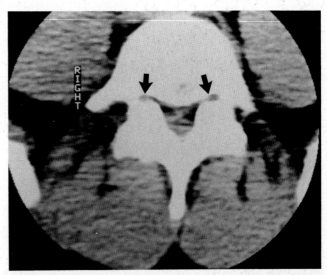

Figure 31.26. The lateral recess in this patient with a trefoil spinal configuration have been narrowed pathologically by overgrowth of the SAP, and the L5 nerve roots are being compressed pathologically and flattened (*arrows*).

The attenuation value of epidural fibrosis is similar to that of the nerve roots, epidural veins, and ligamentum flavum. The cerebrospinal fluid-containing thecal sac is of lower density than neural elements or fibrosis. Fortunately, intervertebral disc material is often of higher density than fibrosis, therefore, distinction between recurrent herniated disc and postoperative epidural fibrosis is possible in most cases.

The differentiation between epidural fibrosis and recurrent herniated discs in patients with FBSS and recurrent back pain and sciatica consists of utilization of internal control values for disc material and fibrosis with comparison to the area in question. In most cases, the attenuation values of epidural fibrosis are 30–50 HU less than those of the control measurement of the disc. When the area in question has an attenuation value equal to that of disc and 30–50 HU above the known scar in the posterior aspect of the wound, recurrent disc herniation can be predicted with a high degree of accuracy.

The attenuation value of disc material and fibrosis will vary with the individual patient as well as differing equipment. The attenuation values of a herniated disc using the infant mode calibration on the GE 8800 most commonly range between 90–120 HU, whereas epidural fibrosis is usually in the range of 50–70 HU. The attenuation values are lower when prospective target imaging is utilized, but the same relative difference in attenuation values is maintained. Occasionally, there is overlap due to unusually low attenuation values of fragmented disc material and/or partial volume effect. Visual discrimination of these subtle differences on film and/or CRT viewing is inadequate for differentiation and, therefore, the use of atten-

uation values obtained from region-of-interest viewing is essential (Fig. 31.43).

In a recent prospective study of 290 patients with the HRCT diagnosis of herniated lumbar disc, 161 patients underwent laminectomy and discectomy. The diagnostic accuracy of HRCT was 98.3%, with two false-negative studies and no false-positives. Included within this series were 19 patients with FBSS. Of these 19 previously operated patients, 14 had significant postoperative epidural and perineural fibrosis. In all of these patients, a correct preoperative diagnosis of recurrent herniated disc underlying the fibrosis was made on the basis of the plain, nonmetrizamide-enhanced CT scan.

There are a number of patients in whom herniated disc material is isodense with the surrounding epidural fibrosis. In such patients who have persistent postoperative pain or especially those who were well following surgery and experience recurrent pain in the dermatome involved, it is essential to augment the plain HRCT with a metrizamide-enhanced study. On metrizamide-enhanced CT scans, epidural fibrosis is shown either to envelope the affected nerve root or to retract it toward the disc space or vertebral body. When a recurrent herniated disc is present, it appears as an epidural mass with dorsal displacement of the affected nerve root (Fig. 31.44). A combination of an underlying herniated disc and perineural fibrosis shows both dorsal displacement and a thickened rim of soft tissue surrounding the metrizamide-filled nerve root sheath (Fig. 31.45). Therefore, whereas myelography is often abnormal but nonspecific in those patients in whom plain HRCT cannot distinguish between fibrosis and recurrent herniated disc, a metrizamide-enhanced CT scan is diagnostic (Fig. 31.46).

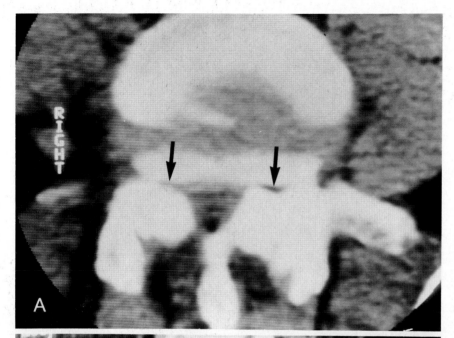

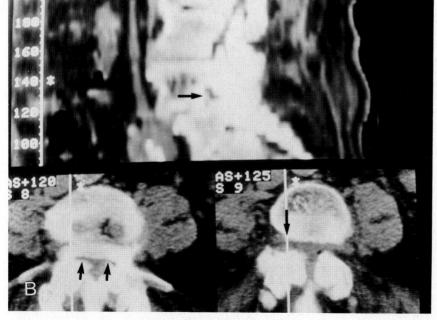

Figure 31.27. A. Degenerative spondylolisthesis with marked constriction of the subarticular recess bilaterally due to anterior subluxation of the inferior articular process (*arrows*). There is also moderately severe central stenosis produced by concomitant anterior subluxation of the lamina as well as thickening of the ligamentum flavum and bulging of the disc anulus. B. Sagittal reconstructed image of severe degenerative spondylolisthesis. Note: Severe bilateral subarticular stenosis (*small arrows*) and central stenosis on the axial images. There is no associated lateral stenosis (*arrows*).

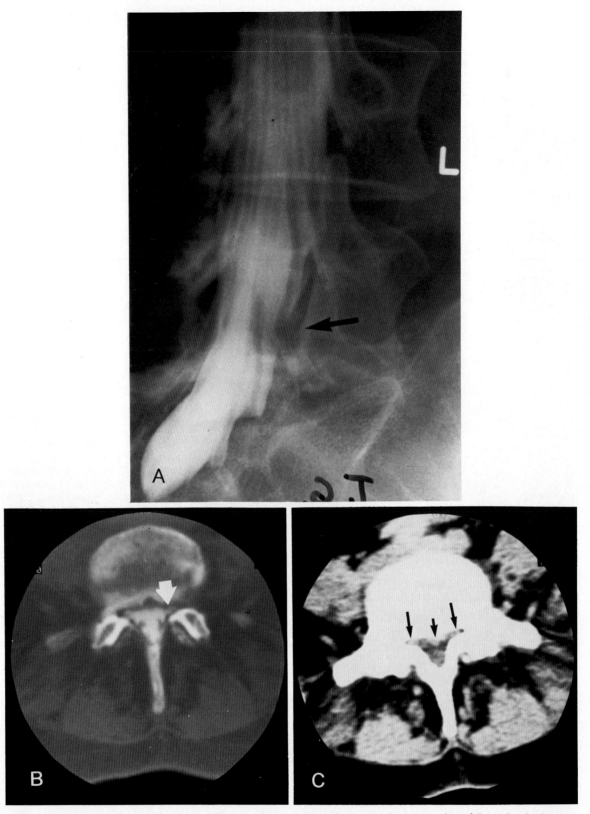

Figure 31.28. Subarticular recess stenosis; A. Metrizamide myelogram demonstrating narrowing of the subarticular recess with impingement on the L5 nerve root as it crosses the disc space and underlies the base of the SAP (*arrow*). In mild cases, only flattening and broadening of the nerve root as it passes beneath the SAP is seen. In more severe cases, amputation of the L5 nerve root sleeve is identified. B. Metrizamide-enhanced CT scan at the L4–5 level demonstrates compression of the L5 nerve root sheath within the subarticular recess (*arrow*). C. Nonenhanced CT scan at the L4–5 level demonstrating constriction of the subarticular recess (*large arrows*). Because of a lack of epidural fat, the L5 nerve root is not imaged directly and, therefore, nerve root impingement must be judged indirectly from the constriction of the subarticular recess itself. In these cases, metrizamide enhancement is required for verification. There is also a central disc herniation (*small arrow*).

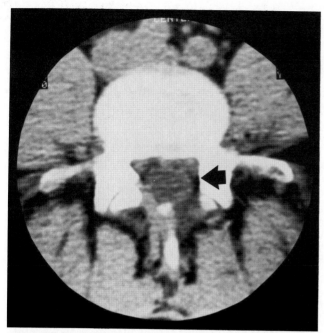

Figure 31.29. Postoperative CT scan demonstrating a (partial) medial facetectomy on the left at the L4–5 level (*arrow*). This operative procedure was described as a foraminotomy on the surgical procedure. The medial facetectomy performed adequately decompresses the subarticular recess and relieved the impingement of the L5 nerve root found at surgery.

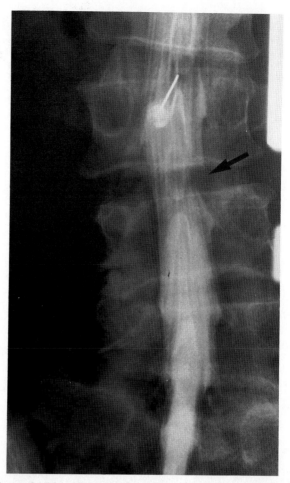

Figure 31.30. Metrizamide myelogram demonstrating compression of the L4 nerve root sheath caused by severe subarticular recess impingement (*arrow*). This myelogram was interpreted as showing findings consistent with an L3–4 herniated disc.

A recent publication reports a series of postoperative patients studied before and after the injection of intravenous contrast material (18). The authors were able to distinguish between epidural fibrosis and recurrent herniated disc with a high degree of accuracy on the basis of contrast enhancement of the epiural fibrosis and the nonenhancing nature of the recurrent disc fragments. This technique, if verifiable, would seem to hold considerable promise as a substitute for metrizamide-enhanced CT scanning in those patients in whom a recurrent recurrent disc underlying epidural fibrosis is suspected (Fig. 31.47). We have, however, been unable to reproduce these results.

Fat Grafts

The use of autogenous fat grafts after spine surgery greatly simplifies interpretation of the postoperative HRCT of the spine because it reduces or prevents postoperative fibrosis. These fat grafts may be pedicle grafts or free-fat grafts. Fat grafts inhibit fibrosis by functioning as an inert mechanical barrier which prevents the collection of serous fluid and blood within the operative space. Therefore, a large-volume fat graft must be placed in order to prevent fibrosis by filling the entire operative defect (Fig. 31.48). Particulate fat grafts harvested from the operative site have been found to be ineffective in preventing fibrosis because of their inadequate volume in patients with large resections. They were associated with signifi-

cant postoperative fibrosis on repeat postoperative HRCT scans (Fig. 31.49).

Burton et al. followed 183 patients with large-volume free-fat grafts with postoperative HRCT. Fifty-three of these patients have been restudied by HRCT up to 2 years after surgery and these fat grafts have been seen to be viable. Immediate postoperative scans show marked compression of the thecal sac (Fig. 31.48B). Over time, they lose approximately one-third of their volume and, in some cases, a pseudomembrane forms dorsal to the fat graft (Fig. 31.48C). Presumably, this is the interface between the fibrotic tissue associated with the scar and the free-fat graft.

The presence of the fat graft greatly simplifies the interpretation of the postoperative HRCT. The structures within the spinal canal retain their interface with fat and are, therefore, well visualized. The structures appear similar to normal patients, and recurrent herniated discs interface with fat and neural elements and are identified

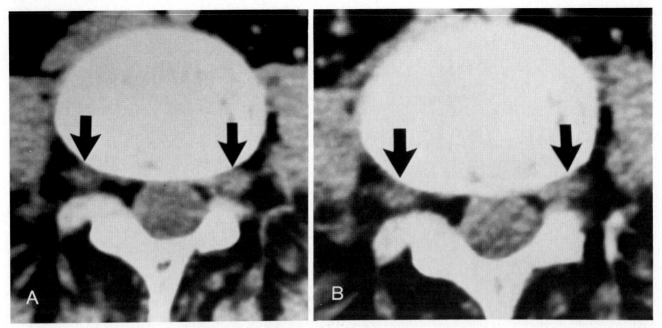

Figure 31.31. Dynamic lateral spinal stenosis: A. Flexion CT spine scan demonstrating mild enlargement of the left L4 nerve root ganglia but no apparent constriction of the left L4–5 nerve root canal. B. Extension view taken at soft-tissue window settings of the same L4–5 nerve root canal shows dynamic instability with anterior subluxation of the SAP of L5. This narrows the AP dimension of the nerve root canal and flattens the L5 nerve root ganglia. (The soft-tissue density posterior to the ganglia represents that portion of the ligamentum flavum which attaches to the superior facet. Bone window settings demonstrated the SAP to better advantage.)

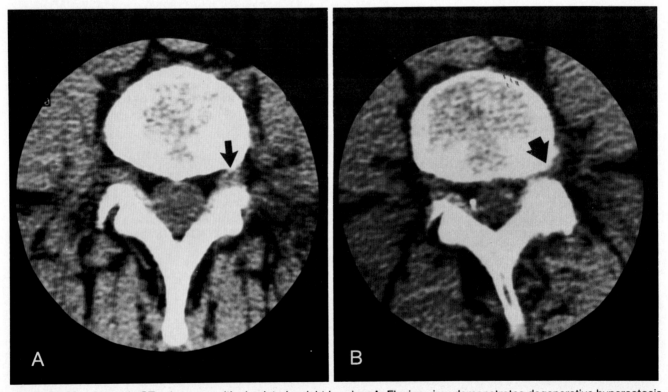

Figure 31.32. Dynamic CT spine scan with simulated weight-bearing: A. Flexion view demonstrates degenerative hyperostosis at L4–5 on the left without stenosis of the nerve root canal. Note the enlargement of the exiting left L4 nerve root (*arrow*). B. Extension and simulated weight-bearing produced by having the patient strain against a continuous strap passed over the shoulders and under the feet. Note the production of left L4–5 lateral spinal stenosis with compression of the left L4 nerve root (*arrow*).

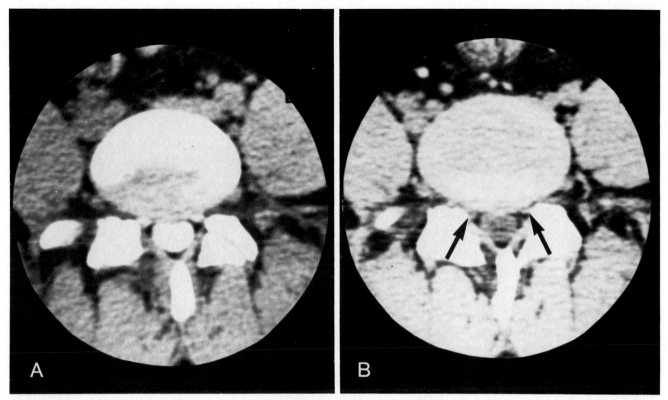

Figure 31.33.   Pathological central disc protrusion with weight-bearing: A. Flexion CT scan of the L4–5 level in a patient with a history of severe sciatica and weakness on extension of the lumbar spine. The scan is essentially normal. There is very minimal central bulging of the disc anulus, but no evidence of impingement on the L5 nerve roots. B. Extended, simulated weight-bearing images of the same L4–5 level demonstrate an additional 5 mm of central disc protrusion and evidence of mild subarticular compression of the L5 nerve roots (*arrows*).

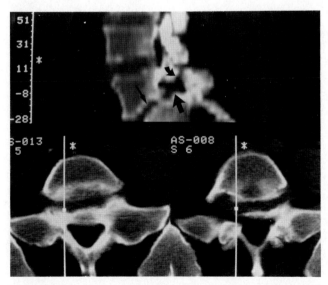

Figure 31.34.   Lytic spondylolisthesis with a mildly decreased L5-S1 disc height. The sagittal reformatted image through the right L5-S1 nerve root canal shows a mildly decreased L5-S1 disc space (*small arrow*), the break in the pars of the L5 vertebra (*curved arrow*) and a nonstenotic L5-S1 nerve root canal (*large arrow*).

easily (Fig. 31.50). Other institutions have also noted long-term viability of free-fat grafts (4, 16, 17). Although fat grafts have not been used widely in this country, experimental and clinical evidence indicates that their use improves clinical results (5, 17). This is presumably due to the noted reduction of nerve root entrapment by epidural and perineural fibrosis.

CHYMOPAPAIN

It is appropriate to conclude this discussion of stenosis and failed back surgery syndrome by relating our experience with chymopapain because it holds the promise of eliminating the necessity for surgical discectomy in some patients.

We were involved in a national study of the efficacy of chymopapain as one of several centers evaluating its use with lumbar HRCT. This was a rigid, double-blind study utilizing preoperative HRCT, myelography, and discography. The patients were injected with either saline or chymopapain in a random double-blind fashion. Patient selection by HRCT required evidence of a herniated disc at only a single level and no other evidence of spine pathology; particularly no evidence of concomitant lateral stenosis. A 6-month follow-up HRCT was performed in

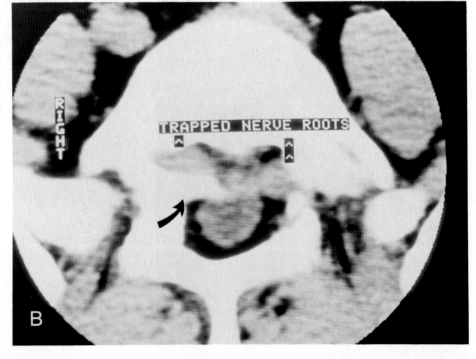

Figure 31.35. Lytic spondylolisthesis with degenerative narrowing of the L5-S1 disc and bilateral lateral spinal stenosis. A. Sagittal reformatted image through the left L5-S1 nerve root canal demonstrates marked narrowing of the posterior aspect of the L5-S1 disc space (*curved arrow*), and marked constriction of the superior-inferior dimension of the left L5-S1 nerve root canal with flattening of the left L5 nerve root ganglia (*arrow*). B. Axial image at the same level as demonstrated in A, demonstrates marked swelling of the L5 nerve roots bilaterally (*arrowheads*). Note the marked medial overgrowth of the right pars which encircles the right L5 nerve root (*curved arrow*).

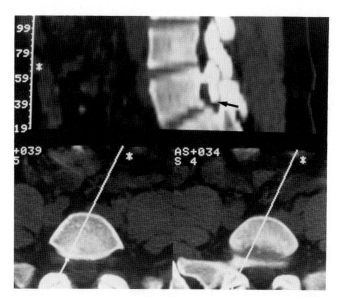

Figure 31.36. Off-axis reconstructed image of the right L5-S1 nerve root canal in a patient with bilateral spondylolisthesis of the pars interarticularis of L5 and minimal spondylolisthesis. Note the normal superior-inferior as well as normal AP dimensions of the nerve root canal and the anterior displacement of the pars of L5 (*arrow*).

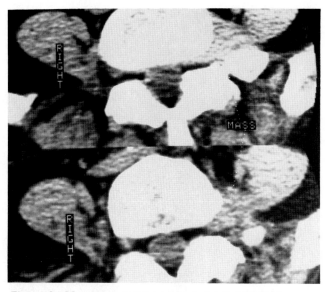

Figure 31.38. Huge lateral herniated left L5-S1 disc produced severe right-sided sciatica. The L5 nerve root is obliterated completely by this disc herniation. The far lateral extension of the disc protrusion produces no mass effect on the thecal sac and the myelogram was normal.

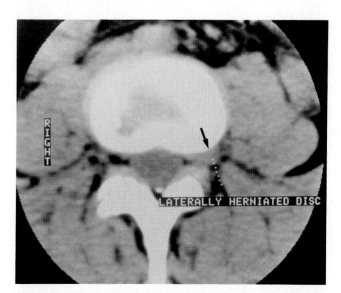

Figure 31.37. Lateral herniated disc at L3–4 on the left. Note the replacement of the normal epidural fat and image of the nerve root by the oval, high-density mass lesion representing a free-fragment extrusion into the intervertebral nerve root canal (*arrow*). The exiting L3 nerve root is displaced superiorly and compressed between the disc fragment and the pedicle of L3. Note the lack of extension into the central spinal canal and absence of mass effect on the thecal sac.

each case. If the patient was unrelieved, and the code was broken, an HRCT was performed. Those patients who had no relief of symptoms after saline injection were then treated with chymopapain.

The efficacy of chymopapain in the combined study was found to be 85%. Disc protrusion failed to retract in all but one of those patients receiving placebo (saline) (Fig. 31.51), but did retract when chymopapain was given subsequently (Fig. 31.52). The study also accurately predicted persistent impingement in those patients who were chymopapain failures. In each case, the cause was due to definite but incomplete retraction of the disc protrusion in patients in whom the incomplete disc retraction produced persistent subarticular stenosis (Fig. 31.53).

The lateral computed radiograph showed marked loss of disc height in those patients injected with chymopapain, however. In no case did lateral stenosis occur after chymopapain injection where CT had shown no evidence of lateral stenosis on the preinjection films (Fig. 31.54). Conversely, two patients who were rejected from this study because they were shown to have concomitant lateral spinal stenosis disregarded our advice, and received chymopapain injections in Canada. In each instance, the patient was unimproved initially and each became significantly worse within a week of the injection of chymopapain. Subsequently, HRCT demonstrated not only a worsening of the lateral spinal stenosis due to acute loss of disc height, but the acute appearance of degenerative spondylolisthesis in one of the patients (Fig. 31.55). We have seen one other patient injected with chymopapain 13 years prior in whom severe degenerative spondylolisthesis had developed at the injected L3–4 level.

On the basis of this limited experience, it is our belief that HRCT should be obtained on all patients considered for injection of chymopapain because of its high degree of accuracy in the diagnosis of herniated disc disease and also to exclude concomitant bony stenoses. We believe

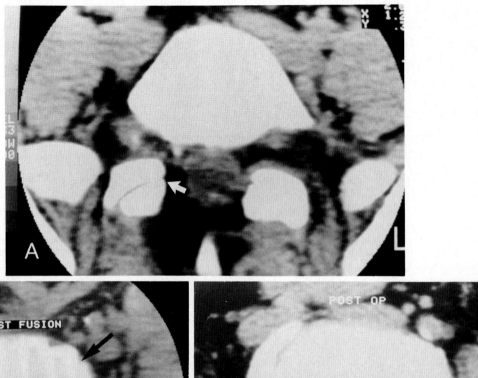

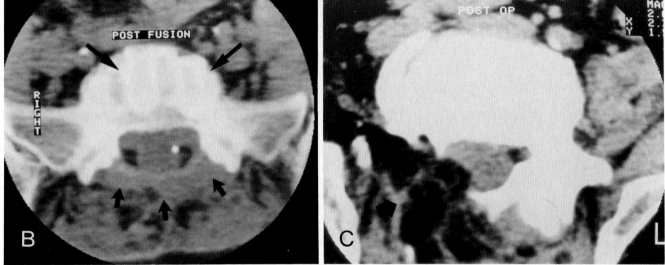

Figure 31.39. Postoperative CT spine scans. A. Decompressive laminectomy with partial medial facetectomy at L5-S1 on the right (*arrow*), and a large volume free-fat graft. Note the absence of postoperative epidural fibrosis. B. Postoperative decompressive laminectomy with marked epidural fibrosis extending onto the posterior aspect of the thecal sac (*arrows*) and onto the left S1 nerve root. Note the posterior interbody fusion as evidenced by several large dense bone plugs overlying the vertebral body (*large arrows*). C. Hemilaminectomy and total facetectomy at L5-S1 on the right with placement of a large volume of free-fat graft (*arrow*).

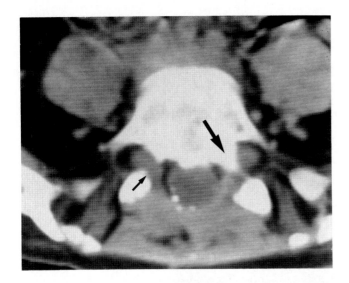

Figure 31.40. Postoperative posterior interbody fusion with posterior displacement of a bone plug into the left L5-S1 nerve root canal (*large arrow*). Note the extensive postoperative epidural and perineural fibrosis extending onto the right L5 nerve root and ganglia (*small arrow*).

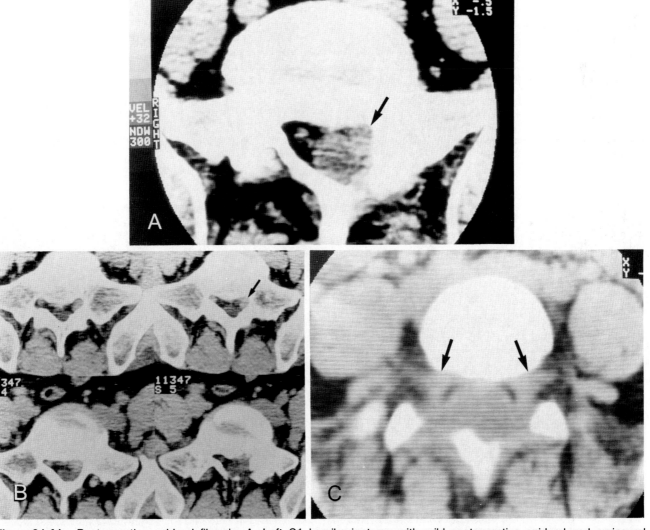

Figure 31.41. Postoperative epidural fibrosis: A. Left S1 hemilaminotomy with mild postoperative epidural and perineural fibrosis. The perineural fibrosis envelopes the left S1 nerve root, however the nerve root can be seen through the fibrosis. Note the loss of epidural fat on the left and enlargement of the outline of the left S1 nerve root (*arrows*). B. Left-sided epidural and perineural fibrosis producing enlargement of the left S1 nerve roots (*arrow*). C. Severe epidural and perineural fibrosis in a patient with posterior interbody fusion. The severe epidural and perineural fibrosis envelopes the thecal sac and extends onto the exiting L5 nerve roots (*arrows*).

that in properly selected patients, chymopapain will be an appropriate therapeutic modality and should decrease the necessity for laminectomy and discectomy considerably.

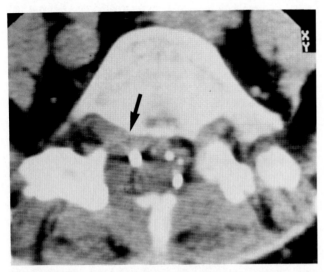

Figure 31.42. Marked epidural fibrosis extending into the central canal at the L5-S1 level which obscures the margin of the L5-S1 disc and extends onto the exiting L5 nerve roots (*arrow*). There are residual droplets of Pantopaque within the lumbar subarachnoid space.

NEW SURGICAL TECHNIQUES

The excellent anatomical depiction of the bony anatomy of the lumbar spine and the causes of nerve root impingement of HRCT allow the surgeon and radiologist to collaborate in planning the surgical procedure. The key to successful surgical technique is successful decompression of the bony impingements noted without producing instability. CT is very useful in both preoperative surgical planning and evaluation of postoperative FBSS patients to determine the exact etiology of the persistent symptomatology. Inadequate decompression is easily determined (Fig. 31.56). This use of CT has led to innovative and individualized approaches to specific pathological entities and impingement syndromes. It allows the surgeon to determine whether a more extensive procedure is indicated. In general, the experience gained in our institution has tended to lead toward a more extensive operative approach with laminectomy and bilateral medial facetectomy for the treatment of lateral stenosis. Preoperative HRCT also should be a valued modality for proper patient selection by those surgeons utilizing microsurgical technique for discectomy. CT scanning can identify easily and accurately those patients who have a small, limited disc protrusion and no associated bony nerve root impingement. These would seem to be the only candidates in whom microsurgical approach would be indicated, because this approach could not address the more extensive lesions noted in other patients with large herniations and/or bony stenosis.

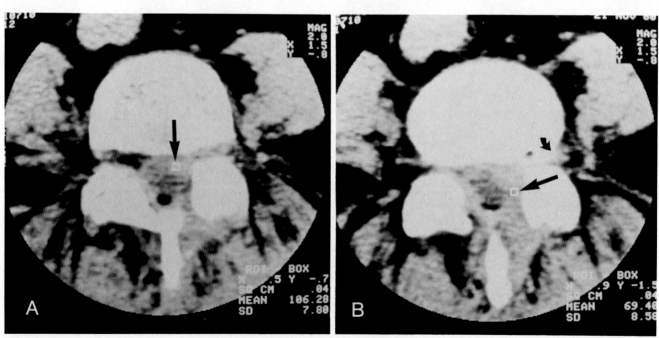

Figure 31.43. Attenuation values of epidural fibrosis and recurrent herniated disc. Surgically confirmed recurrent herniated left L4–5 disc underlying postoperative epidural fibrosis. Attenuation values (*small boxes*) (*arrow*) indicative of disc (A) and of fibrosis (B) were 106 and 69 HU, respectively. Note swelling of the left L4 nerve root due to concomitant lateral spinal stenosis at L4–5 on the left (*curved arrow*).

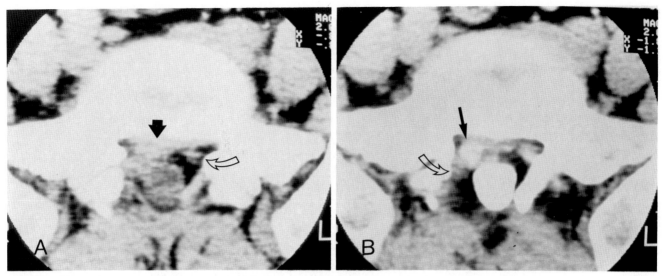

Figure 31.44.   A. A large triangular soft-tissue density anterior to the thecal sac on the right obliterates the epidural fat and right S1 nerve root. There is definite epidural fibrosis posteriorly within the central canal which is of a similar density to the area in question. On the basis of the plain CT scan, one cannot differentiate between recurrent herniated disc and fibrosis (*arrow*). Note the normal epidural fat and S1 nerve root on the left (*curved arrow*). B. Metrizamide-enhanced CT scan showing epidural fibrosis (*curved arrow*) surrounding the distorted right S1 nerve root sheath (*arrow*).

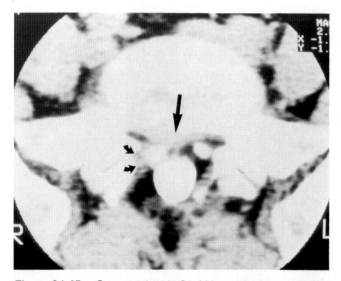

Figure 31.45.   Same patient in 31.44A and B. An underlying recurrent herniated right L5-S1 disc displaces the S1 nerve root sheath posteriorly (*large arrow*). Note the surrounding perineural fibrosis (*small arrows*).

A lateral approach to decompressive foraminotomy has been found to be unsuccessful in decompressing bony stenosis of the intervertebral nerve root canal because of the inaccessability of the medial aspect of the SAP (Fig. 31.57).

A lateral approach to the removal of true lateral herniated discs (foraminal discs) which lie within the lateral nerve root canal has been performed with success. Disc removal and discectomy can be achieved without need

for a hemilaminectomy, pediculectomy, or facetectomy (Fig. 31.58). For this group of patients, the surgical procedure is simplified and no possible instability can occur because of the lack of bony resection.

A prediction of stable and unstable configuration of the Z-A joints is also possible (Fig. 31.59). Visualization of the plane and configuration of the Z-A joints on the preoperative scans is utilized to plan the surgical approach for the plane of the facetectomy. The optimal bony resection which will allow decompression of the bony nerve root impingement and maintain adequate facet joints for maintaining stability can be determined.

SUMMARY

HRCT evaluation of the bony spinal canal in FBSS patients with low back pain and sciatica provides a definitive radiographic evaluation of the diverse bony nerve root impingement syndromes. This clear and complete depiction of the bony and soft-tissue anatomy which the surgeon will be encountering provides a detailed understanding of the exact location and extent of the pathology present, as well as its contribution to lumbar nerve root impingement. This permits a complete, reasoned, preoperative surgical plan for decompression. This increased knowledge and improved diagnostic accuracy before the first surgical procedure will decrease the number of FBSS patients and has improved the salvage rate in those patients already suffering from this entity, as evidenced by the following statistics.

Between 1977 and 1982, 250 patients with FBSS were operated on by Burton et al. (2). All patients had preoperative HRCT scans and had an average of two prior surgical

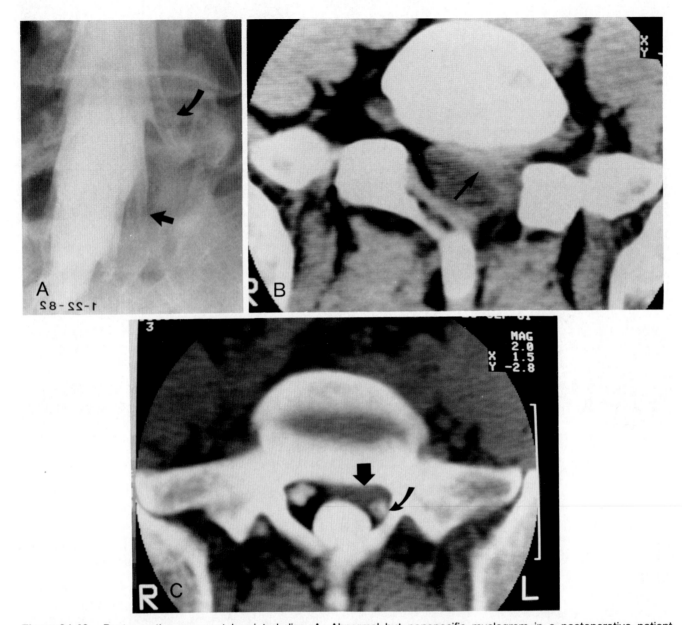

Figure 31.46. Postoperative recurrent herniated disc: A. Abnormal but nonspecific myelogram in a postoperative patient suspected of recurrent disc herniation and known epidural fibrosis (*arrows*). B. Axial unenhanced CT scan of L5-S1 with a large triangular uniform soft-tissue density occupying the anterolateral aspect of the central canal and causing posterior displacement of the thecal sac (*arrow*). One cannot differentiate clearly between recurrent disc herniation and fibrosis, although the mass effect favors a recurrent herniated disc. C. Metrizamide-enhanced CT scan shows a large-soft-tissue density (*arrow*) causing posterior displacement of the metrizamide-filled left S1 nerve root sheath (*curved arrow*), thus, confirming the suspicion of recurrent herniated disc.

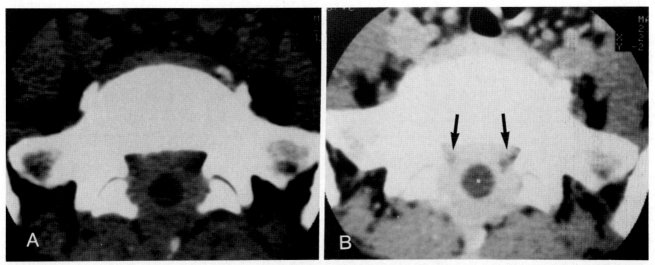

Figure 31.47.   A. Unenhanced CT spine scan with posterior decompressing laminectomy and very extensive postoperative epidural and perineural fibrosis. B. CT scan of the same image following contrast enhancement. Note the delineation of the S1 nerve roots (*arrows*) as well as the low density of the dural contents with respect to the enhancing fibrotic mass. Note that the fibrosis enhances relative to the spinous musculature which was similar in attenuation values to the fibrosis before enhancement. (Contributed by Jack Melamed, Director of Radiology, Grant Hospital, Chicago, IL).

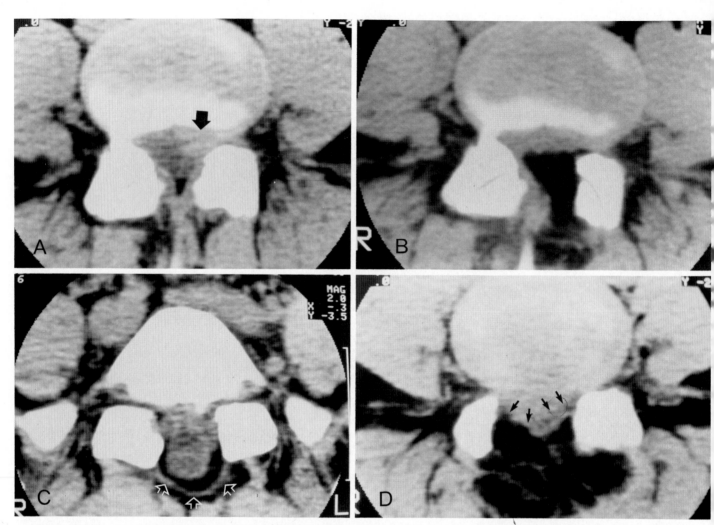

Figure 31.48. Large-volume free-fat grafting: A. Preoperative CT scan showing a large, free-fragment herniated left L4–5 disc (*arrow*). B. Postoperative CT scan showing resection of the herniated disc, placement of a large fat-graft which is causing marked compression of the thecal sac. Despite considerable compression of the thecal sac by these large-volume fat grafts immediately after surgery, no symptoms referrable to nerve root compression is appreciated. C. Postoperative free-fat grafting. The formation of a pseudomembrane simulates the ligamentum flavum (*arrows*). Note the underlying viable free-fat graft and absence of postoperative fibrosis. D. Postoperative patient with laminectomy and bilateral partial facetectomy with a large-volume free-fat graft and no evidence of postoperative epidural fibrosis. There is a large recurrent disc herniation which is of relative low density and nearly obliterates the volume of the thecal sac at this level which makes its appreciation difficult (*arrows*).

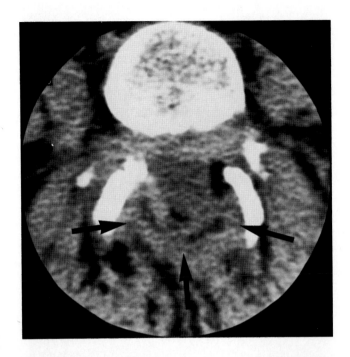

Figure 31.49. Postoperative wide decompressive laminectomy with particulate fat grafting. The particulate fat grafting technique has shown to be ineffective in preventing epidural fibrosis (*arrows*). This is presumed to be due to the small volume of fat able to be harvested at the operative site which results in the fat "floating" away from the neural elements. The fluid and blood which collects in the operative site anteceeds the formation of fibrosis.

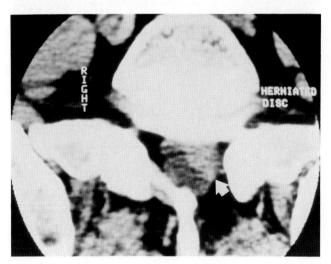

Figure 31.50. Postoperative recurrent herniated disc in a patient with a previous left hemilaminectomy and discectomy. Because of the epidural fat graft and lack of epidural fibrosis, the diagnosis of the recurrent disc herniation is no more difficult than in a previously unoperated patient (*arrow*).

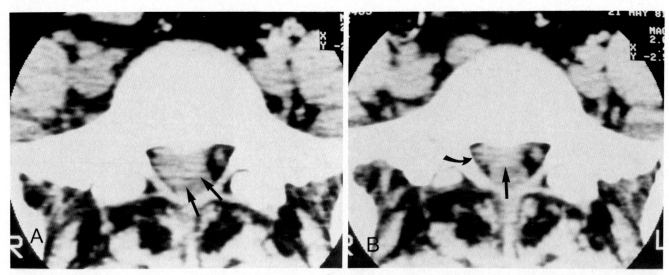

Figure 31.51.   Chymopapain in the treatment of herniated disc disease: A. Very large herniated right L5-S1 disc (*arrows*) with marked compression of the thecal sac and displacement and compression of the right S1 nerve root. B. Repeat CT scan 3 months after placebo (saline) shows a large residual disc herniation (*large arrow*) and persistent compression of the right S1 nerve root (*curved arrow*). There has been some regression in the size of the disc herniation in the 3-month interval. The patient remained symptomatic.

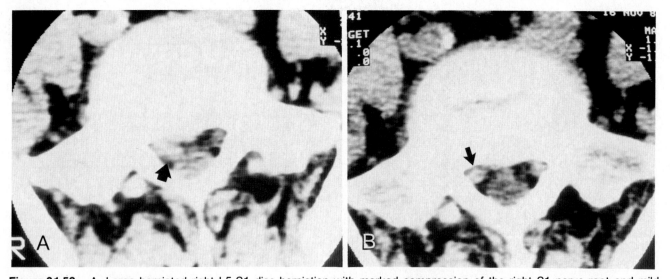

Figure 31.52.   A. Large herniated right L5-S1 disc herniation with marked compression of the right S1 nerve root and mild indentation of the thecal sac (*arrow*). B. Same patient 6 months after Chymopapain injection. There has been complete regression of the disc herniation and the right S1 nerve root is now normal in appearance (*arrow*).

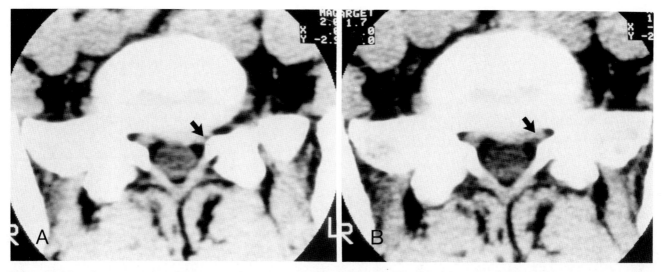

Figure 31.53.   Chymopapain failure: A. Moderate-sized herniated left L5-S1 disc with moderately severe compression of the left S1 nerve root between the disc protrusion and the base of the SAP (*arrow*). B. Six months after Chymopapain injection study. There has been definite regression of the herniated L5-S1 disc, however, persistent protrusion continues to produce mild subarticular recess stenosis with compression of the left S1 nerve root (*arrow*).

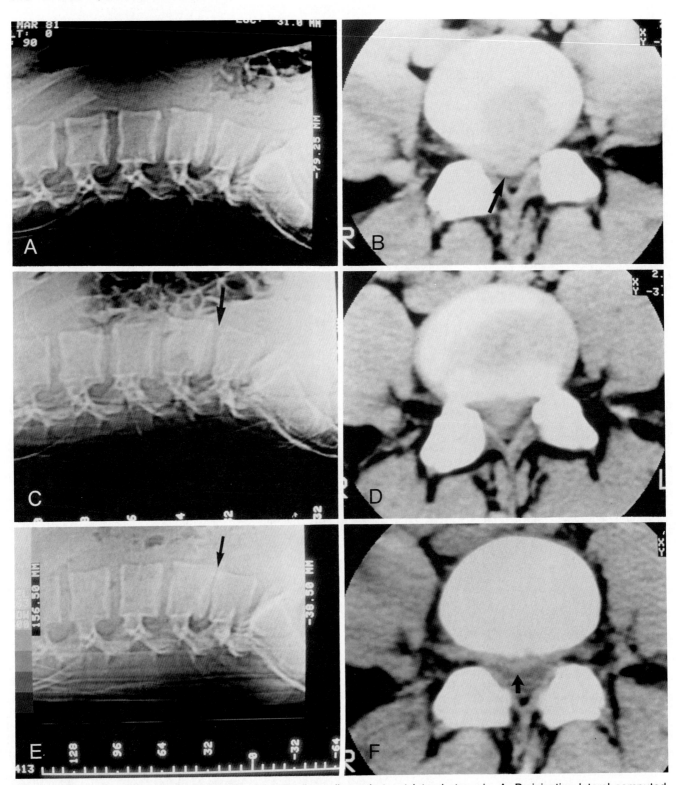

Figure 31.54.   Results of Chymopapain in producing disc collapse but not lateral stenosis. A. Preinjection lateral computed radiograph demonstrating mild disc space narrowing at both the L3–4 and L4–5 levels. B. Axial scan demonstrating a huge central herniated L4–5 disc (*arrow*). C. Lateral computed radiograph 2 months after injection of placebo (saline). No loss of disc height at the injected L4–5 level has occurred (*arrow*). D. Axial CT image at the L4–5 level demonstrates a persistent large disc herniation without apparent regression. The patient remained symptomatic. E. Six-month follow-up after Chymopapain injection shows marked loss of disc height at the injected L4–5 level (*arrow*). F. Six-month after Chymopapain injection follow-up CT scan shows marked regression of the large centrally herniated disc. There is mild residual deformity of the disc anulus (*arrow*).

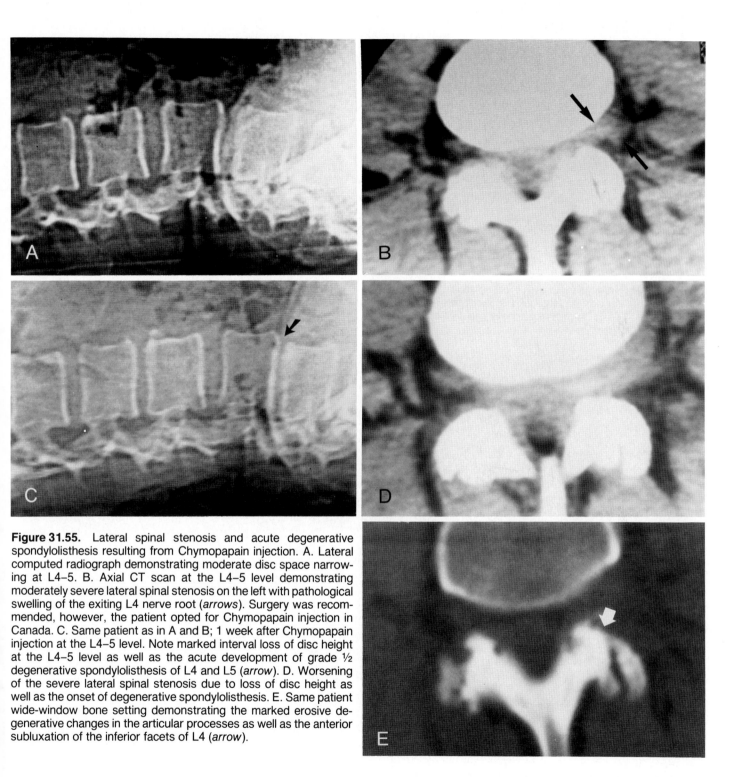

Figure 31.55. Lateral spinal stenosis and acute degenerative spondylolisthesis resulting from Chymopapain injection. A. Lateral computed radiograph demonstrating moderate disc space narrowing at L4–5. B. Axial CT scan at the L4–5 level demonstrating moderately severe lateral spinal stenosis on the left with pathological swelling of the exiting L4 nerve root (*arrows*). Surgery was recommended, however, the patient opted for Chymopapain injection in Canada. C. Same patient as in A and B; 1 week after Chymopapain injection at the L4–5 level. Note marked interval loss of disc height at the L4–5 level as well as the acute development of grade ½ degenerative spondylolisthesis of L4 and L5 (*arrow*). D. Worsening of the severe lateral spinal stenosis due to loss of disc height as well as the onset of degenerative spondylolisthesis. E. Same patient wide-window bone setting demonstrating the marked erosive degenerative changes in the articular processes as well as the anterior subluxation of the inferior facets of L4 (*arrow*).

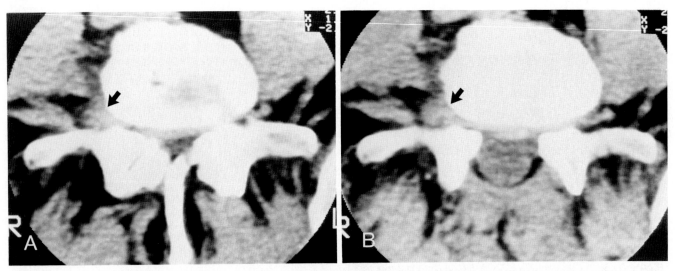

Figure 31.56. A. Preoperative CT spine scan demonstrating severe central spinal stenosis at the L5-S1 level as well as severe lateral spinal stenosis at L5-S1 with marked pathological swelling of the right L5 nerve root (*arrow*). B. Postoperative CT spine scan after central decompressive laminectomy. The patient had residual right L5 radiculopathy. Note the successful decompression of the central spinal canal, but persistent severe right lateral spinal stenosis due to failure to address the lateral spinal stenosis. There is persistent edema of the right L5 nerve root (*arrow*).

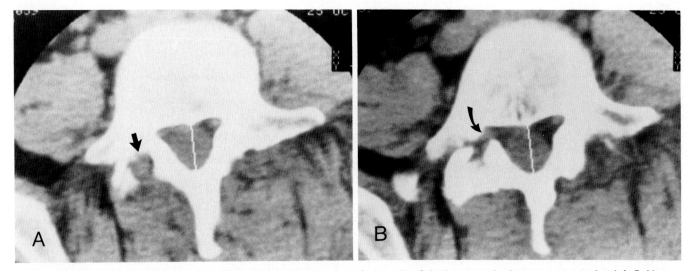

Figure 31.57. A. Lateral approach to attempted decompression of stenosis of the intervertebral nerve root canal at L4–5. Note the rounded surgical resection of the posterior aspect of the inferior articular facet (*arrow*). B. Same patient as A showing the operative defect at the caudal end of the resection. Note persistent swelling of the right L5 nerve root (*arrow*) when compared to the left. Adjacent images demonstrated persistent lateral spinal stenosis. The failure of this operative procedure was easily demonstrated by CT. Inability to resect the medial aspect of the impinging superior articular process with this lateral approach was due to inability to visualize the area with this approach.

procedures. Salvage rates of 80% objective improvement and 70% subjective improvement were obtained in a patient population of whom 30% were workmen's compensation patients. This contrasts radically with prior statistics for success rates quoted at 70% for the first surgical procedure, 30% for the second, and 5% for the third (19–21).

Although the etiology of the FBSS is complex and varied, CT now can provide an accurate preoperative diagnosis of the anatomical etiologies of this syndrome. Prior literature suggests that nonphysiological considerations such as psychological, occupational, social, monetary, motivational, and educational factors played a large role in this syndrome. However, the salvage rates described above indicate that these factors are much less prevalent and causative than supposed, and that the most significant cause of FBSS was inadequate preoperative knowledge of the pathology producing the patients' symptoms, which re-

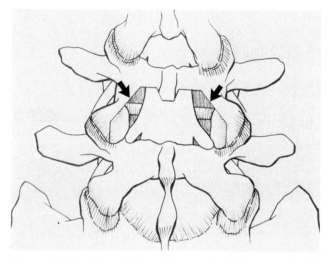

Figure 31.58. A technique of removal of the posterior elements consisting of en block removal of the lamina and inferior facets allows rapid attainment of wide exposure for decompressive laminectomy in patients with severe bilateral stenotic disease (*arrows*). (Contributed by Charles Ray, M.D., Institute for Low Back Care, Minneapolis, MN.)

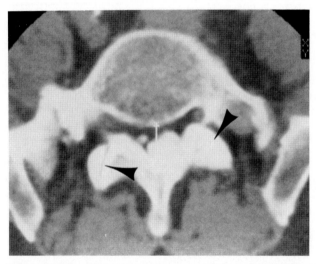

Figure 31.59. Marked asymmetry of the zygoapophyseal joints at L5-S1 with an unstable nearly sagittal orientation of the right zygoapophyseal joint and normal orientation of the left zygoapophyseal joint (*arrowheads*).

sulted in an inadequate or inappropriate surgical treatment. Because of its ability to provide this needed information, HRCT has emerged as the primary modality for assessment of the physiological causes of FBSS. The ability of HRCT to evaluate totally the gross morphology of the lumbar spine in a noninvasive manner with specific and direct imaging of nerve root compression makes it the diagnostic procedure of choice in the study of lumbar spine patients suffering from low back pain and sciatica.

For the future, the most important contribution of HRCT in patients with low back pain and sciatica will be an accurate and precise preoperative diagnosis before the first surgical procedure which should produce a marked decrease in the number of FBSS patients.

References

1. Burton CV: Lumbosacral arachnoiditis. *Spine* 3:24–30, 1978.
2. Burton CV, Kirkaldy-Willis W, Yong-Hing K, et al: Causes of failure of surgery on the lumbar spine. *Clin Orthop Relat Res* 1981.
3. Heithoff KB, Burton CV: The role of high-resolution computed tomography in the salvage of the failed back surgery syndrome patient. Presented at the International Society for the Study of the Lumbar Spine, Toronto, Canada, May, 1982.
4. Heithoff KB: High-resolution computed tomography of the lumbar spine. *Postgrad Med* 70:193–213, 1981; *In*: Genant HK, Chafetz N, Helms CA: *Computed Tomography of the Lumbar Spine.* San Francisco, University of California, Printing Department, 1982.
5. Spangfort EV: The lumbar disc herniation. A computer-aided analysis of 2504 operations. *Acta Orthop Scand* (Suppl) 142, 1972.
6. Naylor A: The late results of laminectomy for lumbar disc prolapse. *J Bone Joint Surg* 56B:17029, 1974.
7. Burton CV: Symposium: The role of spine fusion. *Spine* 6:291, 1981.
8. Crock HV: Observations on the management of failed spinal operations. *J Bone Joint Surg* 58B:193–199, 1976.
9. Kirkaldy-Willis WH, Paine KWE, Caughoix J, et al: Lumbar spinal stenosis. *Clin Orthop* 99:30–50, 1974.
10. Verbiest H: The significance and principles of computerized axial tomography in idiopathic developmental stenosis of the bony lumbar vertebral canal. *Spine* 4:369–378, 1979.
11. Postacchini F, Pezzeri G, Montanaro A, et al: Computerized tomography in lumbar stenosis. *J Bone Joint Surg* 62B:6–10, 1980.
12. White JG, et al: Surgical treatment of 63 cases of conjoined nerve roots. *J Neurosurg* 56:114–117, 1982.
13. Frymoyer JW, Hanley EN, Howe J, et al: A comparison of radiographic findings in fusion and nonfusion patients 10 or more years following lumbar disc surgery. *Spine* 4:435–440, 1979.
14. Tunturi T, Kataja M, Keski-Nisula L, et al: Posterior fusion of the lumbosacral spine—evaluation of the operative results and the factors influencing them. *Acta Orthop Scand* 50:415–425, 1979.
15. Keller JT, Dunsker SB, McWhorter JM, et al: The fate of autogenuous grafts on the spinal dura. *J Neurosurg* 49:412–418, 1978.
16. Jacobs RR, McClain O, and Neff J: Control of postlaminectomy scar formation. *Spine* 5:223–229, 1980.
17. Yong-Hing K, Reilly J, deKorompay V, et al: Prevention of nerve root adhesions after laminectomy. *Spine:* 5:59–64, 1980.
18. Schabiger O, Valavanis A: CT differentiation between recurrent disc herniation and postoperative scar formation. *Neuroradiology* 22:251–254, 1982.
19. Wedell G, Kummel EG, McCulloch JA: Failed lumbar disc surgery and repeat surgery following industrial injuries. *J Bone Joint Surg* 61-A:201–207, 1979.
20. Spangforth EV: The lumbar disc herniation. A computer-aided analysis of 2,504 operations. *Acta Orthop Scand. Suppl.* Vol. 142: pgs. 1–6, 1972.
21. Nachemson A: Pathomechanics and treatment of low back pain and sciatica. In: Stanton-Hicks M, Boas R. Editors. *Chronic Low Back Pain.* Raven Press, New York, 1982.

CHAPTER THIRTY-TWO

Lumbar Spondylosis and Stenosis: Correlation of Pathological Anatomy with High-Resolution Computed Tomographic Scanning

W. H. KIRKALDY-WILLIS, M.A., M.D., F.R.C.S. (E and C), K. B. HEITHOFF, M.D., S. TCHANG, M.D., F.R.C.P.(C), C. V. A. BOWEN, M.B., Ch.B., F.R.C.S.(C), J. D. CASSIDY, D.C., F.C.C.S.(C), and R. SHANNON, M.B., Ch.B. B.A.O., F.R.C.S.(C)*

THE CT SCAN

Transverse axial tomography represented a great advance but now is replaced by CT which permits a clear demonstration of the cross-sectional anatomy of the spine (1–4). Superb bone detail of the vertebral bodies and posterior elements that border the vertebral canal and nerve root canals can be obtained. With CT, the full spectrum of pathology contributing to central and lateral stenosis of the spine can be studied (5, 6). It is our intent to demonstrate the excellent correlation between the CT findings and those shown by dissected specimens.

The normal transaxial anatomy of the spine has been described in detail by Gargano and others (1, 2, 4), and will not be dealt with here. Previous reports of CT images of the lumbar spine have appeared in the literature (7). Our efforts have been directed to correlate pathological findings demonstrated by dissection showing central, lateral, and dynamic stenosis, as well as instability of the posterior joints with their CT counterparts, based on our radiological experience in over 600 examinations of patients suspected of having lumbar stenosis and/or spinal instability (8–11).

Technique

Preliminary lateral radiographs of the spine in flexion and extension are obtained. Scans are then obtained using a General Electric CT/T 8800 scanner with 3.3-msec pulse width, 10-second scan time, infant mode, 400 mA. Contiguous 5-mm sections are made from S1 to L3, unless a higher level must be included. The patients are scanned from below upward, because the lumbosacral junction is characteristic in appearance and allows adequate localization of sequential scans without the necessity of markers. The ScoutView has made the identification of S1 faster and more accurate. The patients are imaged in the supine position in neutral flexion. When indicated, extension and extension-rotation views are added. Routine magnification of the images is performed to enhance visualization and lineal measurement. Sagittal and coronal reconstructions are made when indicated.

Because of the 5-mm thickness of each CT slice, one must remember the thickness averaging effect in interpreting CT images of the spine. What has been described as a "partial volume" effect is present when a given structure occupies only a portion of the scan thickness, and produces a density which averages out with adjacent structures included in the slice. This effect is especially problematic in spine imaging, because bone is of much greater density than the adjacent soft tissues of the spinal canal and nerve root canals. Therefore, if 1 or 2 mm of the 5-mm slice thickness is bone and the remainder is nerve root canal, there will be an increased density of the soft-tissue structures of the nerve root canal, as well as apparent narrowing of the canal. It is for this reason that we now often rescan one particular level of interest with 5-mm, 600-MA scans overlapping every 3 mm to obtain a more accurate image.

Accurate patient repositioning is necessary for scanning of the spine in extension and extension-rotation for the evaluation of possible dynamic stenosis in order to obtain scans at comparable levels. This is facilitated greatly by using the ScoutView. The entire sequence of scans of a foramen must be evaluated, utilizing the greatest anteroposterior AP dimension of the canal for comparison, because comparison of selected single images can lead to erroneous conclusions.

Illustrative examples have been chosen at positions as nearly identical as possible, given the change in alignment of the elements of the spine relative to the incident beam with change in patient posture.

It is expected that further technological advances allowing faster reformed images in any desired projection will improve the diagnostic capabilities in the future (12).

PATHOLOGICAL CHANGES

The lumbar spine is made up of a series of vertebrae, each of which is linked to its neighbor anteriorly by an

* The authors acknowledge the early work done by Dr. K. Yong Hing and Dr. J. Reilly in the collection and preparation of pathological specimens; the authors also extend thanks to Mr. J. Junor and Mr. R. van den Buecken, Ms. Cecile Mason, and Ms. Cindy Nelson for much help with the illustrations.

intervertebral disc and posteriorly by two facet joints—
the three-joint complex. Due to the rigidity of the vertebrae, changes in any one component of this three-joint
complex must be reflected by changes in the other two
components. Thus, it is essential to consider changes in
the posterior joints and disc together in every case.

The spectrum of pathological changes in the lumbar
spine is illustrated in Figure 32.1.

Degenerative change begins at a young age. Repetitive
minor trauma, incorrect posture, and faulty or weak muscle actions produce minor compressive, shear, and rotational strains to the three-joint complex. Initially, the
lowest two lumbar levels most commonly are affected
because of the anatomical alignment of the facet joints
and wedging of the discs (13, 14).

Pathology
FACET JOINT PATHOLOGY (FIG. 32.2)

The posterior facet joint is a small diarthrodial joint
formed by the union of the convex surface of the inferior
articular process and the concave surface of the superior
articular process, which are bound together by a fibroelastic joint capsule. The relatively thin posterolateral
capsule is composed mainly of collagen fibers, whereas
the anteromedial capsule is formed by a thicker lateral
extension of the ligamentum flavum which is 80% elastin
and 20% collagen. These small joints play an active role
in resisting rotational, shear, and some compressive forces.
With repeated strains, these joints may undergo a sequence of events characteristic of degeneration in any
synovial joint, including: 1) inflammation with synovial
proliferation; 2) fibrillation and erosion of articular cartilage; 3) fibrous tissue infiltration of the joint space with
adhesion formation, 4) laxity of the joint capsule with

Progressive Changes
in Facet Joints

Dysfunction	Synovitis Hypomobility Continuing
Unstable phase	Degeneration Capsular laxity Subluxation
Stabilization	Enlargement of articular processes Osteophytes

Figure 32.2. Progressive changes in facet joints.

subluxation of the articular surfaces accompanying loss of
disc height; 5) destruction of articular cartilage with the
formation of subperiosteal new bone and osteophytes
causing enlargement of the articular processes. It is during
the later stages of this sequence of events that the posterior
joints may contribute to nerve entrapment. Pronounced
laxity of the articular capsule with facet subluxation narrows the nerve root canals which may result in lateral
spinal stenosis or nerve root entrapment. Degenerative
enlargement of the superior articular process may aggravate this condition further by causing more narrowing of
the nerve root canal. The enlarged inferior articular process protrudes posteromedially into the central canal and
may compress the cauda equina contributing to central
spinal stenosis (15, 16) (Fig. 32.3A–D, and Fig. 32.4).

INTERVERTEBRAL DISC PATHOLOGY (FIG. 32.5)

This begins with small circumferential tears in the anulus fibrosis. With time, these coalesce to form large
circumferential tears and then radial tears. At this stage,
any increase in intradiscal pressure may cause a radial
tear from the nucleus pulposus to the posterior aspect of
the disc to produce herniation of the nucleus pulposus.
With further coalescence of tears, internal disruption of
the disc occurs. Discograms show that initially this is not
accompanied by loss of disc height. Herniation of the
nucleus pulposus is now less likely to occur as the intradiscal pressure has decreased. Instability, however, is increased, leading to more straining of the posterior joints.
Later, with more loss of proteoglycans and water from the
disc, loss of disc height does occur, so that eventually the
vertebral end plates become approximated closely. Crock
calls this stage isolated disc resorption. The narrow disc
space is filled with fissured fibrous tissue and the adjacent
vertebral body bone is sclerotic. Stability is regained now,
sometimes to such an extent that true bony ankylosis can
occur (8, 10, 16–18). (See section on Soft-Tissue Pathology.)

COMBINED PATHOLOGY (FIG. 32.6)

The three-joint complex concept emphasizes that facet
joint pathology affects the disc, and disc pathology affects

Dysfunction	Dysfunctional problems	Minor rotational strains and compression injury
Unstable phase	Herniation of nucleus pulposus	Recurrent or dynamic entrapment
Stabilization	Lateral and central stenosis one level, multilevel	Fixed or static entrapment

Figure 32.1. Spectrum of change.

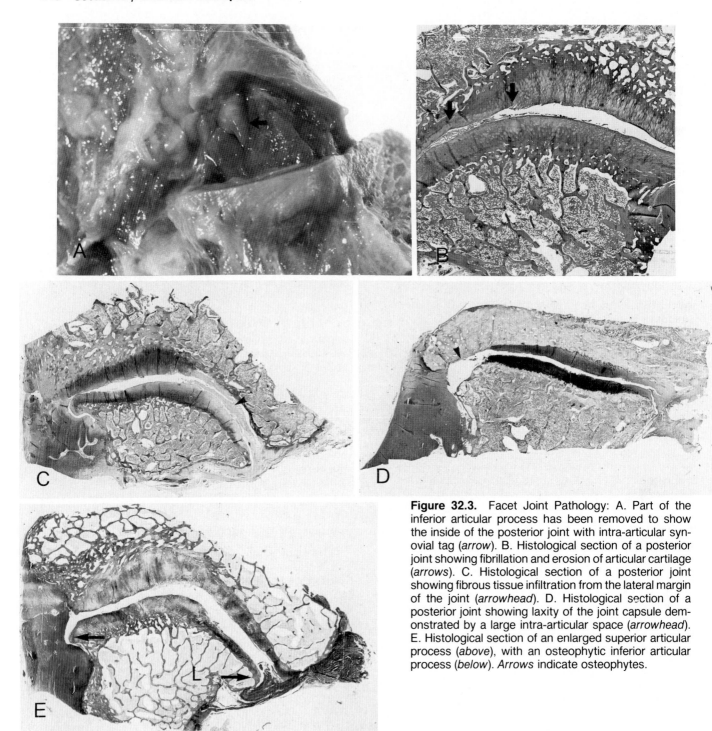

Figure 32.3. Facet Joint Pathology: A. Part of the inferior articular process has been removed to show the inside of the posterior joint with intra-articular synovial tag (*arrow*). B. Histological section of a posterior joint showing fibrillation and erosion of articular cartilage (*arrows*). C. Histological section of a posterior joint showing fibrous tissue infiltration from the lateral margin of the joint (*arrowhead*). D. Histological section of a posterior joint showing laxity of the joint capsule demonstrated by a large intra-articular space (*arrowhead*). E. Histological section of an enlarged superior articular process (*above*), with an osteophytic inferior articular process (*below*). *Arrows* indicate osteophytes.

the facet joints. Thus, clinically, combined pathological changes involving both the disc and the facet joints usually are seen—although the patient's symptoms may arise predominantly from one or the other. For example, when there is disc resorption and loss of disc height, the facet joints sublux. The superior facet moves upward and anteriorly toward the pedicle above. This causes a narrowing of the foramen and lateral recess of the nerve root canal or "lateral spinal stenosis." The inferior articular process is medial to the superior articular process and when this enlarges, the result is "central spinal stenosis."

Over a period of time, an involved spinal segment will pass through three phases as illustrated in Figure 32.1.

The initial phase is one of dysfunctional problems as-

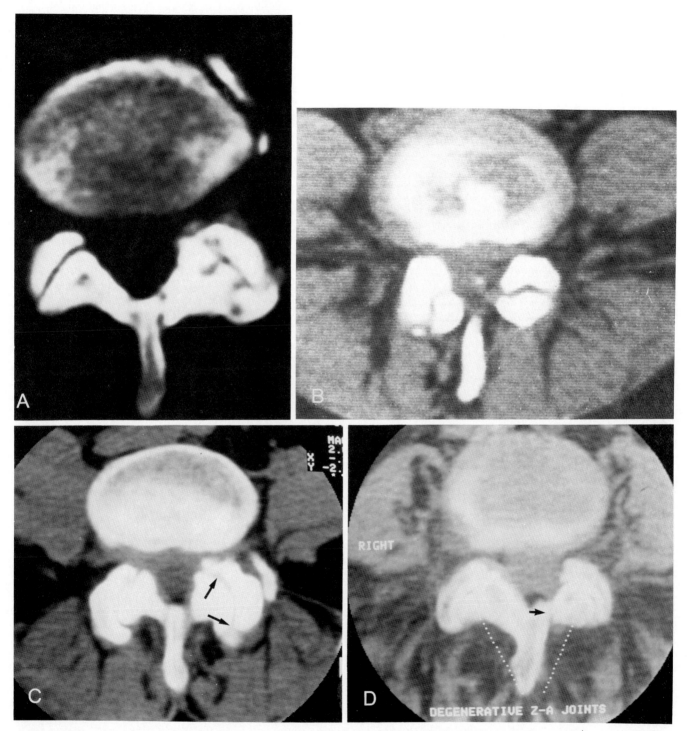

Figure 32.4.   CT Images of Facet Changes: A. Compression injury to the left facet joint with evidence of fracture of the inferior articular process, injury to articular cartilage and osteophytic enlargement of both articular processes. Note: predominantly unilateral. B. Tropism of facets. The right facet is sagittal and the left facet is coronal. C. There are healing fractures of the margins of the left superior articular process (*arrows*). D. Healed fracture of lamina on left (*arrow*). The left lamina is shorter than the right. Enlargement of the right superior facet has narrowed the lateral canal.

sociated with minor rotational strains and compression injuries.

In the second phase (internal disc disruption), the affected segment is unstable. One vertebra moves on the other in flexion/extension or rotation and causes intermittent nerve root compression—recurrent or dynamic compression. *Extension* normally narrows the foramina, but in this phase of instability, this movement may cause the superior articular process to slide sufficiently foward to narrow both the foramen and nerve root canal medial to it to such a degree that the nerve is entrapped. *Rotation* also narrows the recess, this time with anterior displacement of the superior articular process.

In the third phase (with further loss of disc height, more facet subluxation, and enlargement of the articular process), the nerve roots may be entrapped without movement, a fixed or static compression. At the L5-S1 level, lateral stenosis caused by enlargement and subluxation of the superior facet involves the L5 nerve root. Central stenosis, resulting from enlargement of the inferior articular proc-

ess or a medial osteophyte from the superior articular process may involve the S1 root at this level (19–23).

Herniation of the nucleus pulposus occurs late in the dysfunctional phase or early in the unstable phase whereas lateral and central stenosis at one level occurs later in the degenerative process.

Multilevel Pathology

The end result of changes at one level is known as one level central and/or lateral stenosis. Pathological changes at one level places the level above and below at risk. Further minor rotational strains and compression injuries affect these levels resulting in progressive degenerative changes and eventual multilevel spinal stenosis (24).

Enhancing Factors

There are other factors involved which may modify the main line of pathological change.

Developmental changes occasionally are seen in the lumbar spine. These are of two general types:

1. Developmental Narrowing. This usually affects both the sagittal and the coronal dimensions of the canal. More commonly, the whole canal is narrow, but sometimes narrowing only involves the L2 and L3 segments or the L4 and L5 segments.

2. Facet Joint Tropism. This may take several forms. Either one facet joint is in a different plane from the other or there is asymmetry of the superior articular processes— one being larger or more anteriorly placed than the other.

It is unlikely that developmental changes alone produce symptoms, but it does follow that smaller disc herniations and milder developmental changes will compromise the canal sufficiently to produce symptoms and signs of nerve entrapment (11, 24).

Direct Factors

Direct Factors also may cause or augment the stenosis.

Dysfunction	Circumferential tears Radial tears
Unstable phase	Internal Disruption Disc Resorption
Stabilization	Osteophytes

Figure 32.5. Progressive changes in intervertebral disc.

Phase	Facets	Disc	Combined pathology
Dysfunction	Synovitis Hypomobility Continuing	Circumferential tears Radial tears	Three-joint complex dysfunction Herniation
Unstable phase	Degeneration Capsular laxity Subluxation	Internal disruption Disc resorption	Herniation One level central
Stabilization	Enlargement of articular processes Osteophytes	Osteophytes	or lateral stenosis Multilevel spondylosis/stenosis

Figure 32.6. Progressive pathology of the three-joint complex.

Isthmic Spondylolisthesis

There is a mass of new bone and fibrocartilage on that part of the pars interarticularis just proximal to the fracture. This mass causes compression either on the cauda equina or on the nerve exiting at the same level (9, 25).

Degenerative Spondylolisthesis

Degeneration sometimes produces marked erosion of the superior articular process and this usually occurs at the L4 level. The inferior articular process, thus, is allowed to slip forward till it comes to rest near the posterior aspect of the vertebral body of the level below. The nerve exiting one level lower is compressed laterally between the inferior articular process and the back of the vertebral body (25–27).

Trauma

After fracture, the canal may be narrowed by new bone formation.

Paget's Disease

This may cause stenosis by vertebral enlargement.

Fluorosis

Often seen in India, this produces a great deal of new bone around the spinal canal leading to a florid type of spinal stenosis.

Postoperative changes

Postfusion (anterior or posterior)—stenosis may result in two ways: new bone formed beneath the fusion mass; at the level just above the fusion where strains are concentrated.

Postlaminectomy—fibrosis may lead to stenosis particularly if the defect is wide.

THE CT IMAGE OF THE PATHOLOGICAL CHANGES
Central Spinal Stenosis

DEVELOPMENTAL STENOSIS

At skeletal maturity the spinal canal may be narrower than normal. Coronal diameter narrowing is more troublesome than sagittal diameter narrowing. Narrowing most frequently involves the whole canal, but segmental narrowing sometimes is seen. Although developmental stenosis itself may give rise to no symptoms, a small herniation of the nucleus pulposus or a minor degree of degenerative change superimposed on diminished canal measurements may be significant (11, 24).

CT provides accurate and easily obtained measurements of the sagittal, interpedicular, and interfacet measurements of the central canal. Gargano's work indicates that the interfacet measurement is the most accurate for measuring central spinal stenosis (1, 2, 4) (Fig. 32.7A–C).

DEGENERATIVE CHANGES

Whether at one level, usually L4-L5, or many levels, this is the most common cause of central stenosis. The cauda equina is compressed both by osteophytes from the margins of the vertebral body adjacent to the disc and the enlarged osteophytic and encrusted inferior articular process that bulge posteromedially into the canal (11, 22, 24).

CT scans of central spinal stenosis caused by degenerative lesions demonstrate sclerosis and enlargement of the inferior articular processes (Fig. 32.8A and B). These encroach on the posteromedial aspect of the canal, with formation of a posterior recess and narrowing of the interfacet distance. Osteophytes from the vertebral body may be seen projecting posteriorly into the central canal. The hypertrophic changes of the inferior articular facets often are associated with thickening and sclerosis of the lamina. Patients with previous hemilaminectomies often show remodeling of the lamina on the side opposite the surgical defect, with the lamina becoming orientated more transversely, resulting in flattening of the dorsolateral aspect of the canal on that side.

SPONDYLOLISTHESIS

Degenerative. In some cases of severe degenerative change, the superior articular process, as well as becoming enlarged and craggy with osteophytes, erodes in such a way as to allow the inferior articular process to slip anteriorly. This spondylolisthesis continues until the inferior articular process comes to lie against the back of the vertebral body below. There is no defect in the pars interarticularis. Degenerative spondylolisthesis is normally seen at the L4-L5 level, but may be present at the L3-L4 or L5-S1 levels. The nerve that exits at the level below may be entrapped laterally or centrally by the marked local degenerative changes. Asymmetric facet changes lead to a rotational deformity that enhances the nerve entrapment (23, 26).

CT scans in degenerative spondylolisthesis show severe hypertrophic degenerative changes of both the superior and inferior articular processes at that level. The anterior displacement of the inferior articular process causes narrowing of the superior aspect of the lateral nerve root canal. Associated narrowing in the vertical direction due to degenerative loss of disc height distorts the margins of the nerve root canal and visualization of the emerging nerve root is difficult as it is similar in attenuation values to the adjacent disc and fibrous tissue. When this question is raised, it can be resolved with image reformating (coronal, sagittal, and off-axis reconstruction) or rescanning with overlapping images. Marked degenerative changes also may involve the superior articular facet which may also narrow the canal (Fig. 32.9A–D).

Isthmic. When the slip is of a marked degree, kinking of the dura, as it passes posteriorly at the level of the defect, may produce cauda equina compression. Degenerative changes just above the defect may produce central stenosis (9, 23).

CT scans in isthmic spondylolisthesis demonstrate the break in the pars, and elongation of the AP dimension of the central canal at the level of the slip. A transverse band of lower density, which appears to bisect the vertebral body on transverse scans, is produced by transverse imaging of the obliquely angulated disc space at the level of the slip. The vertebral body is imaged anteriorly to this band, and the posterior superior portion of the caudal vertebral body is imaged posteriorly to it. If the slip is

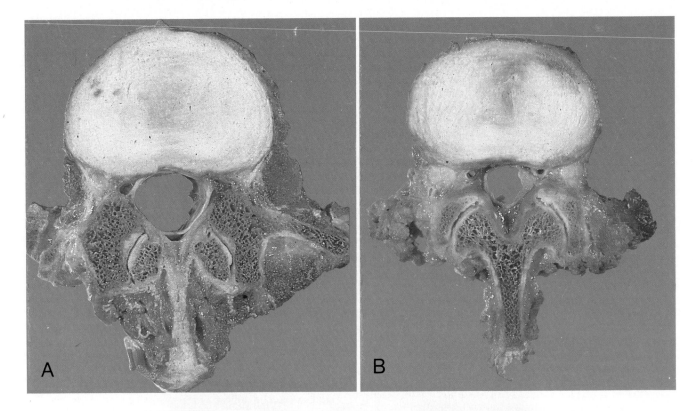

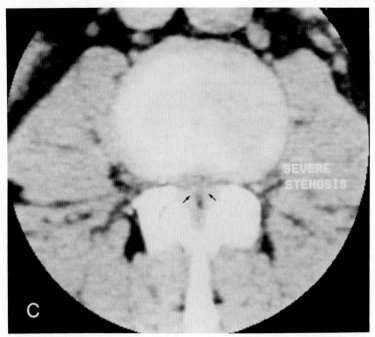

Figure 32.7. Central Developmental Stenosis: A. Normal canal at L3–4. (Reproduced with permission from Kirkaldy-Willis WH, Heithoff K, Bowen CVA, et al: Pathological anatomy of lumbar spondylosis and stenosis, correlated with the CT scan. In: Post MJD: *Radiographic Evaluation of the Spine: Current Advances with Emphasis on Computed Tomography.* New York, Masson Publishing, USA, Inc., 1980, pp. 33–55.) B. Narrow canal at L4–5 (same autopsy case) (Reproduced with permission from Kirkaldy-Willis WH, Heithoff K, Bowen CVA, et al: Pathological anatomy of lumbar spondylosis and stenosis, correlated with the CT scan. In: Post MJD: *Radiographic Evaluation of the Spine: Current Advances with Emphasis on Computed Tomography.* New York, Masson Publishing, USA, Inc., 1980, pp. 33–55.) C. CT image of narrow canal at L4–5 (*arrows*). Thickening of the ligamentum flavum and mild disc bulging produce the characteristic triangular concave outward configuration of the thecal sac seen in central spinal stenosis.

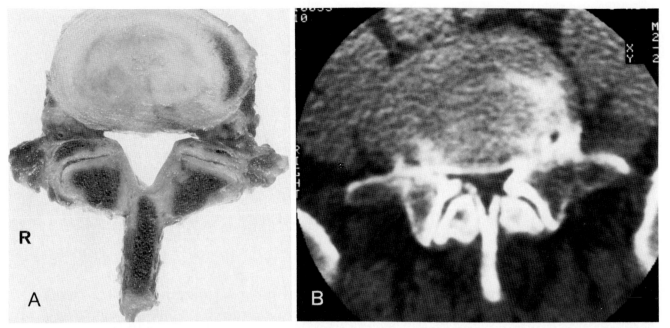

Figure 32.8.   Central Degenerative Stenosis: A. The central canal is small and trefoil in shape, due to enlargement of inferior and superior articular processes on both sides. (Reproduced with permission from Kirkaldy-Willis WH, Heithoff K, Bowen CVA, et al: Pathological anatomy of lumbar spondylosis and stenosis, correlated with the CT scan. In: Post MJD: *Radiographic Evaluation of the Spine: Current Advances with Emphasis on Computed Tomography.* New York, Masson Publishing, USA, Inc., 1980, pp. 33–55.) B. CT image of central stenosis at L4–5. Both inferior and superior articular processes bulge toward the midline on both sides.

marked, the apparent elongation of the central canal is extreme and may be bisected by a thin rim of bone representing the posterior-superior rim of the vertebral body below (Fig. 32.10A–C).

POST-TRAUMA

With fractures in the lumbar spine, immediate cauda equina compression may result if the posterior aspect of the vertebral body is driven backward. Later changes include new bone formation narrowing the central canal from the front and degenerative changes resulting from instability at the level of injury.

In acute fractures, the CT scan clearly delineates the size and location of displaced body fragments, shows the presence or absence of posterior element fracture, and demarcates the extent of local hemorrhage.

Post-traumatic degenerative changes produce either the appearance of narrowing of the anterior aspect of the spinal canal by dense sclerotic bone projecting from the posterior aspects of the vertebral body or sclerosis and enlargement of the posterior articular process due to instability or secondary spondylotic changes (Fig. 32.11A–C).

POSTFUSION STENOSIS

New bone formation beneath the laminae (in the case of posterior fusion) or at the back of the vertebral bodies (after anterior fusion) may cause canal narrowing. More frequenty, however, postfusion degenerative stenosis is

seen one level above the fusion mass as a result of a concentration of strains at this level. The enlarged articular processes protrude posteromedially into the canal to compress the cauda equina. There is also internal disc disruption (23, 25).

CT scans, in patients with postfusion stenosis at the level above the fusion, show narrowing of the canal produced by sclerosis and enlargement of the posterior articular processes and, also, osteophyte formation from the vertebral body. New bone under the fusion mass often obliterates anatomical detail of the posterior articular processes and laminae. Bony overgrowth produces narrowing of the posterolateral aspect of the spinal canal (Fig. 32.12A–C).

Lateral Spinal Stenosis. Nerve root entrapment in the lateral recess may occur in one of two ways:

1. Dynamic or recurrent compression by either extension or rotation.
2. Fixed or static compression at one or more levels.

Recurrent or dynamic compression occurs during Phase II (unstable phase) and fixed or static compression during Phase III (stabilization). It is easier, however, to understand the process by reviewing the changes seen in the static type first.

Fixed or Static Lateral Stenosis

DEVELOPMENTAL STENOSIS

Just as the central canal can be narrow at the end of development, so can the lateral recess. Often it is difficult

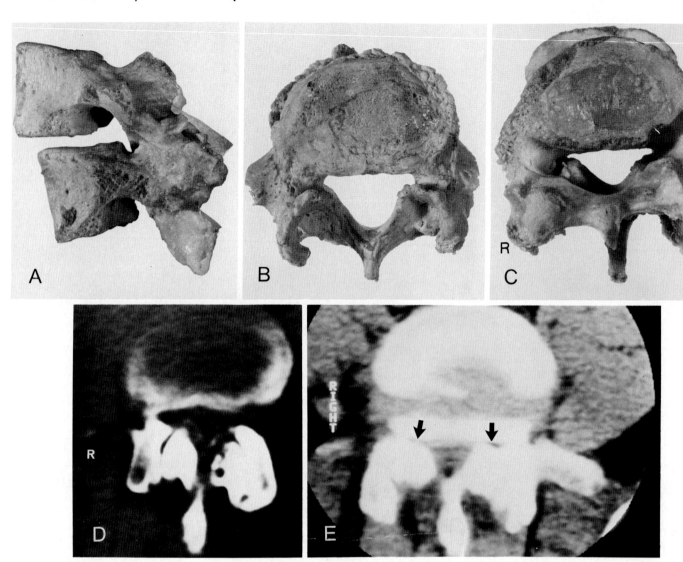

Figure 32.9. Degenerative Spondylolisthesis: A. Lateral view of L4 and L5 vertebrae, L4 has slipped forward on L5 to a marked degree. The anterior aspect of the inferior articular process of L4 is almost touching the posterior aspect of the body of L5. B. Transverse view of the L5 vertebra seen from above. There is marked erosion of the superior articular processes. C. Transverse view of L4 and L5 seen from below. The inferior articular processes of L4 almost touch the back of the body of L5, especially on the right. (Courtesy of Dr. H. F. Farfan) (Reproduced with permission from Kirkaldy-Willis WH, Heithoff K, Bowen CVA, et al: Pathological anatomy of lumbar spondylosis and stenosis, correlated with the CT scan. In: Post MJD: *Radiographic Evaluation of the Spine: Current Advances with Emphasis on Computed Tomography.* New York, Masson Publishing, USA, Inc., 1980, pp. 33–55.) D. CT image of L4–5 in a patient with marked degenerative spondylolisthesis. This specimen shows marked erosion of the superior articular facets with forward slipping of the inferior articular facet on the right side. E. CT image at L4–5 in a patient with degenerative spondylolisthesis. Note the marked erosion of the superior processes and narrowing of the lateral recesses due to erosion of the superior and forward displacement of the inferior processes (*arrows*).

on radiological examination, at operation, and even at autopsy to decide whether changes at any given level are due to developmental or degenerative causes. From the studies of Verbiest and Huisinga in Holland, it seems likely that developmental changes are more important than generally recognized. Sometimes marked asymmetry of the two posterior facet joints at one level causes narrowing of the lateral recess on one side and it seems likely that developmental anomalies are the cause.

In the CT scan, lateral stenosis, caused by developmen-

tal anomalies with marked asymmetry of the two posterior joints at one level, demonstrates sclerosis and hypertrophic enlargement on the side of the stenosis. This may involve the lamina and the inferior and superior articular processes. A continuation of central and lateral stenosis may result (Fig. 32.13).

DEGENERATIVE STENOSIS

In the later stages of degeneration, Crock's isolated disc resorption is seen (19). Anteriorly, there is loss of disc

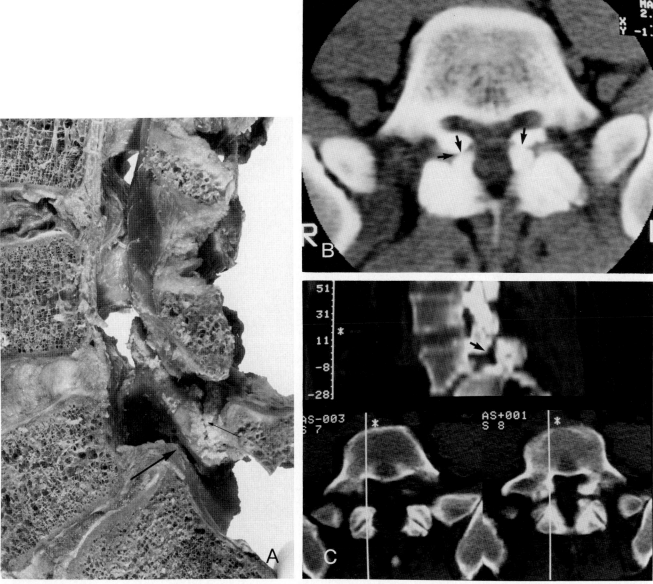

Figure 32.10. Isthmic Spondylolisthesis: A. Sagittal section. Note the defect in the pars articularis (*left arrow*). The pars above the defect (*right arrow*) is enlarged and displaced forward to narrow the lateral recess. (Reproduced with permission from Kirkaldy-Willis WH, Heithoff K, Bowen CVA, et al: Pathological anatomy of lumbar spondylosis and stenosis, correlated with the CT scan. In: Post MJD: *Radiographic Evaluation of the Spine: Current Advances with Emphasis on Computed Tomography.* New York, Masson Publishing, USA, Inc., 1980, pp. 33–55.) B. Axial CT image of lytic spondylolisthesis at L5-S1 shows elongation of the central canal at the level of the slip and the lytic defects of the pars (*arrows*). The L5-S1 Z-A joints lie dorsal to the pars of L5. C. Sagittal and axial CT images of lytic spondylolisthesis. Note the ample size of the lateral nerve root canals. The lytic defect is well visualized (*arrow*).

height, approximation of the vertebral end plates and local bony sclerosis. Posteriorly, the articular processes are enlarged and craggy with osteophyte formation. The joints with their lax capsules are subluxed. The superior articular process moves upward and forward, and there is slight retrospondylolisthesis as the vertebral body above moves slightly backward. The result is narrowing of the lateral foramen and lateral recess (20–22, 25).

This type of stenosis is seen most frequently at the L5-S1 level. Nerve entrapment can occur in two ways:

1. The L5 nerve, between the superior facet and the pedicle.
2. The S1 nerve; medially in a narrow recess between the superior facet and the back of the vertebral body and disc or from medial osteophytic enlargement of the superior facet.

Osteophytes from the back of the vertebral bodies enhance this entrapment.

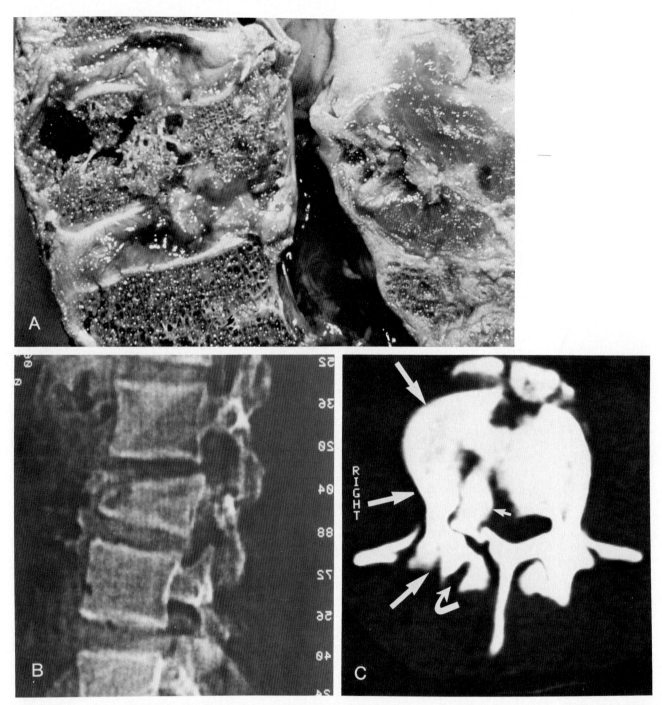

Figure 32.11.   Central Stenosis after Trauma: A. Sagittal section: the crushed vertebral bodies have been displaced backward to narrow both the central and lateral canals. B. Lateral Computed Radiograph: the crushed fracture of the vertebral body is visualized, but the full extent of the fracture and disruption of the spinal canal is not appreciated. C. The CT scan clearly depicted the severity of the injury; the fracture involves both vertebral body and the posterior arch. There is posterior displacement and counterclockwise rotation of a large right-sided fragment which consists of vertebral body, pedicle, and Z-A joint (*three large arrows*). This causes the superior and inferior articular facets to lie posterior to the associated lamina, disrupting the central canal. The posterior fractures involve the lamina at the base of the inferior articular process, the right midlamina, and the right transverse process. There is diastasis of the right Z-A joint (*curved arrow*), and a large fragment of the posterior aspect of the vertebral body extends into the right anterolateral aspect of the central canal (*small arrow*).

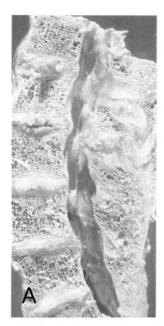 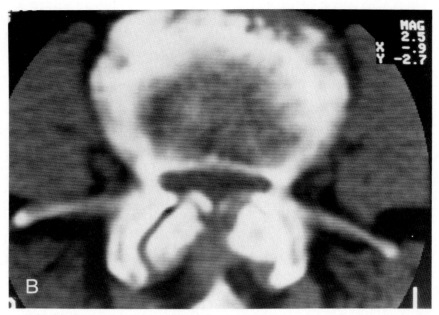

Figure 32.12. Postfusion Stenosis: A. Sagittal section showing a solid posterior fusion from L3 to sacrum; the discs beneath the fusion are normal; the posterior joints and disc at L2–3 have undergone degenerative change and this has produced stenosis. B. CT image at L4–5 showing a solid posterior fusion: the central and lateral canals are very markedly reduced in size.

CT scan experience shows that lateral stenosis is more common than central stenosis. Narrowing of the disc space and associated degenerative changes in the vertebral bodies and posterior joints produce both AP and vertical narrowing of the lateral recess, nerve root canal, and nerve root foramen. The most common abnormality is hypertrophy of the superior articular facet, which narrows the lateral recess medial to the foramen as well as the nerve root canal laterally. Resorption of the disc, resulting in upward and forward movement of the superior articular process, produces apparent narrowing in the AP plane at the upper aspect of the foramen. This may extend as far as the pedicle above. Degenerative enlargement of the articular process further narrows the canal. Anteromedial enlargement of the superior facet narrows the lateral recess medial to the foramen. Vertebral body sclerosis is not infrequent, and often osteophytes project posterolaterally to produce greater narrowing and entrapment. (Fig. 32.14)

SPONDYLOLISTHESIS

Degenerative

Occasionally in degenerative spondylolisthesis, the nerve root that exits one level lower may be entrapped laterally by marked local degenerative changes or in a narrow recess between the superior articular process and the back of the vertebral body and the disc (26).

Isthmic

Here the spinal nerve that exits at the level of the slip is entrapped by anterior displacement and enlargement of that part of the pars interarticularis that lies immediately above the defect. The loose fragment (inferior pars lamina

and inferior articular processes) rarely, if ever, causes nerve entrapment. Degenerative changes at the level above the defect may lead to nerve entrapment at this higher level but this is not common (9).

On the CT scan, the nerve root canal is poorly defined in isthmic spondylolisthesis because of anterior and inferior displacement of the superior aspect of the pars interarticularis above the defect into the nerve root canal. On transverse imaging, the upper part of the pars interarticularis is seen to be displaced anteriorly. When nerve root compression is present, the exiting nerve roots are compressed between the pedicle and pars of the vertebra above and the vertebral body of the vertebra below. Nerve root compression, flattening, and/or pre- and poststenotic swelling are direct signs of nerve root involvement. (Figs. 32.10A–C).

POST-TRAUMATIC

Lateral stenosis may result from trauma in much the same way as central stenosis.

POSTOPERATIVE

After Laminectomy

Dense scar tissue may form posteriorly in the laminectomy defect. This is particularly marked after a wide laminectomy. Postoperative fibrosis is a uniform accompaniment of surgery unless free-fat grafts are placed.

After Fusion

Lateral stenosis may be seen at the level above a fusion. It is seen most commonly after a posterior fusion (Fig. 32.15).

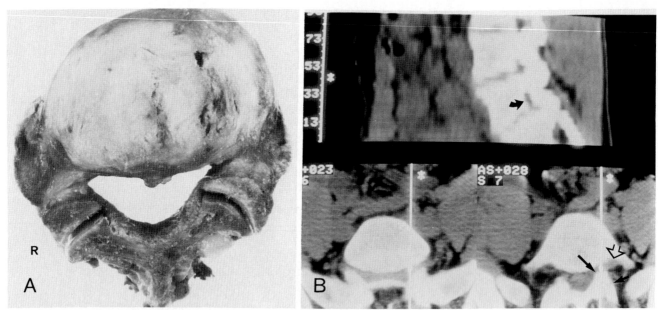

Figure 32.13. Lateral Developmental Stenosis: A. Transverse section at L5-S1. The pedicle on the left is shorter than that on the right. There is asymmetry of the neural arch. This may be a developmental abnormality or possibly the result of trauma. (Reproduced with permission from Kirkaldy-Willis WH, Heithoff K, Bowen CVA, et al: Pathological anatomy of lumbar spondylosis and stenosis, correlated with the CT scan. In: Post MJD: *Radiographic Evaluation of the Spine: Current Advances with Emphasis on Computed Tomography.* New York, Masson Publishing, USA, Inc., 1980, pp. 30–55.) B. Composite axial and sagittal CT images at L5-S1: The axial images show asymmetry of the neural arch, developmental hypoplasia of the left SAP (*small arrow*), and compensatory enlargement and forward subluxation of the IAP (*large arrow*) causing lateral stenosis. Note poststenotic enlargement of the left L5 nerve root (*open arrowhead*). The sagittal reformatted image shows the constructed AP dimension of the lateral nerve root canal (*curved arrow*).

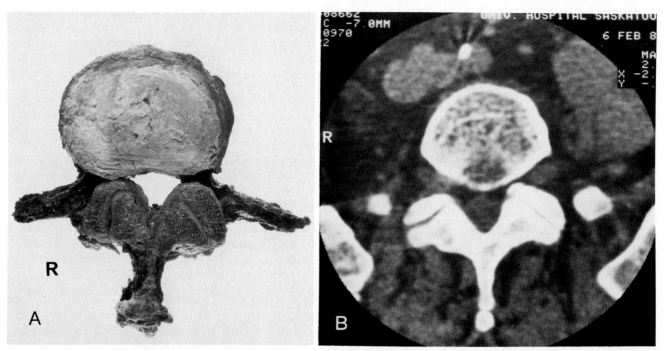

Figure 32.14. Lateral Degenerative Stenosis: A. The lateral canal on the right is narrowed markedly by forward subluxation of the articular process. (Reproduced with permission from Kirkaldy-Willis WH, Heithoff K, Bowen CVA, et al: Pathological anatomy of lumbar spondylosis and stenosis, correlated with the CT scan. In: Post MJD: *Radiographic Evaluation of the Spine: Current Advances with Emphasis on Computed Tomography.* New York, Masson Publishing, USA, Inc., 1980, pp. 30–55.) B. CT image at L4–5: there is marked stenosis of the left lateral canal.

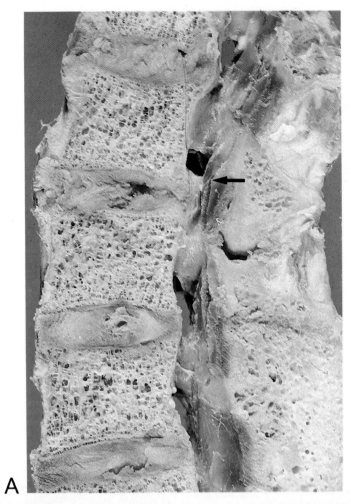

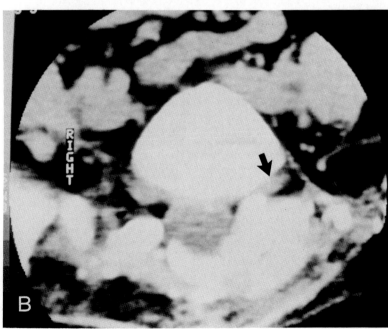

Figure 32.15. Lateral Postfusion Stenosis: A. Sagittal section from L2–4. This shows a solid posterior fusion from L3 downward. The L2–3 disc is disrupted internally. The L2–3 posterior joints are enlarged and have caused lateral stenosis at this level (*arrow*). B. CT images at L5-S1 shows a solid posterior fusion, but the lateral canal on the left is narrow—stenosis after fusion. Note relationship of fusion overgrowth to the L5 nerve root (*arrow*).

Transverse imaging on CT clearly depicts the structures of the spine to which the bony fusion is attached. With this perspective, the underlying spine is not obliterated as it is on plain radiographs and central and lateral stenosis can be evaluated easily. This may lead to the discovery that the fusion is bridging an area of instability without fusing it, or that the fusion is actually contributing to central or lateral stenosis. Not infrequently, after a posterior fusion, bony overgrowth of the fusion may spill over into the foramen and cause marked narrowing.

OTHER CAUSES OF LATERAL STENOSIS

The manner in which central stenosis is produced in Paget's disease and fluorosis has been described already. These conditions also may produce lateral stenosis (Fig. 32.20).

Dynamic or Recurrent Lateral Stenosis

When degeneration has reached the unstable phase, one vertebra is able to move on another. As increased abnormal movement occurs, the superior articular process moves forward and causes narrowing of the lateral recess. Movement is small, not commonly recognized, and difficult to measure. Each time narrowing occurs, the nerve is entrapped in the lateral recess.

Three types of recurrent entrapment are recognized: 1) from flexion/extension; 2) from rotation; 3) combined.

ENTRAPMENT RESULTING FROM ABNORMAL FLEXION/EXTENSION MOVEMENT

This kind of entrapment is seen most frequently at the L4-L5 level. Flexion images are produced with the patient supine and extension with the patient prone. Normally, in extension, the size of the foramina and lateral recess becomes smaller than in flexion. Instability at the L4-L5 level allows the superior facets to move forward to a point at which the nerve exiting at this level may be entrapped intermittently. Oblique radiographs may demonstrate that in extension the posterior joint surfaces are malaligned. Lateral radiographs in flexion and extension may show that in extension the foramen almost is obliterated by anterior displacement of the superior articular process.

When present, the displacement can be seen in transverse CT imaging. Some diminution of the AP dimension of the lateral recess occurs normally with extension. When such narrowing is pathological, however, movement on the side of the abnormality is greater because of the causative instability. In addition to the superior articular process being displaced anteriorly and narrowing the lateral recess, the facet joint space is widened (Fig. 32.16A–D).

ENTRAPMENT RESULTING FROM ABNORMAL ROTATIONAL MOVEMENT

This is seen most often at the L4-L5 level and also at that stage of degenerative change when instability is a marked feature. Rotational images are obtained with the patient supine. A pillow is placed first under one side of the pelvis and then under the other. There is internal disruption of the disc. The anulus bulges around its periphery. The capsule of the posterior joints is lax. Abnormal rotational movement takes place. At the L4-L5 level, as the spinous process of L5 rotates to the side, the superior articular process moves anteriorly on the same side. The lax posterior joint opens. At the same time, the recess is narrowed by this displacement of the superior articular process toward the back of the L4 vertebral body and the disc in front. The L5 nerve becomes entrapped laterally.

On the CT scan, it is difficult to differentiate between recurrent deformity produced by abnormal rotation and that produced by excess extension. With patients carefully positioned either in extension or rotation, it has been possible to reproduce the narrowing of the lateral recess at the unstable level, thus, confirming our clinical and pathological studies (Fig. 32.17A–E).

ENTRAPMENT RESULTING FROM COMBINED ABNORMAL ROTATIONAL MOVEMENT WITH EXCESS EXTENSION

Careful examination of autopsy specimens with L4-L5 instability suggests that the recurrent nerve entrapment often has both rotational and flexion/extension components causing narrowing of the lateral recess. When a transverse CT image is made with these patients rotated and extended simultaneously, the demonstrated narrowing is often greater than with either of these maneuvers alone. Extension may show minimally increased narrowing and extension plus rotation may show marked narrowing with excessive anterior displacement of the superior articular process. On neutral flexion CT images, the foramen demonstrating dynamic stenosis actually may be the larger of the two foramina because of greater fixed changes on the opposite side. In two such cases, the patient was asymptomatic on the side of the greater fixed changes and, at operation, was confirmed as having marked narrowing on the side of dynamic stenosis.

Combined Central and Lateral Spinal Stenosis. Central stenosis most often is caused by posteromedial protrusion of enlarged osteophyte-coated articular processes into the canal. This usually occurs late in the degenerative process. Thus, if central stenosis is present, lateral stenosis is also likely. On the other hand, lateral stenosis, particularly of the recurrent or dynamic type, occurs earlier in the overall process and is often present without involvement of the central canal (25).

Soft-Tissue Pathology and Complications. With the advent of more advanced CT technique, thinner slices are diminishing the problems associated with partial volume effect. This, in conjunction with improved resolution, is enabling local soft-tissue structures to be examined more carefully. Measurements of tissue densities allows differentiation between disc, fat, fibrosis, nerve, and fluid. Knowledge of the precise anatomical location of a soft-tissue mass plus information as to its density has enhanced our diagnostic abilities and also enables planning of operative approaches to be as extensive as necessary.

In cases of nerve root compression, not only can central and lateral entrapment be visualized, but also any asso-

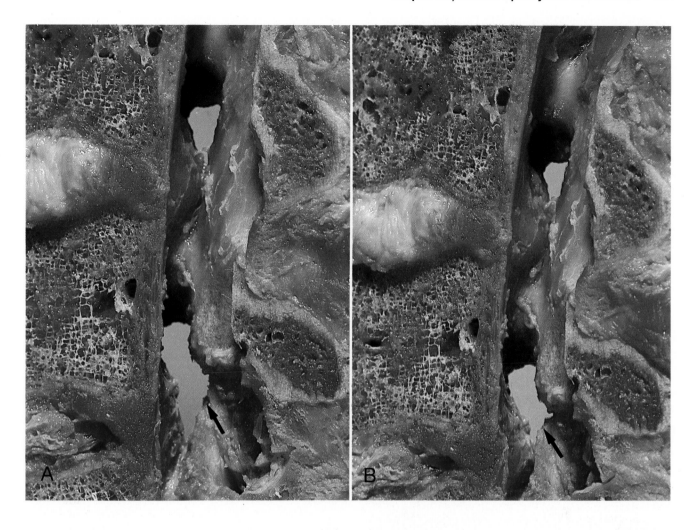

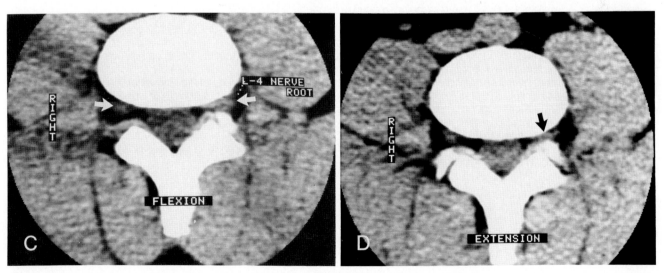

Figure 32.16.   Dynamic Lateral Stenosis in Extension: A. Sagittal section in flexion: note the size of the foramen (*arrow*). B. The same in extension: note the size of the foramen (*arrow*). Extension has narrowed the foramen. C. CT image at L4–5 in flexion: the left lateral canal is narrow. Note enlargement of the left L4 nerve root when compared to the right (*arrows*). D. The same in extension: there is further narrowing of the left lateral canal, and flattening of the L4 nerve root ganglion.

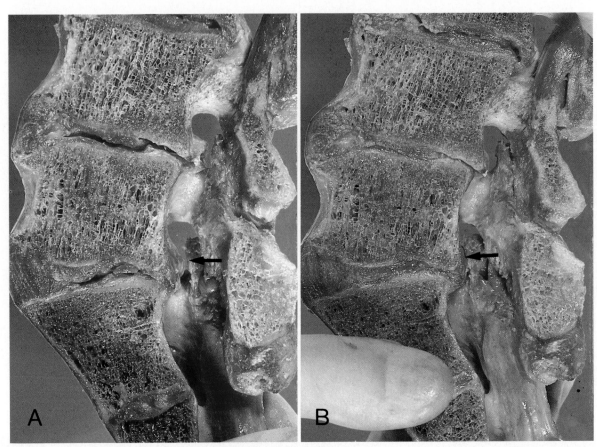

Figure 32.17. Dynamic Lateral in Rotation: A. Sagittal section from L3 to sacrum in the neutral position. There is internal disruption of the L4–5 and L5-S1 discs. At both levels, the foramina are small. B. The same in rotation. The foramina at L4–5 and at L5-S1 are even smaller. C. Transverse section at L4–5. The lateral canal on the left is narrow and that on the right appears normal. (Reproduced with permission from Kirkaldy-Willis WH, Heithoff K, Bowen CVA, et al: Pathological anatomy of lumbar spondylosis and stenosis, correlated with the CT scan. In: Post MJD: *Radiographic Evaluation of the Spine: Current Advances with Emphasis on Computed Tomography.* New York, Masson Publishing, USA, Inc., 1980, pp. 30–55.) D. The same in rotation. The lateral canal on the left has narrowed markedly as the left posterior joint has opened due to instability. (Reproduced with permission from Kirkaldy-Willis WH, Heithoff K, Bowen CVA, et al: Pathological anatomy of lumbar spondylosis and stenosis, correlated with the CT scan. In: Post MJD: *Radiographic Evaluation of the Spine: Current Advances with Emphasis on Computed Tomography.* New York, Masson Publishing, USA, Inc., 1980, pp. 30–55.) E. CT scan of the same patient as in Figure 32.16C, in rotation. There is further narrowing of the canal on the left (*arrow*).

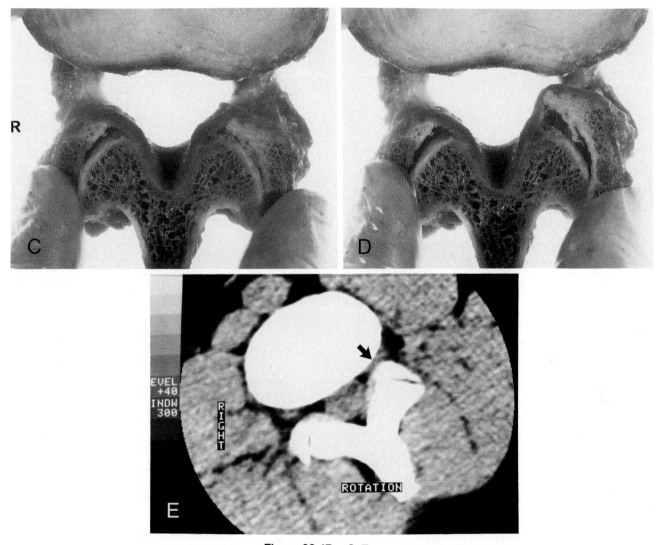

Figure 32.17.   C–E.

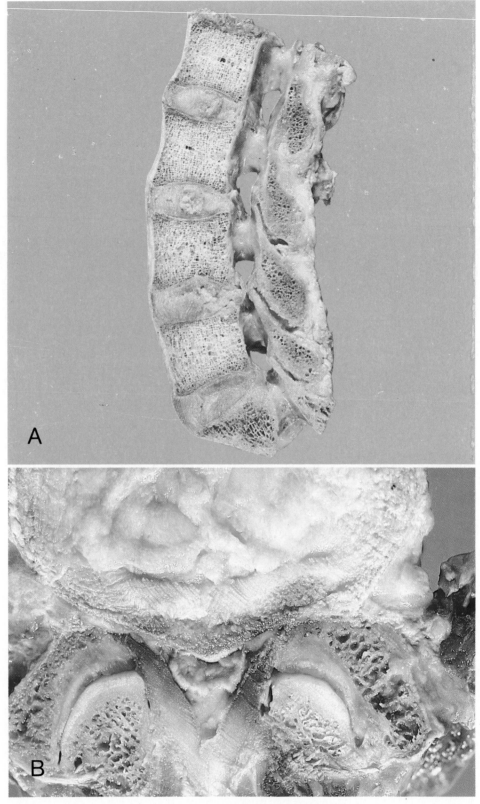

Figure 32.18.   A and B.

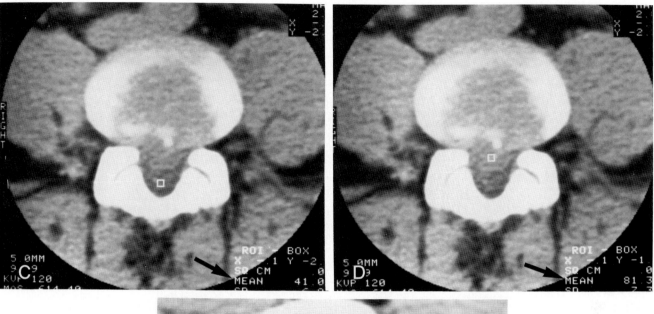

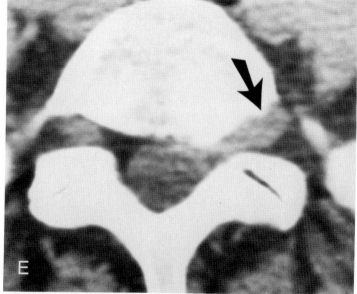

Figure 32.18. Soft-Tissue Pathology: A. Parasagittal section. Note the presence of a disc herniation with extrusion at L4–5 and the small foramen. B. Transverse section at L4–5 showing the presence of a central disc herniation with protrusion only. The central canal is narrow. There is early posterior joint cartilage degeneration. C. CT image at L4–5. The cursor is placed over the cauda equina; mean density 41.0. D. CT image of the same patient at L4–5. The cursor is placed over a large central disc herniation; mean density 81.3. E. CT image at L5–S1. Another patient. The *arrow* points to a lateral disc herniation, mean density 119. This would not be seen in a myelogram. F. CT image at L5–S1. A disc herniation was suspected, but the mean density of the soft-tissue shadow (*arrows*) was 59. At operation, a fibrous nodule was found adherent to the L5 nerve. G. CT image at L4–5 after operation and demonstrating extensive anterior and posterior epidural fibrosis extending into the central canal and onto the L4 nerve roots. Note enlargement of the L4 nerve roots caused by perineural fibrosis. Lateral stenosis on the left results from an osteophyte arising at this site. H. CT image at L5–S1. Postoperative fat graft (*black area*). Note the large size of the graft with flattening of the thecal sac, and the absence of postoperative fibrosis.

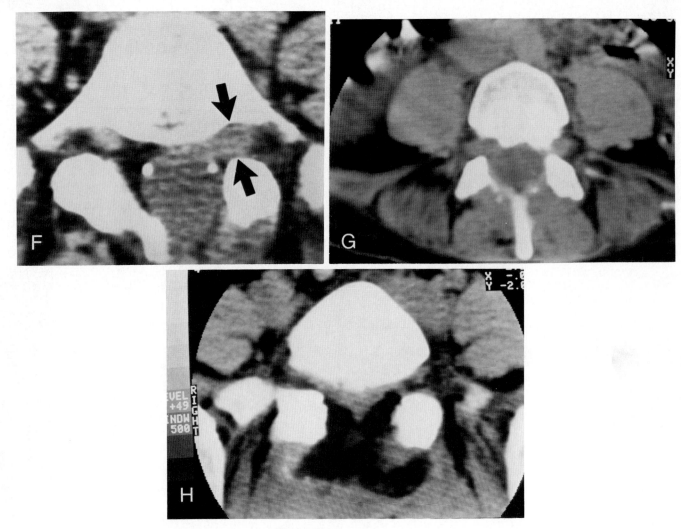

Figure 32.18.   F–H.

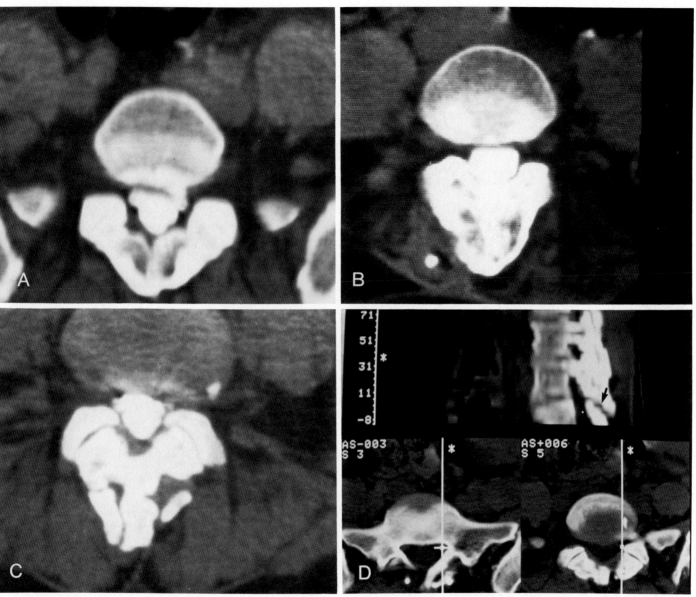

Figure 32.19.   A. CT image at L5-S1 after a posterior fusion. The fusion appears solid. The facet joints are fused. B. The same patient. Scan at L4–5. Again the posterior fusion is solid and the facet joints are fused. C. CT image at L4–5 after posterior fusion. The facet joints are not fused. There is only a small amount of graft posterior to the laminae on each side. Failure of fusion. D. Composite axial CT scans at L5-S1, and sagittal reformatted image. (The plane of the sagittal image is defined by the *white lines* on the axial images.) Note the solid fusion at L4–5 and the failure of fusion at L5-S1. The sagittal reconstructed image clearly shows that the fusion bone overlying the lamina of S1 on the left is not fused to the lamina (*arrow*). Pseudarthroses and failure of fusion are confirmed more easily by sagittal reformatted images than axial images.

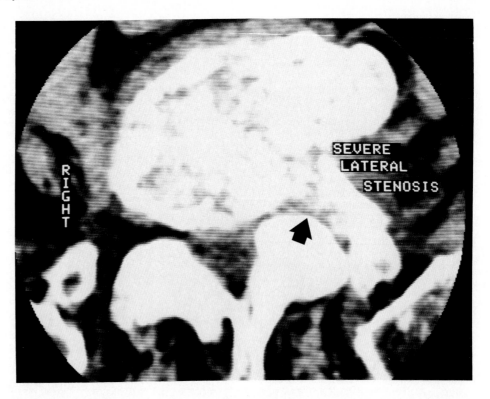

Figure 32.20. CT image of L5-S1: Paget's disease of the Lumbar Spine: There is marked expansion and sclerosis of the L5 vertebral body and left pedicle. This produces severe lateral stenosis on the left (*arrow*). Surgery confirmed marked impingement of the L5 nerve root within the lateral canal. The bone was very vascular with excessive oozing at surgery.

ciated herniation of the nucleus pulposus or thickening of the ligamentum flavum can be taken into consideration.

The image of the cauda equina can be enhanced further by a combination myelogram/CT scan. Sometimes individual nerve root ganglia also can be seen on the CT image (Fig. 32.18A–F).

Assessment of Fusion. The detection of pseudarthrosis after a fusion has been a longstanding problem. The CT scan gives detailed information as to the thickness and anatomical location of the fusion mass at any particular level. Sometimes it also has revealed that the fusion has bridged an area of instability without fusing it. Central or lateral entrapment under a fusion mass may be present. This may either result from new bone formed by the fusion or may have originally been the cause of symptoms for which fusion was used as treatment. Assessment of the upper level of the fusion may reveal that fusion is incomplete or that degenerative changes above the solid bony mass are producing stenosis (Fig. 32.19A–D).

CONCLUSION

The CT scan is now a proven diagnostic aid for the evaluation of lumbar spinal disorders. The cross-sectional images enable accurate measurement of the canal and lateral recesses. Thus, developmental anomalies or central and lateral stenosis, caused by the hypertrophic changes associated with degeneration, can be assessed qualitatively and quantitatively. More recently, techniques to measure dynamic lateral stenosis, in extension and rotation, have been developed. With the more recent high-resolution scans and the advent of contrast enhanced

scans after metrizamide lumbar myelography, soft tissues can be visualized better. The contribution to narrowing by postoperative fibrosis, herniation of the nucleus pulposus, and thickened ligamentum flavum can be evaluated. Equipment capable of providing readouts of density measurements enables bone, disc, fat, fibrosis, nerve, and fluid to be differentiated.

Experience with the CT imaging of lumbar spinal pathology has shown that for correct interpretation of the detailed information produced, the whole scan sequence must be reviewed. The pathological changes may be multiple and so the clinical history and examination of the patient remains vitally important in assessing the significance of the CT findings.

References

1. Gargano FP, Jacobson R, Rosomoff H: Transverse axial tomography of the spine. *Neuroradiology* 6:254–258, 1974.
2. Gargano FP, Jacobson R: Transverse axial tomography of the spine; Part III, The lumbar spine. *CRC Crit Rev Clin Radiol Nuclear Med* 8:311–328, 1976.
3. Hammerschlag SB, Wolpert SM, Carter BL: Computed tomography of the spinal canal. *Radiology* 121:361–367, 1976.
4. Jacobson R, Gargano FP, Rosomoff HL: Transverse Axial Tomography of the Spine, Parts 1 and 2. *J Neurosurg* 42:406–419, 1975.
5. Lee BCP, Kazam E, Newman AP: Computed tomography of the spine and spinal cord. *Radiology* 128:95–102, 1978.
6. Sheldon JJ, Sersland T, Leborgne J: Computed tomography of the lower lumbar vertebral column. *Radiology* 124:113–118, 1977.
7. Carrera GF, Haughton VM, Syvertsen A, et al: Computed tomography of the lumbar facet joints. *Radiology* 134:145–148, 1980.

8. Harris RI, Macnab I: Structural changes in the intervertebral disc. *J Bone Joint Surg* 36(B):304, 1954.
9. Newman PH: Stenosis of the lumbar spine in spondylolisthesis. *Clin Orthop* 115:116, 1976.
10. Richie HJ, Fahrni WH: Age changes in lumbar intervertebral discs. *Can J Surg* 13:65, 1970.
11. Verbiest H: Further experiences on the pathological influence of a developmental narrowness of the bony lumbar vertebral canal. *J Bone Joint Surg* 37B:576, 1955.
12. Hirschy SC, Leue WM, Berringer WH, et al: CT of the lumbosacral spine: importance of tomographic planes parallel to vertebral end plate. *AJNR* 1:551–556, 1980.
13. Farfan HS: *Mechanical Disorders of the Low Back*. Lee and Febiger, Philadelphia, 1973.
14. Yong-Hing K, Reilly J, Kirkaldy-Willis WH: The ligamentum flavum. *Spine* 1:226, 1976.
15. Farfan HS: Effects of torsion on the intervertebral joints. *Can J Surg* 12:336, 1969.
16. Farfan HS, Sullivan JD: The relation of facet orientation to intervertebral disc failure. *Can J Surg* 10:179, 1967.
17. Crock HV: A reappraisal of intervertebral disc lesions. *Med J Australia* 1:983, 1970.
18. Hirsh C, Schajowicz F: Studies on structural changes in the lumbar anulus fibrosus. *Acta Orthop Scand* 22:184, 1953.
19. Crock HV: Isolated lumbar disc resorption as a cause of nerve root canal stenosis. *Clin Orthop* 115:109, 1976.
20. Schlesinger PT: Incarceration of the 1st sacral nerve in a lateral bony recess of the spinal canal as a cause of sciatica. *J Bone Joint Surg* 37A:115, 1955.
21. Schlesinger PT: Low lumbar nerve root compression and adequate operative exposure. *J Bone Joint Surg* 39A:541, 1957.
22. Williams PC: Lumbar spine, reduced lumbo-sacral joint space. Its relation to sciatic irritation. *JAMA* 99:1677, 1932.
23. Wiltse LL, Kirkaldy-Willis WH, McIvor GWD: The treatment of spinal stenosis. *Clin Orthop* 115:83, 1976.
24. Verbiest H: A radicular syndrome from developmental narrowing of the lumbar vertebral canal. *J Bone Joint Surg* 36B:236: 1954.
25. Kirkaldy-Willis WH, Paine KWE, Cauchoix J, et al: Lumbar spinal stenosis. *Clin Orthop* 99:30–50, 1974.
26. Cauchoix J, Benoist M, Chassaing V: Degenerative spondylolisthesis. *Clin Orthop* 115:122, 1976.
27. Kirkaldy-Willis WH, Heithoff K, Bowen CVA, et al: Pathological Anatomy of Lumbar Spondylosis and Stenosis, Correlated with the CT Scan. In: Post MJD: *Radiographic Evaluation of the Spine: Current Advances with Emphasis on Computed Tomography*. New York, Masson Publishing Inc., 1980, pp. 33–55.

CHAPTER THIRTY-THREE

Computed Tomography of Central Lumbar Stenosis

JEROME J. SHELDON, M.D. and JUAN-MARTIN LEBORGNE, M.D.

A common etiology of low back pain is due to cauda equina compression and nerve root entrapment, secondary to discogenic disease, and/or spinal stenosis, secondary to hypertrophic degenerative spondylosis (1–3). The history, physical examination, and perhaps other diagnostic tests having excluded other etiologies of low back pain, the plain lumbosacral spine roentgenogram is usually the first radiographic procedure. This will reveal the number of lumbar vertebrae, their alignment, the interpedicular distances, the height of the lumbar vertebral bodies and intervertebral disc spaces, the presence of abnormal calcifications, and the presence of hypertrophic osteophyte formation. There is usually poor correlation with this examination and actual encroachment on the spinal canal and intervertebral foramina (4).

The transverse axial projection provides a cross-sectional visualization of the vertebrae, and hence an axial projection of the central spinal canal and its surrounding bony vertebral margins (5–9). This allows direct visualization of the cross-sectional area of the spinal canal, and the epidural fat surrounding the dura (10). This projection obtained on CT directly demonstrates encroachments secondary to hypertrophied bone and soft tissue, and currently is considered the best method for evaluating patients suspected of having spinal stenosis (9).

METHODS

The CT examinations represented here were performed using a General Electric 8800 Scanner with lateral ScoutView. The patient is positioned supine on the gantry table with knees slightly flexed, with one or two folded sheets underneath the sacrum. This procedure tilts and elevates the pelvis in an attempt to decrease the normal lumbar lordosis so that the plane of the intervertebral disc spaces will be parallel to the plane of the axial image. A digital lateral scout radiograph then is obtained and utilized in planning and localizing the computed axial images (Fig. 33.1).

Unless otherwise indicated by the clinical history and review of lumbosacral spine radiography, our routine examination consists of an evaluation of the L5-S1, the L4-L5, and the L3-L4 levels (9). Higher levels are examined if indicated. The examination consequently is planned as well as diagnostically evaluated as a separate, distinct examination, one for each anatomical level. The gantry angulation for each level is determined by overlying an electronic linear cursor, parallel to the disc space on the lateral scount radiograph projected on the television monitor (Fig. 33.2). Images 5-mm thick with 3-mm spacing and the appropriate angulation is obtained at each level from pedicle to pedicle (Figs. 33.3 and 33.4). Sagittal and coronal reformatted images are not routinely obtained as the resultant images would be distorted, secondary to the different gantry angulations at each segment level. If reformatted images are desired, the examination is planned to obtain contiguous images with 3-mm spacing through the appropriate levels without gantry angulation.

The axial images are obtained using a 20-cm diameter scanning circle, with the vertebral body positioned in its center (Fig. 33.5A). The images are magnified two times (Fig. 33.5B) and evaluated on the monitor through a range of center and window settings. However, we have found that a center of 140–150, and a window setting of 1000–1200 (expanded scale) yields the maximum information for transparency display. A level of 50–100, and a window setting of 400–600 demonstrates herniated discs to best advantage. The total patient time for the examination, including review of the images on the monitor to assure that the appropriate levels are evaluated accurately, is approximately 45–50 minutes.

NORMAL ANATOMY

Our routine CT examination of the lumbosacral region, unless otherwise clinically indicated, covers the L3-L4, the L4-L5, and the L5-S1 segments. The normal anatomical description, therefore will be confined to this region (Figs. 33.6–33.8). However, the general anatomical principles can be applied to other areas.

The vertebral column can be considered to be composed of multiple repetitive osseous (Figs. 33.6A, 33.7E, and 33.8E), and articular (Figs. 33.6B–E, 33.7A–D, and 33.8A–D) segments (5–9). The osseous segment is composed of the vertebral body, pedicles, lamina, and the dorsal and transverse spinous processes. Its vertical height is much smaller than the articular segment. The latter segment posteriorly, is formed by the articular facets, the capsular ligaments, and the ligamentum flavum. Laterally, it is bounded by the intervertebral foramina. The cartilaginous intervertebral disc and the vertebral body inferior to the pedicle forms the anterior boundary.

The dura containing the cauda equina and spinal fluid, appears as a homogeneous density, outlined by the more lucent epidural fat. The dural contour is triangular in shape, with the base anterior. The anterior lateral margins of the triangle are rounded, except where the nerve roots exit (Figs. 33.6E, 33.7A and B, and 33.8A), where they

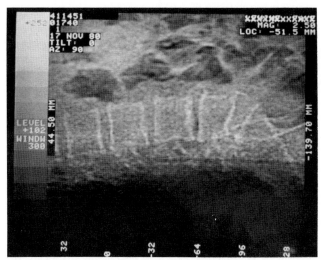

Figure 33.1. Lateral digital radiograph of the lumbar vertebral column. This is the lateral scout projection taken with the x-ray tube and detectors in a lateral position, and the patient cycled through the scanning gantry. The examination is planned from this projection.

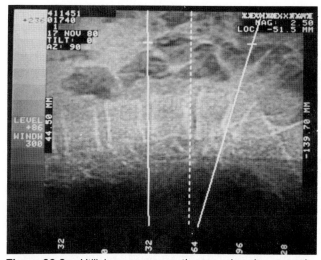

Figure 33.2. Utilizing a cursor on the scanning view console, the angle of the L5-S1, L4–L5, and the L3–L4 intervertebral discs with the perpendicular is obtained. The scanning gantry, thus, is angulated appropriately so that the images will be parallel to the intervertebral disc spaces.

have a more angular configuration. The exiting nerve roots as well as the local expansions of the dorsal root ganglia can be seen in the epidural fat, ventrolateral to the dura (Figs. 33.6A, 33.7D, and 33.8D). The dorsal root ganglia are usually identified as soft tissue densities just inferior to the pedicle in the upper portion of the intervertebral foramina (Gray H: In: Goss CM: *Anatomy of the Human Body.* 27th Ed. Lea and Febiger, Philadelphia, 1960, p. 997) (Figs. 33.7D and 33.8D). However, in the sacral region, the dorsal root ganglia are located within

the spinal canal just medial to the lateral recess (Fig. 33.6A). The overall appearance of the posterior bony contour of the spinal canal has a wineglass configuration at the L5-S1 level (Fig. 33.6), a slight anterior medial convexity at the L4–L5 level (Fig. 33.7), and a more exaggerated anterior medial convexity at the L3–L4 level (Fig. 33.8). The plane of the facet joints are angled greater than 45° to the midsagittal plane (Figs. 33.6B, 33.7B, and 33.8B).

The cartilaginous intervertebral disc has a density slightly greater than surrounding muscle, and much less

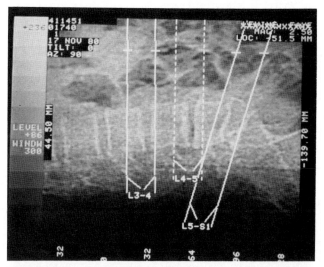

Figure 33.3. The beginning and end of the scanning sequence at each articular segment is plotted on the lateral scout radiograph. This usually extends from pedicle to pedicle with the appropriate gantry angulation at each level.

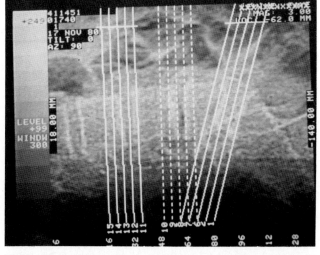

Figure 33.4. The computer projects each of the obtained 5-mm thick images with 3-mm spacing at each level. This is a typical three-level evaluation. By comparing the image number of the axial image, to the number on the lateral digital radiograph, the anatomical level, and relationship to the anatomical structures easily can be obtained.

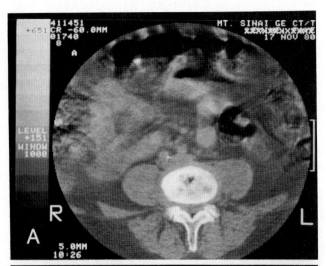

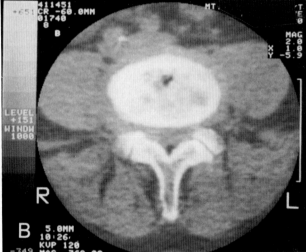

Figure 33.5. A. The 20-cm diameter scanning circle is used to obtain the axial images. B. The vertical segment is then magnified two times for analysis and final hard copy imaging.

than the adjacent bone. If the plane of the image is directly through the intervertebral disc, without averaging of the adjacent bony vertebral body margins, it will appear as an almost water-density structure, slightly greater than the adjacent muscle (Fig. 33.8B). If the plane of the image averages some of the adjacent vertebral body, or if the angle of the image is not exactly parallel to the plane of the disc space, the CT representation of the disc will be denser, and will appear to have various degrees of bone projecting within it (Figs. 33.6B and 33.7B). The surface of the intervertebral disc that borders the spinal canal should be slightly convex anteriorly at the L4–L5, and the L3–L4 levels (Figs. 33.7B and 33.8B). At the L5-S1 level (Fig. 33.6B), its contour should be either convex anteriorly, or flat. If the intervertebral discs do not have the above-described configurations, then one must consider either a bulging anulus if the contour is diffusely abnormal, or a herniated disc (12) if it is focally abnormal (Fig. 33.6B).

The cross-sectional images at each anatomical level are visualized as to normal contour and to determine if there are focal encroachments. As in other areas of radiology, actual measurements are not obtained routinely, except in borderline situations. In these cases, the most useful measurement is that of the cross-sectional area where, for the lower three lumbar levels we accept 1.6 cm^2 as the lower limits of normal (13). However, a normal cross-sectional area may be present, with a narrowed lateral recess or intervertebral foramina. The lateral recess is that region bordered laterally by the pedicle, anteriorly by the vertebral body, and posteriorly by the root of the superior facet (Fig. 33.7A). A vertical measurement of 5 mm is considered normal, 3–5 mm borderline, and less than 3 mm, a narrowed lateral recess (14).

PATHOLOGY

Spinal stenosis implies narrowing of the spinal canal (2). In its broadest sense, this implies not only narrowing due to bony overgrowth, and ligamentum flavum hypertrophy, but also intervertebral disc herniation and other soft-tissue space-occupying lesions (2). Through common usage, however, the term spinal stenosis has come to mean narrowing of the spinal canal, secondary to bony and/or soft-tissue hypertrophy of its surrounding walls.

The most common clinical presentation is that of back pain, which may radiate into one or both lower extremities. Walking and standing may aggravate the symptoms. Coughing, straining, or straight leg raising may or may not exacerbate symptoms. Associated motor deficits, sensory deficits, and neurogenic bladder have been described (15). A syndrome of neurogenic intermittent claudication also may occur (16). The observed CT findings must be correlated with the patient's symptoms and the neurological examination as there may be multiple levels of stenosis, only some of which are causing the patient's clinical problems.

Spinal stenosis usually is not confined to the central portions of the spinal canal, but also involves the intervertebral foramina. This chapter will be concerned primarily with central spinal stenosis, and the intervertebral foramina will be mentioned only secondarily.

The etiologies for spinal stenosis are varied (4), the most common being degenerative, secondary to degenerative disc disease. Discogenic disease also accounts for degenerative retrolisthesis and spondylolisthesis. Congenital, postsurgical, spondolytic spondylolisthesis, and post-traumatic etiologies also will be discussed.

DEVELOPMENTAL SPINAL STENOSIS

Developmental spinal stenosis may be diffuse, involving all levels or focal, involving only one or two levels (17, 18). When focal, the most common levels involved are that of the lumbosacral junction and the immediate superior segment (i.e., the L4–L5, and the L3–L4 level). Early in life, these patients are usually asymptomatic, as the cross-sectional area of the spinal canal is just large enough to contain comfortably the cauda equina and exiting nerve

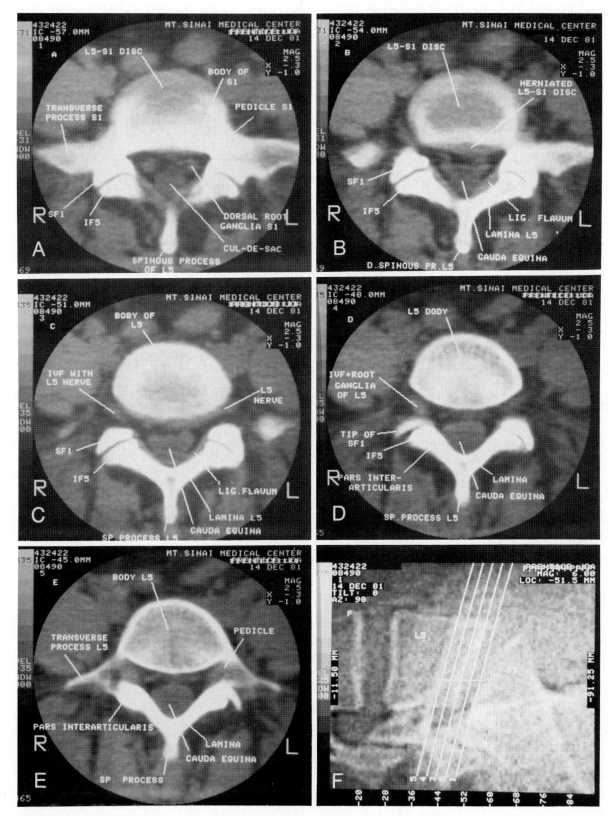

Figure 33.6. Normal L5-S1 level: A. S1 osseous segment. B, C, and D. L5-S1 articular segment. Note the small left lateral herniated disc at the L5-S1 level. E. Beginning of the L5 articular segment. F. Lateral digital radiograph showing the levels of the axial images obtained at the L5-S1 level. SF1 = Superior facets S1, IF5 = Inferior facets of L5, D = Dorsal, Sp = spinous.

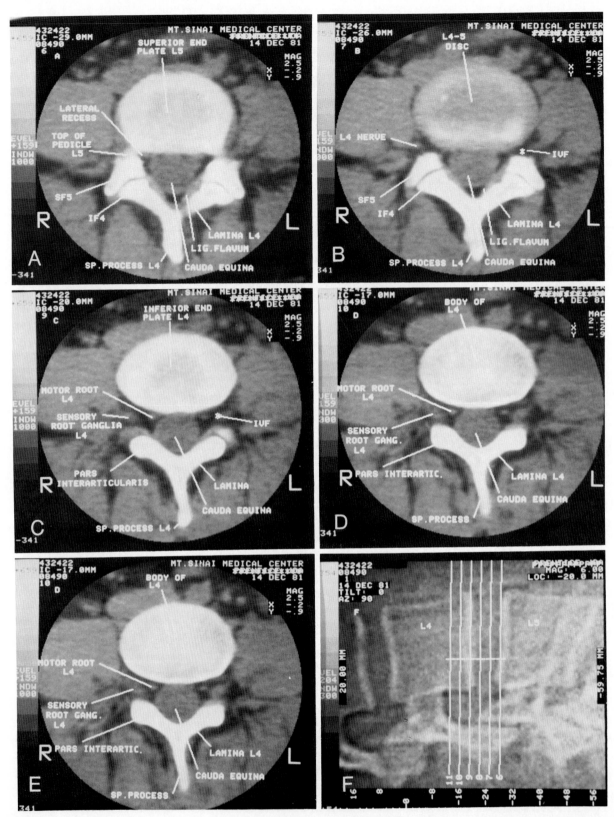

Figure 33.7. Normal L4–L5 level: A. Superior portion of the L5 osseous segment. B and C. L4–L5 articular segment level. D. Axial image through the level of the pars interarticularis portion of the articular segment level. E. Inferior aspect of the L4 osseous segment level. F. Lateral digital radiograph demonstrating the location of the axial images at the L4–L5 level. SF5 = Superior facet of L5, IF4 = Inferior facets of L4, Sp = spinous.

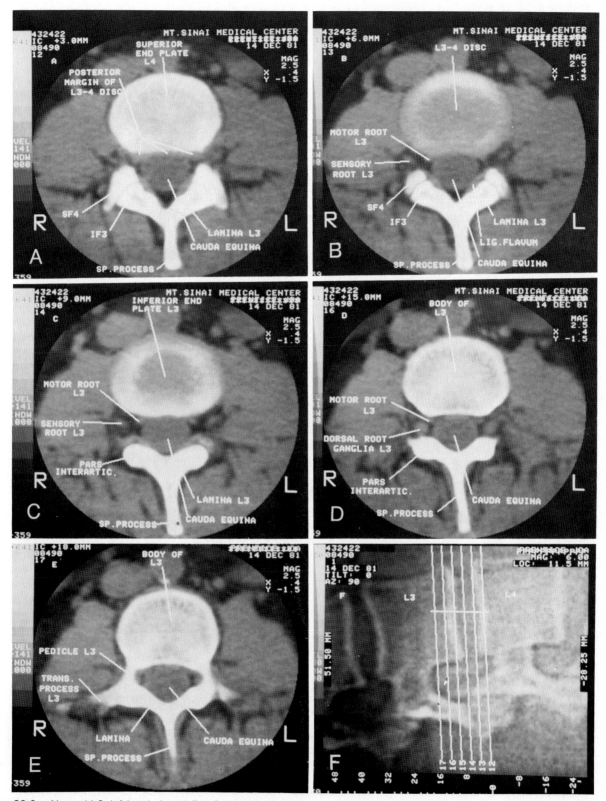

Figure 33.8. Normal L3–L4 level: A and B. L3–L4 articular segment level. C and D. Axial images through the level of the pars interarticularis at the L3–L4 articular segment level. E. Beginning of the L3 osseous segment level. F. Lateral digital radiograph demonstrating the location of the axial images at the L3–L4 level. SF4 = Superior facets of L4, IF3 = Inferior facets of L3, Sp = spinous process.

roots. As these patients get older, the usual degenerative changes, concomitant with increasing age (i.e., bony facet and lamina hypertrophy, ligamentum flavum hypertrophy, bulging anulus, etc.) are superimposed on an already small canal, compressing the cauda equina. Symptoms, therefore, occur at an earlier age than in patients with more capacious spinal canals.

The CT examination on these patients (Fig. 33.9) demonstrates a symmetrically small canal, usually with short, thickened pedicles. Bulbous lamina and facets are present, with a thickened ligamentum flavum. This causes narrowing of the posterior portion of the spinal canal, with ab-

sence of the usual wine-glass configuration at the L5-S1 level. Thickening of the ligamentum flavum causes further encroachment on the cross-sectional area. If the superior facets are also prominent, the canal can have a trilobed appearance. Slight irregularities in contour are usually secondary to superimposed degenerative changes (Fig. 33.9B and D). A bulging anulus can compromise the spinal canal further (Fig. 33.9B).

DEGENERATIVE SPINAL STENOSIS

The intervertebral disc loses its hydroscopic properties

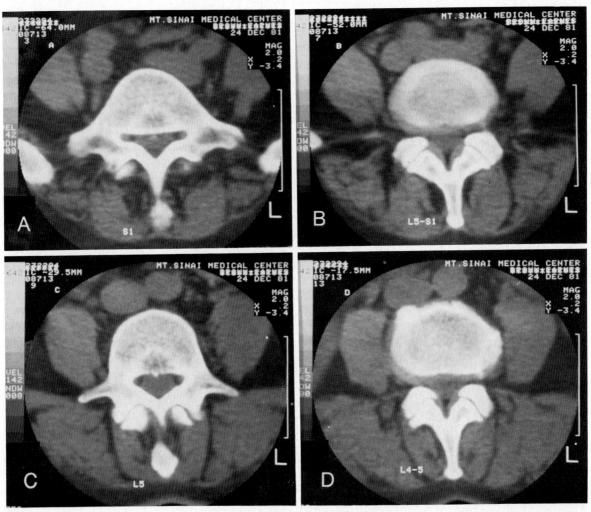

Figure 33.9. A 53-year-old male presents with developmental spinal stenosis. A. Osseous segment of S1, with symmetrical lamina hypertrophy. B. Articular segment L5-S1 with hypertrophy of the superior facets of S1 and the inferior facets of L5. The ligamentum flavum is thickened bilaterally, and there is a bulging anulus. These soft-tissue structures can be seen to encroach on the more central soft-tissue density of the dural sac. There is also encroachment on the intervertebral foramina, bilaterally, with deep lateral recesses. The overall appearance of the spinal canal is trilobed. There is slight focal hypertrophy of the lamina on the left, posteriorly. C. The L5 osseous segment shows short, thickened pedicles and a small spinal canal. D. The articular segment of L4–L5 shows hypertrophy of the inferior facets of L4, and the superior facets of L5, with a narrowed posterior portion of the spinal canal, and deep lateral recesses. Thickening of the ligamentum flavum is also present, and there is slight bulging of the anulus. Degenerative osteophytes from the facet joints are seen bilaterally, extending posterior to the spinal canal. However, a small osteophyte can be seen to extend medially on the right from the medial lip of the superior facet of L5. This latter, along with the bulging annulus are superimposed degenerative changes.

with increasing age. The disc becomes progressively desiccated, and loses its shock-absorber qualities. This causes abnormal stresses on the ligamentum flavum, the capsular ligaments, and the articular facets. These changes most commonly occur at the L4–L5 and L5-S1 levels, and are seen in patients with advancing age (4, 5).

The plain lumbosacral spine examination may show the arthritic changes of the apophyseal joints, and the degenerative hypertrophic facets (Fig. 33.10A and B). However, it does not show the relationship of these facets to the cross-sectional area of the spinal canal (4, 9). Indeed, the demonstrated hypertrophic changes may extend posteriorly, with an intact cross-sectional area of the spinal canal (Fig. 33.10C) or anteriorly, and cause spinal stenosis (Fig. 33.10D). The etiology of the back pain in these individuals could be the arthritic changes in the facet joints, and not cauda equina compression (4).

The plain film findings as demonstrated at the L4–L5 level in the above example may be indistinguishable from plain x-rays taken on patients with spinal stenosis as at the L3–L4 level in the same above patient. In this latter group of patients, the sclerotic, hypertrophied facets, and lamina bulge anterior medially, and encroach on the posterior portion of the spinal canal (1–3). Concomitant hypertrophy of the superior facets causes a deep lateral recess and encroachment on the intervertebral foramina. The spinal canal can have a fleur-de-lis configuration. Associated hypertrophy of the ligamentum flavum further compromises the cross-sectional area of the spinal canal.

Figure 33.11 is a composite of several axial images from different patients with spinal stenosis at the L4–L5 and the L5-S1 levels. Note the calcified centrally and right laterally herniated disc, with bulbous superior facets, narrowing the intervertebral foramina in Figure 33.11A. Figure 33.11B demonstrates a central bulging anulus with associated medial lipping of the superior and inferior facets, more marked on the left than on the right. Osteophytes extending posteriorly also are present. Concomitant bulging anuli, or herniated discs are not unusual as discogenic disease is considered to be the underlying etiology of the hypertrophy and arthritic changes (4). Figure 33.11C–F shows increasing severity of degenerative changes with narrowing and encroachment on the spinal canal by both bony and soft-tissue changes. These changes can be seen to encroach, and even obliterate the peridural fat and deform the contour of the dura, compressing its contents. These changes correlate well with the defects seen on myelography (Fig. 33.12) which currently is performed usually if the patient is to have surgical treatment. Occasionally, a herniated disc not seen on the CT examination because of problems with volume averaging, secondary to bony lipping of the vertebral body margins, or lack of epidural fat will be demonstrated.

RETROLISTHESIS

With advancing age, the cartilaginous intervertebral disc becomes less hydroscopic. With increasing desiccation, there is loss of height of the intervertebral disc space

(4). The plane of the facet joints in the lumbar region has an anterior superior, to a posterior inferior orientation. With a decreasing height of the intervertebral disc space, the superior vertebrae follow the posterior, inferiorly oriented plane of the facet joints and migrate posteriorly. Usually concomitant hypertrophic and erosive arthritic changes occur, and the vertebral bodies remain in alignment. If the erosive changes are excessive, degenerative anterior slippage can occur (see next section). Our preliminary observation suggests that retrolisthesis occurs when there is a relative absence of associated arthritic changes of the facet joints.

In the example shown in Figure 33.13, there is retrolisthesis of L2 on L3. There is encroachment of the retrodisplaced body of L2 on the superior facets of L3. The posterior subluxation of the inferior facets of L2 on the superior facets of L3 are easily identified. There is relative absence of arthritic or hypertrophic degenerative changes.

DEGENERATIVE SPONDYLOLISTHESIS

Spondylolisthesis refers to the anterior slippage of one vertebral segment on its inferior neighbor. The neural arch may or may not be intact. If the neural arch is intact, the term pseudospondylolisthesis (20) or degenerative spondylolisthesis (21) has been used to apply to this process. The term pseudospondylolisthesis was used to infer that the process is not due to a neural arch defect. The term degenerative spondylolisthesis (21) implies the underlying etiology, and hence is more descriptive and is the preferred term for this disorder.

Degenerative spondylolisthesis usually occurs in the 5th or 6th decade of life, and most commonly affects the L4–L5 level, although any level may be involved (22). There is increasing desiccation of the intervertebral discs with increasing age, with a resultant loss of height of the intervertebral disc spaces (4). This causes abnormal stresses and strains on the apophyseal joints with resultant osteoarthritic changes. This process is accentuated by an excessive lumbar lordosis. The osteoarthritis can become excessively erosive, with reorientation of the plane of the facet joints in a more sagittal direction. This facilitates the anterior slippage. Slippage is not greatly excessive, and usually is less than 30% of the superior surface of the inferior vertebral body. Exuberant hypertrophic osteophyte formation from the facet joints usually occurs in an attempt to stabilize the slippage (9).

The slippage is identified easily on plain radiographs (not shown here). CT demonstrates the more sagittal orientation of the plane of the facet joints (Fig. 33.14B), the anterior slippage of the lamina arch, and especially the inferior facets of L4 can be seen to encroach upon the body of L5, narrowing the central portion of the spinal canal and the intervertebral foramina. The hypertrophic osteoarthritic changes also are seen easily. A transverse lucent band representing the L4–L5 disc space between the anterior slipped body of L4 and the more posteriorly positioned body of L5 also is discernible. This finding is very suggestive of an anterior slippage, but also has been

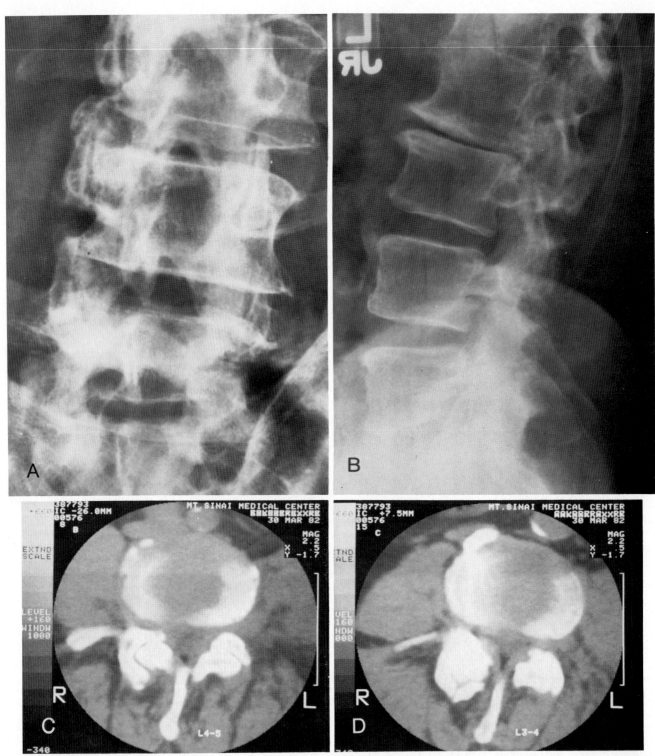

Figure 33.10. An 80-year-old male presents with low back pain. A. The AP radiograph shows similar findings at the L3–L4 and the L4–L5 levels. There is hypertrophy of the superior and inferior facets at the L4–L5, and the L3–L4 levels, respectively. This occurs bilaterally, predominately on the right. B. The lateral radiograph shows the bulbous superior facets of L4, apparently narrowing the intervertebral foramina. This occurs to a much lesser degree at the L3–L4 level. C. The computed axial projection demonstrates the arthritic changes of the facet joints, bilaterally, with prominent hypertrophic osteophyte formation arising from the superior facet of L4 on the right extending posteriorly away from the facet joint. Although there are deep lateral recesses, there is no evidence of central spinal stenosis. D. At the L3–L4 level, there are hypertrophic arthritic changes of the facet joints, bilaterally, more marked on the right than on the left. Although some of these hypertrophic changes extend posteriorly, especially on the right, there is marked medial convexity to the inferior facets of L3. The latter, associated with hypertrophy of the ligamentum flavum, causes spinal stenosis. In this single patient, there is demonstrated how the routine radiographic findings may not necessarily correlate with the actual changes of spinal stenosis as demonstrated on axial imaging.

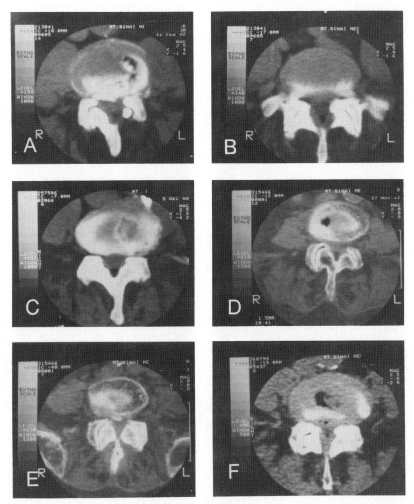

Figure 33.11. Degenerative spinal stenosis. Representative images of several different patients demonstrating encroachment on the cross-sectional area of the spinal canal. A. L4–L5 level: there is a vacuum disc phenomenon. A calcified posterior right lateral herniated disc fragment is present. Hypertrophy of the superior facets of L5 causes a deep lateral recess and stenosis of the intervertebral foramina. Hypertrophy of the inferior facet of L4 and the adjacent lamina encroaches on the right lateral aspect of the posterior portion of the spinal canal. B. L5-S1 level: a central bulging anulus is present. There is marked hypertrophy of the superior facets of S1 and the inferior facets of L5. The facet joints are arthritic, with osteophytes extending posteriorly away from the spinal canal. In addition, more anterior medial osteophytes are noted, especially on the left, encroaching on the spinal canal, causing deep lateral recesses. Hypertrophy of the ligamentum flavum is also present. These areas of hypertrophy can be seen to encroach on the posterior lateral portions of the dural sac. C. L4–L5 level: hypertrophy of the lamina and inferior facets of L4, narrow the posterior portion of the spinal canal. Hypertrophied superior facets of L5 narrow the intervertebral foramina. D. L4–L5 level: there is hypertrophy of the superior facets of L5 and the inferior facets of L4, bilaterally, but much more marked on the right. Arthritic changes of the facet joints are present, with a vacuum facet joint on the right. There is a deep lateral recess on the right, with stenosis of the intervertebral foramina. A vacuum disc is noted anteriorly. E. L5-S1 level: a calcified central bulging anulus is present. Arthritic changes of the facet joints with bulging inferior facets of L4 and superior facets of S1 are present. This causes a deep lateral recess and narrowed posterior portion of the spinal canal. F. L4–L5 level: a vacuum disc is present with a central bulging anulus. Hypertrophy of the ligamentum flavum is also present. Arthritic changes of the facet joints are present, with a vacuum facet on the right. The superior facets of L5 are markedly bulbous and there is marked hypertrophy of the inferior facets of L4 and the adjacent lamina. The ligamentum flavum is also markedly hypertrophied. The cross-sectional area of the spinal canal has a fleur-de-lis configuration. The dura has a vertical anterior posterior linear configuration, being markedly compressed by the hypertrophied ligamentum flavum and adjacent bone.

demonstrated in patients with excessive lumbar lordosis (9). The myelogram (Fig. 33.14C and D) in this patient demonstrates the anterior slippage, and the hourglass deformity, and kinked, Pantopaque-filled dural sac, secondary to the slippage and hypertrophic bony changes.

POSTFUSION STENOSIS

Patients who have had a spinal fusion may have a recurrence of their symptoms. This can progress to the point where further surgical treatment may be warranted

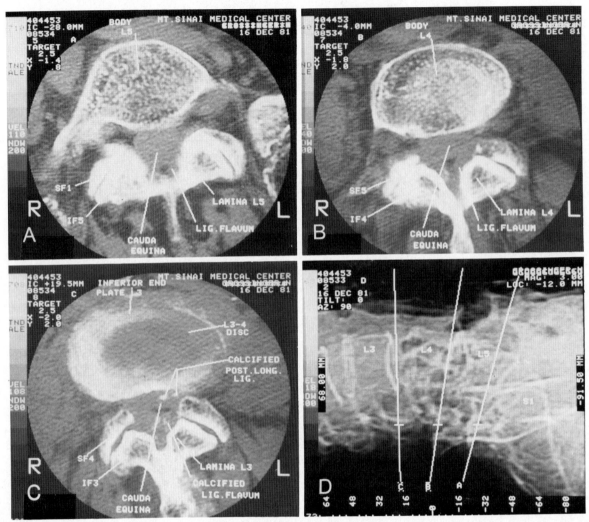

Figure 33.12. A 74-year-old male presented with spinal stenosis at the L3–L4, L4–L5, and L5-S1 levels, correlated with myelography. A. L5-S1 level: There is hypertrophy of the superior facets of S1, causing a medial bulging and loss of the normal wine-glass configuration usually seen at this level. This finding, along with slight hypertrophy of the ligamentum flavum, narrows the posterior portion of the spinal canal. B. L4–L5 level: There is hypertrophy and increased medial convexity of the inferior facets of L4, and the adjacent lamina. Prominent hypertrophy of the ligamentum flavum also is noted. These changes narrow the posterior portion of the spinal canal, obliterating the posterior peridural fat and encroach on the central soft tissue density representing the cauda equina. C. L3–L4 level: Hypertrophy of the ligamentum flavum, lamina, and adjacent inferior facets of L3, narrowing the posterior portion of the spinal canal. There is a bulging anulus, with calcification of the posterior longitudinal ligament. These findings narrow and obliterate the epidural fat and encroach on the cauda equina. D. Lateral digital radiograph demonstrating the location of the above described axial images. E. Lateral myelogram demonstrating encroachment on the posterior portion of the Pantopaque-filled subarachnoid space at the L3–L4, L4–L5, L5-S1 levels. A bulging anulus at the L3–L4 level, and the L5-S1 level also is noted. F. The frontal myelographic projection demonstrates hour-glass deformities at the above described levels. The above described findings correspond to the encroachments on the posterior portion of the spinal canal, as described on the axial images.

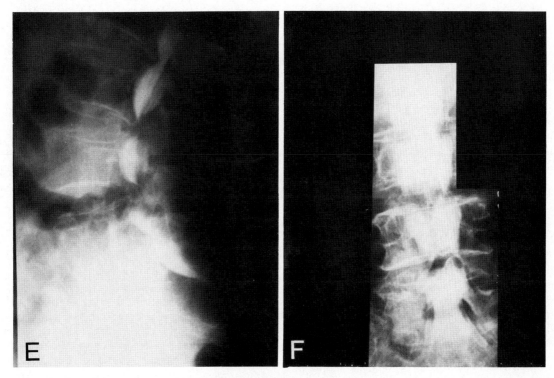

Figure 33.12.   E–F.

(1–3). In some patients these symptoms may be due to an unrecognized developmental or degenerative spinal stenosis, existing before the original surgery. In others, the recurrence of symptoms can be due to overgrowth of the bony fusion (7).

The usual surgical procedure for a medial posterior spinal fusion consists of stripping the periosteum off of the posterior portion of the lamina arch, before the positioning of the bone graft. This allows for the eventual fusion of the bone graft to the lamina arch. However, it also stimulates new periosteal bone growth on the spinal canal surface of the lamina. This lamina overgrowth, coupled with overgrowth of the bone graft is the cause of the spinal stenosis (7–9).

Routine plain roentgenograms (not shown here) demonstrate the vertical extent of the bone graft. Flexion and extension views can demonstrate if there is motion at the level of surgery, and if the fusion mass is intact. A pseudoarthrosis also may be a cause of pain and is demonstrated best by the flexion and extension radiographs, and may not be seen in the axial projection of CT. CT demonstrates the relationship of the bony fusion mass and lamina to the spinal canal and intervertebral foramina (Fig. 33.15).

SPONDYLOLISTHESIS

Spondylolisthesis refers to the slippage of the superior vertebral segment on its inferior member, secondary to a pars interarticularis defect. The etiology of this defect can be developmental or traumatic. A familial incidence has been reported (4, 23). This slippage may occur at any level. However, the L5-S1 level is the most common (23). It usually is discovered during the 2nd decade of life. A pars defect may be present without evidence of slippage. The slippage when present can be minimal, to a complete anterior dislocation of the superior vertebral body on its subjacent inferior neighbor (4). The pedicles, superior facets, and transverse processes slip forward with the vertebral body. The lamina arch, dorsal spinous process, and inferior facets retain their normal relationship to the superior facets of the inferior vertebral segment.

A lateral radiograph (Fig. 33.16A) can demonstrate the slippage of the pars interarticularis defect in this example at the L5-S1 level. Oblique radiographs (not shown here), may show the pars defect to better advantage. A computed axial image (Fig. 33.16C) through the level of the facet joints demonstrates a normal relationship between the superior facets of S1 and the inferior facets of L5. The double density through the posterior portion of the vertebral body usually caused by a slippage is present. The anteriormost portion of the density is caused by the slipped vertebral body of L5, the lucency by the disc space, and the posterior density by the superior border of S1. A slightly higher axial image (Fig. 33.16D) passes through the superior portion of the facet joints, as well as the pars interarticularis defect. The superiormost tip of the superior facet of S1 still is identified in normal relationship with the inferior facet of L5 and the lamina arch. An extra

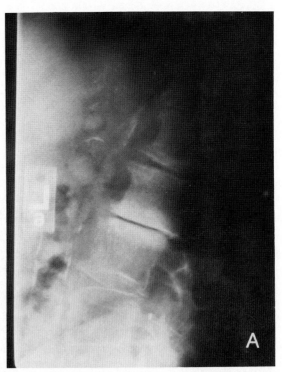

Figure 33.13.   A.

lucency, however, is now present, where the lamina arch in the region of the pars interarticularis usually attaches to the bone of the pedicle. This extra lucency is the pars defect, and the extra bone is usually a hypertrophied spur arising from the pedicle. An axial image (Fig. 33.16E) through the pedicle and lamina arch demonstrates the pars interarticularis defect. Prominent hypertrophied bone and cartilage arising from the pedicle and lamina arch margins of the defect are usually present. This can impinge on the medial posterior portion of the spinal canal and cause deep lateral recesses. The actual slippage itself will kink the dura anteriorly over the superior posterior border of the superior end plate of S1. Exiting nerve roots also could be compromised conceivably by the hypertrophied bone and cartilage in the region of the pars defect, extending into the intervertebral foramina (2). If surgical treatment is contemplated, the above findings at this time usually are confirmed by myelography.

FRACTURES

The most common mechanism of traumatic injury is usually due to acute, forceful hyperflexion (4, 24). The most common location is at the thoracolumbar junction, and the L1–L2 levels. In our complex society, the etiologies causing the hyperflexion are varied and multiple. The more common would be hyperflexion injuries, secondary to contact sports, and seat-belt injuries. The latter type of injury tends to be particularly severe, as the lap belt focuses the force, which results in a severe hyperflexion. The routine roentgenogram demonstrates a decrease in the vertical height of the vertebral body, secondary to the

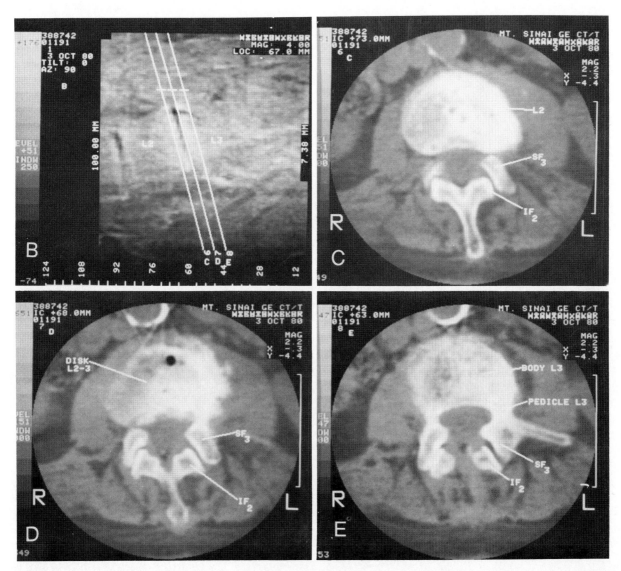

Figure 33.13. Retrolisthesis of L2 on L3 of a 70-year-old female with persistent low back pain. A. A lateral radiograph demonstrates marked loss of height with end plate sclerosis at the L2–L3 level. There is mild retrolisthesis of L2 on L3. B. Lateral digital radiograph demonstrating the location of the demonstrated axial images. C. Axial image at the superiormost aspect of the facet joints. The retrolisthesed vertebral body of L2 impinges on the intervertebral foramina and encroaches on the superior facets of L3. The inferior facets of L2, along with the lamina and dorsal spinous process have migrated posteriorly along with the retrolisthesed L2 vertebral body, demonstrating posterior subluxation at the level of the facet joints. D. Axial image through the midpoint of the L2–L3 facet joints at the level of the cartilaginous intervertebral disc. A vacuum disc is identified anteriorly. The retrolisthesed posteriorly subluxed inferior facets of L2 on the superior facets of L3 is again demonstrated. E. Inferiormost aspect of the facet joints, again demonstrating the retrolisthesed inferior facets of L2 on the superior facets of L3. F. Reformatted sagittal image through the plane of the facet joints on the right. The retrolisthesed vertebral body of L2 on L3 and a narrowed right intervertebral foramina. G. Reformatted sagittal image at the level of the midsagittal plane. L2 is retrolisthesed on L3. H. Reformatted sagittal image at the level of the midsagittal plane, with level and window settings set for soft tissue. The retrolisthesed L2 is again demonstrated on L3. L2 is impinging upon the dura and its contents which are kinked posteriorly at the level of the retrolisthesis. I. Sagittal reformatted image at the level of the inferior facets on the left. L2 is retrolisthesed on L3. There is distraction of the facet joint, with the inferior facet of L2 subluxed posteriorly on the superior facet of L3. This is more marked than on the right side, indicating a rotary component to the retrolisthesis.

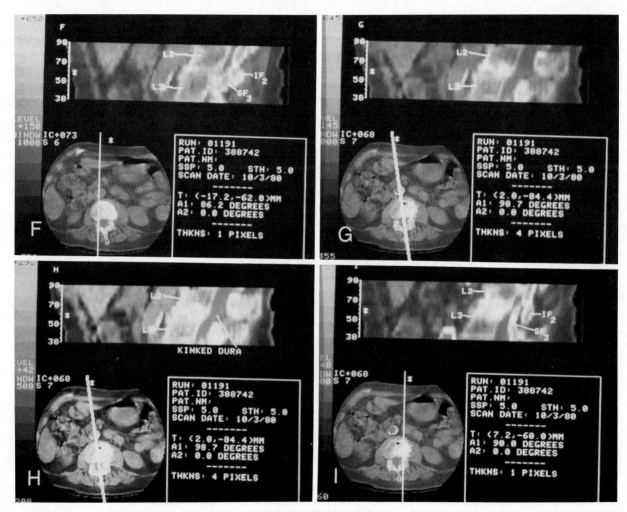

Figure 33.13. F–I.

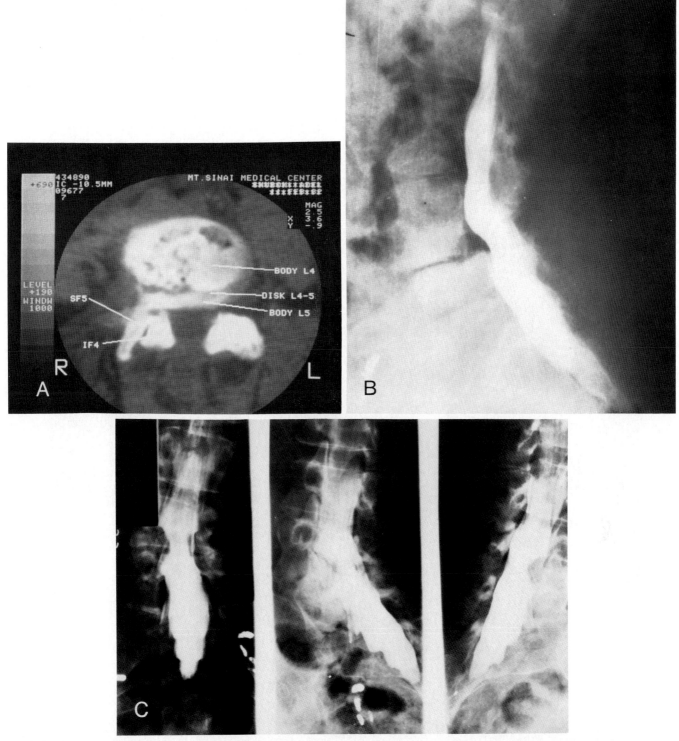

Figure 33.14. Degenerative spondylolisthesis at the L4–L5 level in a 57-year-old female with low back pain extending into both buttocks and the back of the thighs. A. Computed axial image at the L4–L5 articular segment level. This demonstrates a reorientation of the plane of the facet joints, with hypertrophic osteophyte formation arising from the superior and inferior facets of L5 and L4, respectively. The encroachment of the posterior portion of the body of L5 on the anterior slipped inferior facets of L4 is demonstrated. This narrows the central portion of the spinal canal, anteriorly, as well as the intervertebral foramina. The transverse lucent band representing the L4–L5 intervertebral disc is demonstrated between the posterior portion of the body of L5, and the most anteriorly located body of L4. B. Transtable lateral of a Pantopaque myelogram demonstrates the anterior slippage of L4 on L5, and the kinked Pantopaque-filled dura, with posterior encroachment at the L4–L5 level, secondary to the hypertrophied, and anteriorly slipped inferior facets and lamina arch of L4. C. Frontal and oblique views demonstrate the hour-glass deformity, secondary to the slippage at the L4–L5 level. SF5 = superior facets of L5, IF4 = Inferior facets of L4.

585

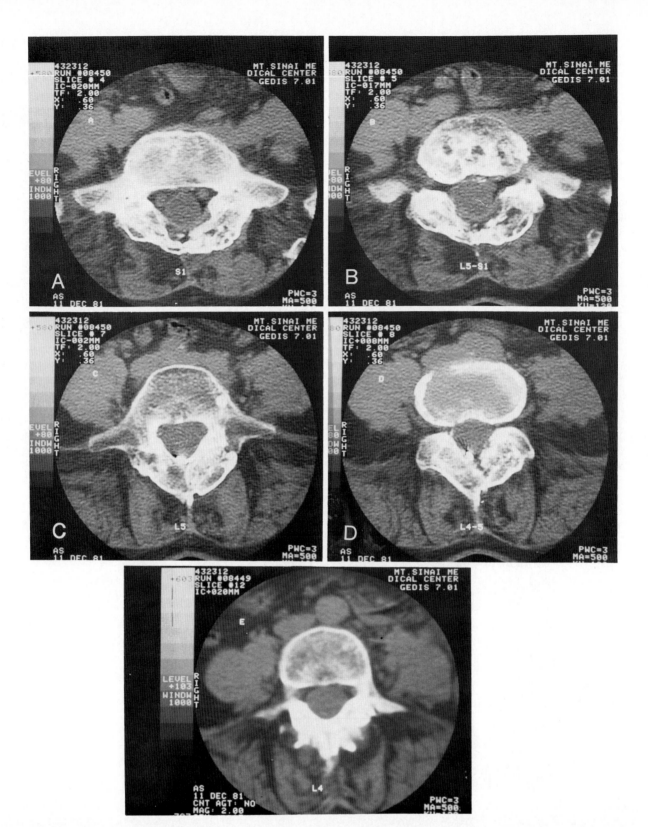

Figure 33.15. Postfusion stenosis (L4-S1). A. S1 osseous segment demonstrates the irregular thickened posterior border of the spinal canal. This is composed of the thickened lamina and the bone graft, forming a mature fusion mass. B. L5-S1 articular segment demonstrating the bony fusion mass and the fused facet joints. Slight overgrowth ventrally causes deep lateral recesses and slight narrowing of the intervertebral foramina. C. L5 osseous segment demonstrates a markedly thickened lamina arch and fusion mass, narrowing the spinal canal. A small amount of Pantopaque is present in the posterior portion of the spinal canal. D. L4–L5 articular segment. A posterior bony fusion mass is demonstrated along with bony fusion and ankylosis of the facet joints. There is marked overgrowth ventrally, causing marked stenosis of the intervertebral foramina. A small amount of Pantopaque is noted in the posterior portion of the spinal canal. E. Osseous segment L4. This is the upper end of the bony fusion. A normally contoured spinal canal is present.

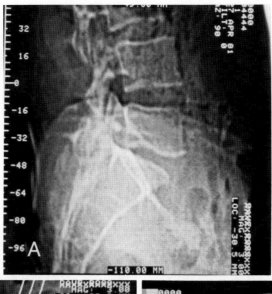

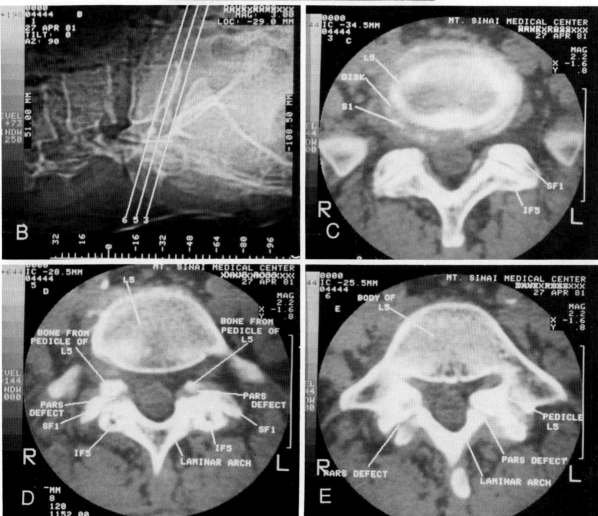

Figure 33.16. Spondylolisthesis, secondary to a pars interarticularis defect at L5-S1. A 40-year-old male presents with low back pain radiating into the right leg. A. Lateral digital radiograph demonstrating slight anterior slippage of L5 on S1, with a pars interarticularis defect demonstrated just inferior to the attachment of the pars to the pedicles of L5. B. Lateral digital radiograph demonstrating the location of the subsequent axial images. C. Computed axial image of the inferior most portion of the articular segment, demonstrating a normal relationship between the superior facets of S1 (SF1) and the inferior facets of L5 (IF5). The double density with central lucency through the anterior vertebral segment consisting of the anterior slipped body of L5, the lucent disc, and the posteriorly positioned body of S1 is demonstrated. D. Computed axial image at the upper portion of the facet joints and the pars interarticularis defect. The superior most aspect of the superior facets of S1, and its articulation with

587   (*Legend continued on next page*)

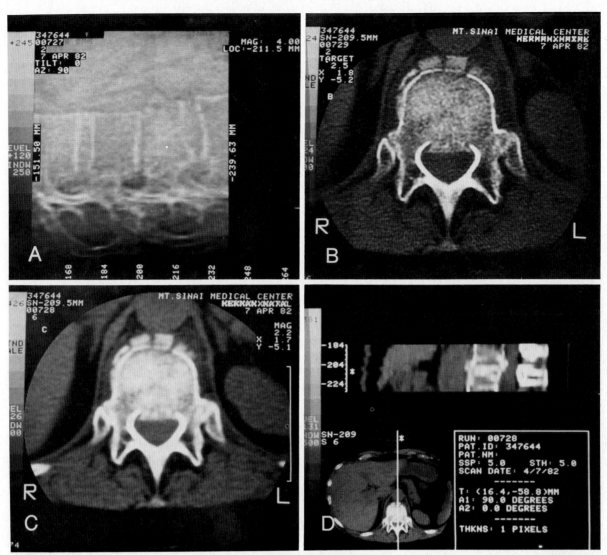

Figure 33.17. Old compression injury of T12 with central spinal stenosis. A 52-year-old male was in an auto accident several months before current examination. A. Digital lateral radiograph demonstrates the compression of T12, with irregularity of the superior end plate and anterior buckling of the anterior cortex. The vertebral body is sclerosed, secondary to the compression and endosteal new bone formation. B. Axial image through the midportion of the vertebral body, with level and window set to show bone to best advantage. There is absence of the cortical margin of the anterior portion of the bony spinal canal. A flat wedge of mature bone contiguous with the spongiosa of the adjacent vertebral body obliterates the anterior portion of the spinal canal. There is hyperdense endosteal new bone within the vertebral body and the adjacent bone within the spinal canal. New bone formation also is noted contiguous with the anterior portion of the vertebral body, with an intact anterior cortex. This is probably secondary to an ossification of hematoma beneath the anterior longitudinal ligament. C. Same axial image as above, with level and window set for soft tissue. There is effacement of the epidural fat and encroachment on the dura and its contents by the bone within the spinal canal. D. Sagittal reformatted image demonstrating the bony encroachment on the spinal canal impinging on the dura and its contents.

the origin of the inferior facets of L5, are demonstrated. The beginning of the pars interarticularis defect also is noted. Hypertrophied bone from the lamina and the pedicle in the region of the pars defect is demonstrated, narrowing the intervertebral foramina, encroaching on exiting nerve roots, especially on the right. E. Computed axial image through the lamina arch and the pars defect. Hypertrophied bone arising from the margins of the pars defect on both the lamina arch side, and the pedicle side is demonstrated. This causes a fleur-de-lis configuration to the spinal canal. Fortunately, most of the bone along with the hypertrophied cartilage extends posteriorly away from the spinal canal. However, a degree of spinal stenosis is present.

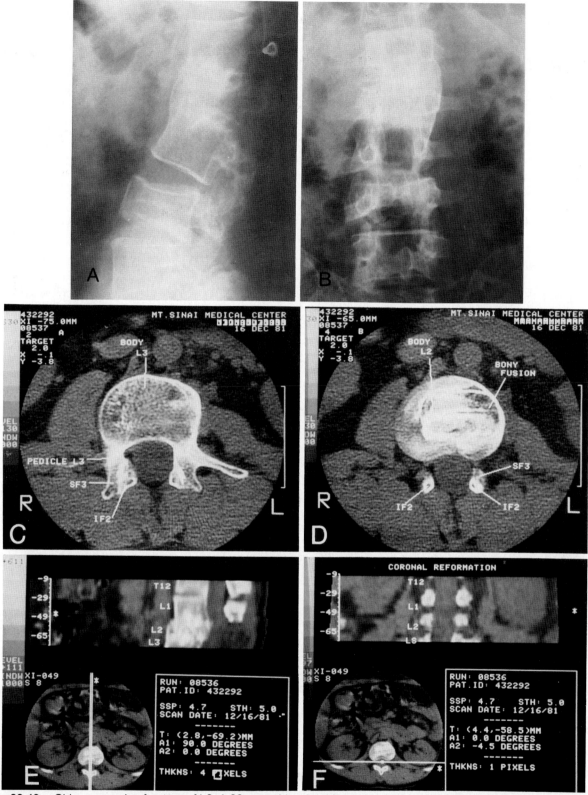

Figure 33.18. Old compression fracture of L2. A 28-year-old male with an old injury to the lumbar vertebral column was treated by surgery. The patient now returns with a high cauda equina compression syndrome. A. A lateral radiograph demonstrates partial compression of L4, with a more severe compression, and bony ankylosis of L2. L2 is fused to the adjacent L1 and L3. B. A laminectomy of L2 and L3 is present. The bony ankylosis of the vertebral bodies can be seen to be predominately on the left, bridging L1, L2, and L3. C. An axial image at the level of L3 demonstrates the laminectomy in a capacious spinal canal. D. An axial image through L2 demonstrates the sclerosis of the L2 vertebral body, secondary to the compression and endosteal new bone formation. The spinal canal is capacious, and the inferior facets of L2 and the superior facet of L3 on the left is diminutive, secondary to the previous facetectomy. E. A sagittal reformatted image demonstrates the compressed L2 with its bony ankylosis with the adjacent L1 and L3. In addition, the posterior kyphosis at the level of L2 is present, as well as the posterior kinking of the dura. The narrowed sagittal diameter of the spinal canal between the compressed L2 and the lamina arch of L1, not apparent on other views, now is demonstrated. F. A coronal reconstruction is unremarkable.

compression. This is usually at the expense of the superior end plate. The anterior cortex of the vertebral body may be buckled (4). With increasing severity of the hyperflexion, the vertebral body can become collapsed completely. The pedicles may be fractured at their attachments to the vertebral bodies. The lamina arch usually is spared. Fractures of the dorsal spinous processes and transverse processes may occur, and these are evulsion type injuries, secondary to the pull of the attached strong erectae spinae and psoas muscles.

Our usual protocol for evaluation of the patients with an acute thoracolumbar spine injury is to obtain a routine plain AP and transtable lateral radiograph performed with the patient on the rigid "spine board" (9). The alignment of the spinal canal and the presence of fractures are determined from these films. If the roentgenograms are normal, the appropriate oblique views are obtained. If any of these films demonstrates a fracture, the patient, still on the spine board is cycled through the CT scanner for computed axial tomograms at the level of the fracture (9, 25). This allows evaluation of the integrity of the spinal canal and the relationship of the bone fragments to the cross-sectional area (Fig. 33.17). Sagittal and coronal reconstructions can demonstrate the relationship of the encroaching bone fragments to the vertical axis of the spinal canal, as well as the displacement of the dura and its contents (Fig. 33.17D).

The reformatted images, in some instances, may be the only images demonstrating the spinal stenosis. The patient demonstrated in Figure 33.18 had an old compression injury at the level of L4 and L2. The latter healed with bony ankylosis of L1–L3. A laminectomy of L2 and L3 was performed at the time of the original injury. Several months later, the patient returned with symptoms. The axial images of the L2–L3 level (Fig. 33.18C and D), demonstrate the laminectomy and partial facetectomy, with no significant bony encroachment. However, the sagittal reformatted image (Fig. 33.18E) demonstrates the kyphosis at the level of the collapsed L2, causing a sharp angulation and posterior displacement of the dura and its contents at this level. In addition, it demonstrates the relative narrowing of the spinal canal between the kyphosis and the lamina arch of L1. This latter is not appreciated on the axial images.

SUMMARY

Computed axial tomography and the axial projection is the method of choice for evaluating the cross-sectional area of the lumbar vertebral column. With current technology, the bony structures of the osseous and the articular segments can be identified, as well as the intervertebral disc, the ligamentum flavum, the peridural fat, and the homogeneous dural sac containing spinal fluid and the cauda equina. Bony soft-tissue encroachments on the spinal canal can obliterate the peridural fat focally and can encroach and deform the dural sac containing the cauda equina.

The computed axial projection directly demonstrates the spinal canal and the effect of the different etiologies of spinal stenosis on the cross-sectional area.

References

1. Jones RAC, Thomson JLG: The narrow lumbar canal. *J Bone Joint Surg* 50:595–605, 1968.
2. Kirkaldy-Willis WH, Paine QWE, Cauchoix J, et al: Lumbar spinal stenosis. *Clin Orthop* 99:30–71, 1974.
3. Schatzker J, Pennal CV: Spinal stenosis, a cause of cauda equina compression. *J Bone Joint Surg* 50:606–618, 1960.
4. Epstein BS: *The Spine. A Radiographic Text and Atlas.* 3rd Ed. Lea and Febiger, Philadelphia, 1969.
5. Gargano FP, Jacobson R, Rosomoff H: Transverse axial tomography of the spine. *Neuroradiology* 6:254–258, 1974.
6. Jacobson RE, Gargano FP, Rosomoff HL: Transverse axial tomography of the spine. Part 1: axial anatomy of the normal lumbar spine. *J Neurosurg* 42:406–411, 1975.
7. Jacobson RE, Gargano FP, Rosomoff HL: Transverse axial tomography of the spine. Part 2: The stenotic canal. *J Neurosurg* 42:412–419, 1975.
8. Sheldon JJ, Russin LA, Gargano FP: Lumbar spinal stenosis. Radiographic diagnosis with special reference to transverse axial tomography. *Clin Orthop* 115:53–67, 1978.
9. Sheldon JJ, Sersland T, Leborgne J: Computed tomography of the lower lumbar vertebral column. *Radiology* 124:113–118, 1977.
10. Haughton WM, Silversten A, Williams AL: Soft tissue anatomy within the spinal canal, as seen on computed tomography. *Radiology* 134:649–656, 1980.
11. Williams AL, Haughton WM, Meyer GA, et al: Computed tomographic appearance of the bulging annulus. *Radiology* 142:403–408, 1982.
12. Williams AL, Haughton WM, Sylversten A: Computed tomography in the diagnosis of herniated nucleus pulposus. *Radiology* 135:95–99, 1980.
13. Ullrich CG, Binet EF, Sanecki MG, et al: Quantitative assessment of the lumbar spinal canal by computed tomography. *Radiology* 134:137–143, 1980.
14. Mikhael MA, Ciric I, Tarkington JA, et al: Neuroradiological evaluation of lateral recess syndrome. *Radiology* 140:97–107, 1981.
15. Epstein JA, Epstein BS: Lumbar and cervical spinal stenosis, with related cauda equina radiculopathy and myelopathy. In: Post MJD: *Radiographic Evaluation of the Spine: Current Advances with Emphasis on Computed Tomography.* Masson Publishing USA, Inc., New York, 1980, pp. 648–671.
16. Verbiest H: Neurogenic intermittent caudication in cases with absolute and relative stenosis of the lumbar vertebral canal (A.S.L.C. & R.S.L.C.) in cases with narrow lumbar intervertebral foramina, and in cases with both entities. *Clin Neurosurg* 20:204–214, 1972.
17. Verbiest H: A radicular syndrome from developmental narrowing of the lumbar vertebral canal. *J Bone Joint Surg* 36:230–237, 1954.
18. Verbiest H: Further experiences on the pathological influence of a developmental narrowness of the bony lumbar vertebral canal. *J Bone Joint Surg* 37:576–583, 1955.
19. Epstein BS, Epstein JA, Jones MD: Lumbar spinal stenosis. *Radiol Clin North Am* 15:227–239, 1977.
20. Junghanns H: Spondylolisthesis, pseudospondylolisthesis und wirbelverschiebung nach hinten. *Beitr 2 Klin Chir* 151:376, 1931.
21. Newman PH, Stone KH: The etiology of spondylolisthesis. *J Bone Joint Surg* 45:39–59, 1963.
22. Epstein BS, Epstein AJ, Jones MD: Degenerative spondylolisthesis with an intact neural arch. *Radiol Clin North Am* 15:275–287, 1977.
23. Epstein BS, Epstein JA, Jones MD: Lumbar spondylolisthesis with isthmic defects. *Radiol Clin North Am* 15:261–273, 1977.
24. Hanafee W, Crandall P: Trauma of the spine and its contents. *Radiol Clin North Am* 4:365–382, 1966.
25. Colley DP, Kunsker SB: Traumatic narrowing of the dorsolumbar spinal canal demonstrated by computer tomography. *Radiology* 129:95–98, 1978.

CHAPTER THIRTY-FOUR

Spondylolysis and Spondylolisthesis

STEPHEN L. G. ROTHMAN, M.D. and WILLIAM V. GLENN, Jr., M.D.

INTRODUCTION

This chapter will describe the multiplanar computed tomographic (CT/MPR) findings in a series of patients with either spondylolysis without dislocation, or spondylolisthesis. Spondylolisthesis may occur with pars interarticularis defects or without, producing two discrete symptom complexes, which will be described in detail.

SPONDYLOLYSIS—CLEAVAGE ABNORMALITIES OF THE PARS INTERARTICULARIS

Spondylolysis is a common condition found in approximately 5% of the general population (1). A fibrous cleft within the pars interarticularis divides the vertebral arch into two segments. The anterosuperior segment consists of the pedicle, the transverse process, and the superior facet. The posterior inferior segment consists of the inferior facet, the lamina, and the spinous process.

Two-thirds of pars interarticularis defects are found at L5 and approximately 30% at L4. The remainder of the lumbar spine accounts for only a very small percentage of the total.

Clefts occur bilaterally far more often than unilaterally. Infrequently, more than one level may be involved, usually at the lowest two lumbar segments.

The etiology of spondylolysis has been the source of much controversy in the literature. The main point of contention is whether the pars interarticularis defect is developmental in nature or an acquired cleft.

Currently, the most popular theory is that spondylolysis is due to repeated minor trauma, similar to stress fractures. The evidence revolves around the fact that the incidence of pars defects is very low in young children and continues to increase with age until it reaches approximately 6% in the adult population. Also, in some children with acute back pain, nuclear bone scans will be positive, suggesting the acute nature of the fracture.

SPONDYLOLISTHESIS

Isthmic spondylolisthesis is a condition whereby there is true anterior slippage of one vertebra on its next lowest mate due to a defect in the pars interarticularis. As is obvious from the previous discussion, isthmic spondylolisthesis most commonly occurs at dislocation of the vertebral body of L5 on the sacrum. Its clinical significance, aside from the obvious malalignment and malformation, rests mainly on the extent of functional disability and impairment of activity.

CLASSIFICATION

The following classifications of spondylolisthesis have been published by Wiltse et al. (2, 3).

Dysplastic

A congenital abnormality of the upper sacrum and/or the neural arch of L5 allows the lower lumbar vertebra to slide forward on the sacrum. The pars interarticularis is elongated and the facets dislocate. This is a very rare entity.

Isthmic

TYPE A

This is the most common type. The lesion tends to appear between the ages of 5½ to 6½ and has a definite familial propensity. It is not clear whether the lesion is due to flexion or extension trauma.

TYPE B

In Type B, the pars interarticularis is not fractured, but elongated. This, too, is thought to be due to repeated but healed stress fractures. The deformity is found occasionally in a family whose other members show signs of classical pars defects.

TYPE C

This is an acute, severe, traumatic injury to the vertebrae. It is the least common type of the group.

Degenerative

This disorder occurs at middle age. It is due to severe degeneration of the facet joints and disc and is caused by intervertebral joint instability. The affected segment may be subluxed forward or backward, with concomitant cauda equina compression.

Traumatic

This type is due to acute, severe fracture and is an unstable injury.

Pathological

In this type, slippage occurs because of some generalized disorder of bone, such as Paget's disease.

Iatrogenic

Dislocation of vertebrae may occur as a sequel to laminectomy with facetectomy, with subsequent loss of stability.

In his comprehensive study of the etiology of spondylolisthesis Wiltse (4) formulates a concept of pathogenesis. He suggests that the defect in the pars is caused by two factors: first, a hereditary propensity, or dysplasia of the pars, probably present at more than one anatomical level;

and second, unusual stress on the pars interarticularis in the lower lumbar spine due to the erect stance and lumbar lordosis in man. He further suggests that, in most cases, stress will not produce dissolution of the pars without the familial dysplasia. The character of the dysplasia has not been elucidated completely, but the effect of the dysplasia appears to be an incomplete or inappropriate attempt at healing these microstress fractures.

In the support of the fracture theory, Wiltse et al. (5) presented a series of 17 patients with lumbar radiographs that were thought to be normal, but later radiographs revealed pars interarticularis defects. All but one of these patients had been involved in some type of vigorous physical exercise. In 5 of these patients, the defect progressed to significant spondylolisthesis. A number of patients in this series were treated with body casts or corsets, and some were followed to complete healing.

MATERIALS AND METHODS

All patients in this study were examined on General Electric 8800 CT scanners with the gantry perpendicular to the plane of the x-ray table (zero gantry angle). Overlapping 5.0-mm thick sections were performed with 3.0 mm of overlap. A standard study extended from the top of the sacrum through the lower end plate of the L3 vertebral body. All the cases were reformatted routinely into sagittal and coronal planes, and the images were magnified to actual life-size for measuring the amount of disc herniation. Two sets of radiographs were made: one taken for soft tissue and the other for bone detail (6).

One hundred consecutive cases of pars interarticularis defects with or without spondylolisthesis were reviewed and the abnormalities were quantitated on a scale of 1–5. The amount of forward slippage was measured on midsagittal reformations, except where the dislocation was asymmetric. In those cases, the largest dislocation was measured on the appropriate sagittal image.

The amount of foraminal stenosis also was measured on the appropriate sagittal films. A value of 1 was assigned to a normal foramen, and 5 was allotted to a foramen reduced in both height and transverse diameter.

The amount of soft-tissue or bony callus at the site of the pars defect was estimated from the axial images and specified as either absent, present but probably not significant, or prominent and likely to be significant. These abnormalities will be discussed in detail in a later section.

RESULTS

In our clinical series, we had no examples of the rare congenital lumbosacral dysplastic type or of the acute traumatic types.

Isthmic defects with or without significant dislocation were noted in 100 patients: 94% were at L5 and 6% were at L4. Unilateral clefts were demonstrated in 13 patients. Disc protrusion or herniations defined as an anterior extradural defect of 5.0 mm or more, as seen on sagittal reformatted images, were noted in 28 levels in 26 patients. Significant herniation was noted far more frequently at

L4–5 than at L5-S1, and was rare at the level of the pars defect. Characteristic deformity of the neural foramina, best described as a flattening of the foramen with anteroposterior deformity, was encountered in 44% of the patients.

Congenital anomalies of the upper sacrum or the affected vertebral arch were noted in 36% of cases. The actual incidence may be slightly higher because the posterior elements of the sacrum were not visualized in many of the examinations. Lateral indentation or compression due to soft-tissue or bony callus was demonstrated in 51 patients, in one-half of whom it was thought to be potentially significant. Bony stenosis of the lateral recesses was defined in 8 cases.

DISCUSSION

The CT appearance of noncomplicated spondylolysis in the axial and sagittal planes is demonstrated in Figure 34.1. The nondisplaced pars fracture lies just anterior to the facets and is seen as horizontal lucencies extending into the spinal canal. In the sagittal plane, a jagged defect separating the vertebral body and superior facet from the inferior facet is noted.

As L5 slips forward on the sacrum, the axial scans take on a "double-canal" appearance. This is a geometric distortion of the canal due to the increase in lordosis that accompanies spondylolisthesis. The L5 disc space is so anteriorly angled that even maximal gantry tilt is unable to produce scans parallel to the disc. Sagittal images are most useful in these patients in evaluating the diameter of the spinal canal (Fig. 34.2).

In our series, unilateral pars defect was seen in 13% of cases. Frequently, they are asociated with anomalies of the neural arch or sacrum. Assuming the microfracture hypothesis is also correct in this category, then one must explain why a fracture occurs in only one pars. It has been suggested that there may have been fracture of the opposite pars with healing or with attempted healing. Some support for this hypothesis is found in patients similar to the one in Figure 34.3. This shows a typical right-sided pars defect, but the left pars and lamina are hypertrophied and sclerotic. The sagittal reformations demonstrate loss of definition of the corticomedullary junction of the pars on the enlarged side. This is thought to represent healing of microfractures and hypertrophy of bone along lines of stress.

Disc Herniation

The most sensitive radiographic procedure for the estimation of disc protrusion or herniation is CT. Sagittal reformations allow one to measure bulging of the anulus, which is invisible on myelography, especially in patients with wide epidural space. Definite disc protrusion is thought to have occurred when there is anterior epidural bulge of 5.0 mm or more. That is not to say that severe symptoms of disc herniation may not occur with lesser degrees of herniation, or that all 5.0-mm bulges cause symptoms. Clinically, however, our experience has shown that patients operated for 5.0-mm discs have significant

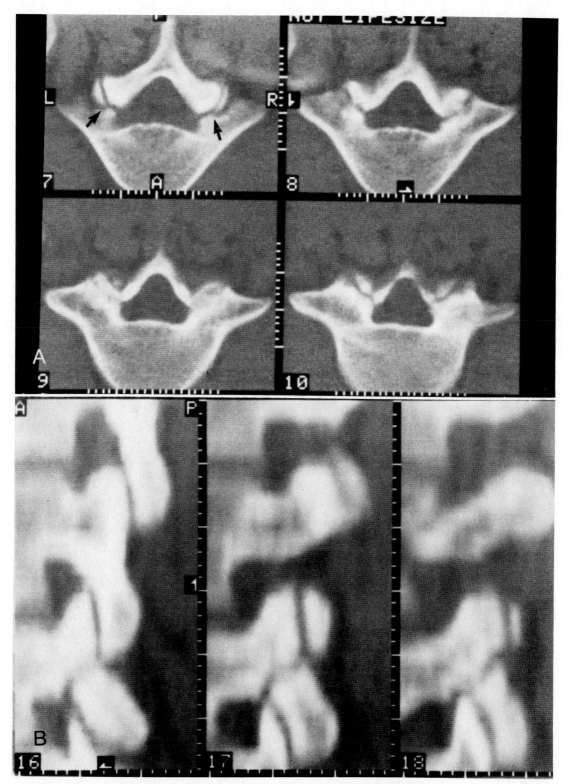

Figure 34.1.   A. Axial scans displayed for bone detail, demonstrating bilateral nondisplaced pars interarticularis defects (*arrows*).
B. Sagittal reformatted image through the pars interarticularis defect.

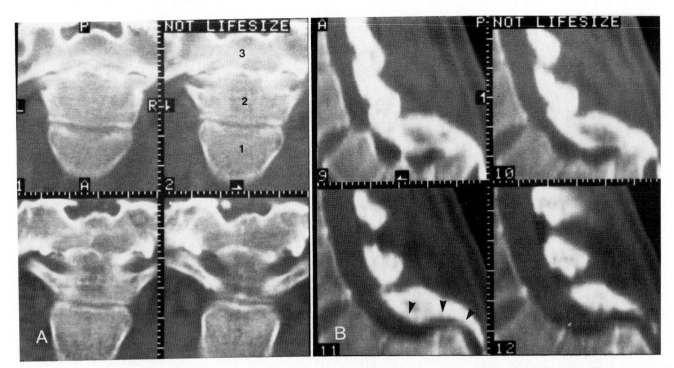

Figure 34.2. A. Axial and sagittal scans performed on a patient with a very severe juvenile spondylolisthesis. Three vertebral bodies are partially visualized on each of the axial sections. B. Sagittal reformatted images clearly demonstrate the remarkable deformity of the spinal canal (*arrowheads*).

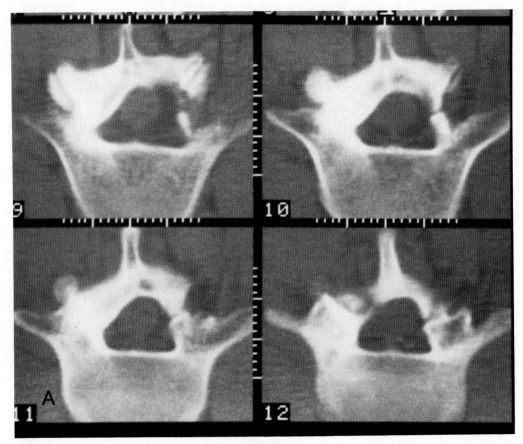

Figure 34.3. A.

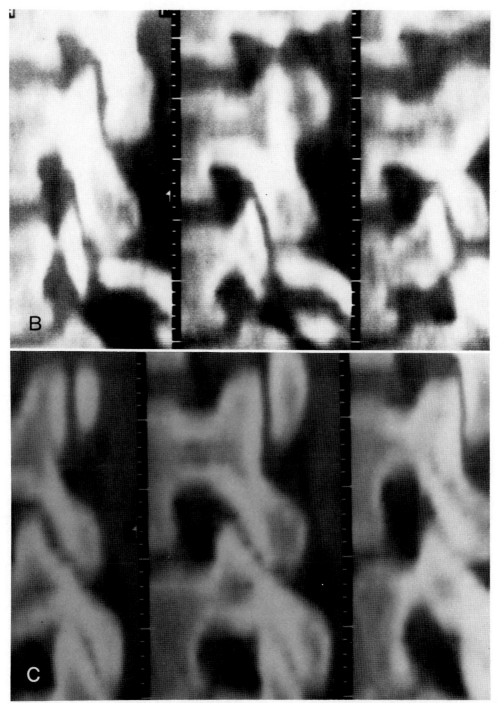

Figure 34.3. A. Axial scans demonstrating a unilateral right pars interarticularis defect. The left lamina is hypertrophied, the neural arch asymmetric, and the spinous process tilted toward the left. B. Sagittal reformatted scan through the right pars defect. The right pars and lamina are somewhat thinned. C. Reformated sagittal view through the thickened pars interarticularis on the left side.

pathology. Twenty-six patients had 5.0 mm or more of disc herniation. Two patients had changes at two levels. Figure 34.4 demonstrates a prominent disc herniation in a patient with a unilateral pars interarticularis defect.

Caution must be used if the amount of disc herniation

is being estimated only from the axial scans. In many of these patients, especially those who display the double-canal artifact, the axial scans tend to overestimate the amount of canal compression by bulging or extruded discs. On the axial view of Figure 34.5, there appears to be a

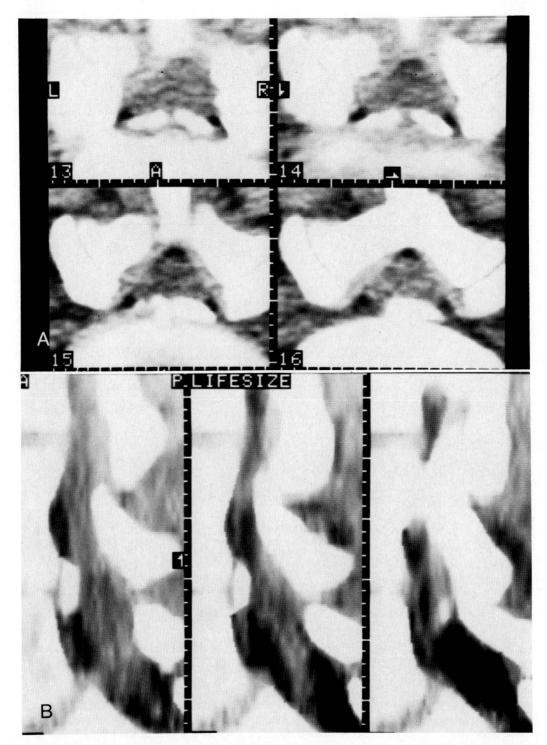

Figure 34.4. A and B. Patient with a unilateral left pars interarticularis defect with prominent disc herniation, noted most obviously on axial 14 and on the sagittal reformatted images.

very prominent extradural defect due to bulging disc. The sagittal images clearly demonstrate that the anulus is distorted, but no disc material bulge is posterior to the plane of the back of the sacrum. True disc herniation at the level of spondylolisthesis is quite rare.

Neural Foramina

Characteristic deformity of the neural foramina was seen in 44% of our patients. The height of the foramen at the involved segment is reduced, and the pedicle forming

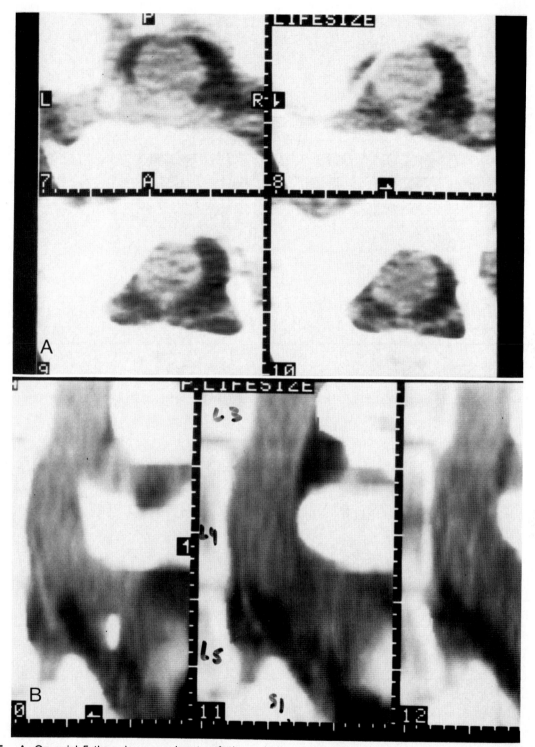

Figure 34.5. A. On axial 5 there is a prominent soft-tissue bulge anterior to the dura. This has the appearance of a large extradural defect. B. The sagittal reformatted image clearly demonstrates that there is no evidence of disc herniation, and that the apparent soft-tissue defect is due to beam angulation artifact.

the roof of the foramen is positioned inferiorly, abnormally close to the sacrum (Fig. 34.6). The orientation of foramen becomes horizontal rather than vertical. This may be noted in patients with little or no forward subluxation, but the degree of flatness of the foramen appears to parallel the amount of slippage in most instances.

Associated with flattening of the foramen is a combination of anterior and posterior bony indentation. Inden-

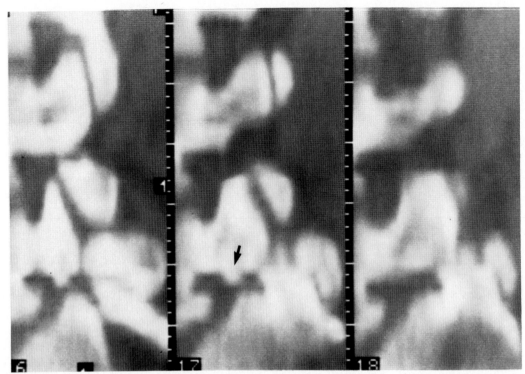

Figure 34.6. Sagittal CT scan for bone detail, demonstrating typical deformity of the neural foramen (*arrow*). The foramen is oriented horizontally rather than vertically and the inferior portion of the fractured pars is displaced downward toward the sacrum.

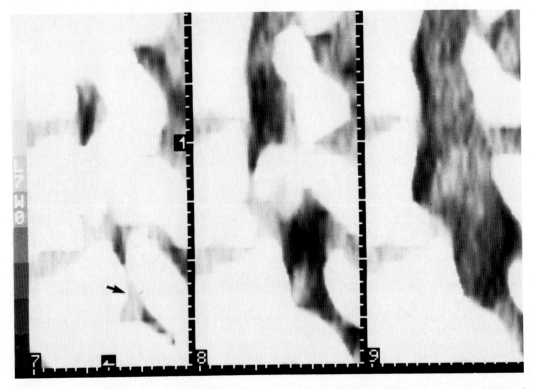

Figure 34.7. Sagittal CT through the neural foramen displayed for soft tissue. In the L4/5 foramen a normal nerve is surrounded by fat. At the level of the spondylolisthesis, the entire foramen is filled with soft-tissue density material, most likely bulging anulus (*arrow*).

tation on the posterior-superior aspect of the foramen is caused by downward displacement of the inferior tip of the base of the fractured pars. This gives the foramen a horizontally bilobed appearance. The descending inferior tip of the fractured pars forms a central bony septum within the horizontally oriented canal. As the amount of spondylolisthesis increases, or the height of the affected disc space decreases, the central indentation on the foramen becomes more severe.

The foramen becomes further compromised by the presence of lateral osteophytes, which occur commonly as changes secondary to the narrowing and deformity of the disc space. On sagittal images optimized for soft tissue (Fig. 34.7), one almost always can see that the deformed foramen is filled with abnormal soft tissue. The perineural fat usually is replaced totally by high-density soft tissue. It is not clear from the scans what this represents. Possibilities include lateral bulging of the anulus fibrosis, "callus" surrounding the pars defect, or a combination of the two. In any case, these findings of a deformed soft-tissue-filled foramen were noted in almost one-half of our cases.

Associated Anomalies

Spondylolysis is associated with a wide variety of congenital vertebral anomalies. The most common include spina bifida, hypoplastic facets, anomalous laminae, and major combinations of the above. A series of axial scans demonstrating a dysplastic left L5-S1 facet joint with a posterior laminar cleft is demonstrated in Figure 34.8. Note the asymmetry of the lamina and abnormal facet and spinous process.

Figure 34.9 shows a more complex anomaly in a patient with bilateral pars defects. A prominent lateral bulge indenting the theca is noted on the soft-tissue views. A prominent cleft is noted through the left half of the neural arch, there is asymmetry of the posterior elements, and a free-floating bone fragment is seen posteriorly on the coronal scans. From these and similar examples, one is tempted to suggest that the pars defect is congenital in origin, at least in patients with major ring anomalies. It certainly is possible, however, that the defect is secondary to minor trauma and congenital weakness due to the anomaly.

Lateral Canal Compression

Soft-tissue or bony indentation or compression of the lateral surface of the spinal canal was noted in 26 patients. This defect has not been emphasized previously in the radiological literature, but is described frequently in surgical articles as a fibrocartilaginous mass. Typically, there is a prominent soft-tissue bulge projecting medially from the site of the pars defect (Fig. 34.9B). In some patients, there may be calcification or true ossification within or abutting the pars defect. These lateral soft-tissue or bony masses may indent the dura, and occasionally severely compromise the spinal canal. These changes can be thought of as callus formed at the fracture site; the soft-tissue or bony sequel to pseudarthrosis formation. The axial plane is best for evaluating the presence and extent of this deformity.

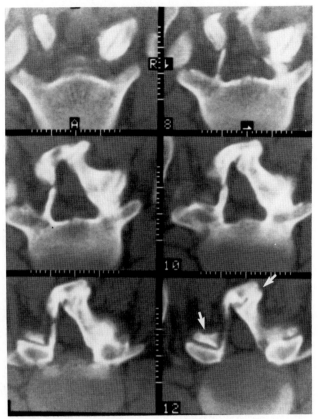

Figure 34.8. A series of axial scans on a patient with an anomalous L5 neural arch. The left lumbosacral facet is hypoplastic (*bottom arrow*) and the laminae asymmetric. The right hemilamina is thickened (*top arrow*), the left is diminutive. A posterior cleft is seen just to the right of the spinous process.

Lateral Recess

Osseous indentation of the lateral recesses was seen in 8% of cases (Fig. 34.10). When present, the compression usually was at the site of the pars defect, and frequently, but not always, associated with callus formation.

CAUSES OF PAIN IN SPONDYLOLISTHESIS

Many patients with spondylolysis and spondylolisthesis demonstrate radiographic abnormalities without ever having significant back pain. It is clear, therefore, that the mere demonstration of the defect on CT scanning does not necessarily indicate that the anatomical deformity is the cause of the patient's pain. According to Wiltse (3), pain in children is due either to degeneration of the disc at the level of the spondylolisthesis or to the acute pars fracture. He suggests that many, but certainly not all, degenerating discs are painful.

Degenerating disc at the level of the isthmic defect is more likely to be a cause of pain in adults. It appears that there may be many causes for back pain in adults with spondylolisthesis. It behooves us to seek out diligently the anatomical causes for each of these potential sources of back pain.

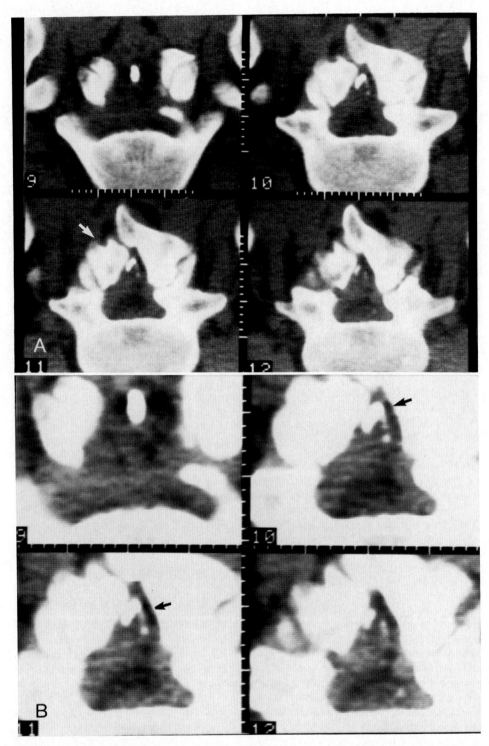

Figure 34.9.   A. Axial scan demonstrating a major anomaly of the posterior arch of L5 (*arrow*), associated with bilateral pars interarticularis defects. B. Soft-tissue axial scan demonstrating prominent calcified fibrocartilaginous mass compressing the dura (*arrows*). C. Coronal reformation: a free-floating bone fragment is visualized on the left side extending medially into the canal (*arrows*).

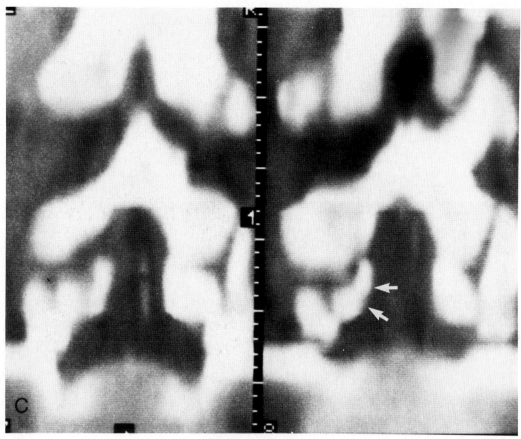

Figure 34.9. C.

It is noteworthy that true disc herniation is quite uncommon at the level of the pars defect; Briggs and Keats (7) report an incidence of 4%. Removal of the offending disc in these patients with or without concomitant spine fusion may be curative. Back pain also may be due to degeneration and abnormal motion at the disc space and abnormal traction on the anulus fibrosis.

Disc herniation at the interspace above the pars defect occurs much more frequently. MacNab (8) found abnormal L4 disc in 31% of patients with spondylolisthesis. Significant disc herniation on the CT scan may signify that the pars defect is asymptomatic and simple L4 discectomy will be curative. This is probably the most common cause of L5 radiculopathy.

L5 nerve-root compression may be caused by a prominent build-up of fibrocartilage at the site of the pars defect (9). This was seen clearly in many of the CT scans and should be brought to the attention of the surgeon. When the vertebral body slips forward on the sacrum, the neural arch can rotate on the pivot formed by its articulation with the sacrum, thereby compressing the foramen. Multiple small bone fragments at the upper end of the defect are said to add to the compression. Symptomatic nerve-root entrapment is more likely to occur if osteophytes have formed secondary to the disc degeneration.

In many of our cases, it appears that the foraminal narrowing primarily is due to downward herniation of the inferior pole of the fractured pars rather than to the floating neural arch. This deformity looks more ominous as the disc space narrows and the spondylolisthesis increases.

It is important that the radiologist be aware of the many causes of pain and neurological deficit in these patients. The CT/MPR study is probably the single most effective diagnostic test for determining the presence and severity of the majority of the abnormalities herein described.

DEGENERATIVE SPONDYLOLISTHESIS

Degenerative spondylolisthesis with intact neural arch is an important clinical condition. Although this entity was known to exist in the last century, it was Junghanns (10) who studied it carefully in 11 spines and described the pathological changes in detail. He coined the term "pseudospondylolisthesis." The terms "degenerative spondylolisthesis" or "degenerative spondylolisthesis with intact neural arch" (11) are more correct linguistically and descriptively since "spondylolisthesis" really means downward vertebral sliding.

The L4–5 intervertebral joint is the most commonly affected, followed by L3–4 and L5-S1. The amount of anterior slippage usually is less than 1 cm, but the effect on the neural elements may be devastating because the pars always is intact and the slipped vertebral body draws

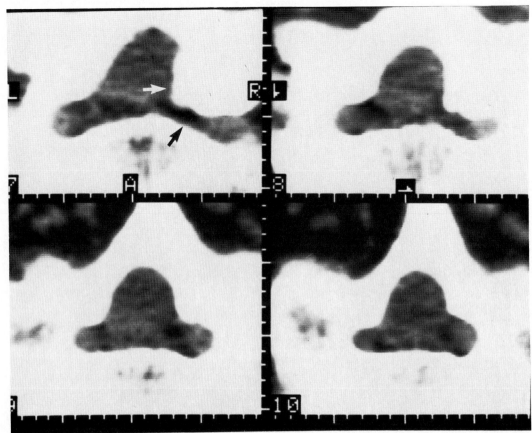

Figure 34.10.   Prominent osseous compression of the lateral recess in a patient with bilateral pars interarticularis defect (*arrow*).

its lamina with it. The cauda equina may become compressed between the anteriorly displaced lamina and the unusually stable L5 vertebral body (Fig. 34.11). Sacralization of L5 is four times more common in these patients than in the general population. This suggests that a relatively immobile L5-S1 articulation tends to predispose L4–5 to added stress. The incidence of degenerative spondylolisthesis is more common in blacks, almost exactly paralleling the increased incidence of sacralization of L5. The disorder is seen in patients under the age of 40 only rarely and in patients under the age of 50 only occasionally. Females are affected four times as frequently as males.

The weight of the upper half of the body is transmitted to the L5 level, producing a forward and downward vector force. This is resisted by the muscles, ligaments, and posterior articulations of the vertebrae. When the plane of the facets is oriented sagitally there is relatively less bony resistance to this force than when the orientation is oblique or coronal (Fig. 34.12). Because the L4–5 joints only occasionally lie in true sagittal orientation, this must be a relatively rare contributing factor. More commonly, the joint surfaces are curved so that they are sagittal posteriorly, but curved like a "J" anteriorly. This forms hooklike retaining surfaces which resist forward displacement similar to more oblique or coronal joints (Fig. 34.13).

MacNab (12) suggests that articular tropism at L5 may be very important in predisposing to dislocation. In these cases, the angle between the pedicle and the facet tends to be closer to 180° than to 90°, the more usual case (Fig. 34.14).

Increasing degeneration of the disc coupled with congenital malalignment leads to increasing mobility at the affected level. Anterior displacement is increased by flexion. On flexion and extension of the spine, therefore, the usual rocking of the joint is accompanied by forward and backward sliding. This abnormal motion adds to the eroding stress on the facets, further aggravating the slippage. It has been suggested that the anterior slippage is due only to disc generation. This seems very unlikely because narrowing of the disc with normal facet orientation should lead to downward and posterior subluxation.

Severe symptoms requiring surgery are relatively uncommon. Only 10 of Rosenberg's (13) 200 cases required surgical intervention. The most common clinical presentation is that of prolonged, chronic, central, low back pain; intermittent at first, but more persistent and severe as time goes on. Symptoms may be present for a matter of months or for many years. Unilateral or bilateral sciatica may be present and associated with motor neuropathy and weakness and atrophy of the lower extremities. Pain

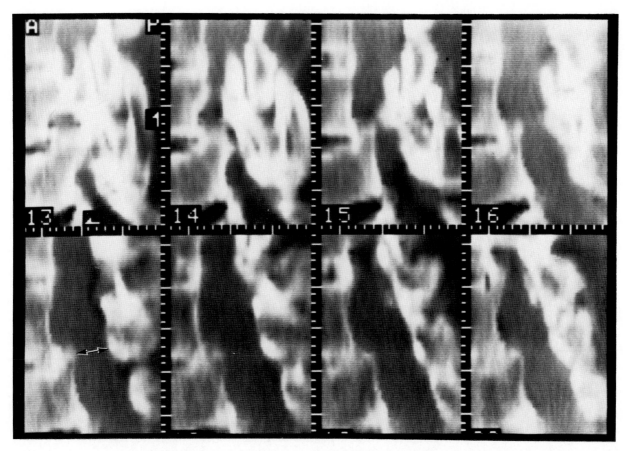

Figure 34.11.   A series of sagittal reformatted CT scans on a patient with degenerative spondylolisthesis. Vacuum disc effect is seen at L4–5 and L5-S1. The sagittal diameter of the spinal canal is severely compromised. The narrowest diameter is between the posterior border of the superior end plate of L5 and the base of the L4 lamina (*arrows*).

on straight leg raising (Lasegue's sign) commonly is not present.

Intermittent neural claudication is a relatively common sign in severe cases. Pain and paresthesia tend to increase upon walking or even standing with the back straight or extended. This pain is relieved by rest and by lying supine. The major reason for surgical intervention is evidence of cauda equina compression, which is similar to that produced by any other type of severe spinal stenosis.

CT ANALYSIS

Routine radiographs will demonstrate the amount of forward dislocation. Flexion-extension views on fluoroscopy are necessary to demonstrate the amount of abnormal motion at the intervertebral segment. Myelography has always been required for complete assessment of cauda equina and nerve-root compression. Multiplanar CT can replace myelography in the majority of these patients. It allows excellent visualization of the bony and soft-tissue deformity. CT analysis must include the following: 1) assessment of the amount of sagittal canal reduction; 2) evaluation of the amount of disc or anulus anterior, soft-tissue, extradural mass; 3) delineation of the anatomy of the facet surfaces and osteophytes; 4) notation of the

lateral or rotary laminar subluxation; 5) assessment of the amount of ligamentum flavum hypertrophy; and 6) evaluation of foramina for bony or soft-tissue encroachment.

Assessment of Spinal-Canal Compression

Figure 34.15 is a sagittal scan of a patient with a relatively wide spinal canal. The amount of subluxation was approximately 5.0 mm, as measured on the sagittal view. The narrowest area of this patient's spinal canal is an oblique line drawn from the tip of the lamina of L3 to the posterior rim of the superior end plate of L4. It is this forward dislocation of the lamina of the upper vertebral body that produces cauda equina compression. In this typical case there is no significant bulge of anulus material or disc herniation.

Disc herniation less commonly is associated with degenerative spondylolisthesis than with isthmic spondylolisthesis. Narrowing of the disc space and anulus degeneration, however, are noted very frequently. These facts correlate well with the overall incidence of disc herniation, which is higher through the 4th decade of life and then tends to decrease. Free-fragment herniation is more likely to occur in the young where the nucleus retains more of its gel-like character. Collapse of the desiccated

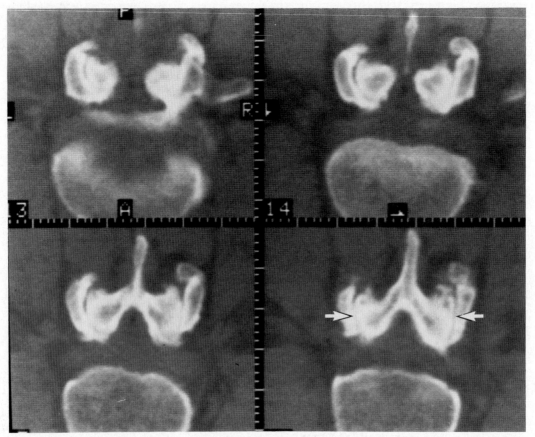

Figure 34.12. A series of axial scans on a patient with sagittally directed facets. There is very severe degeneration of the cartilaginous surfaces. Spurs are noted anteriorly and posteriorly, and there is forward subluxation (*arrows*).

disc space usually occurs without free-fragment herniation in the middle-aged and elderly.

The example in Figure 34.16 reveals severe stenosis of the spinal canal, predominately due to bulging of the disc or anulus at the site of spondylolisthesis. Of note in this patient is that both neural foramina, while relatively normal in size, are filled almost completely with abnormal disc or anulus material.

Assessment of Facet Pathology

Spondylolisthesis with intact neural arch is due primarily to severe erosion and degeneration of facet joints. These changes may be manifest in many different ways. The example in Figure 34.17 shows severe erosive osteoarthritic deformity of the facet joints, especially the left facet. The cartilaginous space appears unusually widened because of the severe irregular erosions that are present on both sides of the joint. This also can be seen to advantage on the sagittal and coronal views. There is a relative paucity of hypertrophic spondylitic spurs.

Not uncommonly, a vacuum joint effect is noted in this disorder. The patient in Figure 34.14 demonstrates very severe hypertrophic degenerative changes of the facets, with a prominent vacuum effect in the right joint. In all three projections, expansion and gas are seen within this

abnormal joint. The axes of the two facets vary considerably in these scans. The left facet is oriented more coronally than the right, and acts as a check to prevent marked subluxation. Although there is severe osteoarthritic erosion of the joints, there is only 3.0 mm of forward subluxation.

The most severe clinical symptoms may occur when there is unrestricted anterior dislocation of the inferior facet of the upper vertebral body, beyond the confines of the anterior limb of the superior facet. This may occur bilaterally, causing forward dislocation. More commonly, this occurs asymmetrically, producing rotatory subluxation. Rotatory subluxation can produce severe compression of the lateral recess and marked narrowing of the neural foramen on the affected side.

The least common type of dislocation is lateral dislocation, and this tends to occur when the joint surfaces are oriented more in the coronal plane. The sagittal diameter of the canal is spared, although there may be compression of the lateral surface of the dura.

Ligamentum flavum hypertrophy and joint-capsule expansion and swelling are findings frequently associated in patients with severe arthritis of the facet joints (Fig. 34.18). In these patients, an already severely compromised bony canal may be occluded totally by these soft-tissue hyper-

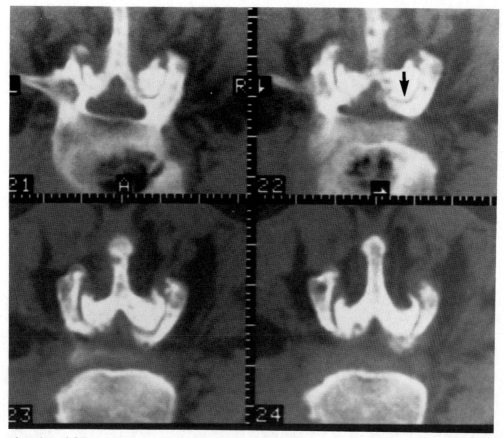

Figure 34.13. A series of CT scans on a patient with severe degenerative spondylolisthesis. The facets are oriented coronally (*arrows*), but there is a prominent anterior J-shaped hook of the facet on the left. Severe degeneration of the joint surfaces with cyst formation is visualized clearly, as well as gas within the disc space.

trophic masses. On occasion, the ligamenta flava may calcify. When this calcification is unduly thick, it also may cause posterolateral spinal-canal compression.

The neural foramina may be compromised by prominent osteoarthritic spurs or by bulging of the anulus fibrosis laterally into the neural foramen. These changes may account for some patients' severe radiculopathy.

RETROLISTHESIS OR REVERSE SPONDYLOLISTHESIS

Reverse spondylolisthesis is another condition that is manifested by abnormal vertebral alignment. Radiographically, one vertebra is seen to be displaced backwards on its next lowest neighbor. This condition is yet another manifestation of disc degeneration and narrowing (Fig. 34.19).

As discs thin and lose turgor, the vertebral end plates come closer to one another. If the facet joints have not been damaged by degenerative arthritis and are relatively normal, the weight of the body displaces the inferior facet of the upper vertebra, down the inclined surface of the superior facet of the lower vertebra, producing true retrospondylolisthesis. Traction of the erector spinatus

muscles and the ligamentum flavum may play some role in this displacement. The most mobile portions of the lumbar spine are more commonly affected. In our series, the usual areas of abnormality are L3–4 and L4–5. The cartilaginous surfaces of the facet are relatively normal in these patients, allowing downward slipping. Cartilage erosion is less evident than in cases of forward degenerative spondylolisthesis. At the involved interspace all the signs of disc degeneration will be present: disc narrowing, spur formation, sclerosis and erosion of the end plates, and facet-joint laxity. One of the important features of retrospondylolisthesis is the resultant foraminal stenosis. The inferior-posterior margin of the upper vertebral body moves backward into the foramen while the superior articular process of the lower vertebra glides upward and forward into the foramen. Frequently there is prominent lateral anulus bulge, further compromising the already diminished foramen.

CT EXAMINATION

CT examination of these patients should include the following: 1) assessment of the amount of sagittal canal reduction; 2) evaluation of the amount of soft-tissue com-

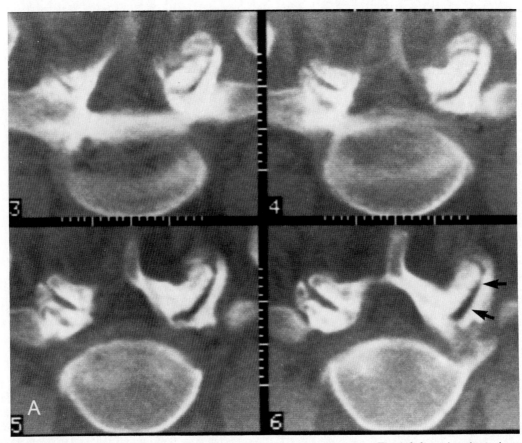

Figure 34.14.   A. A series of axial CT scans on a patient with marked facet tropism. The left facet is oriented coronally and the right facet is oriented sagittally. Note the large right facet spurs and vacuum effect in the right facet joint (*arrows*, A–C). B. and C. Sagittal and coronal of same.

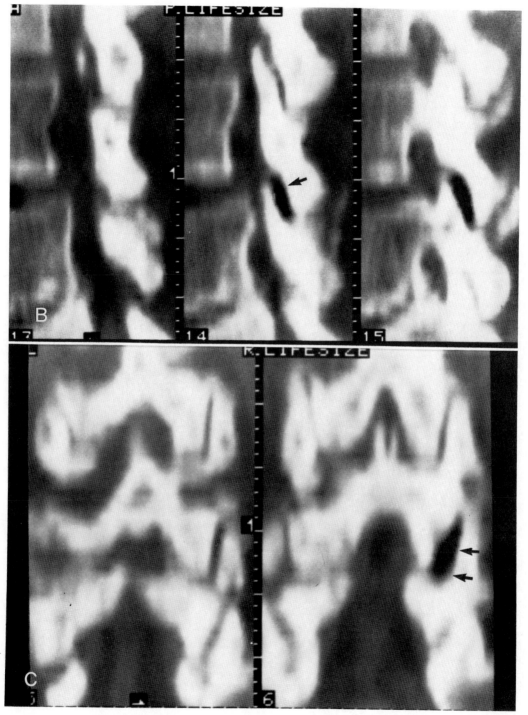

Figure 34.14.   B and C.

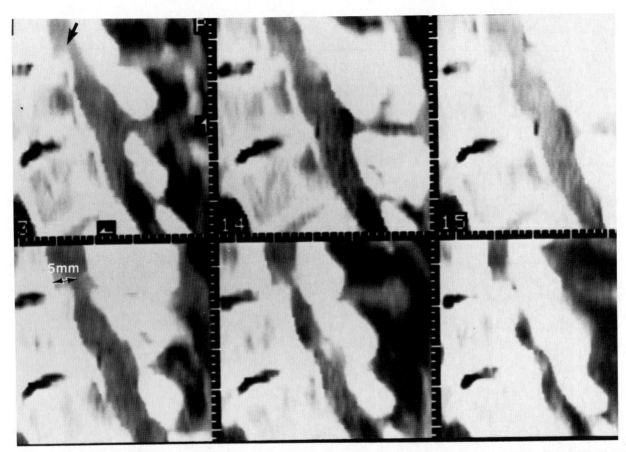

Figure 34.15. Composite set of sagittal reformatted images on a patient with 5.0 mm of degenerative spondylolisthesis.

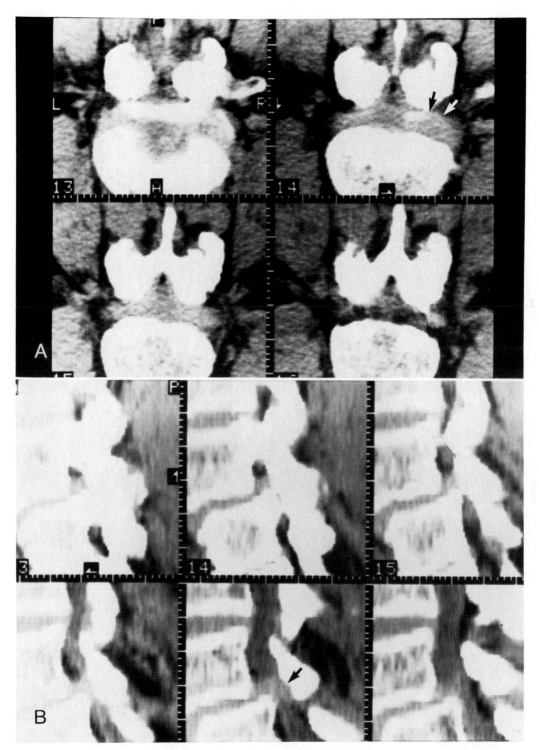

Figure 34.16.   A and B. Axial and sagittally reformatted image on a patient with severe spinal stenosis, due in part to degenerative spondylolisthesis. There is a very prominent bulge of the anulus, which fills the neural foramina bilaterally and severely compresses the cauda equina (*arrow*).

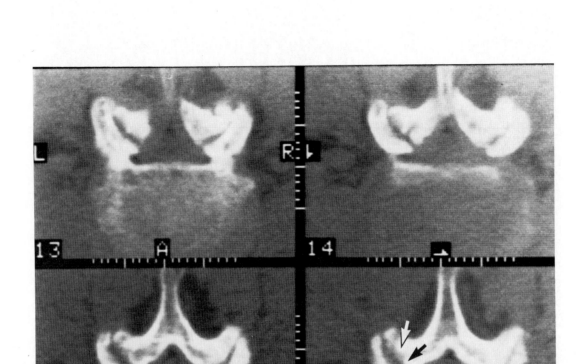

Figure 34.17. A–C. Axial CT scan and sagittal and coronal reformations demonstrating severe destructive arthritis of the left facet. The joint space apparently is widened, due to the severe erosive degenerative change (*arrows*).

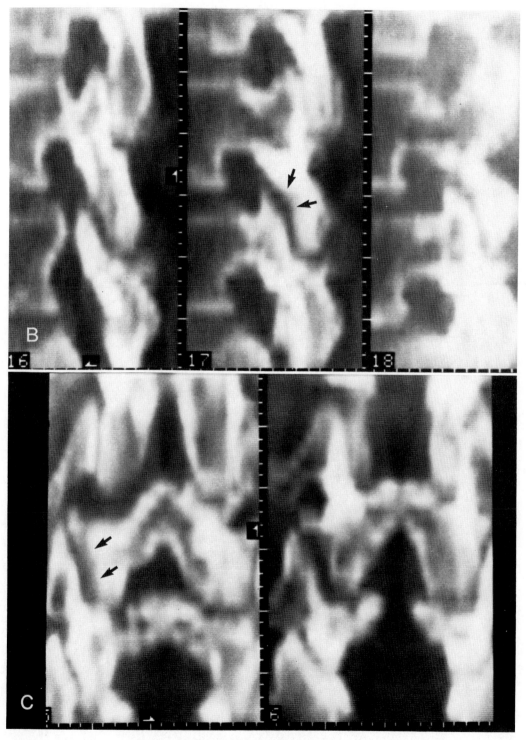

Figure 34.17.   B and C.

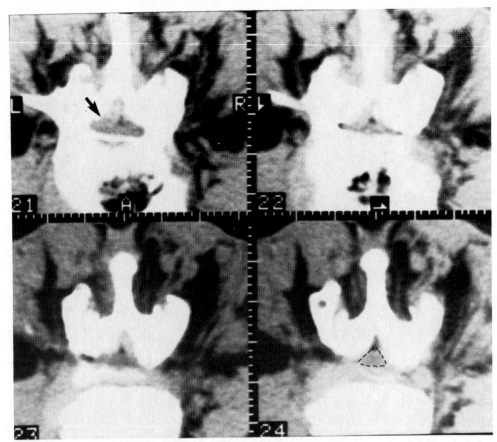

Figure 34.18. Composite axial scans on a patient with severe spinal stenosis. Note the prominent posterolateral indentation on the canal by prominent ligamenta flava (*arrows*).

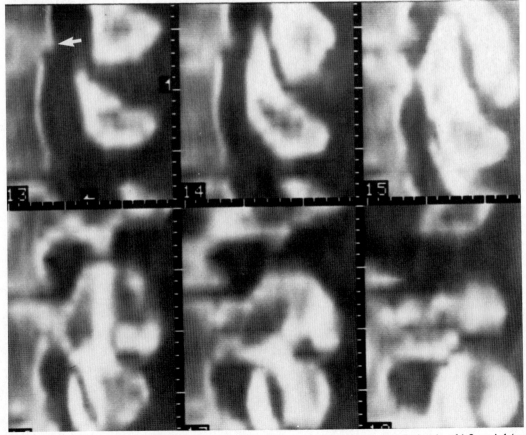

Figure 34.19. Composite of sagittally reformatted images on a patient with retrolisthesis of L3 on L4 (*arrow*).

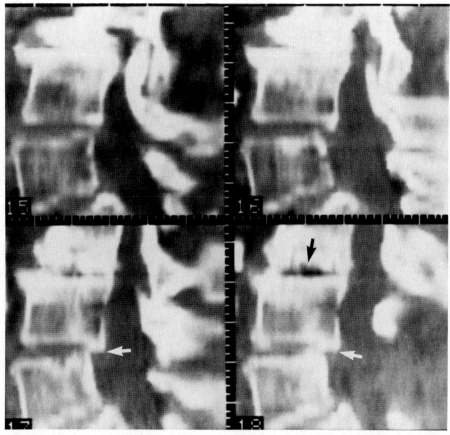

Figure 34.20.   A series of sagittally reformatted images on a patient with spondylolisthesis of L5 on the sacrum and retrolisthesis of L4 and L5 (*white arrow*). Note the severe destruction of the L3–4 disc space (*black arrow*) and the narrowing of the L4–5 disc space. There is minimal bulge of the anulus at L4–5.

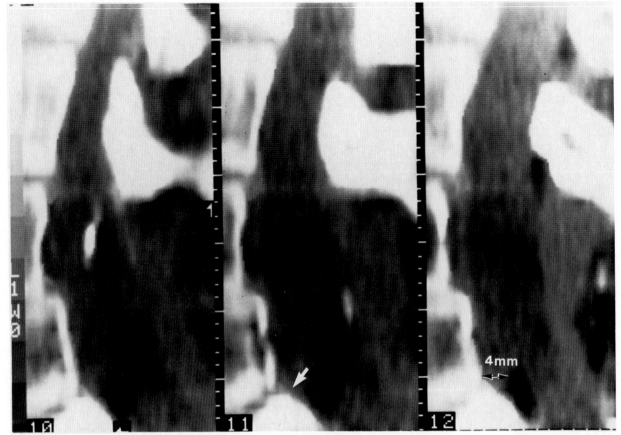

Figure 34.21. Sagittal reformatted CT on a patient with laminectomy at L4 and L5. There is approximately 4.0 mm of anterior dislocation of L4 on L5, due to the previous surgery (*arrows*).

pression; 3) evaluation of foraminal patency.

Marked reduction in the size of the spinal canal is relatively uncommon in patients with retrolisthesis. When present, compression occurs between the inferior end plate of the superior vertebra and the lamina on the inferior vertebra. Figure 34.20 is a sagittal reconstruction on a patient with isthmic spondylolisthesis of L5 and degenerative spondylolisthesis at L4. This is a relatively rare phenomenon. Note that there is only minimal indentation on the spinal canal.

As in degenerative spondylolisthesis with forward subluxation, disc herniation is relatively rare. However, when it does occur, the stenosis may be more severe because of the relatively narrow spinal canal.

IATROGENIC SPONDYLOLISTHESIS

We will clump into this group two distinctly different types of lesions. The first is known as "spondylolisthesis acquisita." It is believed to be a stress fracture of the pars at a level immediately above the spine fusion. Many patients with this lesion have had their fusions because of spondylolisthesis. This suggests an underlying predisposition to pars fracture. It is not clear whether surgical dissection of the muscles or vascular disturbance to the lamina and pars predispose to the fracture or whether it

is totally due to abnormal stress above the fusion. There usually is abnormal stress above or below spine fusion. This is most obvious in patients with congenital fusion who devleop severe degenerative arthritis adjacent to the fused vertebra.

There were no examples of this rare phenomenon in our series. This probably is due to the fact that most spine fusions performed in our geographical area are transverse process and lateral mass fusions, which tend to buttress the pars, protecting them from fracture.

The second disorder in this group is due to overzealous posterior and posterolateral decompression. Classically this is termed "iatrogenic spondylolisthesis." Radical decompression of the spine with facetectomy removes most of the bony support for the posterior elements (Fig. 34.21). We have studied 4 patients with this disorder. Two demonstrated posterior subluxation and 2 demonstrated anterior subluxation. The largest amount of displacement was 13 mm, the smallest was 7.0 mm. The lack of bony support in these patients accounts for the unusual degree of slippage.

SUMMARY

Spondylolysis and spondylolisthesis are common disorders that present to surgeons frequently because of severe back or radicular pain. As CT becomes more popular, it undoubtedly will become the primary diagnostic modality for the preoperative evaluation of these patients. It is important to assess the extent of foraminal encroachment, lateral recess stenosis, and posterolateral compression due to callus, as well as accompanying disc herniation. Myelography is unnecessary in most cases because all the significant pathology is extradural and well seen on the multiplanar CT examination.

References

1. Roche MB, Rowe GG: Incidence of separate neural arch and coincident bone variations. *Anat Rec* 109:233–55, 1951.
2. Wiltse LL: Spondylolisthesis: classification and etiology. *American Academy of Orthopaedic Surgeons Symposium on the Spine.* C.V. Mosby, St. Louis, 1969, pp. 143–167.
3. Wiltse LL: Spondylolisthesis and its treatment. In: Ruge D, Wiltse LL: *Spinal Disorders.* Lea & Febiger, Philadelphia, 1977, pp. 193–217.
4. Wiltse LL: The etiology of spondylolisthesis. *J Bone Joint Surg* 44A:539–569, 1963.
5. Wiltse LL, Widell EH Jr, Jackson DW: Fatigue fracture the basic lesion in isthmic spondylolisthesis. *J Bone Joint Surg* 57A:17–22, 1975.
6. Glenn WV Jr, Rothman SLG, Rhodes ML: Computed tomography/multiplanar reformatted (CT/MPR) examinations of the lumbar spine. In: Genant HK, Chafetz N, Helms CA: *Computed Tomography of the Lumbar Spine.* University of California Printing Department, San Francisco, 1982.
7. Briggs H, Keats S: Laminectomy and foramenotomy with chip fusion. Operative treatment for the relief of low back pain and sciatic pain associated with spondylolisthesis. *J Bone Joint Surg* 29:328–334, 1947.
8. MacNab I: The management of spondylolisthesis. *Progr Neurol Surg* 4:246–276, Basel Karger, 1971.
9. Gill GG: Spondylolisthesis and its treatment: Excision of loose lamina and decompression. In: Ruge D, Wiltse LL: *Spinal Disorders: Diagnosis and Treatment.* Philadelphia, Lea & Febiger, 1977, pp. 218–222.
10. Junghanns H: Spondylolisthese, pseudospondylolisthese und wirbelverschiebung nach hinten. *Beitr Klin Chir* 151:376, 1931.
11. Epstein BS, Epstein JA, Jones MD: Degenerative spondylolisthesis with intact neural arch. *Radiol Clin North Am* 15:2:275–287, 1977.
12. MacNab I: Spondylolisthesis with an intact neural arch—the so-called pseudo-spondylolisthesis. *J Bone Joint Surg* 32B:3:325–333, 1950.
13. Rosenberg NJ: Degenerative spondylolisthesis. Surgical treatment. *Clin Orthop Relat Res* 117:112, 1976.

CHAPTER THIRTY-FIVE

Computed Tomography of Ossification and Calcification of the Spinal Ligaments

KAZUO MIYASAKA, M.D., HIROSHI NAKAGAWA, M.D., KIYOSHI KANEDA, M.D., GORO IRIE, M.D., and MITSUO TSURU, M.D.*

Ossification and calcification of the spinal ligaments frequently may cause pressure upon the spinal cord and nerve roots. Since the first autopsy report of cervical myelopathy due to ossification of the posterior longitudinal ligament (OPLL) in 1960 (1), much attention has been given to this condition as a cause of progressive spinal cord and nerve root deterioration (2–11). Although OPLL of the cervical spine has been seen more frequently among Japanese (1–3% of plain radiographs), increasing numbers of cases have been reported in Western countries (12).

OPLL may affect the thoracic and lumbar regions and may or may not be associated with cervical involvement (13). According to the Japanese Ministry of Health and Welfare (14), about 10% of Japanese with cervical OPLL also had OPLL of the thoracic and lumbar spine. In the recent investigation by Ono et al., the prevalence of thoracic OPLL was 0.6%, with three times as many women as men being affected, compared with cervical OPLL which occurs predominantly in men (13).

In contrast, ossification and calcification of the ligamentum flavum (OLF) frequently is observed in both autopsy specimens and on plain radiographs of the thoracic spine (15–17). Therefore, it has not been considered to be a pathological state but has long been regarded as a normal anatomical process or as an aging change. However, since the first description by Yamaguchi et al. in 1960 (18) and by Tsurumi et al. (19) in 1964, both OLF and OPLL of the thoracic spine have received attention as causes of radiculomyelopathy (20, 21).

Such lesions in the spinal ligaments can be detected by lateral plain spinal radiographs. Nevertheless, some problems arise in the diagnosis of these conditions.

Firstly, plain films even combined with tomograms in sagittal and coronal planes, cannot always accurately define the full extent of ligamentous ossification. Definition in the upper thoracic spine is difficult because of the overlapping thoracic cage and shoulder girdle.

Secondly, because ossification sometimes involves different spinal levels and ligaments, it is not easy to determine which lesions are causing the patient's symptoms and which are asymtomatic. There is the question whether the patient's symptoms are brought on by ligamentous ossification or by associated lesions such as disc herniation and spondylosis.

With recent technical refinements, CT has advanced the delineation of both bone and paraspinal soft tissues greatly. In fact, effectiveness of CT in the diagnosis and management of spinal ligamentous ossification has been described in several reports (12, 13, 21–25). The purpose of this article is to present the CT findings of ligamentous ossification occluding the spinal canal.

MATERIALS AND METHODS

For a 15-month period beginning in 1981, 350 patients with spinal cord symptomatology have been examined by high-resolution CT. Of these, 36 patients were found to have ossification and calcification of the ligaments of the spinal canal. CT scans were performed on a Somatom 2 (Siemens), with the patient in the supine position. Four-millimeter thick sections with a 0.5 × 0.5 mm^2 pixel size were used routinely.

All 36 patients had had plain films of the spine taken before CT scanning. In 9, CT was performed after myelography using metrizamide via the lumbar route.

RESULTS AND DISCUSSION

The distribution of ligamentous ossification in 36 patients is shown in Table 35.1. In 9 patients, the symptoms and signs could not be attributed to ligamentous ossification, but to other causes such as herniated discs, spondylosis, and spondylolisthesis. The main cause of myelopathy or radiculomyelopathy in the remaining 27 patients was ossification of the spinal ligaments.

Twenty-nine patients had OPLL. The ossification was limited to the cervical region in 18 patients. In 10, OPLL involved both the cervical and the thoracolumbar spine, whereas in the remaining 1, it only involved the lumbar spine.

Association of OLF with OPLL was found in 7 patients; isolated involvement of the ligamentum flavum was seen in 7 other patients, 2 at the cervical level and 5 at the thoracic level.

OPLL

CT shows that the ossification is quite variable in shape and extent, and that it compromises the spinal canal to varying degrees. An ossifying mass as dense as compact bone is observed dorsal to the vertebral bodies and discs, which is consistent with the continuous type in the plain radiographic classification of cervical OPLL (26) (Fig. 35.1).

---

* We gratefully thank Hidetoshi Takei, MD, Satoru Abe, MD, and Toyohiko Isu, MD for their help in evaluating the patients.

Table 35.1.
Distribution of Spinal Ligamentous Ossifications[a]

Case	Sex/Age	Spinal level / Type	Associated lesion
1.	M/58	cont.	
2.	F/57	cont.	
3.	M/63	seg.	cd
4.	M/68	seg.	cd
5.	M/72	seg.	cd
6.	M/50	mix.	cd
7.	M/54	mix.	cd
8.	M/56	seg.	cd
9.	M/73	mix.	cd
10.	F/54	cont.	
11.	M/58	mix.	cd
12.	M/69	seg.	cd
13.	M/56	mix.	cd
14.	M/59	seg.	cd
15.	F/58	cont.	cd
16.	F/57	cont.	cd
17.	M/62	cont.	
18.	M/51	mix.	cd, OALL
19.	M/72	mix.	cd, OALL
20.	M/58	cont.	
21.	M/56	seg.	cd
22.	M/46	seg.	cd
23.	F/59	seg.	cd
24.	F/53	cont.	ld
25.	F/55	cont.	OALL
26.	F/51	cont.	ld, OALL
27.	F/65	cont.	
28.	F/62	cont.	ld
29.	M/49		
30.	M/50		
31.	M/36		cd
32.	M/58		
33.	M/49		
34.	M/56		
35.	F/62		cd
36.	F/70		cd

Spinal level columns: C. 1–7, T. 1–12, L. 1–5.

[a] Thin and thick lines show the levels of involvement of OPLL and OLF, respectively. Abbreviations: cont., continuous type of cervical OPLL; seg., segmental type of cervical OPLL; mix., mixed type of above two types (see text); OPLL, ossification of the posterior longitudinal ligament; OLF, ossification of the ligamentum flavum; OALL, ossification of the anterior longitudinal ligament; cd, cervical disc disease; ld, lumbar disc disease.

In some instances, however, the ossification is seen mainly dorsal to the vertebral bodies with little ossification adjacent to the discs, which is designated as the segmental type (26) (Fig. 35.2). As has been described previously, the former type favors the upper cervical spine or is distributed along long segments of the cervical spine, whereas the latter affects the lower cervical spine and is often associated with degenerative disc disease (Table 35.1). Both of these types can coexist in one subject as well.

Occasionally, the posterior longitudinal ligament is ossified asymmetrically in the spinal canal and the ossification extends laterally toward the intervertebral foramen along the intervertebral disc (Figs. 35.1 and 35.3). This extension follows the anatomy of the ligament which is relatively narrower over the bodies and wider over the discs (27, 28); although excessive bony overgrowth sometimes expands in thickness and width beyond the anatomical limits (29). OPLL can extend not only along the intervertebral disc but also along the dural sac (Fig. 35.4). This pattern again can be explained by the anatomy of the ligament. The superficial layer of the ligament extends laterally to cover the intervertebral discs and at the same time some of the other fibers of the layer merge into the dura mater (28).

Either a laminated pattern of dense ossification with an intervening translucent area (Fig. 35.3) or a soft-tissue density between the vertebral body and the ossified mass (Fig. 35.2) is seen on CT. The former pattern is probably

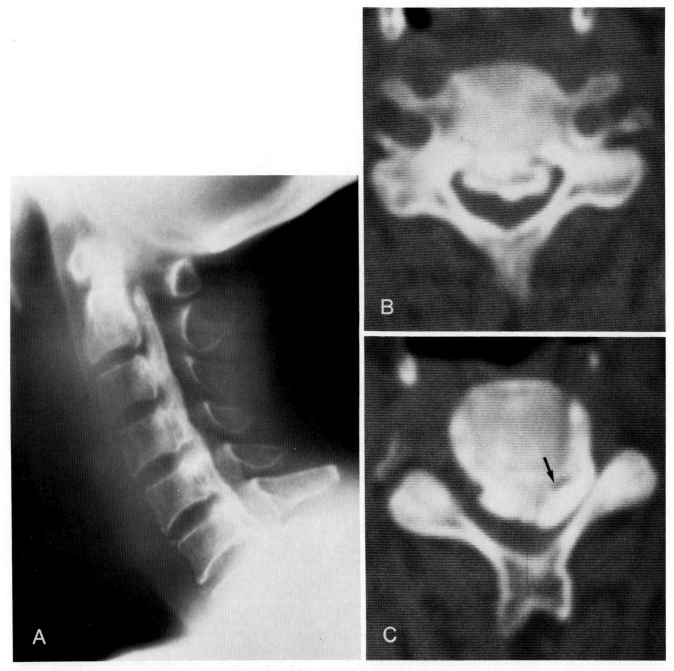

Figure 35.1. Continuous type of cervical OPLL. This 57-year-old female who, 12 years ago, started complaining of tingling pain and numbness in her right hand was admitted because of progressive tetraparesis over a 2-year period (Case 2 in Table 35.1). A. Lateral plain-film of the cervical spine. A long strip of ossification is seen dorsal to the vertebral bodies and discs extending from the base of the odontoid to C7 continuously. B. CT at C5 level. The ossification with a mushroom-like configuration markedly reduces the dimension of the spinal canal. C. CT at C4–5 shows the ossification extending laterally to compromise the left intervertebral foramen. A less dense area is seen posterior to the intervertebral space (*arrow*).

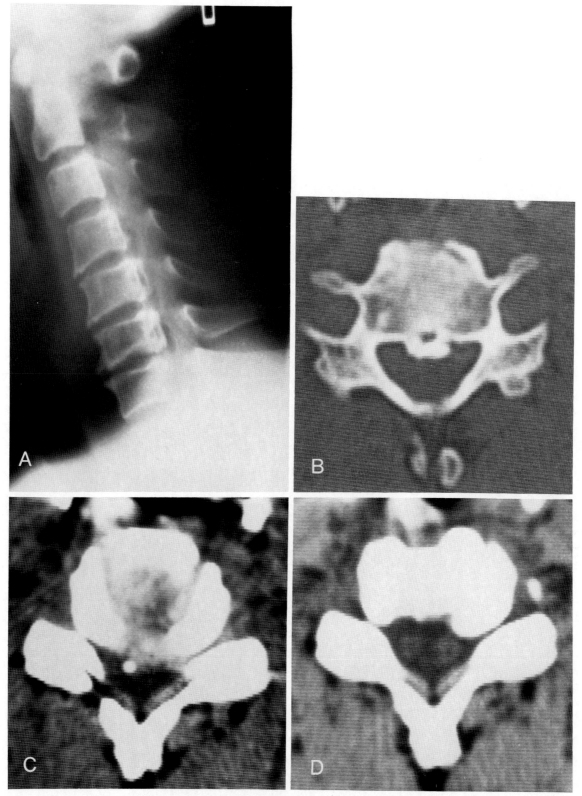

Figure 35.2. Segmental type of cervical OPLL. A 56-year-old male with a 5-month history of numbness in his upper extremities was admitted because of recent onset of gait disturbance (Case 8). A. Lateral plain film of the cervical spine shows ossified strips seen on the posterior aspect of the C5 and C6 vertebral bodies. B. CT image at C5 level which reconstructed by high-resolution bone mode shows the ossified mass on the posterior aspect of the vertebral body. A lucent area is seen between the spinal body and the ossification. C. CT at C5–6 level. Instead of OPLL, a soft-tissue density bulges posteriorly and left posterolaterally from the intervertebral space; which is consistent with a disc herniation. The spinal canal is constricted by the disc herniation ventrally and the thick ligamenta flava dorsally. D. CT at same level as C after anterior corpectomy with fusion. The spinal cord which was not seen preoperatively is now outlined by the subarachnoid space. This finding indicates the adequacy of epidural decompression.

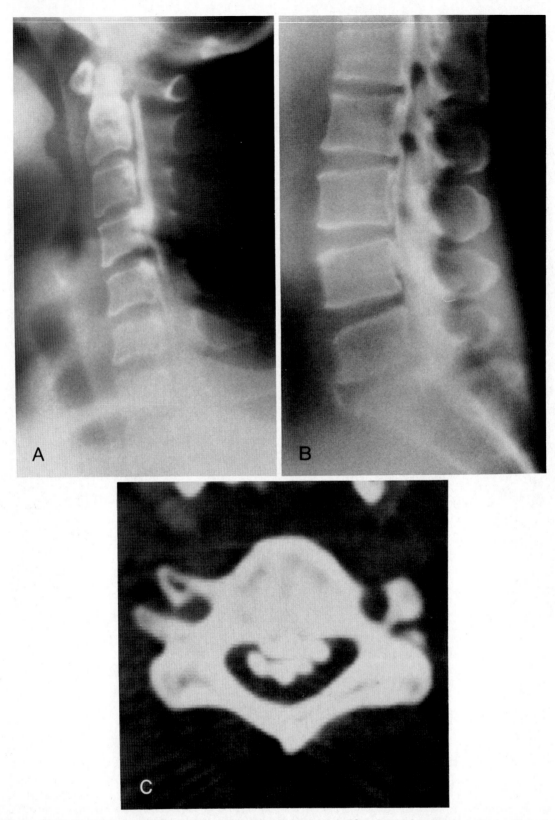

Figure 35.3. OPLL involving the cervical, thoracic, and lumbar spine. A 53-year-old female presented with gait disturbance which had been present for 2 years. A and B. Lateral plain films of the cervical and lumbar spine, respectively. There are OPLLS from C1 to C7 and from T12 to L4. C. CT at C6 level shows OPLL consisting of two ossified masses with an intervening translucency. D. CT at L3 level shows OPLL which is separated from the vertebral body by a radiolucent gap. E. CT at L3–4 level. The ossification extends along the intervertebral disc bilaterally (*arrow*) (Case 24 in Table 35.1).

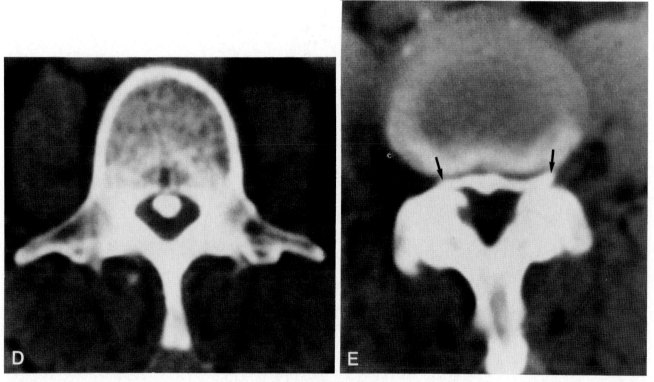

Figure 35.3. D and E.

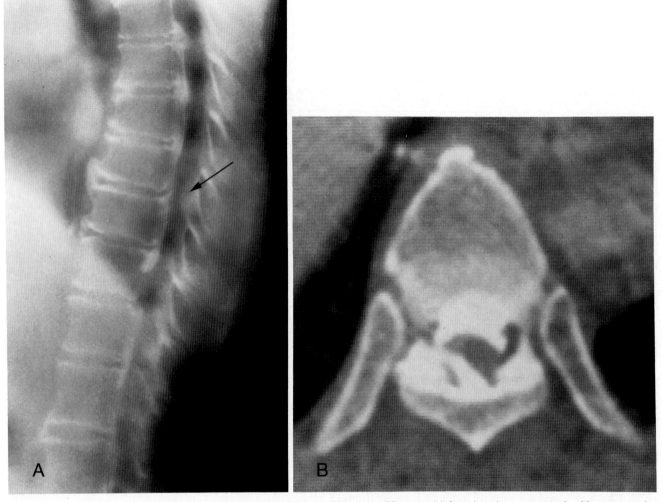

Figure 35.4.   Association of OPLL and OLF at T8–9 level. This is a 55-year-old female who presented with progressive weakness of the lower extremities for a 1-year period. Physical examination showed diminished sensation below T8 (Case 25). A. Thoracic plain film in lateral view shows a band-like OPLL involving the entire thoracic spine. Bony excrescence consistent with OLF is seen arising the lamina at T8–9 level (*arrow*). Also noted is hyperostosis of the ventral aspect of the vertebral bodies. B. CT at T8–9 level shows OPLL extending posteriorly to demarcate the dural sac. The ossified mass of OLF is seen in front of the right lamina and effaces the posterior epidural fat. The spinal canal is markedly reduced in size by these lesions.

due to ossification in both the superficial and the deep layers of the ligaments, and the latter is caused by the unossified deep layer (29). The ligament may be patchily (Fig. 35.5) or less densely calcified (Fig. 35.6); or even may remain as a mere thickening of soft tissue (29) (Fig. 35.5).

Postmortem examinations in cervical OPLL have shown that the bony overgrowth originates in the posterior longitudinal ligament and is composed of lamellar bone with well-developed Haversian canals and marrow cavities (9, 29).

Correlation of severity of neurological symptoms with the degree of spinal canal occlusion has been studied by several authors (24, 26, 29). Although cervical myelopathy can occur when the anteroposterior diameter is reduced by more than 40% (26), there is not always a close correlation with the degree of OPLL (2); or with the degree of reduction in canal size (13, 24, 26). Mobility of the cervical spine or of associated soft-tissue elements such as disc tissue and hypertrophic ligaments may be another prerequisite for neurological deterioration. Although the former factor is difficult to evaluate without myelography performed in flexion and extension position, the latter is well-delineated by CT (Fig. 35.2).

Cervical OPLL causing myelopathy unresponsive to conservative therapy may be operated on either by a posterior decompression with laminectomy or by an anterior decompression with fusion. The latter procedure has been described in detail by one of us (30). The effect of epidural decompression is well evaluated by CT (Fig. 35.2).

OPLL in the thoracic spine may or may not be associated with cervical OPLL, but it usually causes myelopathy in association with OLF (Fig. 35.4). OPLL in this region is distributed predominantly in the upper and midthoracic

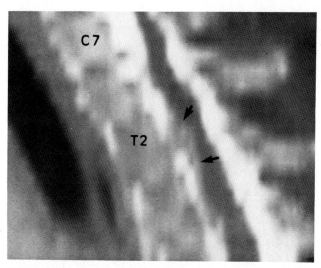

Figure 35.6.   Incomplete ossification of the posterior longitudinal ligament. Same case as in Figure 35.1. Reconstructed image in sagittal plane shows the lesion is less dense at the levels from T2 to T4 (*arrow*); although it also markedly compromises the spinal canal. Conventional tomography does not well delineate such a lesion, particularly when it involves the thoracic spine.

spine (13, 21). The shape of the ossification in the thoracic spine is slightly different from that in the cervical (13) (Fig. 35.4). Frequently seen is a type in which the ossification bridges over the adjacent vertebrae with maximal protrusion at the level of the intervertebral disc (Fig. 35.4).

OLF

The ligamentum flavum is affected in its lateral part, the capsular portion merging into the joint capsule; and also in its medial part, the interlaminar portion; and results in a mound-like excrescence ventral to the lamina (Figs. 35.4 and 35.7). CT optimally defines the location and extension of dense OLF. Often, a translucent area is seen between the ossification and the lamina (Figs. 35.4 and 35.7). OLF usually occurs bilaterally (Fig. 35.7). The lesion seen in OLF may not be as dense as compact bone. It may even have a soft tissue component associated with it. Although one can easily observe the presence of the lesion by employing CT, deformity of the spinal cord is demonstrated clearly by CT with intrathecal enhancement (Fig. 35.7).

We recently stressed the clinical significance of this condition (21). Myelopathy attributed to OLF, which favors the lower thoracic spine, was misdiagnosed for years, because myelography usually is performed with the patient in the prone position and the lesion is located posterolaterally in the spinal canal. It is important to keep in mind, therefore, that meticulous attention should be directed to the lateral plain film of the spine, where the bony excrescence arising from the lamine can be observed. Once this observation is made, the necessity of a CT scan for diagnosis will be obvious (Fig. 35.7).

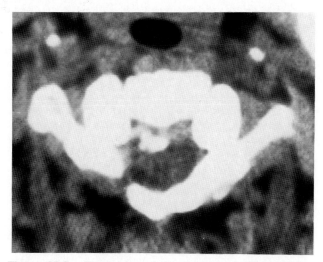

Figure 35.5.   Thickening of the posterior longitudinal ligament with patchy calcification. Same case as in Figure 35.3. CT at the C1 level shows thickening of the posterior longitudinal ligament in the membrana tectoria. Calcified deposits are seen in the ligament.

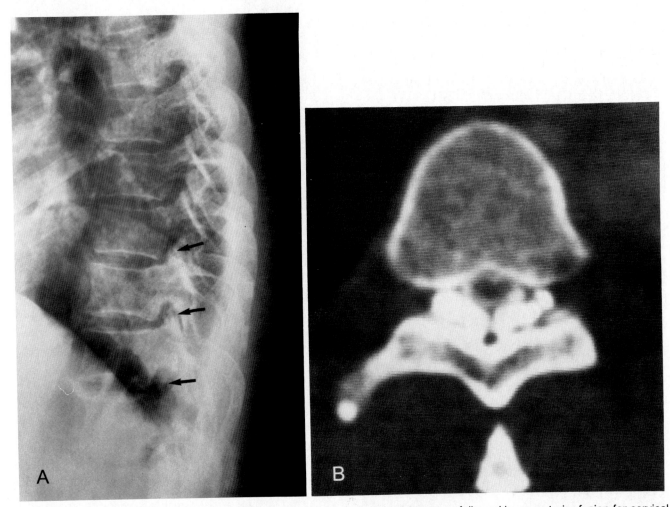

Figure 35.7. OLF at T9–10. A 50-year-old male who 3 years ago had a laminectomy followed by an anterior fusion for cervical OPLL at C3 and C4 was readmitted because of progressive weakness of his lower extremities for several months (Case 30). A. Lateral plain film of the thoracic spine shows bony excrescences in the intervertebral foramen arising from the laminae (*arrow*). B. CT at T9 level with intrathecal introduction of metrizamide. Bone excrescences are seen ventral to the laminae extending laterally toward the intervertebral foramen. The spinal cord is deformed by these lesions. A heavily ossified ligament extending to the pedicles was surgically removed.

In the cervical spine, ossification and calcification of the ligament are rare, but also are observed (Fig. 35.8).

Histopathological examinations of the ligamentum fla-

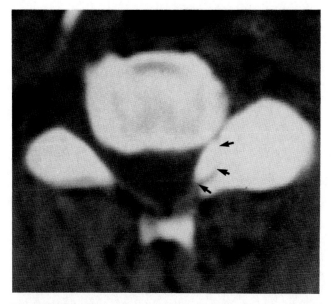

Figure 35.8. OLF at C4–5. A 63-year-old male was referred because of weakness and pain of his right arm (Case 3). CT at C4–5 level shows extensive ossification of a thickened ligamentum flavum on the left side (*arrow*). This OLF is separated from the hypertrophic facet joint by a lucent strip.

vum in the thoracic spine have shown mature bone extending along ligamentous fibers with no evidence of inflammation (21, 31). However, ligamentous calcification may be a feature of endemic fluorosis (32). We also have histologically confirmed calcification in the ligamentum flavum in the cervical spine.

Ossification of Other Ligaments and Differential Diagnosis

Although of little neurological significance, ossification of ligamentous structures outside the spinal canal can occur. The anterior longitudinal ligament, paravertebral connective tissue, and the joint capsules can ossify. Excellent delineation of these ossified ligaments can be achieved with CT.

Ankylosing spinal hyperostosis (ASH) (Forestier's disease (33), diffuse idiopathic skeletal hyperostosis (34)) occurs in middle-aged and elderly patients characterized by bone proliferation along the anterior aspect of the spine, particularly along the anterior and right lateral aspects of the thoracolumbar region (35). Association of ASH and OPLL, however, has been observed recently (13, 29, 36). Therefore, the question still remains as to whether these conditions are inter-related or, in other words, whether a common ossifying diathesis may involve the anterior aspect of the vertebral bodies or the posterior aspect or both. Radiological and histological evaluations described by Ono et al. (29) show that the pathological findings and the mode of development and growth of OPLL are quite distinct from that of syndesmophytes seen in ASH.

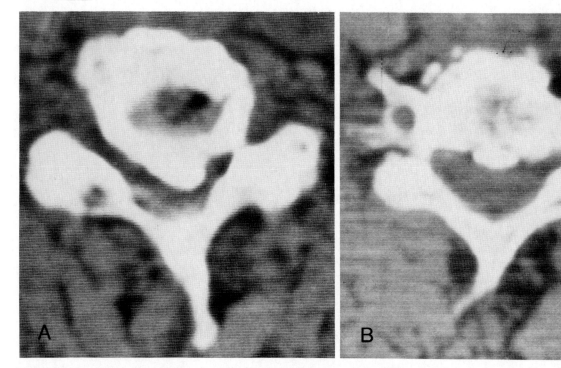

Figure 35.9. Probable herniated disc with calcification at C5–6. A 72-year-old male with a 1-year history of numbness in his left hand was admitted because of recent onset of weakness in all extremities (Case 19). A. CT at C5–6 level shows a calcified lesion dorsal to the intervertebral space. There is a low density area in the intervertebral disc space which is consistent with a vacuum phenomenon. B. CT at C6. Small OPLL is associated with the calcified disc.

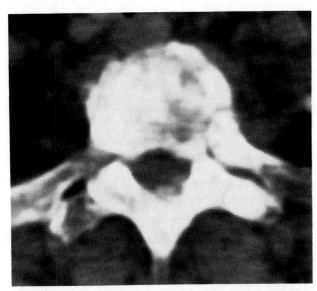

Figure 35.10. Metastatic adenocarcinoma of the spine. A 61-year-old female who 3 years ago had anterior corpectomy with fusion for metastatic tumor of the cervical spine was referred for acute onset of weakness of the lower extremities. CT at T1–2 level shows a high density mass ventral to the lamina which is irregular in outline. The vertebral body also has irregular margins and is of inhomogeneous density. These findings are consistent with metastatic disease of the spine with intrusion of destroyed bone fragments into the spinal canal.

The differential diagnosis of spinal ligamentous ossification shown on CT includes osteophytes in spondylosis, a calcified herniated disc (Fig. 35.9), degenerative hypertrophy of the intervertebral joint and lamina, and a calcified meningioma; and bone tumors such as osteochondroma, chordoma, benign osteoblastoma, and metastasis (Fig. 35.10); and subluxation with or without burst fracture of the spinal elements; and rarely extramedullary hematopoiesis, and Paget's disease. Ligamentous ossification is differentiated easily from most of these conditions because the ossification usually is confined to the anatomical boundaries of the ligament and is not associated with bone destruction.

SUMMARY

This study has shown that CT can demonstrate the extent of ligamentous ossifications causing radiculomyelopathy and can delineate associated soft-tissue abnormalities. CT shows that the posterior longitudinal ligament not infrequently ossifies along the intervertebral disc laterally and along the dural sac. CT also reveals that ossification of the ligamentum flavum often extends to the intervertebral foramen and pedicle. These CT findings are important for surgical intervention, whether an anterior or posterior approach is used. CT also demonstrates hypertrophic and incompletely ossified ligaments and disc degeneration including herniated or bulging discs and osteophytes. Pre- and postsurgical evaluation as to effectiveness of epidural decompression is atraumatically made by CT.

References

1. Tsukimoto H: Pathological case reports of hyperostosis in the cervical spinal canal which caused myelopathy (abstr.). *J Jpn Orthop Assoc* (Tokyo) 34:107, 1960.
2. Onji Y, Akiyama H, Shimomura Y, et al: Posterior paravertebral ossification causing cervical myelopathy. A report of eighteen cases. *J Bone Joint Surg* 49A:1314–1328, 1967.
3. Yanagi T, Yamamura Y, Ando K, et al: Ossification of the posterior longitudinal ligament of cervical spine. Analysis of 37 cases. *Clin Neurol* (Tokyo) 7:727–735, 1967.
4. Okamoto Y, Yasuma T: Ossification of the posterior longitudinal ligament of cervical spine with or without myelopathy. *J Jpn Orthop Assoc* 40:1349–1360, 1967.
5. Minagi M, Gronner AT: Calcification of the posterior longitudinal ligament: A cause of cervical myelopathy. *AJR* 105:365–369, 1969.
6. Forcier P, Morsey WJ: Calcification of the posterior longitudinal ligament at the thoracolumbar junction. Case report. *J Neurosurg* 32:684–685, 1970.
7. Hiramatsu Y, Nobechi T: Calcification of the posterior longitudinal ligament of the spine among Japanese. *Radiology* 100:307–312, 1971.
8. Palacios E, Brackett CE, Leary DJ: Ossification of the posterior longitudinal ligament associated with a herniated intervertebral disk. *Radiology* 100:313–314, 1971.
9. Nagashima C: Cervical myelopathy due to ossification of the posterior longitudinal ligament. *J Neurosurg* 37:653–660, 1972.
10. Takahashi M, Kawanami H, Tomonaga M, et al: Ossification of the posterior longitudinal ligament. A roentgenologic and clinical investigation. *Acta Radiolol* 13:25–36, 1972.
11. Nakanishi T, Mannen T, Toyokura Y, Sakaguchi R, Tsuyama N: Symptomatic ossification of the posterior longitudinal ligament of the cervical spine. Clinical findings. *Neurology* 24:1139–1143, 1974.
12. Murakami J, Russell WJ, Mayabuchi N, et al: Computed tomography of posterior longitudinal ligament ossification: Its appearance and diagnostic value with special reference to thoracic lesions. *J Comput Assist Tomogr* 6:41–50, 1982.
13. Ono M, Russell WJ, Kudo D, et al: Ossification of the thoracic posterior longitudinal ligament in a fixed population. Radiological and neurological manifestations. *Radiology* 143:469–474, 1982.
14. Tsuyama N, Kurokawa T: Posterior longitudinal ligament ossification in the thoracic and lumbar spine. Statistical report of posterior longitudinal ligament ossification for all of Japan. *Clin Orthop Surg* (Tokyo) 12:337–339, 1977.
15. Shore LR: A report on the nature of certain bony spurs arising from the dorsal arches of the thoracic vertebrae. *J Anat* 65:379–387, 1931.
16. Bakke SN: Spondylosis ossificans ligamentosa localisata. *ROEFO* 53:411–417, 1936.
17. Oppenheimer A: Calcification and ossification of vertebral ligaments (spondylitis ossificans ligamentosa): roentgen study of pathogenesis and clinical significance. *Radiology* 38:162–173, 1942.
18. Yamaguchi M, Tamagake S, Fujita S: A case of ossification of the ligamentum flavum causing thoracic myelopathy. *Orthop Surg* 11:951–956, 1960.
19. Tsurumi K, Hashimoto K, Niwa G, et al: Unusual cases of ankylosing spondylitis causing myelopathy. *Jahreber Kurashiki Zentral Hosp* 33:327–340, 1964.
20. Yanagi T, Kato H, Yamamura Y, Sobue I: Ossification of the spinal ligaments with special reference to the relationship between ossification of the ligamenta flava of the thoracic spine and the posterior longitudinal ligament of the cervical spine. *Clin Neurol* (Tokyo) 12:571–577, 1972.

21. Miyasaka K, Kaneda K, Ito T, Takei H, Sugimoto S, Tsuru M: Ossification of spinal ligaments causing thoracic radiculo-myelopathy. *Radiology* 143:463–468, 1982.
22. Hyman, RA, Merten CW, Liebeskind AL, et al: Computed tomography in ossification of the posterior longitudinal ligament. *Neuroradiology* 13:227–228, 1977.
23. Kadoya S, Nakamura T, Tada A: Neuroradiology of ossification of the posterior longitudinal spinal ligament—Comparative studies with computer tomography. *Neuroradiology* 16:357–358, 1978.
24. Yamatomo I, Kageyama N, Nakamura K, Takahashi T: Computed tomography in ossification of the posterior longitudinal ligament in the cervical spine. *Surg Neurol* 12:414–148, 1979.
25. Hanna M, Watt I: Posterior longitudinal ligament calcification of the cervical spine. *Br J Radiol* 52:901–905, 1979.
26. Seki M, Tsuyama N, Hayashi K, et al: Calcification of the posterior longitudinal ligament of the cervical spine. A clinical study of 185 cases. *Orthop Surg* (Tokyo) 25:704–710, 1974.
27. Davies DV, Coupland RE (Eds): *Gray's Anatomy.* Longmans, 1967, pp. 496–511.
28. Suzuki Y: An anatomical study on the anterior and posterior longitudinal ligament of the spinal column. Especially on its fine structure and ossifying disease process. *J Jpn Orthop Assoc* 46:179–195, 1972.
29. Ono K, Ota H, Tada K, Hamada H, Takaoka K: Ossified posterior longitudinal ligament A clinicopathological study. *Spine* 2:126–138, 1977.
30. Abe H, Tsuru M, Ito T, Iwasaki Y, Koiwa M: Anterior decompression for ossification of the posterior longitudinal ligament of the cervical spine. *J Neurosurg* 55:108–116, 1981.
31. Furuya M, Hachisuka A, Ogino M, et al: Three cases of paraparesis caused by ossification of the ligamentum flavum. *Clin Orthop Surg* 10:535–542, 1975.
32. Singh A, Dass R, Hayreh SS, Jolly SS: Skeletal changes in endemic fluorosis. *J Bone Joint Surg* 44:802–814, 1962.
33. Forestier J, Lagier R: Ankylosing hyperostosis of the spine. *Clin Orthop* 74:65–83, 1971.
34. Resnic D, Niwayama G: Radiographic and pathologic features of spinal involvement in diffuse idiopathic skeletal hperostosis (DISH). *Radiology* 119:559–568, 1976.
35. Epstein BS: *The Spine. A Radiological Text and Atlas.* Lea & Febiger, Philadelphia, 1976, pp. 382–385.
36. Resnic D, Guerra Jr. J, Robinson CA, et al: Association of diffuse idiopathic skeletal hyperostosis (DISH) and calcification and ossification of the posterior longitudinal ligament. *AJR* 131:1049–1053, 1978.

CHAPTER THIRTY-SIX

Computed Tomography of the Narrowed Spinal Canal

SEIKO HARATA, M.D. and SHUJI TOHNO, M.D.*

INTRODUCTION

In 1941, the authors reported on the application of transverse axial tomography (TAT) (1) to the spine. This procedure provided a cross-sectional view of the spine which allowed osseous abnormalities to be detected (2, 3). In recent years, the introduction of computed tomography (CT) has enabled a cross-sectional view of the spine to be obtained with greater contrast resolution than with TAT (4, 10). CT also has resulted in visualization of the spinal cord. Reconstruction of axial views into coronal and sagittal projections has provided three-dimensional views of the spine which have been very useful for determining the size and position of spinal lesions before surgical intervention.

Before the advent of high-resolution CT (HRCT) multiple radiographic studies such as plain films, conventional tomograms, myelograms, and angiograms were needed to establish a diagnosis. With the introduction of HRCT, fewer traditional radiographic studies have been necessary because of the increased diagnostic accuracy of CT.

MATERIALS AND METHODS

Delta 2060 and Delta 2020 Scanners were used for CT imaging. Using this equipment, there were few motion artifacts. Slice thicknesses varied from 2 mm to 5 mm to 10 mm. The thinner sections had less partial volume phenomenon and therefore little image distortion.

CT OF THE NORMAL ADULT CERVICAL SPINE

Standard Transverse Axial Tomographic Image Obtained by CT Scanning

CT technique is critical to the proper evaluation of the spine. As in TAT (6) (Fig. 36.1), it is important to adhere to a method for scanning the spine in cross-section which will allow a symmetrical view of the vertebral body and posterior arch to be obtained at every level. In this way, pathology can be detected when asymmetry of the spine is seen. Varying imaging methods for CT have been reported in the literuatre (7–9, 11–14).

We use a similar technique to TAT. We place the patient

---

* We would like to express our deep appreciation to Drs. M. Murosawa and Kimura for their help.

supine on the table with his face directed vertically. In this position, we obtain a Delta View—a CT scanogram in anteroposterior (AP) and lateral projections. When a Delta View of the atlas is desired, we angle the gantry so that the x-ray beam passes through the line joining the anterior tubercle with the posterior tubercle. For imaging C2–C7, we angle the gantry so that the x-ray beam passes through the line joining the arch with the pedicle. Because faulty positioning results in asymmetric imaging of the spine, we pay careful attention to gantry angulation. We view the final image that is obtained at either bone window or soft-tissue window settings, depending upon the purpose of the scan (Fig. 36.2A and B).

CT Myelography

The purpose of CT-assisted myelography (CTMM) is to provide contrast between the subarachnoid sac and the spinal cord. Since Di Chiro's and Schellinger's report in 1976 (15), the use of metrizamide (Amipaque) for CT of the spine has been reported by many authors (5, 6, 13, 16–22). Injected in the subarachnoid space, metrizamide surrounds the spinal cord and dura, thus, enabling clear differentiation of high-density osseous structures (Fig. 36.3).

To obtain a metrizamide CT scan, we perform a standard myelogram under fluoroscopic control using 10 cc of 250 mg/ml metrizamide via the lumbar route. Thirty minutes after this intrathecal injection, we image the patient on the CT scanner. We use a C1-C2 lateral puncture or a cisternal puncture to supplement the lumbar puncture when there is a complete block.

Figure 36.3 illustrates a normal CTMM. Sagittal reconstruction of axial metrizamide CT scans is beneficial for demonstrating the longitudinal extent of the osseous spine, subarachnoid space, and spinal cord.

Peridurography

Peridurography involves the injection of contrast medium into the epidural space which has a negative pressure. This procedure allows the morphology of the space between the dura and bony spinal canal to the determined (23).

Previously, the authors used a combination of peridurography and TAT to evaluate disease in the epidural space (24, 25). These combined procedures also allowed an accurate measurement of the true bony canal to be obtained. Recently, we have used CT with peridurography

Normal Adult

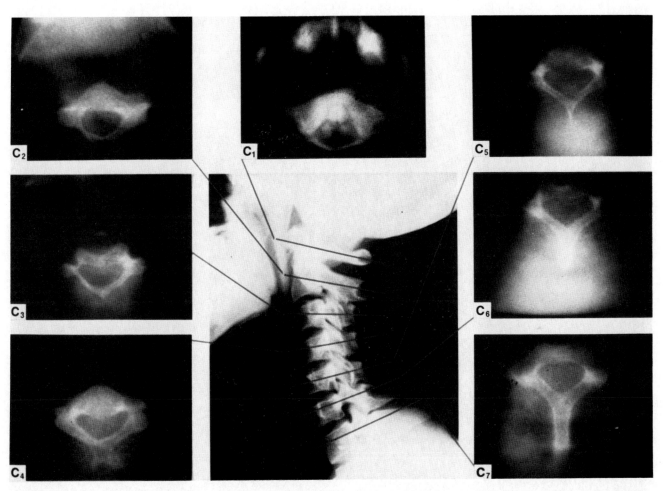

Figure 36.1.   TAT of the cervical spine in the normal adult. The C1–C7 vertebral bodies and posterior arches are symmetrically imaged.

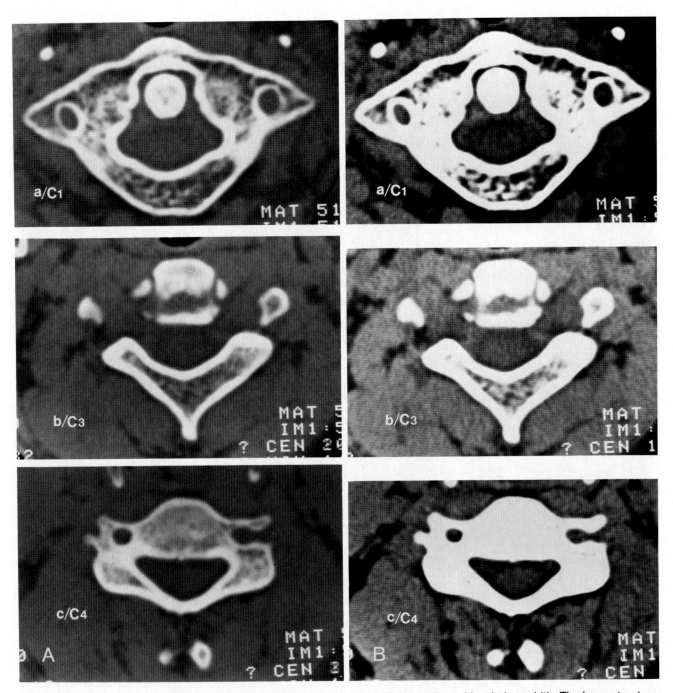

Figure 36.2. Plain CT scans of the cervical spine in the normal adult. A. Taken with a wide window width. The bony structures are imaged with more contrast on the CT scans than on the transverse axial tomograms seen in Figure 36.1. a/C1, b/C3, c/C4. B. Taken with a narrow window width for visualization of the soft tissues, including spinal cord (×), nerve roots (*arrows*), and ganglion, (△).

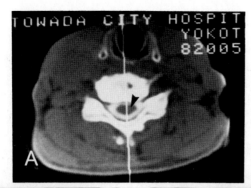

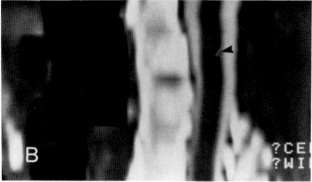

Figure 36.3. CTMM of the normal adult. A. Axial view of the spine clearly delineating the subarachnoid space and spinal cord (*arrowhead*). B. Sagittally reconstructed view of the cervical spine showing the longitudinal extent of the spinal cord (*arrowhead*) and subarachnoid sac to excellent advantage.

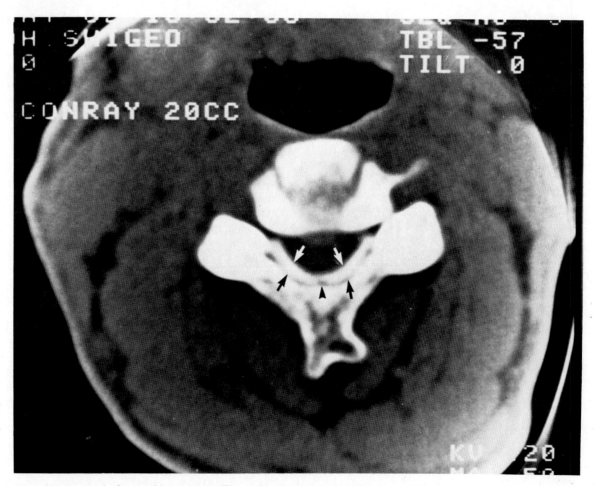

Figure 36.4. CT obtained after peridurography. The yellow ligament (arrowhead) and osseous borders of the spinal canal are delineated clearly because of the contrast in the peridural space (*arrow*).

and have found that the changes in the epidural space are easier to interpret with CT than with TAT. Figure 36.4 shows the CT scan of a normal case obtained after the injection of 20 cc of 20% Conray into the epidural space.

Cervical peridurography is performed with the patient in a sitting position. After palpating the C6 and C7 spinous processes, the operator inserts the needle into the skin and directs the needle toward a point between the C6 and C7 spinous processes. The Tuohy Flower needle is preferred for this procedure. After puncture of the yellow ligament, no resistance is felt thereafter. Physiological salt

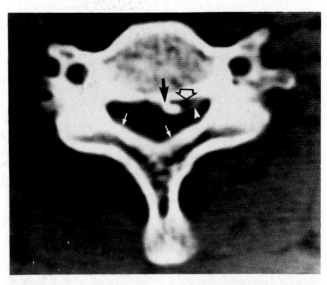

Figure 36.6. CT of peridurography in a case of cervical spondylosis. An osteophyte from the posterior aspect of the vertebral body (*large arrow*) and a disc (*open arrow*) project into the spinal canal. The contrast media introduced during peridurography discriminates clearly the anterior dural space (*arrowhead*) and the osteophyte. Posteriorly the layer of contrast (*short arrows*) is thin, an indication of the narrowed dural space.

water then is injected first. If no contraindications for injection are found, contrast media is then introduced into the epidural space.

CT Discography

There are some limitations to the imaging of disc herniations on plain CT scans (26, 27). The injection of contrast directly into the herniated disc has the advantage of showing the direction of the disc herniation, the size of the herniated disc within the spinal canal, and the degree of compression of the nerve roots and/or spinal cord.

Discography is performed under fluoroscopic control with the patient in the supine position. The operator separates the neck vessels from the trachea and esophagus and thus inserts a 23-gauge blue long needle percutaneously. Aiming slightly downward, he inserts the needle into the intervertebral disc.

If the needle penetrates the anterior longitudinal ligament, a small amount of local anesthetic agent is injected. If then the needle penetrates the intervertebral disc space, 1–2 cc of 60% Conray is injected. Very careful attention should be paid to whether the injected contrast medium leaks in an outwardly direction or in a posterior direction, whether there is radiating pain on injection and where the pain is located. When there are no such occurrences, CT scanning is performed.

DISEASES OF THE SPINE

This section discusses various pathological conditions which cause narrowing of the cervical spinal canal, in-

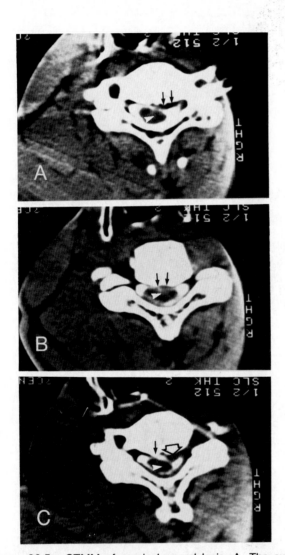

Figure 36.5. CTMM of cervical spondylosis. A. The subarachnoid sac is compressed by an osteophytic spur which is projecting from the posterior aspect of the vertebral body and by a herniated disc (*arrows*). The spinal cord (*arrowhead*) is displaced posterolaterally. B. The anterior aspect of the subarachnoid sac is not seen because of compression by the large osteophyte (*arrows*). C. The spinal cord (*arrowhead*) is compressed by the osteophyte in the midline (*arrow*) and by the disc (*open arrow*) laterally.

cluding cervical spondylosis, cervical disc herniation, ossification of the posterior longitudinal ligament (OPLL), and ossification of the yellow ligament (ligamentum flavum).

Cervical Spondylosis

In cervical spondylosis, osteophytes form and protrude into the spinal canal. Symptoms develop when the spinal cord or nerve roots are compressed by these osteophytes. The cross-sectional view is the best projection to demonstrate this disease process. This view can be accomplished both with TAT and with CT. However, contrast resolution is better with CT. With CTMM, displacement and compression of the spinal cord by osteophytes can be seen to best advantage (Fig. 36.5).

CT combined with peridurography can be used when

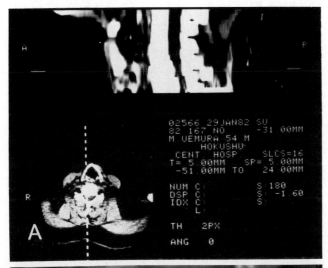

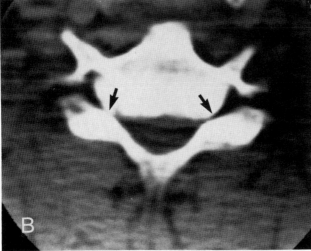

Figure 36.7. Plain CT demonstrating stenosis caused by cervical spondylosis. Sagittally reconstructed (A) and axial (B) views showing protrusion of the osteophytes (*arrows*) into the spinal canal and neuroforamen.

osteophytes deform the epidural space. Differentiation of osteophytic spurring from disc herniation can be accomplished by this procedure (Fig. 36.6).

Plain CT is effective for demonstrating degenerative changes of the joints of Luschka and for showing protrusion of osteophytes into the adjacent neuroforamen. Because osteophytic encroachment on the neuroforamen can cause muscle atrophy of the upper extremities, it is important to recognize this condition radiographically (Fig. 36.7).

Soft cervical disc herniations are not delineated clearly on plain CT. CTMM, however, outlines the disc herniation and also shows the compressed spinal cord. In order to determine the process by which the disc herniates from the disc space, however, or to what degree it extends into the spinal canal, CT discography is the procedure of choice. Figure 36.8A and B demonstrate a soft-disc herniation at the C5-C6 level in a 56-year-old male with intense pain radiating into his upper extremity. The contrast medium injected into the epidural space leaked profusely to the right and posteriorly into the spinal canal. CT discography in axial and coronally reconstructed views demonstrated the leakage of the contrast medium and showed its extension to the right and the compression of the nerve root. As a result of this study, the disc between C5 and C6 was excised and an anterior interbody fusion was performed. The patient's symptoms resolved after surgery.

OPLL

The cross-sectional appearance of OPLL changes with each vertebral body level. Previously, the authors classified the OPLL cross-sectional images into 6 types based on the location of calcification as determined by TAT (28). With CT, it is possible to detect ossification of the dura along with OPLL (29–33). When evaluating cases of OPLL with CT, it is best to take two images at different window settings, one for examining the ossification and the other for examining the condition of the spinal cord (Fig. 36.9A and B). With the use of a narrow window, deformities of the spinal cord caused by the ossification can be appreciated.

A laminectomy is one surgical procedure which can be used in cases of OPLL. With this method, decompression of the spinal cord can be accomplished (32). Figure 36.10A and B shows the CT scan of a patient who underwent a wide posterior arch decompression for OPLL and a posterolateral fusion. Relief of pressure on the spinal cord can be seen.

Ossification of the yellow ligament (OYL) rarely affects the spinal cord (34–36). On CT, however, encroachment on the posterior aspect of the spinal canal can be seen when the yellow ligament extensively ossifies (Fig. 36.11).

The Importance of CT to Adequate Preoperative and Postoperative Evaluation

The availability of CT with its cross-sectional view has made it possible to achieve a better morphological understanding of compressive lesions of the spinal canal than

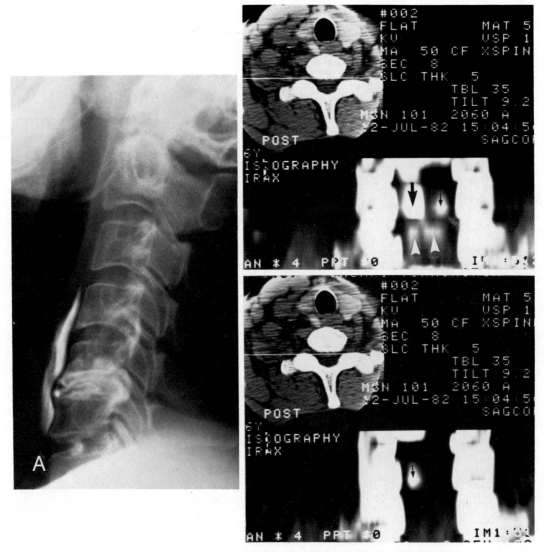

Figure 36.8. CT after discography for cervical disc herniation. A. Left. This lateral view of the cervical spine taken during discography shows a disc herniating into the spinal canal. *Top right*. CT images after coronal reconstruction reveal that the disc herniation is more severe on the right (*long arrow*) and less marked in the midline and to the left (*short arrow*). Leaked contrast medium (*arrowhead*) is seen. *Bottom right*. At a more posterior level than B, the disc (*arrow*) appears smaller. B. Axial section. *Top* and middle. The herniated disc is seen projecting into the spinal canal (*arrows*). *Bottom*. The leaked contrast (*arrow*) also is seen posterior to the vertebral body.

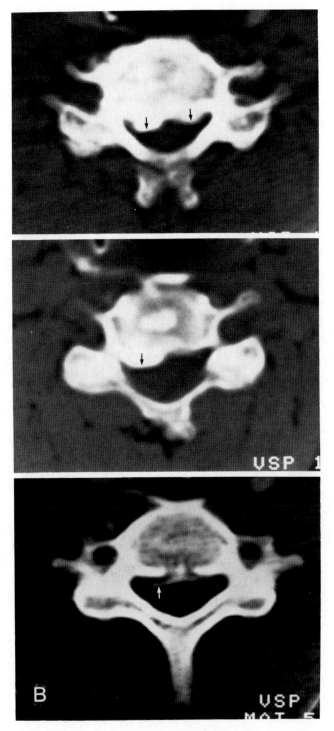

Figure 36.8 B.

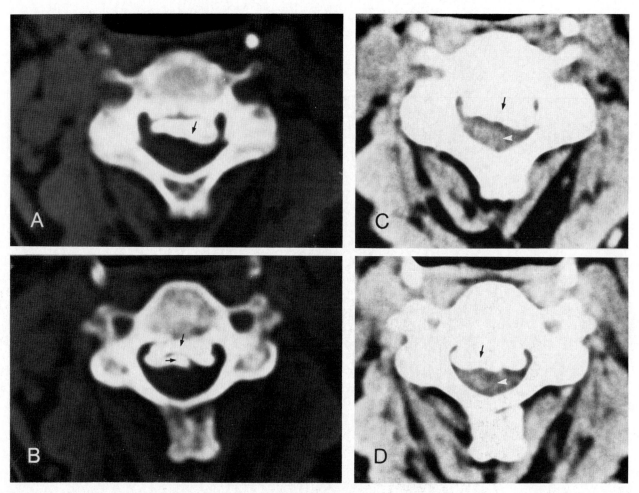

Figure 36.9. CT demonstration of ossification of the posterior longitudinal ligament. A and B. CT images taken at bone windows showing the large ossified posterior longitudinal ligament (*arrow*). In A, notice the separation of this ossified ligament from the vertebral body. C and D. CT images taken at soft-tissue windows of the same sections as A and B, showing compression and deformity of the spinal cord (*arrowhead*) by the ossified ligament (*arrow*).

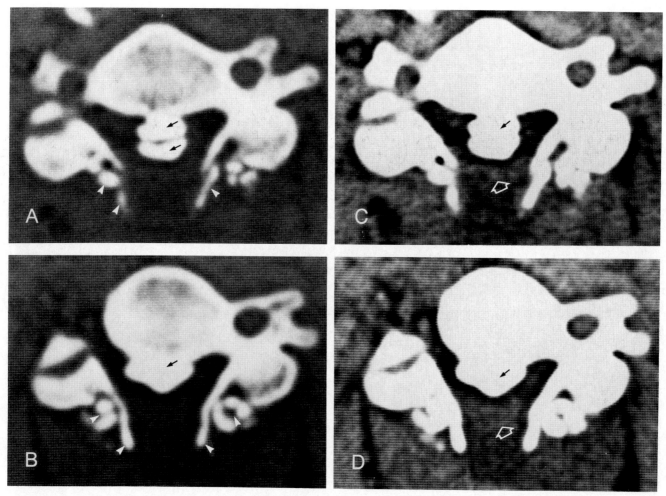

Figure 36.10.   A and B. CT images taken at bone-window settings showing an OPLL (*small arrow*) projecting into the spinal canal. Notice the wide posterior arch decompression and the bone chips for posterolateral fusion (*arrows*). C and D. CT images of the same levels as shown in A and B but taken at soft-tissue window settings. Notice the posterior displacement of the spinal cord (*open arrowhead*) as a result of the decompression. The OPLL (*small arrow*) also is seen.

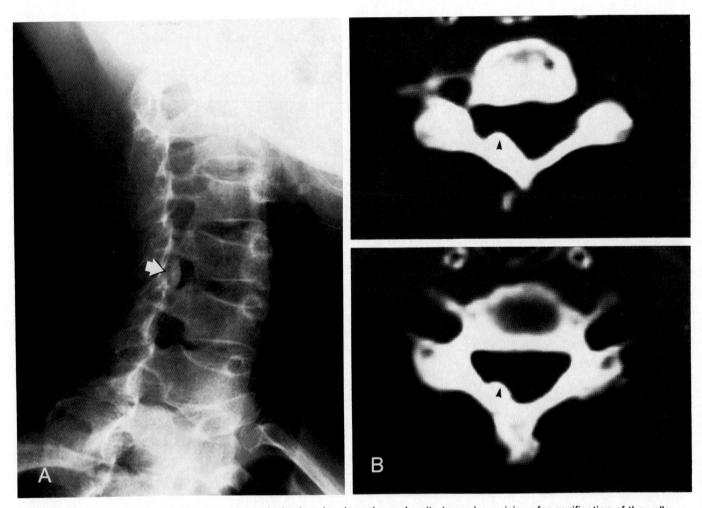

Figure 36.11. A. Oblique plain film of the cervical spine showing a bony density (*arrow*) suspicious for ossification of the yellow ligament. B. Top. CT scan of the inferior aspect of C5 documenting ossification of the yellow ligament (*arrowhead*). *Bottom,* CT scan of the superior aspect of C5 showing the extent of the ligamentum flavum ossification (*arrowhead*).

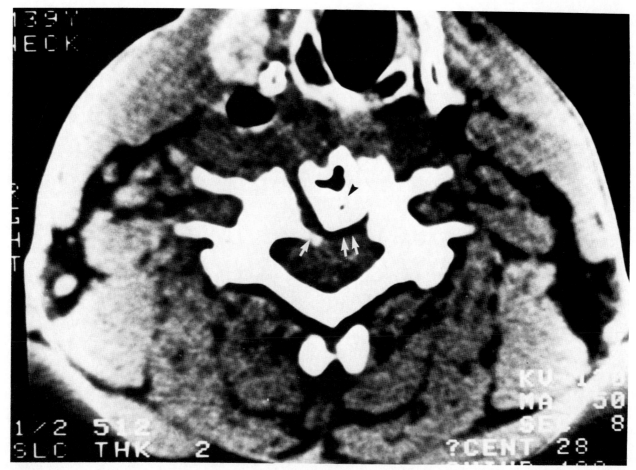

Figure 36.12. Anterior cervical fusion using iliac bone transplantation (*arrowhead*). This CT scan shows that there has been an adequate bony decompression of the spinal canal on the left (*double arrows*). On the right, however, the operation has not been effective because osteophytes still protrude into the spinal canal in this location (*single arrow*).

was possible with conventional radiographic studies. As a result, CT can determine the following more accurately than AP and lateral radiographs obtained during myelography, peridurography, and discography: 1) the size and configuration of the ossified lesion; 2) the presence of osteophytes causing compression; 3) the way in which the spinal canal is being narrowed; and 4) whether the lesion that is compressing the spinal cord is located ventrally or laterally. This determination by CT leads to the selection of the most appropriate surgical procedure for the lesion under evaluation (37).

Postoperatively, CT also plays an important role. CT determines in patients with spondylosis, OPLL, or OYL whether the spinal cord and/or nerve roots have been adequately decompressed (Fig. 36.12).

DISCUSSION

Before the advent of CT, TAT was the best study for demonstrating bony lesions such as cervical spondylosis and OPLL (1, 36). Since the introduction of CT, CT has become the procedure of choice for evaluating these le-

sions. The advantage that CT holds over TAT is that it can demonstrate not only the bony structures and osseous abnormalities but also the intraspinal soft tissues. Compression of the spinal cord by osteophytes and by OPLL, therefore, can be appreciated.

One limitation of CT that should be mentioned, however, is that the thickness of the slice, even when as thin as 2 or 5 mm, is still too thick to be able to calculate an exact measurement of the AP diameter of the canal and of canal area. Thus, even though measurements can be obtained from CT (38, 39), they are approximations. TAT, in contrast, is able to give more precise and accurate canal measurements which more closely approximate the real values, because the slice thickness in this procedure is 0.3 mm (6).

CONCLUSIONS

CT images obtained from high-resolution Delta 2060 and Delta 2020 Scanners were used to provide a cross-sectional view of the spine in cases of cervical spondylosis, OPLL, and OYL. The morphology of these lesions was determined from these scans. Plain scans were supplemented by CTMM, CT-peridurography, and CT discography when soft-tissue abnormalities and spinal cord position needed to be assessed.

References

1. Takahashi S: *An Axial Transverse Tomography and its Clinical Application.* Springer-Verlag, New York, 1969.
2. Harata S: Horizontal rotatory tomography. *J Jpn Orthop Assoc* 44:405, 1970.
3. Harata S: Axial transverse tomography. *Orthop Surg* 28:554, 1977.
4. Alfidi RJ, Hagga J, Meaney TF, et al: Computed tomography of the thorax and abdomen. *Radiology* 117:257, 1975.
5. Post MJD: *Radiographic Evaluation of the Spine:Current Advances with Emphasis on Computed Tomography.* Masson Publishing, New York, 1980.
6. Takahashi S: *Illustrated Computed Tomography.* Springer-Verlag, Heidelberg, 1900.
7. Nakagawa H: Disorders of spinal cord and spinal column. In: Takahashi: *CT in Neurological Disorders.* Nankodo, Tokyo, 505, 1979.
8. Nakagawa H: Spinal CT scan—Part 1, Cervical and thoracic spine. *Clin Orthop Surg* 17:51, 1982. (in Japanese)
9. Nakagawa H: CT Diagnosis of the spinal disorders—Mid and lower cervical spine. *Progr CT* 3:141, 1981.
10. Maehara T: Computed tomography of spine and spinal cord. *Neurol Surg* 9:993, 1981.
11. Hammerschlag SB, Wolpert SM, Carter BL: Computed tomography of spinal canal. *Radiology* 121:361, 1976.
12. Sheldon JJ, Sersland T, Leborgne J: Computed tomography of the lower lumbar vertebral column. Radiology, 124:113, 1977.
13. Thijssen HOM, Keyser A, Horstink MWM, et al: Morphology of the cervical spinal cord on computed myelography. *Neurology* 18:57, 1979.
14. Sha N, Kuihara A, Kataoka O: Application of computed tomography to spinal disorders. *Progr CT* 2:495, 1980.
15. Di Chiro G, Schellinger D: Computed tomography of spinal cord after lumbar intrathecal introduction of metrizamide (computer-assisted myelography). *Radiology* 120:101, 1976.
16. Roberson GH, Brisman J, Weies A, et al: CFS enhancement for computed tomography. *Surg Neurol* 6:235, 1976.
17. Skalpe Ingar O, Sortland O: *Myelography, Textbook and Atlas.* Tanum, Oslo, 1978.
18. Skalpe IO, Srtland O: Cervical myelography with metrizamide (Amipaque). *Neuroradiology* 16:275, 1978.
19. Harwood-Nash DC, Fitz CR: *Metrizamide in Children, New Techniques in Myelography.* Harper and Row Publishers, New York, 1979.
20. Masuzawa H: Usefulness and adverse effects of intrathecal metrizamide instillation. *Brain Nerve* 31:843, 1979.
21. Nagase J, Inoue S: Spinal CT with the use of metrizamide.

Cent Jpn Orthop Traumat 23:442, 1980.
22. Isu T: Computed tomography metrizamide myelography in spinal. *Neurol Surg* 9:483, 1981.
23. Nitta S: Cervical peridurography. In: Hattori: *Orthopedic MOOK,* Kanehara, Tokyo, 6;121, 1979.
24. Fujisawa Y, Tohno S, Harata S: Epidural space in peridurography. *Tohoku Arch Orthop Surg* 11:694, 1976.
25. Fujisawa Y, Tohno S, Harata S: Lumbar spinal canal in lumbar peridurography. *Clin Orthop Surg* 11:694, 1976.
26. Carrera GF, Williams AL, Haughton VM: Computed tomography in sciatica. *Radiology* 137:433, 1980.
27. Williams AL, Haughton VM, Syvertsen A: Computed tomography in the diagnosis of herniated nucleus pulposis. *Radiology* 135:95, 1980.
28. Harata S: Diagnosis fo OPLL of cervical spine by horizontal cross ratatory tomography. *Tohoku Arch Orthop Surg Traumat* 11:63, 1967.
29. Hyman RA, Merten CW, Stein HL: Computed tomography in ossification of the posterior longitudinal spinal ligament. *Neuroradiology* 13:227, 1977.
30. Wakabayashi A: A computed Tomography in OPLL of cervical spine. *J Jpn Orthop Assoc* 53:1387, 1978.
31. Kadoya S: Ossification of the posterior longitudinal ligament—Comparative studies with CT. *Neurol Surg* 7:63, 1979.
32. Shirgu H: CT of the cervical spine following surgical treatment for ossification of the posterior longitudinal ligament. *Orthop Traum Surg* 24:1005, 1981. (in Japanese)
33. Tanaka H, Ishida T: Morphological studies of OPLL by CT. *Nipp Arch Radio* 41:1048, 1981. (in Japanese)
34. Kawano N: Cervical radiculopathy caused by deposition of calcium phyrophosphate dihydrate crystals in the ligament flava. *J Neurosurg* 52:279, 1980.
35. Horhg-ko, Miura Y: Calcification of ligament flava of cervical spine. *Kanto J Orthop Traumat* 12:138, 1981.
36. Matsuda T, Takahashi S: Latest development in the evaluation of the spine with the Toshiba Transaxial Tomographic Unit. In: Post MJD: *Radiographic Evaluation of the Spine: Current Advances with Emphasis on CT.* Masson Publishing USA, New York, 1980, p. 491.
37. Nakagawa H: CT diagnosis of the spinal disorders—CT and various surgical approaches. *Progr CT* 3:659, 1981.
38. Lee Benjamin CP, Kazam E, Newman A: Computed tomography of the spine and spinal cord. *Radiology* 128:95, 1978.
39. Koehler PR, Anderson RE, Baxter B: The effect of computed tomography viewer controls on anatomical measurements. *Radiology* 130:189, 1979.
40. Hirose T: Studies on the measurement of spinal canal by using CT. *Cent Jpn Traumat* 23:1682, 1980.
41. Post MJD: Comparison of radiographic methods of diagnosing constrictive lesions of the spinal canal. *J Neurosurg* 48:360, 1978.
42. Ishimine T: A case of cervical myelopathy caused by calcification of the ligament flavum accompanied with C2-C3 cervical anomaly.

CHAPTER THIRTY-SEVEN

Advanced Cervical Rheumatoid Arthritis

RONALD L. KAUFMAN, M.D., F.A.C.P. and WILLIAM V. GLENN, Jr., M.D.

The cervical spine, via 25 synovial and 6 fibrocartilage articulations, spans the distance from the occipital condyles to the 1st thoracic vertebra. In addition to the osseous and cartilaginous structures, stability is provided by multiple ligamentous structures.

The articulation of the cranium with the atlas (C1) occurs at the occipitoatlantal joint, which is synovial-membrane lined. Additional support is provided by the anterior longitudinal ligament, anterior and posterior atlanto-occipital membranes, and the fibrous capsule of the atlanto-occipital joint. This area is thought to be unstable in children and increasingly stable in adults as ligaments decrease in elasticity. Motion at this joint is a moderate amount of flexion and extension (13°) and lateral bending (8°), but negligible axial rotation.

Atlantoaxial articulation occurs at three synovial-lined areas. There are two atlantoaxial articulations which are located directly below the atlanto-occipital joint and adjacent to the synovial membrane-encased dens. The ligamentous stability at this level is provided by the anterior longitudinal ligament, transverse ligament, tectoral membrane (continuation of posterior longitudinal ligament), posterior atlantoaxial membrane, and the nuchal (interspinal ligament). The dens also is joined to the cranium by apical and alar ligaments. The motion at this area is a moderate degree of flexion and extension (10°), negligible lateral bending, and extensive axial rotation (47°).

The ligamentous attachments in the area between occiput, atlas, and axis do not provide a tremendous amount of stability to this area. There are a number of weak links providing stability and, thus, any distortion or dissolution allows structural instability. This is in contradistinction to the remainder of the cervical spine and axial skeleton in general.

The articulations of the 2nd cervical segment through the 1st thoracic vertebra are accomplished by homologous structures. There are intervertebral discs at each of these levels. The diarthrodial articulations are at the posterior apophyseal joints and at the uncovertebral joints of Luschka, each with fibrous capsule and synovial lining. Ligamentous attachments are the anterior longitudinal ligament, posterior longitudinal ligament, and the very durable ligamentum flavum, which terminates at C3 and becomes the thin posterior atlanto-occipital membrane. Motion in the C2-T1 segment of the cervical spine accommodates a moderate amount of flexion, extension, lateral bending, and axial rotation.

When assessed as an intact unit, there are several anatomical relationships which are constant. The anterior margin of the odontoid process, if extended cephalad by an imaginary line, will meet the anterior margin of the foramen magnum. Similarly, an imaginary line joining posterior arches of the cervical vertebra will meet in a cephalad direction the posterior margin of the foramen magnum. These relationships remain constant with flexion or extension of the cervical spine. The vertical relationship of the occipitoatlantoaxial complex has been defined on both lateral and anteroposterior (AP) projections. In the lateral projection, the tip of the odontoid should not be more than 4.0 mm above Chamberlain's or 4.5 mm above MacGregor's line. In the AP projection, the tip of the odontoid should be within 1.0 mm of a line joining the tips of the mastoid process (bimastoid line). The relationship between the anterior aspect of the odontoid process and the posterior margin of the anterior portion of C1 is no more than 2.5 mm in females or 3.0 mm in males. In addition to the well-known standard measurements relating the components of the occipitoatlantoaxial complex to each other, there are a few large population surveys of the cervical spinal canal and spinal cord, which define these dimensions in the midsagittal plane. The minimum midsagittal diameter of the spinal canal should be 16 mm at the level of the ring of C1 and greater than 12 mm in the remaining segments of the cervical spine. Air myelography has demonstrated the spinal cord to be 10 mm (range 8.0–11 mm) at the 1st cervical segment and tapering to 8.0 mm at C7 (range 7.5–9.0 mm). A more recent CT study demonstrated the spinal cord to be 7.2 ± 1.6 at the C1 level, 6.0 ± 1.5 at C4, and 6.8 ± 2.5 at C7. Pathological studies have measured the postmortem cord at the C1 level to be 10 mm.

Given this historical background, several minimum numbers seem to be useful in evaluating the cervical spine: 1) the canal at the level of the ring of C1 should be at least 16 mm in midsagittal diameter; 2) the cervical canal from C2–C7 should measure at least 12 mm in midsagittal diameter; 3) the spinal cord normally will measure greater than 7.0 mm at all levels within the cervical spine, being maximum in the region of the occipitoatlantoaxial complex.

Compressive cervical myelopathy can be a catastrophic occurrence in patients with chronic inflammatory polyarthritis—most commonly, rheumatoid arthritis. The radiographic incidence of cervical spine involvement in rheumatoid arthritis ranges from less than 25% to 90%, dependent on the disease severity and radiographic criteria evaluated. Radiographic involvement in the rheumatoid cervical spine includes osteoporosis, apophyseal joint and disc-space erosions, and gross subluxations of the atlantoaxial and subaxial articulations. While rheumatoid cervical subluxation is a frequent radiographic finding in severely involved patients, corresponding neurological manifestations occur in less than 10% of these patients. Mathews, at the end of a 5-year follow-up, found that one-third of patients with AP subluxation and one-half of patients with vertical penetration of the dens developed long tract signs. Neurological manifestations of rheumatoid compressive myelopathy are multiple in kind and nature. Nakano has divided these findings into three clinical patterns: 1) slowly progressive spastic quadriparesis, frequently with painless sensory loss of the hands associated with atlantoaxial subluxation; 2) transient episodes of medullary or pontine dysfunction associated with vertical penetration of the dens and probable vertebral artery compression; and 3) occipital neuralgia. Patients with rheumatoid arthritis have many associated problems, making a precise and accurate neurological examination difficult. These patients frequently will have resorption and subluxation of articular structures, tendon attenuation and rupture, rheumatoid myopathy, and peripheral and entrapment neuropathies, all complicating the neurological examination. Additionally, rheumatoid arthritis of the cervical spine as detailed by Bland can involve the occipitoatlantal, atlantoaxial, atlantodental, zygoapophyseal, or uncovertebral (neurocentral, Luschka) joints. Involvement of these various articulations by rheumatoid arthritis would allow encroachment on the spinal cord, nerve roots, vertebral arteries, and the medulla or pons.

Once suspected, the evaluation of compressive myelopathy includes a careful history and physical examination, and a cervical spine radiographic series. These are frequently followed by tomography and myelography to document the areas of spinal cord impingement. There is increasing evidence for the use of CT and CT with multiplanar reconstruction (CT/MPR) in the diagnosis of spine related diseases.

Our initial experience with CT/MPR in the evaluation of rheumatoid cervical myelopathy relates to a compre-

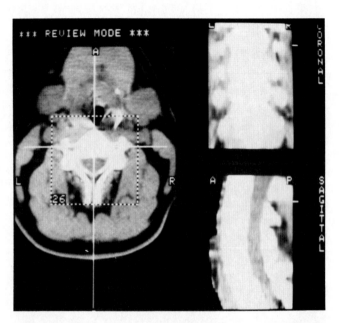

Figure 37.1. Normal cervical spine at the level of C3: Image on left is the axial section of C3 with the axis for the coronal reconstruction intersecting the foramina transversaria and the axis for the sagittal section coursing through the middle of vertebral body, spinal canal, and bifid spine. The level of the axial section is indicated on the coronal and sagittal views by the horizontal tic mark on their right. All three views have only one pixel in common which is on the axial section at the intersection of the coronal and sagittal views.

Table 37.1.
Steinbrocker Functional Class in 14 Patients with RA Myelopathy

Functional class	No.	%
I	0	0
II	1	7
III	7	50
IV	6	43

Table 37.2.
Presenting Complaints in 18 Episodes of RA Myelopathy

Upper extremity clumsiness	9
Occipital Neuralgia	5
Quadriparesis	4

Table 37.3.
Clinical Syndromes in 14 Patients with Rheumatoid Cervical Myelopathy

Patient (Age[a]/sex)	RA duration (years)	Functional class	Medications	Clinical manifestations
OH (65/M)	11	IV	Pred[b] Gold[c] NSAID[d]	↓ADL, L ON, weakness, ↑DTR, L Babinski, UE & LE numbness & paresthesiae, ↓Pos, ↓vib, ↓R temp, alteration in consciousness, Brown-Sequard syndrome
SG (57/F)	15	IV	Pred Gold NSAID	1977 occiput-C4 fusion, neck pain with L shoulder radiation, ↓ADL, UE & LE weakness & ↑DTR, UE & LE numbness & paresthesiae
KN (68/F)	30	III	Pred Gold NSAID CTX[e]	R ON
MS (69/F)	15	III	Pred Gold NSAID	↓ADL, R ON, UE weakness, UE & LE DTR, ↓sensation R C5 dermatome, UE paresthesiae, ext spasms
MD (65/F)	28	III	Pred NSAID	Syncopal episodes, ↓ADL, LE weakness, ↑DTR, numbness & paresthesiae, ↓vib, ↓pos, ↓pin, ↓auditory acuity
AM-1 (58/F)	11	IV	Pred Gold NSAID Pen[f]	↓ADL, weakness, neck pain, ↑DTR, bilateral Babinski, L > R UE paresthesiae, ↓LE pin, dysphagia, dysphonia, auditory acuity
AM-2 (6 mo)				Recurrence of above, ↓alertness, respiratory cycle aberration
AM-3 (17 mo)				Quadriparesis, ext & fl spasms, ↑DTR, ↓pos, no brain-stem signs
MB-1 (74/F)	11	III	Pred Gold NSAID	↓ADL, R ON, UE & LE weakness, UE heaviness, UE & LE paresthesiae
MB-2 (12 mo)				↓ADL, R ON, loss bilateral hand function & progression of above, numbness, dizziness
VS (61/F)	7	II	Pred Gold NSAID	↓ADL, weakness, ↑DTR, ↑UE clumsiness, numbness & paresthesiae
AC (68/F)	20	III	Pred Gold NSAID	↓ADL, L ON, UE ↑DTR, dizziness
RB (85/F)	40	III	Gold NSAID	↓ADL, R ON, UE & LE weakness, L ↑ DTR
JF (41F)	14	IV	Pred Gold NSAID Pen Leukeran	↓ADL, weakness, ↑DTR
JT (62/F)	38	IV	Pred NSAID	1976 Occ-C7 fusion for vertical penetration & C6–7 subluxation, ↓ADL, weakness, Babinski, numbness & paresthesiae, L ON, loss vib & pos, dysphagia, dysphonia, dysarthria, vertigo, respiratory cycle aberration, ↓auditory acuity, loss bowel & bladder continence, ext spasms
DG-1 (63/F)	24	III	Gold Pen Pred NSAID	↑DTR with crossed adductor, UE weakness, L ON with L ear numbness
DG-2 (14 mo)				As above, ↓ADL, weakness, loss triceps DTR, ↓pos, numbness & paresthesiae, ↓hand function
DS (41/M)	25	IV	Gold Pen Pred NSAID	1973 C1–2 fusion, "neck slips", ↓ADL, weakness, ↑DTR with crossed adductor, numbness & paresthesiae, ↓auditory acuity

[a] Age in years or interval in months from first evaluation.
[b] Prednisone.
[c] Myochrysine or Solganol.
[d] Nonsteroidal anti-inflammatory drug including salicylates, ibuprofen, naprosyn, tolmetin, sulindac, indomethacin, fenoprofen.
[e] Cyclophosphamide.
[f] D-penicillamine.
[g] Abbreviations: ↓/↑ = decrease/increase; L/R = left/right; UE/LE = upper extremity/lower extremity; ADL = activities of daily living/general functional abilities; ON = occipital neuralgia; DTR = deep tendon reflexes; pos = position; vib = vibration; temp = temperature sensation; pin = pin prick sensation; ext/fl = Extensor/flexor.

Table 37.4.
Clinical Findings in 18 Episodes of Rheumatoid Cervical Myelopathy

Clinical finding	No.	%
Generalized decreased functions	15	83
Weakness	16	89
Hyperreflexia	14	78
Babinski sign	5	28
Paresthesia	13	72
Hypesthesia	12	67
Vibration alteration	4	22
Position alteration	4	22
Occipital neuralgia	9	50
Post circulation changes	7	39
Extensor spasms	4	22
Bowel/bladder dysfunction	1	6
Previous cervical fusion	5	28

hensively evaluated series of 14 consecutive patients from Rancho Los Amigos Hospital Arthritis Service. These 14 patients with classical or definite rheumatoid arthritis presented a clinical history and physical examination compatible with compressive myelopathy to the Rancho Los Amigos Hospital Arthritis Service between September 1979 and July 1980. Three patients had more than one evaluation and, therefore, clinical data will reflect 18 evaluations on 14 patients. This hospital serves as a tertiary referral center for severely disabled patients with rheumatoid arthritis. During the calendar year 1980, there were 166 adult seropositive patients admitted to the hospital. Seventy-five percent of these patients had cervical spine involvement and seven patients had frank myelopathy.

The demographic data presented include sex, age at presentation, or interval since first evaluation of cervical

Table 37.5.
Radiographic and CT/MPR Evaluation in 14 Patients with Rheumatoid Cervical Myelopathy

Patient	Radiographic (X/R)[a]	CT/MPR[b]	Unsuspected	Surgery
OH	A = 18 mm; B = 8 mm; C = 8.0 mm; dens erosion	Severe dens erosion, asymmetric lateral mass collapse on L with rotation at C1 to 2, C3 to 4 rotational change with L spinal canal compromise	C1–2 & C3–4 rotation	+
SG	A = 3.0 mm; B = 10 mm; C = 17 mm; spine not visualized below C6, fusion occ-C4, C3–4 41% subluxation, C5–6 25%	A = 3.0 mm; B = 8.5 mm; C = 13.5 mm; solid fusion occ-C4, midsagittal diameter at C3–4 6.2 mm, C5–6 6.7 mm, C6–7 8.2 mm (diag 3.7 mm)	C6–7 diagonal of 3.7 mm	+
KN	A = 5.0 mm; B = 12 mm; C = 24 mm	Head tilted L, R lat mass collapse C6–7 osteophytic ridge midsag diam 6.7 mm, rotation at C2, C7	C6–7 ridge	–
MS	A = 0 mm; B = 0 mm; C = 34 mm C4–5 40% subluxation, severe dens erosion	C1–2 rotation with R lat mass loss C4–5 5.4 mm midsag	C4–5 subluxation severity	–
MD	A = 0 mm; B = 25 mm; C = 11 mm; C4 post subluxation on C5 minimal	A = 0 mm; B = 9.0 mm (above FM); C = 11 mm; C4 posterior subluxation on C5–6	C4–5 post subluxation severity	+
AM-1	A = 0 mm; B = 0 mm; C = 21 mm; C3–4 64%, C4–5 55%, C5 compression fx	C3–4 7.5 mm (6.1 mm diag) C4–5 rotated	–	+
AM-2	A = 0 mm; B = 0 mm; C = 21 mm; C3/4 79%, C4–5 69%, C5 compression fx	Lack of fusion, C4–5 rotated C3–4 4.5 mm (1–2 mm diag)	–	+
AM-3	A = 0 mm; B = 0 mm C = 21 mm; C3–4 85%, C4–5 57%, C5 compression fx	Lack of fusion, C3–4 1.5 mm no rotary deformity		
MB-1	A = 10 mm; B = 4.0 mm (bimastoid); C = 14 mm; 33% C3–4 sublux, 29% C4-T1 myelographic block C7-T1	Loss R lat mass CI		
MB-2	A = 8.0 mm; B = 7.0 mm; C = 15 mm; 26% C3–4 sublux, 43% C7-T1	C3–4 midsag 4.8 mm; C5–6 7.1 mm; C7-T1 7.1 mm, C6–7 6.9 mm, midsag diam	C3–4 & C6–7 severity	+
VS	A = 9.0 mm; B = 0 mm; C = 8.0 mm; dens fx free floating, 28% C4–5 subluxation	Dens free between C1–2 10.5 mm, C4–5 midsag 7.3 mm with rotation	C1–2 & C4–5 rotation	+
AC	A = 3.0 mm; B = 17 mm (bimastoid); C = 15 mm	A = 0 mm; B = 12 mm (above FM) C = 12.7 mm; rotation & asym erosion L lat mass, C3 post C4 7.1 mm, C5–6 & C6–7 10 mm, osteophytic ridges C2–3 & C3–4	C3–4 (severity)	– (refused)

Table 37.5—*Continued*

Patient	Radiographic (X/R)[a]	CT/MPR[b]	Unsuspected	Surgery
RB	A = 0 mm; B = 16 mm; C = 9.0 mm; R lat mass loss	A = 0 mm; B = 7.0 mm (above FM); C-6.7 mm; asym lat mass loss of R ring of Cl at C2–3 interspace, lg osteophyte at L C6–7 spinal nerve canal	–	–
JF	A = 0 mm; B = 11 mm; C = 22 mm; C4–5 & C5–6 minor subluxation	A = 0 mm; B = 9.12 mm (above FM); C-20 mm; C4–5 & C5–6 minimal sublux	–	–
JT	A = 3.0 mm; B = 15 mm; C = 14 mm; 25% C2–3 subluxation	B = 10.5 mm; no fusion mass above C2–3, occiput & Cl laminectomy, rotation at C2–4	lack of fusion C2–3	+
DG-1	A = 6.0 mm; B = 20 mm; C = 15 mm; lat sublux with loss L lat mass, C2 lat on C3, C4–5 20%, C6–7 20%	Rotation loss L lat mass, sublux C1–2 R, C6 subluxed on C7	–	– (refused)
DG-2	A = 7.0 mm; B = 15 mm; C = 14 mm	C = 16.6 mm; C4–5 12.2 mm, C6–7 10.9 mm	–	+
DS	A = 5.0 mm; B-11 mm; C = 15 mm; C2–3 33%, C5–6 65%	Fusion mass or solid C5–6 7.5 mm, C7–T1 sublux, foraminal stenosis C6–7	–	+

[a] A = C1–2 subluxation; B = vertical penetration, MacGregor's line unless otherwise stated (bimastoid line on AP film line joining mastoid tips should lie within 1 mm of odontoid tip); C = sagittal measurement from posterior aspect of dens to anterior unless otherwise stated; % = percentage of subluxation in subaxial areas, all are anterior unless otherwise stated.

[b] CT/MPR = Measurements – A, B, C similar to X/R unless otherwise stated; all measurements are in millimeters in the midsagittal diameter unless otherwise stated.

Table 37.6.
Cervical Spinal Canal and Cord Normal Measurements

Vertebral level	Spinal canal radiographic minimum (range)	Spinal cord by gas myelography	Spinal cord by metrizamide CT
C1	21.3 mm (16–30 mm)	10 mm (8.0–11.0 mm)	7.2 ± 1.6 mm
C2	19.2 mm (16–18 mm)	10 mm (8.0–11.0 mm)	6.5 ± 2.0 mm
C3	19.1 mm (14–25 mm)	9.5 mm (7.5–10.0 mm)	6.2 ± 2.2 mm
C4		9.0 mm (7.5–10.0 mm)	6.0 ± 1.5 mm
C5	18.5 mm (14–25 mm)	9.0 mm (7.5–9.0 mm)	6.2 ± 2.3 mm
C6		8.5 mm (7.5–9.0 mm)	6.4 ± 2.7 mm
C7	17.5 mm (13–24 mm)	8.0 mm (7.5–9.0 mm)	6.8 ± 2.5 mm

Table 37.7.
Comparison Between Flexion and Extension Radiographs and CT/MPR in Determining Levels of Subluxation

	X/R		CT/MPR	
	No.	%	No.	%
C1–2	15	83	15	83
AP	11	61	10	56
Vert	13	72	13	72
C2–3	2	11	2	11
C3–4	6	33	9	50
C4–5	9	50	10	56
C5–6	3	17	4	22
C6–7	2	11	5	28
C7-T1	2	11	3	17

myelopathy, duration and treatment of rheumatoid arthritis, and the clinical manifestations of the myelopathy.

All patients had cervical radiographs, including lateral flexion and extension, open-mouth odontoid, and AP views. Conventional tomography was performed when the cervical structures could not be delineated clearly. Standardized measurements were performed on the radiographs; these included C1–2 horizontal subluxation, C1–2 vertical penetration, and percentage of subaxial subluxation. Anterior subluxation of C1 on C2 was present if the distance between the posterior aspect of the anterior ring of C1 and the anterior aspect of the dens was greater than 2.5 mm in a woman or 3.0 mm in a man on a lateral cervical spine radiograph. Vertical penetration had occurred if MacGregor's line, joining the hard palate to the outer table of the occiput, was more than 4.5 mm caudad to the tip of the dens on a lateral radiograph, or if the bimastoid line joining the mastoid tips on an AP film was more than 1.0 mm caudad to the dens. Although subaxial subluxation has many forms of measurement, this form of subluxation was expressed as a percentage of the sagittal breadth of the adjacent vertebra to accommodate for size of our patients. White suggests that a subluxation of greater than 3.5 mm (figure adjusted for radiographic magnification) is beyond physiological range and, therefore, is significant. The usual vertebral body measurement on the lateral radiograph was between 15–25 mm in this group of patients; therefore, 3.5 mm would be between 14–23%, depending on the size of the individual. A last

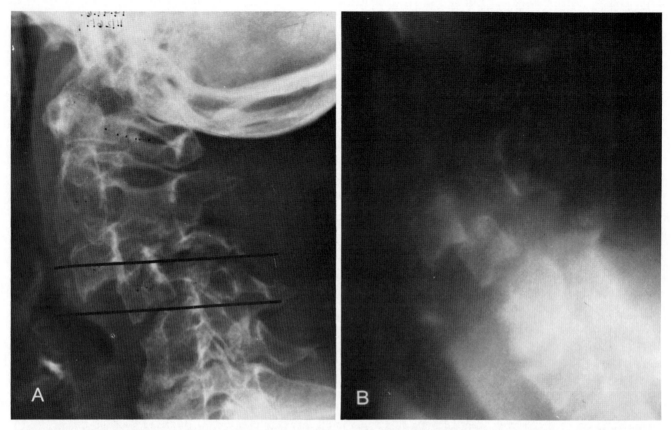

Figure 37.2.   Patient AM-1: A. Lateral cervical radiograph with indication of the CT/MPR levels. B. Tomogram midline section. C. CT/MPR at the upper level indicated in A demonstrating area of compromise on axial section and on sagittal section in midsagittal plane. D. CT/MPR at the lower level indicated in A demonstrating subluxation and rotation of C4 on C5 with probable vertebral artery distortion on the left.

measurement was the distance between the posterior aspect of the dens to the anterior portion of the posterior ring of C1; the radiographic size of the spinal cord at this level is 10 mm in its midsagittal diameter.

In this initial study, 16 of 18 CT/MPR exams were performed using a second generation EMI CT 5005 body scanner, and 2 of 18 studies were performed with the high-resolution, third generation GE CT/T 8800 body scanner. Slice thicknesses were 8.0 mm (EMI) and 5.0 mm (GE), with scan intervals of 3.0 mm. A region-of-interest box can be placed interactively about the spine portion of a representative axial slice. When this box is projected through all the carefully registered axial slices, a three-dimensional data block can be created within the computer. From this data block, a sequence of orthogonal images then is created in the alternative coronal and sagittal planes. For detailed evaluation of a complex problem, various keyboard interactions provide for simultaneous presentation of one slice from each of the transverse, coronal, and sagittal series of images. That single pixel common to all three of these intersecting orthogonal planes can be made to clink as a precise localizing dot in all three views. The three different planes are carefully cross-referenced to each other. An example of this display format can be seen in Figure 37.1, where the transaxial

section is to the reader's left, and both the coronal and sagittal images are seen on the right side of the figure. In this example, the foramina transversaria and the spinal canal are the key points of interest. Other computer programs (software) are available to extract from the data block a plane in virtually any orientation. Measurements can be made with the computer and CT display console or, more recently, from direct measurements on life-size films of the appropriate axial, coronal, and sagittal images of the structure or abnormality in question.

There were 14 patients in this study—12 women and 2 men. The patients' mean age was 62.6 years (range 41–85 years) with a duration of 19.7 years (range 7–40 years). All patients were seropositive and met the ARA criteria for the diagnosis of classical or definite rheumatoid arthritis. All patients were functionally disabled; one was Steinbrocker functional class II, 7 were class III, and 6 were class IV (Table 37.1).

Presenting complaints for the 18 episodes were upper extremity clumsiness in 9, occipital neuralgia in 5, and quadriparesis in 4 (Table 37.2). The clinical findings in 14 patients with 18 episodes of cervical myelopathy were multiple and are detailed in Table 37.3 and summarized in Table 37.4. Fifteen of 18 episodes were described as a recent, progressive, generalized decrease in the patient's

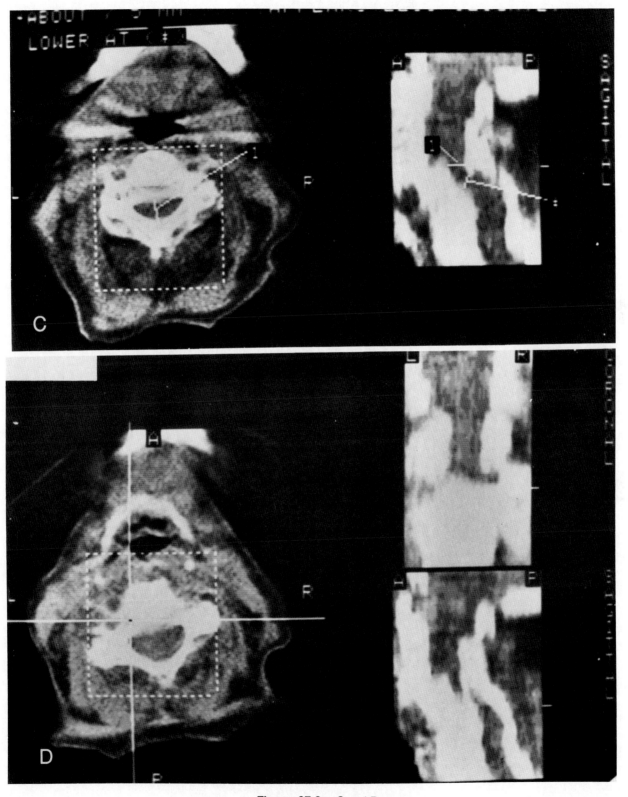

Figure 37.2.   C and D.

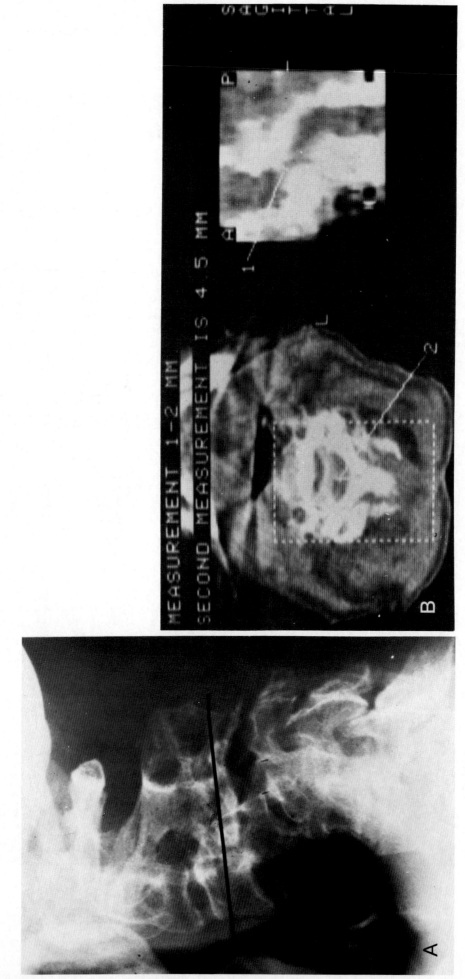

Figure 37.3. Patient AM-2: A. Lateral radiograph with plane of CT/MPR indicated. B. CT/MPR demonstrating lack of fusion and decrease in sagittal diameter when compared with Figure 37.2.

functional abilities. Sixteen claimed progressive loss of motor strength, while 14 were found to have hyperreflexia, and only 5 had Babinski's sign. Nine patients complained of pain in the radiation of the greater occipital nerve. Flexor and extensor muscular spasms, a sign of spinal cord automatism, were present in three episodes in two patients. Only one patient had bowel and bladder dysfunction.

Seven of the eight episodes demonstrated findings of brain stem dysfunction suggesting vertebral artery compromise. Vertebral artery symptoms were dysphagia and dysphonia in 4 patients, and dysarthria in 2. Two patients each had decreased auditory acuity and/or dizziness, and true vertigo was found in one. Four patients demonstrated altered level consciousness and 3 of these 4 patients had respiratory cycle aberrations. These abnormalities of vertebral artery supply were found in a total of 6 separate patients.

The radiographic and CT/MPR on all patients are detailed in Table 37.5, and comparable normal cervical spine measurements are shown in Table 37.6. Radiographs showed all these patients to have severe disorganization of cervical spine architecture secondary to rheumatoid arthritis. The majority of patients had severe osteoporosis and zygoapophyseal joint changes. In addition, there was disc-space narrowing without significant sclerosis or osteophyte formation. All of these changes are characteristic of the involvement described with rheumatoid arthritis. Table 37.7 summarizes the levels of subluxation for the radiographs and CT/MPR. Eighty-three percent of these patients showed involvement at the C1–2 articulations, with 61% having anterior subluxation and 72% having vertical penetration. In this patient group, subaxial subluxations were found as follows: 11% at C2–3, 33% at C3–4, 50% at C4–5, 17% at C5–6, and 11% at C6–7 and C7-T1. Seventy-eight percent of this group of patients with compressive myelopathy had multiple levels of subluxation. Whereas the incidence and severity of cervical spine involvement is selected for by presence of suspected compressive myelopathy, the distribution of the level of involvement was not unlike previous surveys.

CT/MPR confirmed the levels of abnormality in all patients; this comparison is found in Table 37.5. However, review of the patient data reveals several interesting divergences. It became apparent early in this early period that frequently there were surgically significant changes on the CT/MPR exam which were not appreciated on the routine radiographic studies. Of 14 patients, (64%) were found to have unsuspected levels of significant pathology. Of these 9 patients, 7 (78%) had their surgical procedures altered by the addition of this new information. In addition to assessing for presence or absence of subluxation at each level, the quality and severity of the lesion could be assessed. All areas of spinal canal compromise can be measured with computer precision; the critical measurements are detailed in Table 37.5 for each patient. These measurements then can be evaluated in comparison to normal values detailed in Table 37.6.

CT/MPR can reveal rotary changes in the cervical spine and spinal canal which cannot be appreciated on AP or lateral radiographs or tomograms. While these rotary changes at the atlantoaxial level can be suggested by lateral mass asymmetry at C1 or by head rotation and tilt, rheumatoid synovitis can distort the size, shape, and symmetry of the lateral masses, and subaxial levels remain unsuspected. Foramina transversaria are not visualized in the AP or lateral views, but are visualized clearly by CT/MPR (Fig. 37.1). Six patients had clinical syndromes suggestive of vertebral artery compromise (OH, MD, AM, MB, AS, JT), all of these had distortion of the course of the vertebral arteries. This was the interpretation when foramina transversaria (the bony canals wherein the vertebral arteries ascend) of adjacent vertebrae were visualized on a single 3.0-mm axial section. There were two types of compromise, the first being severe vertical penetration of C2 through C1, and the second being rotary and anterior subluxation in the subaxial vertebrae.

CT/MPR allowed complete assessment of five previous fusions and showed three to be incomplete (JT, AM-2, AM-3). Patient VS was shown to have a fracture of the odontoid, the free-floating fragment of which was found between the ring of C1 and the anterior margin of C2. Neural foramina showed areas of compromise, some of which were unsuspected on routine radiographs. CT/MPR clearly shows structural changes at the occipitoatlantoaxial complex. There were 8 patients with occipital neuralgia; all of these had asymmetrical collapse of the lateral masses of C1 with complete correlation between symptoms and CT/MPR assessment.

Patient AM will serve as an illustrative case to demonstrate the use of CT/MPR in the assessment of the rheumatoid cervical spine involvement. The initial referral was prompted by neurological signs and symptoms in a lady with longstanding rheumatoid arthritis. AM, on her first hospitalization (Table 37.3, AM-I), demonstrated clinical findings of compressive myelopathy, hyperreflexia, weakness, bilateral Babinski's signs, paresthesia, and hypesthesia. Additionally, she had involvement in the brain stem with pharyngeal dysfunction, manifested as dysphagia and dysphonia, and decreased auditory acuity. The initial cervical spine film is shown in Figure 37.2A. There was osteoporosis and apophyseal and disc-space erosions without sclerosis or osteophyte formation. The striking findings were a normal atlantoaxial configuration and a 64% subluxation of C3 on C4 and a 55% subluxation of C4 on C5. The AP and lateral tomograms (Figure 37.2B) yielded no further information. The first CT/MPR demonstrated the subluxations at C3–4 and C4–5. Additional information supplied was the degree of narrowing at the C3–4 level (Fig. 37.2C), measuring 7.5 mm in the axial plane, but the critical level of narrowing was in a diagonal plane and was 6.1 mm. Subsequent axial levels demonstrated a rotary subluxation of C4 on C5 with the axis of rotation appearing to be at the right foramen transversarium. Also demonstrated was the tortuous course of the left vertebral artery. The left foramina transversaira at the

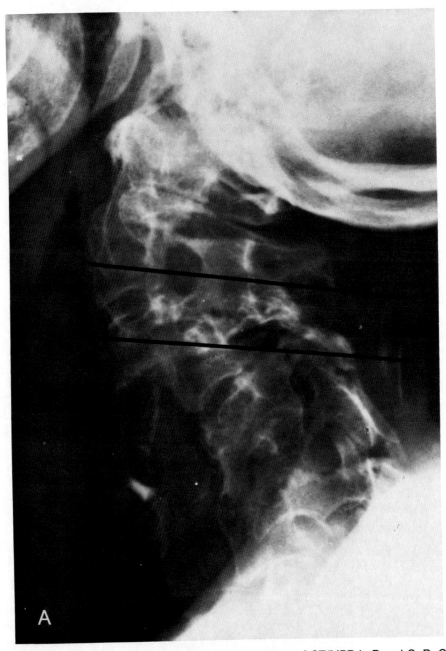

Figure 37.4. Patient AM-3: A. Lateral cervical radiograph indicating planes of CT/MPR in B and C. B. CT/MPR at the upper level in A demonstrating fusion failure. C. CT/MPR at the lower level in A showing severe and progressive subluxation in the midcervical area with a critical midsagittal measurement of 1.5 mm in diagonal plane. Note that foramina transversaria are no longer subluxed in a rotary manner, and the soft-tissue density of vertebral artery.

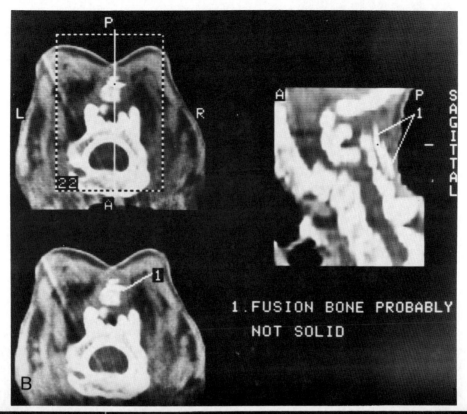

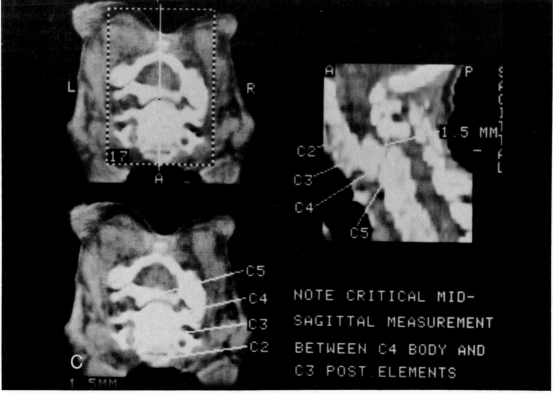

Figure 37.4. B and C.

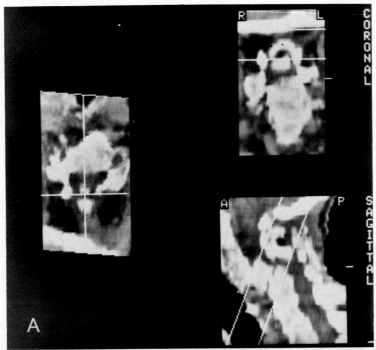

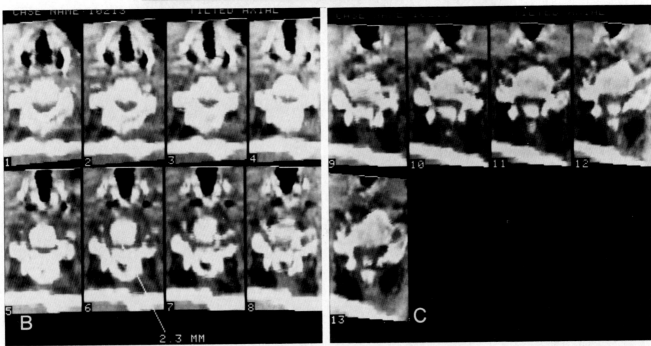

Figure 37.5. Patient AM-3: A. CT/MPR shows the generation of the axial section in the plane of the cervical canal as indicated on the sagittal section. B and C. CT/MPR reconstructed axial sections through the cervical canal section, which is 65° to the long axis of the central canal.

C4 and C5 levels appear on the same 3.0-mm thick axial section (Fig. 37.2D). The patient underwent posterior cervical fusion with halo-jacket immobilization and left the hospital as a household ambulator.

Figure 37.3 reflects the situation six months after the initial presentation when AM returned with progression of her myelopathy. The clinical syndrome at this time (Table 37.3, AM-2) was similar to the first, with the additional findings of alterations in consciousness and aberrations of respiratory cycle, including periods of apnea. Plain radiographs (Table 5, AM-2) demonstrated progression of the C3–4 subluxation to 79% and C4–5 to 69%, and the status of the cervical fusion was not clear (Fig. 37.3A). CT/MPR (Fig. 37.3B) demonstrated progressive narrowing at the C3–4 level to 4.5 mm in the midsagittal plane on the axial view, but 1.0–2.0 mm in the more important sagittal reconstruction in a diagonal plane. Additionally, CT/MPR showed the fusion mass was present and closely adjacent to the laminae, but not fused. Repeat cervical fusion and halo-jacket immobilization again allowed the patient to be discharged as a minimal household ambulator.

Seventeen months after the initial presentation, she was again hospitalized. At this time, the clinical presentation included quadriparesis and typical neurological changes of compressive myelopathy (Table 37.3, AM-3); however, there were no brain stem signs. Radiographs (Fig. 37.4A) demonstrated 85% subluxation of C3 on C4 and 57% subluxation of C4 on C5. The fusion mass was not appreciated. CT/MPR on this final episode was of improved resolution owing to the use of the GE CT/T 8800. It clearly demonstrated the fusion mass to be lying in the posterior soft tissues of the neck (Fig. 37.4B) and the critical area of compromise to be 1.5 mm in a diagonal plane (Fig. 37.4C). Axial sections suggested narrowing, but did not define the actual severity. Figure 37.5 represents the diagonal reconstruction of the spinal canal in the narrowed segment, an area that lies 65° to the long axis of the canal and could not be accommodated with a tilting gantry.

This case demonstrates the clinical usefulness of CT/MPR in assessing the patient with rheumatoid cervical myelopathy. Since these initial 14 patients, and with additional sophistication in both hardware and software, we have evaluated another 40 patients with signs or clinical syndrome suggestive of cervical myelopathy secondary to chronic inflammatory polyarthritis. The following will be examples of the severe but common deformities demonstrated by CT/MPR.

Figure 37.6 is a photograph of a patient with severe psoriatic arthritis. Of note is the rotation of his face to his right so that his chin no longer overlies the sternal notch. Additionally, there is a contralateral head tilt, which frequently is unappreciated by the clinician and is a clue to the presence of underlying cervical pathology. Figure 37.7A–C represent sequential lateral cervical spine radiographs over an 8-year period. Figure 37.7A is a normal cervical spine; Figure 37.7B is the lateral radiograph from 1977, 3 years later, and demonstrates severe and marked progression. The true lateral radiograph may be a misnomer as, while the mandibular rami overlap, the midcervical segment appears as an oblique film. Figure 37.7C from 1982 shows the progressive atlantoaxial subluxation in both horizontal and vertical planes, and marked subaxial cervical subluxation. Figure 37.8A demonstrates the serial 1.5-mm axial sections numbered 1–32 from the upper thoracic region through the atlantoaxial area. Figure 37.8B demonstrates the entire series of axial, sagittal, and coronal sections, which have been reformatted from the initial total-frame CT study. While it is possible to correlate plain radiographs with axial sections, CT/MPR in these complicated cervical cases allows interactive manipulation of

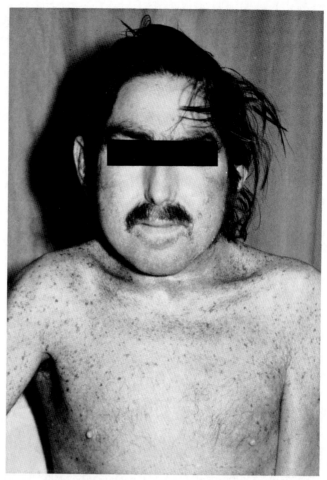

Figure 37.6. The patient shown in Figures 37.7 and 37.8: Of note is the rightward head rotation and leftward head tilt.

sections to identify precisely structures and alterations of the normal architecture. Figure 37.8A and B show axial section 32 with the coronal section indicated by the line intersecting the foramina transversaria of C1. Figure 37.9A clearly demonstrates the vertical penetration of C2 through the ring of C1 and the 12° of rotation that has occurred between the vertebrae. Figure 37.9B shows the identical axial and coronal sections and clearly identifies foramina transversaria of C1 and C2 and, in the absence of radiopaque material, the left vertebral artery. The alteration in the alignment of these foramina, which are the bony canals wherein the vertebral arteries lie, suggests potential for alterations in blood flow. Figure 37.9C demonstrates the C3–4 subluxation seen on the radiographs in the axial and sagittal planes. In this neutral cervical position, the largest midsagittal canal diameter is 8.1 mm—an area where the normal cervical spinal cord is 7.0 mm. Additionally, if Figure 37.9A is referred to with regard to the orientation of C1, Figure 37.9C continues to demonstrate the rotary subluxation of these midcervical vertebrae. If an imaginary radiographic beam were directed perpendicular to the sagittal plane indicated on the axial

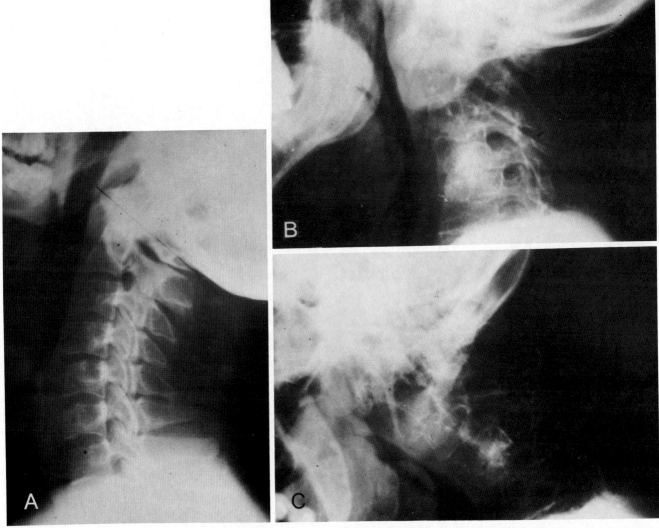

Figure 37.7. A. The initial lateral radiograph done in 1974, which is essentially normal. B. Lateral cervical radiograph done in 1977, which shows marked progression in cervical subluxation. Of note is the aberrant location of the C3–4 apophyseal articulation overlying the vertebral body and the appearance of the neural foramina on a true lateral film. C. Lateral cervical radiograph in 1982 shows marked progression at atlantoaxial and subaxial levels, in addition to severe osteoporosis.

section in Figure 37.9C it would become obvious that the right neural foramina would become visible and the left apophyseal joint would overlap the vertebral body at this level. Figure 37.9D demonstrates the compensatory level of subluxation at the C5–6 level with anterior, lateral, and slight rotary subluxation shown in the axial and coronal planes. This precise delineation of architectural abnormalities can be accomplished only when the cervical spine is viewed in three dimensions.

Figures 37.10A–D continues the demonstration that CT/MPR can aid clearly in the identification of structures in severe inflammatory cervical spine disease. Figure 37.10A demonstrates the lateral flexion radiograph of a patient with severe changes. This radiograph shows severe osteoporosis, structural shortening, loss of disc and apophyseal

joint spaces, and marked vertical penetration. The anterior portion of the C1 ring is at the C2 inferior margin; the posterior aspect is overlapping the occiput. Figure 37.10B clearly shows dense penetration into foramen magnum and measures 19.2 mm above the ring of C1. Figure 37.10C identifies the compressed, overlapping structures of C1, C2, and C3, and the foramina transversaria of C2 within C1 and at the same level as the right C1 foramen. Figure 37.10D, in addition to showing the rightward nonrotational head tilt of C1, shows the adequacy of the cervical canal in this patient.

Before surgical fusion, the previous standard has been suggested to be myelography to document the severity of cord impingement. The results of this study would be a myelographic block or encroachment on the contrast col-

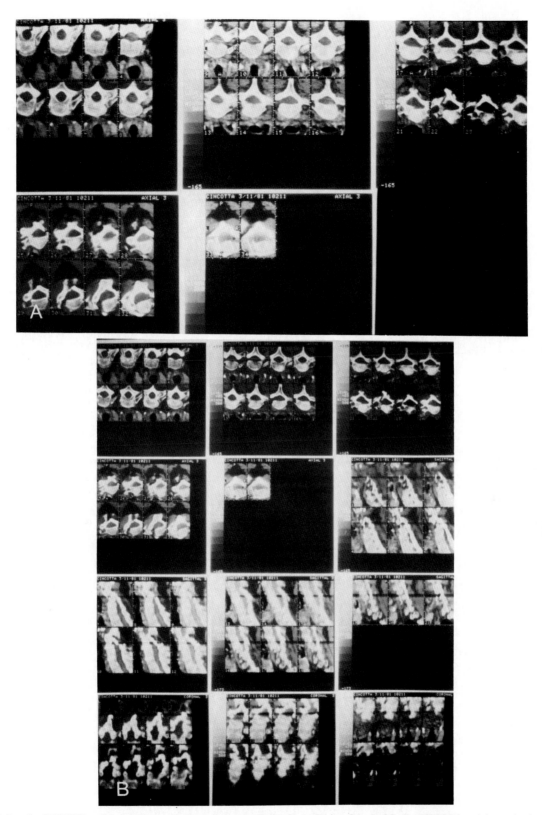

Figure 37.8.   A. CT/MPR axial sections numbered sequentially, from T1 to C1, 1–32. B. CT/MPR axial, sagittal, and coronal sections available for interpretation and interactive display.

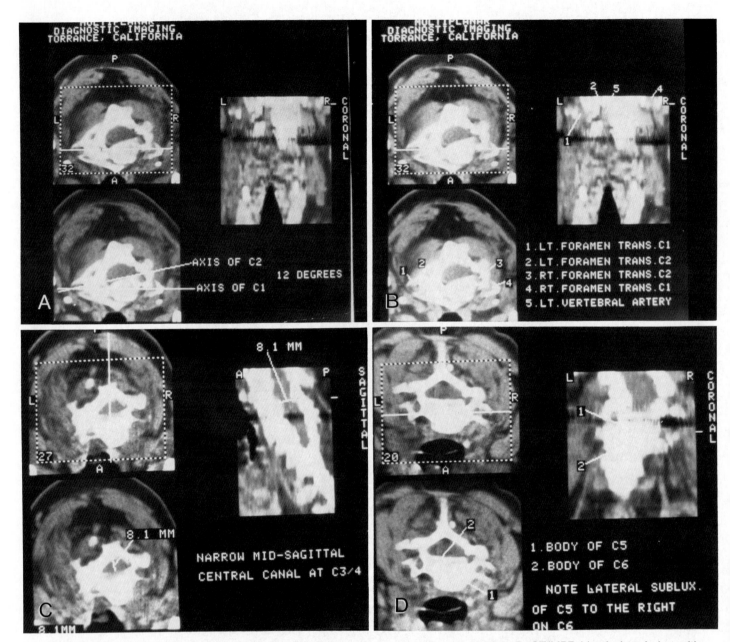

Figure 37.9.   A. CT/MPR at the atlantoaxial level demonstrating the 12° axial rotation. B. CT/MPR identical to A, but with annotations demonstrating the foramina transversaria and the left vertebral artery. C. CT/MPR at the C3–4 level demonstrating the patency of the spinal canal, 8.1 mm in the largest diameter, and the rotary orientation comparable to that of C2 in A and B. D. CT/MPR at the C5–6 level demonstrating the compensatory lesion at this level for the rotation at the atlantoaxial level. Of note is the anterior, lateral, and slight rotary subluxation.

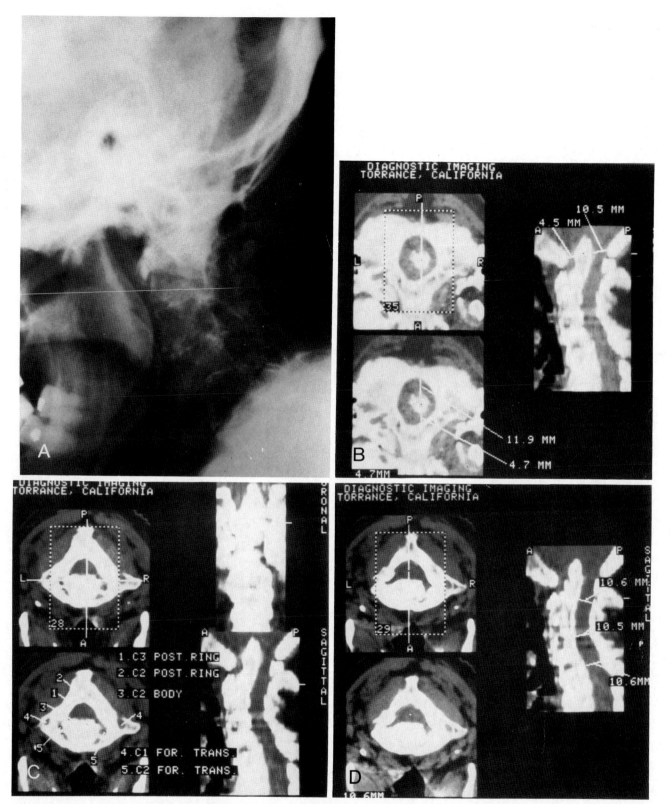

Figure 37.10. Lateral radiograph demonstrating severe osteoporosis, loss of disc and apophyseal joint spaces, and distorted occipitoatlantoaxial complex in the flexion posture. B. CT/MPR with two identical axial views to the left and a sagittal view labeled to the right. The upper axial section demonstrates the slice number 35, the sagittal plane, and the delineation of the field of interest from which sagittal, coronal, or alternative views can be reconstructed. The lower axial section is annotated with a measurement from the anterior margin of foramen magnum to the dens, 4.7 mm, and the posterior margin of foramen magnum to the dens. Sagittal section also has tick marks along right margin indicating level of axial section. C. CT/MPR axial, coronal, and sagittal sections with annotation of structures. The coronal and sagittal planes are shown on the axial sections, and the tick marks on the right margin of the coronal and sagittal indicate the axial section level. The pixel at the intersection of coronal and sagittal planes is the only pixel in common with all three sections and it appears as black dot on all three views and four images. D. CT/MPR demonstrating spinal canal patency.

657

umn. Previous studies have suggested that myelography, in addition to its recognized morbidity (headache, arachnoiditis, allergy) and expense (hospitalization mandatory), is especially difficult to perform on patients in this category because of the need for alternative positions. The difficulty stems from the general debility and multiple articular involvement that makes alternative positioning difficult. The advantage of CT is that it can be performed in all these patients on an inpatient or outpatient basis. Furthermore, CT/MPR requires only one position and no contrast material.

CT has several advantages which make it complementary to plain film tomography. Our entire patient group was severely osteoporotic on the basis of their age, menopausal status, longstanding rheumatoid arthritis, and previous corticosteroid therapy. While the study is done at settings chosen by the technician, the final interpretation is done by video screen with adjustable contrast. Frequently, there is a loss of cervical height because of vertical penetration, loss of apophyseal and disc space, and increased cervical lordosis. Plain films and standard tomography are encumbered by superimposition of cranium and shoulders. CT is unimpeded unless there is a shoulder prosthesis or multiple dental fillings. The addition of CT/MPR format to standard CT augments diagnostic accuracy and detail. The CT/MPR representation of a severely disorganized cervical spine allows the detailed description of the quality and severity of all levels of subluxation in any direction. Vertical penetration and anterior or posterior subluxation can be recognized at the occipitoatlantoaxial complex, as can anterior, posterior, or lateral subluxation at the subaxial levels. A new dimension of interpretation is revealed by the transaxial sections, which show clearly areas of rotatory subluxation at any level of the cervical spine. Additionally, the foramina transversaria, which trace out the course of the vertebral arteries, can be followed and areas of skeletal compromise of these arteries become obvious. All of this information is visualized by a study done with the patient in one position and without contrast material injection. It is our observation that CT/MPR is sufficiently sensitive to delineate clearly areas of disease which should be taken into consideration when the surgical procedure is planned.

We conclude that CT/MPR should be performed on all patients with cervical spine involvement from rheumatoid arthritis and neurological manifestations suggestive of a cervical origin. The diagnostic accuracy of CT/MPR has been found to compare very favorably with myelography in the lumbar spine for disc/annulus abnormalities as well as for stenotic changes of both the central canal and foramina. In view of this, noninvasive CT/MPR as an outpatient procedure has become an attractive alternative to myelography in terms of diagnostic accuracy as well as patient morbidity and expense. For severe cervical spine involvement by rheumatoid arthritis, CT/MPR is considered mandatory before surgery in order to plan a procedure which will include all levels of central-canal or foraminal compromise.

References

1. Bland JH, Davis PH, London MG, et al: Rheumatoid arthritis of the cervical spine. *Arch Intern Med* 112:892, 1963.
2. Bland JH: Rheumatoid arthritis of the cervical spine. *J Rheum* 1:319–342, 1974.
3. Conlon PW, Isdale IC, Rose B: Rheumatoid arthritis of the cervical spine. *Ann Rheum Dis* 25:120–126, 1966.
4. Martel W: Pathogenesis of cervical discovertebral destruction in rheumatoid arthritis. *Arthritis Rheum* 20:1217–1225, 1977.
5. Bywaters: Origin of cervical disc disease in rheumatoid arthritis (letter). *Arthritis Rheum* 21:737, 1978.
6. Smith PH, Benn RT, Sharp J: Natural history of rheumatoid cervical luxations: *Ann Rheum Dis* 31:431–439, 1972.
7. Mathews JA: Atlanto-axial subluxation in rheumatoid arthritis: A 5 year follow-up study. *Ann Rheum Dis* 33:526–531, 1974.
8. Nakano KK, Schoene WC, Baker RA, et al: The cervical myelopathy associated with rheumatoid arthritis: Analysis of 32 patients with 2 postmorten cases. *Am Neurol Assoc* 3:144–151, 1978.
9. Decker JL, Plotz PH: Extra-articular rheumatoid disease. In: McCarty DJ: *Arthritis and Allied Conditions.* Philadelphia, Lea & Febiger, 1979, pp 479–480.
10. Meijers KAE, Van Beusekom G, Luyendijk W, et al: Dislocation of the cervical spine with cord compression in rheumatoid arthritis. *J Bone Joint Surg* 56B:668–680, 1974.
11. Dirheimer Y, Babin E: Upward atlantoaxial dislocation in rheumatoid arthritis. *Neuroradiology* 7:229–236, 1974.
12. Glenn WV Jr, Rhodes ML, Altschuler EM, et al: Multiplanar display computerized body tomography applications in the lumbar spine. *Spine* 4:282–352, 1979.
13. Martel W: The occipito-atlanto-axial joints in rheumatoid arthritis and ankylosing spondylitis. *AJR* 86:223–240, 1961.
14. Meschan I: *An Atlas of Anatomy Basic to Radiology.* Philadelphia, W. B. Saunders, 1975.
15. White AA, Johnson RM, Panjabi MM, et al: Biomechanical analysis of clinical stability in the cervical spine. *Clin Orthop* 109:85–96, 1975.
16. Lowman RM, Finkelstein A: Air myelography for the demonstration of the cervical spinal cord. *Radiology* 39:700–706, 1942.
17. Wholey MH, Bruwer AJ, Baker HL Jr: The lateral roentgenogram of the neck. *Radiology* 71:350–356, 1958.
18. Thijnssen HJM, Keyser A, Horstink MWM, et al: Morphology of the cervical spine on computed myelography. *Neuroradiology* 18:57–62, 1979.
19. Ranawat CS, O'Leary P, Pellicci P, et al: Cervical fusion in rheumatoid arthritis. *J Bone Joint Surg* 61A:1003–10, 1979.
20. White AA, Panjabi MM: Clinical biomechanics of the spine. Philadelphia, J. B. Lippincott, 1978.

D. SPINAL TUMORS

CHAPTER THIRTY-EIGHT

The Diagnosis of Spinal Column and Spinal Cord Tumors with Emphasis on the Value of Computed Tomography

BARTH A. GREEN, M.D., ROSENDO D. DIAZ, M.D., and M. JUDITH DONOVAN POST, M.D.*

INTRODUCTION

Tumors of the spinal cord and spinal column occur in both sexes and in all age groups. The advent of CT, especially the new generation of high-resolution scanners with faster scanning times, thin slice thicknesses, ScoutView devices, and multiplanar reconstruction capabilities, has added a new dimension of accuracy and effectiveness to the diagnosis and treatment of these lesions. In addition to affording better three-dimensional imaging of these tumors, the CT scan can act as a visual guide for percutaneous biopsy and can provide the clinician with serial noninvasive measures of monitoring the effectiveness of surgical therapy, chemotherapy, and radiation therapy.

One must approach the differential diagnosis of these tumors with a basic understanding of their classification according to location, histopathological characteristics, and predeliction regarding age or sex. These lesions may be divided into tumors of the spinal column and those of the spinal cord. The spinal cord tumors may then be subdivided into intramedullary, intradural-extramedullary, and extradural. These categories may be differentiated further into primary lesions originating from within these compartments and secondary lesions presenting as metastases from distant primary sources or by direct extension. This simplistic manner of classifying tumors is valid for most lesions, although certain tumors are known to involve more than one compartment.

CLINICAL ASSESSMENT

The diagnostic approach to these lesions must begin with a history and general physical examination to iden-

tify any evidence of systemic disease. The physical examination should localize any areas painful to palpation and any obvious spinal deformities. The neurological assessment must be most thorough and include a careful rectal examination of both motor and sensory functions. Care must be taken to differentiate between deficits of the various sensory modalities which may localize spinal cord parenchymal involvement. The sensory examination also may aid in determining the extent of a lesion, and may expose characteristic deficits such as suspended sensory level often associated with intramedullary tumors or with syrinxes. The Brown-Sequard syndrome with pain and temperature loss on the opposite side of a touch, vibration, position sense, and motor deficit may provide the examiner with valuable lateralizing information and often may be seen in lesions such as meningiomas and neurofibromas. Stocking feet and glove distribution sensory loss may make one suspicious of a peripheral neuropathy or a hysterical conversion reaction. Motor examination includes the strength of various muscle groups as well as evaluation of motor tone which characteristically can be increased or decreased with lesions depending on level and extent of involvement. Observation of abnormal muscle activity such as fasiculations is of diagnostic value as is the distribution and extent of muscle atrophy. Examination of deep tendon and superficial reflexes are not as reliable as motor and sensory assessments but can provide one with valuable information especially if asymmetry exists as opposed to a generalized increase or decrease in responses. Pathological reflexes such as the Babinski and Hoffman signs usually are indicative of direct spinal cord involvement. Skin areas of excessive sweating or discoloration as well as other signs such as a Horner's syndrome may provide evidence of autonomic nervous system involvement. Distinction between upper motor neuron and lower motor neuron dysfunction is important in localizing lesions although a combination of these signs may be observed in certain lesions such as those involving the

* Appreciation is expressed to Paula Garcia, Yolanda Marin, Tamera Johnson, Maria Gajardo, and Louise Rhodes for the excellent secretarial assistance and to Chris Fletcher for the fine photographic prints.

conus medullaris. Lesions at these levels often are characterized by loss of sensation in a saddle distribution and abnormalities of sphincter function.

Electrophysiological testing has traditionally been based on the use of electromyography and nerve conduction velocities and the use of the "H" reflex. These examinations may be valuable in determining the levels and degrees including central (spinal cord) versus plexus versus peripheral versus primary myopathies. More recently, these tests have been supplemented by the refinement of computer averaged evoked responses in the form of somatosensory evoked responses and spinal cord evoked responses. These electrophysiological examinations can be utilized diagnostically as well as for intraoperative monitoring. Urodynamic testing provides another electrophysiological tool for evaluation of bladder and sphincter function. This test is of special value in differentiating level of nervous system involvement (i.e., upper motor neuron versus lower motor neuron lesions).

Laboratory tests available range from the serum sedimentation rate (increased in certain infections and tumors) and the serum CEA test used to screen and monitor patients with colon or breast cancer to more specific assays such as an acid phosphatase determination valuable in monitoring cases of prostatic carcinoma. All patients should have a multisystem blood chemistry analysis. Abnormalities can be characteristic in certain malignancies. Blood chemistry analyses should include: complete blood count, platelet count, LDH, CPK, SGOT, SGPT, alkaline phosphatase, acid phosphatase, blood urea nitrogen, creatinine, total and fractionated proteins, electrolytes (NA, K, CA, CL), glucose, and clotting profiles. Many of these assays can be obtained in samples on spinal fluid and urine if indicated. Skin tests for tuberculosis and other systemic diseases should be utilized when indicated because often malignancies may be complicated by an infectious disease. Invasive procedures such as bone marrow aspirations often can provide valuable information in suggested myelogenous malignancies. Radioisotope studies including bone scan, gallium scan, liver-spleen scan, brain scan, and vascular and cerebrospinal fluid (CSF) dynamic flow studies, chest films, and contrast examinations including gastrointestinal and gallbladder series and intravenous pyelograms can provide valuable information in selected cases. Added to this lengthy list of diagnostic tools must be the use of ultrasound technology which recently has been sophisticated to provide valuable information especially as a real-time instrument during open operative procedures.

RADIOLOGICAL ASSESSMENT

The radiological evaluation of both spinal column and spinal cord tumors should begin with plain films of the spine. The computed radiographs of the spine obtained for localization purposes before CT scanning currently do not provide sufficient detail to replace conventional plain films. Routinely, anteroposterior (AP), lateral, and oblique views of the spine should be obtained of the level of clinical interest. These projections can be supplemented when deemed clinically necessary by stress views. These films can be taken in positions of extreme flexion, extension, and lateral bending which may be enhanced by weight bearing. These studies are of particular value in cases involving malignancies destroying spinal column elements where a question of stability exists. These maneuvers should be performed under careful supervision by the consulting neurological and/or orthopaedic surgeon.

Plain films can provide valuable etiological clues. Distortion of the normal curvature of the spine including scoliosis and/or kyphosis can raise the suspicion for intraspinal mass. Such spinal deformities most commonly are associated with more chronic benign processes such as lipomas or neurofibromas but also may be related to more aggressive pathology. The plain spine survey can reveal congenital anomalies such as spina bifida and diastematomyelia, abnormalities which can be clues to the presence of associated spinal tumors. Enlarged neuroforamen and vertebral body scalloping can suggest neurofibromatosis. Widening of the spinal canal and thinning of the pedicles can point to slowly growing intraspinal tumors. Diffuse lytic and blastic lesions in the spine can speak for metastatic disease.

Radionuclide studies are also indispensable tools for the investigation of certain types of spinal tumors. In patients with known or suspected metastatic disease, the bone scan should be used to detect and localize sites of spinal involvement. The bone scan is much more sensitive than plain films in diagnosing osseous metastases. In patients with neck, chest, or back pain without neurological deficit with unremarkable or equivocal plain films, the bone scan should be used to detect lesions of the vertebral column, such as osteoid osteomas. Destructive lesions of the sacrum which are notoriously difficult to discern on plain films can be discerned on bone scans. Gallium scans should supplement the radiographic investigation when deemed appropriate such as in cases of lymphoma.

Conventional tomograms should not be obtained routinely but rather only in selected cases. With the advent of high-resolution CT scanning (HRCT) with multiplanar reconstruction, the need for this modality has been decreased substantially. Nevertheless, when computer scan time is not available and when sufficient information concerning osseous detail has not been obtained from other radiographic studies, complex motion tomograms with 3- to 5-mm thick sections can be used to provide very useful diagnostic information.

Although the role of myelography has changed after the introduction of HRCT, at our institution we believe that myelography is still an essential component of the radiological work-up of patients with spinal cord tumors. In those with spinal column tumors and neurological deficits, especially cord compression, we also believe that myelography is necessary. Because visualization of the spinal cord is still limited on plain HRCT scans, especially when pathology is present which is distorting normal anatomy, we believe that intrathecal contrast is needed to assess tumors completely that may be deforming, displacing, or arising within the spinal cord. When there is the suspicion for intradural or subarachnoid tumor(s), we also believe that intrathecal contrast is necessary. Even when those tumors may be suspected at levels below the cord, we still believe that subarachnoid contrast is required for the detection of these neoplasms. This is because plain HRCT scans often fail to reveal neoplasms within the dura and subarachnoid sac, especially when they are small and at multiple sites.

If there are no contraindications such as allergy to iodine, metrizamide should be used as the myelographic agent of choice because high-quality CT scans can be obtained after this procedure. When significant neurological deficit or complete blocks are suspected, the patient should be prepared to be moved immediately to the operating room for open decompression in the rare event of a sudden loss of neurological function. Therefore, it is mandatory that a neurosurgical consultant be available in all of these high-risk cases. If a complete myelographic block is encountered, both lumbar and cervical subarachnoid punctures should be performed to outline the extent of the lesion(s). If radiation therapy is anticipated, the level(s) of the tumor should be outlined by pen marks on the patient's skin.

Critical information that is obtained from myelography includes the following: 1) localization of the level(s) of pathology; 2) determination of the longitudinal extent of the tumor; 3) determination of the effect of the tumor on CSF flow—i.e., is there a block or not?; 4) determination of the type of spinal tumor present—i.e., intramedullary, intradural-extramedullary, or extradural.

In those patients with spinal tumors who have been chosen for myelographic evaluation, a metrizamide CT scan of the area of clinical and myelographic interest should be obtained within 4 hours of the standard myelogram. For this study, the use of 5-mm or less thick sections is preferable unless very long segments of the spine need to be evaluated. Multiplanar reconstructed views should supplement the axial projection in selected cases. Permanent hard copies of the metrizamide CT scan should be recorded at both bone and soft-tissue window settings. In this way, neither osseous nor soft-tissue pathology will be missed. The images taken at narrow windows for visualization of the soft tissues of the spine should be magnified(X2).

Among the advantages of the metrizamide CT scan are the following: 1) spinal pathology can be evaluated in areas beyond or between myelographic blocks (frequently even small amounts of metrizamide will be detected on CT beyond the region of myelographic block); 2) spinal tumors can be delineated more completely because cross-sectional views can be obtained as well as oblique, coronal, and sagitally reconstructed views; 3) the size, position, and configuration of the spinal cord and cauda equina can be assessed accurately, information valuable for determining the compartment from which the tumor is arising as well as for planning surgical therapy; 4) tumor extension can be determined precisely not only within the spinal

canal but also within the paraspinal spaces; 5) related pathology in other organs can be detected; 6) 4-hour delayed CT scans can visualize cord cysts filled with metrizamide; 7) percutaneous needle biopsies can be monitored under CT control.

In those patients not undergoing standard myelography, a number of other CT modalities can be chosen for the evaluation of spinal tumors. They include: 1) the plain; 2) the intravenously enhanced, and 3) the primary metrizamide HRCT scan. The noncontrast HRCT scan can be used to investigate tumors confined to the vertebral column (such as osteoid osteomas) and paraspinal spaces. A plain scan also can be employed to evaluate those tumors not causing cord compression. An intravenously enhanced HRCT scan can be used to detect enhancing nodules within certain spinal cord tumors, such as astrocytomas either initially or on a follow-up basis. This modality also can be utilized when vascular tumors are suspected. Additionally, it can be used in conjunction with a metrizamide CT scan to enhance the visibility of certain neoplasms between myelographic blocks, such as neurofibromas. A primary metrizamide CT scan, can be chosen for certain tumor work-ups such as those in children where a standard myelogram might be considered unnecessary. When this modality is selected, a small volume (usually about 4 cc) of metrizamide in a low concentration (170 mg/ml) is used. Scanning commences immediately after the intrathecal injection.

The protocol we have outlined above for the radiographic investigation of spinal tumors is based upon current technology. In the future, we anticipate that we will be able to alter this radiographic protocol, decreasing the number of invasive studies needed. This change will be made possible because of new advances in computed technology and because of the development and sophistication of nuclear magnetic resonance.

SPECIFIC SPINAL TUMORS—THEIR CLINICAL AND RADIOGRAPHIC FEATURES
Tumors of the Spinal Column

The best way to classify tumors of the vertebral column is by histological characteristics rather than by location. Therefore, we will discuss these tumors by dividing them into benign tumors of the spine and malignant tumors of the spine, with the first two groups representing primary lesions and then a brief discussion of secondary malignant bone tumors of the spine.

BENIGN

Hemangiomas

Hemangiomas are classified as angiogenic tumors which are benign and usually occur in the lower thoracic or upper lumbar level usually involving just one vertebra. They are slightly more frequent in females and usually are noted to occur in the middle decades. Histologically, these may be capillary or cavernous but do not communicate with the systemic circulation. Clinically, these patients may present with pain and muscle spasms, which may be secondary to microfractures or rarely to gross vertebral body collapse. Often these lesions are found as incidental findings, but occasionally patients with hemangiomas may present with a neurological deficit.

Radiographically, these tumors display radiodense vertical striations which represent thick bony trabeculae extending from the superior aspect of the vertebral body to the inferior aspect. They may be associated with a paravertebral mass. Plain CT shows these characteristic dense thick trabeculae and any adjacent paraspinal mass to excellent advantage (Fig. 38.1). CT with intrathecal contrast best delineates any epidural extension and cord compression, (Fig. 38.2).

In the past, radiotherapy was considered a reasonable treatment for these lesions but, more recently, conservative management has gained general acceptance and radiotherapy is reserved for more malignant lesions. In cases where the findings are incidental and are not associated with collapse or neurological deficit, periodic radiographic monitoring is recommended. If the involved vertebral body collapses resulting in an unstable spinal column, with or without neural element compression, the procedure of choice is surgical removal of the lesion and simultaneous interbody stabilization by whatever techniques are indicated according to the size and extent of the lesion (1–5).

Osteoid Osteomas

Osteoid osteomas are small solitary benign tumors that may develop anywhere in the skeletal system with about 5.7% occurring in the spinal column (1, 2). The lesions

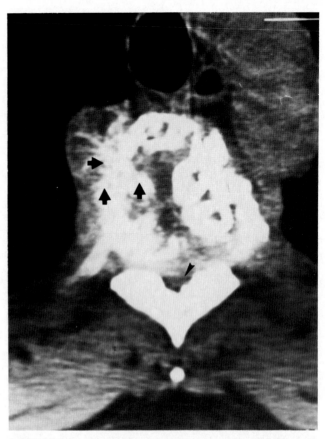

Figure 38.2. Thoracic Hemangioma: A 43-year-old male was admitted with a 6-month history of progressive paraparesis. He had multiple operations for decompression of a thoracic hemangioma. His paraparesis, however, worsened. CT shows evidence of a partial corpectomy and an anterior interbody fusion. It also demonstrates residual hemangioma within the vertebral body and spinal canal. Thickened trabeculae (*arrows*) in the vertebral body are seen along with a soft-tissue mass (*arrowhead*) encroaching on the spinal canal.

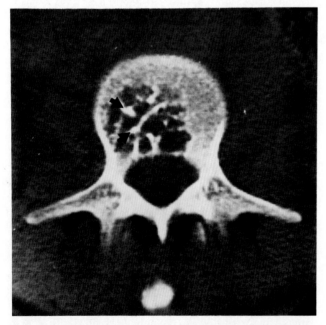

Figure 38.1. Hemangioma of L3: A teen-aged female presented with low back pain and sciatica. While being evaluated for disc disease an L3 hemangioma was found incidentally. CT shows the classical thickened vertical trabeculae (*arrows*) on the right dorsal aspect of the vertebral body.

may be associated with a significant amount of pain, which typically is relieved by aspirin. Onset is usually between the ages of 5 and 24. Lesions are characterized by a peripheral formation of dense periosteal bone or reactive bone which often may obscure the nidus of the tumor itself. Within the vertebral column, osteoid osteomas usually occur in the posterior elements: in the neural arch adjacent to or in a facet joint or in a lumbar transverse process. On gross examination, these tumors often appear as small, spherical, reddish-brown lesions.

Radiographically, osteoid osteomas are characterized by a typical radiolucent ring delineating the tumor and a central nidus. These changes may be difficult to detect on plain films (6). Bone scans and CT scans, however, demonstrate the nidus clearly (Fig. 38.3). In addition to demonstrating the lucent nidus, CT may reveal a dense calcification within the nidus.

Treatment is surgical removal. Radiation therapy is not indicated. In the painful scoliosis syndrome, the pain will

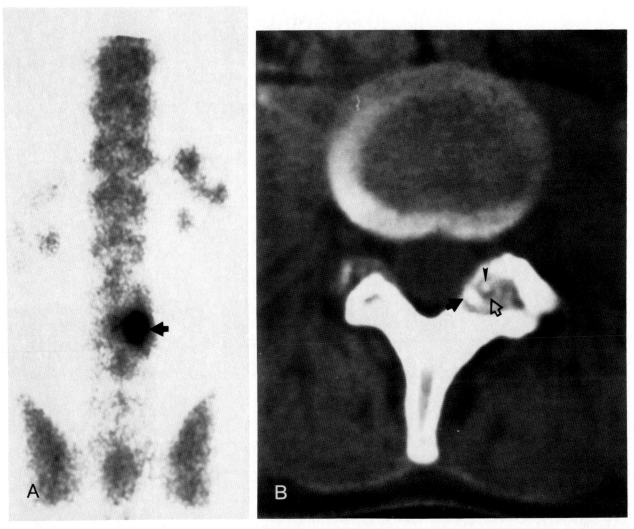

Figure 38.3. Osteoid Osteoma of the Lumbar Spine: The radionuclide bone scan (A) shows a localized area of intense uptake in the region of L3 on the left (*arrow*). The CT (B) reveals the lucent nidus (*open arrow*) with surrounding sclerosis (*arrow*) and a calcific density in the center of the nidus (*arrowhead*) in the posterior arch, establishing the diagnosis of osteoid osteoma. (Case courtesy of John Mani, M.D. of San Francisco, CA).

resolve after resection of the tumor. Rare cases are associated with a self-limiting history with spontaneous resolution over a course of several years (2, 3, 6).

Osteoblastomas

Osteoblastomas usually occur between the ages of 10–35. They are twice as common in males as in females. Forty percent occur in the spine with 60% of those limited to the posterior elements (1). The lamina and pedicles are the most common sites of posterior arch involvement. Vertebral body involvement is usually secondary to direct extension by the tumor. Histologically, these lesions are characterized by numerous osteoblasts, tumor bone, and tumor osteoid and can be confused with osteosarcoma.

Plain films of these tumors show lucent lesions with thin reactive margins and punctate calcifications. When the tumor matrix is lucent, it is difficult to differentiate

from an aneurysmal bone cyst. When the tumor matrix is calcified, differentiation from an osteochondroma is difficult. CT shows an expansile bone lesion in the posterior arch and demonstrates extension into the adjacent soft tissues or spinal canal (Fig. 38.4). Because CT defines the extraosseous extension of this tumor, it is a valuable tool in planning surgical approach.

Surgical removal is the treatment of choice. Radiotherapy is reserved for inoperable lesions or for those that recur after removal because of the possibility of sarcomatous change (3,7).

Osteochondromas

Osteochondromas involving the spine (6% of cases) usually affect the spinous processes or transverse processes and occur at the cervical or thoracic level. They may extend into the extradural space. They commonly are

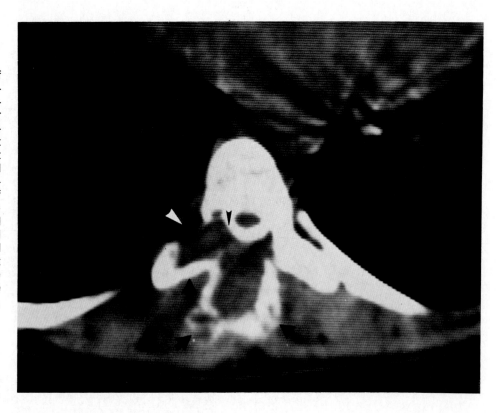

Figure 38.4. Osteoblastoma of Midthoracic Spine: Postmetrizamide CT demonstrates an expansile lesion with radiolucent tumor matrix involving the spinous process, both laminae (the right greater than the left), and the right pedicle of a midthoracic vertebral body (*arrows*). The lesion is well-outlined except in the region of the right pedicle (*white arrowhead*) in which there is cortical breakthrough. There is minimal encroachment on the dorsolateral subarachnoid space on the right (*black arrowhead*) by a soft-tissue mass. (Case courtesy of C. Barrie Grossman, M.D., of Indianapolis, IN).

associated with multiple exostoses, (Ehrenfried's disease). Symptoms of osteochondromas include radiculopathy and/or myelopathy which can usually be relieved by resection of the bony spur (2, 3).

Plain films may show the bony projection of osteochondroma but they do not outline the cartilaginous cap. CT, however, demonstrates the entire lesion and shows its relationship to the paraspinal and intraspinal tissues. When a radiculopathy or myelopathy is present, metrizamide myelography and CT should be obtained. The intrathecal contrast permits cord compression to be detected on CT.

Eosinophilic Granuloma

Eosinophilic granulomas arise from the reticuloendothelial system and occur most frequently in the 5- to 10-year age group. The majority of patients are under the age of 30. Although the most common locations are skull vault, mandible, and long bones, the vertebrae frequently are involved as well. Lesions are often multiple. When the spine is involved, the cervical level predominates followed by the lower thoracic and upper lumbar levels. Cervical spine disease manifests itself by the sudden onset of neck pain or torticollis. In the lumbar region, low back pain occurs. Although frequently resulting in collapse of the vertebral body, eosinophilic granulomas usually do not cause neurological deficit. The collapsed vertebral bodies may spontaneously reconstitute during the growing years.

Radiographically, eosinophilic granulomas appear as lytic lesions without sclerotic borders. A collapsed single vertebral body—vertebrae plana—is classical for this lesion. Although bone scanning is valuable in identifying multiple sites of involvement in the bony skeleton, CT is useful for demonstrating any spinal canal encroachment and for directing needle biopsy.

When eosinophilic granulomas present as a solitary lesion, biopsy is indicated. Once diagnosis is established with a needle biopsy, these lesions usually can be followed conservatively with serial clinical and radiographic evaluations. Usually they will resolve. External splinting with orthoses can help the pain and correct the deformity while they are resolving. If there are signs of cord compression, however, anterior surgical excision and bone grafting is warranted. Usually surgical exploration reveals a small amount of yellow tissue at the site of the osteolytic lesion which histologically reveals the presence of many eosinophils (2). In rare cases, low-dose radiation (approximately 500 rads) may be useful because these lesions are very radiosensitive.

Aneurysmal Bone Cysts

These osteolytic lesions which can be progressively destructive are neither aneurysms nor cysts. Rather, they are believed to be neoplasms characterized by numerous large vascular channels, rarely possessing endothelial linings. These channels of blood flowing through clefts in a tissue mass possess little cohesion. They are spongelike in appearance. They are not malignant.

Onset is usually in the 1st or 2nd decade of life. There are no reports of sexual predilection. The most common presentation is local pain. However, neurological deficits, commonly including long tract signs, may occur along with radicular symptoms. These lesions usually occur in the metaphyses of long bones or, in about 20% of cases, in the spine (1). When the spine is involved, the spinous processes and transverse processes are affected more commonly than the vertebral bodies. These lesions may advance from one vertebral level to the next through the posterior elements. They may remain intraosseous but characteristically present with a prominent soft-tissue component bulging from the surface of the host bone with a thin margin of fibrous bone overlying the bulge.

On plain films, a lytic expansile lesion is seen with a thin shell of bone usually at the periphery. The posterior elements may be expanded in an eggshell or soap-bubble pattern with vertebral body involvement and partial or complete collapse. CT demonstrates a soft-tissue mass expanding bone with well-defined margins, sometimes extending across the intervertebral disc space or the joints of long bones (8). With intravenous contrast injection, enhancement of the vascular components of the cyst has been seen (9). CT is especially helpful in outlining the extent of the lesion. In the sacrum, it may be difficult to differentiate this lesion radiographically from giant cell tumor, chordoma, myeloma, and metastasis. Elsewhere osteoblastoma may be included in the differential diagnosis.

Because of the vascularity of aneurysmal bone cysts and the risk of severe hemorrhages, biopsy is dangerous. Treatment is surgical removal with block resection. The recurrence rate without radical removal is greater than 20% requiring repeated surgical resection. When indicated, surgical resection should be combined with simultaneous stabilization (fusion). Multiple bodies often are involved. Radiotherapy is recommended only as a last resort, even though these lesions are sensitive to radiation, because of the possibility of the development of secondary sarcoma.

Giant Cell Tumors

These are locally aggressive primary bone tumors which usually are nonmalignant initially but display characteristics of local aggressiveness requiring complete removal to prevent recurrence. They represent from 3–7% of primary bone tumors and mostly present in the 2nd or 3rd decade. They are found in females more than males. Eighty percent of these cases occur in the spine. The most frequent level of involvement is the thoracic area. However, they can occur at all other spinal levels as well. Clinical onset may be associated with local pain and sometimes with spinal cord involvement. Twenty-five percent of patients present with a compression fracture (1, 2).

Conventional radiographs show an expanded radiolucent lesion in the vertebral body; associated compression fracture may be seen as well as posterior element involvement. Differential diagnosis includes aneurysmal bone cysts, Brown tumor, osteoblastoma, and fibrous dysplasia. In older patients, multiple myeloma and metastases should be included.

CT reveals an expanding lucent lesion. In certain areas, such as the sacrum, where the expansion is often difficult

to detect on plain films, CT accurately portrays the amount of expansion. CT also demonstrates spinal canal involvement as well as the extent of the associated soft-tissue mass (10). Furthermore, CT is the best radiographic study for monitoring recurrence (10).

Treatment is surgical removal. Radiation may be added as an ancillary treatment. The prognosis is fair to good with malignant transformation occurring in 10% of cases. This tumor rarely may be associated with solitary lesions in the lung which can be removed, resulting in total cure. Diagnosis may be made by needle biopsy of the osteolytic lesions in the involved vertebral bodies or transverse processes. Resection of the vertebral giant cell tumors should be performed in conjunction with simultaneous fusion when indicated (2, 3).

MALIGNANT

Primary

Chordomas. Chordomas account for between 1–4% of all spinal cord tumors. These lesions originate from intraosseous notochordal remnants and consist of clear cells of variable size with large PAS-positive vacuoles in their cytoplasm called physaliphorous cells. Combinations of dense connective tissue trabeculae result in a lobular appearance. Malignant forms with mitotic figures are rare. These lesions are usually histologically benign but have an unfavorable prognosis because of local invasion being characteristic and the difficulty of obtaining total surgical removal. Ten percent of these lesions metastasize via the bloodstream.

Chordomas are found in males more than females in a 2:1 ratio with the most frequent age group being 50–70 years old. Approximately two-thirds of the central nervous system chordomas occur in the spine and one-third at the base of the skull. In the spine, the sacrococcygeal area is affected most frequently with about 50% of the lesions occurring in this area. The patients presenting with sacrococcygeal lesions are usually older. The cervical level is the next most common site of spinal occurrence, especially near the atlas and axis. Thirty-five percent of spinal chordomas affect the clivus (4, 11–14).

Clinical onset may be associated with pain, especially in the sacrococcygeal region where coccydynia is the most frequent complaint.

On conventional radiographs, areas of bone destruction are seen accompanied by new bone formation and soft-tissue masses. Calcification may occur in 15–30% of chordomas (13, 15). Sacral lesions typically exhibit large areas of bone destruction in the midline associated with presacral soft-tissue masses and, occasionally, calcifications. However, sacral chordomas may be very difficult to discern or to outline completely on plain films. If the tumor does not extend to the level of the caudal sac even myelography may be normal. For these reasons, CT is especially valuable in delineating sacral chordomas. CT demonstrates diffuse sacral destruction with associated anterior and/or lateral soft-tissue mass which extends into the retroperitoneum in advanced cases (13, 16). CT is essential for diagnosing the extent of bone involvement and extra-

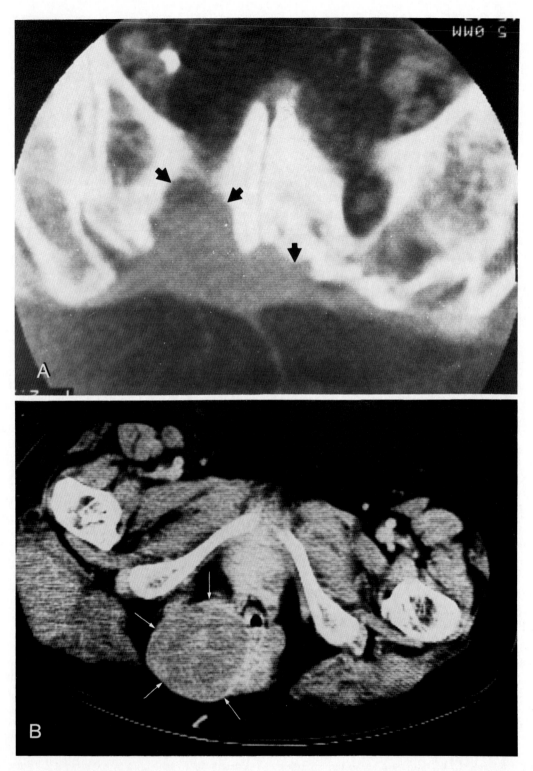

Figure 38.5. Recurrent Sacral Chordoma: A 71-year-old female presented with low back pain 12 years before admission. She was found to have a sacral chordoma. After surgical resection, she was asymptomatic for 6 years. The tumor recurred and a radical resection was performed. For the last 5 years before admission there has been regrowth of the tumor, especially in the right buttocks, associated with weakness and numbness in the right lower extremity and low back pain. On physical examination, there is a large palpable mass in the right buttocks. CT through the area of prior surgery (A) reveals a soft-tissue mass eroding the sacrum posteriorly on the right more than on the left (*arrows*). A more inferior CT slice demonstrates the soft-tissue mass extending into the right ischiorectal fossa (*arrows*, B). Recurrent sacral chordoma proven by subsequent surgery.

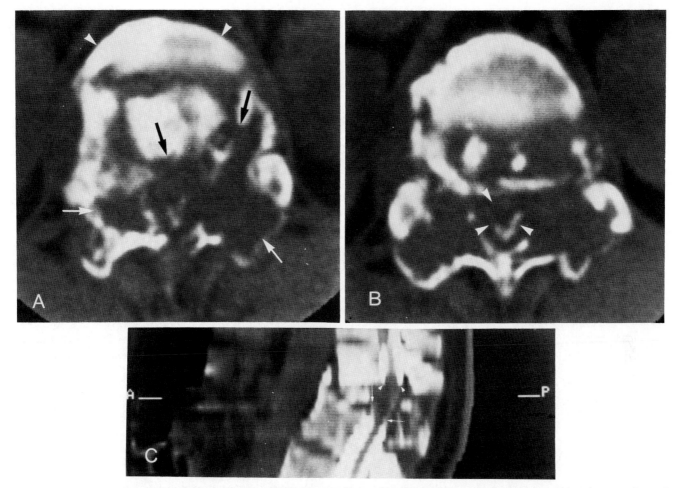

Figure 38.6. Plasmacytoma of T12: A 44-year-old female was in good health until the day of admission when she experienced sudden onset of numbness and weakness in the lower extremities. Plain films of the spine revealed a compression fracture of T12. Postmetrizamide CT through T12-L1 (A) reveals a markedly lytic expansile lesion involving the body and posterior elements of T12 (*arrows*). The anterosuperior aspect of the L1 vertebral body is seen anteriorly (*arrowheads*) because of the compression fracture of T12. A CT slice (B) 5 mm inferior to A shows the subarachnoid space circumferentially compressed by intraspinal tumor extension (*arrowheads*). The sagittal reconstruction (C) demonstrates the complete epidural block outlined from below (*arrows*) and above (*arrowheads*) via a C1-C2 puncture.

vertebral soft-tissue mass (13) (Fig. 38.5). Because chordomas have the tendency to spread to the intradural space, postmetrizamide CT, as suggested by Zito et al, can be used to assess the boundaries of this extension accurately, thereby aiding in patient management (17).

The treament of choice is gross total surgical removal if possible, because radiation and chemotherapy are of questionable value. If indicated, simultaneous fusion procedures should be performed. If diagnosis is made early and total surgical removal accomplished, the prognosis is good. Some patients have had 5-year tumor-free periods. However, if diagnosis is made late and if because of the large size of these tumors only a subtotal resection is possible, the prognosis is much poorer. Nevertheless, long-term survival has been reported from repeated resections (2, 3, 13, 17). However, some of the cases in which metastases

have occurred have been reported after surgery (11, 13, 15, 18).

Ewing Sarcoma (Ewing's Tumor). Ewing sarcoma arises from immature reticulum cells or primitive mesenchyme (2, 19). Histologically, the tumor is composed of closely packed small cells with prominent nuclei. In the 1st decade of life, this lesion has the highest incidence of any primary malignant bone tumor. The peak incidence is in the 2nd decade and the first half of the 3rd decade. It most often presents in extremity bones in the metaphyseal area or in the pelvis or ribs. When found in the spine, Ewing sarcoma is usually metastatic from another primary site (2). As a solitary primary spinal malignant tumor, these lesions are extremely rare, even rarer than osteogenic sarcoma of the spine. When this tumor is located in the spine, it usually is found in the vertebral bodies, although

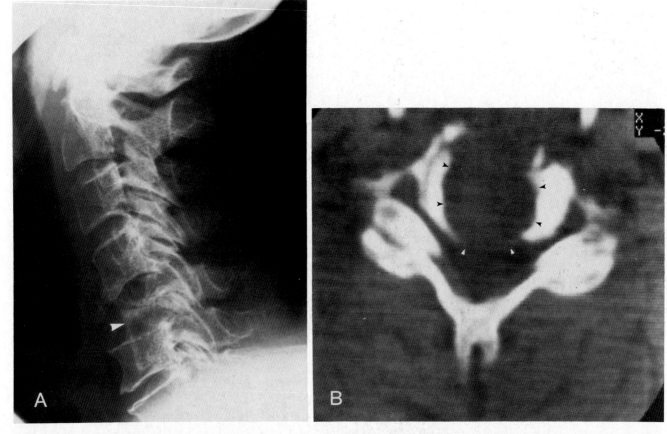

Figure 38.7. Multiple Myeloma of C5: A 58-year-old male with multiple myeloma presented with a 1-year history of numbness in his fingers. On physical exam, he had decreased triceps reflex bilaterally. A lateral view of the cervical spine (A) reveals osteopenia throughout the cervical spine with partial destruction of the C5 vertebra (*arrowhead*). A CT scan through C5 (B) shows extensive destruction of the vertebral body (*black arrowheads*) and demonstrates extension into the epidural space (*white arrowheads*). The patient had a C5 corpectomy and a C4-C6 interbody fusion. He did well postoperatively.

spread to the posterior elements can be seen. In the spine, the sacrum and then the lumbar region are the most common locations. Clinically, onset may be associated with pain and not infrequently with neurological deficit. This lesion rarely metastasizes to other sites in the skeleton. However, lung metastases frequently are noted at the initial presentation or soon thereafter.

Typically, on routine roentgenograms, a sclerotic vertebral body may be seen associated with a large paraspinal mass. This picture may simulate osteogenic sarcoma. CT is the radiographic study of choice, however, for evaluating this tumor because not only will the osseous abnormalities be detected but also the full extent of the extravertebral soft-tissue mass can be seen. In the thoracic region, CT reveals the extra-vertebral intrathoracic extent of the tumor in relation to the heart and also reveals pleural metastases (19). CT, therefore, plays a crucial role in the preoperative evaluation of this lesion.

These tumors are initially very radiosensitive but recurrence is very common. The cure rate for radiation therapy has been reported at 5–10%. However, with the adjunct of chemotherapy and immunotherapy these rates are becoming higher.

Plasmacytoma and Multiple Myeloma (Myelomatosis). Plasmacytoma and multiple myeloma arise from hematogeneous cells in the bone marrow. Plasmacytoma, a solitary lesion, is usually a precursor of multiple myeloma and occurs between the 5th and 7th decades with males more frequently affected than females. Forty percent of the cases present with neurological deficits. On plain films and CT, the plasmacytoma appears as an osteolytic expansile lesion. The vertebral body is involved first with the pedicle being spared in the early stages. Vertebral body collapse follows (Fig. 38.6), often accompanied by soft-tissue masses. CT can guide percutaneous needle biopsies.

Multiple myeloma occurs three time more commonly in males than in females with middle age or later onset. Rarely it presents under age 30. It is a diffuse disease involving a major portion of the skeletal system. Lesions can be seen in the pelvis, ribs, skull, femur, and spine. Vertebral involvement occurs in two-thirds of all cases. Often there is simultaneous onset in multiple vertebrae, more frequently in the thoracic and lumbar areas than in the cervical spine. These lesions may be associated with pathological compression fractures. Vertebral collapse is most severe at the thoracolumbar junction because of the

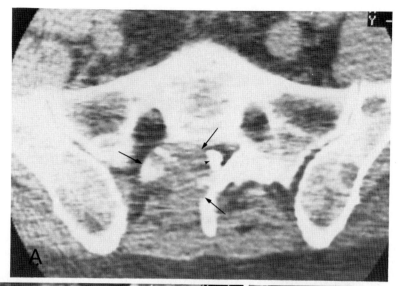

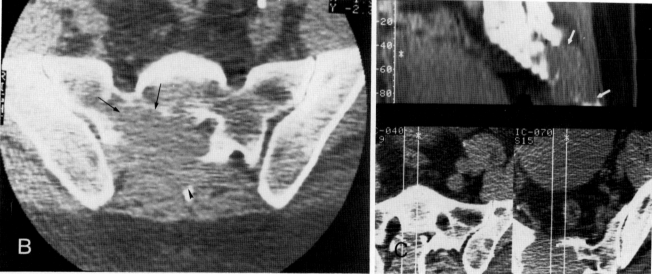

Figure 38.8.   Multiple Myeloma of S1–S2: A 59-year-old male was diagnosed as having multiple myeloma in 1967. In 1974, he had multiple ribs involved with myeloma which were treated with radiation therapy. Now he presents with low back pain. A metrizamide myelogram showed displacement of the caudal sac to the left with questionable bone destruction. The postmetrizamide CT through the lower S1 level (A) reveals destruction of the right intermediate sacral crest and lamina with displacement of the caudal sac to the left (*arrowhead*) by a soft-tissue mass (*arrows*). A CT slice through S1–S2 (B) demonstrates the soft-tissue mass producing widespread destruction of the lateral aspect of the sacrum (*arrows*) and extending posteriorly into the median sacral crest (*arrowhead*). On the sagittally reconstructed view (C), the longitudinal extent of the mass (*arrows*) is shown to good advantage.

mobility and mechanical stress at this level. Pain with-onset is seen in association with these compression fractures or even with microfractures. If epidural extension occurs, neurological deficits can develop.

This disease also is characterized by secondary anemia, elevated blood sedimentation rate, and characteristic electrophoretic patterns in the serum and urinary proteins. In 50% of cases, Bence Jones proteinuria is present intermittently. A sternal puncture, i.e., bone marrow, will confirm the diagnosis in most cases, with plasma cells of 15% or higher. Needle biopsies of the vertebrae may be diagnostic.

Classically, on radiographic studies, the spinal column is seen riddled with osteolytic foci, accompanied by multiple collapsed vertebral bodies. A diffuse loss of bone density as well as circumscribed "punched out" foci in the pelvis, ribs, and skull also are seen. As in cases of solitary plasmacytoma CT shows vertebral body destruction, soft-tissue mass, and extravertebral extension (Figs. 38.7 and 38.8). CT also demonstrates the extraspinal sites of involvement. This radiographic picture may simulate metastatic carcinoma.

Treatment is with radiation therapy, chemotherapy, and

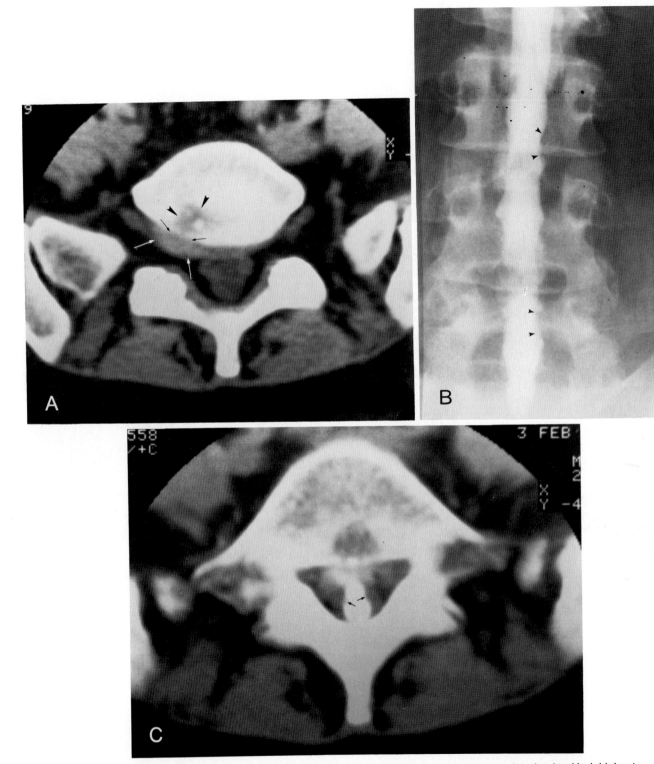

Figure 38.9. Metastatic Hodgkin's to the Lumbar Spine: A 42-year-old female was diagnosed as having Hodgkin's stage III B in 1981. She was found to have metastatic Hodgkin's to the lungs in 1982 (stage IV B). A CT scan through L5-S1 (A) revealed an osteolytic lesion in the body of L5 (*black arrowheads*) eroding the cortex posteriorly (*black arrows*) with some new bone formation and with an associated soft-tissue mass encroaching on the spinal canal and on the right neural foramen (*white arrows*). The AP view from a metrizamide myelogram (B) showed diffuse irregularity of the lumbar subarachnoid sac (*arrowheads*). A post metrizamide CT at S1 (C) and L3 (D) demonstrated soft-tissue epidural masses as well as marked deformity of the subarachnoid sac (*arrows and arrowheads*, C and D) suggestive of intradural involvement as well. At the level of the conus (E) filling defects within the metrizamide-filled subarachnoid sac were clearly seen (*arrowheads*).

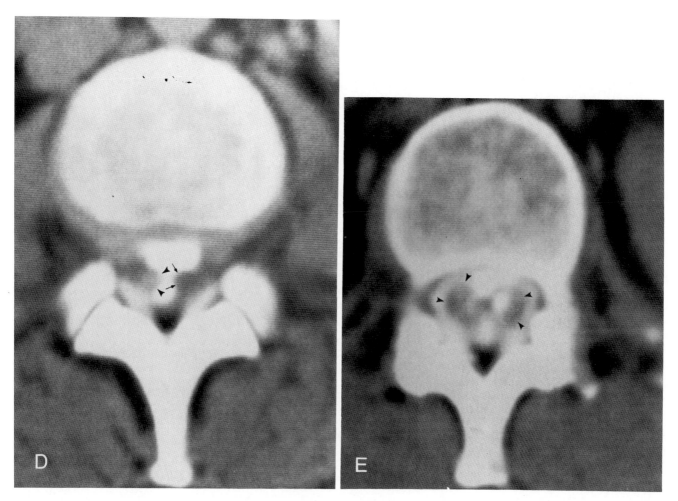

Figure 38.9.   D and E.

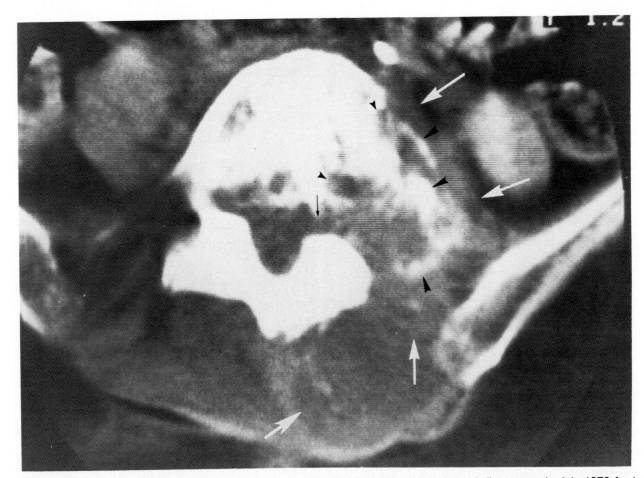

Figure 38.10.   Chondrosarcoma of L3 to S1: A 55-year-old female had a laminectomy and discectomy in July 1979 for low back pain and lower extremity weakness without relief of symptoms. Re-exploration in December 1979 revealed a chondrosarcoma. She was started on chemotherapy. In May 1980 she underwent surgical removal of a left epidural mass from L3 to S1. The patient improved significantly postoperatively and was able to ambulate till 1981. She died of metastatic chondrosarcoma in January 1982. CT performed before the May, 1980 surgery at the level of L4–L5 shows a mass destroying the left posterolateral aspect of the vertebral body and segments of the posterior arch (*small black arrowheads*). It extends into the ventral and left lateral aspect of the spinal canal (*black arrow*) as well as into the paraspinal and retrospinal soft tissues (*white arrows*). Arc-like amorphous calcific densities (*large black arrowheads*) also are evident in this chondrosarcoma.

possibly immunotherapy or a combination. Disseminated multiple myeloma is 100% fatal, although life may be prolonged with therapy. The cure rate may reach approximately 50% when the disease presents as a solitary plasmacytoma (2, 3).

Hodgkin's Disease. Hodgkin's is a disease of the lymphoid reticulum occurring in the 20- to 30-year age group. It is seen more frequently in males than in females. Common sites of involvement include the vertebral bodies, ribs, pelvis, and femurs. Patients often present initially because of symptoms from pathological fractures. Treatment of Hodgkin's disease is a combination of chemotherapy and radiation therapy.

When the spine is involved, plain films show ivory vertebrae and varying degrees of vertebral body collapse. Occasionally, scalloping anteriorly of the vertebral bodies may be seen. CT has the advantage of not only demonstrating the increased density within the vertebral bodies

but also associated soft-tissue masses and their epidural extension (Fig. 38.9). CT also reveals any fusiform lobulated paraspinal masses which may be due to enlarged lymph nodes.

Malignant Lymphomas. Malignant lymphomas present in the 40- to 60-year age group. Males are involved more commonly than females.

Lymphomas can produce bone destruction as well as osteosclerosis. Thus, on radiographs of the spine, osteolytic as well as hyperostotic lesions can be seen in the vertebrae. On initial presentation, pathological fractures may be seen. In advanced cases, the osteolytic process may be observed extending to adjacent vertebrae.

CT is very sensitive in detecting subtle vertebral body hyperostosis and destruction. CT also discerns enlarged lymph nodes and any epidural extension of tumor. The epidural extension, which is best seen on metrizamide CT scan, can occur with or without bone involvement. The

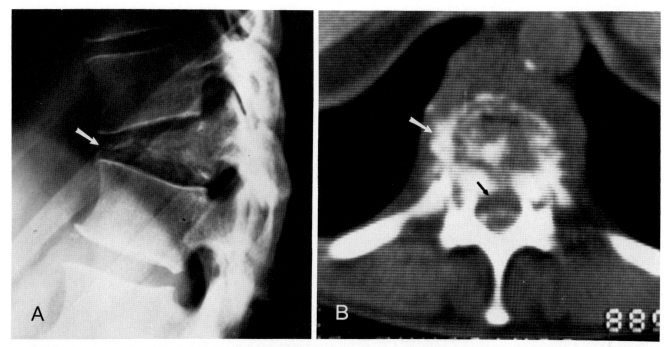

Figure 38.11. Osteogenic Sarcoma of the Thoracic Spine: A young adult male presented with a 6-month history of back pain. Plain lateral film of the thoracic spine (A) demonstrates collapse of the T11 vertebral body. On a metrizamide CT scan (B), the extensive bone destruction, new bone formation (*white arrow*), and paraspinal extension with soft-tissue and calcific components are seen to much better advantage. Involvement of the posterior arch as well as the vertebral body is documented. Also evident is extension of the mass into the epidural space (*black arrow*) with compression of the subarachnoid sac and posterior displacement of the spinal cord. Surgical diagnosis: Osteogenic sarcoma. (This case courtesy of Glenn Morrison, M.D., Miami, FL).

latter occurs when lymphomas extend into the epidural space directly from contiguous prevertebral lymph nodes or hematogeneously from intercostal and epidural veins. This is in contrast to other metastatic neoplasms to the spine in which bone destruction is a precursor or accompanies extradural involvement (20).

Chondrosarcomas. Chondrosarcomas are malignant cartilage tumors arising from bone or from a pre-existing cartilage tumor. They occur mainly in the 4th to 6th decades with males being affected twice as often as females. These tumors present in the pelvis, ribs, femur, humerus, and spine. Their overall incidence in the spine is approximately 6% (2). The posterior and anterior elements of the spine may be involved with local extension from one level to the next. They arise from previous exostoses and initially are associated with pain. They may increase to a very large size. Compression fractures of the involved vertebral bodies are not uncommon. Onset of symptoms usually is associated with pain or spinal cord compression or a mass in the trunk or neck.

Radiographically chondrosarcomas appear as lytic lesions which may be associated with soft-tissue masses which may contain calcifications. Because plain films do not delineate these abnormalities completely, CT is crucial. CT adequately demonstrates the extent of vertebral destruction as well as the extent of the soft-tissue tumor mass and calcifications, important information for deciding surgical approach (Fig. 38.10) (19, 21). Postmetrizamide CT best delineates any intraspinal extension.

The treatment of choice is surgical combining simultaneous resection with stabilization, i.e., fusion, where indicated. Radiation and chemotherapy have only a limited effect. It is often difficult, however, to resect the entire lesion and metastases may occur. The 5-year survival rate is reported as approximately 21% (19, 21).

Osteogenic Sarcoma. Osteogenic sarcoma is a primary malignant bone tumor of mesenchymal origin with tumor osteophytic production. Histology shows osteoid and tumor bone with irregular spicules of bone immersed in the osteoid. The peak age is 10–25 years with a slight male predominance. Seventy-five percent of these tumors occur about the knee, with the spine rarely being affected. Of the approximately 25 cases of osteogenic sarcoma of the spine recorded in the literature, 5 were primary tumors and the rest were metastatic from other primary osteogenic sites. Osteogenic sarcomas also can develop after radiotherapy. A latent period is reported between radiotherapy and sarcoma of 5–30 years, depending whether external (shorter latent period) or internal (longer latent period) radiation was used.

Plain films commonly reveal new bone formation with lytic transition zones. Lesions, however, may be completely lytic. In contrast to osteogenic sarcoma involving the long bones, Codman's triangle and periosteal reaction

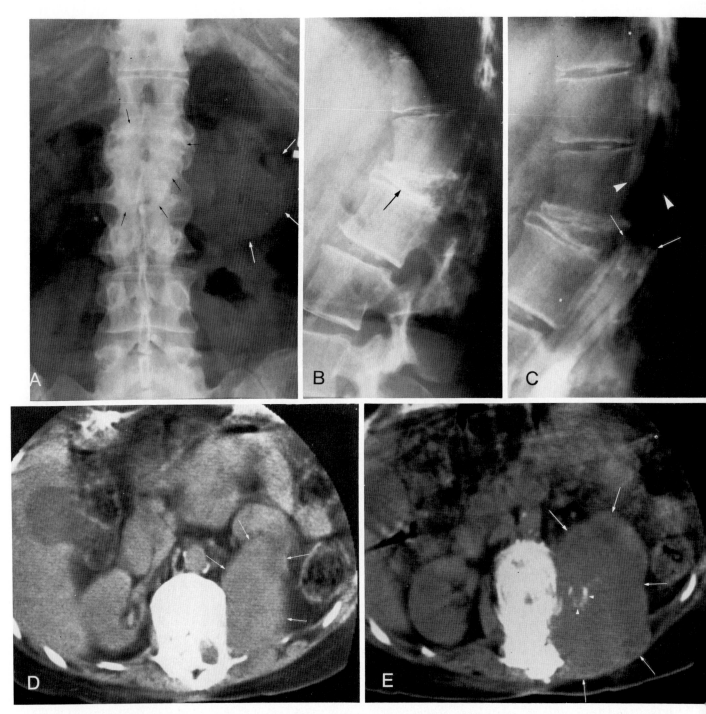

Figure 38.12. Osteogenic Sarcoma of L1 and L2: A 52-year-old female in 1947 had an L1–L2 laminectomy and posterior fusion for a giant cell tumor followed by radiation therapy. She did well for approximately 30 years, until 1½ years before admission when she noticed left sciatica and underwent an L4–L5 discectomy. Her left leg continued to become weaker and new right leg weakness developed as well. An AP view of the lumbar spine (A) demonstrates amorphous new bone formation involving mostly L1 and L2 (*black arrows*) and a paravertebral soft-tissue mass on the left (*white arrows*). The lateral view (B) shows a collapsed L1 vertebral body (*black arrow*). The lateral view from a metrizamide myelogram (C) reveals a complete epidural block at the T12–L1 level outlined from below (*arrows*) and above (*arrowheads*), the latter via a C1–C2 lateral subarachnoid puncture. A postmetrizamide CT demonstrates the paravertebral mass (*arrows*, D and E) with calcific densities in its medial aspect (*arrowheads*, E). New bone formation is noted in the T12 to L2 vertebrae. A magnified view of E with wide window (F) shows displacement of the irregular conus medullaris to the right and anteriorly (*arrowheads*) secondary to intraspinal tumor extension. At the level of T11–T12 (G) the conus medullaris is displaced anteriorly and to the right (*arrowheads*) by the tumor which has extended intradurally (*arrow*). (Operative confirmation of the intradural extension of this osteogenic sarcoma which was presumably radiation induced).

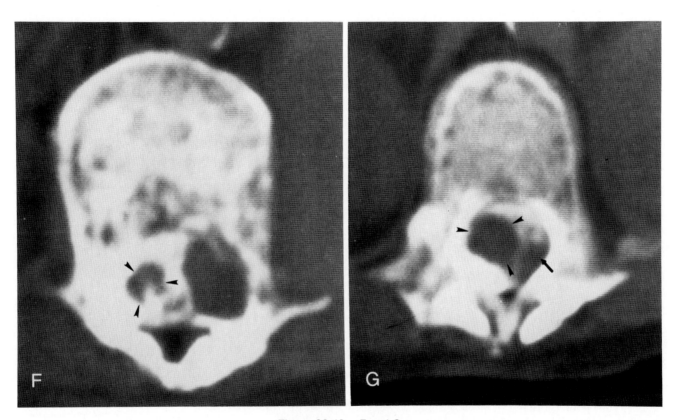

Figure 38.12.   F and G.

are not observed in the spine except in the sacrum. However, a sunburst appearance of bone in the tumor's paravertebral mass has been described. CT shows the osteogenic and osteolytic bone changes to excellent advantage, (Fig. 38.11). When the tumor is radiation induced, CT also can show radiation changes in the adjacent vertebrae (2, 3). More importantly, CT defines the soft-tissue component of the tumor and any associated calcifications (Fig. 38.12A-F). Postmetrizamide CT delineates any epidural extension of tumor and more importantly any intradural extension as well, (Fig. 38.12G). CT also detects metastases, such as those in the lung.

Paget's Disease—Sarcomatous Degeneration. Paget's disease a focal disorder of unknown etiology characterized by excessive resorption followed by excessive bone formation resulting in a mosaic pattern of lamellar bone. These changes often are associated with increased vascular tissue and increased fibrous tissue reaction. Lesions present in older age groups, most commonly in the pelvis, proximal femur, and skull. Plain films and CT show radiolucency and radiopacity plus an abnormally thickened trabecular pattern. In the spine, Paget's may present as a "picture window" with enlarged outer borders of the vertebrae and a radiolucent central body. Differential diagnosis must include that of an ivory vertebrae with Hodgkins and osteoblastic metastasis high on the list of diagnostic possibilities. Paget's disease also may undergo sarcomatous degeneration. When this occurs in the spine, the lumbar level is the most frequent site. CT is the best radiographic study for demonstrating the sarcomatous degeneration with soft-tissue mass and bony changes. The prognosis is poor (2, 3).

Secondary

Metastatic Disease. Metastatic disease represents the most common malignant tumor of bone with 70% of primary malignant tumors having evidence of metastases at the time of autopsy. Bone can be destroyed by the mechanical effects of the tumor or by destructive processes promoted by substances elaborated by the tumor. Metastases generally are not seen distal to the elbows and knees except in breast and lung disease. Vertebrae are the most common bones involved by metastatic disease. The most common level involved is the thoracic spine with T4 and T11 most frequently affected. Mean survival in one review of patients was 8.8 months. The most common tumors to metastasize to the spine are breast, prostate, thyroid, kidney, lung, sarcomas and lymphoma. Age incidence is middle to later decades. Overall there is an equal sex incidence. However, osteoblastic metastases are seen more commonly in males with prostatic carcinoma and osteolytic metastases in females with breast carcinoma. The histological picture is compatible with the primary source of the metastatic disease.

Metastases cannot only involve the osseous spine but also can extend into the epidural space. Primary epidural metastases also can occur either with or without osseous involvement. Intramedullary, intradural, and subarachnoid metastases can be seen too, but they are rare.

At the onset of metastases to the osseous spine, the earliest and most prominent symptom is pain with radicular weakness. The early onset of pain is noted especially in osteolytic lesions. This pain is due to the development of microfractures. In contrast are osteoblastic metastases which remain silent for long periods of time provided reactive bone forms diffusely and is strong enough to give support to the vertebral body preventing collapse.

In 5% of patients with systemic cancer, spinal metastases cause cord compression. The two most common syndromes from cord involvement include: 1) slow steady neurological progression from direct cord compression and 2) a rapid deterioration secondary to ischemic compromise. In patients with metastases to the upper lumbar and lower thoracic spine, symptoms typically include pain, weakness, sensory impairment, bladder dysfunction and in more than three-quarters of the patients, an abnormal gait. These patients have a poor prognosis. Only 20% show motor improvement after treatment. The prognosis is poorest, however, in cases with cord transection or complete paraplegia of longer than 12 hours duration, uncontrolled generalized disease, sphincter loss, and major sensory loss.

Early in metastatic disease to the spine, plain films may be unremarkable. Hematogeneous spread affects the spongiosa primarily which may delay conventional radiographic diagnosis until cortical bone is involved or until an osteolytic focus becomes 1 cm or greater in diameter. Fortunately, radionuclide bone scanning can detect early bone metastases which are not yet apparent on plain films. When bone reaction is seen on spine films it is either osteolytic, osteoblastic, or mixed. Bone reaction depends on the nature of the primary lesion. Breast and prostate tumors are usually osteoblastic whereas thyroid, kidney, and adrenal gland lesions are usually osteolytic (although any combination of these may exist). The pedicles frequently are involved by these osteolytic and/or osteoblastic reactions. Pathological fractures, however, usually occur only in osteolytic metastases and uncommonly in osteoblastic disease. Extension across an intervertebral disc space is unusual for either type of metastasis because the disc acts as a natural barrier to tumor spread (22). Partial to extensive reossification of the sites of osteolytic metastases can occur. Involution and resorption of metastatic tissue can be caused by immunological influence, by the mechanical crushing which can follow vertebral body collapse, by irradiation or chemotherapy or spontaneously without a known cause (2–4, 11, 14, 22–24).

In metastatic disease to the osseous spine and epidural space, CT usually demonstrates bone destruction and/or new bone formation associated with a paraspinal mass and with a soft-tissue mass in the epidural space compressing the dural sac (Figs. 38.13–38.16). Intradural extension rarely is seen because the dura impedes the spread of tumor (22). Epidural compression on the dural sac and spinal cord are shown to best advantage on CT scans with metrizamide. Although some metastases enhance with intravenous contrast on CT (8), and although some metastases can be seen invading the epidural space on plain

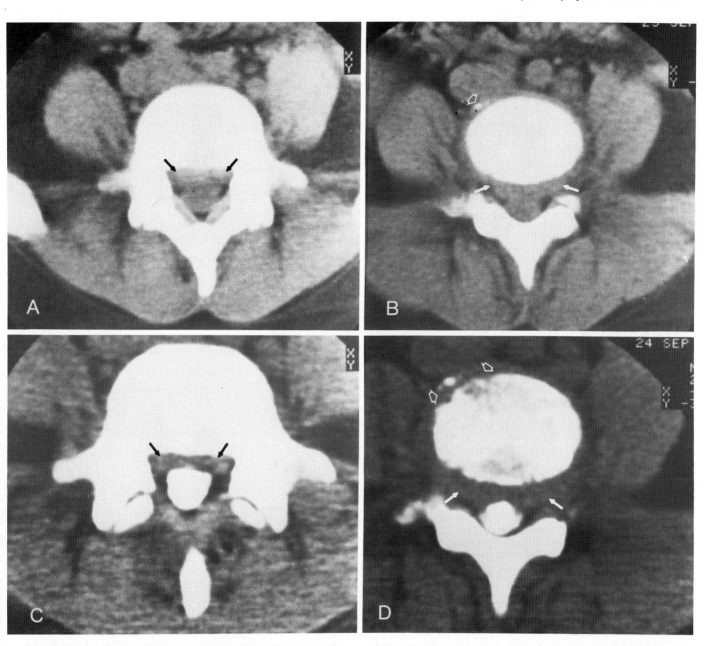

Figure 38.13.   Breast Carcinoma Metastatic to the Lumbar Spine: A 32-year old black female with Stage IV left breast carcinoma developed bilateral proximal lower extremity weakness progressive over the 2 weeks before admission. A plain CT scan showed ventral and lateral soft-tissue lesions in the epidural space at multiple sites in the lumbar spine, including L-5 (*arrows*, A) and L-3 (*arrows*, B). At soft-tissue window settings, it was difficult to appreciate the bony involvement (*arrowhead*, B). A metrizamide CT scan delineated well the compression of the subarachnoid sac by these epidural masses, (the latter indicated by the *black arrows* in C and the *white arrows* in D). Bone destruction (*arrowheads*, D) and mild adjacent paraspinal soft-tissue extension were nicely shown too.

HRCT, some lesions go undetected or are delineated incompletely with these modalities. This is particularly true in the thoracic and cervical spine where there is less abundant epidural fat to provide sufficient contrast to outline soft-tissue lesions in the epidural space.

In patients presenting with sciatica and having normal myelograms, CT may be the only modality to diagnose a metastasis. The majority of patients having myelograms for spinal metastases, however, have a complete block (2). In these cases, if surgery is contemplated, a postmetrizamide CT through the area of block is beneficial in planning the surgical approach. Often CT will detect metrizamide in the areas beyond or between myelographic blocks, thus, enabling a complete assessment of the tumor to be made.

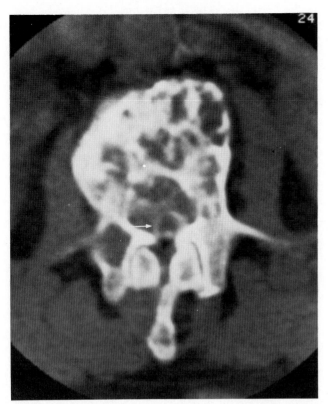

Figure 38.14. Metastatic Breast Carcinoma to L2: A 39-year-old female presented after left mastectomy 3 years before admission for intraductal breast carcinoma. She did not receive radiotherapy or chemotherapy after the surgery. One month before admission, she noticed severe low back pain radiating down the right lower extremity and difficulty walking. On physical examination she had proximal weakness in the right lower extremity. A postmetrizamide CT through L2 showed extensive mottled destruction of the vertebral body, both pedicles and right superior articular process. The conus medullaris was compressed and displaced posteriorly and to the left (*arrow*) by tumor which had extended into the epidural space. The patient was started on chemotherapy and radiotherapy.

Other advantages to CT in metastatic spine disease include the following: 1) CT can identify lymphadenopathy, 2) CT can detect metastatic disease in other organs, 3) CT can be used to guide percutaneous needle biopsies of spinal lesions when the diagnosis of metastasis is in doubt, and 4) CT can be used to monitor the effectiveness of various treatment modalities.

The treatment of metastatic disease is primary radiation therapy and in certain cases, chemotherapy. However, if progressive neurological deficit is associated, surgical decompression may be indicated if radiation and steroid therapy do not halt or reverse this deterioration of function. When this disease is associated with spinal column instability, surgical decompression should be accompanied by a stabilization procedure, i.e., fusion with metal instrumentation and/or bone grafts. Occasionally, acrylic

may be a useful adjunct in these stabilization procedures (2, 3, 11).

Tumors of the Spinal Cord and Nerve Roots

A review of 1322 spinal cord tumors at the Mayo Clinic revealed that 29% were neurilemmomas, 25.5% meningiomas, 22% gliomas, 11.9% sarcomas, 6.2% vascular tumors, 4% chordomas, and 1.4% epidermoids. Of the intramedullary lesions, 56.2% were ependymomas, and 28.6% astrocytomas, with epidermoid, dermoid, and teratomas together accounting for 3.3%, hemangioblastomas 3.3%, oligodendrogliomas 2.6%, lipomas 2%, and other, approximately 4% (12). Others have reported that, in adults, the incidence of intramedullary tumor ranges from 7–22%, extramedullary-intradural tumors 53–65%, extradural tumors from 28–30% with 11% of the tumors (mostly dumbbell neurilemmomas and a few meningiomas), extending both intradurally and extradurally (25).

NEURILEMMOMAS AND NEUROFIBROMAS

Neurilemmomas (schwannomas) and neurofibromas are the most common spinal cord tumors and are estimated to represent between 16–30% of all spinal tumors with 72% being intradural and extramedullary, 14% ex-

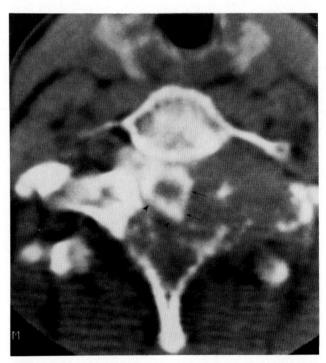

Figure 38.15. Metastatic Breast Carcinoma to C7–T1: A 68-year-old female in 1978 had a right modified radical mastectomy with negative axillary nodes. In February 1982, she developed weakness in the left arm and in the fingers. A postmetrizamide CT through C7 reveals destruction of the posterior elements on the left and spinous process by a soft-tissue mass which extends into the spinal canal and compresses the dural sac on the left (*arrows*) and dorsally (*arrowheads*). The patient received radiotherapy to the lower cervical-upper thoracic spine.

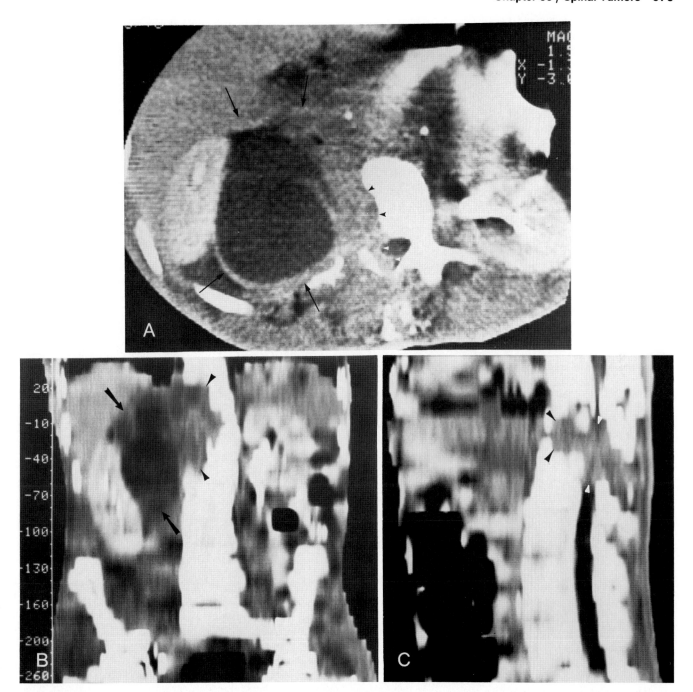

Figure 38.16.   Metastatic Lung Carcinoma to T12–L1: A 58-year-old male had history of severe back pain for 8 months before admission. He had lost 25 pounds and had suffered generalized weakness, lethargy, and productive cough over the two months prior to admission. Chest x-ray revealed a cavitary mass. An intravenously enhanced CT scan in axial (A), coronal (B), and sagittal (C) views demonstrated destruction of the right aspect of the L1 and L2 vertebral bodies (*black arrowheads*, A-C) and posterior arch by a large soft-tissue mass which was extending into the spinal canal (*white arrowheads*, A and C) as well as into the right paraspinal space (*arrows*, A and B). Notice that this mass has a large low density component which is displacing the kidney inferiorly and to the right. Surgical biopsy revealed metastatic lung carcinoma.

tradural, 13% dumbbell, and 1% intramedullary. They show no sexual predilection and present primarily in the 4th and 5th decades. These are benign tumors arising from schwann cells. They are located on spinal nerve roots,

commonly in the thoracic area, but also at cervical and lumbar levels where they are situated on the cauda equina. They most frequently arise from the dorsal sensory nerve roots, but also have been reported as arising

Figure 38.17. Neurofibroma of T4-T5: A 10-year-old male developed pneumonia in the right lung and was treated with antibiotics. The right middle lobe infiltrate resolved but a right paraspinal mass persisted. Closer inspection of the chest x-rays revealed erosion of the right 4th and 5th ribs posteriorly. On physical examination, there were no neurological deficits. A plain CT scan through T4-T5 (A) shows a right paraspinal mass (*white arrows*), enlarging the right intervertebral foramen (*black arrow*), eroding the posterior portion of the right 4th rib (*black arrowheads*), and extending slightly into the spinal canal. The CT slice just inferior to A with wider windows (B) demonstrates erosion of the right 5th rib (*arrowheads*) as well. Diagnosis of neurofibroma confirmed at surgery.

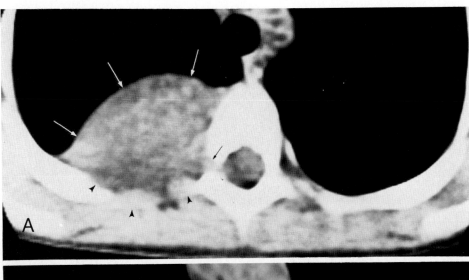

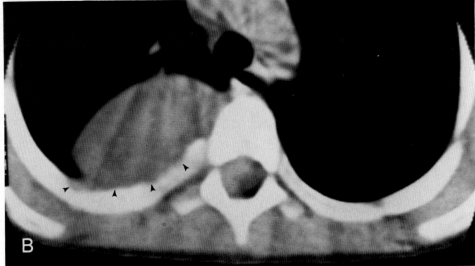

from the ventral motor nerve roots. They are firm, well-circumscribed encapsulated tumors of variable size which displace and do not invade the nerves from which they originate. The nerve sheath tumors tend to be larger than meningiomas sometimes involving two or more vertebrae (25).

Neurilemmomas are usually single solitary lesions in contrast to von Recklinghausen's disease. They are composed of two types of tissues: dense fibrillary Antoni type A tissue and loose reticular Antoni type B tissue. These masses are surrounded by a connective tissue capsule and rarely are reported to undergo malignant changes or be malignant from the onset. These tumors rarely calcify. Clinically, they may be associated with a spinal column deformity, i.e., kyphoscoliosis.

Neurofibromas are different tumors than neurilemmomas. They form multiple tumors of nerve roots and peripheral nerves as part of von Recklinghausen's neurofibromatosis. Examination with both light and electron microscopy reveals the same constituents that normal nerves possess in contrast to schwannomas, which are true be-

nign tumors arising from schwann cells. Neurofibromas are considered a form of hyperplasia of the schwann cells and fibroblastic supporting elements of the nerves, i.e., a benign proliferation. The likelihood of malignant changes are extremely rare in neurofibromas just as they are in neurilemmomas (4, 26, 27).

Bony changes in cases of neurilemmomas and neurofibromas are more frequent than in meningiomas and usually occur with dumbbell tumors which extend out of the spinal canal along the nerve roots into the paraspinal region. Changes include pedicle erosion with widening of the interpediculate distance, enlargement of the foramen, scalloping of the posterior surfaces of the vertebral bodies, thinning of the lamina, rib erosion, and kyphoscoliosis. Some of these changes may occur without the tumor in the same location, i.e., as part of the mesenchymal defect (dural ectasia). Paraspinal soft-tissue masses may accompany these bony changes.

CT demonstrates a soft-tissue mass often denser than the spinal cord, which homogeneously enhances with intravenous contrast (8, 28, 29). It is unusual to see calcifications (8, 30). CT will show bone involvement and extraspinal extension more effectively than plain films (31) (Figs. 38.17 and 38.18). With small neurilemmomas or neurofibromas, CT may be the only modality to demonstrate the lesion (29). Postmetrizamide CT best determines the margins of the spinal cord and tumor (Figs. 38.19). Epidural angiomas can simulate neurolemmomas and neurofibromas radiographically (Fig. 38.20).

The treatment of these lesions is surgical removal using the illumination and magnification of the operating microscope and microneurosurgical technology. With these advances, total removal often may be accomplished without removal of the nerve root of origin of the tumor. In von Recklinghausen's disease, these lesions often are located at multiple levels within the spinal canal. Surgical intervention is performed only when symptomatically indicated and usually is limited to the lesion or lesions responsible for the symptoms (11, 27).

MENINGIOMAS

Meningiomas are the second most common spinal cord tumors; accounting for approximately 22% of the lesions. They have a predilection for females (80%) in their 4th through 6th decades of life. Although they can occur anywhere within the spinal canal, two-thirds occur in the thoracic region. Often they seem to be attached to the dentate ligament insertion and may extend either superiorly or inferiorly. More commonly, they are located in the lateral compartment of the subdural space. Eighty-five percent are intradural and extramedullary, 15% extradural. These tumors are usually single but can be multiple. If multiple meningiomas do occur, it is usually in von Recklinghausen's disease. These tumors only rarely undergo malignant changes.

In contrast to neurilemmomas and neurofibromas which usually present primarily with nerve root symptoms, meningiomas usually present first with long track signs. In contrast to the neurofibromas, bony changes occur in only about one-third of the cases (11, 12, 18, 27). Histological characteristics vary between endotheliomatous, fibroblastic, and psammomatous types. They are usually well-circumscribed, firm, rubbery, or granular lesions and under the microscope are made up of meningothelial cells with whorl formations and frequently with psammoma bodies (26, 32). They commonly contain microscopic calcifications. If the calcifications are gross, they can be recognized by plain films (25). If minute in nature, however, only CT can detect these calcifications.

On CT, meningiomas are usually solid masses, hyperdense, and sometimes calcified (8, 30). Hyperostosis typically is seen in meningiomas and more frequently is recognized by CT than by conventional films. The tumor may enhance markedly with intravenous contrast. Postmetrizamide CT demonstrates the extramedullary location of the tumor as a metrizamide surrounded mass displacing the spinal cord (26) (Fig. 38.21). Seven percent of meningiomas extend into the extradural space (25)—this extension also is detected best by postmetrizamide CT (8). When meningiomas are located in a difficult position for surgical

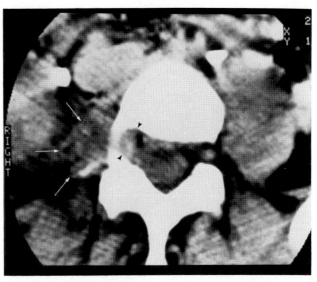

Figure 38.18. Neurofibroma of L-3: A 30-year-old female with von Recklinghausen's disease presented with a 2-year history of progressive weakness in the right lower extremity, especially proximally, decreased sensation in the L1 to L3 dermatones, and absent right knee jerk. A CT scan through L3 shows a soft-tissue mass within an enlarged foramen (*black arrowheads*). The mass is extending outside of the foramen into the right paraspinal region (white arrows). An L2–L3 laminectomy revealed a large, intradural and extradural, right lateral neurofibroma involving several nerve roots. The mass was totally removed. The patient gradually improved over several months following surgery.

removal, such as in the anterior aspect of the spinal canal, CT is of great benefit in planning the surgical approach (33).

Treatment of meningiomas is surgical removal using microneurosurgical techniques. Total removal often requires excision of the involved meninges and application of a dural graft either from autogenous tissue or from a cadaver tissue bank. As in neurofibromas and neurilemmomas, radiation and/or chemotherapy are of no proven value (11).

GLIOMAS

Over 95% of intramedullary spinal cord tumors are gliomas which often cause widening of the spinal canal at multiple levels. They must be differentiated from non-neoplastic lesions such as traumatic contusions or hematomyelia, syringomyelia, hydromyelia, and rarely, intramedullary metastatic lesions (34–37). Over 95% of the gliomas are either ependymomas or astrocytomas (11, 14, 25).

Ependymomas are the most common of all intramedullary tumors and account for approximately 13% of all spinal cord tumors. They are located most commonly in the cauda equina (conus medullaris and filum terminale). They occur more frequently in males, especially in the 4th decade, and account for 60% of spinal cord gliomas.

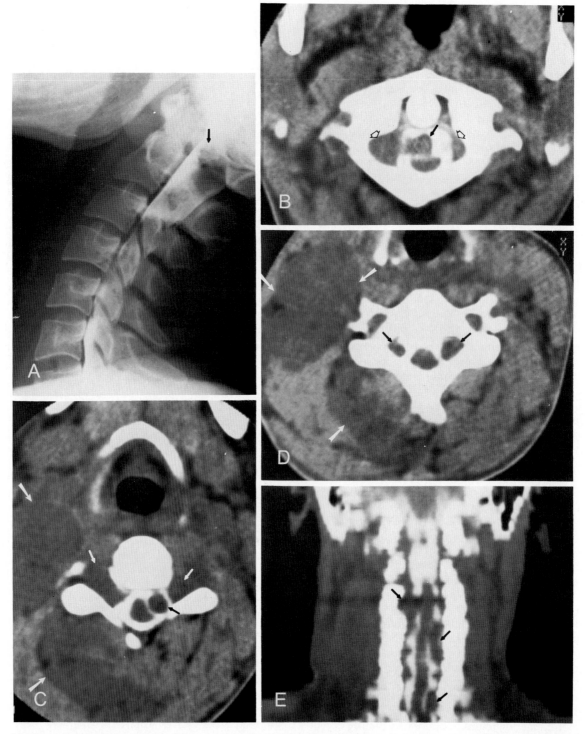

Figure 38.19. Multiple Cervical Neurofibromas: A 26-year-old black female with Von Recklinghausen's disease noted an enlarging right neck mass and neck pain. A metrizamide myelogram (A) showed a lesion at C1 (*arrow*) displacing the cord posteriorly. The true number of cervical lesions and their precise location, however, were not satisfactorily defined. A metrizamide CT scan in axial (B-D) and coronal (E) views localized the intradural neurofibromas (*black arrows*, B-D) and showed their intraspinal extradural extension (*arrowheads*, B; *arrows*, D) as well as their extension through enlarged neuroforamen (*small white arrows*, C). Displacement and deformity of the cervical cord (B-D) and the position of the neurofibromas in the soft tissues of the neck (*large white arrows*, C and D) were also shown.

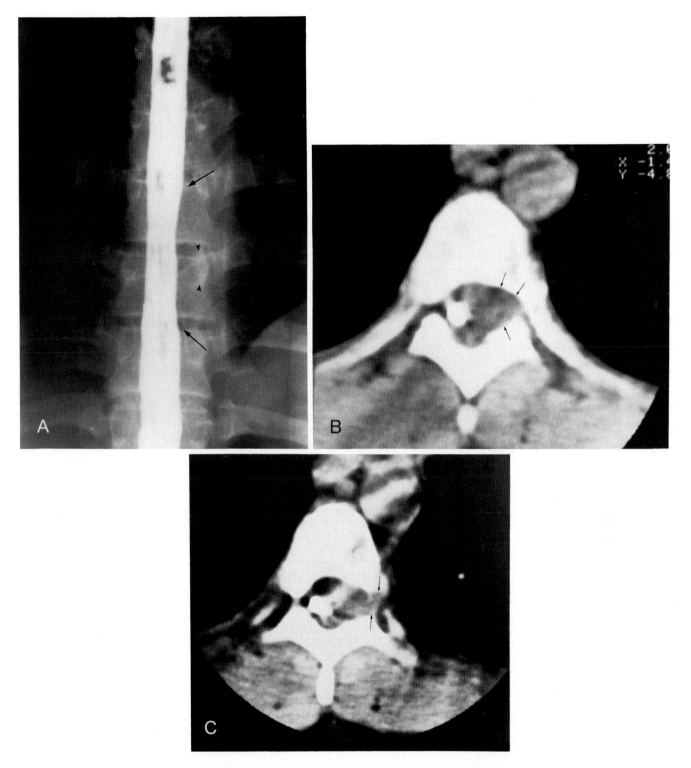

Figure 38.20.   Angioma of T7–T9: A 41-year-old male had progressive left leg weakness for 2 years, a sensory level at T-8 and spastic paraparesis. The supine AP view from a Pantopaque myelogram (A) demonstrates erosion, medially, of the left pedicle of T8 (*arrowheads*) and epidural compression, laterally, on the left from T7 to T9 (*arrows*). The CT scan through T7–T8 (B) shows a deformed and widened spinal canal on the left (*arrows*). A slice inferior to B (C) reveals an enlarged left intervertebral foramen (*arrows*). (Residual Pantopaque is noted.) The preoperative diagnosis was neurofibroma. A T7–T9 laminectomy was performed and a reddish, cystic epidural mass was found involving the dura. There was no intradural component, although the spinal cord was distorted from the chronic pressure. The final pathological diagnosis was an epidural angioma.

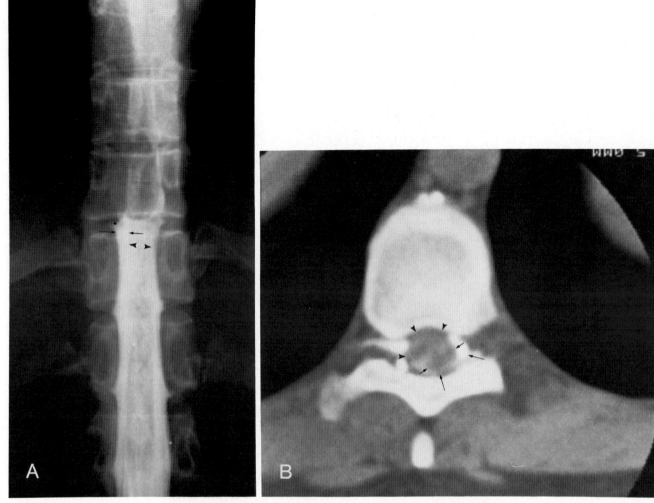

Figure 38.21.   Meningioma of T10–T11: A 38-year-old female developed numbness and tingling in both feet without weakness 1 year before admission. The numbness gradually extended upward to include her calves, thighs, and abdomen. She experienced weakness in both legs 3 months before admission, which progressively worsened to the point where on admission she had difficulty walking. She also had bladder and bowel incontinence. On physical examination, she had point tenderness over T11 and T12 with paraspinal tenderness especially on the right. The AP view from the metrizamide myelogram (patient's head down) (A) shows an almost complete block at T10–T11 with the spinal cord being displaced to the left (*arrowheads*) and with widening of the subarachnoid space on the right (*arrows*) compatible with an intradural mass. The postmetrizamide CT through T10–T11 (B) better delineates the displaced spinal cord (*small arrows*) encircled by metrizamide (*medium arrows*) as well as the intradural mass in the right ventral aspect of the spinal canal (*arrowheads*) flattening the right ventral aspect of the spinal cord. The patient underwent a thoracic laminectomy with gross total removal of an intradural meningioma at T10–T11. Postoperatively, she only has some residual numbness in the right lower extremity with a normal motor examination.

They usually have the appearance of a reddish, nodular, lobulated well-circumscribed mass. They grow by local extension although rarely they may present with distant metastases through CSF pathway spread. They are often highly cellular and composed of closely grouped polygonal cells in the cytoplasm. Blepharoplasts can be seen if stained with Mallory's phosphotungistic acid-hematoxylin. Features which are highly diagnostic but not always present are ependymal tubules and perivascular pseudorosettes. Especially characteristic of spinal cord and filum terminale tumors are papillary lesions with cells arranged as a simple epithelium covering central cores made up of connective or gliovascular tissue. Characteristic of only filum terminale lesions are most myxopapillary ependymomas in which the stroma is characterized by mucinous degeneration.

Malignant ependymomas rarely occur, and are highly invasive undifferentiated tumors (11, 12, 26, 32, 38). These tumors most often occur in the conus medullaris and filum terminale (Fig. 38.2) as large lesions producing thinning and erosions of the pedicles, and enlargement of the spinal canal over several vertebrae.

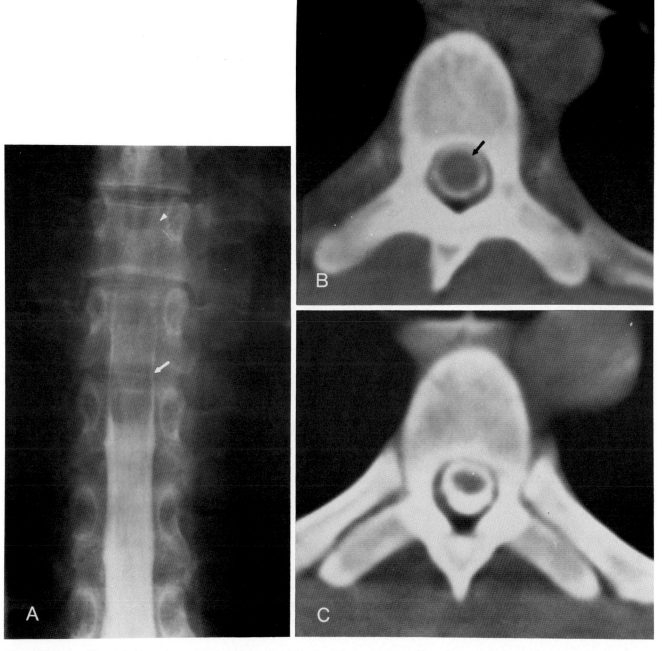

Figure 38.22.   Thoracic Ependymoma: An 18-year-old black male presented with a 6-month history of progressive weakness of the right and then the left leg. A recent rapid increase in severity of the leg weakness prompted hospital admission. Physical examination additionally revealed an incomplete sensory loss from T6 down. A metrizamide myelogram (A) showed a partial intramedullary block at T4–T5 (*arrow*). The superior extent of the lesion could not be determined because of the small amount of metrizamide (*arrowhead*) above the site of incomplete block. A subsequent metrizamide CT scan, however, not only documented the intramedullary nature of the lesion (*arrow*, B) but determined its true extent from T3–4 to T4–5 by demonstrating the level at which the cord returned to normal size (C). At surgery, an ependymoma was removed which resulted in considerable improvement in the patient's neurological deficit.

Clinically, ependymomas usually present with extremity weakness and pain. Cord and cauda equina lesions are often associated with sphincter disturbances. They may sometimes present with an acute onset of subarachnoid hemorrhage and sciatica (Fincher's syndrome).

Bony changes may be associated with 15–36% of reported cases especially with increased interpediculate distance and vertebral body scalloping. Calcification is rare. Bone erosions or enlargements are most easily detected with CT. CT demonstrates a hypodense mass (8). Areas of

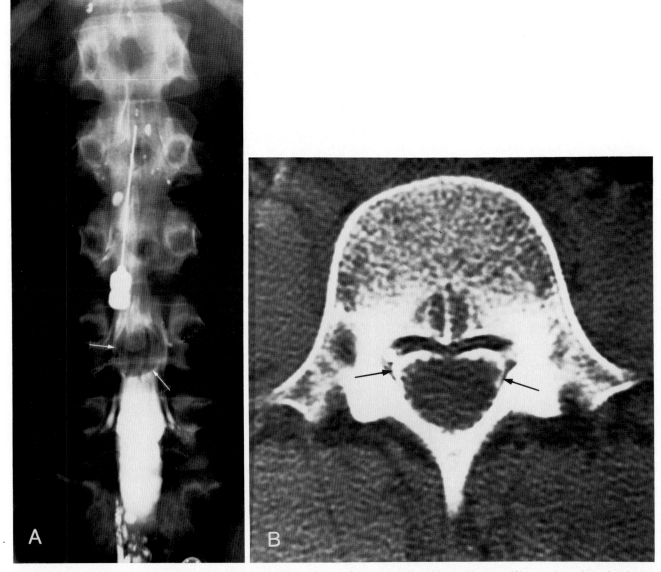

Figure 38.23. Ependymoma of the Filum Terminale: The AP view from a metrizamide myelogram (A) reveals an intradural round filling defect (*arrows*) with well-outlined margins inferior to the emergence of the L4 nerve roots. The postmetrizamide CT (B) shows a large soft-tissue mass filling the subarachnoid sac (*arrows*). (Case courtesy of Robert H. Dowart, M.D. of San Antonio, TX and John Mani, M.D. of San Francisco, CA).

increased density may be noted if there is an associated hematoma (39). Intravenous contrast enhancement near the central canal is highly suggestive of ependymoma (8). Postmetrizamide CT shows an enlarged spinal cord or sac with a markedly thin subarachnoid space (Figs. 38.22–38.24) or an intramedullary block in advanced cases.

Treatment is primary surgical gross total removal. Radiation therapy is reserved most often for subtotally removed lesions or those with more aggressive histological characteristics. Chemotherapy also is considered systemically and/or intrathecally in certain cases (11, 18).

Astrocytomas account for about 30% of the gliomas of the spinal cord. The most common of these lesions are well-differentiated Grade I and II astrocytomas which are more prevalent in males. The more aggressive Grades III and IV, i.e., malignant astrocytomas and glioblastomas, have equal sex incidence. Intramedullary cysts often are associated with these tumors and are found most commonly at the cervical and thoracic level where they result in a fusiform swelling (11, 12). Histologically they appear similar to fibrillary astrocytomas which are often pilocytic and may undergo malignant changes. Grossly, they are pale, grey lesions which tend to blend in with the normal spinal cord tissue and may be solid or cystic.

The lower grade astrocytomas are relatively acellular with essentially normal-appearing cells in larger than

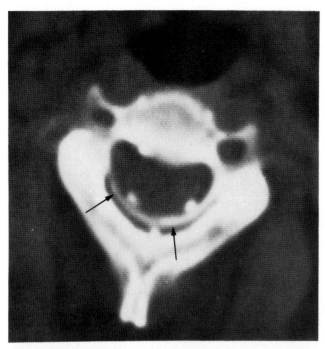

Figure 38.24. Ependymoblastoma of C3 to T3: A 46-year-old female was in good health until 1966 when she developed right-sided weakness. An intramedullary mass was found on myelography. Lower cervical-upper thoracic laminectomy revealed an ependymoma. She received 5000 Rads postoperatively. The patient did well for 14 years when she developed right-sided weakness again. An exploration at that time only revealed scar tissue and no recurrence. She continued to deteriorate and 6 months after the surgery a myelogram revealed a large intramedullary mass from C3 to T3. The postmetrizamide CT demonstrated an intramedullary mass compressing the subarachnoid space (*arrows*). A posterior exploration was performed with gross total removal of a recurrent malignant ependymoblastoma. Her quadriplegia partly resolved with extensive radiation therapy. She did well for approximately 18 months at which time she became weaker and lost the use of her extremities. A myelogram showed recurrence. Again a gross total removal was carried out, followed by chemotherapy and radiation therapy. The most recent pathological diagnosis is a mixed glioblastoma/ependymoblastoma.

normal numbers. In Grade II, a larger number of cells are seen with larger hyperchromatic nuclei. Vascular changes are also present, including thickening of the walls. Grade III is considered a malignant variety with multinucleated giant cells and a few mitotic figures with increased vascularity and necrosis, although there are still many recognizable astrocytes. In Grade IV, the most malignant (glioblastoma multiforme), there are few recognizable astrocytes with many multinucleated cells and frequent mitoses, vascular proliferation and extensive necrosis (26, 32).

Clinically, these patients most often present with long tract involvement, including weakness, associated sensory loss and sphincter disturbance, especially if they are located in the thoracolumbar area.

Astrocytomas will produce the same bony changes as ependymomas because they both are slow-growing tumors, namely, enlargement of the spinal canal, erosion of the medial aspect of the pedicles (Fig. 38.27A), scalloping of the posterior margins of the vertebral bodies and thinning of the laminae. On CT, astrocytomas appear isodense (31) or as inhomogeneously hypodense lesions (8). Cystic components may be seen (31), although the cysts may be difficult to recognize because they may have the same density as the tumor. Marked intravenous contrast enhancement was demonstrated in one case report (36). Postmetrizamide CT shows a compressed subarachnoid space (Figs. 38.26–38.27) and may outline the nodular mass and an enlarged spinal cord (39).

Until recently, the treatment of astrocytomas primarily has been biopsy and drainage of cysts followed by radiation therapy. More recently, with the sophistication of microneurosurgical technology, gross total removal often is being attempted depending on the extent and characteristics of the lesion. HRCT after metrizamide myelography has significantly improved the preoperative evaluation of these lesions and their associated cysts. More recently, the introduction of ultrasound technology in the operating room has allowed more accurate intraoperative delineation of these lesions and, therefore, a better chance of successful surgical removal. Subtotal surgical excision is most often followed by radiation therapy. One-half of these lesions are located in the thoracic area. Treatment of the malignant glioblastoma is essentially the same as the lower grade gliomas with the exception of patients with total paralysis with isolated lesions of the distal cord which extend cephalad in spite of radiation therapy. In these cases, radical cordectomy can be performed, although no series are large enough to make conclusions regarding this treatment (11, 18, 38).

Oligodendrogliomas occur most frequently in the 4th and 5th decades and account for 4.1% of spinal cord intramedullary tumors. Most often they appear as well-circumscribed, grayish-pink lesions characterized by areas of mucoid change resulting in gelatinous consistency and zones of necrosis, cystic degeneration, hemorrhagic areas, and calcifications. Microscopically they appear as uniformly swollen and closely packed oligodendrocytes, exhibiting small, round, darkly stained nuclei surrounded by a clear halo giving a honeycomb appearance. Mitotic figures are rare. Metastases through the cerebrospinal pathways have been reported and these may undergo malignant changes into glioblastoma. Treatment is the same as for other spinal cord gliomas (11, 12, 18, 26, 32).

LIPOMAS

Intraspinal lipomas are composed of adipose cells in which connective tissue and vascular elements coexist to variable degrees (26, 32). Sixty percent are intradural and forty percent extradural. They have equal sex incidence. Intradural spinal lipomas often present in the first three decades of life, usually near puberty. Excessive weight

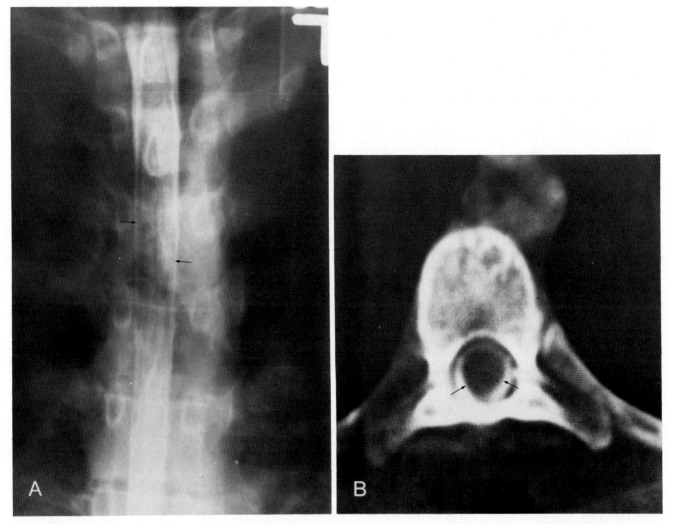

Figure 38.25. Low Grade Glioma of T3–T4: A 34-year-old male fell and hit the back of his head 10 months before admission. Afterward he noted right chest wall pain, "abnormal" sensations in his left lower extremity, impotence, decreased flow during micturition, and loss of control during urination. In addition, he had difficulty discriminating between hot and cold in the left lower extremity. Physical examination revealed mild weakness and clonus in the left lower extremity with a suspended midthoracic sensory level from T4 inferiorly on the left. An AP view from a metrizamide myelogram (A) demonstrated a widened spinal cord maximal at T4 (*arrows*). The metrizamide CT (B) clearly delineated the intramedullary mass (*arrows*). A T2–T5 laminectomy was performed and biopsy at T3–T4 was compatible with a low grade glioma.

gain and pregnancy may be precipitating factors. Intraspinal lipomas are most commonly located in the thoracic spine followed by the cervical region. However, they also occur in the lumbar-sacral region. In fact, they represent the most commonly occurring tumor of the filum terminale (8).

Intraspinal lipomas often extend over four or five segments of the cord. They are found commonly in the dorsal half of the spinal canal (25) and lie within the pia often cavitating the posterior columns, i.e., subpial in location. They may be multiple and may be associated with other tumors such as teratomas and dermoids. Extradural lipomas occur primarily in the middle and lower thoracic segments with onset usually in the 5th decade with a short history of symptomatology. They may present as either

angiolipomas or fibrolipomas and often adhere loosely to the dura (11, 18, 26, 32).

Because they are slow-growing tumors, they will manifest the same vertebral body changes as intramedullary tumors. They also may be associated with bony abnormalities of the spine, especially spina bifida occulta and with adjacent subcutaneous lipomas. Because they consist mostly of fat and fibrous tissue, they are easily recognizable by CT as a homogeneous hypodense mass with characteristic absorption coefficients (Fig. 38.28) (6, 8, 30). Lipomas do not enhance with intravenous contrast (8). Postmetrizamide CT is of benefit in delineating cord displacement as well as in evaluating any associated congenital anomalies such as meningocele and/or tethered cord (8).

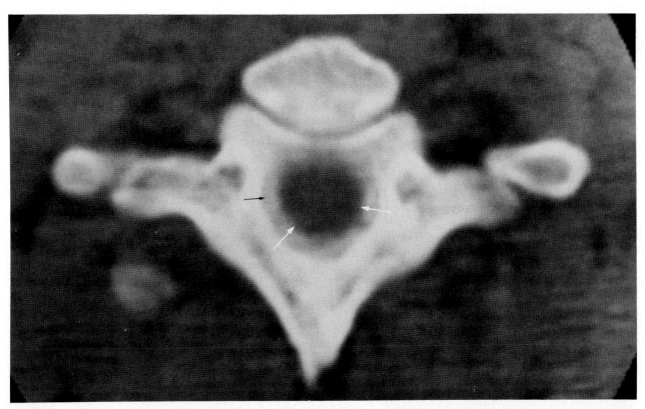

Figure 38.26. Presumed Glioma of C7–T1: A 53-year-old male had a 1-year history of pain radiating into both upper extremities. A myelogram performed 1 year before admission was normal except for a ''cervical bar'' which was removed. A postmetrizamide CT through the lower cervical spine reveals an enlarged spinal cord (*white arrows*) with a compressed subarachnoid space (*black arrow*). Because his neurological exam was normal, no surgery was performed.

Surgical removal is the treatment of choice and because of the slow growth pattern, whether complete or incomplete removal is accomplished, it often results in long-term symptom free survial.

HEMANGIOBLASTOMAS

Hemangioblastomas represent between 1–3.3% of spinal cord tumors. These lesions have no sex predeliction. Onset of symptoms is usually in the 4th decade. They are most often solitary lesions located in the cervical and thoracic cord with 60% being intramedullary and most located in the dorsal half of the spinal cord. Between 43–67% have been reported to be associated with syringomyelia and 33% with von Hippel-Lindau's disease. Histologically there are numerous capillaries and blood vessels of different sizes separated by trabeculated sheets of varying dimensions composed of clear cells with round or elongated nuclei. These tumor cells lack all cytonuclear abnormalities and often present a spongy appearance caused by the abundance of intracytoplasmic vacuoles that have been emptied of their lipid content as a result of the embedding procedure. A fine network of reticulum fibers separates the capillary blood vessels and the individual tumor cells. These lesions are histologically benign, although postoperative recurrences are possible. They appear, grossly, as well-circumscribed, often cystic lesions and, at times, ap-

pear as a small mural nodules attached to the wall of a larger cyst with a yellow color due to abundant lipid content (26, 32).

On plain films as well as CT, one may see enlargement of the interpediculate and anterior-posterior diameters of the spinal canal secondary to the slow growth of this intraspinal mass. One-half of cases show meningeal varicosities on myelography and spinal angiography. On CT, the hypodense tumor markedly enhances, usually homogeneously, with contrast injection (4, 8, 14, 30). In addition, intravenous contrast may reveal dilated veins adjacent to the intramedullary mass which would suggest the diagnosis. A delayed postmetrizamide CT demonstrates a syrinx if it is part of the lesion (34).

Treatment is surgical removal using microneurosurgical technology with total excision usually possible (11, 12, 18, 40).

DERMOIDS, EPIDERMOIDS AND TERATOMAS

Dermoids, epidermoids, and teratomas account from 1–3.3% of all spinal cord tumors and are of congenital origin. They usually occur in the lumbosacral area involving the conus medullaris and cauda equina, however, they may occur anywhere in the spinal canal. They often are associated with other congenital defects especially dermal sinus tracts and spina bifida, but also hypertrichosis, skin

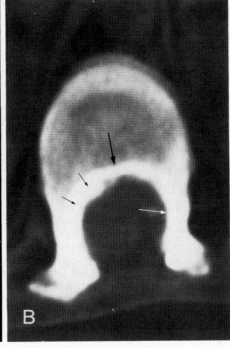
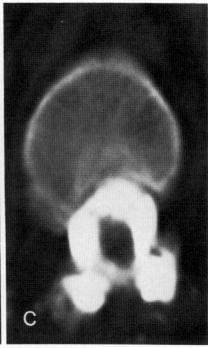

Figure 38.27. Astrocytoma of the Lower Thoracic Spine: A 22-year-old male sustained low back pain and left leg weakness 8 years before the present admission. At the time, a myelogram showed an intramedullary mass in the lower thoracic spine which was surgically explored. An intramedullary cystic astrocytoma from T9–T12 was found. The patient received postsurgical radiation (5000 rads). Two years later, the symptoms recurred and a surgical decompression for a recurrent astrocytoma was carried out. He had brief relief of symptoms, followed by rapid deterioration. In 1 year, he was totally paraplegic below T10 with loss of bowel, bladder, and sexual function. An AP view of the lower thoracic spine (A) in addition to showing the posterior arch decompression revealed erosion of the medial portions of the pedicles (>left), most marked at T11 (arrow) with widening of the interpediculate distance. A postmetrizamide CT through the lower thoracic spine (B) showed enlargement of the spinal canal, erosion of the left pedicle (*white arrow*), and scalloping of the posterior margin of the vertebral body (*large black arrow*). The subarachnoid space was thinned (*small black arrows*) by the intramedullary mass. The lesion extended to the conus, (C). Laminectomy defects from the prior surgeries were also noted. A third operation was performed which showed recurrent tumor extending to the high thoracic area. A cordectomy to T3 was done along with resection of the cauda equina. The patient is 1 year after the latest surgery with no evidence of tumor recurrence.

pigmentation, and cutaneous angiomas (4, 11, 12, 38). Dermoids and epidermoids often are called cholesteatomas or pearly tumors. These are cystic neoplasms resulting from the inclusion of epithelial elements in areas where they are normally absent. This process may take place in the fetal period or later as a result of mechanical trauma such as a lumbar puncture. Epidermoid cysts have walls composed of a thin connective tissue capsule upon which lies stratified squamous keratinized epithelium. Their contents are a granular material arranged in layers as in an onion bulb which is rich in cholesterol crystals formed by the breakdown products from these desquamating epithelial cells (26, 32). Dermoid cysts contain epidermal epithelium like epidermoid cysts and also an underlying layer similar to dermis which may contain hair follicles, sebaceous glands, and sweat glands. The cyst contents may include glandular secretory products and matted hair in addition to desquamated keratinizing cells (26, 32).

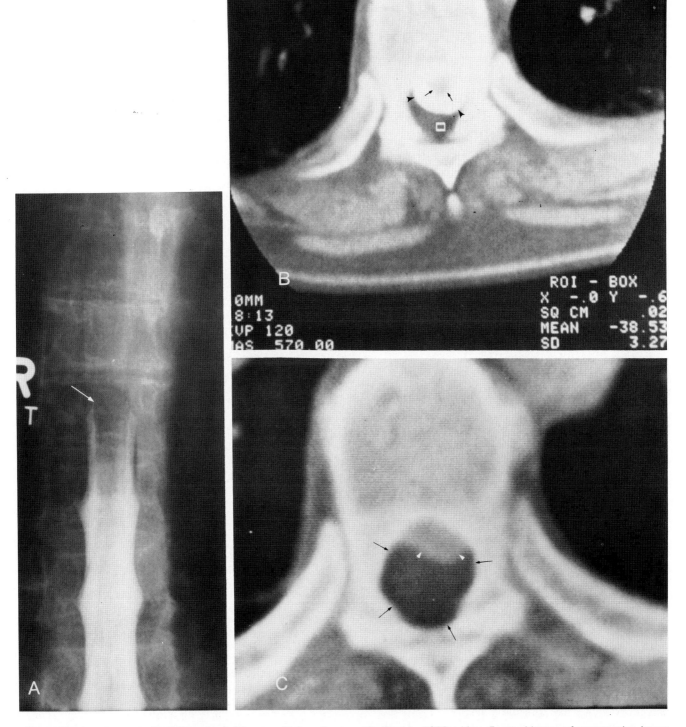

Figure 38.28. Thoracic Angiolipoma: A 61-year-old female was admitted in 1979 with a 5-year history of progressive lower extremity numbness, frequent falls, and spastic paraparesis. The AP view from a metrizamide myelogram (A) reveals a high-grade extradural thoracic block (*arrow*). The postmetrizamide CT through this area (B) shows displacement of the thoracic spinal cord (*arrows*) and dural sac (*arrowheads*) ventrally by a low-density mass in the dorsal aspect of the spinal canal having absorption coefficients compatible with fat (−76 HU). A CT slice slightly superior to B (C) demonstrates more clearly the homogeneously hypodense mass (*black arrows*) compressing the dural sac ventrally (*white arrowheads*). A thoracic laminectomy from T3–T9 was performed with gross total removal of an epidural mass pathologically diagnosed as an angiolipoma. Postoperatively the patient's neurological deficits have resolved.

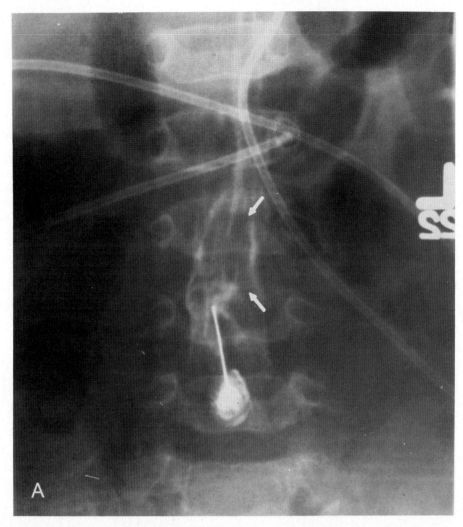

Figure 38.29.   Drop Metastases from a Primitive Neuroectodermal Tumor: A 10-month-old male presented with a progressively enlarging head for 8 months. He had a CT scan of the brain which showed hydrocephalus. The child was shunted. A follow-up CT scan of the brain without contrast again failed to reveal the etiology of the hydrocephalus. The patient subsequently developed a 7th nerve palsy and a third CT scan of the brain with contrast demonstrated a large mass with some contrast enhancement in the posterior fossa, extending into the subarachnoid cisterns. Biopsy revealed a primitive neuroectodermal tumor. He underwent radiation therapy. Within 1 month after the biopsy, the patient became paraplegic. A metrizamide myelogram with 2 cc of contrast was performed (A). It revealed multiple filling defects in the lumbar subarachnoid sac (*arrows*) and a high-grade block. The postmetrizamide CT scan documented the multiplicity of lesions in the lumbar subarachnoid sac (*arrows* and *arrowheads*, B and C). More importantly, it showed their extension into the thoracic (*arrowheads*, D and E) and lower cervical spine. A small amount of tissue that had been found on the spinal needle during myelography was sent for histological analysis. It revealed primitive neuroectodermal tumor, confirming the myelographic diagnosis of drop metastases to the spinal subarachnoid space.

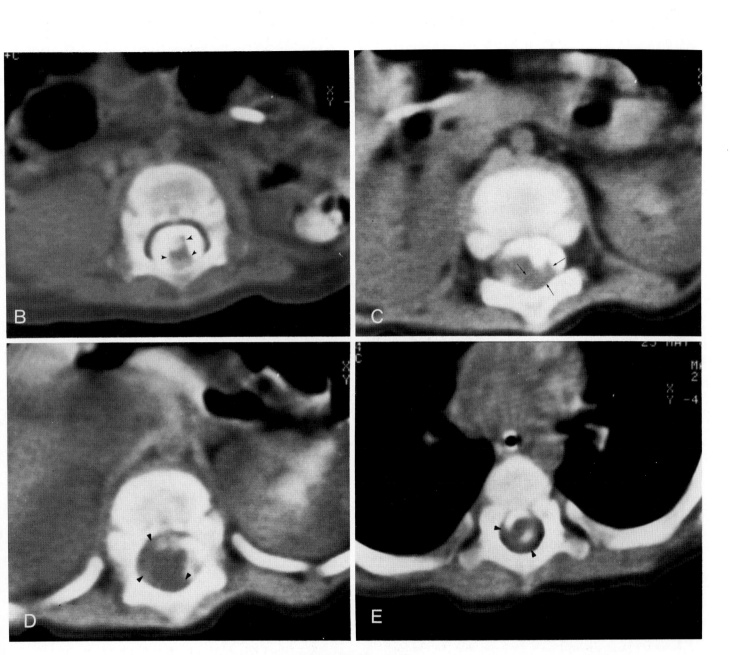

Figure 38.29.   B–E.

Treatment of epidermoids and dermoids is surgical removal which in many cases is most difficult without causing increasing neurological deficit. The contents of the cyst should always be kept away from the adjacent neural tissues to prevent a chemical arachnoiditis from spillage on aspiration (11, 18).

Teratomas usually occur within the 1st decade of life and tend to favor the midline. They commonly occur in the sacrococcygeal area and often are associated with spina bifida (38, 39). They are composed of various derivatives of the three primitive germ cell layers, with epidermal, dermal, vascular, cartilaginous, glandular, and muscular elements. They may well circumscribed and encapsulated. They are histologically benign. However, they seem to have a predisposition towards malignant change. Radiographically, one typically sees a presacral soft-tissue mass with irregular calcification or ossification. Therapy of these lesions is a combination of surgical removal plus chemotherapy (26, 32, 38, 39).

METASTATIC DISEASE

As discussed in the section on spinal column tumors, the epidural compartment is a frequent site of metastatic disease to the spine. The epidural neoplasms may be primary or may be the result of direct extension from bone or adjacent soft tissues. In contrast, intramedullary metastases are rare. CT in intramedullary metastases may demonstrate a low density cavitary lesion (37). Postmetrizamide CT will reveal an enlarged spinal cord (8) with minimal bony changes because of the rapid growth. Besides tumor, the differential diagnosis of an enlarged spinal cord includes myelitis, intramedullary granuloma, intramedullary hematoma, and syringomyelia. CT may be able to diagnose hematomyelia by its increased density (37) and a syrinx with a delayed postmetrizamide scan (34), narrowing the differential diagnosis of a widened spinal cord. Metastases to the extramedullary intradural compartment are usually secondary to primary brain tumors—cerebellar medulloblastomas, ependymomas, and supra- and infratentorial gliomas. These tumors metastasize to the spinal cord and cauda equina via cerebral spinal fluid. Metastatic implants occur more often in the dorsal half of the spinal cord and may invade the cord without displacing it, as opposed to other extramedullary lesions, because the entire periphery of the cord is involved (25). Tumor nodules, however, will displace and thicken nerve roots in the cauda equina. Postmetrizamide CT reveals filling defects within the dural sac in the cauda equina (2, 12, 22, 39).

SPINAL TUMORS IN THE PEDIATRIC AGE GROUP

Although discussed in general in the text above, spinal cord tumors in children deserve special consideration because of the unique characteristics of many of these lesions. In a series of 80 spinal cord tumors in children, 51 were males and 29 were females and they occurred in a ratio of 1:10 spinal cord to brain tumors in the pediatric

population examined. The greatest number of cases occurred between the ages of 1–3 years (38, 41). The most common signs included reflex changes, motor weakness, and sensory disturbances accompanied by muscle wasting, sphincter involvement, local tenderness, and spinal posture deformity.

Congenital tumors often are accompanied by cutaneous stigmata including subcutaneous lipomas, abnormal hairy patch in the midline, capillary hemangiomas, sacral dimples, sinus tracts, and cafe au lait spots. They often are associated with congenital spinal abnormalities with 70% of the patients having plain spine film abnormalities. Of the developmental or congenital tumors, the most common are dermoids predominately in the lumbosacral area followed by neurenteric and teratomatous cysts in the upper thoracic area and by teratomas, extradural cysts, and lipomas. Neurenteric and teratomatous cysts are mainly upper thoracic and the teratomas thoracolumbar. The results of treatment of patients with these tumors are considered good to excellent (38).

Other pediatric tumors include the intrinsic or primary cord tumors with the most frequent being astrocytomas in the cervical region with a 50/50 chance of there being either excellent or fair treatment results (38). Ependymomas of the filum terminale or the thoracolumbar area have good to excellent prognosis after treatment (38).

CSF-borne metastases also affect the pediatric group with the most common being glioma followed by melanoma and ependymoma. Gliomas occur at multiple levels, melanomas at the sacral level, and the ependymomas in the basal regions. Prognosis is poor in this group of gliomas and melanomas but good for ependymomas (38). Drop metastases (Fig. 38.29) from central nervous system tumors and blood-borne metastases also occur in children. Blood-borne metastases, usually affecting the thoracic spine, have a poor prognosis.

Another group of tumors seen in children are those that cause compression by direct extension. They include tumors such as ganglioneuromas, in the thoracic area, neuroblastomas, neurofibrosarcomas at the various levels, and neurofibromas and schwannomas in the cervical area. The ganglioneuromas, neurofibromas, and schwannomas have excellent outcomes and the fibrosarcomas have a poor outcome. The bone tumors have a prognosis varying between these two groups. If treated in the age group under 18 months, neuroblastomas have a good prognosis as compared to a poorer prognosis when treated after this time period. CT metrizamide myelography has proven to be an excellent diagnostic tool for use in these intra- and paraspinal neoplasms, both in infants and children (26, 32, 38, 39).

References

1. Beabout JW, McLeod RA, Dahlin DC: Benign tumors. *Sem Roentgen* 14:33–43, 1979.
2. Herkowitz HN: Neoplasms of the spine: A synopsis of the more common lesions. Presented at the Spine Study Group course on Spine Disorders, Snowmass, Colorado, March 9–13, 1981.

3. Luck JV, Monsen DCG: Bone Tumors and tumor-like lesions of vertebrae In: Ruge D, Wiltse L: *Spinal Disorders, Diagnosis and Treatment.* Lee and Febiger, Philadelphia, 1977, pp. 274–286.

4. Schecter MM, Sajor E: Radiology of the spine. In: Yeomans WR: *Neurological Surgery.* 2nd ed., W. B. Saunders Co., Philadelphia 1982, Vol. 1:487–550.

5. Unni KK, Ivins JC, Beabout JW, et al: Hemangioma, hemangiopericytoma, and hemangioendothelioma (angiosarcoma) of bone. *Cancer* 27:1403–1414, 1971.

6. Schroeder S, Lackner K, Weiand G: Lumbosacral intradural lipoma. *J Comput Assist Tomogr* 5:274, 1981.

7. Epstein N, Benjamin V, Pinto R, et al: Benign osteoblastoma of a thoracic vertebra. Case report. *J Neurosurg* 53:710–713, 1980.

8. Haughton VM, Williams AL: *Computed Tomography of the Spine.* The C. V. Mosby Co, St. Louis, 1982.

9. Bret P, Confavreaux C, Thouard H, et al: Aneurysmal bone cyst of the cervical spine: Report of a case investigated by computed tomographic scanning and treated by a two-stage surgical procedure. *Neurosurgery* 10:111–115, 1982.

10. Schwimer SR, Bassett LW, Mancuso AA, et al: Giant cell tumor of the cervicothoracic spine. *AJR* 136:63–67, 1981.

11. Connolly EF: Spinal cord tumors in adults. In: Yeomans WR: *Neurological Surgery.* 2nd ed., W. B. Saunders Co., Philadelphia, 1982, Vol. 5:3196–3214.

12. Kurland LT: The frequency of intracranial and paraspinal neoplasms in the resident population of Rochester, Minnesota. *J Neurosurg* 15:627–41, 1958.

13. Sundaresan N, Galicich JH, Chu FCH, et al: Spinal chordomas. *J Neurosurg* 50:312–319, 1979.

14. Taveras J, Woods E: *Diagnostic Radiology.* 2nd ed., Vol. 2:1168–1206, Williams & Wilkins Co., Baltimore, 1976.

15. Subbarao K, Jacobson HG: Primary malignant neoplasms. *Sem Roentgen* 14:44–57, 1979.

16. Ciappetta P, Di Lorenzo N, Delfini R: CT Evaluation of sacral tumors with neural involvement. *J Neurosurg Sci* 25:89–94, 1981.

17. Zito JL, Davis KR: The role of computed metrizamide myelography in evaluation of extradural extension from vertebral chordoma. CT: *J Comput Tomogr* 4:38–42, 1980.

18. Austin G: *The Spinal Cord Basic Aspects and Surgical Consideration.* 2nd ed. Charles C Thomas, Springfield IL, 1972, pp. 281–346.

19. Verbiest H: Neurosurgical use of spinal CT. In: Post MJD: *Radiographic Evaluation of the Spine: Current Advances with Emphasis on Computed Tomography.* Masson Publishing, New York, 1980, pp. 139–185.

20. Abdel-Dayem HM, Oh YS: Treated stage IIb Hodgkin's Disease complicated by late paraplegia. In: Kagan AR, Steckel RJ: Diagnostic oncology case studies. *AJR* 132:265–266, 1979.

21. Camins MB, Duncan AW, Smith J, et al: Chondrosarcoma of the spine. *Spine* 3:202–209, 1978.

22. Davis JM, Zimmerman RA, Bilaniuk LT: Metastases to the central nervous system. In: Libshitz HI: Symposium on Metastatic Disease. *Radiol Clin North Am* 20:417–435, 1982.

23. Bassett LW: Lytic spine lesion and cold bone scan. In: Kagan AR, Steckel RJ: Diagnostic oncology case study. *AJR* 136:129–131, 1981.

24. Schoter VI, Wappenschmidt J: Computer assisted myelography in the investigation of intraspinal space-occupying lesions. *Fortschr Rontgenstr* 133:527–530, 1980.

25. Shapiro R: *Myelography.* Year Book Medical Publishers, Inc. Chicago, 1975.

26. Escourolle R, Poirier J: *Manual of Basic Neuropathology.* W.

B. Saunders Co., Philadelphia 1978, pp. 18–59.

27. Nittner K: Spinal meningiomas, neurinomas, and neurofibrous and hourglass tumors. In: Vinker PJ, Brayan BW: *Handbook of Clinical Neurology.* Vol. 20:177–322, Amsterdam, North Holland Publishing Co., New York, American Cr., Inc., 1976.

28. Balériaux-Waha D, Terwinghe G, Jeanmart L: The value of computed tomography for the diagnosis of hourglass tumors of the spine. *Neuroradiology* 14:31–32, 1977.

29. Yang WC, Zappulla R, Malis L: Case report. Neurolemmoma in lumbar intervertebral foramen. *J Comput Assist Tomogr* 5:904–906, 1981.

30. Nakagawa H, Huang YP, Malis LI, et al: Computed tomography of intraspinal and paraspinal neoplasms. *J Comput Assist Tomogr* 1:377–390, 1977.

31. Nakagawa H, Malis LI, Huang YP: Computed tomography of soft tissue masses related to the spinal column. In: Post MJD: *Radiographic Evaluation of the Spine: Current Advances with Emphasis on Computed Tomography.* Masson Publishing, New York, 1980, pp. 320–352.

32. Russell DS, Rubenstein LJ: *Pathology of Tumors of the Nervous System.* 3rd ed., Williams & Wilkins Co., Baltimore, 1971.

33. Memon MY, Schneck L: Ventral Spinal Tumor: The value of computed tomography in its localization. *Neurosurgery* 8:108–111, 1981.

34. Bonafe A, Manelfe C, Espagno J, et al: Evaluation of syringomyelia with metrizamide computed tomographic myelography. *J Comput Assist Tomogr* 4:797–802, 1980.

35. Browne TR, Adams RD, Roberson GH: Hemangioblastoma of the Spinal Cord. Review and report of five cases. *Arch Neurol* 33:435–441, 1976.

36. Handel S, Grossman R, Sarwar M: Computed tomography in the diagnosis of spinal cord astrocytoma. *J Comput Assist Tomogr* 2:226–118, 1978.

37. Zumpano BJ: Spinal intramedullary metastatic medullo-blastoma. Case report. *J Neurosurg* 48:632–635, 1978.

38. Hendrick EB: Spinal cord tumors in children. In: Yeomans WR: *Neurological Surgery.* W. B. Saunders Co., Philadelphia, 1982 Vol. 5:3215–3221.

39. Resjo IM, Harwood-Nash DC, Fitz CR, et al: CT metrizamide myelography for intraspinal and paraspinal neoplasm in infants and children. *AJR* 132:367–372, 1979.

40. Sloof J, Kernohan J, MacCarty C: Primary intramedullary tumors of the spinal cord and filium terminale. W. B. Saunders Co., Philadelphia, 1964.

41. Aubin ML, et al: Computerized tomography in 32 cases of intraspinal tumor. *J Neuroradiol* 6:81–92, 1979.

42. Arii H, Takahashi M, Tamakawa Y, et al: Metrizamide spinal computed tomography following myelography. *Comput Tomogr* 4:117–125, 1980.

43. Balériaux-Waha D, Osteauz M, Terwinghe G, et al: The management of anterior sacral meningocele with computed tomography. *Neuroradiology* 14:45–46, 1977.

44. Federle MP, Moss AA, Margolin FR: Role of computed tomography in patients with "sciatica". *J Comput Assist Tomogr* 4:335–341, 1980.

45. Miki T, Oka M, Shima M, et al: Spinal angiolipoma. A case report. *Acta Neurochirurg* 58:115–119, 1981.

46. Sartor VK: Computer tomography for spinal tumors. *Fortschr Rontgenstr* 132:391–398, 1980.

47. Scotti LM, Marasco JA, Pittman TA, et al: Computed tomography of the spinal canal and cord. *Comput Tomogr* 1:229–234, 1977.

48. Wedge JH, Tchang S, MacFadyen DJ: Computed tomography in localization of spinal osteoma. *Spine* 6:423–427, 1981.

CHAPTER THIRTY-NINE

Efficacy of Intravenous Contrast Medium in the Computed Tomographic Demonstration of Spinal Cord Neoplasms

WEN C. YANG, M.D., JAN J. SMULEWICZ, M.D., ROSARIO ZAPPULLA, M.D., and LEONARD I. MALIS, M.D.*

The value of intravenous contrast medium administration in cranial computed tomography (CT) has been well recognized. Only a few reports have appeared in the literature to indicate the usefulness of intravenous contrast medium in the CT evaluation of spinal lesions, and in particular spinal cord neoplasms (1–3). This is understandable because of the limited resolution of the early CT scanners. With the advent of high-resolution CT (HRCT), soft-tissue structures within the spinal canal can be differentiated (4). As a result, demonstration of contrast-enhanced lesions within the spinal canal is possible.

Until recently, delineation of the spinal cord as well as of intramedullary lesions either by conventional radiographs or CT scans required the introduction of intrathecal contrast which had to be accomplished through spinal puncture. However, with high resolution, it is now possible to detect spinal cord neoplasms by CT without resorting to myelography.

We wish to demonstrate the efficacy of intravenous contrast medium in the CT evaluation of spinal cord masses and the potential of differentiating the various types of mass lesions.

MATERIAL AND METHODS

From July 1979 to March 1981, 13 spinal cord masses were studied with spinal CT with intravenous contrast medium administration (Table 39.1). These included 5 cases of astrocytoma, 4 cases of ependymoma, 1 case of hemangioblastoma, 1 case of myelitis, 1 case of ependymal cyst, and 1 case of hydromyelia. All patients had previous myelography and surgery at the time of spinal CT, except the case of ependymal cyst. The diagnosis in each case was established at previous or subsequent surgery. In the case of hydromyelia, the metrizamide CT demonstrated the spinal cord pathology.

As a control group and to assess the effect of intravenous contrast medium administration on the normal spinal cord, 10 patients scheduled for a CT examination of the neck for various lesions other than intraspinal pathology were included in this project.

A General Electric CT/T 8800 scanner was utilized with the following techniques: 120 kV, 5-mm scan slices, 9.6-second scanning time, 25-cm calibration field, and 0.75 mm pixel size.

The contrast material used was 150 cc Conray 60% (Mallinckrodt Inc, St. Louis), which is equivalent to 42.3 g of iodine.

Initial precontrast CT scanning was performed to evaluate the spinal region of interest. The contrast material was then given intravenously by drip infusion. Upon completion of one-half of the infusion, CT scanning was resumed to evaluate the same spinal region of interest.

Abnormal contrast enhancement was apparent on visual inspection by using the appropriate window and by comparing with the precontrast scan. To determine the degree of contrast enhancement of the mass lesion, we used the tissue-blood ratio of enhancement which was obtained as follows:

$$\text{Tissue-Blood Ratio} = \frac{\text{enhancement of tissue}}{\text{enhancement of blood}} \times 100$$

The mean CT numbers of the spinal cord mass were taken on the pre- and postcontrast CT scans. The difference of the mean CT numbers represented the enhanced value of the tissue. To determine the enhancement of blood, the major vessels such as internal jugular vein, carotid artery, descending aorta, and abdominal aorta on the axial CT scans were identified. The mean CT numbers then were taken from the major blood vessel on the pre- and postcontrast CT scans. The difference of these two CT numbers represented the enhanced value of the blood. The tissue-blood ratio was expressed in percentage as the enhanced value of tissue in relation to the enhanced value of blood.

In 4 cases, metrizamide myelography was performed in conjunction with spinal CT. In Case 6, only a small amount of metrizamide was injected intrathecally for the purpose of outlining the cervical spinal cord.

Spinal angiography was done in 1 patient to evaluate the spinal cord hemangioblastoma.

* We are grateful to our CT technologists of Beth Israel Medical Center, Mr. Nastor Grant, Ms. Nereida Gonzales, and Ms. Carol Hansen for their technical assistance, to Mrs. Pat Gorman for typing the manuscript, and to Dr. Yun Peng Huang of Mt. Sinai Medical Center for his help in the preparation of this paper.

RESULTS

All 10 cases with a normal spinal canal showed no significant contrast enhancement in the area of the spinal cord (Fig. 39.1).

Table 1 shows the results of contrast enhancement in the spinal cord masses and their respective tissue-blood ratios.

Astrocytoma—All 5 cases were operated upon previously. Significant contrast enhancement was evident in all the residual tumors (Fig. 39.2). The tissue-blood ratios ranged from 63–87.3%. After the CT examinations, 3 patients went on to have repeat spinal surgery with confirmation of the diagnosis of spinal cord tumor and 2 patients received radiotherapy and chemotherapy.

Ependymoma—There were 3 cases in the thoracic cord and 1 case in the cervical cord. All showed significant enhancement with the tissue-blood ratio ranging from 42.1–100%. In Case 6, a recurrent ependymoma was located in the left side of the cervical cord (Fig. 39.3) which was successfully removed at subsequent surgery. In Cases

Table 39.1.
Contrast Enhancement And Tissue-Blood Ratios in Spinal Cord Masses

Patients			Diagnosis	Contrast enhancement		Tissue-blood ratio (%)
				Lesion (HU)	Blood (HU)	
1.	BM	F/52	Astrocytoma, C1–4	38.6	46.8	82.4
2.	PE	F/40	Astrocytoma, C4-T1	80.9	92.8	87.3
3.	BN	M/63	Astrocytoma, C3–5	29.0	35.6	81.5
4.	LE	M/44	Astrocytoma, C2–7	31.4	50.0	63.0
5.	MB	F/40	Astrocytoma, C5–6	56.4	77.4	72.8
6.	WS	M/56	Ependymoma, C3–4	21.7	51.7	42.1
7.	AA	M/10	Ependymoma, T9-L1	30.5	30.5	100.0
8.	NA	F/14	Ependymoma, T12-L1	29.2	60.0	48.6
9.	SA	F/54	Ependymoma, T12	19.5	40.1	48.4
10.	GJ	F/65	Hemangioblastoma, T10-L2	49.3	44.1	111.7
11.	KI	F/36	Myelitis, C3–7	7.9	72.0	11.0
12.	LP	M/12	Ependymal cyst, T12-L1	0	40.0	0
13.	MN	F/54	Hydromyelia, C2–4	0	30.8	0

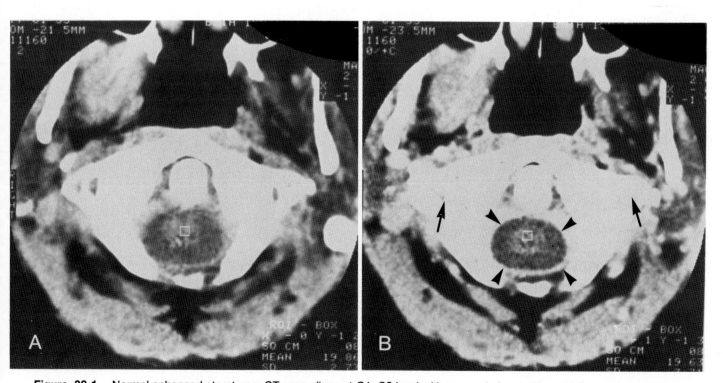

Figure 39.1.   Normal enhanced structures: CT scan slices at C1–C2 level with same window setting. (A) Precontrast scan. (B) Postcontrast CT scan. The dura matter (*arrowheads*) is enhanced. The spinal cord remains unenhanced. The vertebral arteries (*arrows*) in the transverse foramina are enhanced.

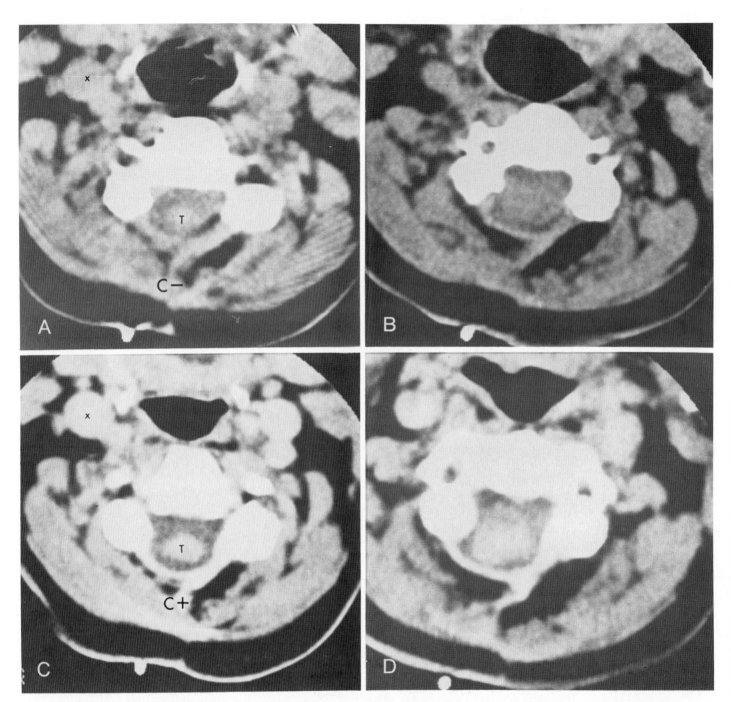

Figure 39.2. Case 1: Astrocytoma of C1–C4 cord: A 52-year-old female had a cervical laminectomy 2 years previously for biopsy of a spinal cord astrocytoma. Radiotherapy was given. She developed further neurological deficits and diagnostic work-up was again initiated. CT scans at C3 level: A and B. Precontrast CT scans. C and D. Postcontrast CT scans. Spinal cord astrocytoma (T) is enhanced. * Indicates internal jugular vein. E. Midsagittal reformated image of cervical CT scans shows an enhanced astrocytoma (*arrows*) in the central portion of the spinal canal. F. Metrizamide cervical myelogram in lateral projection shows an enlarged cord at C1–C4 level.

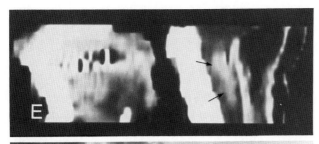

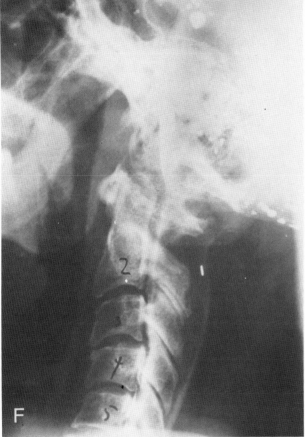

Figure 39.2. E and F.

7 (Fig. 39.4) and 8, surgery also confirmed the CT findings.

Hemangioblastoma—(Fig. 39.5) Homogeneous enhancement was noted within the enlarged spinal canal. The tissue-blood ratio was high and measured 111.7%, suggesting increased vascularity and considerable extravascular accumulation of contrast material. Spinal angiography revealed abundant tumor vascularity and a tumor stain. The diagnosis was confirmed by autopsy.

Myelitis—The enhancement was low and the ratio was only 11.0%.

Ependymal Cyst and Hydromyelia—No enhancement was evident.

DISCUSSION

CT of the spinal cord with intravenous contrast medium administration is easy to perform and less invasive than

myelography. This CT study can be carried out on an outpatient basis. The capability of intravenous contrast medium to enhance and localize spinal cord neoplasms is important in surgical planning, especially in cases of recurrent or residual tumors. As demonstrated in this series, it is useful in the postoperative assessment of spinal cord tumors.

Early experiences with intravenous contrast injection in the CT evaluation of the spinal cord masses were unrewarding (5–8). The unfavorable results can be attributed to the poor resolution of the CT scanners and suboptimal amounts of contrast medium injected.

The measurement of tissue-blood ratio in this report is different from the method used by Gado et al. (9, 10) in cranial CT. The method we used is simple and easier to follow. There were 2 cases with tissue-blood ratios measured at 100% and above, suggesting considerable extravascular accumulation of contrast material. This is in conformity with the previous observations for cerebral lesions (9–11).

The CT number within the spinal canal may not be an accurate measurement of the absorption coefficient, and is affected by the surrounding bony tissues (6, 12). With similar settings before and after intravenous contrast injection the enhanced value and the tissue-blood ratio are considered a better expression of contrast enhancement than the absolute CT numbers.

The current CT scanner has been equipped with the reformation computer program. One now can visualize the craniocaudal extent of the neoplastic process within the spinal cord in dimensions comparable to myelography (Fig. 39.2). Rather than simply showing the enlarged cord, the reformated image is able to demonstrate the actual neoplastic core in longitudinal dimension.

The contrast enhancement noted in spinal cord neoplasms may be used to differentiate neoplastic from other spinal cord lesions. As noted in this study, astrocytoma, ependymoma, and hemangioblastoma were enhanced significantly, whereas the ependymal cyst was not enhanced. The case of myelitis also showed minimal enhancement presumably because it was in the chronic stage. The patient had surgery 1 year earlier, and had been on steroid therapy before CT scanning. As expected, hydromyelia did not show enhancement.

Although the tissue blood ratio may be used to differentiate benign from malignant spinal cord masses, its predictive value for specific histological diagnosis remains to be seen and a larger series is needed to substantiate this diagnostic criterion.

In spite of the proven capability of intravenous contrast medium to detect spinal cord neoplasms on HRCT scans, it would be inappropriate at this point in time to replace myelography completely with this modality. Myelography is still essential in the initial investigation of patients without previous surgery who are suspected of having spinal cord lesions. Myelography is also important in surgical planning. Myelography identifies intramedullary masses, distinguishes them from intradural extramedul-

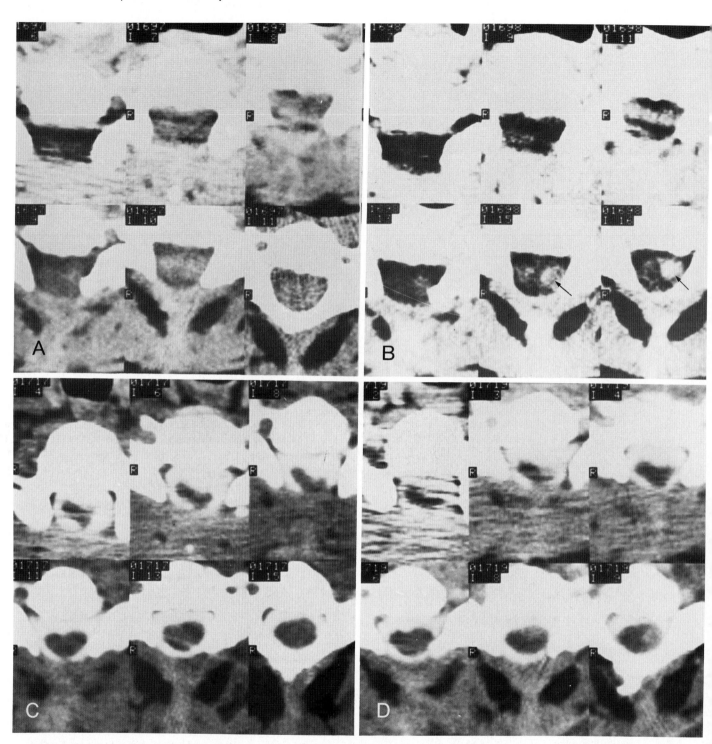

Figure 39.3.   Case 6: Recurrent ependymoma at C3–C4 level: A 56-year-old male was operated 2 years earlier for a spinal cord tumor at C3–C6 level. Postoperatively, he was stable neurologically with left hemiparesis until a few weeks before admission when he developed right hand numbness. A. Plain CT scans at multiple cervical levels. B. CT scans after intravenous contrast infusion at corresponding levels. An enhanced lesion is demonstrated (*arrows*) in the left side of the C3–C4 spinal canal. C. Metrizamide CT scans. D. Metrizamide CT scans after intravenous contrast infusion. The enhanced lesion is noted in the spinal cord which is clearly defined by metrizamide. The lower cervical cord is collapsed from previous surgery. The enhanced ependymoma was removed successfully at surgery.

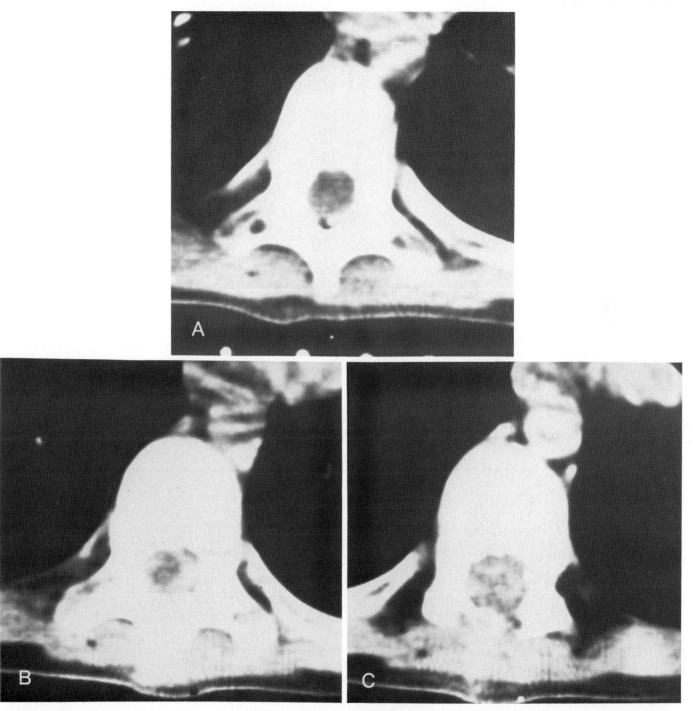

Figure 39.4.   Case 7: Ependymoma at the T9 level: A 10-year-old boy presented with paraparesis and myelography demonstrated an enlarged cord from C2 to L1. A. Precontrast CT scan. B and C. Postcontrast CT scans at corresponding levels. Note the abnormal irregular enhancement within the spinal canal. The tumor was removed completely and the patient's neurological status improved. He was ambulating unassisted at the time of discharge.

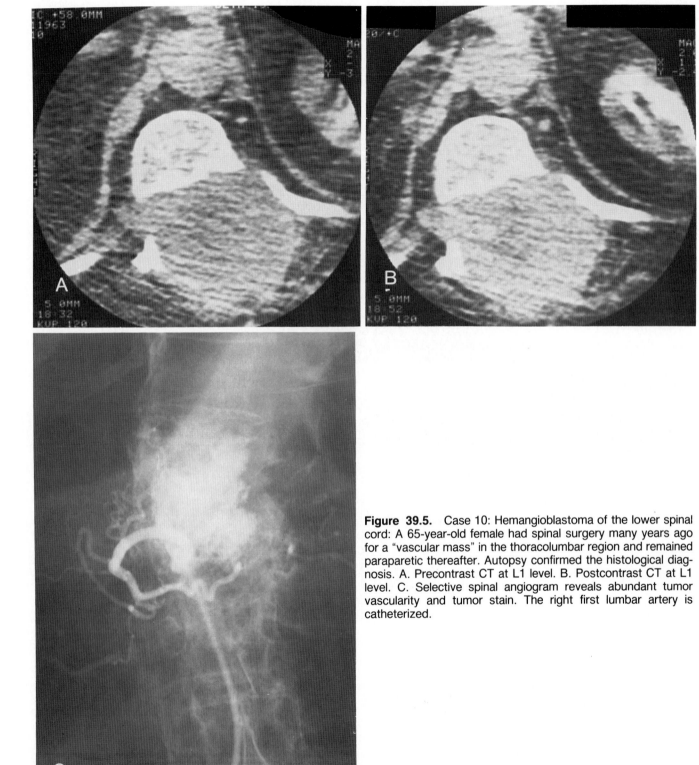

Figure 39.5.   Case 10: Hemangioblastoma of the lower spinal cord: A 65-year-old female had spinal surgery many years ago for a "vascular mass" in the thoracolumbar region and remained paraparetic thereafter. Autopsy confirmed the histological diagnosis. A. Precontrast CT at L1 level. B. Postcontrast CT at L1 level. C. Selective spinal angiogram reveals abundant tumor vascularity and tumor stain. The right first lumbar artery is catheterized.

lary and from extradural lesions, and demonstrates their longitudinal extent. However, one can take advantage of the intravenously enhanced CT scan after myelography to determine the nature of the spinal cord mass by the type of contrast enhancement which is seen. Most importantly, one can use this modality in the postoperative evaluation of spinal cord tumors. In those patients who are reluctant to return to the hospital for myelographic assessment, this procedure can be used on an outpatient basis to identify those with tumor recurrence. As for those patients with recurrent tumors which are amenable only to radiation therapy, this study might be used as the definitive diagnostic procedure.

As the efficacy of intravenous contrast injection in the CT evaluation of spinal cord masses is recognized, applications of this modality with modified techniques are to be expected. Although not yet employed due to limitation of facility and time, expanded high iodine dose and delayed CT scanning which have been applied in cranial CT (13, 14) may be useful in the further appraisal of spinal cord tumors.

CONCLUSIONS

With HRCT, intravenous contrast medium administration is a valuable adjunct for the demonstration of spinal cord neoplasms. It makes possible the precise localization of spinal cord neoplasms which is very helpful in surgical planning. The postoperative assessment of spinal cord neoplasms can be made by performing spinal CT with intravenous contrast injection, without resorting to myelography.

Spinal cord neoplasms had visible contrast enhancement on HRCT scan with high tissue-blood ratios whereas chronic myelitis, ependymal cyst, and hydromyelia had low or no enhancement. The result of measuring tissue-blood ratios of enhancement in spinal cord masses suggests that, as in cerebral lesions, there is an extravascular component of contrast enhancement.

References

1. Handel S, Grossman R, Sarwar M: Computed tomography in the diagnosis of spinal cord astrocytoma. *J Comput Assist Tomogr* 2:226–228, 1978.
2. Nakagawa H, Huang YP, Malis LI, et al: Computed tomography of intraspinal and paraspinal neoplasms. *J Comput Assist Tomogr* 1:377–390, 1977.
3. Baleriaux-Waha D, Terwinghe G, Jeanmart L: The value of computed tomography for the diagnosis of hourglass tumors of the spine. *Neuroradiology* 14:31–32, 1977.
4. Haughton VM, Syvertsen A, Williams AL: Soft tissue anatomy within the spinal canal as seen on computed tomography. *Radiology* 134:649–655, 1980.
5. Aubin ML, Jardin C, Bar D, et al: Computerized tomography in 32 cases of intraspinal tumor *J Neuroradiol* 6:81–92, 1979.
6. Post MJD: Computed tomography of the spine: its value and limitations on a nonhigh resolution scanner. In: Post MJD: *Radiographic Evaluation of the Spine: Current Advances with Emphasis on Computed Tomography.* Masson Publishing, Inc., USA, New York, 1980, pp. 180–258.
7. Ethier R, King DG, Melançon D, et al: Diagnosis of intra- and extramedullary lesions by CT without contrast achieved through modifications applied to the EMI CT 5005 Body Scanning. In: Post MJD: *Radiographic Evaluation of the Spine: Current Advances with Emphasis on Computed Tomography.* Masson Publishing, Inc., USA, New York, 1980, pp. 377–393.
8. Lee BP, Kazan E, Newman AD: Computed tomography of the spine and spinal cord. *Radiology* 128:95–102, 1978.
9. Gado MH, Phelps ME, Coleman KE: An extravascular component of contrast enhancement in cranial computed tomography. Part I: The tissue-blood ratio of contrast enhancement. *Radiology* 117:589–593, 1975.
10. Gado MH, Phelps ME, Coleman KE: An extravascular component of contrast enhancement in cranial computed tomography. Part II: Contrast enhancement and the blood tissue barrier. *Radiology* 117:595–597, 1975.
11. Handa J, Matsuda I, Handa H, et al: Extravascular iodine in contrast enhancement with computed tomography. *Neuroradiology* 15:159–163, 1978.
12. McCullough EC: Factors affecting the use of quantitative information from a CT scanner. *Radiology* 124:99–107, 1977.
13. Davis JM, Davis KR, Newhouse J, et al: Expanded high iodine dose in cranial computed tomography: a preliminary report. *Radiology* 131:373–380, 1979.
14. Norman D, Stevens EA, Wing SD, et al: Quantitative aspects of contrast enhancement in cranial computed tomography. *Radiology* 129:683–688, 1978.

CHAPTER FORTY

The Diagnosis and Surgical Management of Spinal Tumors Using Computed Tomography

CHARLES C. EDWARDS, M.D.*

A wide range of tumors can affect the spine. Because of the spine's central location—adjacent to viscera and the great vessels and containing the spinal cord—spine tumors may be of greater consequence to the patient than similar tumors involving other bones. However, this central location and the architectural complexity of the spine make early diagnosis and effective management of these tumors particularly difficult for the treating physician. The use of computed axial tomography can simplify this task. Obscure lesions can be diagnosed more rapidly and accurately. Of even greater importance, the extent of tumor involvement usually can be delineated clearly, making it possible to effectively resect tumors formerly thought "inoperable."

TUMORS AFFECTING THE SPINE: INCIDENCE

Tumors and tumor-like conditions affecting the spine (C1-S5) can be divided conveniently into three broad categories: In order of frequency of occurrence, these include: 1) metastatic lesions, 2) primary spinal column tumors, and 3) primary intradural tumors.

Metastatic Lesions

Metastases account for the great majority of tumorous lesions present in the spine. Jaffe estimates that 70% of malignancies eventually metastasize to bone (1). Cancer cell emboli ordinarily reach the skeleton via the blood stream. The direct passage of cells from viscera to vertebrae was studied by Batson. His injections demonstrated a valveless vertebral vein system (Batson's plexus) about the spine characterized by sluggish flow. Hence, emboli from nearby viscera can drain directly into vertebrae, bypassing the liver and lungs. This phenomenon may explain why the spine is the most common bony recipient of metastases (2).

The most likely origin of a metastatic spine lesion is the breast in the female and the lungs in the male patient. These are followed in frequency by metastases from the prostate, gastrointestinal tract, kidney, and thyroid (1, 3). The bone lesions which occur in roughly 15% of Hodgkins disease also concentrate in the vertebrae (4). Considering the location of the viscera most frequently seeding the spine, it is not surprising that the thoracic, followed by the lumbar segments, are affected most frequently (1). Metastases to the cervical spine and sacrum are less common and metastases to the cord are extremely rare (3).

Primary Spinal Column Tumors

Myeloma is by far the most common primary tumor of bone to appear within the spine (5). It accounts for about one-half of all spine tumorous lesions (4, 6), although vertebrae may not be the first manifestation of myeloma in many of these cases. Including myeloma (6%), almost 11% of all primary bone tumors develop in the spine.

An appropriate index of suspicion facilitates prompt diagnosis. It is well known that different tumors predominate in the spine than in the extremities. What is the relative frequency of primary bone tumors presenting within the spine? In an effort to provide at least a rough answer to this question, the author combined and extrapolated data for Table 40.1 from the published reports of Schajowicz (6), Huvos (4), Dahlin (7), and others. The table lists the 10 most common vertebral tumors.

Less common spinal tumors include reticulum cell sarcoma, osteosarcoma, and Ewing's sarcoma which each represent 2%. Fibrosarcoma accounts for only 1.5% of spinal tumors (4, 6–8). It is noteworthy that such common bone tumors as osteosarcoma and Ewing's sarcoma comprise such a small fraction of the primary tumors found within the spine.

Spinal Canal Tumors

Tumors arising within the spinal canal are less common than either metastatic or primary vertebral lesions. Four tumor types account for 77% of all intrathecal tumors. In order of frequency these include: neurofibromas (27%), meningiomas (23%), intramedullary gliomas encompassing both astrocytomas and ependymomas (17%), and various sarcomas (10%). Numerous other lesions, each comprising less than 2% each account for the remaining 23% of all intradural tumors (3).

TUMORS AFFECTING THE SPINE: CHARACTERISTICS

The diagnosis and management of spinal tumors is based upon the clinical and radiographic characteristics of var-

* The author wishes to express appreciation for: the permission to use the pathology example radiographs in Figures 40.1, 40.2, 40.4, and 40.5 from cases treated primarily by Dr. Alan Levine; the University of Maryland residents and fellows who contributed to the treatment of all cases mentioned; the cooperation of Dr. Joseph Whitley and the Department of Radiology; and the efforts of my research assistant, Margaret Weigel, in collecting data and helping to prepare the manuscript.

Table 40.1.
Ten Common Vertebral Tumors (C1-S5)

Order of Frequency	% of Spinal Tumors	"Tumor"
1	45%	Myeloma
2	8	Chordoma
3	6	Giant cell
4	5	Osteoid osteoma
5	5	Aneurysmal bone cyst
6	4.5	Chondrosarcoma
7	4	Hemangioma
8	4	Osteochondroma
9	3	Eosinophilic granuloma
10	3	Osteoblastoma

ious tumor types. Before discussing tumor diagnosis and management in more detail, a brief summary of the most common primary spinal column tumors seems in order. The definition, clinical characteristics, vertebral location, and radiographic features of each tumor are outlined in the following section according to the order of the tumor's frequency in the spine.

Myeloma

Myeloma is a malignant tumor of marrow plasma cells which usually progresses to multiple sites throughout the skeleton (multiple myeloma). The disease typically afflicts patients between 50–70 years of age. It primarily involves red marrow so the first lesions usually originate in the axial skeleton. Back pain from a vertebral lesion is the first symptom in about one-third of myeloma patients (9). With growth of the myeloma lesion, vertebral body collapse occurs, associated with severe pain and occasionally with neurological deficit from cord compression. Although myeloma may present as a solitary lesion, skeletal dissemination almost always follows; hence, marrow aspiration biopsies usually will make the diagnosis.

Myeloma plasma cells produce immunoglobulins. This aids diagnosis, because an (M-component) spike or other abnormalities occur in the globulin range on protein electrophoresis in over 90% of myeloma patients (10). The excessive globulins often cause renal dysfunction. When abundant light-chain globulins are produced, they pass through the glomerulus where they can be detected in the urine as Bence-Jones proteins.

Myeloma cells invoke a markedly osteolytic response. Osteolysis contributes to hypercalcemia and its clinical sequelae of lethargy, anorexia, and thirst. Plasma cell proliferation crowds out other marrow cells and compromises the patient's resistance to infection. Chemotherapy and prednisone can slow the progression of the disease significantly (4). Radiation of vertebral lesions often will arrest tumor growth. However, no treatment regimen has succeeded yet in diverting the ultimate fatal outcome of multiple myeloma.

The vertebral body is the most frequent site for myelomatous lesions (Fig. 40.1A and B). Myelomas usually present as punched-out lesions, but the destruction may be diffuse—mimicking osteoporosis. Because there is little if any bone reaction, the affected vertebral body eventually collapses. Unlike metastatic carcinoma, myeloma rarely obliterates the pedicles (4) (Fig. 40.1A). Hence, the pattern of flattened vertebrae with preservation of pedicles and endplates in an older patient without other bone disease is considered to be almost diagnostic of multiple myeloma (5).

Chordoma

Chordoma is a malignant tumor arising from vertebral body remnants of the fetal notochord. Cancerous transformation of the notochord remnant typically occurs in the 50- to 70-year-old age bracket, with a 2:1 male predominance (11). The tumor grows slowly and metastasizes late so it is often quite large and "unresectable" when discovered (Fig. 40.2A–C). In its usual sacral location, its presence is signaled by dull pain or bladder/bowel incontinence from compression of sacral roots. The tumor responds poorly to chemotherapy, radiation, and/or incomplete resection (12). The only chance for cure is with complete resection—prompting recommendations for hemicorporectomy in selected cases (13). Although only perhaps 20% of the tumors eventually metastasize, they cause death in over 96% of the reported cases (4, 14).

The majority of chordomas develop about the sacrum, making it by far the most common sacral tumor (8, 12). Another 15% of chordomas occur in the vertebral column and the remainder in the spheno-occipital area (4). The tumor is osteolytic and may destroy one or more adjacent vertebral bodies. It usually forms a large soft-tissue mass anterior to the spine causing rectal displacement (Fig. 40.2A) and also may protrude posteriorly into the canal. Occasionally, calcified necrotic tumor can be seen within the mass and a thin calcific shell may develop around it (5).

Giant Cell Tumor

A giant cell tumor is a borderline malignant bone tumor of osteoclast-like giant cells and histiocytic cells in a well-vascularized stroma (15). Spinal giant cell tumors tend to occur earlier in life than giant cell tumors elsewhere with a peak incidence in the 2nd and 3rd decades. There also appears to be a strong (2:1) female predominance in giant cell tumors of the spine (7). Like chordomas, spinal giant cell tumors often grow quite large before back and root pain or neurological deficit focuses medical attention on the tumor (16). Tumor recurrence after radiation or surgical treatment approaches 50% for sacral lesions (8, 17–19). However, recurrence is less likely (20%) in the thoracic and lumbar vertebrae where the prognosis appears more favorable than for giant cell tumors in other parts of the skeleton (7, 20, 21).

Approximately 8% of giant cell tumors are thought to be malignant when first diagnosed but up to about 30% eventually undergo malignant transformation (22, 23). The great majority of tumors which become malignant have a history of radiation therapy (4, 6). Hence, although some giant cell tumors are radiosensitive, surgical resection is

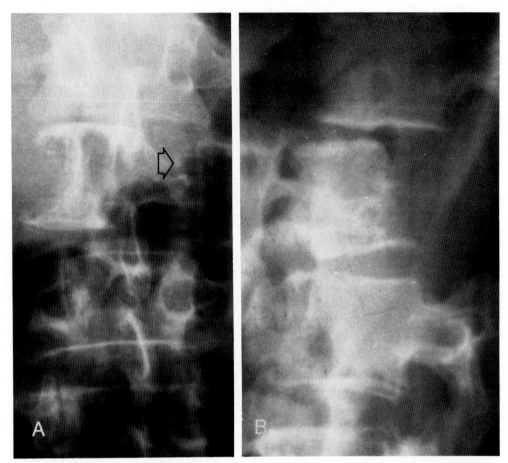

Figure 40.1. A and B. Multiple myeloma presenting in the vertebral body as a discrete, highly lytic lesion with little reactive bone. In contrast with metastastic adenocarcinoma, there is still preservation of a faint pedicle outline (*arrow*) despite significant destruction of the posterolateral vertebral body.

preferable. If complete resection cannot be accomplished, supplemental radiation warrents consideration.

Spinal giant cell tumors mostly occur in the sacrum (17, 18, 20, 24) making it the second most common sacral tumor (8). The osteolytic giant cell tumor arises within the vertebral body, occasionally involving the pedicle or transverse process (7). It produces a cyst-like initial lesion with eventual cortical expansion (Fig. 40.3A and B) followed by vertebral body collapse or disappearance. The tumor frequently extends out of the vertebral body to form a large paravertebral soft-tissue mass (Fig. 40.3A). Unfortunately, the radiographic appearance provides no help in differentiating between the benign and malignant varieties of this most unpredictable of spinal column tumors (5).

Osteoid Osteoma

Osteoid osteoma is a benign, self-limiting tumor of bone in which a small (<5 mm), central, well-vascularized nidus is surrounded by reactive bone. This condition usually occurs under the age of 30 with a 2:1 male predilection (4). It presents with backache, sometimes associated with scoliosis (25). As with other locations, the constant pain from osteoid osteoma of the spine is relieved with aspirin. The tumor neither causes neural compression nor jeopardizes spine stability. However, because of persisting pain and the unpredictable timing of possible spontaneous regression, most patients require surgical resection. Surgery should be performed under radiographic control to verify removal of the nidus. Pain is alleviated with removal of the nidus; however, with removal of most sclerotic bone, but without the nidus, pain resolves in only 50% of cases (26).

Spinal osteoid osteoma characteristically occurs in the posterior arch. It centers about the facet, often involving the adjacent pedicle or lamina (9, 27). Osteoid osteoma seems to evoke less reactive bone in the spine than in the extremities (5, 9). Accordingly, tomograms, CT, or a Technetium Pyrophosphate scan may be needed to localize the lesion if plain films are negative.

Aneurysmal Bone Cyst

An aneurysmal bone cyst is a benign, but expanding, bone cyst containing blood-filled spaces and osteoclastic

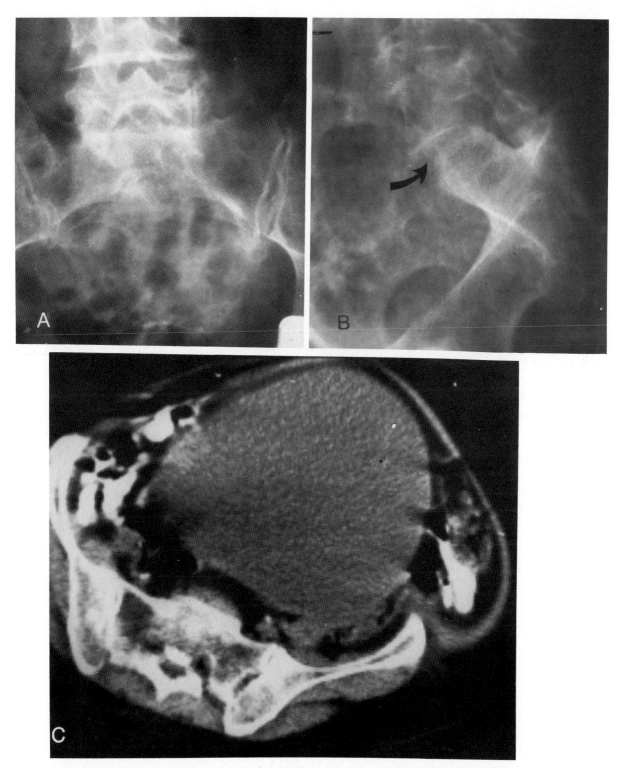

Figure 40.2. A and B. Chordoma of the sacrum: Dull low back pain and intermittent incontinence prompted lumbosacral radiographs in this 77-year-old white female. Only subtle changes in sacral architecture were observed. Note, however, the L5-S1 disc space involvement suggestive of chordoma (*arrow*). C. CT demonstrated a massive presacral soft-tissue extension of the chordoma which could not be appreciated on the plain radiographs (A and B). Oral contrast administered before CT helped identify the position of the bowel.

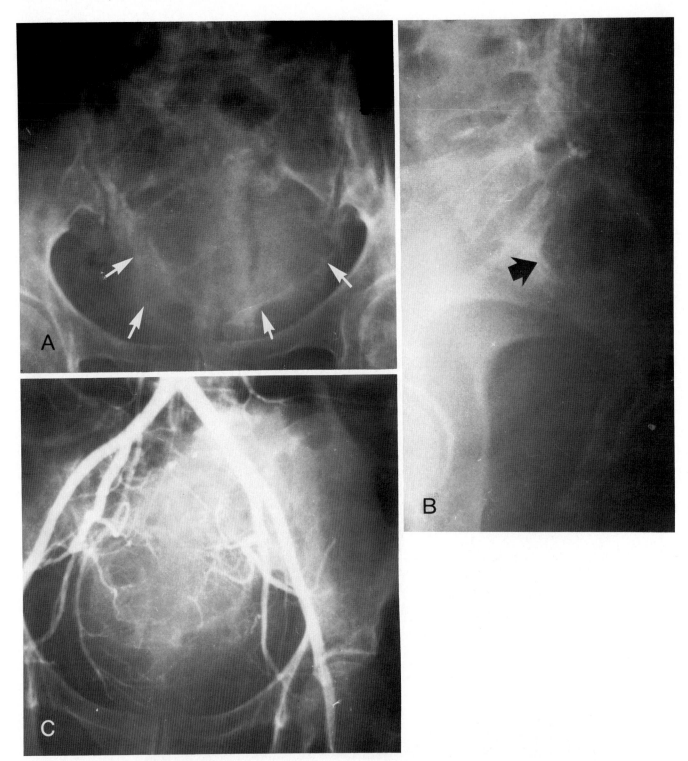

Figure 40.3.   A and B. Sacral giant cell tumor: Unexplained severe low back pain and progressive lower extremity weakness after treatment for a failed fusion prompted repeat radiographs for this 60-yr-old white female. A characteristic lytic lesion (*arrow*) within the body of the sacrum is seen on the sagittal film (B). The anterior projection (A) demonstrates considerable cortical expansion (*arrows*) with distortion of the sacral shape. C. Both the angiogram and CT demonstrated a large soft-tissue mass anterior to the sacrum. C shows the typical round and well-defined shape and vascularity of the giant cell tumor mass.

giant cells. The lesion usually affects patients under age 30. Up to 20% of aneurysmal bone cysts may develop in association with such pre-existing lesions as giant cell tumors, hemangiomas, or sarcomas, but the great majority are independent lesions (6). This radiolucent cyst may grow rapidly causing vertebral cortical margins to balloon out. Neurological deficit often develops from compression of the expanding cyst wall or from pathological fracture of the vertebrae. Surgical resection successfully eliminates the lesion and curettage with grafting has only a 16% recurrence rate (28). The aneurysmal bone cyst is also very radiosensitive and can be obliterated with as little as 2000–3000 rads (9). However, there have been several reports of sarcomatous change after radiation (6, 24). Accordingly, radiation should be reserved for those rare spinal cysts so large and/or inaccessible that the expected blood loss from curettage or resection would represent undue risk for the patient.

Fortunately, aneurysmal bone cysts arise within the posterior spinal elements (5, 29). Aside from the difference in location, they have a similar radiographic appearance to the giant cell tumor. Typically, aneurysmal cysts are osteolytic with a soap-bubble appearance from trabeculae crossing the cyst and a thin, sclerotic margin.

Chondrosarcoma

A chondrosarcoma is a malignant tumor in which cartilage is formed by a sarcomatous stroma. Although only a small proportion of chondrosarcomas begin in the spine, this tumor still represents one of the 10 most common tumor-like lesions to present in the spine (8). It typically affects patients in the middle years of life. The more differentiated grades of chondrosarcoma grow slowly but eventually will metastasize. They are only mildly radiosensitive; incomplete surgical resection is notorious for tumor "seeding" within the wound and local recurrence. Hence, early en bloc resection with a good margin of normal tissue is the only effective treatment. With various forms of surgical treatment, average 5-year survival for axial chondrosarcoma ranges between 4% and 15%, depending on the tumor grade (30). Supplemental chemotherapy and earlier, more extensive surgery may extend survival times further.

Spinal chondrosarcoma usually develops within a vertebral body. The tumor is osteolytic but central portions may show almost diagnostic "punctate calcifications" (Fig. 40.7). The more differentiated lesions often have well-defined margins (Fig. 40.6A) and can appear quite benign. Chondrosarcomas are confused easily with the chordoma; however, the disc space usually is affected by chordoma (Fig. 40.2B) but preserved in chondrosarcoma (5).

Hemangioma

An hemangioma is a benign tumor of proliferating capillaries or blood vessels. The spine, especially the thoracolumbar junction, is the most common site for hemangiomas. Their incidence increases with age (4). At autopsy, 10% of spines will evidence small and asymptomatic hemangiomas (1). At times, the hemangioma extends through the vertebral cortex to grow within the spinal canal causing direct cord compression. Spinal hemangiomas can be asymptomatic until the expanding lesion causes neurological deficit or vertebral body collapse. Treatment is symptomatic. Malignant transformation is rare, although hemangioendothelial sarcoma of bone has been reported years after radiation therapy for benign hemangiomas (10).

Most hemangiomas occur within the vertebral body where capillaries and sinusoids replace cancellous bone. The remaining trabeculae thicken to produce exaggerated, parallel vertical striations crossing the radiolucent hemangioma on x-ray. The vertical striations are not diagnostic, however, because they also may be seen with myeloma, lymphoma, and some cases of metastatic carcinoma (5). Like metastatic carcinoma, the pedicle outline may become distorted. However, unlike carcinoma, the vertebral body is not completely destroyed and a thin rim of bone surrounding the hemangioma is often apparent until vertebral collapse (4) (Fig. 40.4).

Osteochondroma

An osteochondroma is a benign and well-defined bony protrusion formed by an aberrant growth plate cartilage cap (31). Spinal osteochondromas may represent solitary lesions or may be a manifestation of hereditary multiple osteochondromatosis. Because osteochondromas arise from aberrent foci of epiphyseal plate cartilage, their development is related to skeletal growth in general; they typically become symptomatic during adolescence but stop growing at skeletal maturity. Osteochondromas arise adjacent to secondary ossification centers. Hence, they usually emanate from the posterior spinal arch (4), particularly about the pedicles (32).

Most osteochondromas are asymptomatic and require no treatment. However, there are three exceptions: 1) occasionally osteochondromas grow into the spinal canal causing cord compression and paraparesis (32–34), 2) posterior arch lesions sometimes cause angulation of the spine (4), and 3) rarely, malignant transformations of the cartilage cap occurs, signaled by resumed growth of the exostosis after skeletal maturity. Osteochondromas have a characteristic radiographic picture with continuity between the tumor's cortex and trabeculae and those of the underlying bone. However, osteochondromas projecting into the canal or foramina may be difficult to delineate unless CT is used (32).

Eosinophilic Granuloma

An eosinophilic granuloma is a benign and self-limiting lesion composed of eosinophils and histiocytes. Eosinophilic granuloma occurs in children and young adults as a solitary bone lesion or in a disseminated form. Both forms present with constant localized pain (9). The osteolytic lesions tend to spontaneously regress, often within months. If treatment is required, either curettage or low-dose radiation under 600 rads are both said to be curative. Chemotherapy may be helpful in the multifocal form of eosinophilic granuloma (4).

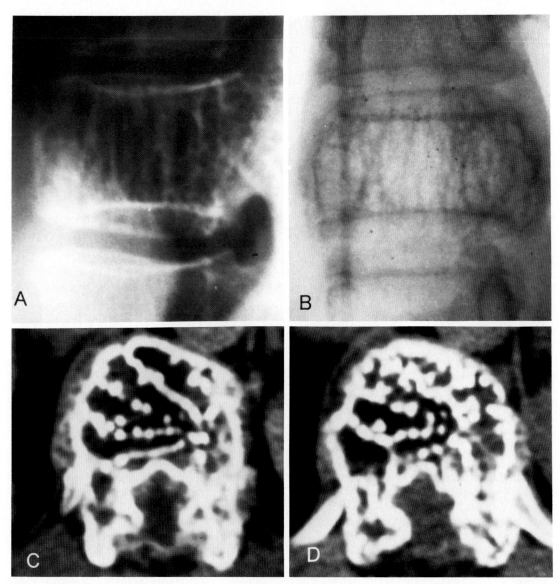

Figure 40.4. A and B. Hemangioma. This 52-year-old white female presented with L-1 radicular pain. Radiographs A and B demonstrate the classic striated appearance of a hemangioma in its characteristic thoracolumbar location. Despite involvement of both anterior and posterior elements, the cortex remains intact and a pedicle outline is still vaguely apparent. C and D. The enlarged and confluent remaining trabeculae, separated by sinusoids, are responsible for the vertical striations seen on the plain films and the "constellation of stars" appearance on CT. The expansion of the pedicle and body cortex seen on CT explain the patient's radicular symptoms. E. Selective arteriography was used to determine the hemangioma's vascular pattern before embolization and surgical resection. Arteriography showed a well-collateralized supply and confluent sinusoids involving the body and pedicle.

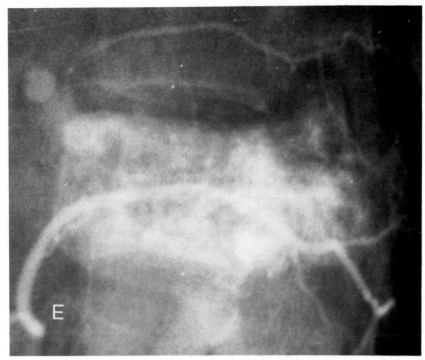

Figure 40.4.   E.

Radiographically, the granuloma causes oval, osteolytic, punched-out bony defects without peripheral sclerosis. The ovoid lesions may be superimposed in a vertebral body to produce the "hole-within-a-hole" sign (35). As the vertebral body granulomas grow and coalesce, vertebral collapse occurs to produce wedging or the characteristic "vertebral plana" (flattened vertebral body) in children. Spontaneous or treatment-induced healing is signaled by the appearance of sclerotic margins which become ill-defined as the granuloma ossifies.

Osteoblastoma

An osteoblastoma is a benign but progressively enlarging and locally aggressive lesion histologically similar to the nidus of an osteoid osteoma. The tumor affects patients under age 30 with a 2:1 male predominance (4) and arises most often in the spine. The tumor exceeds 2 cm in diameter and expands the vertebral cortex, eventually breaking through to form a soft-tissue mass. Cord or root compression occurs in 26% of spinal cases (36). Osteoblastoma contains a highly vascular stroma which can complicate surgical removal. Probably due, in part, to occasional incomplete removal, osteoblastoma recurrence approximates 10–20% overall, but is certainly higher in the spine (4, 37). Rather large radiation doses are required for reliable cure (4, 9). Accordingly, optimal treatment may be complete removal of the tumor and use of supplemental radiation if excision of large or recurrent spinal tumors is incomplete.

Osteoblastoma usually occurs in the posterior elements, and may involve the spinous or transverse processes. Radiographically, the tumor can mimic an aneurysmal bone cyst (36). It presents as a well-defined, radiolucent expansile lesion, often with a thin sclerotic rim (38). However, unlike the aneurysmal cyst, the lytic area often contains granular or mottled opacities representing spotty calcification of osteoid matrix (4).

Sarcomas

The next four most common tumor-like lesions to occur in the spine are all sarcomas. Reticulum cell and most, but not all, Ewing's sarcomas are highly osteolytic and tend to form paraspinous soft-tissue masses (5) (Fig. 40.8C). However, Ewing's occurs mostly in children and reticulum cell sarcoma usually develops beyond childhood. Osteosarcoma of the spine is rare and generally associated with either Paget's disease or after radiation of other lesions (4).

Spinal Canal Tumors

Neurofibromas, meningiomas, and gliomas account for the great majority of tumors arising within the spinal canal.

NEUROFIBROMAS

These are benign tumors of the nerve root. They typically arise within the vertebral foramen and may protrude both inside and/or outside the canal to form a dumbbell shape. They produce a marked increase in spinal fluid protein (3). Radiographically, neurofibroma cause widening of the affected nerve root foramen.

MENINGIOMAS

These are benign, fibrous tumors arising from the arachnoidal meninges. They are found most often in the cervical spine (81%) (39) and tend to occur in middle-aged women (3). These tumors are visualized best by myelogram and by CT scan where fine calcification within the tumor can be detected (40). Once delineated they usually can be resected successfully with significant neurological recovery.

GLIOMAS

These are malignant intramedullary spinal cord tumors, most often occurring within the cervical cord. They arise from either astrocytes or the ependymal cells which line the ventricular system. These intramedullary tumors grow insidiously until producing neurological deficits. Radiographs may show narrowing of pedicles or neural canal cortical thinning. The myelogram will demonstrate fusiform swelling of the spinal cord shadow and eventually complete myelographic block. Significant neurological recovery can follow meticulous tumor resection before the establishment of complete paraplegia. After tumor excision, radiation often is recommended to depress recurrent central nervous system metastases (3).

Metastatic Tumors

Metastatic lesions afflict the spine far more often than primary tumors. Unlike most primary tumors, the therapeutic goal is palliative and supportive rather than curative. To this end, radiation therapy will halt progression and relieve pain for most carcinomatous spine metastases. Bracing also may be needed to help prevent vertebral collapse.

Typically, spine metastases locate in the vertebral bodies and are osteolytic. As the tumor expands through the vertebral cortex, cord or root compression occurs with resulting neurological deficit. If the cord or roots are decompressed, some degree of neurological recovery occurs unless complete paralysis has been present for over 48 hours. Maximal decompression requires surgery (41) although limited decompression sometimes can be achieved with radiation. One important, but sometimes overlooked, goal in decompression is to correct kyphotic angulation. Motor deficit usually is due to pressure against the anterior cord by tumor. However, this pressure is compounded by kyphosis secondary to vertebral collapse because the cord then is tethered over and forced against the anterior lesion. Hence, more important than posterior laminectomy is the elimination of anterior angulation and subsequent stabilization of the diseased portion of the spine in an anatomical, or preferably slightly hyperlordotic posture. With improved posterior fixation techniques and radiation, the morbidity of more extensive anterior surgery can be avoided in most cases.

Metastatic spinal tumors produce a wide array of radiographic patterns. Carcinomas typically locate in vertebral bodies and often cause resorption of the base of the pedicles. This produces the missing pedicle sign on an anteroposterior (AP) radiograph which suggests metastatic disease (Fig. 40.5). Breast metastases are lytic and usually cause extensive lesions. Kidney and thyroid metastases

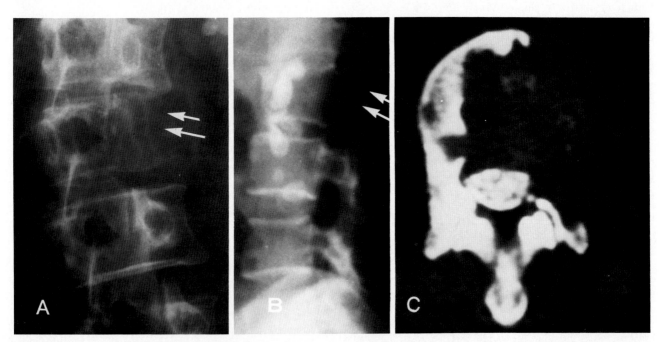

Figure 40.5. A, B, and C. Metastatic renal cell carcinoma: This 46-year-old Oriental female sought treatment for progressive myelopathy. CT localized the center of the osteolytic lesion at the pedicle-body junction, explaining the "absent-pedicle-sign" (*arrows*) characteristic of metastatic carcinoma. Metrizamide was placed intrathecally before CT and shows mild anterior and lateral compromise of the subarachnoid sac. Because of progressive spinal instability and radiculopathy, the patient was treated with spinal rod-sleeve reduction and stabilization followed by a second-stage vertebral body resection/reconstruction. The neurological deficit resolved and the patient returned to ambulatory status. (Case courtesy of Dr. A. Levine).

are lytic but tend to be solitary; however, they often will extend past the vertebral cortex to produce a soft-tissue mass. Lung carcinoma and Hodgkins granuloma are primarily lytic but sometimes incite bone formation. Prostatic carcinoma and often tumors from the gastrointestinal tract evoke an osteoblastic response; occasionally, these tumors elevate the vertebral periosteum, giving rise to a "sunburst pattern" (5).

THE DIAGNOSIS OF SPINAL TUMORS

Tumor Localization with CT

The central location and architectural complexity of the spine make the early diagnosis of spinal column lesions far more difficult than most other skeletal locations. The central location and numerous interacting segments also mute the accuracy of clinical signs and symptoms. The spatial complexity of the bony structures and the amount of soft tissue surrounding the spine strain the capabilities of standard radiography. Hence, the early diagnosis of spinal lesions must often rest heavily on special imaging techniques and early biopsy.

The first spine tumor symptom is either localized pain or neurological deficit. Unlike most causes of back pain, tumor pain begins as a constant dull pain not alleviated by bedrest. There may be local tenderness, but the straight leg raising test is usually negative (9). The pain often becomes severe after pathological fracture or rapid tumor growth. Likewise, initial neurological symptoms from cord compression may be subtle with gradual impairment of balance, premature tiring of the legs when walking, and/or occasional urinary incontinence (3).

If spine pain persists without explanation in the face of negative radiographs, a Technetium Pyrophosphate bone scan should be considered. The scan will identify areas where there is increased bone turnover and blood flow well in advance of sufficient bone destruction or formation for radiographic detection. Subsequent conventional tomography, focused on the area of abnormal Technetium-Pyrophosphate uptake often will reveal the lesion. Axial polytomography also may be useful for early lesion identification. However, we have not achieved sufficient resolution with our unit (General Electric model 8800) to employ this technique for early tumor detection routinely.

For patients with reproducible neurological signs, conventional myelography serves to localize the lesion and characterize it to some extent. For example, extradural lesions deviate the cord shadow and produce a "paint brush" pattern where the contrast column thins adjacent to the tumor (3). Neurofibromas and meningiomas usually project into the contrast column causing distinct lobulations. Intramedullary gliomas produce fusiform widening of the cord shadow.

There are some areas of the spine and certain clinical circumstances where standard radiography, tomography, and/or myelography are known to be frequently inadequate and misleading. Detailed visualization of the sacral and lower lumbar vertebrae are obscured by the ilea on the lateral projection and bowel gas or fecal matter on the AP. A similar problem exists near the craniocervical junction where the dense bony processes about the base of the skull can overshadow early lesions (42). Identification of small lesions also can be complicated by pre-existing osteosclerotic conditions that obscure new adjacent lesions, such as Pagets disease (43, 44), spinal stenosis (42), and bone fusions.

Failure to recognize the limitations of standard radiographic techniques in these areas and circumstances often has significant consequences. For example, in both the literature and the author's experience, sacral tumors are missed on initial radiographs in about one-half of all cases (Fig. 40.2) (8, 40, 45). Chordomas and giant cell tumors account for over half of all sacral tumors. They both tend to form presacral soft-tissue masses before symptoms become pronounced (Figs. 40.2, 40.3, 40.16). These soft-tissue masses, surrounded by the bony pelvis and viscera, often escape radiographic detection. Unless diagnosed early enough to permit complete resection, chordomas have a fatal outcome and sacral giant cell tumors, in particular, are prone to recurrences and malignant transformation (17, 23, 44, 46).

A negative myelogram can be equally misleading in the search for early spinal tumors. Neurofibromas appear to be one of the most likely spine tumors to escape detection—particularly if located near the upper end of the spine or where there is already bony pathology (42). In these cases, subtle signs of foraminal or pedicle deformity are not seen on plain radiographs and they often are missed on myelography until the tumor is large enough to protrude into the contrast column (42, 47). Likewise, sacral tumors often escape myelographic detection if they are located below the variable termination of the caudal sac or if there is pronounced tapering of the lower dural sac (45). Unnecessary laminectomy for presumed disc disease is another consequence of failure to appreciate the major limitation of plain radiographs or myelography in detecting lumbosacral spine tumors (44, 45).

Accordingly, in sacral or craniocervical locations and in cases with pre-existing spinal disease, it seems reasonable to employ CT early, perhaps before tomography or standard myelography, if radiographs fail to delineate a suspected lesion. CT offers two important advantages in identifying early spinal tumors: the axial projection and the ability to represent subtle differences in soft-tissue density. The ability to visualize the spine in axial cross-section clarifies such potentially difficult radiological diagnoses as early chondrosarcoma in an arthritic or upper thoracic spine (Fig. 40.6A) or osteochondroma projecting into the spinal canal (43, 34). The axial view separates the anterior, posterior, or lateral bony structures and local pathology from the areas or lesion under study.

Secondly, CT is able to discern much smaller gradations in tissue density than standard tomography by recording 100-fold smaller differences in the attenuation of x-ray beams than conventional x-ray (48). Accordingly, CT can demonstrate presacral masses associated with giant cell tumors and chordomas nicely (Fig. 40.2C); it also shows derangements in pelvic visceral anatomy which may suggest more subtle prespinal lesions (44). CT is now more reliable than other imaging techniques for diagnosing most primary and metastatic sacral tumors (44, 45) and high-resolution scanners are at least comparable for detecting meningiomas (40, 42) and perhaps neurofibromas (47).

In order to enhance the accuracy of CT in diagnosing spinal canal lesions, many have advocated CT in conjunction with metrizamide myelography (49–51). For this technique, metrizamide is moved to the level of the lesion under fluoroscopic control and CT is performed immediately (50) (Fig. 40.6B). Until recently, CT equipment did not have sufficient soft-tissue resolution to discern non-calcified lesions reliably within the spinal canal. For example, Nakagawa reported that using a 1975 scanner with 8- to 13-mm slices, 8 of 19 intraspinal tumors were not seen clearly with CT alone (40). Certainly, if the available scanner cannot delineate normal canal soft-tissue structure clearly, metrizamide should be employed if tumors within the canal are suspected. Metrizamide with sequential CT scanning may be especially useful if syringomyelia is in question. The metrizamide naturally refluxes to the 4th ventricle and can be seen within a connected spinal cord syrinx if a sequential CT is performed between 6 and 24 hours after injection (50).

With current and certainly future high-resolution scanners and soft-tissue enhancement techniques, it may be possible to achieve comparable accuracy detecting canal lesions without the use of metrizamide. This would have the diagnostic advantage of eliminating any chance that excess contrast could obscure a small lesion (52) and would obviate the need for intrathecal injection and repeated sequential scans. Several authors already have collected sufficient cases to state that high-resolution CT can supplant the need for myelography in nearly all spinal cases (32, 53) and cite diagnostic accuracy rates as high as 98% in detecting herniated discs (53).

Tumor Characterization with CT

Once a spinal tumor is discovered, CT can play a key role in characterizing the gross pathology. Its great advantage over other imaging techniques is the ability to display bone and soft-tissue architecture simultaneously and represent small gradations in tissue density. Hence, CT can be particularly helpful in diagnosing bone tumors which break through the vertebral cortex to form a paraspinous soft-tissue mass. Among more common spine tumors these include the giant cell tumor (Fig. 40.3C and 40.16), chordoma (Fig. 40.2C), osteoblastoma, reticulum cell sarcoma (Fig. 40.8), and Ewing's sarcoma (54), occasionally multiple myeloma (Fig. 40.1), and rarely hemangiomas (5). CT has largely replaced the need for arteriography to delineate these soft-tissue tumor extensions.

CT also surpasses plain or tomographic radiography in its ability to detect fine calcifications (40, 55). Calcifications are present in chondrosarcomas (Figs. 40.6A, 40.7), most meningiomas (40), osteoblastomas (5), and the soft-

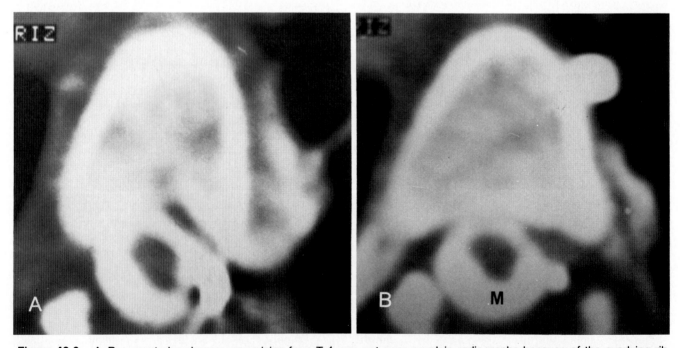

Figure 40.6. A. Recurrent chondrosarcoma arising from T-4 was not seen on plain radiographs because of the overlying rib cage. On CT, the mottled pattern suggestive of chondroid calcification is seen both within and adjacent to the vertebral body. B. Metrizamide (M) surrounding the spinal cord demonstrated canal encroachment to explain the patient's mild but progressive myelopathy.

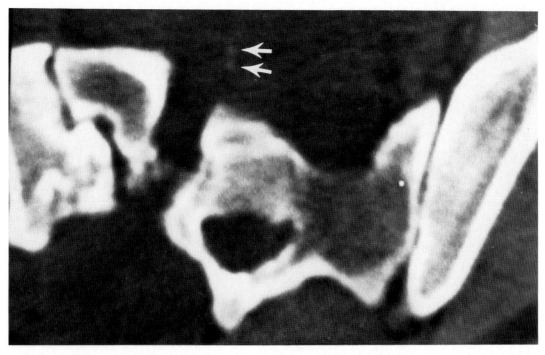

Figure 40.7. Sacral chondrosarcoma: CT of the upper sacrum demonstrates a typical pattern of focal lytic bone destruction and punctate calcifications (*arrows*) within the presacral tumor mass.

tissue extensions of some chordomas (4). The thin bony rim surrounding an expanded aneurysmal bone cyst also is easier to see on CT than with plain films (5).

A third advantage of CT is the ability to exaggerate contrasting densities; this feature provides a diagnostic advantage in lesions forming cystic cavities such as syringomyelia, aneurysmal bone cyst or the giant cell tumor (Fig. 40.9A and B). It facilitates finding the nidus in osteoid osteoma (6, 56). The reduced density of a lipoma also makes this lesion easier to spot on CT (40). The radiographic density patterns of other common spinal tumors were outlined in the second section of this chapter.

As mentioned earlier, a fourth advantage of CT is the axial projection. This makes it possible to characterize the bony pattern of small tumors projecting within the canal or foramina. One example is the osteochondroma. With overlying bony shadows out of the way, it projects as a sharply outlined rounded mass of bone with adjacent scattered calcifications (32). Another example is the neurofibroma. Nerve root foramina are not always seen clearly in thoracic and lumbar spine x-rays. By eliminating overlapping bony shadows, the CT axial projection can demonstrate subtle erosion of foramina and pedicles. In addition, with high-resolution scanners, soft tissues within the spinal canal often can be differentiated. With these findings, the often-missed paraspinous neurofibroma portion of a dumbbell neurofibroma often can be seen projecting from the neural foramina (40).

The combination of clinical factors, radiographic ap-

pearance, and laboratory studies may be sufficient to confirm the diagnosis of myeloma, osteoid osteoma, osteochondroma, some intradural tumors, metastatic disease, and occasionally other tumors. However, final diagnosis for other common spinal tumors usually requires biopsy. Because the course of treatment will vary considerably among these different tumors and tumor-like conditions, the importance of this procedure cannot be overemphasized. Open midline biopsies, usually excisional biopsies, are most effective for posterior arch or sacral lesions. Vertebral body lesions in the cervical spine are approached best openly through the interval just medial to the carotid sheath (57). The costotransversectomy approach will lead the surgeon to most anterior lesions in the upper thoracic spine. The lower thoracic and lumbar vertebral bodies are accessible to Craig needle biopsy. We, as many others, have found this to be a safe and productive procedure for lesions contained within the vertebra. The biopsy is done with the patient prone on a radiolucent table under image intensification. The author prefers local anesthesia with sedation, but general anesthesia can be used. The technique is well outlined in Craig's original article (58). After correct position of the trochar is achieved, one or more core biopsies are taken until a good specimen of abnormal tissue is obtained. After biopsy of very vascular lesions, gelfoam or Avitine can be pushed into the biopsy hole before removing the Craig cannula. Using this technique, adequate biopsy material can be obtained in over 90% of cases.

RESECTION OF SPINAL TUMORS

Indications for Surgical Treatment

Various combinations of curettage, radiation, chemotherapy, and complete resection are advocated for tumors commonly affecting the spine. Either thorough curettage or local removal is adequate treatment for osteoid osteoma, aneurysmal bone cyst, hemangioma, or osteochondroma. For each of these conditions, recurrence rates are low and rarely associated with malignant transformation.

Other tumors are responsive to radiation and chemotherapy and seem to do as well (or poorly) after these treatments as they do after surgical resection. This group includes eosinophilic granuloma and the marrow-origin tumors: multiple myeloma, Ewing's, and reticulum cell sarcomas. Solitary eosinophilic granulomas in the spine can be halted routinely if not eliminated by low-dose radiation. Solitary lesions of multiple myeloma likewise are arrested by radiation, although the disease almost always progresses elsewhere. However, due to the diffuse nature of myeloma, there is no reason to expect that radical resection of a spine lesion would deter progression of the disease unless the lesion was very early, well-contained, and all other studies including distant marrow aspirations and bone scanning were still negative. Most reports suggest that Ewing's, reticulum cell, and lymphosarcoma respond as well to combined radiation and chemotherapy alone as when surgical resection is added (59). However, if an early and well-defined lesion could be removed completely, preceded by chemotherapy for shrinkage, and followed by radiation therapy (60), it seems reasonable that the chance of survival might be enhanced. For these marrow tumors, the surgeon must weigh the often considerable risks associated with complete resection of each spinal tumor against the speculation of improved survival (Fig. 40.8).

Whereas radiation therapy may be the most efficacious treatment for most marrow-origin tumors in the spine, its risk/benefit ratio of radiation therapy should be weighed carefully before using it in other spine tumors. Like major surgery, full-dose radiation of the spine is sometimes associated with major complications. These include possible fibrosis of subcutaneous skin and muscle which complicates subsequent surgical wounds (60), sarcomatous transformation of benign lesions, aggravation of cord compression by postradiation edema, and spinal cord radionecrosis with permanent deficit (61, 62).

There is good evidence that complete surgical resection is the treatment of choice for the primary bone tumors: chordoma (9, 12), giant cell tumor (1, 7, 17, 18, 20, 46, 63, 64), chondrosarcoma (9, 30), osteoblastoma (4, 9, 37), and for the most common intradural tumors including neurofibromas, meningiomas, and gliomas, as well (3). If surgery fails to remove these tumors completely, supplemental radiation is probably indicated (65).

Although chordoma carries a 96% chance of eventual fatality despite radiation and surgical treatment (4), this is usually from local compression and invasion because only 10% of chordomas metastasize (9). Moreover, they typically grow slowly and metastasize late. Hence, the tumor should be an ideal candidate for early and complete resection (Fig. 40.14).

Giant cell tumors above the sacrum may do well with currettage, incomplete resection, and/or radiation although up to a 20% recurrence rate is reported (2, 7, 20). In the sacrum, the tumor is probably more advanced when discovered and these treatments lead to a 50% recurrence rate with occasional fatalities (8, 17–19). In general, at least 10–15% of giant cell tumors become malignant, often after irradiation (7, 20). Like the chordoma, giant cell tumors grow slowly and metastasize late (17, 18, 66, 67). Hence, early complete resection probably represents the treatment of choice for giant cell tumors of the spine (63, 64) (Figs. 40.9 and 40.16). Cryotherapy, using freezing from liquid nitrogen to kill peripheral tumor cells, has been used in the spine (6), but is usually logistically impractical.

Chondrosarcoma is not very responsive to radiation and is notorious for local seeding and recurrence after incomplete resection. Treatment of this tumor should, therefore, consist of en block resection through normal tissue planes and encompassing the initial biopsy site (Fig. 40.17).

As discussed earlier, osteoblastomas are benign but over 20% of spinal osteoblastomas recur if excision is not complete (4, 9, 37). Because most osteoblastomas arise in the posterior elements, complete removal should be a practical goal in most cases.

Radical resection of metastatic lesions in the spine is unwarranted, save perhaps a solitary hypernephroma metastasis, because radiation therapy—occasionally supplemented with stabilization procedures—provides satisfactory palliation in most cases without neurological deficit (65). However, resection may be indicated in cases with associated incomplete neurological deficit. Some surgeons prefer initially approaching vertebral body lesions directly in order to relieve tumor and bone cord compression and then stabilize anteriorly (41). This reduces tumor bulk which is said to make subsequent radiation therapy more effective (41, 68). We have had less morbidity with initial restoration of spinal lordosis and rigid posterior fixation combined occasionally with laminectomy followed by radiation therapy. If sufficient resolution of the deficit does not occur, we then proceed anteriorly to remove the tumor. This sequence has not been associated with the subsequent failure of fixation we have occasionally seen with anterior corporectomy and grafting alone.

The Limits of Resectability

As discussed above, complete resection of such tumors as chordoma, chondrosarcoma, and malignant giant cell tumor, is considered best for the patient, but generally has been dismissed as surgically "impossible or unfeasible" (4, 7–9, 20, 69). This is because these tumors tend to occur in such inaccessible locations as the anterior sacrum or vertebral bodies and proceed to form soft-tissue extensions encasing the spine. Hence, conventional surgical approaches usually fail to effect complete tumor removal,

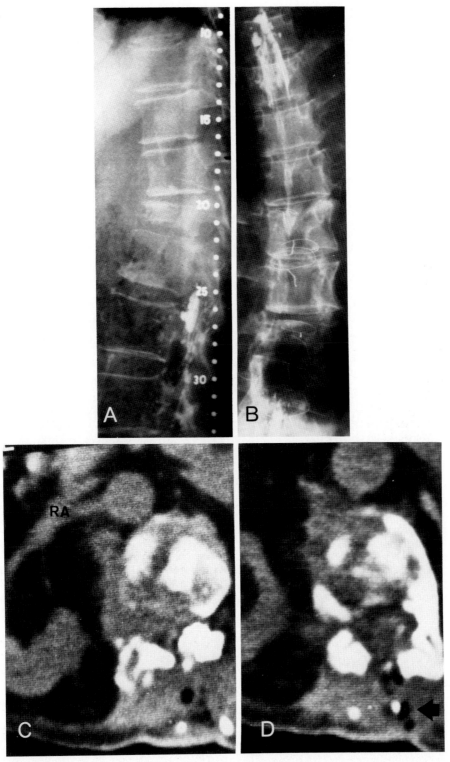

Figure 40.8. A and B. Inoperable reticulum cell sarcoma: This 40-year-old Iranian male was referred for possible spine resection due to progression of tumor size and paralysis despite laminectomy, chemotherapy, and radiation treatments. In addition to T-12 collapse, there is lysis of L-1 and L-2 and complete blockage of myelographic contrast introduced from both above and below the lesion to determine the limits of tumor extension in the spinal canal. C and D. CT of L1-L2 shows diffuse extension of the tumor around the aorta and renal artery (RA) not visible on the plain films. In addition, there is a large posterior sinus tract emanating from a previous laminectomy (*arrow*). The extent of tumor infiltration precluded tumor-free margins and the residual deep infection jeopardized subsequent reconstruction; we did not recommend resection.

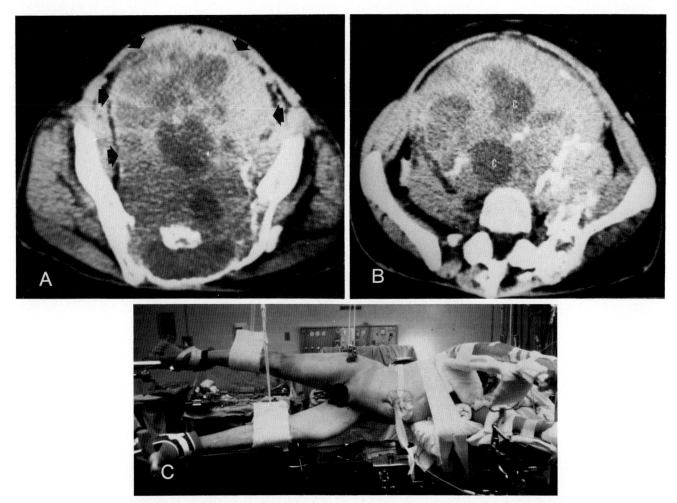

Figure 40.9.   A. Terminal spine resection: This massive giant cell tumor from the sacrum had already necessitated ureteroileostomy and caused paralysis of the patient's left leg. CT demonstrates considerable expansion of the posterior sacral cortex, but preservation of the spinal canal. The well-defined presacral mass fills the entire pelvis (*arrows*). B. The presacral mass extends cephalad adjacent to L-4 and L-5. Characteristic areas of cystic degeneration (C) are seen within the giant cell tumor. C and D. The lateral suspension position uses femoral external fixation and permits simultaneous anterior and posterior surgery for removal of large lumbosacral spine tumors. The sterile pan collects blood for autotransfusion. E. The buttocks are reflected distally on their vascular pedicles to permit complete resection of the sacrum and tumor mass. F. Postoperative radiograph of the patient on a Stryker frame following en bloc resection of L4-S5 together with the giant cell tumor depicted in A and B.

are fraught with major complications including the risk of fatal hemorrhage, and raise concerns over a mechanically unreconstructable spine following radical resection (8, 20, 70). Accordingly, subtotal resection with supplemental radiation has become the clinical standard by default. When these tumors recur, they, unfortunately, then are judged inoperable with fatal consequences.

Chordoma, malignant giant cell tumors, and chondrosarcoma form large paraspinous masses which eventually pull or compress adjacent structures, causing severe pain (Fig. 40.9A and B). Death usually comes slowly, not from distant metastases, but from local destruction and compression. Experience with this dismal scenerio has led isolated surgeons to a second look at the "inoperability" of these tumors. In the 1950s, MacCarty and Hays both

achieved unprecedented resection of large tumors involving the distal four sacral vertebrae (65, 71). Hemicorporectomy for large, otherwise "unresectable" tumors below L2 was described in 1966; it was a mutilating procedure but one compatible with a painless, if inconvenient, existence (13, 72).

Removal of one or more vertebral bodies to extirpate tumors was introduced for the cervical spine by Scoville (73) and extended to the lumbar spine with complete, although piecemeal removal of an entire lumbar vertebra reported by Lievre et al. in 1968 (74). Another important step was the use of staged anterior then posterior approaches to permit better anterior tumor dissection and vascular control before posterior removal. Using this approach, successful resection of tumor masses up to 10 cm

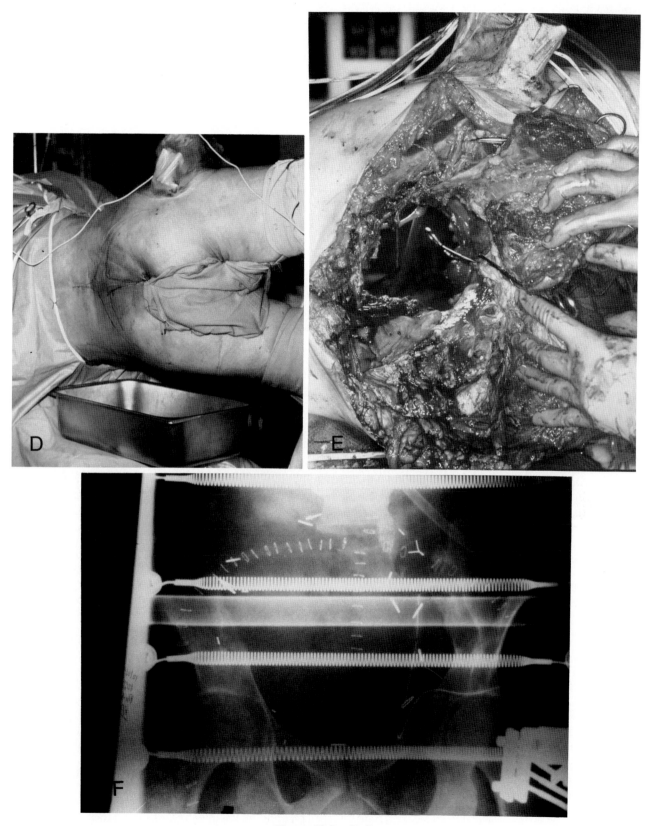

Figure 40.9. D–F.

affecting the lower sacral vertebrae was reported in 1967 by Localio (14). In 1971, Stener reported the use of a staged approach and both anterior and posterior exposure to remove the T11, T12, and L1 vertebrae in order to excise a giant cell tumor (75). Despite the failure of fixation, a cure was effected and the patient maintained the ability to function on her own. In 1979, we performed a 3½-level (T12-L3) complete resection of the spine to remove a 14-cm diameter malignant giant cell tumor (76, 77).

Despite these advances, tumors affecting the L4-S2 region remained a dilemma (8). Both biomechanical studies and clinical opinion held that removal of the entirety of S1 would not permit sufficient skeletal stability or neurological function for ambulation (78), leaving hemicorporectomy as the only alternative. In 1980, we were fortunate to effect complete removal of the entire sacrum and lower lumbar vertebrae (terminal spine resection) in several tumor cases with the use of simultaneous anterior and posterior approaches. We found that reasonable function could be preserved postoperatively, including ambulation (16, 77).

Current Resection Techniques

It now appears that large primary spine tumors in virtually any location can be resected, although the risks and complications may be considerable. If resection is judged to be in the patient's best interests, we have found the following surgical approaches and techniques of value: The key to complete resection of spinal tumors is good surgical exposure. Good access is needed for circumferential vascular control and in order to dissect the great vessels and viscera away from the tumor safely. For tumors involving the posterior arch, a long posterior midline incision is satisfactory. The most utilitarian anterior cervical approach is anterior to the sternocleidomastoid muscle proceeding just medial to the carotid sheath to the vertebral bodies. In the thoracic spine, a thoracotomy incision is extended to intersect with a midline posterior incision to achieve simultaneous anterior and posterior exposure. Although the author and others have excised thoracic vertebrae with preservation of the cord (79), incomplete or complete paraplegia is a frequent complication due to the precarious vascularity of the thoracic cord. For thoracolumbar tumors, a "T" incision also can be used with the lower leg of the T extending from the umbilicus, posteriorly across one of the lower ribs. The spine is approached retroperitoneally, detaching an edge of the diaphragm if necessary (57). From this approach, an involved paraspinous or psoas muscle can be resected with the specimen.

Lumbosacral area tumors can grow quite large before detection. Safe and complete removal of these most challenging tumors requires simultaneous anterior and posterior surgical approaches. To accomplish this, we introduced the "lateral suspension position" (77) (Fig. 40.9C). Three transfixion pins are placed through the femur at the trochanteric level and attached to an external fixation frame. The patient's torso then is suspended in the lateral

position by a rope from the external frame to either a ceiling hook or the overhead beam on a Chick-Langren table. The patient's chest is supported by the upper portion of the table and the feet are placed in traction stirrups. The area between the rib cage and midthighs then can be prepped, permitting circumferential surgical access (Fig. 40.9D).

For lumbar lesions, midline anterior and posterior incisions are used. When total sacrectomy is planned for very large tumors, the author recommends a lower abdominal "U" incision and a T posteriorly. The leg of the T is over the midline of the sacrum and the upper arms are just caudal to the iliac wings. The buttocks with overlying skin are raised off the sacrum as two flaps on their superior gluteal vascular pedicles (Fig. 40.9E). Through the abdominal incision the tumor mass is dissected anteriorly and feeding vessels are ligated. Simultaneous with the anterior surgery another team operates posteriorly. They dissect the functional portions of the spinal cord, roots, cauda equina, and the sacral plexus by removing bone posterior to these neural structures. Thereafter, the tumor and resected spine and/or sacrum can be rotated anteriorly, away from the preserved cord or roots (Fig. 40.9E and F).

For small tumors confined to the lower sacrum, a longitudinal posterior midline approach may be satisfactory (71). For large tumors, separate abdominal paramedian and posterior transverse sacral incisions should be considered (14). The lateral suspension position offers advantages in both sterility and versatility over the former practice of turning the patient from supine to prone midway during the operation.

SPINAL RECONSTRUCTION

Concerns over reconstructing a stable spine often compromise adequate tumor resection. With recent developments in the techniques of spine stabilization, virtually any portion of the spine either can be stabilized, replaced, or bypassed. Hence, resection of malignant or borderline malignant spine tumors now should be aimed at complete en bloc removal with adequate margins whenever possible. With this approach, large malignant giant cell tumors, chordomas, and chondrosarcomas and a solitary myeloma have been removed from the spine without recurrence (3, 39, 63, 75, 77, 80).

Stabilization of the spine may require either posterior fixation or anterior fixation or both, depending on the resection and previous surgery to the spine. In general, if resection of the vertebral body is not essential and the facets are intact, as in the case of most patients with metastatic disease, posterior stabilization alone will suffice. The affected spinal segments are fixed in relative lordosis so as to transmit axial loads through the facets (lateral masses) rather than the vertebral bodies. On the other hand, if the vertebral body must be resected and no posterior laminectomy has been performed, anterior reconstruction alone will suffice. However, combined anterior and posterior reconstruction is necessary in cases where both anterior and posterior bone and/or ligamentous structures have been removed or previously injured.

Reconstruction After Partial Vertebral Destruction or Resection

In the cervical spine, posterior wiring methods can achieve secure fixation and the desired amount of lordosis. For fixation following multiple-level vertebral body destruction or subluxation the author combines: a) tight interspinous wiring with b) "guy-wires" from every other facet laterally to the lowest spinous process to be fused to prevent rotation (81) and c) a flexion tension-band from the uppermost lamina to the lowermost spinous process (82). If a laminectomy has been performed, a Southwick lateral rib strut or curved metal rod (83) can be substituted for the interspinous wire portion of the fixation (81) (Fig. 40.10). The ribs or rods are wired to each facet to maintain the desired lordosis and provide rotatory fixation.

For patients with a life expectancy of more than 2 years, iliac bone grafting is added to the constructs described above to achieve lasting stability. For patients with more limited life expectancy, methyl methacrylate bone cement can be used for supplemental fixation to decrease the need for postoperative external immobilization (Fig. 40.11). However, if methacrylate is used in place of bone graft in patients with very short life expectancy, it is important to make numerous drill holes through the cortex of each segment (Fig. 40.11B) and/or to insert multiple K-wires or facet wires (Fig. 40.11B) so the cement will achieve reliable fixation at each level. It has been demonstrated clearly that simply pressing cement over lightly decorticated lamina and a single interspinous wire achieves no better fixation after several months than use of the wire alone (84–86).

After resection of a cervical vertebral body, either bone or methacrylate (73, 85, 87) reconstruction has proven satisfactory if there is close attention to technical detail. Bone should be used after removal of primary tumors and where life expectancy of 3 years or more is anticipated. A bicortical iliac graft is cut to shape and longitudinally transfixed with one or two Steinman pins. These pins fit

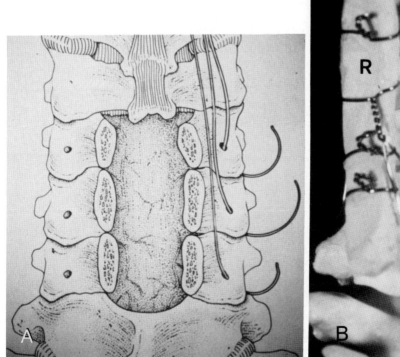
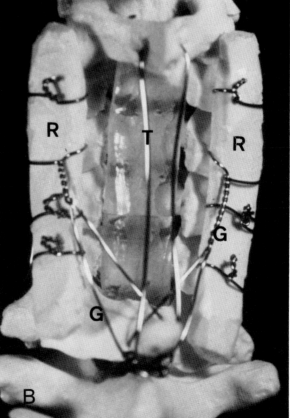

Figure 40.10.   A and B. Multiple wire cervical spine stabilization can maintain anatomical position of the neck following either extensive laminectomy or tumorous destruction of multiple vertebral bodies. a) Drill holes are placed through the inferior facets. Wire is then passed through the holes and out the facet joints. b) The facet wires are twisted around bilateral rib (R) strut grafts. Selected guy-wires (G) are extended to the distal spinous process. A posterior tension band (T) is used to counteract the flexion movement of the head.

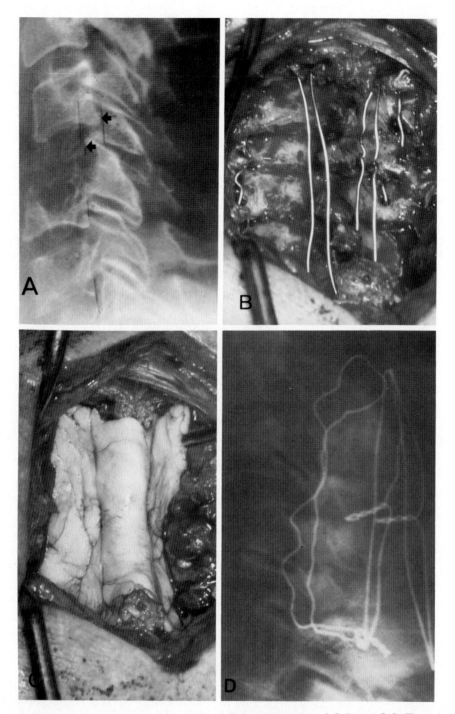

Figure 40.11.   A. Metastatic breast carcinoma obliteration of C-4 and invasion of C-5 and C-6. There is posterior subluxation of C-3 on C-4 (*arrows*). The patient had incapacitating pain and early myelopathy. B. After reducing the spine, wires were placed through the facets, multiple drill holes were made in the cortex, and a wire tension band was passed between C-2 and C-7. C. The construct described in B was encased in methyl methacrylate cement for immediate stability. D. This temporary methacrylate fusion eliminated the patient's pain and progressive myelopathy for the remaining 8 months of her life.

into holes predrilled in the normal body above and slots in the body below; the anterior slots are plugged with cement to fix the pin position (88). Alternatively, a small plate on the anterolateral spine can be used to fix the graft and the position of adjacent vertebrae (89). A similar technique using methacrylate to replace the body was first recommended by Scoville for patients with short life expectancy in order to minimize the need for postoperative immobilization and eliminate the added surgery of obtaining iliac graft (73). Anterior cement loosening and postoperative dislodgement can be reduced by embedding within the cement, wires, or other fixation devices connecting the normal bodies on either side of the defect (41, 85, 90). For removal of multiple cervical vertebral bodies, prosthetic replacements have been used successfully in China (91) and Japan (92). Japanese workers recently reported that a polyethylene prosthesis cemented in place of multiple cervical bodies is less prone to loosening than when methacrylate alone if used (93).

Because the forces traversing the thoracic and lumbar spine are much greater, different techniques are needed. In the thoraco-lumbar spine, posterior rod-sleeve fixation alone will reliably maintain reduction into relative lordosis after kyphotic angulation due to metastatic collapse of one or more vertebral bodies and/or laminectomy. Double distraction rods afixed to the spine with hooks restore vertebral height. Rod Sleeves placed over the rods push anteriorly through the pedicles to provide local lordosis and wedge between the facet masses and spinous process for rotary stability as well (94) (Fig. 40.12). After laminectomy, a pair of sleeves is placed over the first intact lamina above and below the laminectomy defect (82, 95) (Fig. 40.13). An alternative method is use of segmental wiring. In 1971, Stener reported the use of AO plates wired to thoracic transverse processes (79). A more satisfactory method is now available in which (Luque) rods are bent to conform to the desired lordosis and wired to the lamina of each segment after spine length is restored by a distraction outrigger. Spinal rod sleeves also can be placed over the Luque rods to enhance rotary stability and provide more precise control over localized lordosis. Iliac bone graft is used after either fixation method for longrange security of fixation.

After vertebral body resection in the lower thoracic or lumbar spine, the reconstruction must be able to maintain vertebral space height. Otherwise, late collapse will likely occur with the partial graft resorption that accompanies the normal creeping substitution phase of bone graft healing. This can be accomplished with posterior rod-sleeve fixation and/or anterior devices. Various acceptable anterior fixation alternatives include plates, the Dunn distraction device (96), distraction rods encased within cement (41), or custom prosthetic devices featuring axially directed screws (80) or intramedullary rods (76, 82). If there has been a previous laminectomy or ligamentous injury at the same level as the vertebral resection it is important to supplement the anterior fusion with 1-level posterior compression rod fixation. When anterior bone

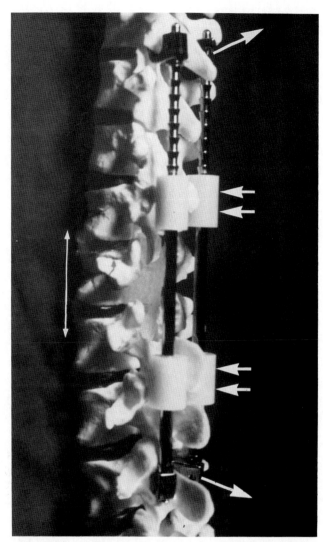

Figure 40.12. Model of the rod-sleeve construct for reconstructing the thoracic and/or lumbar spine after cancerous destruction of the vertebral bodies or laminectomy. Sleeves surrounding Harrington distraction rods are placed over the first intact posterior elements on either side of the laminectomy. They push anteriorly (*arrows*) and hold the spine in a relatively lordotic posture to unload the vertebral bodies; they wedge between the spinous process and the facets to provide rotatory stability and rigid fixation.

grafting alone is used in such cases, eventual loss of anterior fixation with pain and deformity often result (41).

Reconstruction After Complete Vertebrectomy

The reconstruction plan after complete vertebrectomy varies with the level and extent of spinal resection. In the upper and midthoracic spine, the protection of the rib cage and lack of major forces acting against the spine permit the use of conventional anterior grafting (fibular, rib, or iliac bone struts screwed or slotted into place) over several consecutive levels. In order to obtain anatomic alignment

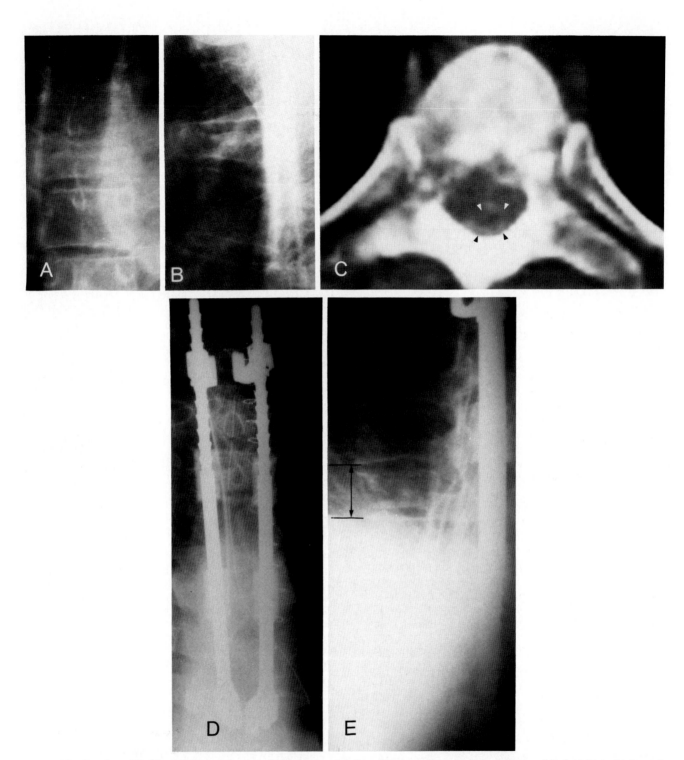

Figure 40.13. A and B. Metastatic carcinoma of unknown origin in a 52-year-old male with collapse of T-4, right radicular pain, and paraparesis. C. CT of T-4 after metrizamide myelogram shows tumor involvement of the right pedicle and vertebral body, disruption of the posterior body cortex, and tumor in the canal pressing the cord against the lamina. The cord is outlined faintly by residual metrizamide (*arrows*). D and E. Treatment consisted of laminectomy and rod-sleeve stabilization. The rod-sleeve construct provides enough stability so that no anterior fusion is needed. Note restoration of T-4 height despite over 3½ months of pre-existing vertebral collapse. The patient's pain and strength improved immediately after surgery.

initially and prevent late angulation, it is advisable to use posterior rod-fixation as well for multiple-level reconstructions (Fig. 40.14).

Reconstruction after complete vertebrectomy in the thoracolumbar or upper lumbar spine requires both secure anterior and posterior internal fixation. Although meticulously constructed interconnected bone grafts have succeeded anteriorly (63), use of bone grafts without anterior implant fixation is likely to result in late graft collapse and angulation, especially following multiple level vertebrectomies (75). Without a versatile and rigid posterior fixation system, accurate spinal alignment is difficult to achieve and maintain (75, 80) (Fig. 40.14). Accordingly, we have used a custom prosthesis anteriorly combined with double distraction rod-sleeve fixation posteriorly. This fixation method has been successful in replacing up to 3½ vertebrae (T12-L3) although length of follow-up is short (76, 77, 82). The prosthesis features retractable intra-

medullary rods which can be jacked into methacrylate-lined holes within the vertebrae above and below the defect. The prosthesis should be constructed to permit addition of a fibular strut and/or cancellous bone graft. As discussed above, the posterior rod-sleeve fixation using bridging sleeves above and below the defect; shields the anterior prosthesis from flexion and rotation moments (Fig. 40.15).

There are three situations after complete vertebral resection where spine reconstruction can be simplified greatly or even bypassed. First, shortening should be considered after 1-level lumbar vertebrectomies if the roots of the resected segment are already sacrificed or afunctional. The inferior facets of the body above the resection will articulate with those below. Reconstruction then merely requires conventional anterior and posterior grafting combined with posterior single-level compression rods.

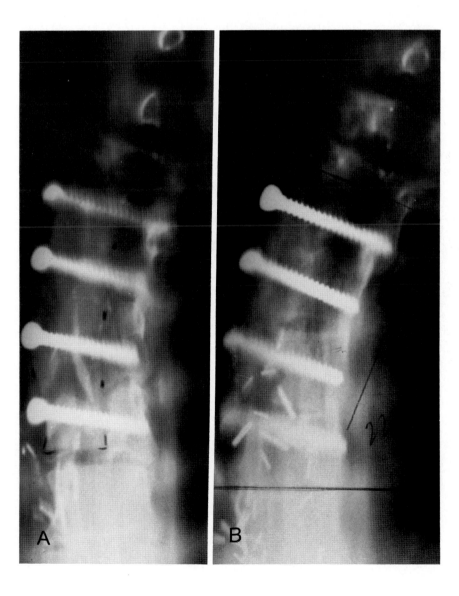

Figure 40.14. A. Anterior iliac graft reconstruction (outlined) after subtotal resection of T3-T6 including the posterior elements. B. Due to the absence of posterior instrumentation, scoliosis progressed postoperatively until union occurred.

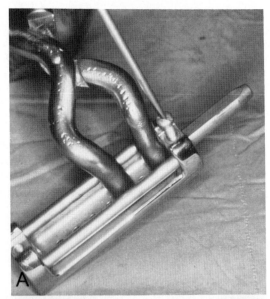

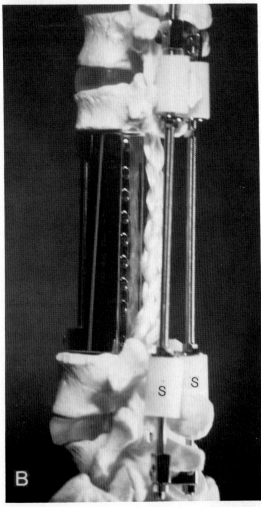

Second, Gunterberg has shown that there is sufficient mechanical strength of the lumbosacral connection to permit ambulation after resection of all sacral vertebrae below the superior half of S1 if the proximal half of the sacral ala are not disturbed (97).

Third, we have found that it is not necessary to reconstruct the spine after terminal spine resection (complete removal of the sacrum plus one or more lumbar vertebrae) (77). We place the patient on a rotating bed (Rotobed) for 3 months. This allows gradual shortening, prevents excess motion across the unprotected cauda equina, and yet provides the position changes needed to support respiratory physiology. Axial stability is finally achieved via the natural development of a "biologic sling" (16); this sling is formed by muscles attaching the pelvic ring to the distal lumbar vertebrae and from associated scar. A removable plastic orthosis provides angular support. This concept has been used in 2 of the author's patients, 1 of whom achieved full ambulatory status with the use of a cane (Fig. 40.22).

It should be noted that the largest of the spine resections or reconstructive procedures discussed in this article are associated with significant risk and postoperative complications. Due to the magnitude of surgery, some major complications are unavoidable, but others can be prevented with good preoperative planning. For example, it is well established that preoperative radiation greatly complicates dissection and aggravates bone graft and wound healing (41). Hence, radiation should be deferred until after surgery whenever possible. Postoperative chemotherapy markedly depresses incorporation of bone grafts. Accordingly, any spine stabilization construct which depends on a bone graft for early fixation should be avoided if chemotherapy is anticipated (60).

Considering the risks associated with complete vertebrectomy, these procedures should be undertaken only after careful study of the tumor and surrounding structures to determine if complete removal is an achievable goal. There is little point in performing a massive resection for a malignant tumor unless there is a reasonable possibility of achieving tumor-free margins. Without the use of CT, it would be impossible to make this determination in most cases. If CT demonstrates that a malignant tumor has not only destroyed the spine but also has invaded the mediastinum or vena cava, resection might not be feasible (Fig. 40.8), but the spatial data obtained still can be used to establish radiation portals. The question of resection is often more one of philosophy and value-judgement than technical capability. For example, CT with or without metrizamide myelography may show a grade I chondrosarcoma at L1 surrounding the dura with equivocal intrathecal penetration in a patient with minimal neurolog-

Figure 40.15. A. Segmental spine replacement of multiple thoracolumbar vertebrae. The anterior spine prosthesis features retractable rods for fixation in adjacent vertebral bodies. After the prosthesis is in place, the rods are jacked out to length with a special tool. B. The posterior construct combines compression rods to protect the anterior prosthesis from flexion forces with rod-sleeves (S) for rotatory stability.

ical deficit. Should the cord be transected above the tumor to permit en bloc resection and probable cure or should the involved dura be removed and grafted to preserve neurological function, but risk probable recurrence and possible death?

SURGICAL PLANNING FOR TUMOR RESECTION WITH IMAGING TECHNIQUES

Tumor Margins

Once the decision is made to attempt complete removal of a primary spine tumor, how much normal tissue margin is necessary? Osteoid osteoma, osteochondroma, and hemangioma require no tissue margins. Complete currettage and grafting will eliminate all but a few aneurysmal bone cysts (28). Normal tissue margins are not necessary for successful removal of spinal osteoblastomas or giant cell tumors either, but excision must be complete or recurrence is likely (98). Because of the more aggressive nature of sacral giant cell tumors, a thin margin of normal tissue should be taken. Malignant giant cell tumors and and chondrosarcomas should be removed en bloc with a margin of normal tissue. Attempts to scrape these tumors off the dura or vessel walls frequently will cause recurrence so tissues adjacent to the tumor must be removed together with the tumor if the goal is cure rather than palliation. Failure to remove these tumors en bloc, including former biopsy sites, can seed the wound and initiate recurrence.

Chordoma and less differentiated chondrosarcoma or other sarcomas tend to invade adjacent tissues. They are best resected en bloc with sufficient normal tissue to include the next fascial or periosteal or perichondral plane and perhaps 3 cm of uninvolved longitudinal muscle or iliac bone. The bodies of any affected vertebra should be excised completely through the adjacent disc and midpedicle. For instance, if CT shows a chordoma or malignant giant cell paravertebral soft-tissue mass, the adjacent paraspinous or psoas muscle should be resected along with the tumor from 3 cm proximal to 3 cm distal to the known tumor. For myeloma, if all studies indicate a truly solitary lesion, it may be worthwhile to remove the intact affected bone since myeloma arises from and quickly spreads through the marrow.

Unfortunately, Enneking's radical resection guidelines for sarcomas are not applicable to the spine (59, 99). Due to its axial location, paraspinous muscle resection from origin to insertion would be impossible. Likewise, the thickness of tissue margins are often compromised due to the immediate presence of the aorta, vena cava, and spinal cord. However, judging from experiences with extremity tumors (60), with postoperative chemotherapy such borderline resections may still be worth undertaking (Fig. 40.16).

Surgical Approach

CT and plain radiographs with markers are used to plan the surgical approach. Preoperative CT is worthwhile for all spinal tumors located near the neural canal in order to determine whether to approach the tumor from anteriorly, posteriorly, or both (56). For example, in one case, failure to obtain a preoperative axial scan resulted in the recurrence of an osteoblastoma because it extended too far anteriorly for access from a posterior laminectomy approach. After CT, the lesion was reapproached from both sides with successful resection (98). Accurate location of the anterior and posterior extent of all tumors is particularly important for neurofibroma which may project posteriorly into the canal or anteriorly along a root or even into the vertebral body (51). In the naturally kyphotic thoracic spine, small lesions extending as far anterior as the vertebral body are often accessible from the posterior midline or paraspinous costotransversectomy approach. However, in the cervical, lumbar, and sacral spine, access for proper resection requires an anterior or anterolateral approach if CT shows tumor extension anteriorly into the pedicles (57) (Fig. 40.16). Conversely, vertebral body tumors which extend posterior to the pedicles require a supplemental posterior or paraspinous incision for good control and access.

In order to determine how much muscle should be resected about a malignant tumor, one must look closely at the axial scan. Tumor infiltrations may evoke an inflammatory response and edema, which together with invading tumor, will expand the cross-section of the involved muscle. Hence, an asymmetrically enlarged muscle should be viewed with suspicion (44) and probably should be included within the tumor specimen (Fig. 40.17).

Once the surgical approach and circumferential margin is determined, the proximal-distal extent of the resection must be decided. This can be done most efficiently by using a CT scan with a sagittal reconstruction which specifies the vertebral level for each cut (Fig. 40.18). Accordingly, to permit accurate planning for any spinal operation, spinal scans should always be done with a sagittal reconstruction. We have not found axial view anatomical markings characteristic enough to determine accurately the vertebral level when the sagittal reconstruction is omitted and there is no digital radiograph available.

A helpful technique in planning the surgical incision is to tape needles over designated skin blemishes near the intended upper and lower margins of the tumor. By including the needles on the CT scan or preoperative radiograph, the accuracy of the incision placement may be enhanced. During the surgical resection of large tumors, it is important to place Kirschner wires at the intended levels for proximal and distal transection. Intraoperative radiographs then are taken to be sure that no more or less than the intended margin of spine and muscle are removed with the tumor.

Blood Loss Control

After designing the surgical approach(es), resection of large spinal tumors requires careful planning to control blood loss. The spine and tissues anterior to it are highly vascular. There are segmental arteries and veins from the

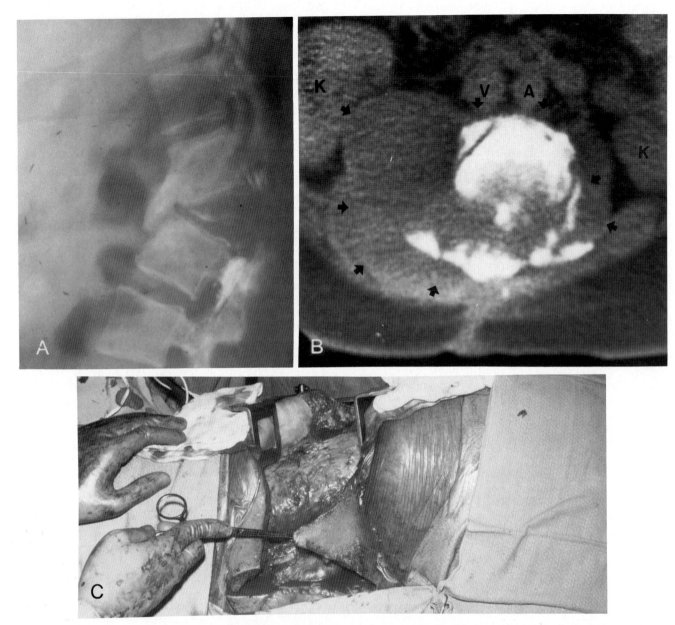

Figure 40.16.   Resection of malignant giant cell tumor with second-stage prosthetic replacement of T12-L3: A. Acute paraplegia after a fall prompted this radiograph suggesting recurrence of a giant cell tumor irradiated 7 years previous. There is dissolution of the L-2 body and signs of chronic kyphosis, but no clear evidence of the large soft-tissue tumor mass (outlined). B and C. CT of L-2 demonstrates the actual extent of the giant cell tumor (*arrows*) and its relationship to the kidneys (K), aorta (A), and vena cava (V). Because the bulk of the tumor extended to the right of the midline, a right anterolateral approach was used to permit dissection of the tumor from the kidney and great vessels. Because the CT scan showed infiltration of the right but not the left posterior paraspinous muscles, the spinal cord was approached posteriorly from an incision to the left of midline. D. The tumor, the T12-L3 spine, and the involved paraspinous muscles were resected en bloc. E, F, and G. After resection of one-half T-12 and all of L-1, L-2, and L-3, the patient was treated on a Stryker frame. The upper lumbar spine was subsequently replaced with an anterior prosthesis and posterior compression rod-sleeve construct (see Fig. 40.15 for details). The reconstruction provided spine stability and enabled the patient to be discharged and ambulate in a wheelchair.

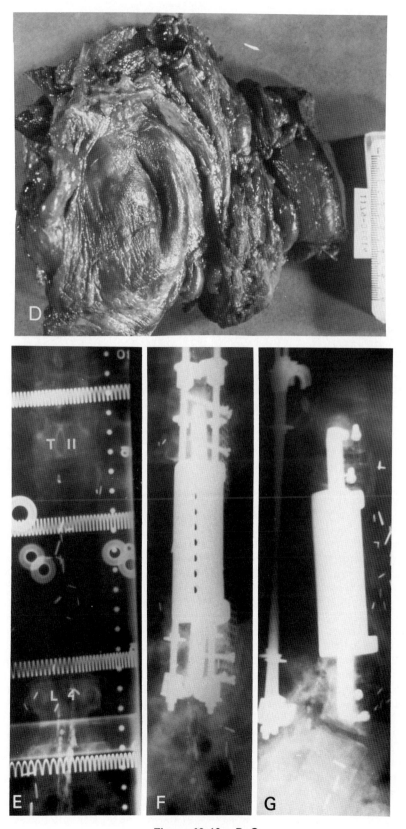

Figure 40.16.   D–G.

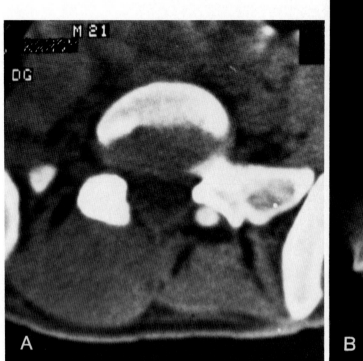 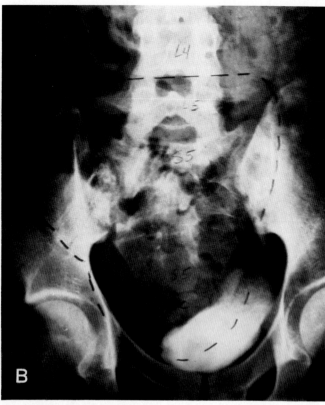

Figure 40.17.   A. Asymmetry of the paraspinous muscles in this L-5 cut suggests infiltration of the sacral chondrosarcoma proximally into the right paraspinous muscles. B. Accordingly, the proximal margin of resection was established at the L4–5 disc space. The *dotted line* outlines the extent of tumor resection necessary to achieve even thin normal tissue margins. A late postoperative radiograph is displayed in Figure 40.20C.

aorta and vena cava at every level; these segmental vessels collateralize within the vertebral bodies. A host of large vessels from the internal iliacs engulf the presacral area. Despite good access and careful planning, resection of large spinal tumors, especially with vertebrectomy, is associated with substantial blood loss (14).

To minimize the risk of fatal hemorrhage, arteriography should be obtained before major spine tumor resections. Principal vessels can then be embolized preoperatively or the surgical approach can be ordered so as to dissect out the vessels to the specimen and ligate them before attempting resection. Without arteriography, the location of even major vessels might not be obvious. For example, in treating large intrapelvic spinal tumors, we have found the normal position of the internal and external iliacs to be substantially deviated by the tumor (Fig. 40.19A). If arteriography shows multiple feeding vessels, the author has detoured blood flow around a lumbar or sacral surgical field. This is accomplished by cross-clamping the great vessels and shunting arterial and venous blood flow to the legs via plastic tubes placed into the great vessels (Fig. 40.19B). For shorter procedures, the lower aorta can simply be cross-clamped before actual transection of the spine (75). To minimize extensive blood loss from vertebral

bodies, spine transection should be done through the intervertebral discs.

When operating on the thoracic spine, care must be taken to avoid compromising the artery of Adamkiewicz which is often critical to the vascular sufficiency of the lower thoracic cord. Preoperative selective angiography is needed to identify the level and side of this variable artery. Assessment of the segmental blood supply to the cord is difficult but also important. Tumor, previous surgery, or congenital anatomy may result in asymmetric radicular blood supply to the thoracic cord. If particular radicular vessels are seen to be dominant on selective angiography, the surgical approach should be designed to preserve those vessels if at all possible to avoid cord ischemia and resultant paraplegia. Likewise, any deviation in the path of the vertebral arteries caused by the tumor must be discovered preoperatively to avoid catasrophe.

Bowel and Ureteral Management

Before treating large lumbar or sacral tumors of the spine, the ureters and rectum need to be evaluated. We have found it especially useful to perform an intravenous pyelogram immediately followed with CT. Because most lower spine primary malignancies form large prespinal

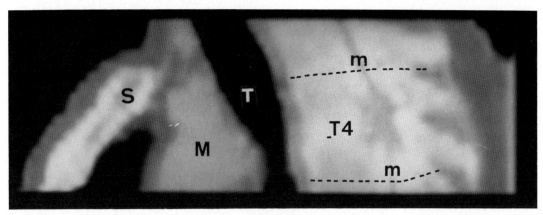

Figure 40.18. Plain films suggested tumor involvement only of T-4. This sagittal reconstruction demonstrated irregularity of the posterior vertebral bodies of T-3 through T-5 and blockage of metrizamide (m) adjacent to the midportions of T-3 and T-5. For orientation, the sternum (S), mediastinum (M), and trachea (T) are also labeled. The tumor was subsequently diagnosed as possible chordoma. A T3–5 complete vertebrectomy was performed with margins roughly at the level of the *dotted lines*.

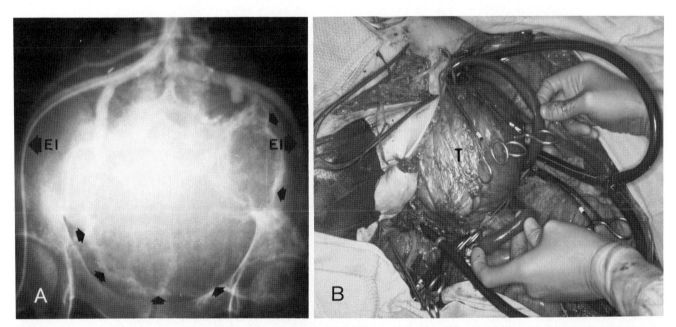

Figure 40.19. A. Preoperative aortography shows the remarkably lateral location of the internal and external iliac (EI) arteries. The normal position of the vessels has been altered by chronic pressure from the large intrapelvic extension of a sacral giant cell tumor (*arrows*). B. In order to decrease intrapelvic blood pressure prior to the resection of the tumor (T) the great vessels were cross-clamped. Heparinized "Y" tubes were then used to shunt blood from the cross-clamped aorta and vena cava to the legs.

soft-tissue masses, displacement of the ureters is common. If the scan is performed while Renographin is still being excreted, the position of the ureters relative to the tumor is determined easily (Fig. 40.20A and B). This will aid in deciding whether to perform an ileoureterostomy and in protecting the ureters during surgery.

If a malignant tumor is immediately adjacent to the rectum or ureters, or if complete terminal spine resection is planned, a diverting ileostomy and/or colostomy should be performed. Otherwise, tumor margins are compro-

mised, the chance of inadvertent bowel or ureteral injury during tumor resection is high, and kinking or scar constriction of the ureters is likely if they traverse the massive dead space after vertebrectomy and/or sacrectomy. The author recommends doing the diversions at least 2 weeks in advance of the tumor resection. This will permit healing of the ureteral and bowel anastomoses before the massive catabolic insult of spine resection; it also will reduce the time and blood loss of the tumor resection operation.

Another factor to consider in the ileostomy/colostomy

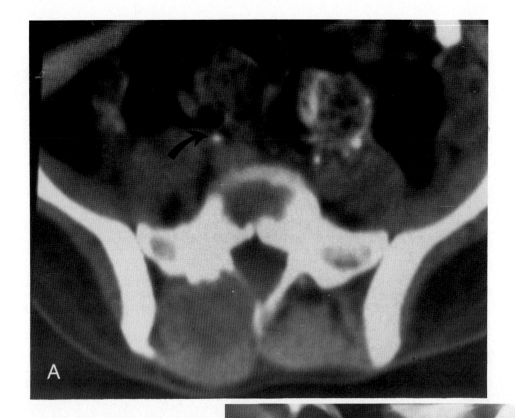

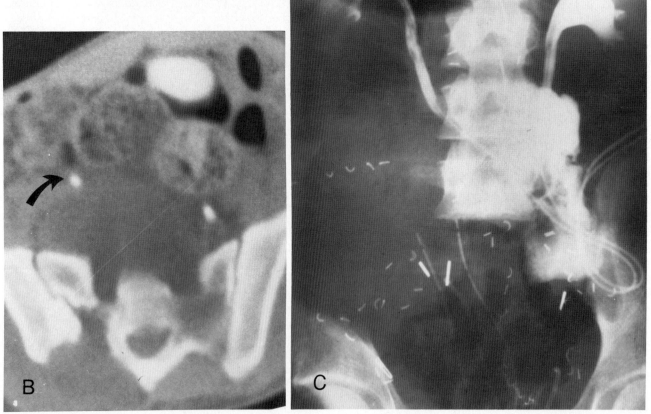

Figure 40.20. A and B. A CT with intravenous contrast was used to determine the position of the ureters before tumor surgery. The anterior extension of this sacral chondrosarcoma displaces the right ureter (*arrow*) from a relatively normal position adjacent to L-5 (A) to an anteriorly displaced position at the level of the midsacrum (B). Resection of the distal ureters along with the entire sacrum, therefore, was necessary to achieve adequate tumor margins. C. A retrograde pyelogram demonstrates a ureteroiliostomy which was performed before terminal spine resection.

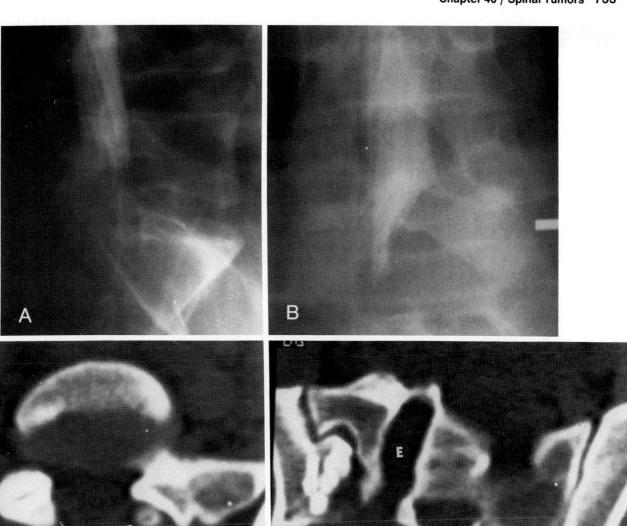

Figure 40.21. A and B. Metrizamide myelogram demonstrates extradural compression from the lobular superior extension of a sacral tumor. There were no L-5 bone changes on the plain film or CT to suggest this tumor extension up the spinal canal. C. metrizamide CT scan near the L5-S1 disc space localizes the caudal end of the dural sac (*arrow*) which has been compressed and pushed laterally by the tumor. D. Upper sacral CT shows well-demarcated bone erosion and anterior extension of the sacral chondrosarcoma. Note the erosion (E) which opens into one of the posterior paraspinous muscle groups; the muscle is enlarged from tumor infiltration, yet the spinal canal remains intact and the opposite paraspinal muscle appears normal. Accordingly, the canal was approached from the left side (*dotted line*) to liberate the functioning S-1 root.

decision is the postresection status of the bladder and rectum. The third sacral root is responsible for the micturation reflex and bladder and rectal continence (78). Adequate continence is often possible after unilateral but not bilateral sacrifice of this root. Hence, tumor or probable surgical destruction of both S3 roots would influence the decision toward a preliminary diversion procedure (Fig. 40.20C).

Dissection of Neural Structures

Another essential step before surgery is to determine the extent of cord and root involvement and to plan the dissection of neural structures. Either CT alone or myelography alone is often satisfactory for tumor localization and characterization. However, the combination in the form of a metrizamide CT scan is helpful for planning the resection in cases where tumor involves the neural canal

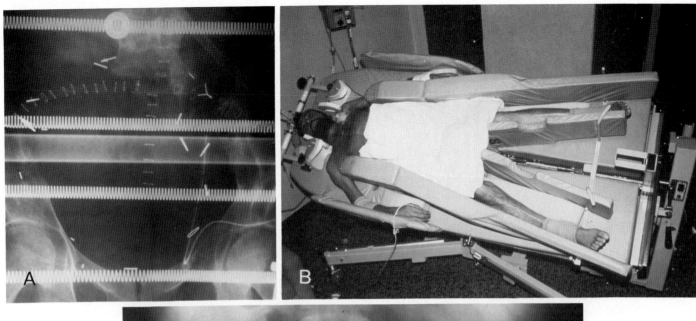

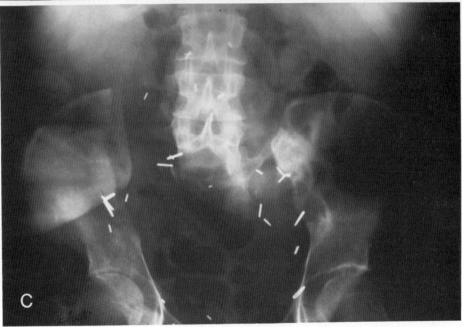

Figure 40.22. A. Terminal spine resection (L-4, L-5, and the entire sacrum) for removal of a massive giant cell tumor, but with dissection and preservation of the right cauda equina and lumbosacral plexus. B and C. The patient was treated on a rotating bed for 2½ months to permit shortening until the spine achieved a stable position—suspended by a biologic sling of muscle and scar from the pelvic rim. D. Good strength and sensation remained in the right leg. A brace was required for the left leg which had been previously paralyzed by the tumor. At 2-year follow-up, the patient was able to walk with a cane.

or roots. Because dura and root positions may be distorted by tumor, metrizamide is needed to localize the intradural space, as well as areas of tumor impingement. The metrizamide axial scan provides the third dimension which makes it possible for the surgeon to develop a three-dimensional perspective of the tumor before surgery (Fig. 40.21). Only with the spatial relationships clearly fixed in his mind can the surgeon select the best approach and order of dissection.

In the case of malignant tumors, it is important to scrutinize the metrizamide myelogram and metrizamide CT to determine if tumor has penetrated through the dura. If this is the case, it may be necessary to transect the cord and suture the dura above the site of tumor invasion. Fortunately, the dura mater serves as a natural barrier for most malignancies (3). This often permits salvage of at least some cauda equina and roots despite the presence of tumor adjacent to the dura.

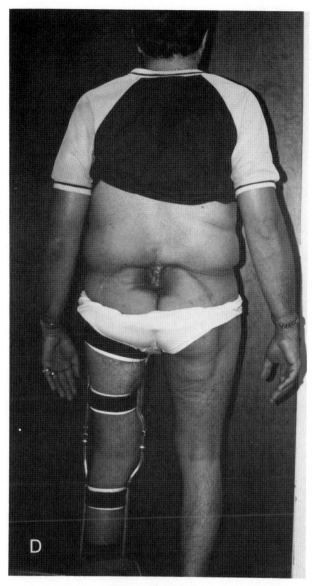

Figure 40.22. D.

Large tumors that require complete vertebrectomy or sacrectomy generally arise in the vertebral bodies and form anterior masses which tend to encircle the spine. However, even these large tumors usually have a tumor-free interval between the skin and posterior elements which can be identified on the CT scan. After approaching the spine through this interval, the tumor-free posterior bone is removed to expose the cord/cauda equina. Key nerve roots which pass through normal tissue then are unroofed laterally to a point beyond the anticipated margins of the specimen (Fig. 40.21). At the lumbosacral level, this task is considerable because channels must be cut through the entire thickness of the posterior ilium and sacral ala to free the sacral plexus. Due to the time and risk of retaining residual tumor that is associated with root/plexus lateral dissection, lateral dissection is only recommended for roots with essential motor function such

as C5–8, L2–S1, and S3 (bowel and bladder continence). Roots or portions of the cauda equina to be salvaged are dissected away from those entrapped by tumor. If the dura must be cut to separate specimen from retained structures, the free edge is oversewn. The transected spinal tumor specimen then is moved anteriorly away from the preserved cord/roots/plexae.

Is it possible for neurological function to remain after circumferential removal of the spine? Stener reported three vertebrectomy cases each of which succeeded in preserving sufficient neurological function to permit ambulation and bladder control. His T7 vertebrectomy patient developed spastic paresis postoperatively (79) but his T11 and T11-L1 vertebrectomy cases showed significant improvement over their preoperative status (63, 75). After terminal spine resection (L4-S5 inclusive) we have recorded postoperative function in two cases. Despite circumferential dissection of approximately 9 inches of cauda equina and sacral plexus, one of these patients recovered near normal strength and was able to walk (77) (Fig. 40.22). Hence, the tedious dissection of neural structures from the spinal specimen is certainly worthwhile. From the cumulative experience of Stener and the author, the chances of retaining neurological function appear to rise as one proceeds caudally from T3 to S1. Neurological function can even improve postoperatively in incomplete paraplegia with compressive neuropathy.

CT has dispersed the fog of spatial obscurity surrounding large spinal tumors. This spatial obscurity has long restrained clinicians from timely therapeutic intervention and left too many patients with hopeless, inoperable tumors. CT makes possible efficient localization, characterization, and three-dimensional reconstruction of virtually all spinal tumors. When used together with Renographin and metrizamide, CT will elucidate the tumor's relationship to adjacent urological and neurological structures. Armed with these data, and some recent advances in surgical techniques and biomechanical understanding, surgeons now have the necessary tools to undertake resection/reconstruction of virtually any spinal tumor where there is still a good chance of preserving functional existence. With increasing use of CT to elucidate suspicious spinal radiographs, it may now be possible to spot spinal tumors earlier, diagnose them more accurately, resect selected tumors while still small, and provide spinal tumor patients with a more favorable prognosis.

References

1. Jaffe HL: *Tumors and Tumorous Conditions of the Bones and Joints.* Philadelphia, Lea & Febiger, 1958.
2. Batson OV: The function of vertebral veins and their role in the spread of metastases. *Ann Surg* 112:138, 1940.
3. Simeone FA: Intraspinal neoplasms. In: Rothman RH, Simeone FA: *The Spine.* (Vol. II) Philadelphia, W. B. Saunders Co., 1975.
4. Huvos AG: *Bone Tumors: Diagnosis, Treatment, and Prognosis.* Philadelphia, W. B. Saunders Co., 1979.
5. Edeiken J: *Roentgen Diagnosis of Diseases of Bone* (3rd ed). Baltimore, Williams & Wilkins, 1981.
6. Schajowicz F: *Tumors and Tumorlike Lesions of Bones and Joints.* New York, Springer-Verlag, 1981.
7. Dahlin DC: Giant-cell tumor of vertebrae above the sacrum.

Cancer 39:1350–1356, 1977.

8. Smith J, Wixon D, Watson RC: Giant-cell tumor of the sacrum: Clinical and radiologic features in 13 patients. *J de L'Association Canadienne des Radiologistes* 30:34–39, 1979.

9. Francis KC: Tumors of the spine. In: Rothman RH, Simeone FA: *The Spine*. Vol. II. Philadelphia, W. B. Saunders Co., 1975.

10. Spjut HJ, Dorfman HD, Fechner RE, et al: *Tumors of Bones and Cartilage: Atlas of Tumor Pathology*. Washington, D.C., Armed Forces Institute of Pathology, 1971, Series 2, Fasc. 5, pp. 325–340.

11. Higinbotham NL, Phillips RF, Farr HW, et al: Chordoma: 35 year study at Memorial Hospital. *Cancer* 20:1841, 1967.

12. Sundaresan N, Galicich JH, Chu FCH, et al: Spinal chordomas: A clinical review. *J Neurosurg* 50:312–319, 1979.

13. Maroske D, Hupe K: Sacrococcygeal chordoma: Radical operation, a problem. *Chirurgica* 48:118–112, 1977.

14. Localio SA, Francis KC, Rossano PG: Abdominosacral resection of sacrococcygeal chordoma. *Ann Surg* 166:394–402, 1967.

15. Jaffe HL, Lichtenstein L, Portis RB: Giant cell tumor of bone: Its pathologic appearance, grading, supposed variants, and treatment. *Arch Path* 30:993–1031, 1940.

16. Edwards CC, DeSilva JB: Total resection of multiple lumbar and sacral segments in tumor surgery. *Proceedings of the 16th Annual Scoliosis Research Society*. 1981, p. 140.

17. Dahlin DC, Cupps RE, Johnson EW, Jr.: Giant cell tumor: A study of 195 cases. *Cancer* 25:1061–1070, 1970.

18. Goldenberg RR, Campbell CJ, Bonfiglio M: Giant-cell tumor of bone: An analysis of 218 cases. *J Bone Joint Surg* 52A:619–663, 1970.

19. Mnaymneh WA, Dudley HR, Mnaymneh LG: Giant-cell tumor of bone: An analysis and follow-up study of 41 cases observed at Massachusetts General Hospital between 1925 and 1960. *J Bone Joint Surg* 46A:63–75, 1964.

20. DiLorenzo N, Spallone A, Nolletti A, et al: Giant cell tumors of the spine: A clinical study of six cases, with emphasis on the radiological features, treatment, and follow-up. *Neurosurgery* 6:29–34, 1980.

21. Larsson SE, Lorentzon R, Boquist L: Giant-cell tumors of the spine and sacrum causing neurological symptoms. *Clin Orthop* 111:210–211, 1975.

22. Shamsuddin AKM, Varma VA, Toker C, et al: Ultrastructural features of a malignant giant cell tumor of bone with areas of osteogenic sarcoma. *Mt Sinai J Med* 46:297–308, 1979.

23. Hutter RVP, Worcester JN, Francis KC, et al: Benign and malignant giant cell tumors of bone: A clinicopathological analysis of the natural history of the disease. *Cancer* 15:653–690, 1962.

24. Dahlin DC: *Bone Tumors*. 3rd Ed. Springfield, IL, Charles C Thomas, 1978.

25. MacLellan DI, Wilson FC, Jr.: Osteoid osteoma of the spine. *J Bone Joint Surg* 49:111–121, 1967.

26. Sim FH, Dahlin DC, Beabout JW: Lesions which simulate osteoid osteoma (Abstract) *J Bone Joint Surg* 56:1541, 1974.

27. Sabanas AO, Bickel WH, Moe JH: Natural history of osteoid osteoma of the spine. *Am J Surg* 91:880–889, 1956.

28. Clough JR, Price CHG: Aneurysmal bone cyst: Pathogenesis and long-term results of treatment. *Clin Orthop* 97:52–63, 1973.

29. Hay MC, Paterson D, Taylor TKF: Aneurysmal bone cysts of the spine. *J Bone Joint Surg* 60B:406–411, 1978.

30. Marcove RC, Mike V, Hutter RVP, et al: Chondrosarcoma of the pelvis and upper end of the femur: An analysis of factors influencing survival time in 113 cases. *J Bone Joint Surg* 54:561–572, 1972.

31. Lichtenstein L: *Bone Tumors*. 4th Ed. St. Louis, C. V. Mosby Co, 1972.

32. Spallone A, DiLorenzo N, Nardi P, et al: Spinal osteochondroma diagnosed by computed tomography: Report of two cases and review of literature. *Acta Neurochirurg* 58:105–114, 1981.

33. Bradford FK: Intraspinal tumors: Report of twelve cases. *Dis Nerv System* Feb:55–60, 1954.

34. Loftus CM, Rozario RA, Prager R, et al.: Solitary osteochondroma of T4 with thoracic cord compression. *Surg Neurol* 13:355–357, 1980.

35. Moseley JE: *Bone Changes in Hematologic Disorders (Roentgen Aspects)*. New York, Grune & Stratton, 1963, pp. 161–179.

36. McLeod RA, Dahlin DC, Beabout JW: The spectrum of osteoblastoma. *AJR* 126:321–335, 1976.

37. Jackson RP: Recurrent osteoblastoma: A review. *Clin Orthop* 131:229–233, 1978.

38. Pochaczevsky R, Yen YM, Sherman RS: The roentgen appearance of benign osteoblastoma. *Radiology* 75:429–437, 1960.

39. Drobni S. Kudasz J: Abdominoperineal resection for enormous presacral cysts and tumors. *Am J Protocol* Oct:33–36, 1975.

40. Nakagawa H, Huang YP, Malis LI, et al: Computed tomography of intraspinal and paraspinal neoplasms. *J Comput Assist Tomogr* 1:377–390, 1977.

41. Harrington KD: The use of methyl methacrylate for vertebral-body replacement and anterior stabilization of pathological fracture-dislocations of the spine due to metastatic malignant disease. *J Bone Joint Surg* 63A:36–46, 1981.

42. Vancoillie P, Kaiser MC, Veiga-Pires JA: Computed tomography in the diagnosis of space occupying lesions of the occipito-cervical junction. *J Neuroradiol* 8:335–341, 1981.

43. Hoeffken W, Traupe H, Heiss WD: CT-visualization of an intraspinal osteomalike mass in Paget's disease. *Neurosurg Rev* 3:179–182, 1980.

44. Naidich DP, Freedman MT, Bowerman JW, et al: Computerized tomography in the evaluation of the soft tissue component of bony lesions of the pelvis. *Skeletal Radiol* 3:144–148, 1978.

45. Federle MP, Moss AA, Margolin FR: Role of computed tomography in patients with "sciatica." *J Comput Assist Tomogr* 4:335–341, 1980.

46. McGrath PJ: Giant-cell tumor of bone: An analysis of 52 cases. *J Bone Joint Surg* 54B:216–229, 1972.

47. Yang WC, Zappulla R, Malis L: Neurilemmoma in lumbar intervertebral foramen. *J Comput Assist Tomogr* 5:904–906, 1981.

48. Hounsfield GN: Computerized transverse axial scanning (tomography): Part I. Description of the system. *Br J Radiol* 46:1016–1022, 1973.

49. Di Chiro G, Schellinger D: Computed tomography of spinal cord after lumbar intrathecal introduction of metrizamide (computer-assisted myelography). *Radiology* 120:101–104, 1976.

50. Arii H, Takahashi M, Tamakawa Y, et al: Metrizamide spinal computed tomography following myelography. *Comput Tomogr* 4:117–125, 1980.

51. Kamano S, Amano K, Machiyama N, et al.: The contribution of computed tomography in the choice of an anterolateral approach, for treating cervical dumb-bell tumours. *Neurochirurgica* 23:121–125, 1980.

52. Roberson GH, Taveras JM, Tadmore R, et al: Computed tomography in metrizamide cisternography—Importance of coronal and axial views. *J Comput Assist Tomogr* 1:241–245, 1977.

53. Heithoff KB: High-resolution computed tomography of the lumbar spine. *Postgrad Med* 70:193–213, 1981.

54. Whitehouse GH, Griffiths GJ: Roentgenologic aspects of spinal involvement by primary and metastatic Ewing's tumor. *J Assoc Can Radiol* 27:290–291, 1976.

55. Turner ML, Mulhern CB, Dalinka MK: Lesions of the sacrum: Differential diagnosis and radiological evaluation. *JAMA* 245:275–277, 1981.

56. Wedge JH, Tchang S, MacFadyen DJ: Computed tomography in localization of spinal osteoid osteoma. *Spine* 6:423–427, 1981.

57. Southwick WO, Robinson RA: Surgical approaches to the

vertebral bodies in the cervical and lumbar regions. *J Bone Joint Surg* 39A:631–643, 1957.

58. Craig FS: Vertebral-body biopsy. *J Bone Joint Surg* 38A:93–102, 1956.
59. Enneking WF, Dunham WK: Resection and reconstruction for primary neoplasms involving the innominate bone. *J Bone Joint Surg* 60A:731–746, 1978.
60. Watts HG: Introduction to resection of musculoskeletal sarcomas. *Clin Orthop* 153:31–38, 1980.
61. Berman HL: The treatment of benign giant cell tumors of the vertebrae by irradiation. *Radiology* 83:202–207, 1964.
62. Verbiest H: Giant-cell tumours and aneurysmal bone cysts of the spine. *J Bone Joint Surg* 47B:699–713, 1965.
63. Stener B: Total spondylectomy for removal of a giant-cell tumor in the eleventh thoracic vertebrae. *Spine* 2:197–201, 1977.
64. Schwimer SR, Bassett LW, Mancuso AA, et al: Giant cell tumor of the cervicothoracic spine. *AJR* 136:63–67, 1981.
65. Hays RP: Resection of the sacrum for benign giant cell tumor: A case report. *Ann Surg* 138:115–120, 1953.
66. Johnson EW, Dahlin DC: Treatment of giant-cell tumor of bone. *J Bone Joint Surg* 41A:895–904, 1959.
67. Murphy WR, Ackerman LV: Benign and malignant giant-cell tumors of bone: A clinical-pathological evaluation of 31 cases. *Cancer* 9:317–339, 1956.
68. Bucy PC: The Treatment of malignant tumors of the spine: A review. *Neurology* 13:938–944, 1963.
69. Kambin P: Giant-cell tumor of the thoracic spine with pathological fracture and paraparesis: A method of stabilization: A case report. *J Bone Joint Surg* 48A:779–782, 1966.
70. MacCarty CS, Waugh JM, Coventry MD, et al: Sacro-coccygeal chordoma. *Surg Gynecol Obstet* 113:551, 1961.
71. MacCarty CS, Waugh JM, Mayo CW, et al: The surgical treatment of presacral tumors: A combined problem. *Proceedings of the Staff Meetings of the Mayo Clinic* 27:73–84, 1952.
72. Miller TR, Mackenzie AR, Randall HT, et al: Hemicorporectomy. *Surgery* 59:988–993, 1966.
73. Scoville WB, Palmer AH, Samra K, et al: The use of acrylic plastic for vertebral replacement of fixation in metastatic disease of the spine. A technical note. *J Neurosurg* 27:274–279, 1967.
74. Lievre JA, Darcy M, Pradat P, et al: Tumeur a cellues géantes du rachis lombaire spondylectomie totale en deux temps. *Revue du Rhumatisme et des Maladies Osteo-articulaires* 35:125, 1968.
75. Stener B, Johnsen OE: Complete removal of three vertebrae for giant-cell tumour. *J Bone Joint Surg* 53B:278–287, 1971.
76. Elliott J: Orthopedist is pioneer in prosthetic design. *JAMA* 242:1831, 1979.
77. Edwards CC, DeSilva JB: Resection of the sacrum and multiple lumbar vertebrae in tumor surgery. *J Bone Joint Surg Orthop Trans* 7:000, 1983.
78. Gunterberg B: Effects of major resection of the sacrum: Clinical studies on urogenital and anorectal function and a biomechanical study on pelvic strength. *Acta Orthop Scand* (Suppl) 162:9–38, 1976.
79. Stener B: Total spondylectomy in chondrosarcoma arising from the seventh thoracic vertebra. *J Bone Joint Surg* 53B:288–295, 1971.
80. Hamdi FA: Prosthesis for an excised lumbar vertebra: A preliminary report. *Can Med Assoc J* 100:576–580, 1969.
81. Robinson RA, Southwick WO: Indications and technics for early stabilization of the neck. *South Med J* 53:565, 1960.
82. Edwards CC, Levine AM, Murphy JC, et al: *New Techniques in Spine Stabilization* (technical monograph). Warsaw, Indiana, Zimmer USA Publications, 1982.
83. Murphy MJ, Southwick WO: Spinal instrumentation for stabilization and fusion of the cervical spine. *J Bone Joint Surg Orthop Trans* 7:119, 1983.
84. Panjabi MM, Hopper W, White AA, et al: Posterior spine stabilization with methylmethacrylate: Biomechanical testing of a surgical specimen. *Spine* 2:241–247, 1977.
85. Dunn EJ: The role of methyl methacrylate in the stabilization and replacement of tumors of the cervical spine. A project of the Cervical Spine Research Society. *Spine* 2:15–24, 1977.
86. Whitehill R, Reger SI, Barry JS, et al: A biomechanical analysis of the use of methylmethacrylate as in instantaneous posterior fusion mass: A canine in vivo experimental model. *J Bone Joint Surg Orthop Trans* 7:119, 1983.
87. Cantu RC: Anterior spinal fusion using methylmethacrylate. *Internat Surg* 59:110–111, 1974.
88. Barrasso JA, Keggi KS: Vertebral body excision in the treatment of cervical disc disease, spondylosis and spinal stenosis. *J Bone Joint Surg Orthop Trans* 7:114, 1983.
89. Tscherne H: Operative treatment of cervical spine injuries. *J Bone Joint Surg Orthop Trans* 6:389, 1982.
90. White, AA, Panjabi MM: *Clinical Biomechanics of the Spine.* Philadelphia, J.B. Lippincott Co., 1978.
91. Dept. of Orthopedics, First Medical College of Shanghai: Treatment of tumors of the cervical spine by excision and prosthetic replacement: Report of 5 cases. *Chinese Med J* 1:5, 1974.
92. Ono K, Tada K: Metal prosthesis of the cervical vertebrae. *J Neurosurg* 42:256, 1975.
93. Ono K, Fuji T, Okada K: Pathologic basis of surgical salvaging of the spine with metastases or invasion of cancer. *J Bone Joint Surg Orthop Trans* 7:118, 1983.
94. Edwards CC: The spinal rod sleeve: Its rationale and use in thoracic and lumbar injuries. *J Bone Joint Surg Orthop Trans* 6:11, 1982.
95. Edwards CC, DeSilva JB, Levine AM: Early results using spinal rod sleeves in thoracolumbar injury. *J Bone Joint Surg Orthop Trans* 6:345–346, 1982.
96. Dunn HK: The operative correction of congenital kyphoscoliosis. *J Bone Joint Surg Orthop Trans* 6:13, 1982.
97. Gunterberg B, Romanus B, Stener B: Pelvic strength after major amputation of the sacrum. *Acta Orthop Scand* 47:635–642, 1976.
98. Epstein N, Benjamin V, Pinto R, et al: Benign osteoblastoma of a thoracic vertebra: Case report. *J Neurosurg* 53:710–713, 1980.
99. Simon MA, Enneking WF: The surgical management of soft tissue sarcomas of the extremities. *J Bone Joint Surg* 58A:317, 1976.

CHAPTER FORTY-ONE

Value of Computed Tomographic Scanning in Infectious Disease of the Spine

ROBERT M. LIFESO, M.D., F.R.C.S.(C)

Infectious disease of the spine is among one of the oldest known afflictions of mankind. Tuberculous changes have been found in the vertebrae of Egyptian mummies dating from 3000 BC (1). Tuberculosis-causing paraplegia has been described by both Hippocrates and Sir Percival Pott (2). It was Sir Percival Pott who suggested the application of a hot poker to tuberculous abscesses in cases of tuberculous paraplegia in hopes of draining the abscess and relieving pressure on the spinal cord.

As long as treatment was only supportive, and paraplegia and death the not unusual sequelae, early diagnosis of spinal sepsis was of little importance. Fortunately, this situation has improved and early treatment depends upon early and accurate diagnosis.

Spinal infections differ from other musculoskeletal infections in a number of significant ways:

1. The difficulty in the early stages of making a diagnosis especially in the very young and the very old;
2. The dangerous complications of spinal cord involvement. This occurs in about 20% of all cases of spinal tuberculosis (3). It is of interest that the paraplegia rate has not been affected significantly by the introduction of antituberculous chemotherapy.
3. The problem of late spinal instability with the possible complication of late neurological impairment.
4. The difficulty in differentiating spinal sepsis from spinal tumor with possible catastrophic results.

Saudi Arabia still suffers from the endemic diseases now rarely seen in North America and Northern Europe. Tuberculosis (TB), brucellosis, hydatid disease, and the like are all prevalent. Unlike most of Asia, Africa, and China, tuberculosis in Saudi Arabia is primarily a disease of adulthood (4–6). In Hong Kong, for example, 69% of cases of TB of the spine occur in patients less than 10 years of age (6). In Europe and North America, as in Saudi Arabia, the disease is almost exclusively one of adults (7, 8). Our average age for the presentation of spinal tuber-

culosis in the King Faisal Specialist Hospital is 38 years. This is similar to the average age seen in the United Kingdom and Ireland (7, 8).

In the past 4 years, approximately 250 cases of suspected spinal infections have been referred to the author at the King Faisal Specialist Hospital in Riyadh. One hundred and forty of these cases have proven to be tuberculosis with 25 infections due to other organisms. The remainder of the cases were tumors, 55 primary and the rest metastatic. All of these patients presented with the presumptive diagnosis of TB of the spine with failure to respond to conservative treatment.

Diagnosis in these cases always is preplexing on clinical grounds alone. The histories are usually extremely similar: the main referring complaint is usually back pain with varying degrees of neurological impairment. Hematological work-up usually shows a normal white blood count and a normal hemoglobin. Erythrocyte sedimentation rates usually are elevated in all cases, regardless of etiology. Tuberculin skin tests in our setting are often positive and may only be helpful if negative. Serological testing for Brucella is useful in some instances but occasionally may yield false-negatives especially if the tube dilution technique is not utilized. Blood cultures are occasionally positive if the patient is cultured during the febrile episode but most of our patients unfortunately present in later stages of the disease. Specific tests for TB, such as urine and sputum cultures, are generally negative and require an 8-week incubation period before one can be certain. Serological testing for Staphylococcus is, unfortunately, not constantly reliable (9, 10). Biochemical investigations of the various tumors, i.e., acid phosphatase, serum thyroid, and the like may be helpful in specialized cases.

Conventional radiology and the various isotope studies are helpful in localizing a lesion but, unfortunately, usually give no other information as to etiology. Tomography and myelography are useful in delineating the extent of disease, but again seldom yield clues as to etiology. Myelography is mandatory in any case with neurological impairment or in any case where surgery is contemplated but, again, is seldom diagnostic.

Technetium scanning is valuable in identifying tumors and nongranulomatous infectious disease and in differentiating active from quiescent disease but in TB we have found bone scanning occasionally to be falsely negative, not only in the early stages of the disease, but also in the later stages when gross radiographic changes are apparent. Similarly, we have found gallium scanning especially in spinal TB to have a high incidence of false-negatives, especially early in the course of disease.

The most difficult cases to diagnose are those with a short clinical history and a high index of suspicion and where plain roentgenograms show little, if any, appreciable changes. It is important to realize that in early septic disease there are often no abnormalities seen on plain films. In fact, in some of these cases CT scanning and conventional tomography may be nondiagnostic. However, because CT is much more sensitive than conventional studies in discerning soft-tissue and early bony changes, it can detect disease when other radiographic studies are negative or equivocal. Nevertheless, if no abnormalities are seen on any radiographic study early in

the course of disease, repeat x-rays must be taken at regular intervals as long as clinical suspicion of disease still exists. It is in these cases that bone scanning and gallium scanning are most valuable as long as one realizes that both may be falsely negative in early spinal TB.

Plain roentgenograms taken in early vertebral sepsis due to nongranulomatous organisms are usually quite nonspecific. Initially, on plain films one may see an increase in soft-tissue density in the paraspinal spaces. This is usually followed by diffuse porosis and rarefaction of contiguous vertebral end plates. Occasionally, a small lytic defect in the vertebral end plates is the earliest bony defect (Fig. 41.1). Intervertebral disc narrowing is often a relatively late finding and often occurs only weeks or months after the onset of disease. With progression of disease there are variable degrees of vertebral body destruction, increasing disc collapse, and often total disc obliteration and spontaneous fusion (Figs. 41.2 and 41.3). Sclerosis and kyphosis often are seen in varying degrees in the later stages.

In pyogenic disease, a smaller abscess usually is seen than in TB. Bone destruction is much less than with TB

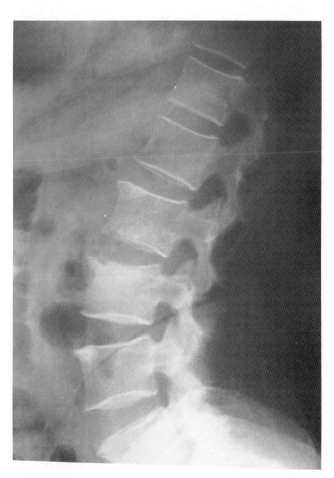

Figure 41.1. L2–3 Enterobacter infection. Early rarefaction of end plates. Note preservation of disc space.

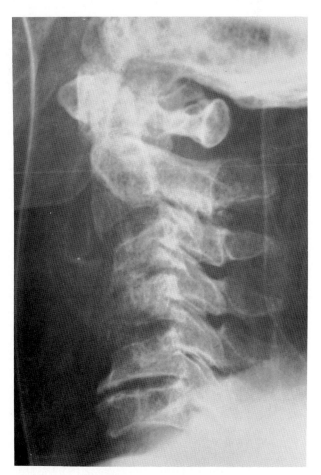

Figure 41.2. Plain film showing anterior erosion of C3 and C3–4 disc space narrowing and a prevertebral soft-tissue mass in a 65-year-old male with *E. coli* osteomyelitis 2 months after prostate surgery.

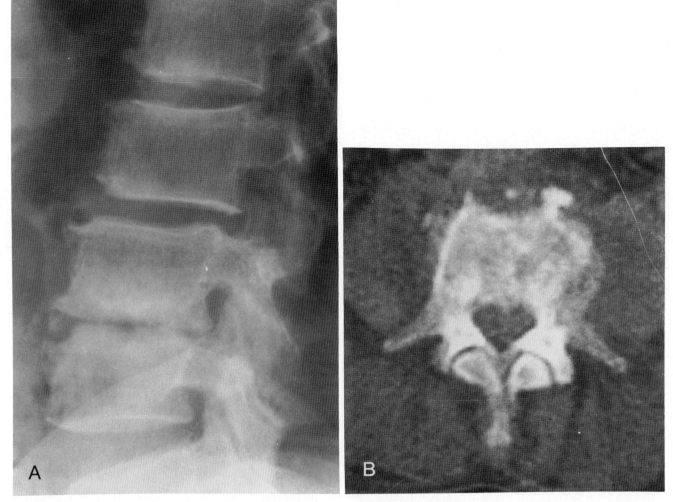

Figure 41.3. A. L3–4 staphylococcal osteomyelitis of 3 months' duration with disc narrowing and sclerosis seen on plain film. B. CT scan in same patient showing small soft-tissue abscess and minimal bone destruction. Hazy bone outline.

and usually confined to contiguous bodies only. There is little, if any, calcification in the adjacent paraspinal abscess, a fact apparent with CT scanning. Posterior elements rarely are involved.

Rapid progression of disease and complete disc collapse suggest pyogenic discitis. Paraspinal soft-tissue abscesses are often not apparent initially and this is most often a problem in the patient with postoperative discotomy pain where a septic discitis is suspected. In these cases a rising sedimentation rate, an increasing soft-tissue abscess, increasing pain, and a high index of suspicion are necessary to make the diagnosis. On clinical grounds pain, especially night pain, plus a relatively rapid clinical course help differentiate sepsis from normal postoperative pain.

Brucellosis is still endemic in many areas of Saudi Arabia. It is a small, Gram-negative coccobacilli and the predominant species affecting the spine in this country is Brucella melitensis found primarily in goats. This is in contrast to the United States where the predominant species is Brucella abortus found most commonly in cattle or

Brucella suis found in swine. It usually is accompanied by a very small soft-tissue abscess and by a marked degree of sclerosis, more so than what one sees in either TB or nongranulomatous infection. One always is impressed by the degree of bone destruction in brucella. There is often a delay of months between the onset of disease and the appearance of radiological signs. Osteoporosis of the contiguous vertebral end plates is followed by end plate erosions and usually a very small, if any, soft-tissue abscess. Sclerosis occurs rapidly and in a more marked degree than with other septic conditions or tumors (Fig. 41.4).

Diagnosis in these cases often can be made on a serum agglutination test where a titer of 1:160 or higher is suspicious of recent disease on the tube agglutination test. Serum titers often will rise as high as 1:1200 or higher and then fall to 1:160 over a year. The serum agglutination test is often strongly positive before radiographic signs are apparent but false-negatives have occurred due to the "Prozone" phenomenon especially with the slide test.

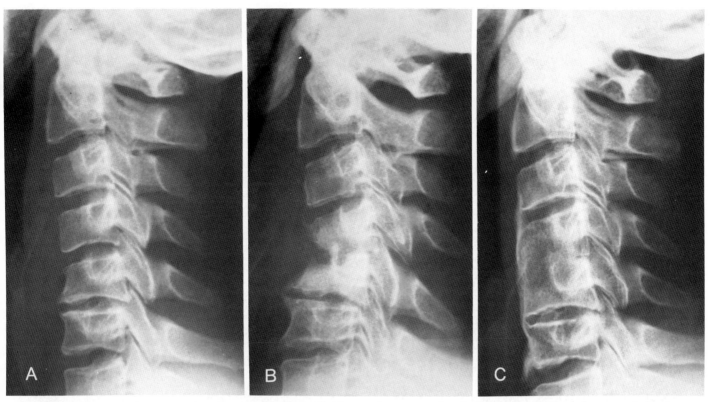

Figure 41.4. A. A 39-year-old Saudi male with a 2-month history of severe neck pain. B. Same patient repeat x-rays 2 months after A. Gross destruction C4–5 with sclerosis and destruction C4–5 disc space. C. Three months after anterior decompression and fusion. Pathology revealed Brucella.

TB of the spine generally exhibits a great deal of bone destruction with two, three, or more vertebral bodies involved (Figs. 41.5–41.7). The paraspinal abscess is usually large and occasionally shows soft-tissue calcification (Figs 41.8 and 41.9). It usually involves vertebral bodies as opposed to the posterior elements, but posterior elements can be involved both in granulomatous disease and in tumors (Figs 41.10 and 41.11). Pyogenic sepsis generally involves anterior structures only. In TB, the presence of a paraspinal abscess usually indicates active disease and the absence of an abscess, quiescence. However, this is not invariably true and I have operated on cases with no clinical or radiological evidence of a paraspinal abscess and found active TB. Sequestered avascular bone can often be seen on CT scan and a common finding is to find that the cancellous bone of a body has been totally destroyed, leaving the cortex intact. As with other causes of spinal osteomyelitis, the earliest x-ray changes are osteoporosis of the body or bodies adjacent to a disc space followed by erosion and disc narrowing, and at this stage, differentiation from other causes of disc narrowing is difficult.

Tumors, generally speaking, are more sharply outlined than septic conditions and often exhibit well-demarcated lytic areas. These usually involve one vertebral body tending not to cross the disc space above or below. The soft-tissue component is of variable size. Usually, the vertebral body is primarily involved, but the posterior elements can be affected as well (Figs. 41.12–41.14). Soft-tissue calcifications rarely may be seen but they are not the frequent occurrence that they are in TB. Tumors presenting as purely osteoblastic or osteolytic lesions may make the diagnosis a little simpler but securing tissue is usually necessary to make a definitive diagnosis (Figs. 41.15 and 41.16).

Retroperitoneal and pelvic tumors or abscesses often can give a history very compatible with spinal sepsis (Fig. 41.17). Routine x-ray examination often will show the effects of external compression on vertebral bodies and often anterior vertebral body erosion may appear very similar to that seen on conventional radiographs of patients suffering from spinal TB. CT scanning is the most useful diagnostic test in these cases to evaluate both possible retroperitoneal and pelvic masses and the anterior vertebral body erosions.

The final problem in differential diagnosis is with the various metabolic diseases affecting the spine. Often severe osteoporosis, osteomalacia, or Vitamin D deficiency rickets will mimic many of the changes seen with tumors or TB (Fig. 41.18). Anterior vertebral body erosions, symmetrical vertebral body collapse of multiple levels or localized compression fractures often look very similar to TB or occasionally to multiple myeloma. Generalized spinal osteoporosis and osteoporosis at other sites are usually indicative of the correct diagnosis, but often in

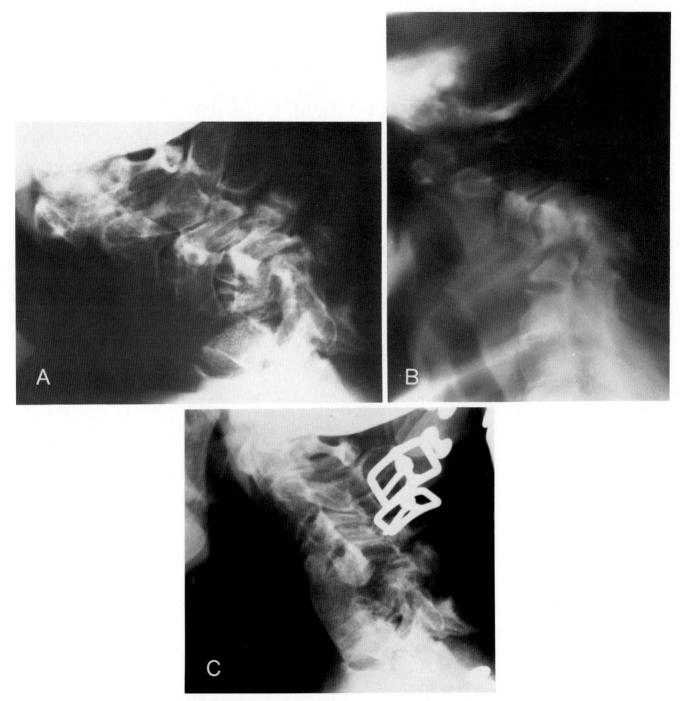

Figure 41.5. A and B. Four years after cervical TB and 3 years after completing course of antituberculous chemotherapy. Severe kyphus at C5–6 seen on plain film (A) and tomogram (B). C. After correction and fusion.

partially treated Vitamin D deficiency rickets with vertebral collapse and kyphosis, the diagnosis is much more difficult. The absence of a soft-tissue abscess, the usual preservation of disc spaces and the generalized nature of disease combined with a normal erythrocyte sedimentation rate and the biochemical profile usually simplify the diagnosis.

Unfortunately, the overlap between the various features of septic infection, TB, tumors, and metabolic disease as seen on conventional radiology is such that it is almost impossible to be certain of diagnosis without bone biopsy. Accurate diagnosis usually depends upon obtaining material for bacteriological and microscopic examination. Even when one is certain on x-ray that the disease is a septic process, material for culture and specific sensitivities is required before treatment can be begun.

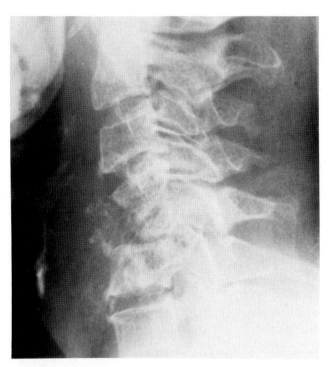

Figure 41.6. Plain film showing destruction of C4 and C5 with disc space collapse and with prevertebral soft-tissue mass with calcification in a patient with TB of the spine and adjacent abscess.

CT scanning at this stage, once the disease is localized accurately with conventional radiology, is of help in certain specific instances:

1. In areas difficult to visualize with conventional radiology, CT is superb in showing both the extent and amount of bone destruction. It is also very accurate in depicting paraspinal soft-tissue abscesses. This is particularly important in the upper cervical spine region and also at the cervicothoracic junction (Figs. 41.19 and 41.20). However, because CT is the best radiographic examination for evaluating the paraspinal spaces, it is also important in every other region of the spine. Axial and coronal views are unequalled in their ability to demonstrate the extent of paraspinal disease (Fig. 41.21).

2. CT shows not only the extent of bone and soft-tissue involvement but also the location of adjacent vital structures which may be distorted by soft-tissue involvement.

3. CT detects soft-tissue calcifications which may not be evident on plain films.

4. CT in spinal sepsis aides in the detection of associated nonspinal sites of disease. For example, CT shows intracranial tuberculomas that might exist in association with spinal TB (Fig. 41.22).

5. High-resolution CT often is able to demonstrate the intraspinal soft tissues without the need for enhancement except where previous arachnoiditis, previous surgery, or extensive disease has considerably distorted the normal anatomy. However, in parients with neurological deficit and in those in whom surgical intervention is planned intrathecal contrast should be used. A conventional myelogram should be obtained in these cases followed by a metrizamide CT scan. The latter procedure will optimally delineate intraspinal disease and determine whether it is of a bony or soft-tissue nature (Figs. 41.23 and 41.24).

Another major benefit of CT scanning is in the planning of operative procedures. It is here that CT scanning, at least to the practicing orthopaedic surgeon, has its greatest practical application. CT scanning allows the accurate evaluation of the extent of the disease, the amount of soft-tissue involvement and the location of other structures in relation to the primary disease pathology. In TB, the vertebral bodies may look surprisingly normal on conventional radiology and yet the entire cancellous bone may be replaced by granulation tissue.

CT scanning allows planning of percutaneous needle biopsies with a high degree of accuracy and with little risk to the adjoining structures (Figs. 41.25 and 41.26). Similarly, in planning the operative approach, CT scanning is valuable in deciding whether to approach the spine from anterior or posterior. The choice of a right or left approach can be made accurately on the CT scan. In the anterior approach, the spine should be approached from the side most involved, leaving as much viable bone intact on the opposite side as possible. This partially helps to stabilize the spine and to allow more rapid incorporation of bone graft.

Surgical Indications in Spinal Sepsis

Surgery in the patient with vertebral sepsis takes one of two forms. The first is needle aspiration of the body or disc involved. This can be done in two ways. The simplest is fine-needle aspiration without utilizing anesthesia. An 18- or 20-gauge spinal needle is introduced into the soft-tissue abscess or disc space involved and material aspirated for culture, sensitivity, and pathology. This is most applicable where a soft-tissue abscess exists or where the disc space primarily is involved. This does not require admission to the hospital; it has not been associated with morbidity or mortality; and it has been very accurate in cases where aspiratable soft tissue exists. This usually is done under image intensifier control but can be done with ultrasound where a large abscess exists and also with CT.

The second operative approach requires general anesthesia and the use of image intensification. A large trocar or trephine biopsy with a 2- to 3-mm trocar is introduced about 6–7 cm lateral to the midline posteriorly usually under general anesthesia. Four to five cores at different sites in the body are taken for pathology, culture, and sensitivity and special studies. This is most valuable where disease is localized to a vertebral body and where fine-needle aspiration does not yield sufficient tissue. Fine-needle aspiration has a negligible morbidity and can be done as an outpatient procedure. Large bore trocar biopsies do require admission to hospital, do require general anesthesia, but to date we have had no serious morbidity nor mortality from that procedure. The yield from trocar biopsy has been very good and diagnosis usually can be made in these cases. We now reserve open biopsy for those cases where biopsy is to be combined with

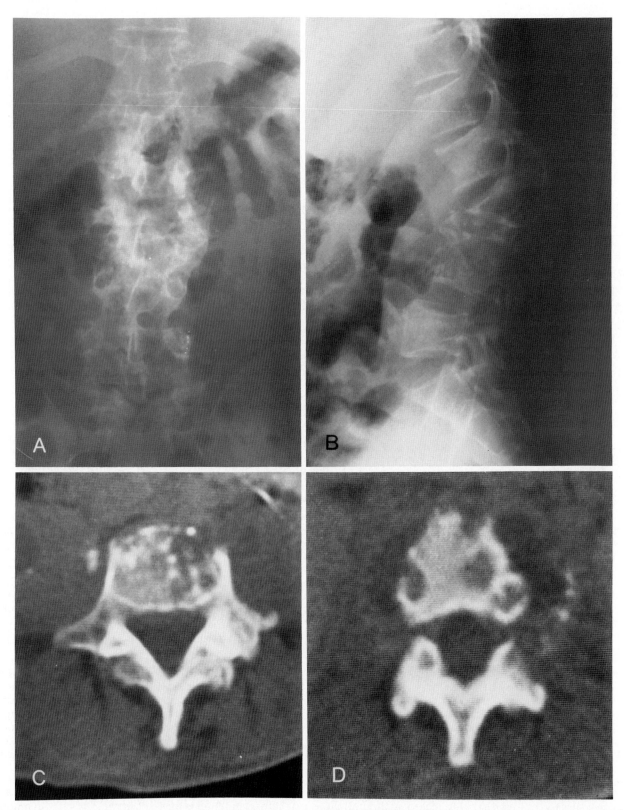

Figure 41.7. A and B. AP and lateral plain films showing destruction of multiple vertebrae, disc space collapse, and marked gibbus deformity in a patient with TB of the lumbar spine. C and D. CT images demonstrating bilateral paraspinal abscesses with calcifications as well as bone destruction. (Case courtesy of M.J.D. Post, M.D., Miami, FL).

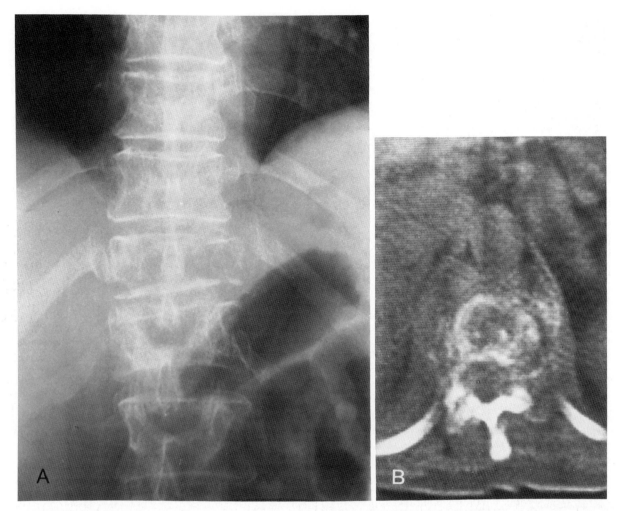

Figure 41.8. A. TB affecting body of T11 and T12 in a 70-year-old lady. Paraparetic on admission. Myelogram showed a complete extradural block. B. CT scan of 11th thoracic body. Soft-tissue paraspinal abscess with new bone in abscess. Aorta pushed anteriorly. Soft-tissue granulation tissue around cord. No evidence of sequestered bone. Complete recovery on antituberculous medications without surgery.

another operative procedure. Generally, this occurs in those cases where decompression and stabilization are to be performed at the same time. It is in these cases that CT scanning is most helpful both in planning the operative procedure and in deciding which cases should and should not undergo surgical decompression.

My personal treatment protocol in spinal sepsis:

1. Fine-needle aspiration is performed now almost routinely as an outpatient procedure in patients presenting with spinal sepsis where the diagnosis is still in doubt after the above-mentioned hematological, biochemical, and radiographic investigations.

2. Large bore trocar biopsy under general anesthesia or neuroleptic using image intensification when a patient presents with a spinal lesion, the etiology of which is still in doubt after fine-needle aspiration and the above investigation. These patients usually present with minimal or no neurological impairment and on presentation are not likely to suffer from spinal instability in the future. Spinal instability covers a whole spectrum of presentations but

generally disease at the C1-C2 level or at the cervicothoracic junction with a great deal of bone loss are areas where the risk of subsequent instability and/or kyphus is so high that in my opinion these lesions should be stabilized primarily.

3. Open biopsy is reserved for those cases where—a. there is severe neurological impairment and biopsy is being combined with anterior decompression and fusion; b. where spinal instability either exists or is a threat in the near future. This is most important in the upper cervical spine where instability occurs rapidly and often with fatal results. c. where there has been a failure of adequate medical treatment either because of persisting abscesses or because of sequestered bone or disc.

There is a tremendous debate in the literture now as to whether spinal TB is treated best with or without anterior decompression and fusion. I personally believe that if paraparesis or paraplegia is due to sequestered bone or disc, then no amount of conservative treatment will alleviate this bony block and correct the cause of the neuro-

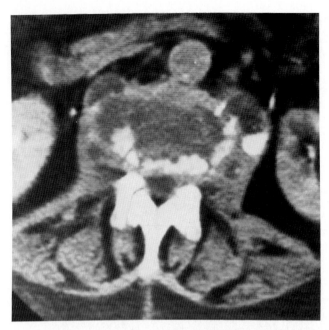

Figure 41.9. CT scan showing paraspinal abscesses with calcification, bone destruction, and disc space involvement at the L2-L3 level in a patient with biopsy proven TB (Case courtesy of M.J.D. Post, M.D., Miami, FL).

logical impairment. In these cases, CT scanning has been extremely valuable in identifying those cases presenting with paraplegia due to granulation tissue or pressure from an abscess alone. In this group, conservative treatment is generally very successful. If CT scanning reveals that there is posteriorly displaced pieces of bone or disc, then in this group I recommend immediate anterior decompression. Before the introduction of CT scanning in this group, myelography usually revealed a total block but gave no information as to the etiology of that block. It would show the extent but not the etiology of the disease. CT scanning is extremely valuable in showing bone and disc protrusion back into the canal and in differentiating these from other causes of obstruction. Sagittally reconstructed views also show the extent of this block. In those cases presenting with paraparesis without complete paraplegia and where CT scanning suggests the cause is soft-tissue abscess rather than mechanical obstruction due to sequestered bone and disc, then a supervised trial of chemotherapy alone often leads to rapid resolution of neurological deficits.

Many of our patients in their 7th or 8th decades present not only with spinal disease but also with severe osteoporosis. The risks of thoracotomy in these patients is appreciable and the chance of graft failure is high. Many of these patients present with severe neurological impairment and spinal sepsis, although suspected, is often but one of a list of possible diagnoses including metabolic disease, primary and secondary tumors, and the like. After the routine hematological and biochemical examinations, CT scanning, metrizamide myelography, and tomography as indicated, we have been able to predict with a high degree of accuracy which patients will or will not require

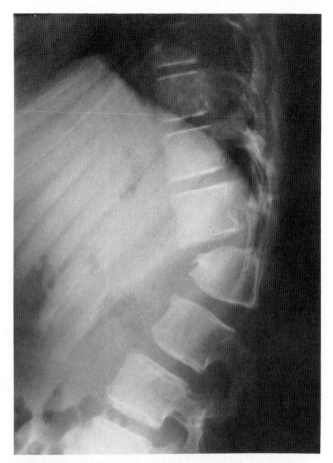

Figure 41.10. Plain film showing anterior deformity and complete loss of the posterior elements of T12, subluxation, and kyphus in a 13-year-old female with spinal TB.

surgical decompression. Trocar needle biopsy is the usual diagnostic procedure of choice in those cases where open surgical biopsy is not indicated and is of greatest value in the elderly patient with spinal TB and minimum neurological impairment.

CT scanning with its almost negligible risk of complications is now widely used in the follow-up of the patient with spinal sepsis. It is of greatest value in those areas most difficult to see with conventional radiography, e.g., at the cervical-thoracic junction and upper cervical spine.

Secondly, it is of great value in areas where myelography is of little value, specifically in patients with previous arachnoiditis, patients with allergy to contrast, and in those patients with previous surgery or disease that make it difficult to interpret a myelogram. With CT scanning, the size of soft-tissue abscess can be assessed to quantitate response to treatment and to assess the decompression achieved at surgery. Its greatest postoperative value is where there is some question as to the adequacy of anterior decompression or where there is a doubt as to the position of the strut graft. This is most important in cases which respond slowly after surgical decompression and where the graft placement and adequacy of decompression are in question.

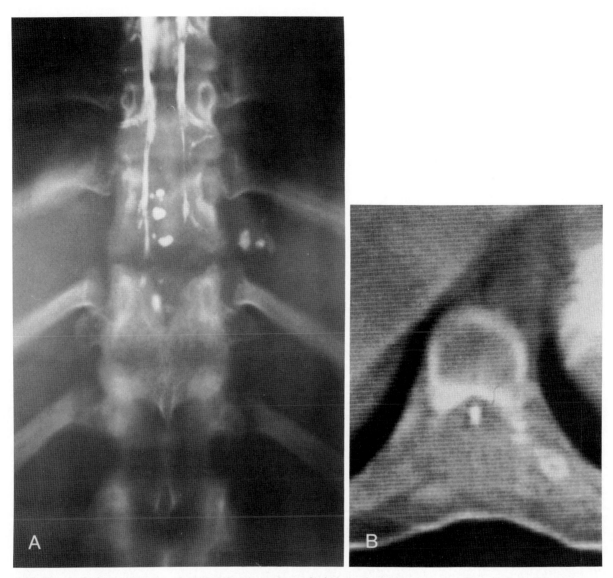

Figure 41.11. A. Ewings sarcoma—tomography shows loss of inferior articular facets and pedicles T10. B. CT scan—complete loss of posterior elements of T10. Surgical approach posteriorly for biopsy.

One of the most difficult problems facing the clinician is the patient presenting following discotomy with increasing back pain. The specter of postoperative discitis is always present but the diagnosis is often difficult to confirm. All the changes seen on conventional roentgenograms can be attributed to postsurgical changes. Suspicion often is raised by persistent or increasing pain and a rising sedimentation rate. CT scanning in these cases will show an enlarging soft-tissue abscess which may not be apparent on plain roentgenograms. Often, only repeat films or repeat CT scanning will establish the diagnosis but the final diagnosis, specifically the causative organisms, usually depends upon the securing of tissue for microscopic and bacteriological examination, (Fig. 41.27).

A suggested protocol for the investigation of the patient with spinal sepsis:

1. A complete history with emphasis on recent surgery

or trauma to the gynecological or urological systems. The high association between pyogenic spondylitis and urinary tract manipulation is well-documented (4, 12, 13).

2. Physical examination directed toward the spine, specifically pain, abscesses, sinuses, kyphosis, etc. Complete assessment of the neurological status to ascertain the spinal level involved. This will act as a baseline for future follow-up, both in the surgical and nonsurgically treated patient.

3. Hematological work-up to include complete blood count, sedimentation rate, SMAC 20. Tuberculin skin testing, febrile agglutinins for Brucella and Salmonella, sickle cell test as indicated, and the like. Blood cultures are taken during the febrile stage. Serological testing for Salmonella and Staphylococcus as indicated. Special tests as indicated, e.g., acid phosphatase, serum thyroid, etc. if tumor is clinically suspected.

4. Plain roentgenograms are taken of the involved area, augmented by CT scanning and tomography as required.

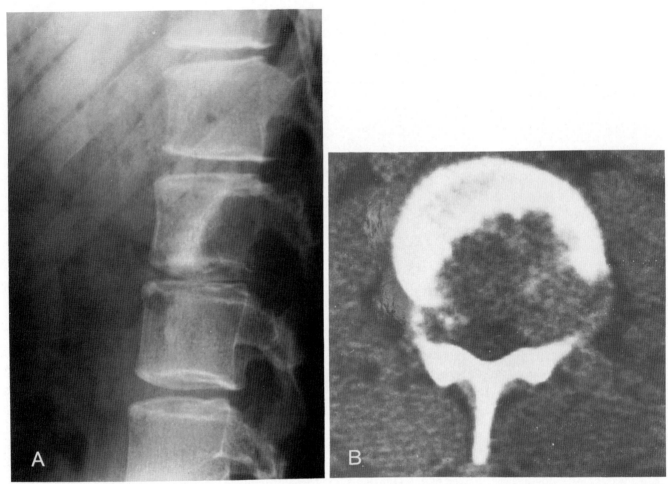

Figure 41.12. A. plain film showing an aneurysmal bone cyst involving body of L1 with paraparesis. Myelogram both lumbar and cisternal showed complete obstruction. B. CT scan showing destruction of body of L1 plus pedicles.

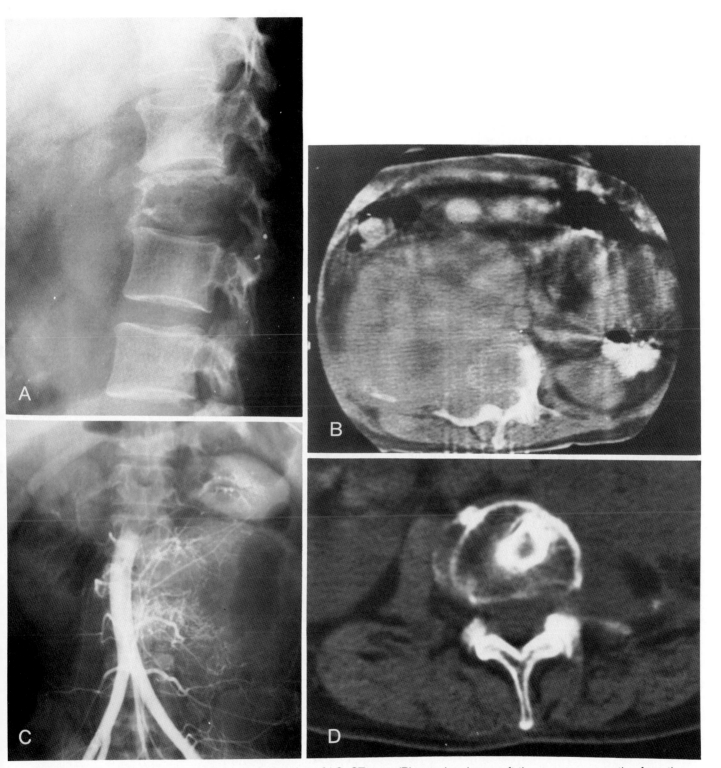

Figure 41.13. Plain film (A) shows bone destruction of L2. CT scan (B) reveals a large soft-tissue mass emanating from the eroded L2 vertebral body and posterior elements. Angiogram (C) shows abnormal vascularity, stretching, and displacement of vessels and deviation of the left kidney superiorly. Surgical diagnosis: Aneurysmal bone cyst. CT scan postoperatively (D) confirms the correct position of a strut graft that was placed between the vertebral bodies for stability.

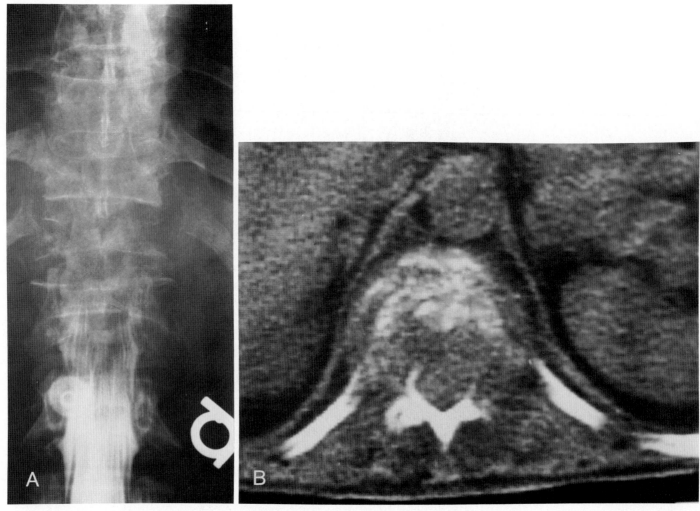

Figure 41.14. Metastatic adenocarcinoma simulating spinal infection. AP myelogram (A) show a complete extradural block and marked bone destruction of T10, T11, T12, and L1. Axial CT scan (B) demonstrates erosion of the vertebral body and posterior elements and extension of the soft-tissue component of the tumor into the spinal canal.

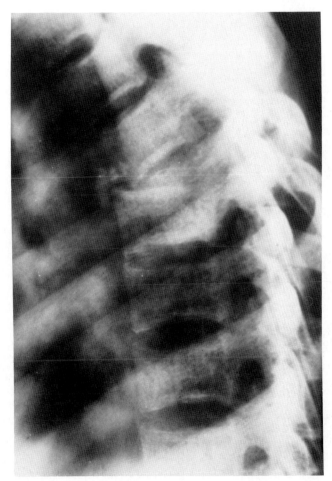

Figure 41.15.   Plain film showing destruction of T6, disc space collapse, and spinal angulation. These abnormalities were not secondary to spinal infection but to a paraganglioneuroma of T6 in a 26-year-old female.

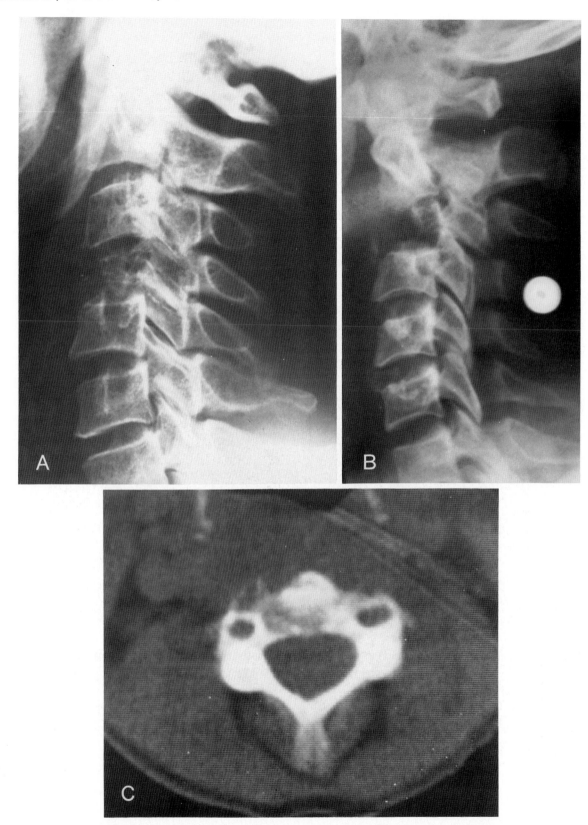

Figure 41.16.   A. Multiple myeloma C4. Difficult to diagnose on plain film alone. B. TB C3. C. CT scan of TB of C3. Same patient as B. Bone erosion, prevertebral abscess. New bone formation indicative of TB seen on other images.

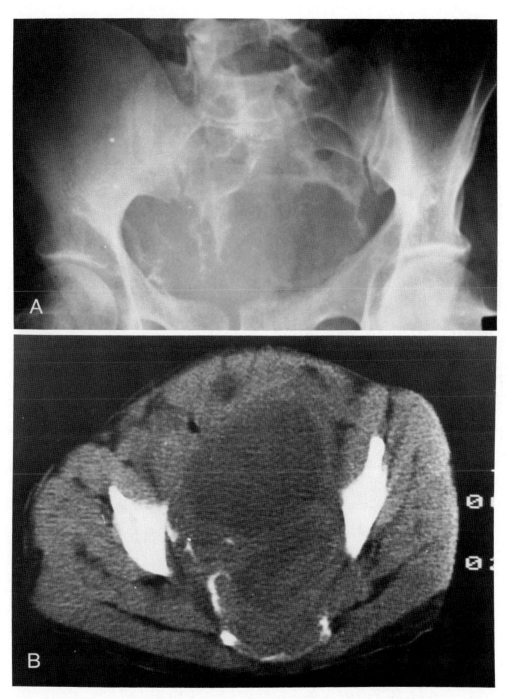

Figure 41.17.   Plain film in a patient with a giant cell tumor of the sacrum. Shows erosion of the sacrum, calcifications, and an increase in soft-tissue density in the pelvis. CT scan (B), however, delineates to much better advantage the soft-tissue mass and the bone destruction.

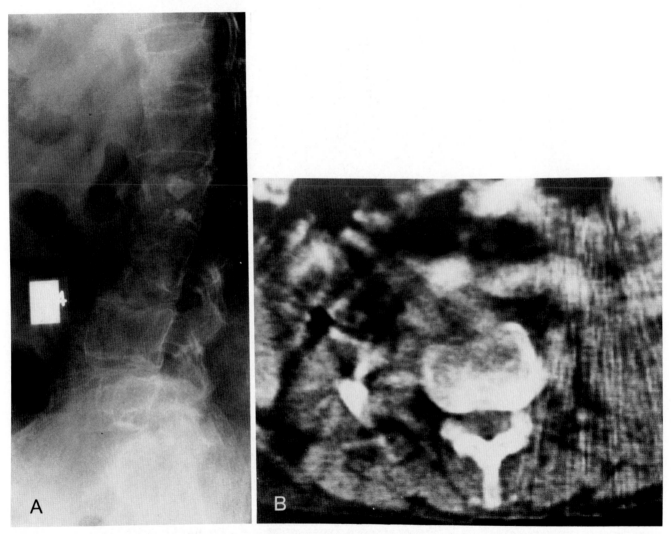

Figure 41.18. A. Severe osteoporosis due to prolonged recumbency after hip fracture. Bodies of L2, L3, and L5 eroded anteriorly. B. CT scan showing minimal anterior changes of lumbar spine.

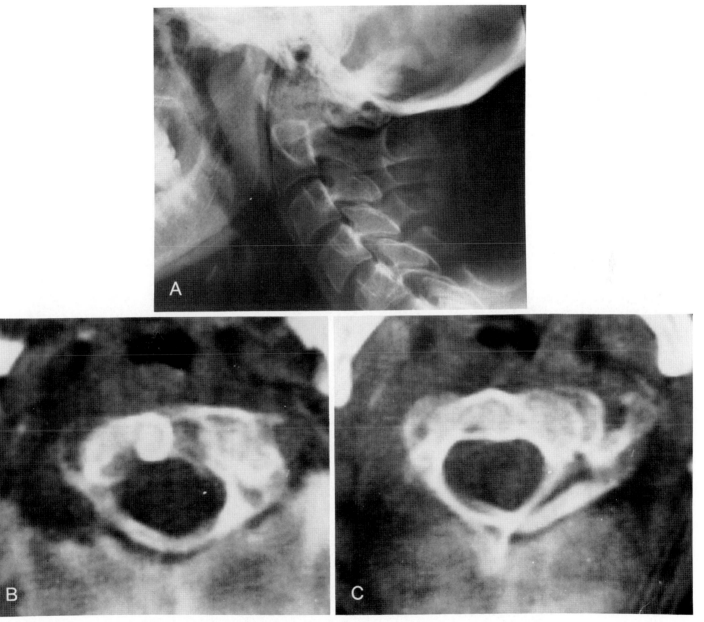

Figure 41.19. Prevertebral soft-tissue swelling adjacent to C1 seen on plain film (A) and on CT scan (B and C). CT also shows rotary subluxation of C1 on C2 in this patient with TB of C1.

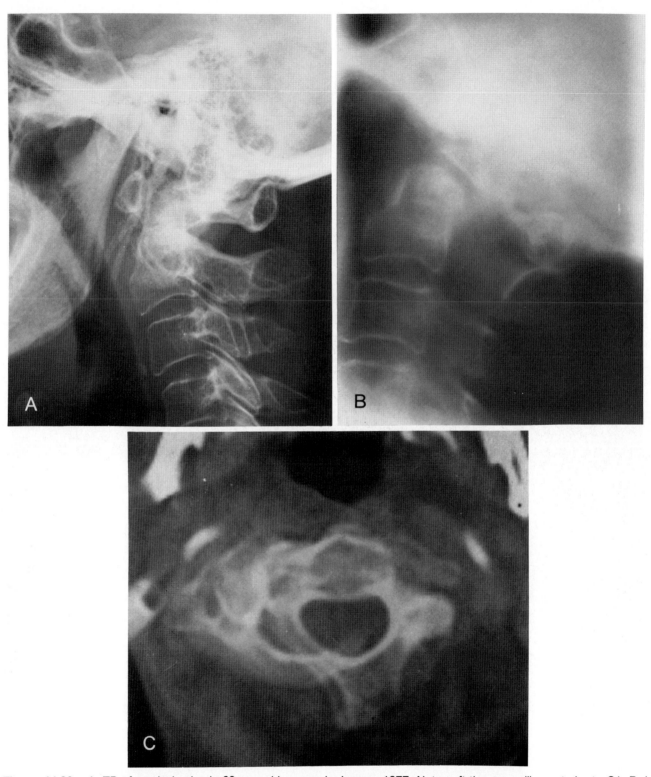

Figure 41.20.   A. TB of cervical spine in 69-year-old woman in January 1977. Note soft-tissue swelling anterior to C1. B. In January 1979, the same patient, 2 years later. Tomograms reveal complete destruction of C1. Patient had received no treatment. C. CT scan showing bone destruction, rotary subluxation, and prevertebral soft-tissue mass.

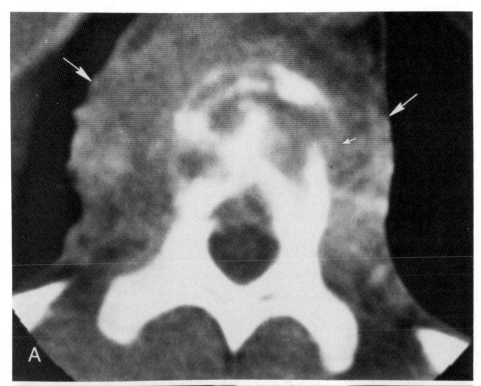

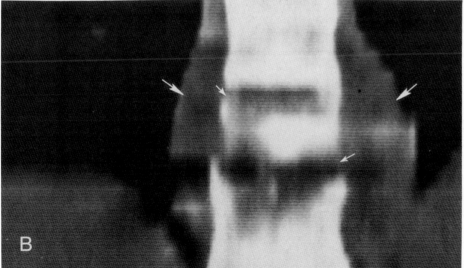

Figure 41.21. Axial (A) and coronally reconstructed (B) intravenously enhanced CT scans show destruction of two contiguous vertebral bodies (*small arrows*) and bilateral paraspinal masses (*large arrows*) consistent with abscesses. Pyogenic osteomyelitis confirmed at surgery. (Case courtesy of M.J.D. Post, M.D., Miami, FL).

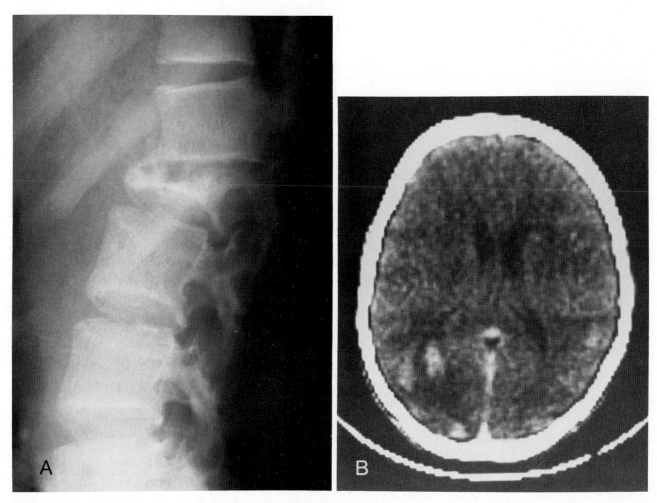

Figure 41.22. A. Plain film of a 16-year-old young lady with tuberculosis L1 who presented with seizure disorder. B. Intracranial tuberculomas posterior parietal-occipital areas.

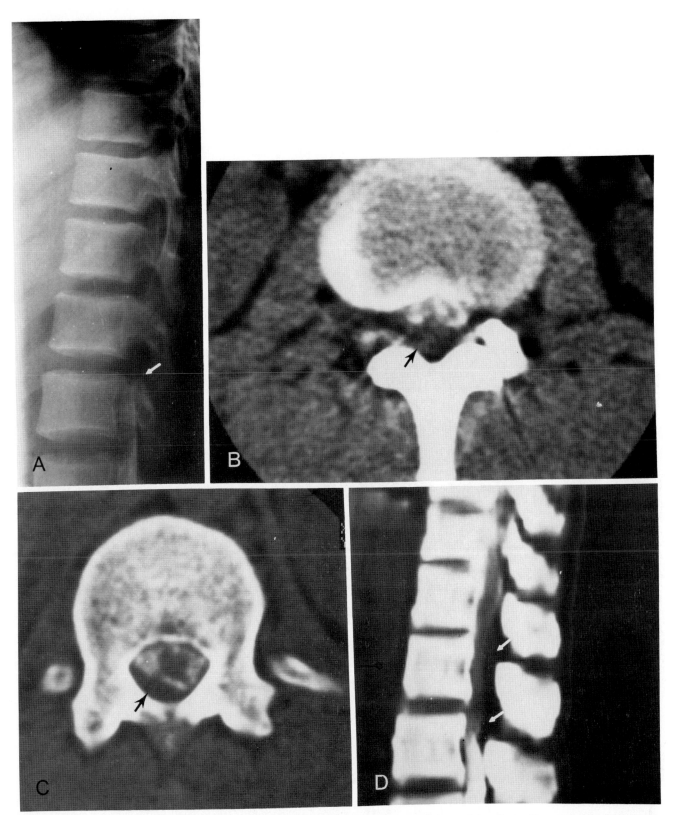

Figure 41.23. A 32-year-old male with a history of intravenous drug abuse with bacterial endocarditis secondary to Staphylococcus aureus and with the sudden onset of weakness in both lower extremities, urinary retention, and fecal incontinence. A metrizamide meylogram (A) revealed a partial right posterolateral extradural block at L2-L3 (*arrow*). No bone destruction or disc space narrowing was seen. A metrizamide CT scan in axial (B and C) and sagittally reconstructed (D) views showed a soft-tissue epidural right posterolateral mass (*arrows*, B–D), compressing the subarachnoid sac and extending from L2–L3 to T10, findings consistent with an epidural abscess from involvement of posterior epidural veins. At surgery, a T10 to L3 Staphylococcal aureus epidural abscess was removed. (Case courtesy of M.J.D. Post, M.D., Miami, FL).

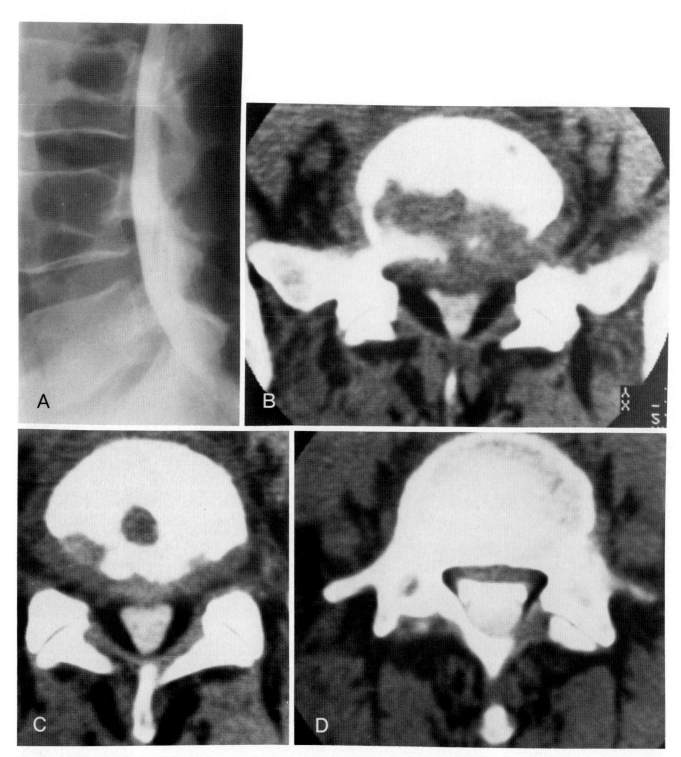

Figure 41.24.   A. Metrizamide meylogram showing a wide insensitive epidural space L4 to S1. Bone erosion at L5 and S1 difficult to appreciate. B–D. Metrizamide CT scans. L5–S1 bone destruction is readily apparent. Soft-tissue component of this chronic Staphylococcal aureus osteomyelitis is seen extending into the capacious epidural space from S1 to L4. (Case courtesy of M.J.D. Post, M.D., Miami, FL).

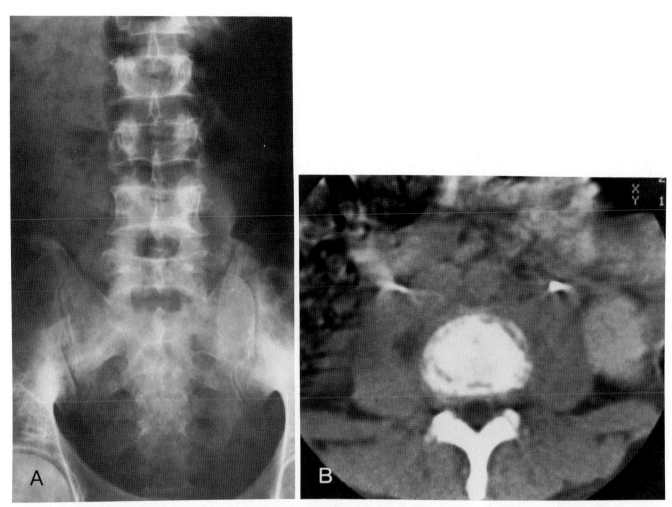

Figure 41.25. A. Loss of height of L3 and L5 seen on the plain film of a sickler with fever, chills, and back pain. B. Plain high-resolution CT showing L3 bone destruction with bilateral paraspinal abscesses. Guided by CT findings biopsy was obtained of paraspinal abscess and of bone. Diagnosis: Salmonella, type B osteomyelitis. (Case courtesy of M.J.D. Post, M.D., Miami, FL).

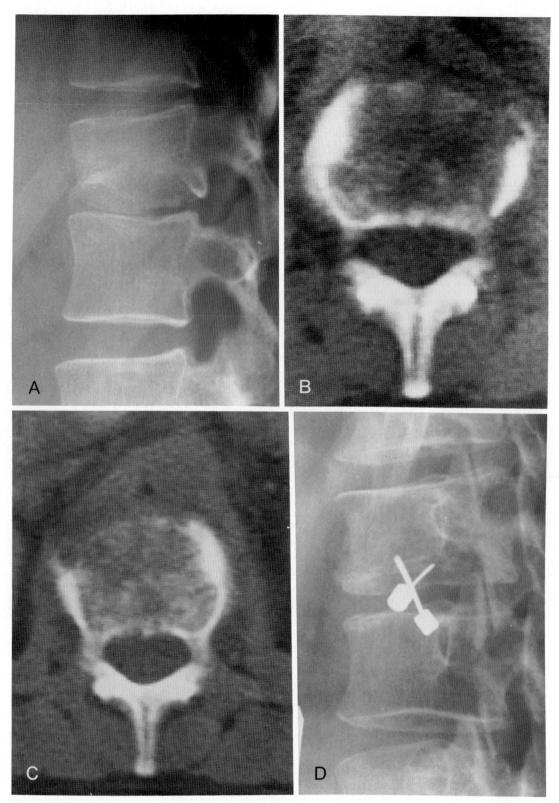

Figure 41.26. A. Early tuberculous changes at L1. B and C. CT Scans of L1 showing destruction of cancellous body of L1. D. Biopsy under fluoroscopic control.

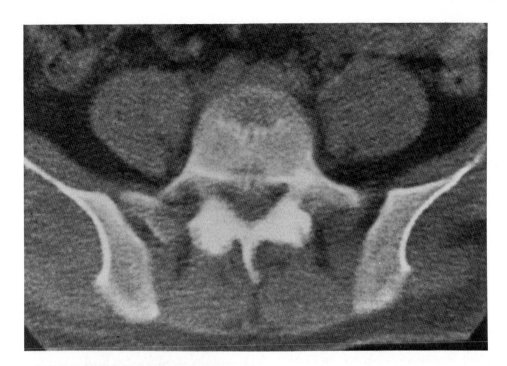

Figure 41.27. Postdiscotomy sepsis—Staphylococcal aureus. Minimal soft-tissue abscess and bone erosion.

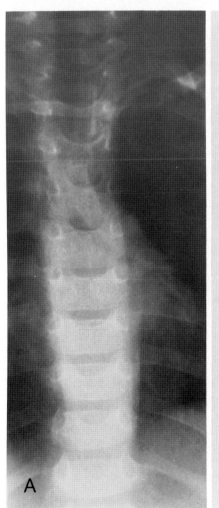

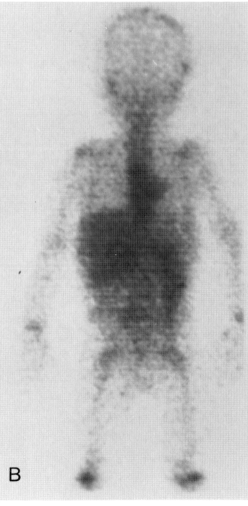

A

B

Figure 41.28. Plain film (A) and gallium scan (B) in a 4-year-male with Staphylococcal aureus septicemia. A small paraspinal abscess in the thoracic spine is detected on the gallium scan.

A plain CT scan is usually sufficient if the patient has no neurological deficit. Myelography is performed for all cases with neurological impairment or where surgery is contemplated. After myelography, a metrizamide CT scan is obtained. Bone scanning is only utilized if there is a suspicion of other bone foci or if no definite bone foci can be seen on conventional radiographs. In our hands, gallium scanning has been only very occasionally rewarding (Fig. 41.28).

5. After the above work-up, percutaneous fine-needle aspiration is performed under image intensification, usually at the same time as myelography, if the lesion involves a disc space or where a soft-tissue abscess is seen. Fine-needle aspiration, as mentioned previously, is done with an 18-gauge spinal needle introduced lateral to the midline and placed into the abscess. Material then is aspirated for culture, sensitivity, smears, and pathology, if possible.

Surgical intervention, whether by trocar biopsy or by open surgical decompression, is reserved for those cases where:

1. no definite diagnosis can be made after the above investigation;
2. there is severe neurological impairment from disease at any spinal level and CT scanning suggests this is related to either sequestered bone or disc. Occasionally, where CT scanning plus myelography suggests the cause of obstruction is due to tissue granulation or due to pressure from an abscess, we will place the patient on a carefully supervised program of conservative treatment for a period of 3–4 weeks. If the condition worsens in this period of time, or if there is a question as to the adequacy of our diagnosis, then surgery is indicated.
3. when an adequate course of medical treatment has failed to alleviate clinical symptoms in a reasonable period of time;
4. where there is either early or late spinal instability, especially in the cervical and upper thoracic spine and in cases with loss of three or more vertebral bodies;
5. where late kyphosis has developed with increasing neurological sequellae, I suggest this needs immediate correction of the kyphosis, decompression, and anterior fusion.

Conservative treatment is utilized initially for most cases, but all such cases are followed closely for deterioration.

CONCLUSION

CT scanning, especially with the high-resolution CT scanners now available, does have a definite place in the diagnosis, treatment, and long-term follow-up of the patient with spinal sepsis. Its major advantages are:

1. It detects osseous and soft-tissue changes secondary to inflammatory disease of the spine and determines the extent of disease.
2. It delineates paraspinal and intraspinal soft-tissue involvement better than any other radiographic study and shows the effect of inflammatory spine disease on adjacent vital structures.
3. It demonstrates the inflammatory disease in three dimensions and determines whether any decrease in the sagittal or transverse diameter of the spinal canal has been caused by the disease.
4. It helps the clinician plan an accurate surgical approach as to anterior or posterior, right or left, in relation to the vertebral body and in relation to the area of greatest disease involvement. It also shows associated disease in other parts of the body and brain.
5. It allows one to follow the clinical course of treatment accurately both with and without surgical intervention.

References

1. Smith EG, Dawson WR: *Egyptian Mummies.* London, 1924, p. 157.
2. Pott P: *Remarks on that kind of Palsy of the Lower Limbs which is Frequently Found to Accompany a Curvature of the Spine.* London, J. Johnson, 1779.
3. Martin JS: Tuberculosis of the spine. *J Bone Joint Surg.* 52:623–28, 1970.
4. Medical Research Council: A controlled trial of ambulant outpatient treatment and inpatient rest in bed in the management of tuberculosis of the spine in young Korean patients on standard chemotherapy. A study in Masan Korea. *J Bone Joint Surg* 55:678–97, 1973.
5. Medical Research Council: A controlled trial of debridement and ambulatory treatment in the management of tuberculosis of the spine in patients on standard chemotherapy. A Study in Botswano, Rhodesia. *J Trop Med Hyg* 77:72–97, 1974.
6. Medical Research Council: A controlled trial of anterior spinal fusion and debridement in the surgical management of tuberculosis of the spine in patients on standard chemotherapy. A study in Hong Kong. *Br J Surg* 61:853–66, 1974.
7. Martin, NS: Pott's Paraplegia: A report on 120 cases. *J Bone Joint Surg* 53B:596–608, 1971.
8. Kemp VB, Jackson JW, Jeremiah JD, et al: Anterior fusion of the spine for infective lesions in adults. *J Bone Joint Surg* 55:715–34, 1973.
9. Stone DB, Bonfiglio M: Pyogenic vertebral osteomyelitis. *Arch Intern Med* 112:491, 1963.
10. Hodgson AR: In: Rothman-Simeone; *The Spine.* Philadelphia, W. B. Saunders Co, 1975, p. 570.
11. Henrigues, CQ: Osteomyelitis as a complication of urology. *Br J Surg* 46:19–28, 1958.
12. Batson OU: The function of the vertebral veins and their role in the spread of metastasis. *Ann Surg* 112:138, 1940.
13. Henson SW Jr, Coventry MB: Osteomyelitis of the vertebrae as a result of infection of the urinary tract. *Surg Gynecol Obstet* 102:207, 1956.

CHAPTER FORTY-TWO

Computed Tomography of Spinal Trauma

M. JUDITH DONOVAN POST, M.D.*

INTRODUCTION

Computed tomography (CT) should be included as part of the standard radiographic work-up of patients with spinal trauma. It should be used whether or not there is acute or chronic injury, neurological deficit or nonfocal examination, soft-tissue or bony damage, penetrating or closed trauma. Its routine application is warranted because CT maximizes patient safety and comfort while providing information that cannot be obtained with conventional radiographic studies.

ADVANTAGES OF CT

The unique advantages offered by CT include the following:

1. CT requires minimal patient manipulation and, therefore, is safer for the spinal trauma victim than other radiographic procedures.

2. CT is quick, easy to perform, and comfortable.

3. CT is less invasive than myelography.

4. CT provides a cross-sectional view of the spine which is optimal for detecting and localizing bony ring fractures (Figs. 42.1–42.6), displaced bone fragments (Figs. 42.7–42.12), and bullet fragments (Figs. 42.13–42.15) which may be missed on other studies.

5. CT enables multiple projections of the spine to be obtained without additional patient movement or radiation exposure (Fig. 42.7).

6. CT evaluates the osseous spine as well as the paraspinal (Fig. 42.2D) and intraspinal soft tissues.

7. CT examines other parts of the body and brain without necessitating additional procedures.

* Gratitude is expressed to Barth Green, M.D. and Frank Eismont, M.D. from the Departments of Neurological Surgery and Orthopaedics and Rehabilitation, University of Miami School of Medicine; to Chris Fletcher for the fine photographic prints; to Louise Rhodes, Paula Garcia, Maria Gajardo, Yolanda Marin, and Tamera Johnson for the excellent secretarial assistance.

LITERATURE REVIEW

These advantages of CT in spinal trauma and the limitations of traditional radiographic studies have been documented in the literature (1–42). Various reports have cited the ability of CT to detect fractures of the spine, even those missed by plain films and occasionally by tomograms, such as some posterior arch fractures (4, 7, 9, 11, 16, 18–21, 23, 25, 30, 31, 34). In particular, cervical fractures diagnosed by CT, especially at the C1-C2 level, have received considerable attention (2–4, 8, 9, 12, 18, 20–22, 24, 31, 33).

The advantages of CT's cross-sectional view of the spine in assessing the size, configuration, and integrity of the spinal canal also have been described (2, 4, 8, 10, 11, 13, 18, 25, 27, 28, 30, 32). Cases in which CT, often in contrast to conventional radiography, has detected bone fragments displaced into the canal with secondary canal narrowing have served to illustrate the value of the axial projection of CT (4, 6, 7, 10, 11, 16, 18–23, 27, 28, 30–32, 42). So too have diagnoses made by axial CT of spinal instability, facet distraction, rotatory subluxation without or with fixation, and stenosis secondary to fracture-subluxations superimposed on congenital anomalies of the spine (2, 5, 12, 14, 18, 20–22, 28, 31). Although not mentioned often in the literature, the axial view afforded by CT also has been advocated for localizing foreign bodies, such as bullet fragments, within the spinal canal, lateral recesses, and adjacent body and brain (16, 22, 29, 30, 32, 34).

The benefit of other CT projections has not gone unrecognized, however. Sagittal-coronal reconstructions have been found useful in the diagnosis not only of fractures (especially horizontal ones), but also of subluxations, displaced fractured fragments and traumatic kyphoses (6, 14, 18, 20, 22, 25, 28, 34, 35). Canal measurements derived from CT images have also been documented as an aid to the diagnosis of traumatic spinal stenosis (2, 6, 11, 35). Recently, Brant-Zawadzki et al. have described the advantages of multiplanar reformation (23).

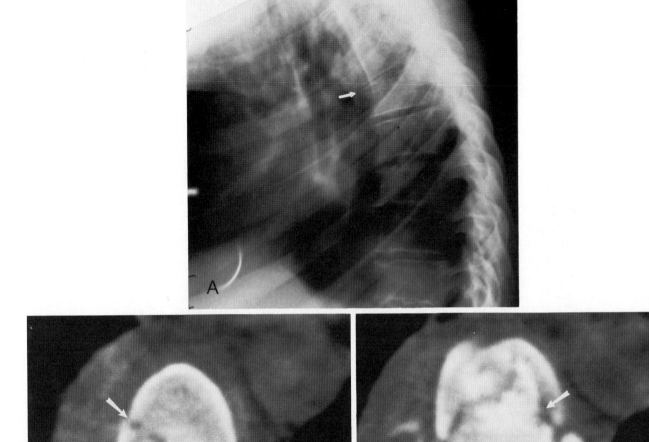

Figure 42.1. Diagnosis of Posterior Arch Fractures by CT: Plain films demonstrated the fracture of the T6 (*arrow*, A) and adjacent vertebral bodies but failed to show the posterior arch fractures. In contrast CT delineated not only the vertebral body compression fractures (*large arrows*, B and C) but also the fractures through the T6 laminae and spinous process (*small arrows*, B and C). CT also demonstrated mild bony impingement on the metrizamide-filled subarachnoid sac (*arrowheads*, B and C), a right paraspinal hematoma, and small pleural effusions.

Although receiving less attention than CT of acute fractures, CT of chronic fractures, and CT of the postoperative spine have been described as well. Faerber et al. (20) reported a case in which the spinal canal was narrowed because of bone proliferation that had occurred about an old fracture of C1. McInerney and Sage (21) reported the CT diagnosis of an old ununited fracture of C1 and the persistence of a bone fragment trapped between the articular mass and the odontoid process. The CT detection of a fracture through a fusion, unrecognized on conventional radiographs, was recorded by Roub and Drayer (19). Other authors have described the use of CT for determining if all bony fragments have been successfully removed from the spinal canal at surgery and for evaluating the position of bone grafts and Harrington rods following surgery for spinal trauma (16, 18, 19, 21, 24, 27, 29, 31, 34).

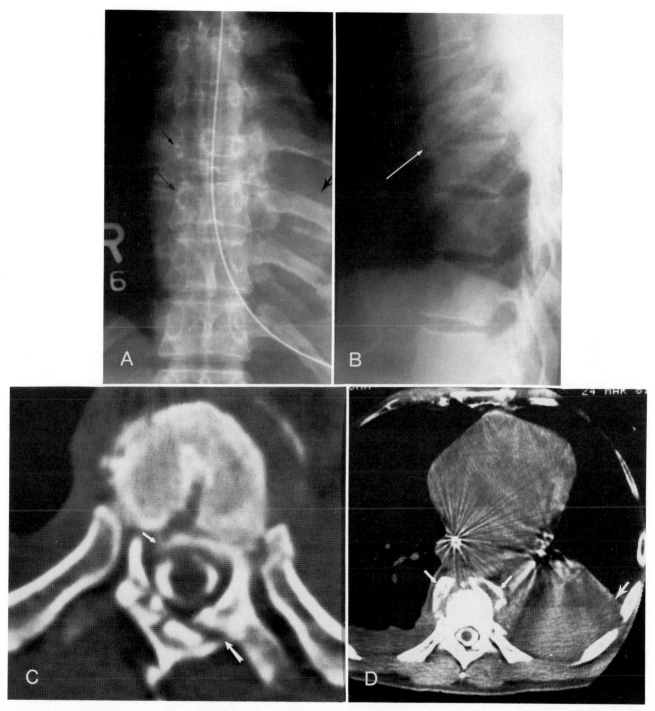

Figure 42.2. Diagnosis of Posterior Arch Fractures and Adjacent Hemothorax by CT: Plain films were reliable in localizing the spinal injury to the T7 and T8 vertebral bodies (*thin arrows*, A and B). They also showed a large left paraspinal density (*thick arrow*, A). The CT scan, however, showed to best advantage the anterior and posterior displacement of the vertebral body fragments (*small arrows*, C and D) and the posterior arch fractures (*large arrow*, C). In addition, it revealed that the left paraspinal mass was being caused by a large left hemothorax. Notice the fluid level (*large arrow*, D) which was caused by degenerating blood several days old. This hemothorax was drained at surgery. (See also Fig. 42.17).

CT also has been cited for its ability in spinal trauma to assess the intraspinal and paraspinal soft tissues. Intramedullary hematomas seen on CT have been reported by Lee et al. (10), by Roub and Drayer (19), and by Post (34). Tadmor et al. (8) thought that because the spinal cord, the

spinal canal, and the adjacent bone could all be imaged simply by altering the window settings, that CT could be used to determine whether or not a hematoma was present. Faerber et al., however, doubted whether all hematomas could be discerned by CT (20). Other authors, on

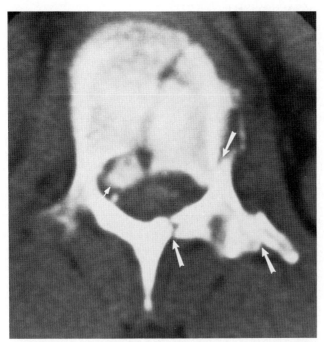

Figure 42.3. CT Demonstration of Posterior Arch Fractures: Axial CT scan demonstrating well not only the lumbar vertical body fractures but also the posterior arch fractures (*large arrows*) and the intraspinal bone fragments (*small arrow*).

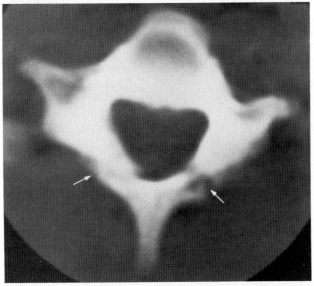

Figure 42.4. CT Demonstration of Cervical Posterior Arch Fractures: Plain CT scan demonstrating fractures of the laminae of C7 (*arrows*) which were not evident on plain films.

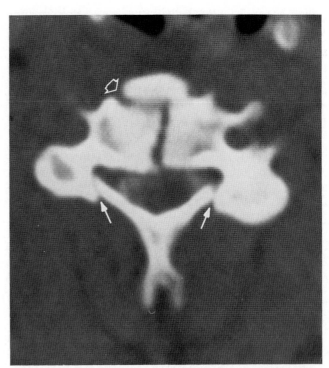

Figure 42.5. CT Demonstration of an Unstable C5 Fracture: Metrizamide CT scan showing fractures of the C5 vertebral body (*arrowhead*) and laminae (*arrows*), the latter not well seen on plain films, with secondary C5-C6 subluxation. Mild compression of the ventral subarachnoid sac secondary to the fracture subluxation as well as some cord swelling also evident. These latter findings were not demonstrated well on the standard myelogram performed in the supine position. [Reproduced with permission from Post et al. (16).]

differentiated from cord hematoma. Seibert et al. reported the use of CT in making the diagnosis of post-traumatic syrinx (26). Colley et al. thought that the spinal cord and cauda equinae could be assessed by CT (11). Miller mentioned that CT could demonstrate the position and configuration of the thecal sac (25). Naidich et al., although describing the limited ability of nonhigh-resolution CT (HRCT) scans to assess intraspinal soft tissues, also reported that the spinal cord and subarachnoid sac could be demonstrated with HRCT and that the diagnostic potential of CT, therefore, was increased in spinal trauma (22). Post similarly mentioned the limitations of non-HRCT scanning in the evaluation of intraspinal soft tissues in trauma (30), but also stressed the ability of HRCT to visualize the intraspinal soft tissues and, therefore, to diagnose traumatic intraspinal soft-tissue abnormalities (34). Roub and Drayer also described limitations to the CT delineation of intraspinal abnormalities (19). They suggested the use of CT gas myelography as a means of discerning the exact cause of myelographic block in trauma. Coin et al. reported a case in which the plain CT nicely delineated a cervical fracture but did not demonstrate an associated herniated disc (18). A subsequent metrizamide CT scan, however, delineated this soft-tissue abnormality. Other authors have also reported on the usefulness of metriza-

the other hand, have reported several different cases of epidural hematomas diagnosed by plain CT (18, 31, 41).

Cord edema on the CT scan of a patient with a cervical fracture was demonstrated by Ethier et al. (33). He believed that the cervical cord could be distinguished routinely by plain CT, that pathological entities such as syrinxes could be discerned, and that cord edema could be

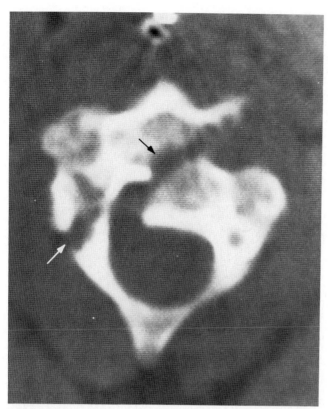

Figure 42.6. C2 Fracture Delineated by CT: Plain CT scan showing a complete fracture separation of the body of C2 (*black arrow*) accompanied by a fracture of the posterior arch (*white arrow*) and subluxation.

mide CT scanning in trauma (16, 29, 30, 34). In general, however, the value of computer assisted myelography (CAM) in trauma has been given very little attention in the literature (16, 18, 22, 29, 30, 34).

As for soft-tissue abnormalities outside the spinal canal, Lee et al. (10), and Faerber et al. (20), have described the ability of CT to detect paraspinal hematomas related to trauma. The CT detection of associated injuries in the body and brain, such as pneumo- and hemothoraxes, also has been mentioned (20).

The fact that CT has diagnosed these sequelae of spinal trauma in a quick, easy, simple, comfortable, relatively noninvasive way, has not gone unnoticed (4, 8, 11, 14, 20–22, 25, 27, 28, 32, 33, 35, 37). The minimal amount of manipulation needed to obtain a CT scan in the supine position in patients with traction has been contrasted to the greater amount of movement needed to obtain plain films in different projections, lateral tomograms, and myelograms. In those patients with unstable spines who run the risk of increasing their neurological deficit with movement, CT has been thought to be especially valuable.

The diagnostic information provided in spinal trauma by CT, especially its magnified views (11, 27), has been compared favorably to conventional radiography. The limitations of plain films and tomograms in detecting osseous and soft-tissue abnormalities in contrast to CT

have been delineated. The higher radiation dose of tomography, its time-consuming nature, the multiplicity of views needed to obtain the same information about the osseous spine as can be provided by direct axial CT images which later can be reconstructed in different planes, the greater patient discomfort, and the higher patient risk from greater patient manipulation have been added to the disadvantages of tomography already mentioned above (4, 8, 11, 14, 18, 23, 25, 28, 35, 37). Ullrich and Kieffer have suggested that because the sagittal-coronal reconstructed views of CT can be considered similar to AP and lateral tomograms that CT can replace tomography in most cases of spinal trauma (35). Reduction or elimination of tomography also has been recommended by Naidich et al. (17, 22), O'Callaghan et al. (28), and Brant-Zawadzki et al. (23).

The inability of myelography to ascertain the exact etiology of a block in spinal trauma, the greater patient manipulation required by this study, and the advent of HRCT have led some authors to suggest that the need for myelography in spinal trauma also might be reduced if CT is available (11, 20, 22, 33).

CT TECHNIQUE

Patient transfer

With clinical guidance, the spinal injury victim is cautiously transferred from his stretcher to the scanning unit on a trauma board. Traction, if warranted, is maintained throughout the procedure. The patient is kept supine for the entire examination. Direct axial views are later reconstructed into other pertinent planes.

Slice thickness

If a latest generation scanner is available and if the field of interest is small, 1.5-mm slices are used to demonstrate fine fractures optimally (42). Spatial resolution is greatly improved with this technique and reformatted images are of higher quality (42). There are drawbacks to these techniques, however. It is impractical to scan more than three adjacent vertebrae with these thin sections; the noise level is increased; and it is time-consuming. Target scanning, another technique for improving the sensitivity of CT, is also time-consuming and is best-suited for the evaluation of short spinal segments.

If 1.5-mm slices are not available for use or if a number of spinal levels need to be examined, overlapping 5-mm thick slices can be employed at 3-mm intervals (42). When reliance is placed on plain CT for diagnosis, this 2-mm superimposition of contiguous sections is, of course, preferable to the use of thicker nonoverlapping sections. Nevertheless, 5-mm thick slices without overlap also can be diagnostic. Even 1.0-cm thick sections can be useful, especially when intrathecal contrast is employed and long segments of the spine need to be examined.

Intrathecal contrast

Metrizamide CT scanning can be used either after conventional myelography or as a primary procedure. If performed as a secondary study, it should be obtained within 4 hours of myelography except in cases of post-traumatic

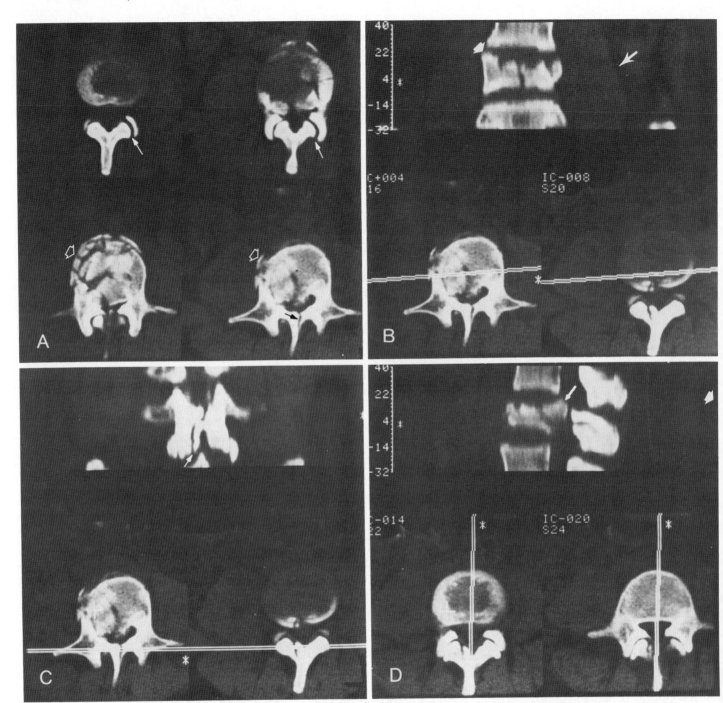

Figure 42.7. Multiplanar Reformation of Lumbar Spine Fractures: Plain CT scan in axial view (A) with multiplanar reformation in coronal (B and C) and sagittal (D) projections showing fractures through the L3 vertebral body (*arrowheads*, A and B) with displacement of the fragments (*white arrow*, D) and canal compromise. Facet separation (*white arrows*, A), posterior arch fractures (*black arrow*, A and *white arrow*, C), and a paraspinal hematoma (*arrow*, B) are also seen. Notice how nicely the coronal reformated image shows the fracture of the L3 inferior facet (*arrow*, C). (Case courtesy of Michael Brant-Zawadzki, M.D., San Francisco General Hospital).

syrinxes (34). This time ensures the optimal delineation of the spinal cord, nerve roots, and subarachnoid sac. Hence, abnormalities related to these structures can be best appreciated within this time frame. If a post-traumatic cord cyst is suspected, however, a 4-hour or more delayed scan is necessary to detect metrizamide within the cord substance.

If metrizamide CT scanning is performed without conventional myelography, the patient should be scanned immediately after the instillation of intrathecal metriza-

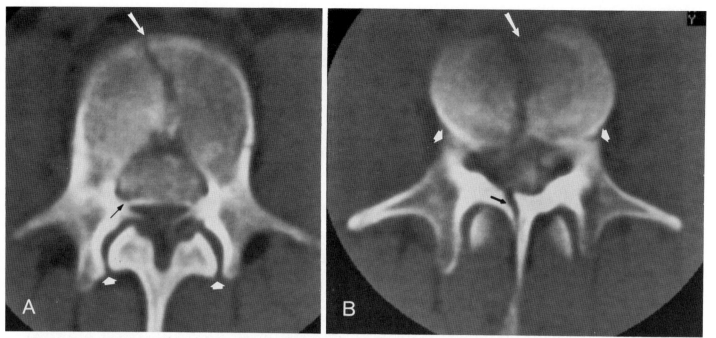

Figure 42.8. Canal Compromise Caused by Displaced Bone Fragments: A large bone fragment displaced into the spinal canal (*black arrow*, A) is shown on CT to be the cause of an L1-L2 myelographic block. Also evident in this 22-year-old male construction worker who fell 15 feet are compression fractures of the L2 vertebral body (*large white arrows*, A and B), mild distraction of the facets bilaterally (*arrowheads*, A), and fractures at the junction of the right lamina and spinous process (*black arrow*, B) and at the pedicles (*arrowheads*, B).

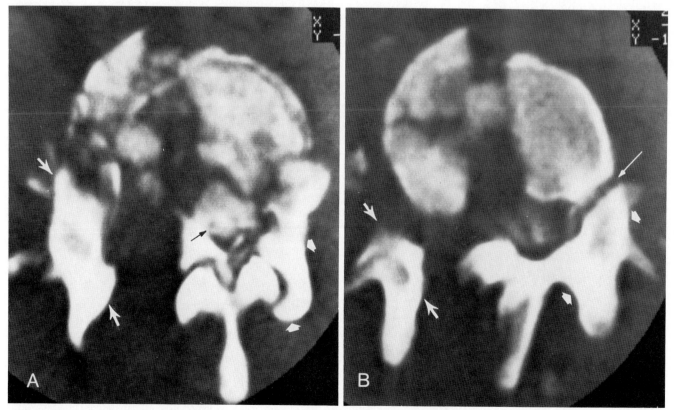

Figure 42.9. L4 Disruption with Compromise of Spinal Canal: CT scan showing complete disruption of L4. Transection and comminution of the vertebral body are evident as well as fracture fragments displaced into the spinal canal (*black arrow*, A). In addition, disarticulation of the vertebral body from the posterior arch is seen. The posterior arch on the left (*arrowheads*, A and B), the spinous process, and part of the right lamina have been separated off by a transpedicular fracture (*long arrow*, B) and by a right laminar fracture. A similar process has occurred on the right isolating off a segment of the right posterior arch (*short white arrows*, A and B).

771

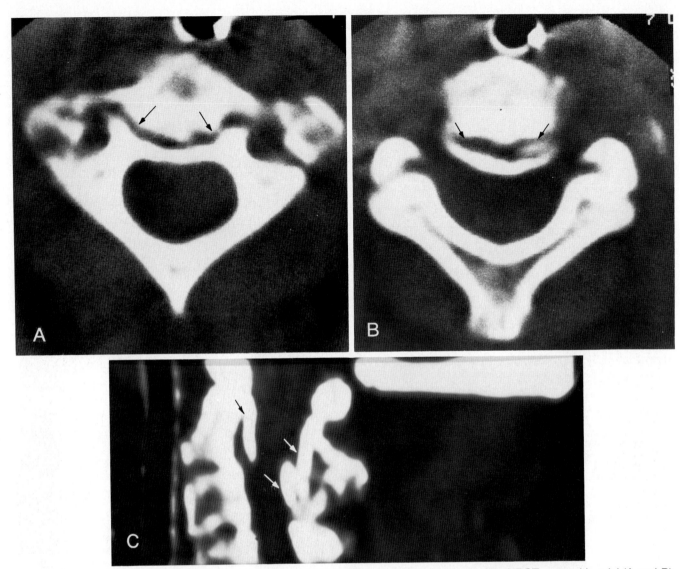

Figure 42.10. Canal Narrowing Secondary to an Avulsion Fracture with Subluxation: A plain HRCT scan with axial (A and B) and sagittally reconstructed (C) views was obtained in a 78-year-old male who fell and developed a central cord injury. This study showed an avulsion fracture through the posterior portion of the C2 vertebral body (*black arrows*, A and B). Also seen was narrowing of the spinal canal caused by this displaced fragment (to which the pedicles were still attached) and by the accompanying posterior subluxation of C2 on C3 (*white arrows*, C). [Fig. 42.10A and 42.10C reproduced with permission of Brant-Zawadzki M, Post MJD: Chapt. 8, Trauma. In: Newton TH, Potts DG: *Modern Neuroradiology.* Vol. 1. *Computed Tomography of the Spine and Spinal Cord.* San Anselmo, CA, Clavadel Press, 1983.]

mide. This timing is necessary because small volumes of dilute metrizamide are used in this procedure. Four to six cc of 170 mg/ml concentration of metrizamide are sufficient for the delineation of intraspinal pathology. An advantage of this technique is that it reduces the patient morbidity that can be associated with the use of large volumes of more concentrated metrizamide. A disadvantage is that overhead films in anteroposterior (AP) and lateral views which are so helpful in surgical planning cannot be obtained.

Multiplanar reformation

Multiplanar reformation is a technique which should be used routinely in the evaluation of spinal trauma pa-

tients if machine time is available. Sagittal, coronal, and oblique reconstructions supplement the information provided on axial views and occasionally make possible diagnoses that cannot be established from axial sections alone. These reconstructed images aid in the detection of fractures, especially horizontal ones (Figure 12B), subluxations (Fig. 42.17D), and spinal angulation deformities that may be missed on axial view. They display fractures of the posterior arch, especially of the facets, to excellent advantage (Fig. 42.7C). Oblique reformations optimally show narrowing of the neural foramen by bone fragments and by subluxed facets. Sagittal reconstructions are especially useful in the demonstration of displaced bone fragments and traumatic kyphosis.

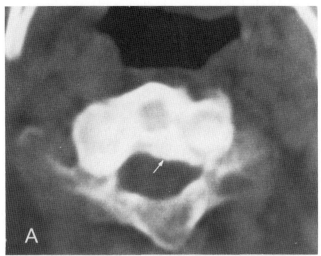

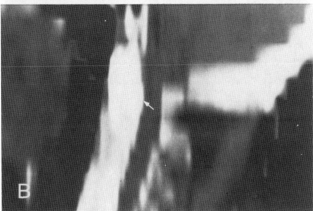

Figure 42.11. Reduction of Canal Size by a Chronic Fracture of C2: Axial (A) and sagittally reconstructed (B) views at C1-C2 showing mild canal encroachment by bony proliferation from an old healed fracture. [Reproduced with permission of Post et al. (16).]

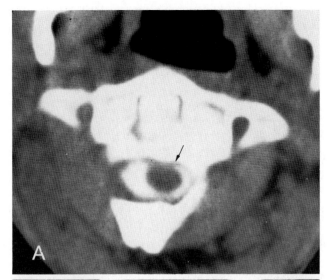

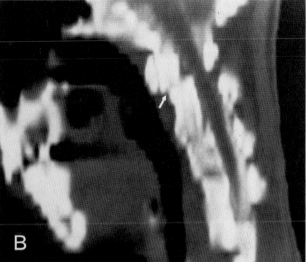

Figure 42.12. Nonunion of a Chronic C2 Fracture with C1-C2 Subluxation: Three months before admission, this 22-year-old white female with a history of trauma complained of pain in her neck and shooting pains radiating into her arms, legs, and back on movement of her neck. Physical examination revealed decreased strength in her upper extremities. Plain films did not show this patient's pathology to good advantage. A subsequent metrizamide CT scan in axial (A) and sagittally reconstructed (B) views demonstrated an ununited fracture of the base of the odontoid (*arrow*, B), anterior subluxation of C1 and on C2, with narrowing of the cervical canal and compression of the ventral subarachnoid sac at C1 and C2. (Notice that the horizontal fracture through the base of the odontoid is best seen on the sagittal view.) With the information provided by CT scan the patient underwent an open reduction and a posterior C1-C2 fusion. [Reproduced with permission of Brant-Zawadzki M, Post MJD: Chapt. 8, Trauma. In: Newton TH, Potts DG: *Modern Neuroradiology*. Vol. 1. *Computed Tomography of the Spine and Spinal Cord.* San Anselmo, CA, Clavadel Press, 1983.]

ScoutView devices

The use of ScoutView devices in the evaluation of trauma patients is extremely beneficial. These computed radiographs which provide AP and lateral views of the spine substantially decrease scan time because the area of interest can be determined precisely before scanning commences. Appropriate gantry angulation can be chosen when necessary, such as in cases of traumatic disc herniation. Most importantly, the ScoutView devices allow for the precise localization of pathology. If ScoutView devices are not available, close correlation with plain films is critical.

Image recording and review

Recording of the CT images should be done at two different window widths. Both wide and narrow windows should be used to ensure detection of both osseous and soft-tissue pathology. Minified views, which are helpful in localization of level when no ScoutView device is available, can be obtained at bone window settings. Magnified views (2.00X) can be taken at narrow window

widths to show soft-tissue structures to best advantage. The practice of obtaining two different sets of hard copies does not obviate the need for reviewing cases of spinal

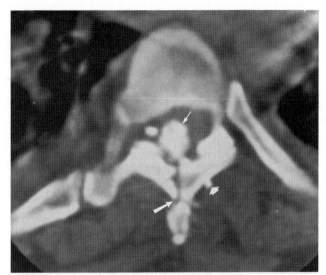

Figure 42.13. Localization of Bullet Fragments by CT: After a gunshot wound had rendered a 60-year-old female paraplegic a plain CT scan was used to localize bullet fragments within (*small arrow*) and adjacent to (*arrowhead*) the thoracic spinal canal. Posterior arch fractures of T7 (*large arrow*) and T6 and bilateral pleural effusions were also detected.

trauma on the oscilloscope. Adjusting the window while viewing the case on the monitor aids in the detection of pathology.

PROTOCOL

HRCT has not obviated the need for plain films of the spine. Plain films should be performed as the initial study in all patients with spinal trauma. These conventional radiographs allow a preliminary survey of the spine to be made. They help to localize the levels of pathology. As a result, other radiographic examinations can be directed toward a specific area of interest. Plain films also provide a longitudinal view of the spine which is useful in treatment planning. At this point in time, the computed radiographs which act as localizing devices for CT scanning do not replace conventional plain films because they do not provide sufficient detail of the bony structures of the spine.

The plain film examination should begin with AP and lateral views in neutral position of the area of clinical interest. Oblique and flexion and extension views should be added only when careful scrutiny of the preliminary films and discussion with the clinician have excluded any contraindications.

The radiographic protocol that follows an initial plain film survey is dependent upon multiple factors: 1) the presence or absence of neurological deficit; 2) the type and severity of neurological deficit; 3) the time interval that has elapsed between the spinal injury and the radiographic work-up; 4) the etiology of the trauma, (whether penetrating or not); 5) the availability of a high-resolution scanner and of machine time; and 6) the institutional approach to spinal cord injury victims.

The multiplicity of factors involved makes a rigid radio-

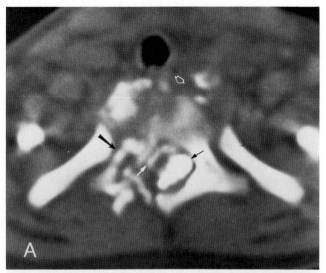

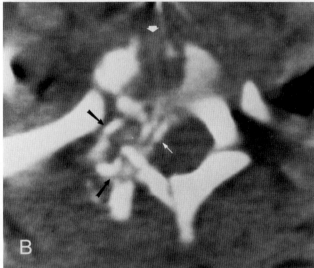

Figure 42.14. Localization of Bullet and Bone Fragments by CT: In this child with quadraplegia secondary to a gunshot wound, a CT scan revealed that the bullets had shattered the T1 vertebral body (*arrowheads*, A and B) and posterior arch (*large black arrows*, A and B). It also showed that the spinal canal was compromised by displaced fracture fragments (*white arrows*, A and B) and residual bullet fragments (*small black arrow*, A).

graphic protocol impossible and impractical. For example, in patients with acute or chronic injury without neurological deficit, either CT scanning or conventional tomography can be used for evaluation of the osseous spine. The choice would depend upon the type of equipment available and upon CT accessibility. Similarly, in spinal trauma victims with neurological deficit, different radiographic work-ups can be used.

The particular protocol which we have chosen for our institution is outlined in Tables 42.1 and 42.2. Its details are described in another publication (16). This protocol, which might not be applicable for all hospitals, reflects our attitude that an aggressive approach to the evaluation

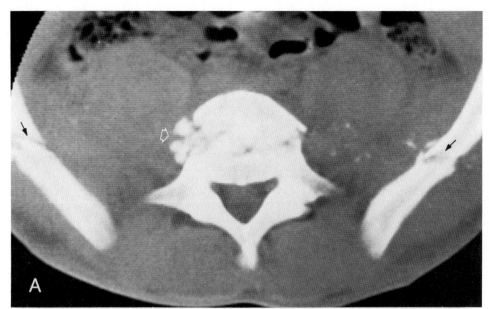

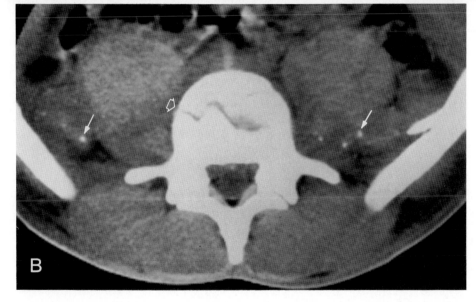

Figure 42.15. Extraspinal Disruption of the L4 Nerve from a Gunshot Wound: In this patient with a gunshot wound to the pelvis and an L4 plexopathy, a plain CT scan identifies the entrance and exit sites of the bullet as well as its tract. It shows fractures traversing both iliac bones (*arrows*, A) as well as the L5 vertebral body (*arrowheads*, A and B). It also demonstrates residual bullet fragments (*arrows*, B) in the extraspinal soft tissues. The enlargement and distortion of the iliopsoas and psoas muscles that is seen is secondary to hemorrhage and contusion.

and treatment of spinal trauma victims with neurological deficits is justifiable by the potentially devastating nature of many of the lesions and by the belief that complete or partial reversal of these lesions can be achieved in some cases (43).

Although the management of patients with spinal injuries is quite controversial (43–60), numerous reports in the literature have documented improvement or resolution of neurological deficits in patients operated upon in the acute and chronic stages of their injuries (18, 24, 58–60). Those individuals who in our opinion might be benefited by surgery include those with extrinsic lesions severely compressing the spinal cord and/or nerve roots that cannot be corrected by conservative means, those with foreign bodies which are compromising the spinal canal, and those with symptomatic posttraumatic syrinxes. To identify those individuals who might be benefited by surgical

intervention, we perform standard myelography and follow this procedure with a metrizamide CT scan of the area of clinical and myelographic interest. Our frequent use of CAM in patients with neurological deficit of recent onset or in those with incomplete or progressive neurological deficit or intractable pain is because of this procedure's many advantages and because of the limitations of conventional myelography.

Among the limitations of myelography are the following (16):

1. In acute spinal trauma victims whose mobility must be restricted, the spinal cord and subarachnoid sac are frequently not completely delineated (Figs. 42.26 and 42.30). Metrizamide, introduced via the cervical route with the patient supine and semierect, frequently outlines well only the posterior aspect of the spinal canal when no obstruction is present.

Table 42.1.
Radiographic protocol for acute spinal trauma victims[a]

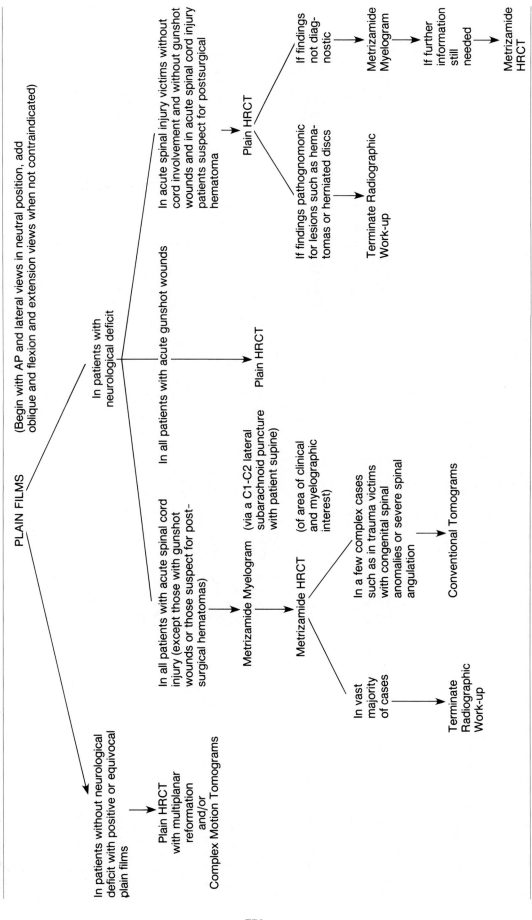

[a] Modified with permission from Post et al. (16).

Table 42.2.
Radiographic protocol for subacute and chronic spinal trauma victims[a]

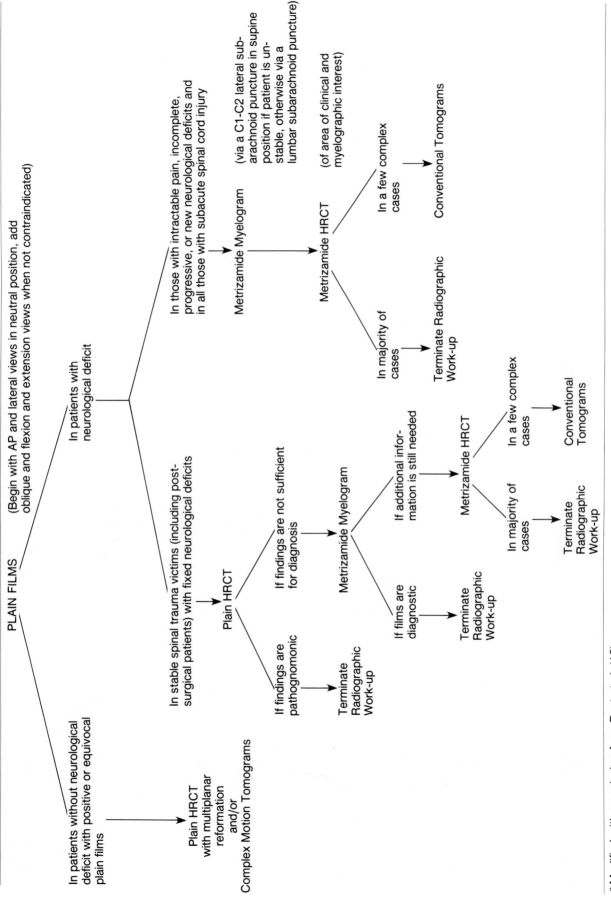

[a] Modified with permission from Post et al. (16).

777

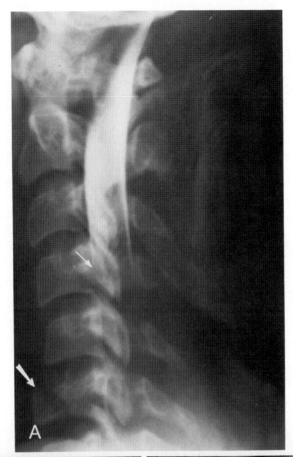

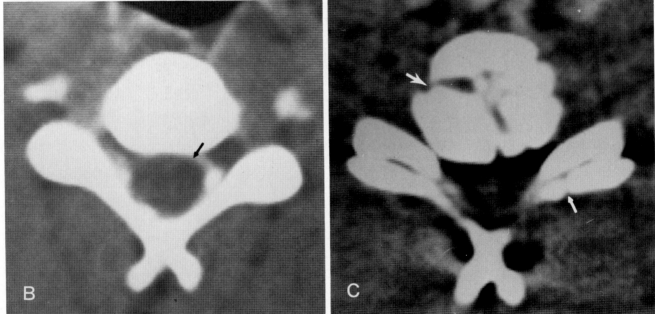

Figure 42.16. Cord Swelling: The lateral view of a metrizamide myelogram (A) demonstrates a complete block at C4 (*small arrow*), two levels above the acute C6 fracture-subluxation (*large arrow*). The metrizamide CT scan (B and C) verifies that the block is intramedullary and secondary to marked cord swelling (*arrow*, B). The CT also demonstrates well the fractures of the C6 vertebral body (*large arrow*, C) and left inferior facet (*small arrow*, C) and encroachment on the canal by fracture fragments.

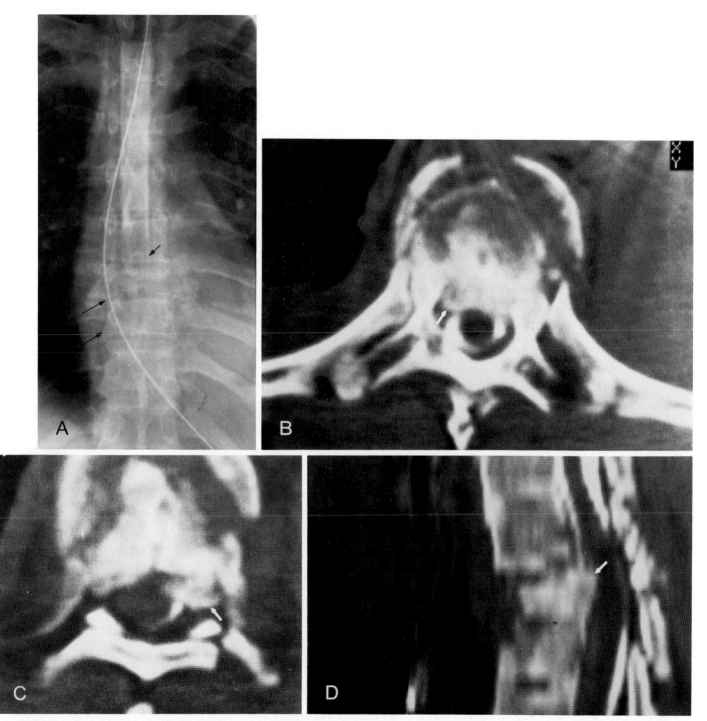

Figure 42.17. Canal Compromise Caused by Displaced Bone Fragments: In this 37-year-old white male who was rendered paraplegic by a fall from a 2-story building, an emergency myelogram performed via the cervical route demonstrated a complete extradural block (*short arrow*, A) just above the fractured T7 and T8 vertebral bodies (*long arrows*, A). A subsequent metrizamide CT scan in axial (B and C) and reconstructed sagittal (D) views clarified the etiology of this block. It was being caused by displaced bone fragments (*arrows*, B and C) which were compressing the subarachnoid sac and spinal cord. The metrizamide CT scan also showed to better advantage the comminuted T7 and T8 vertebral body fractures. [Reproduced with permission of Brant-Zawadzki M, Post MJD: Chapt. 8, Trauma. In: Newton TH, Potts DG: *Modern Neuroradiology*. Vol. 1. *Computed Tomography of the Spine and Spinal Cord.* San Anselmo, CA, Clavadel Press, 1983.]

2. Myelography is not always able to determine the exact etiology of a block or the precise nature of a non-obstructing defect.

3. Myelography is not able to demonstrate directly intraspinal soft-tissue abnormalities—it can only show their secondary effects.

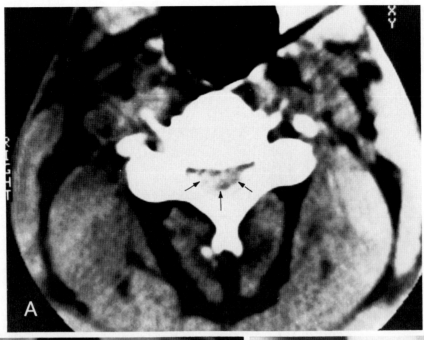

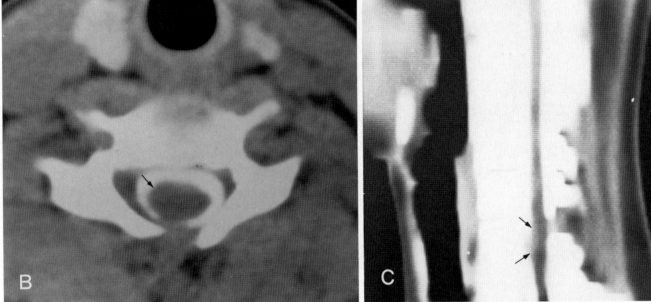

Figure 42.18. CT Differentiation in Acute Trauma of Extradural From Intramedullary Lesions: Metrizamide CT scans in two different patients with acute spinal cord injury. In the first patient, the CT scan demonstrates a large ventral extradural soft-tissue lesion (*arrows*, A) compressing the cervical cord consistent with an acute soft-disc herniation. This CT finding prompted surgical decompression. In the second patient, the metrizamide CT scan demonstrates enlargement of the cervical cord in axial (*arrow*, B) and sagittally reconstructed (*arrows*, C) views. This finding was consistent with cord edema. Conservative therapy followed. [*A* reproduced with permission of Post et al. (16).]

4. Myelography is not able to evaluate well the areas beyond or between myelographic blocks (Figs. 42.16 and 42.17).

Myelography, however, should not be eliminated from the diagnostic work-up of all patients with spinal trauma. As has been reported in the past, this procedure can be useful in evaluating patients with acute or chronic spinal injury (61–73). Both gas and opaque myelograms via either the lumbar or cervical route, have been shown to be beneficial to patient management. Diagnoses such as cord swelling, cord transection, cord atrophy, extradural hematomas, epidural abscesses, disc herniations, bony impingement on the spinal canal, scar formation, nerve root avulsions, CSF leaks, and spinal pleural fistulas have been reported. In addition, in patients with closed as well as penetrating spinal trauma, some have used the demonstration of a myelographic block to indicate the need for

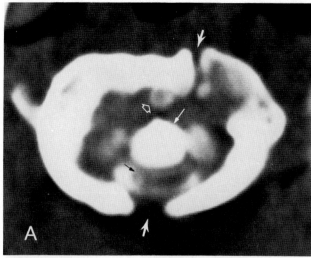

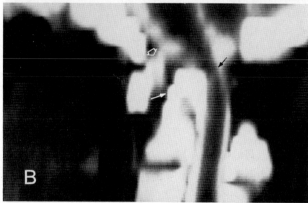

Figure 42.19. C1-C2 Subluxation and Cord Compression in a Trauma Patient with Congenital Spine Anomalies: Axial (A) and sagittally reconstructed (B) views of a metrizamide CT scan showing marked cord compression (*black arrows*) at the C1-C2 level in this 11-year-old boy who fell off a skate board and aggravated a C1-C2 subluxation. This study also showed a hypoplastic odontoid (*small white arrows*), an os odontoideum (*arrowheads*), incomplete ossification of the arch of C1 (*large white arrows*) and failure of segmentation of C2 and C3. [Reproduced with the permission of Post et al. (16).]

surgery (44, 45, 62).

Recently, Leo et al. suggested that metrizamide myelography via a C1-C2 lateral puncture be used to evaluate patients with acute injuries to the cervical cord (74). According to these authors, this procedure was simple and safe and gave diagnostic information not available by more traditional methods or agents. The metrizamide myelogram was able to determine whether an extradural lesion such as a herniated disc or a hematoma was causing spinal cord compression and whether surgical decompression was therefore necessary.

The value of performing metrizamide CT scanning after myelography is that this procedure complements the standard myelogram. It overcomes the limitations of myelography in the following ways:

1. It determines the etiology of myelographic defects, whether obstructive or nonobstructive. Thus, it distinguishes extrinsic lesions such as disc herniation (Fig. 42.18A) from intrinsic lesions such as cord edema (Fig. 42.18B and C).

2. It directly demonstrates certain intraspinal soft-tissue abnormalities such as intramedullary hematomas, cord fissures, and cord cysts.

3. It occasionally detects contrast beyond an area of myelographic block.

4. Its cross-sectional view allows optimal delineation of compressive lesions of the spine.

5. It demonstrates dural leaks and nerve root avulsions which may not be appreciated by myelography.

SPECIFIC TRAUMATIC LESIONS OF THE SPINE AND THEIR CT APPEARANCE

Bony lesions

The various types of osseous injury of the spine and the mechanisms responsible for them have been extensively described in the literature and, thus, will not be dealt with in this chapter. The CT appearance of these lesions also has been previously reported (42, 75).

It is worth emphasizing however, CT's vital role in the detection of bony or calcific lesions which are the cause of acute or chronic neurological deficit. CT detects not only displaced bone fragments and fracture subluxations but also any coexistent pathology which may be aggravating the spinal trauma such as congenital anomalies of the spine (Fig. 42.19), spinal stenosis, posterior longitudinal ligamental calcification, and ankylosing spondylitis (Fig. 42.20). CT also demonstrates complications of surgical intervention such as displaced bone plugs, displaced or broken surgical wires with secondary subluxation (Fig. 42.21) and osteomyelitis (Fig. 42.22).

Figures 42.23–42.25 serve as an illustration of CT's ability to diagnose bony compressive lesions of the spine in acute trauma. Figures 42.26–42.28 illustrate how CT benefits the managment of subacute and chronic spinal injury victims. These illustrations are of particular interest because the information on CT led to surgical intervention which resulted in improvement of these patients neurological deficits. One of these cases will be summarized below.

In the patient illustrated in Figure 42.28, a 31-year-old white male with ankylosing spondylitis who fell off his horse and sustained a C6-C7 fracture-subluxation, a complete motor-sensory quadraplegia was originally present. Surgery was performed only for vertebral column stabilization. A posterior spinal fusion was done. However, within 6 months of injury, the patient showed neurological improvement. The development of an incomplete quadriplegia led to a new radiographic work-up. A myelogram demonstrated a C6-C7 posterior extradural defect. The etiology of this defect was shown subsequently by a metrizamide CT scan. It revealed compression of the subarachnoid sac and spinal cord by a subluxed and fractured spinous process and laminae. These findings led to a second surgical procedure. Decompression of the

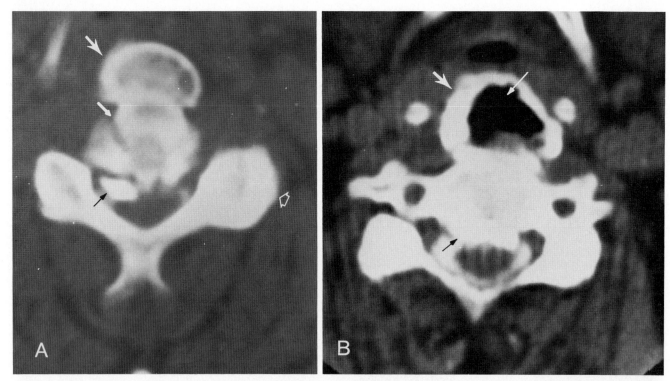

Figure 42.20. Ankylosing Spondylitis with Traumatic Cord Compression and Fracture-Separation of C3-C4: Injury to the spine in a 68-year-old male with ankylosing spondylitis resulted in incomplete quadriplegia. A metrizamide CT scan performed 4 months later after transfer to our institution demonstrated cord compression caused by a fractured and displaced calcified posterior longitudinal ligament (*black arrow*, A). Pre-existing canal stenosis from the extensive ligamental calcification (*black arrow*, B) contributed to this cord compression. A fracture-separation of C3-C4 was also evident. The fracture extended through the calcified anterior longitudinal ligament between C3 and C4. The collection of air (*thin white arrow*, B) between the calcified anterior longitudinal ligaments of C3 and C4 (*large white arrows*, A and B) was evidence of this traumatic separation. A fracture of the C3 vertebral body (*small white arrow*, A) also was seen in this patient with facet fusion (*arrowhead*, A) secondary to the ankylosing spondylitis.

spinal canal was undertaken. This resulted in improvement of the patient's neurological deficit.

Intraspinal Soft-tissue Lesions

CORD EDEMA

Swelling of the cord occurs frequently after spinal cord trauma and may peak during the first several weeks after acute injury. Because this is an intrinsic lesion which should be treated by conservative means, it is important to recognize this condition radiographically.

Myelography can be used to diagnose this condition. However, in cases of myelographic block, differentiation between intrinsic and extrinsic lesions can prove difficult. Furthermore, the spinal levels below the area of block, which might be the site of additional pathology, will not be evaluated well by this procedure (Fig. 42.29A).

CT scanning also can be used in the evaluation of cord edema. Swelling of the cord has been detected on some plain HRCT scans (33). However, generally speaking, a noncontrast study is not sufficient for diagnostic purposes. The marked distortion of intraspinal anatomy that occurs in patients with severe trauma usually makes it impossible to discern the spinal cord and to recognize any increase

in its size. However, with the use of metrizamide, the cord can be outlined and its diffuse symmetrical enlargement in cases of cord edema can be seen (Figs. 42.16B, 42.18B and C, and 42.29B).

HEMATOMYELIA

A hematoma within the cord substance can be the cause of a traumatic neurological deficit. Although the cord often is enlarged in this condition as well as in cord edema, these two entities can be distinguished by CT. If the bleeding is acute and of sufficient quantity, it can be recognized on a plain HRCT scan or on a metrizamide CT as a focal area of hyperdensity within the cord parenchyma, generally measuring from approximately 40–100 HU (Fig. 42.30). On CAM, this hyperdensity can be differentiated from the intramedullary collections of metrizamide which occur in cord cysts or fissures because the latter will usually have absorption coefficients greater than 140 HU.

Compared to an extradural hematoma the intramedullary hematoma will be more centrally located in the spinal canal and will be more irregular and less sharply defined. The diagnosis of hematomyelia on CT results in conservative therapy. For this reason, this diagnosis is especially

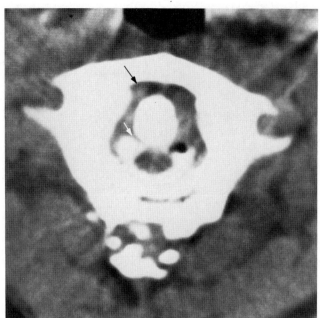

Figure 42.21. C1-C2 Subluxation in a Postoperative Chronic Spinal Injury Patient: The above metrizamide CT scan was performed in a 22-year-old male with neck pain who had undergone a Brooks fusion for a traumatic C1-C2 subluxation 4 years ago. It demonstrated recurrence of the C1-C2 subluxation (*black arrow*) and secondary compression of the ventral subarachnoid sac (*white arrow*) and spinal cord. Other images demonstrated breakage of the surgical wires. (Postmyelographic air is seen incidentally in the subarachnoid space).

important to make in trauma patients who have undergone recent surgical intervention and who display increasing neurological deficits. The exclusion by CT of any surgically correctable extradural lesion and the detection by CT of intramedullary hemorrhage obviates the need for further surgical intervention (Fig. 42.31).

CORD FISSURES

A large rent in the spinal cord after severe acute trauma can be recognized on an immediate metrizamide CT scan. It appears as a collection of metrizamide within the cord.

Figure 42.32 is an illustration of such a case. The hyperdensity seen within the cervical cord in this patient with an acute fracture-subluxation of C2 and quadriplegia had an absorption coefficient compatible with metrizamide. This traumatic cord fissure was no longer recognized radiographically on a follow-up metrizamide CT scan 1 week later, suggesting gross "closure" or marked approximation of the rented portions of the cord.

CORD MACERATION AND TRANSECTION

When severe trauma occurs to the spinal cord, maceration of the cord substance can occur. This severe disruption of cord anatomy which probably rarely results in a true cord transection can be diagnosed on a metrizamide CT scan. It is recognized by absence of the cord shadow and by the presence of metrizamide diffusely throughout the subarachnoid sac (Fig. 42.33B). Immediately above and below the levels of cord transection or maceration a cord shadow will be seen. (Fig. 42.33A and C).

CORD ATROPHY

One of the complications of spinal trauma is an atrophied cord. This abnormality is seen in those with chronic spinal injury. Its radiographic diagnosis, just as in cases of cord edema, is made best on a metrizamide CT scan. However, the significance of cord atrophy must be based on clinical findings, because there can be a discrepancy between the severity of the CT picture and that of the clinical presentation. Spinal cord atrophy is recognized on CAM by a reduction in spinal cord size and by a concomitant increase in size of the subarachnoid sac (Fig. 42.34B). Typically, a uniformly small spinal cord is seen over several levels. When associated with a posttraumatic syrinx, atrophy of the spinal cord has a different CT appearance. The spinal cord not only appears small but flattened as well (Fig. 42.35B). In these cases, the cord cyst that accompanies the small cord will be seen on images taken at narrow window widths (Fig. 42.35C).

DURAL LEAKS AND NERVE ROOT AVULSIONS

A metrizamide CT scan is the radiographic study of choice for detecting dural leaks and nerve root avulsions. Although myelography may diagnose these conditions, they may be missed by this procedure, especially if the lesions are small. They also may be missed or incompletely evaluated on plain CT scans (16). This is especially true of small CSF leaks and those which diffuse freely into the retroperitoneal space.

A noncontrast HRCT scan, however, can detect large well-contained collections of CSF outside the dural sac. In these cases, these traumatic pseudomeningocoeles will appear as hypodense lesions silhouetted against the denser soft tissues. A plain CT also will discern osseous abnormalities that may develop as a result of complications of dural leaks. Sachdev et al. described a patient with a posttraumatic pseudomeningomyelocele which had developed over an extended period of time within a fractured L1 vertebral body (60). The plain CT revealed an area of bone destruction involving the L1 vertebral body which had a sclerotic margin and which was in direct continuity with the spinal canal. However, a myelogram was needed to diagnose the cause of this bony defect, namely the traumatic pseudomeningomyelocele.

Because of the limitations of plain CT in evaluating dural leaks, it is recommended that a metrizamide CT scan be performed immediately after myelography. This procedure will demonstrate even small amounts of contrast that have extended beyond the confines of the thecal sac, (Fig. 42.36). It will also show the site of dural tear (Fig. 42.37) and any herniation of the cauda equinae through the defect and possible nerve root entrapment within bony fragments (43).

Nerve root avulsions which commonly occur in the lower cervical spine can also be best delineated on a metrizamide CT scan. They will appear as abnormal col-

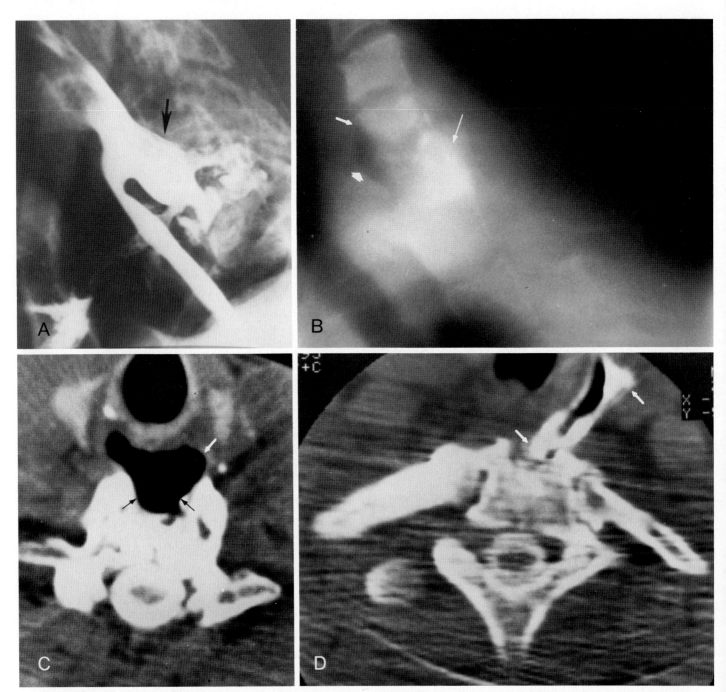

Figure 42.22. Osteomyelitis and Fistula Formation in a Patient with Prior Trauma and Cervical Fusion: Thirteen months ago, this patient became quadriplegic from a motor vehicle accident in which he sustained a C6–7 dislocation. At an outside hospital, his injury was treated by a laminectomy and later by an anterior cervical fusion. He was transferred to our institution when he became infected and developed a draining cutaneous fistula after a surgical tear of his esophágus. A barium swallow (A) demonstrated extravasation of barium (*arrow*) into the spine and skin. A conventional tomogram (B) showed extensive destruction of C6 (*short arrow*) and C7, residual barium at the site of the eroded C7 vertebral body (*long arrow*), air in the prevertebral soft tissues (*arrowhead*) and laminectomy defects. A metrizamide CT scan (C and D) excluded compression of the subarachnoid sac and cervical cord. It also showed extension of the prevertebral air (*white arrow*, C) into the osteomyelitic cavity (*black arrows*, C). In addition, it delineated nicely the fistulous tract filled with barium extending from the vertebral body to the skin (*arrows*, D). After this study, the infected bone was removed.

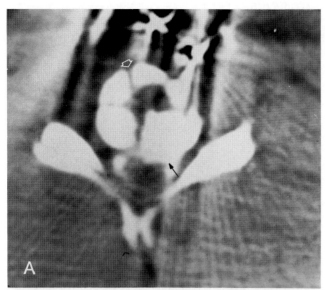

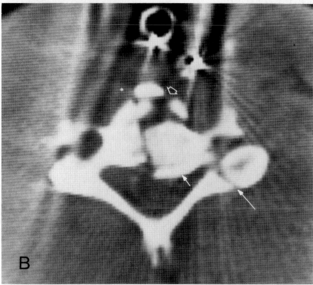

Figure 42.23. Cord Compression Caused by Displaced Fracture Fragments from a Swimming Accident: Metrizamide CT scan in a quadriplegic male showing comminuted fractures of C5 (*arrowheads*, A and B), fractures of the posterior arch (*long arrow*, B), and ventral subarachnoid sac and cord compression caused by displaced bone fragments (*black arrow*, A; *short white arrow*, B).

lections of metrizamide extending out the neural foramina (Figs. 42.38 and 42.39). However, if clot and fibrosis are associated with the root avulsion, an extradural defect will be seen instead.

SPINAL EPIDURAL HEMATOMA

Trauma can result in the development of a spinal epidural hematoma, (SEH). The trauma can be severe or minimal in nature. SEHs have been reported even after such minor activities as coughing, sneezing, or twisting (41). These lesions also can be the result of iatrogenic trauma and can follow lumbar punctures, epidural spinal

anesthesia, spinal surgery, and anticoagulation therapy (41). They can be spontaneous or they can result from coagulopathies, neoplasm, infection, pregnancy, and rupture of epidural varicose veins, arteriovenous malformations, and venous angiomas.

SEHs are seen in all age groups but have a predilection for the elderly hypertensive atherosclerotic patient (41). The thoracic spine is affected most frequently. Involvement of multiple spinal levels, however, is common.

When this lesion causes severe pain and rapidly progressive neurological deficits, it should be considered a neurosurgical emergency. Under these circumstances, immediate decompression usually is required to prevent irreversible quadriplegia, paraplegia, or death. In these emergency cases, CT provides the means for prompt diagnosis (Fig. 42.40).

It should be mentioned, however, that with the increased use of CT in spinal trauma that cases of epidural bleeding similar to those in Figures 42.41 and 42.42 undoubtedly will be detected on CT which are not associated with a devastating prognosis or are not the primary cause of the patient's neurological deficit. Close clinical CT correlation will be imperative in these cases.

Acute SEHs appear on plain HRCT scans as smoothly outlined, sharply marginated biconvex hyperdense collections which approximate the osseous margins of the spinal canal (41) (Fig. 42.40A). Most commonly, they are located posteriorly or posterolaterally, a factor which helps to differentiate these lesions from those which typically have a ventral location, such as disc herniations. However, occasionally SEHs may be circumferential in nature. Oscilloscopic review is mandatory in cases of SEH. These lesions easily can be missed when hard copies alone are relied upon for diagnosis. Use of the monitor allows absorption measurements to be made which will demonstrate coefficients compatible with fresh blood in acute cases. Use of the monitor also ensures selection of a window width appropriate for the display of this type of pathology. We have found that narrow window widths are optimal for demonstrating SEHs on plain CT scans. They enhance detection of the interface between these extradural lesions and the subarachnoid space.

When an acute SEH involves either the cervical or thoracic spine, it may be impossible to discern the compressed spinal cord on a plain HRCT scan. Under these circumstances, the subarachnoid sac and the spinal cord will appear together as a relative radiolucent area silhouetted against the more dense SEH.

If plain HRCT with 5-mm or less thick sections in axial and sagittally reconstructed views fail to demonstrate the position of the spinal cord or if it fails to show the true extent of a SEH, intrathecal contrast is necessitated. A discrepancy between the level of involvement determined by clinical examination and that ascertained by CT scan indicates the need for a metrizamide CT scan also.

A SEH appears on CAM as a very well-delineated peripheral extradural lesion that compresses the subarachnoid sac and displaces the spinal cord (Figs. 42.40C, 42.41, and 42.42). In comparison to the high-density metriza-

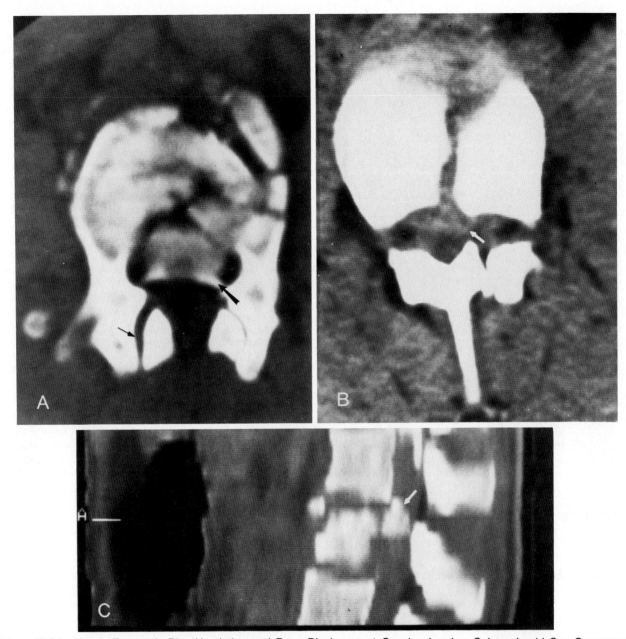

Figure 42.24. Acute Traumatic Disc Herniation and Bone Displacement Causing Lumbar Subarachnoid Sac Compression: Metrizamide CT scan in axial (A and B) and sagittally reconstructed (C) views demonstrating in a patient with a myelographic block a large bone fragment within the spinal canal at L1-L2 (*large black arrow*, A; *arrow*, C), comminuted fractures of the L2 vertebral body, facet distraction (*small arrow*, A) and posterior arch fractures. A soft-tissue traumatic disc herniation also is seen (*arrow*, B).

mide-filled subarachnoid sac, it appears as a relative radiolucent defect. However, close scrutiny of the lesion on the monitor will show that it is of variable soft-tissue density, depending upon the age of the hematoma.

SPINAL SUBARACHNOID BLEEDING

Subarachnoid bleeding may be seen in association with epidural and/or subdural hematomas. It may result from trauma, which may be direct or iatrogenically induced. If iatrogenic in nature, subarachnoid bleeding is usually secondary to a spinal tap, either alone or in conjunction with anticoagulant therapy or thrombocytopenia (41).

On a plain HRCT scan subarachnoid blood appears as a hyperdense area silhouetting the spinal cord and/or nerve roots (Fig. 42.40B) (41). Visually, it resembles a metrizamide CT scan. However, by density measurements it is markedly different. Fresh blood in the subarachnoid space has a much lower absorption coefficient than metrizamide.

If the spinal fluid is not grossly blood, it may be very

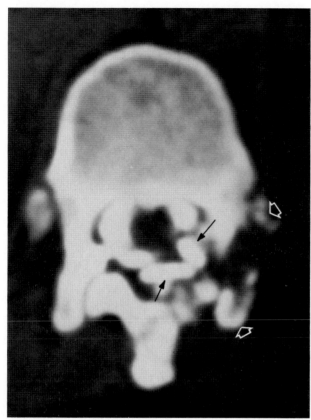

Figure 42.25. CT Localization of Spinal Fractures Caused by a Gunshot Wound: In this 40-year-old female who was rendered paraplegia by a gunshot wound, a metrizamide CT scan demonstrates comminuted fractures of the posterior arch of T11 (*arrowheads*). It also detects bone fragments displaced into the spinal canal (*arrows*) and shows that they are compressing the subarachnoid sac. Swelling of the conus is apparent too.

difficult to discern subarachnoid bleeding on CT. Because subarachnoid blood can readily diffuse throughout the CSF pathways, it becomes diluted by the spinal fluid. As a result, in modest quantities it may be impossible to detect on CT.

POSTTRAUMATIC SYRINX

Cystic degeneration of the spinal cord is a delayed complication of spinal cord injury (66, 76). In this entity, progressive cavitation of the spinal cord occurs and results in an upward extension of spinal cord dysfunction (66). These cysts which may be single or multiple, may develop because of contusion, myelomalacia and/or hemorrhage in the cord (76). They begin in segments of the cord adjacent to the level of injury, forming glial-lined cavities not in communication with the central canal or subarachnoid space. Adhesions which tether the cord and subject it to excessive stress during changes in spinal extramedullary pressure cause these cysts to extend (76). The alterations in spinal pressure can be caused by coughing, sneezing, or straining. As these cysts expand and extend,

compression of previously unaffected neural tissue occurs. A progressive ascending myelopathy results. The patients frequently experience increased spasticity, hyperhidrosis, disassociated sensory loss, severe automotive hyperflexia, and the onset of new pain (76). Diagnosis is critical because shunting of the expanding cyst to the subarachnoid sac can arrest the progression of neurological deficit.

Whereas diagnosis of a posttraumatic syrinx previously rested on the results of a myelogram and a percutaneous cyst puncture and cystography, it now is based upon the findings of a myelogram and a delayed metrizamide CT scan (76). Whereas a plain HRCT scan occasionally can demonstrate hypodense areas within the cord (Fig. 42.43A), it usually does not show the entire extent of the lesion. Intrathecal contrast is necessary for complete delineation of this lesion before surgical intervention (Figs. 42.43B and C, and 42.44). The value of contrast CT scans in patients with intraspinal soft-tissue abnormalities recently has been recognized by Seibert and coauthors and Aubin et al. (76, 77). These authors have demonstrated the value of the delayed metrizamide CT scan in establishing the diagnosis of posttraumatic syrinxes.

When a myelogram is performed it occasionally may show cord enlargement. However, it more usually reveals a normal sized or even a small spinal cord (33, 76) (Fig. 42.35A). In 11 of the 25 patients presented by Seibert et al., the spinal cord was of normal size (76). Adhesions interfered with an accurate myelographic assessment of cord size. Due probably to transneural migration of metrizamide into the cyst, the metrizamide scan when performed between 2–5 hours after myelography (and even up to 24 hours) shows metrizamide filling the syrinx cavity. In 22 of the 25 cases reported by Seibert and others, this metrizamide-filled cavity extended cranially from the site of injury whereas in one it extended caudally and in two it extended both cranially and caudally (76). Figure 42.45 illustrates the cranial and caudal extension of posttraumatic syrinx in a patient with a gunshot wound. (See Chapter 43 for an extensive discussion of posttraumatic cord cysts.)

DISC HERNIATION

Both acute and chronic disc herniations are seen after spinal trauma. They may be seen in association with fractures, fracture-subluxation, or gunshot wounds. As mass lesions, they can be the source of progressive neurological deficits. Radiographic recognition of these lesions is critical because they are extradural lesions which are surgically amenable.

On plain HRCT scans disc herniations appear as ventral, ventrolateral or lateral extradural soft-tissue lesions (Figs. 42.24B, 42.46B, and 42.47A). They are sharply delineated and focal in nature. They occur adjacent to disc space levels, except in cases of disc extrusion. They may be accompanied by disc space narrowing. However, especially in acute cases, a normal disc space may be seen. Absorption coefficients will be in the range of disc material at other disc space levels. In patients with chronic disc herniations or in those with underlying degenerative disc

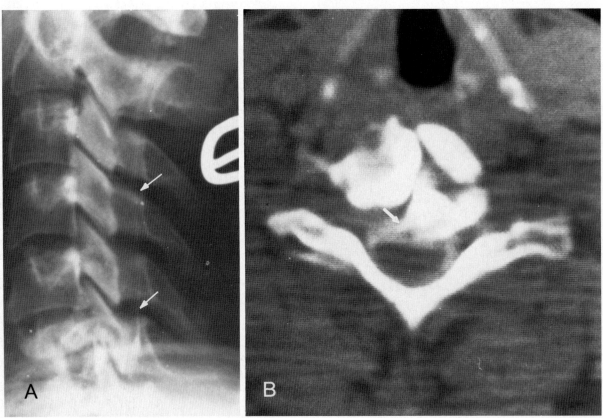

Figure 42.26.   Cord Compression after Chronic Spinal Injury and Cervical Fusion: A metrizamide myelogram via the cervical route outlined only the posterior aspect of the subarachnoid sac (*arrows*, A) because of the absence of a block in this chronic spinal trauma victim with prior surgery. A subsequent metrizamide CT scan, however, delineated the entire subarachnoid sac and demonstrated compression of the sac and flattening and posterior displacement of the cervical cord at the C6 level by a retropulsed bone fragment (*arrow*, B). At surgery, a significant amount of bone was found in the canal, especially on the left which corresponded to the patient's greater neurological deficit. This fracture fragment was removed and bilateral foramenotomies and discectomies at C5–6 and C6–7 were performed as well as an anterior cervical fusion. Neurological improvement followed, consisting of increased strength in the patient's arms and legs and decreased spasticity. [Reproduced with permission of Brant-Zawadzki M, Post MJD: Chapt. 8, Trauma. In: Newton TH, Potts DG: *Modern Neuroradiology.* Vol. 1. *Computed Tomography of the Spine and Spinal Cord.* San Anselmo CA, Clavadel Press, 1983.]

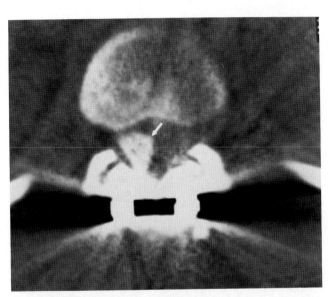

Figure 42.27. Residual Intraspinal Bone Fragment in a Post-operative Patient: In the individual illustrated above, a 19-year-old white male with complete paraplegia and an L3–4 sensory level after a motor vehicle accident, open reduction and Harrington rod instrumentation were performed for an L1 fracture-subluxation. Subsequently incomplete paraplegia was noted. A new radiographic work-up revealed persistence of an extradural myelographic block at T12. It was the metrizamide CT scan however, which demonstrated marked encroachment on the spinal canal at the L1 level by a residual bone fragment (*arrow*). After removal of this fragment, the patient noted increased strength in his lower extremities. [Reproduced with permission of Brant-Zawadzki M, Post MJD: Chapt. 8, Trauma. In: Newton TH, Potts DG: *Modern Neuroradiology*. Vol. 1. *Computed Tomography of the Spine and Spinal Cord*. San Anselmo, CA, Clavadel Press, 1983.]

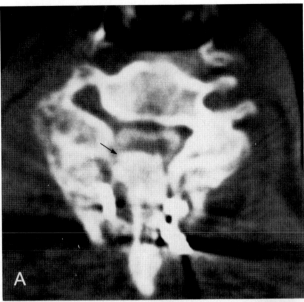

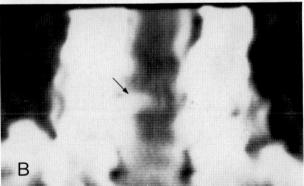

Figure 42.28. Fracture Fragment Causing Cord Compression in a Postoperative Patient with Ankylosing Spondylitis: Axial (A) and reconstructed coronal (B) views from a metrizamide CT scan showing displaced bone (*arrows*) compressing the spinal cord in this spinal injury patient with prior posterior cervical fusion and ankylosing spondylitis. Notice the fusion of the facets.

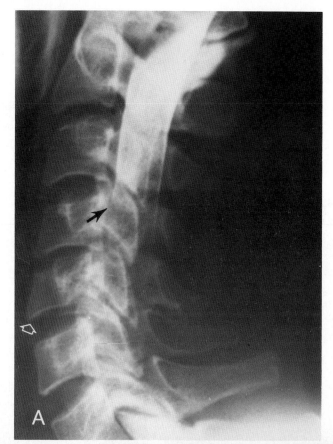

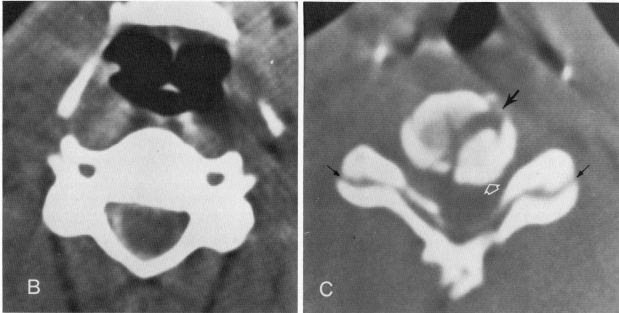

Figure 42.29.   Cord Swelling and C5 Fracture Subluxation: Three weeks after injury in this patient with incomplete quadriplegia, a metrizamide myelogram (A) and CT scan (B and C) were obtained before cervical fusion. The myelogram demonstrated a complete intramedullary block (*arrow*) at a level above the site of fracture-subluxation (*arrowhead*). The CT scan confirmed the cord swelling (B) and also demonstrated comminuted fractures of C5 (*large arrow*, C) with bone fragments displaced into the canal (*arrowhead, C*). Notice the facet subluxation (*small arrows, C*) and posterior arch fractures.

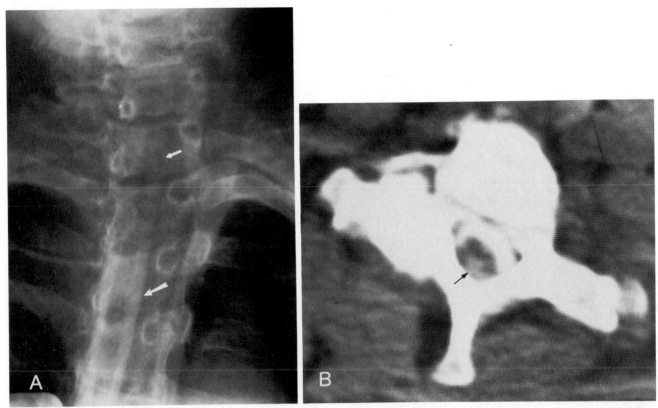

Figure 42.30.   Posttraumatic Hematomyelia: In this 55-year-old black female who had developed flaccid quadriplegia after falling out of bed, an emergency myelogram performed via a C1-C2 lateral subarachnoid puncture revealed no block but poorly delineated the subarachnoid sac in the area of clinical interest (*top arrow,* A). However, a subsequent metrizamide CT scan beautifully outlined the entire subarachnoid sac and demonstrated a hyperdense lesion (*arrow,* B) within the cervical cord compatible with a hematomyelia. As a result of this CT diagnosis, the patient was treated conservatively. [Reproduced with permission of Post et al. (16).]

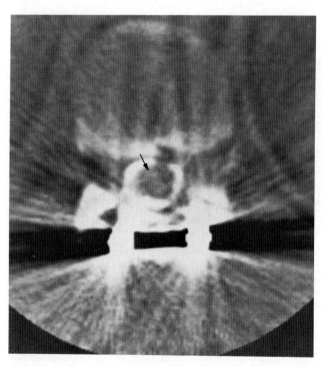

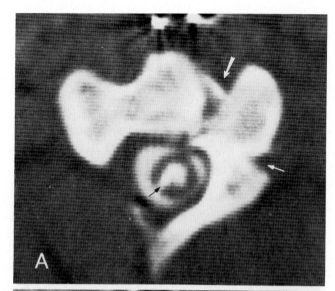

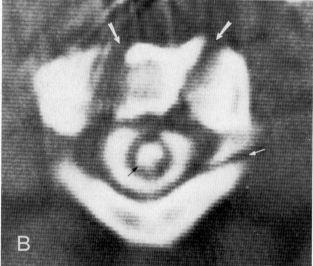

Figure 42.31. Posttraumatic Intramedullary Hemorrhage: On this emergency metrizamide CT scan enlargement of the conus is seen at T11-T12 secondary to hemorrhage (*arrow*). This and other CT images ruled out any significant extradural lesions as the cause of an increasing neurological deficit in a 29-year-old male who had undergone immediate decompression and Harrington rod fixation of an acute T11-T12 fracture subluxation.

Figure 42.32. Acute Traumatic Cord Fissure: In this 31-year-old male with quadripegia after a boating accident, a metrizamide CT scan performed immediately after myelography showed fractures through the body of C2 (*large white arrows*, A and B) and posterior arch fractures (*small white arrows*, A and B). It also revealed a collection of metrizamide (*black arrows*, A and B) within an enlarged cervical cord. This was felt to represent an acute traumatic cord fissure. A follow-up myelogram after a short time interval demonstrated absence of metrizamide within the cord, indicating closure of the acute cord fissure.

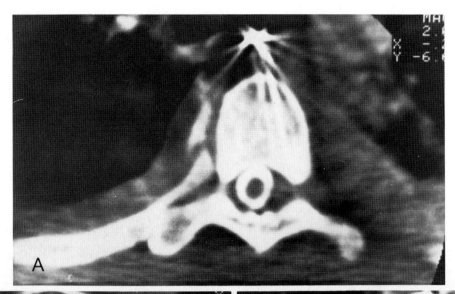

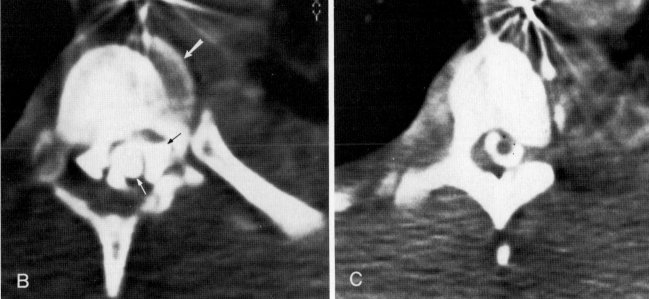

Figure 42.33.   Cord Transection and Avulsed Facet within the Spinal Canal: A 25-year-old black male who was run over by a truck had complete paraplegia and no sensation below the nipple line. A metrizamide CT scan revealed a cord transection at the T4-T5 level. Notice that metrizamide fills the spinal canal (*white arrow,* B) at the level of rotatory and anterior-posterior subluxation of T4 on T5. Metrizamide silhouettes the spinal cord, however, at the levels immediately above and below the cord transection (A and C). Notice also the superior facet of T5 (*black arrow,* B) which is completely avulsed and displaced into the spinal canal. This facet was removed at surgery when the patient underwent a fusion and Harrington rod fixation. [Reproduced with permission of Brant-Zawadzki M, Post MJD: Chapt. 8, Trauma. In: Newton TH, Potts DG: *Modern Neuroradiology.* Vol. 1. *Computed Tomography of the Spine and Spinal Cord.* San Anselmo, CA, Clavadel Press, 1983.]

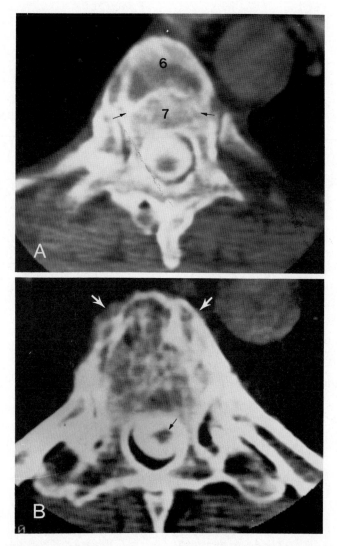

Figure 42.34.   Posttraumatic Cord Atrophy: Because of an incomplete motor deficit in a 46-year-old male who fell 4 years ago, a metrizamide CT scan was performed after a myelogram. It demonstrated old healed compression fractures of T6 and T7 (A and B) with exuberant bone proliferation (*white arrows,* B) and with fusion of the vertebral bodies (*black arrows,* A). Cord atrophy was also apparent (*black arrow,* B).

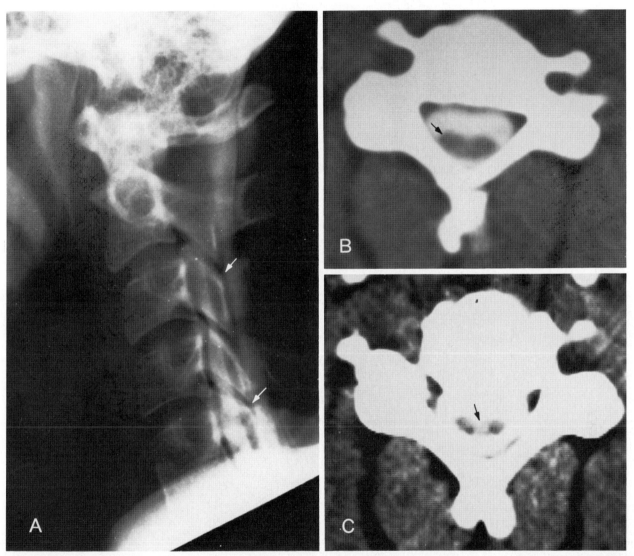

Figure 42.35.   Cord Atrophy and Posttraumatic Syrinx: A metrizamide myelogram demonstrated a small cervical cord (*arrows,* A) in a 28-year-old quadriplegic male with an old anterior cervical fusion for a C5-C6 fracture and with recent onset of hyperhidrosis and blood pressure fluctuations. The delayed metrizamide CT scan demonstrated the cord atrophy (*arrow,* B), and also diagnosed a posttraumatic syrinx. Notice metrizamide filling a cavity within the cervical cord at the C5 level, seen to best advantage on the CT image taken at a narrow window width (*arrow,* C). [Reproduced with permission of Brant-Zawadzki M, Post MJD: Chapt. 8, Trauma. In: Newton TH, Potts DG: *Modern Neuroradiology.* Vol. 1. *Computed Tomography of the Spine and Spinal Cord.* San Anselmo, CA, Clavadel Press, 1983.]

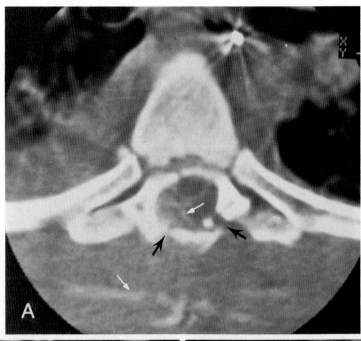

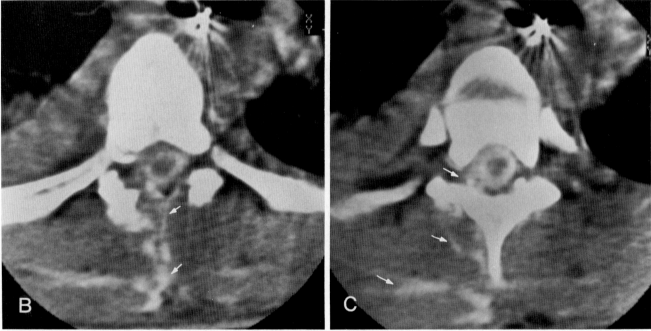

Figure 42.36. Dural Leak: Before surgical reduction and Harrington rod fixation, a metrizamide myelogram and CT scan were performed in a 28-year-old male who had no neurological deficit after a motor vehicle accident. The myelogram showed a partial block at T6-T7, the site of fracture-subluxation. CT delineated well the posterior arch fractures of T6 (*black arrows,* A) which were not optimally seen on the conventional studies. It also demonstrated vertebral body fractures from T6-T9, an epidural hematoma (see Fig. 42.41), pleural effusions, lung contusions, and a small dural leak (*white arrows,* A–C).

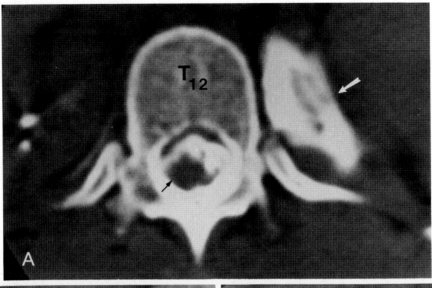

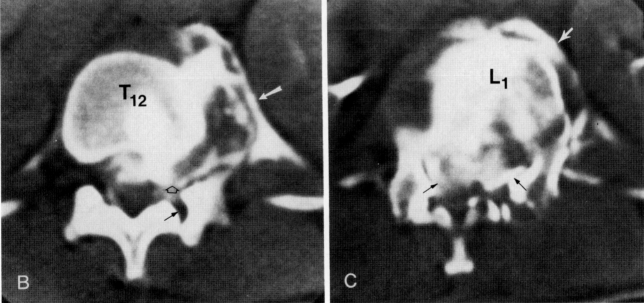

Figure 42.37. Dural Leak: In this 41-year-old male with incomplete paralegia from a motor vehicle accident, a myelogram revealed a high grade block at T12-L1, secondary to a fracture-subluxation. The metrizamide CT scan showed a large dural leak. Notice the extravasation of metrizamide into the paraspinal soft tissues (*white arrows,* A–C). Notice also the swelling of the conus (*black arrow,* A), the facet distraction (*black arrow,* B), the comminuted fracture of L1 (C), and the severe canal compromise caused by the displaced fracture fragments (*black arrows,* C) and marked subluxation. [A and B reproduced with permission of Brant-Zawadzki M, Post MJD: Chapt. 8, Trauma. In: Newton TH, Potts DG: *Modern Neuroradiology.* Vol. 1. *Computed Tomography of the Spine and Spinal Cord.* San Anselmo, CA, Clavadel Press, 1983.]

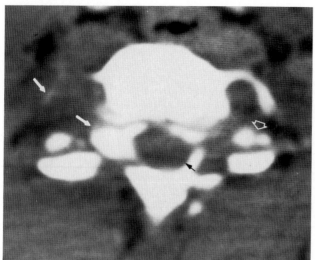

Figure 42.38. Dural Leak: A 23-year-old female was rendered quadriplegic by an automobile accident. Before myelography, an acute C6-C7 fracture-subluxation was reduced. The subsequent CT scan showed metrizamide extending outside the normal confines of the subarachnoid sac into the neural foramen and extraspinal soft tissues (*white arrows*). In addition to this dural leak fractures of the vertebral body and of the superior facets (*arrowhead*) and other posterior elements were seen. Cord swelling (*black arrow*) was also apparent.

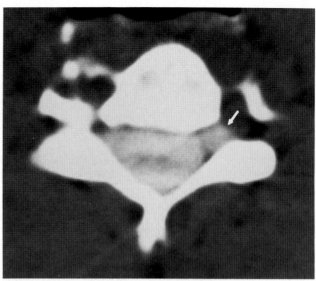

Figure 42.39. Nerve Root Avulsion: A delayed metrizamide CT scan, performed for evaluation of a posttraumatic syrinx, demonstrated a nerve root avulsion. Notice the abnormal collection of metrizamide extending into the neural foramen (arrow). (Same case as shown in Fig. 42.35).

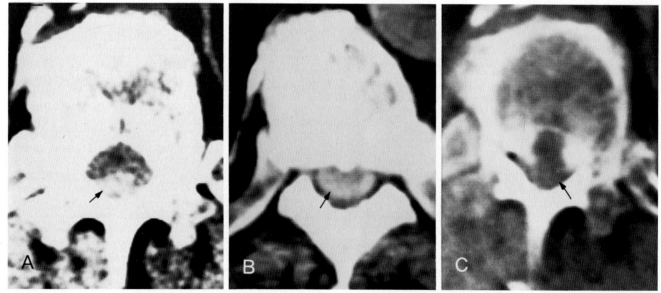

Figure 42.40. Acute Epidural Hematoma: An emergency plain HRCT (A–B) was prompted by the sudden onset of chest pain, flaccid paraplegia, and sensory loss in this 76-year-old white male who had been anticoagulated with heparin 18 hours earlier for posterior fossa transient ischemic attacks. Multiple unsuccessful lumbar punctures had preceded the anticoagulation. An epidural hematoma was diagnosed on the noncontrast study by the sharply demarcated peripheral area of hyperdensity (*arrow*, A). Subarachnoid blood was also seen (*arrow*, B). However, because the true extent of the lesion could not be determined (the hematoma was seen at multiple discontinuous levels), and because the spinal cord could not be discriminated, a myelogram was performed followed by metrizamide CT scan. The latter study (C) demonstrated that the epidural hematoma (*arrow*) extended continuously from L2 to T5. It also delineated the spinal cord and its anterior displacement. (Autopsy confirmation of diagnosis). [Reproduced with permission of Post et al. (41).]

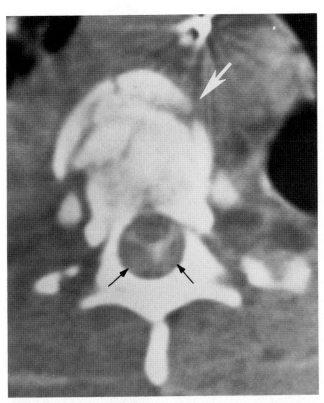

Figure 42.41. Acute Epidural Hematoma: Posterolateral extradural defects (*black arrows*) consistent with epidural hematomas are seen compressing the metrizamide-filled subarachnoid sac at T7 in this patient with multiple acute thoracic fractures (*white arrow*).

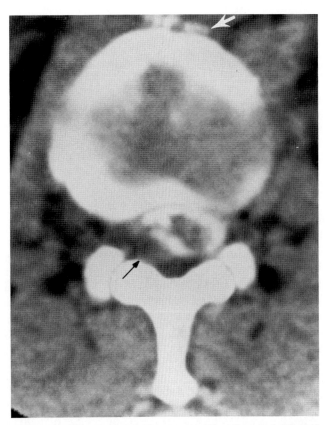

Figure 42.42. Epidural Hematoma After Gunshot Wound: Four days after a gunshot wound to the abdomen, a metrizamide CT scan was obtained. It localized bullet fragments to the soft tissues anterior to L1 and L2 (*white arrow*) as well as to the L1 vertebral body and spinal canal. Immediately above and below the intraspinal bullet fragments posterolateral compression of the subarachnoid sac and displacement of the swollen conus were seen. These mass effects were felt to be secondary to a SEH (*black arrow*).

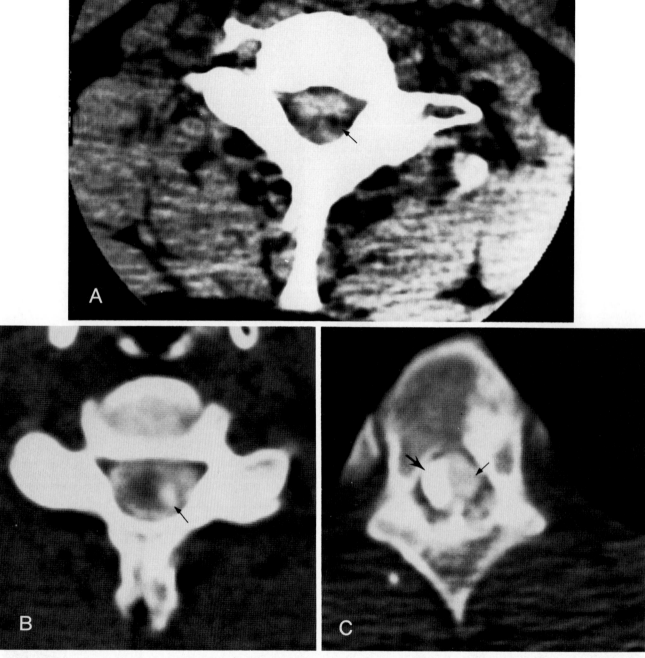

Figure 42.43.   Posttraumatic Syrinx from a Gunshot Wound: In this 41-year-old male with an old gunshot wound to the thoracic spine, a plain HRCT scan was performed because of the development of severe pain, increasing spasms, and upward ascent of neurological deficit. It demonstrated a hypodense lesion within the cervical cord (*arrow,* A). However, a delayed metrizamide CT scan was needed to show the entire extent of this posttraumatic syrinx. It revealed that the syrinx extended from the level of injury in the thoracic cord (*small arrow,* C) to the cervical cord (*arrow,* B). The bullet fragment retained within the thoracic canal (*large arrow,* C) was also apparent. [A and B reproduced with permission of Brant-Zawadzki M, Post MJD: Chapt. 8, Trauma. In: Newton TH, Potts DG: *Modern Neuroradiology.* Vol. 1. *Computed Tomography of the Spine and Spinal Cord.* San Anselmo, CA, Clavadel Press, 1983.]

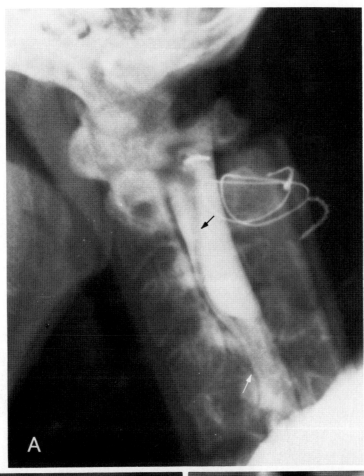

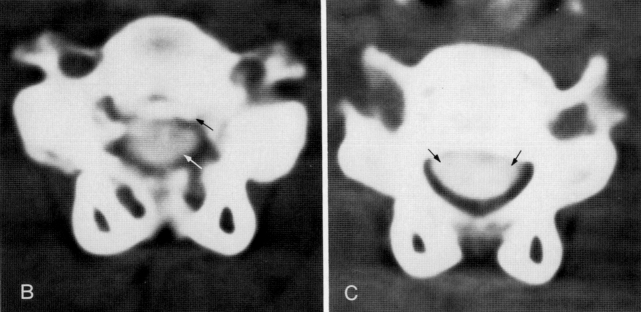

Figure 42.44. Posttraumatic Syrinx: This 26-year-old quadriplegic male with a chronic fracture-subluxation of C4-C5 treated by anterior and posterior cervical fusion developed increasing pain. The metrizamide myelogram (A) demonstrated a very small atrophic cervical cord (*black arrow*) which appeared tethered anteriorly at the C3 level. It also showed considerable compression of the subarachnoid sac at the level of prior surgery (*white arrow*). The delayed metrizamide CT scan confirmed the bony encroachment on the canal (*black arrow*, B) at the C4-C5 level. However, more significantly, it revealed a large posttraumatic cord cyst (*white arrow*, B; *arrows*, C). The patient was shunted as a result of this study.

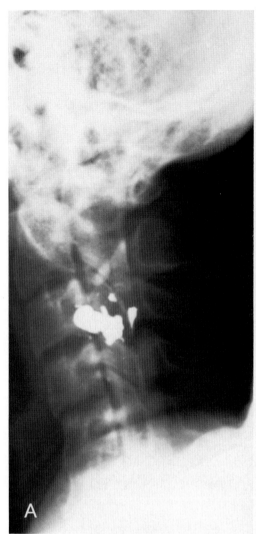

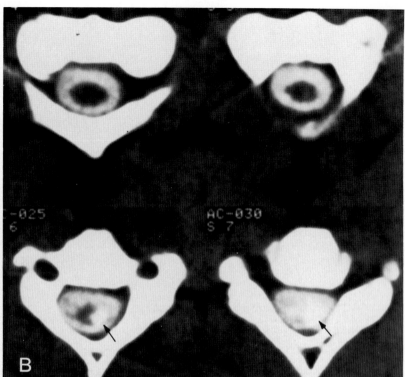

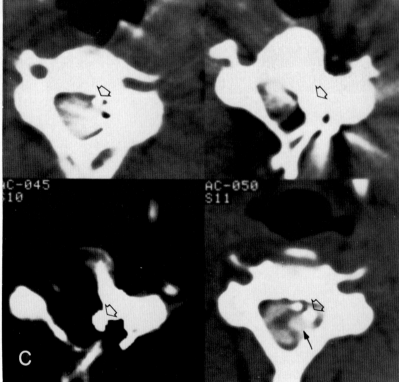

Figure 42.45. Posttraumatic Cyst from a Gunshot Wound: In this 28-year-old male with quadriplegia secondary to a gunshot wound to the C3-4 level 3 months previously, an increase in pain led to a radiographic work-up. The myelogram (A) demonstrated defects secondary to the gunshot wound but no block. The subsequent metrizamide CT scan, however, showed metrizamide filling a portion of the cervical cord both above (*arrows*, B), at and below (*arrow*, C) the level of injury, findings compatible with a post-traumatic syrinx. The streak artifacts in C are being caused by the bullet fragments (*arrowheads*). [Reproduced with permission of Brant-Zawadzki M, Post MJD: Chapt. 8, Trauma. In: Newton TH, Potts DG: *Modern Neuroradiology.* Vol. 1. *Computed Tomography of the Spine and Spinal Cord.* San Anselmo, CA, Clavadel Press, 1983.]

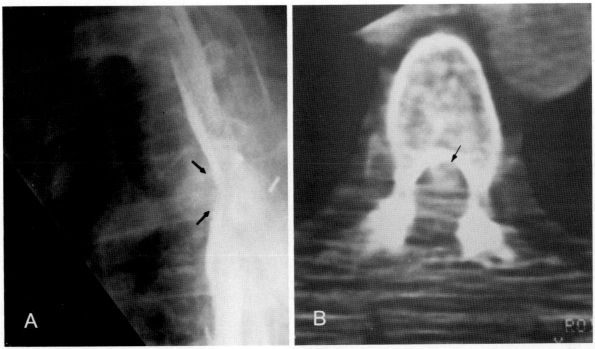

Figure 42.46. Chronic Posttraumatic Disc Herniation: A 48-year-old female with a history of prior trauma had undergone a laminectomy which was unsuccessful at revealing the cause of her incomplete paraplegia. A subsequent myelogram (A) revealed a ventral extradural defect at T5 (*arrows*). An HRCT scan demonstrated the etiology of this myelographic defect: a herniated disc (*arrow,* B). This diagnosis was confirmed at surgery. [Reproduced with permission of Brant-Zawadzki M, Post MJD: Chapt. 8, Trauma. In: Newton TH, Potts DG: *Modern Neuroradiology.* Vol. 1. *Computed Tomography of the Spine and Spinal Cord.* San Anselmo, CA, Clavadel Press, 1983.]

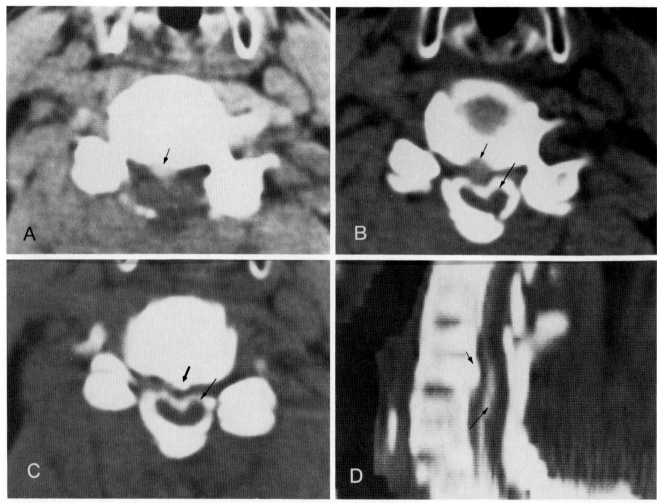

Figure 42.47. Chronic Posttraumatic Disc Hernation: Plain CT scan showing a soft-tissue lesion compatible with a herniated disc (*arrow,* A) projecting into the cervical canal in this chronic trauma victim in whom a prior laminectomy had failed to reveal the source of the patient's weakness. Subsequent myelogram and metrizamide CT scan in axial (B and C) and sagittally reconstructed (D) views demonstrated that this cervical disc had both a soft-tissue (*short arrow,* B) and calcific (*short arrows,* C and D) component. Severe cord compression and deformity (*long arrows,* B–D) were also apparent. Notice too the incidental postsurgical meningocele. [Reproduced with permission of Brant-Zawadzki M, Post MJD: Chapt. 8, Trauma. In: Newton TH, Potts DG: *Modern Neuroradiology.* Vol. 1. *Computed Tomography of the Spine and Spinal Cord.* San Anselmo, CA, Clavadel Press, 1983.]

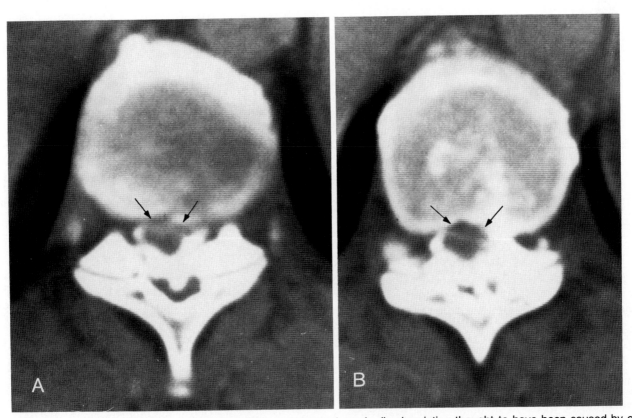

Figure 42.48.   Chronic Posttraumatic Disc Hernation: A chronic thoracic disc herniation thought to have been caused by old trauma is shown on the above metrizamide CT scans. It is seen at the disc space level (*arrows,* A and B) markedly compressing the ventral subarachnoid sac and thoracic cord.

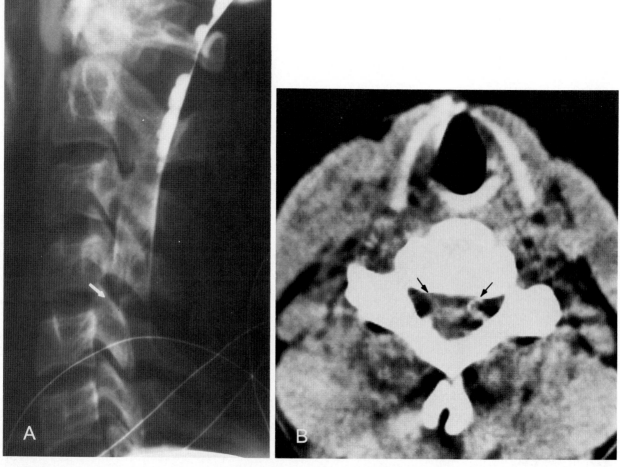

Figure 42.49. Acute Posttraumatic Disc Herniation: Lateral view of a metrizamide myelogram (A) in this acute spinal trauma patient shows a complete extradural ventral block (*arrow*) at the site of mild C4-C5 subluxation. Subsequent CT scan (B) identifies a large soft-tissue disc herniation (*arrows*) as the etiology of the myelographic block. Notice also the cord compression.

disease, calcification within the lesion and/or adjacent osteophytes may be seen (Fig. 42.47C and D).

While plain HRCT may suffice in the evaluation of traumatic lumbar disc herniations, metrizamide CT scanning often is needed for the complete evaluation of thoracic and cervical disc herniations. CAM silhouettes the herniated disc against the metrizamide-filled subarachnoid sac (Fig. 42.48). CAM also demonstrates the position and configuration of the spinal cord (Fig. 42.49B). This is useful information to the surgeon because the spinal cord is often compressed and displaced by disc herniations.

CONCLUSION

CT should be a standard radiographic study in the evaluation of patients with spinal trauma. It provides unique and critical information in the spinal injury victim about the osseous spine and the intraspinal and paraspinal soft tissues. This information directly affects patient management.

References

1. Grossman ZD, Wistow BW, Waldman HA, et al: Recognition of vertebral abnormalities in computed tomography of the chest and abdomen. *Radiology* 121:369–373, 1976.
2. Balériaux-Waha D, Mortelmans LL, Dupont MG, et al: Computed tomography for lesions of the craniovertebral region. *Neuroradiology* 13:59–61, 1977.
3. Coin CG, Chan Y-S, Keranen V, et al: Computer assisted myelography in disk disease. *J Comput Assist Tomogr* 1:398–404, 1977.
4. Kershner MS, Goodman GA, Perlmutter GS: Computed tomography in the diagnosis of an atlas fracture. *AJR* 128:688–689, 1977.
5. Wolpert SM, Scott RM, Carter BL, et al: Manifestations of fractures of the spine as seen on computed tomography. Presented at the *Sixteenth Annual Meeting of the American Society of Neuroradiology*, New Orleans, February-March, 1978.
6. Binet EF, Ullrich CG, Sanecki MG: Computed tomography in the evaluation of post-traumatic impingement on the spinal canal. Presented at the *Sixteenth Annual Meeting of the American Society of Neuroradiology*, New Orleans, February-March, 1978.
7. Nykamp PW, Levy JM, Christensen F, et al: Computed to-

mography for a bursting fracture of the lumbar spine. *J Bone Joint Surg* 60-A:1108–1109, 1978.

8. Tadmor R, Davis KR, Robertson GH, New PFJ, Taveras JM: Computed tomographic evaluation of traumatic spinal injuries. *Radiology* 127:825–827, 1978.

9. Coin G, Keranen VJ, Pennink M, et al: Computerized tomography of the spine and its contents. *Neuroradiology* 16:271–272, 1978.

10. Lee BCP, Kazam E, Newman AD: Computed tomography of the spine and spinal cord. *Radiology* 128:95–102, 1978.

11. Colley DP, Dunsker SB: Traumatic narrowing of the dorsolumbar spinal canal demonstrated by computed tomography. *Radiology* 129:95–98, 1978.

12. Rinaldi I, Mullins WJ Jr., Delaney WF, et al: Computerized tomographic demonstration of rotational atlanto-axial fixation. *J Neurosurg* 50:115–119, 1979.

13. Paul DF, Morrey BF, Helms CA: Computerized tomography in orthopedic surgery. *Clin Orthop* 139:142–149, 1979.

14. O'Callaghan JP, Yuan H, Ullrich CG, et al: Computed tomographic imaging of facet distraction in flexion injuries of the thoracolumbar spine: The "naked facet." Presented at the *Seventeenth Annual Meeting of the American Society of Neuroradiology*, Toronto, May 1979.

15. Sackett JF, Alter AJ, Keene JS, et al: Efficacy of spinal CT to evaluate spinal fractures. Presented at the *Seventeenth Annual Meeting of the American Society of Neuroradiology*, Toronto, May 1979.

16. Post MJD, Green BA, Quencer RM, et al: The value of computed tomography in spinal trauma. *Spine* 7:417–431, 1982.

17. Naidich TP, King DG, Moran CJ, et al: CT of the spine and spinal cord. Presented at the *Seventeenth Annual Meeting of the American Society of Neuroradiology*, Toronto, May 1979.

18. Coin CG, Pennink M, Ahmad WD, et al: Diving-type injury of the cervical spine: Contribution of computed tomography to management. *J Comput Assist Tomogr* 3:362–372, 1979.

19. Roub LW, Drayer BP: Spinal computed tomography: Limitations and applications. *AJR* 133:267–273, 1979.

20. Faerber EN, Wolpert SM, Scott RM, et al: Computed tomography of spinal fractures. *J Comput Assist Tomogr* 3:657–661, 1979.

21. McInerney DP, Sage MR: Computer-assisted tomography in the assessment of cervical spine trauma. *Clin Radiol* 30:203–206, 1979.

22. Naidich TP, Pudlowski RM, Moran CJ, et al: Computed tomography of spinal fractures. In: Thompson RA, Green JR: *Advances in Neurology*. New York, Raven Press, 1979, Vol 22, pp. 207–253.

23. Brant-Zawadzki M, Miller EM, Federle MP: CT in the evaluation of spine trauma. *AJR* 136:369–75, 1981.

24. Light TR, Wagner FC, Johnson RM, et al: Correction of spinal instability and recovery of neurologic loss following cervical vertebral body replacement. *Spine* 5:392–394, 1980.

25. Miller EM: The role of CT in evaluation of spinal trauma. Presented at the *Eighteenth Annual Meeting of the American Society of Neuroradiology*, Los Angeles, March 1980.

26. Seibert CE, Dreisbach JN, Swanson WB, et al: Neuroradiological evaluation in progressive post-traumatic cystic myelopathy (PPCM) (post-traumatic syringomyelia). Presented at the *Eighteenth Annual Meeting of the American Society of Neuroradiology*, Los Angeles, March 1980.

27. White RR, Newberg A, Seligson D: Computerized tomographic assessment of the traumatized dorsolumbar spine before and after Harrington instrumentation. *Clin Orthop* 146:150–156, 1980.

28. O'Callaghan JPO, Ullrich CG, Yuan HA, et al: CT of facet distraction in flexion injuries of the thoracolumbar spine: The "naked" facet. *AJR* 134:563–568, 1980.

29. Post MJD, Quencer RM, Stokes NA: Computed tomography of the spine. In: Margulis A, Gooding CA: *Diagnostic Radiology*. San Francisco, University of California at San Francisco,

1980, pp. 673–702.

30. Post MJD: Computed tomography of the spine: Its values and limitations on a non-high resolution scanner. In: Post MJD: *Radiographic Evaluation of the Spine: Current Advances with Emphasis on Computed Tomography*. New York, Masson Publishing, 1980, pp. 186–258.

31. Coin CG: Computed tomography of the spine. In: Post MJD: *Radiographic Evaluation of the Spine: Current Advances with Emphasis on Computed Tomography*. New York, Masson Publishing, 1980, pp. 394–412.

32. Sheldon JJ, Leborgne J-M: Computed tomography of the lumbar vertebral column. In: Post MJD: *Radiographic Evaluation of the Spine: Current Advances with Emphasis on Computed Tomography*. New York, Masson Publishing USA, Inc., 1980, pp. 56–87.

33. Ethier R, King DG, Melancon D, et al: Diagnosis of intra- and extramedullary lesions by CT without contrast achieved through modifications applied to the EMI CT 5005 body scanner. In: Post MJD: *Radiographic Evaluation of the Spine: Current Advances with Emphasis on Computed Tomography*. New York, Masson Publishing USA, Inc., 1980, pp. 377–393.

34. Post MJD: CT update: The impact of time, metrizamide and high resolution on the diagnosis of spinal pathology. In: Post MJD: *Radiographic Evaluation of the Spine: Current Advances with Emphasis on Computed Tomography*. New York, Masson Publishing, 1980, pp. 259–294.

35. Ullrich CG, Kieffer SA: Computed tomographic evaluation of the lumbar spine: Quantitative aspects and sagittal-coronal reconstruction. In: Post MJD: *Radiographic Evaluation of the Spine: Current Advances with Emphasis on Computed Tomography*. New York, Masson Publishing, 1980, pp. 88–107.

36. Harris JH, Jr: Acute injuries of the spine. *Sem Roentgenol* 13:53–68, 1978.

37. Maravilla KR, Cooper PR, Sklar FH: The influence of thin-section tomography on the treatment of cervical spine injuries. *Radiology* 127:131–139, 1978.

38. Russin LD, Guinto FC, Jr: Multidirectional tomography in cervical spine injury. *J Neurosurg* 45:9–11, 1976.

39. McCall IW, Park WM, McSweeney T: The radiological demonstration of acute lower cervical injury. *Clin Radiol* 24:235–240, 1973.

40. Braakman R, Vinken PJ: Old luxations of the lower cervical spine. *J Bone Joint Surg* 50B:52–60, 1968.

41. Post MJD, Seminer DS, Quencer RM: CT diagnosis of spinal epidural hematoma. *AJNR* 3:190–192, 1982.

42. Brant-Zawadzki M, Post MJD: Trauma. In: Newton TH, Potts DG: *Computed Tomography of the Spine and Spinal Cord*. San Anselmo, CA, Clavadel Press, 1983, pp. 149–186.

43. Green BA, Callahan RA, Klose KJ, et al: Acute spinal cord injury: Current concepts. *Clin Orthop* 154:125–135, 1981.

44. Härkönen M, Lepistö P, Paakkala T, et al: Spinal cord injuries associated with vertebral fractures and dislocations: Clinical and radiological results in 30 patients. *Arch Orthop Trauma Surg* 94:185–190, 1979.

45. Julow J, Szarvas I, Sárváry A: Clinical study of injuries of the lower cervical spinal cord. *Injury* 11:39–42, 1979.

46. Cloward RB: Treatment of acute fractures and fracture-dislocations of the cervical spine by vertebral-body fusion. *J Neurosurg* 18:201–209, 1961.

47. Verbiest H: Anterolateral operations for fractures and dislocations in the middle and lower parts of the cervical spine. *J Bone Joint Surg* 51-A:1489–1630, 1969.

48. Frankel HL, Hancock DO, Hyslop G, et al: The value of postural reduction in the initial management of closed injuries of the spine with paraplegia and tetraplegia. *Paraplegia* 7:179–192, 1969.

49. Holdsworth F: Fractures, dislocations, and fracture-dislocations of the spine. *J Bone Joint Surg* 52-A:1534–1551, 1970.

50. Yashon D, Jane JA, White RJ: Prognosis and management of spinal cord and cauda equina bullet injuries in sixty-five

civilians. *J Neurosurg* 32:163–170, 1970.

51. Norrell HA: Fractures and dislocations of the spine. In: Rothman RH, Simeone FA: *The Spine*. Vol 2, Philadelphia, W.B. Saunders, 1975, pp. 529–566.

52. Flesch JR, Leider LL, Erickson DL, et al: Harrington instrumentation and spine fusion for unstable fractures and fracture-dislocations of the thoracic and lumbar spine. *J Bone Joint Surg* 59-A:143–152, 1977.

53. Dickson JH, Harrington PR, Erwin WD: Results of reduction and stabilization of the severely fractured thoracic and lumbar spine. *J Bone Joint Surg* 60-A:799–805, 1978.

54. Bedbrook GM: Spinal injuries with tetraplegia and paraplegia. *J Bone Joint Surg* 61-B:267–284, 1979.

55. Bohlman HH: Acute fractures and dislocations of the cervical spine. *J Bone Joint Surg* 61-A:1119–1141, 1979.

56. Ducker TB, Russo GL, Bellegarrique R, et al: Complete sensorimotor paralysis after cord injury: Mortality, recovery, and therapeutic implications. *J Trauma* 19:837–840, 1979.

57. Maynard FM, Reynolds GG, Fountain S, et al: Neurological prognosis after traumatic quadriplegia. *J Neurosurg* 50:611–616, 1979.

58. Larson SJ, Holst R, Hemmy D, et al: Lateral extracavitary approach to traumatic lesions of the thoracic and lumbar spine. *J Neurosurg* 45:628–637, 1976.

59. Brodkey JS, Miller Jr CF, Harmody RM: The syndrome of acute central cervical spinal cord injury revisited. *Surg Neurol* 14:251–257, 1980.

60. Sachdev VP, Huang YP, Shah CP, et al: Posttraumatic pseudomeningomyelocele (enlarging fracture?) in a vertebral body. Case report. *J Neurosurg* 54:545–549, 1981.

61. Hinkel CL, Nichols RL: Opaque myelography in penetrating wounds of the spinal canal. *AJR* 55:689–709, 1946.

62. Murtagh F, Chamberlain WE, Scott M, et al: Cervical air myelography: A review of 130 cases. *AJR* 74:1–21, 1955.

63. Alker GL, Jr, Glasauer FE, Zov JG, et al: Myelographic demonstration of lumbosacral nerve root avulsion. *Radiology* 89:101–104, 1967.

64. Kelly DL, Alexander E: Lateral cervical puncture for myelography. *J Neurosurg* 29:106–110, 1968.

65. Zilkha A, Reiss J, Shulman K, et al: Traumatic subarachnoid mediastinal fistula. *J Neurosurg* 32:473–475, 1970.

66. Nurick S, Russell A, Deck MDF: Cystic degeneration of the spinal cord following spinal cord injury. *Brain* 93:211–222, 1970.

67. Raynor RB: Discography and myelography in acute injuries of the cervical spine. *J Neurosurg* 35:529–535, 1971.

68. Heinz ER, Goldman RL: The role of gas myelography in neuroradiologic diagnosis. *Radiology* 102:629–634, 1972.

69. Pear BL: Spinal epidural hematoma. *AJR* 115:155–164, 1972.

70. Shapiro BL: *Myelography*. Chicago, Year Book Medical Publishers, Inc., 1975, pp. 195–224.

71. Paul RL, Michael RH, Dunn JE, et al: Anterior transthoracic surgical decompression of acute spinal cord injuries. *J Neurosurg* 43:299–307, 1975.

72. Miyazaki Y: Selective anterior cervical gas myelography by the lateral approach. *Neuroradiology* 10:151–153, 1975.

73. Pay NT, George AE, Benjamin MV, et al: Positive and negative contrast myelography in spinal trauma. *Radiology* 123:103–111, 1977.

74. Leo JS, Bergeron RT, Kricheff II, et al: Metrizamide myelography through supine lateral C1–2 puncture in early management of acute cervical spinal cord injuries. Presented at the *Sixteenth Annual Meeting of the American Society of Neuroradiology*, New Orleans, February-March, 1978.

75. Haughton VM, Williams AL: *Computed Tomography of The Spine*. St. Louis, The C. V. Mosby Co, 1982, pp. 187–207.

76. Seibert CE, Dreisbach JN, Swanson WB, et al: Progressive post-traumatic cystic myelopathy: Neuroradiologic evaluation. *AJNR* 2:115–119, 1981.

77. Aubin ML, Vignaud J, Jardin C, et al: Computed tomography in 75 clinical cases of syringomyelia. *AJNR* 2:199–204, 1981.

CHAPTER FORTY-THREE

The Radiological and Clinical Features of Posttraumatic Spinal Cord Cysts

ROBERT M. QUENCER, M.D., BARTH A. GREEN, M.D., and FRANK J. EISMONT, M.D.

INTRODUCTION

Among the most depressing events in the life of a spinal cord injured patient is the onset of new and/or progressively worsening neurological symptoms after a period of clinical stability. Because of the large number of spine injured patients hospitalized at the University of Miami/Jackson Medical Center and its regional spinal cord injury center we have had an opportunity of evaluating clinically and radiologically patients with this type of medical history. In these patients, intramedullary cysts have been found by the use of metrizamide computed tomography (MCT) and substantial clinical improvement has been achieved after the shunting of these cysts into the subarachnoid space. It is, therefore, important for clinicians and radiologists alike to appreciate the varied clinical and radiological features of this entity which we have termed "posttraumatic spinal cord cysts" (PTSCC) (1). The material for this chapter is based on our observations of 16 cases of PTSCCs.

OBJECTS

The objects of this chapter are 2-fold. The first is to describe the clinical presentations of PTSCCs and the benefits of the cyst shunting procedure. The second is to demonstrate the radiological features of PTSCCs.

From the clinical standpoint, a number of questions will be attempted to be answered, specifically: 1) Do injuries at certain cord levels have a greater propensity for developing cysts than injuries at other levels and does the development of a PTSCC relate to the severity of the injury? 2) Does the stabilization of the spine soon after the original injury prevent the development of PTSCCs? 3) Under what time frame do PTSCC symptoms develop? 4) What are the most common symptoms of PTSCCs? 5) Is there a relationship between the location and severity of the original spinal cord injury and the time interval within which the symptoms of a PTSCC develop? 6) Are cyst shunting procedures valuable in alleviating the symptoms of PTSCCs?

From the radiological standpoint, we will describe 1) the incidence of single versus multiple cysts, 2) the length and location of the cysts in relation to the site of original injury, 3) the common positions of cysts within the cord, 4) cyst width relative to the size of the cord, and 5) the incidence of associated cord atrophy at levels other than at the cyst level. Combining these findings with the clinical information, the operability of a PTSCC can be determined.

CLINICAL FEATURES

As would be expected, PTSCC occurs predominately in young adult males in whom the major cause for the original injury was a motor vehicle accident. Gunshot wounds, diving accidents, and falls are less common precipitating factors. As a result of their injuries (fractures and/or subluxations), these patients are rendered either completely or incompletely paraplegic or quadriplegic. Quadriplegia is more common because the majority of injuries occur in the midcervical region. We have found that the development of PTSCCs is independent site of the injury—i.e., it may occur either as a result of thoracic trauma or cervical trauma. We have never seen a case of a PTSCC which was a consequence of minor spinal trauma as has been reported as a rare finding (2). In addition, whether the patient had suffered a complete or incomplete injury had no bearing on the eventual development of a PTSCC.

Virtually an equal number of PTSCCs occurred in patients who had spine fusions after the initial injury as those who had no fusion. It appears, therefore, that immediate postinjury fusion surgery had no bearing on the eventual development of PTSCCs.

There are three different circumstances under which PTSCCs may be discovered. The most common circumstance is that the patient has been neurologically stable for a well-defined period of time which, in our cases, has ranged from 3 months to 13 years with an average of 4 years after the original injury. Then there is the onset of a new set of symptoms which become increasingly severe with time. The time intervals we have found are similar to other reported clinical series (3–5). The fact that cysts were found by 3 months postinjury indicates that cysts of significant size may begin to form shortly after the original trauma. In the less common situations, either there is a slowly and progressively worsening of the patients' symptoms right from the time of injury or there is neither the onset of new symptoms nor is there progressive symptomatology. In cases where there are no new or progressive symptoms, a PTSCC may be found incidentally in a patient who is being examined with MCT either in order to see if there are bone fragments in the canal or in hopes of explaining a discrepancy between motor and sensory levels. The fact that not all patients will have progressive symptomatology has lead us to use the more anatomically descriptive term posttraumatic spinal cord cysts rather than the term "progressive posttraumatic cystic myelopathy" which has been used by others (6).

Neck or back pain was the most common complaint in

patients with new or progressive symptoms. The pain frequently was worsened by any Valsalva maneuver such as straining, coughing, or sneezing. In decreasing order of frequency, the other symptoms were increasing spasticity, motor/sensory loss, and hyperhidrosis. Usually there is a presenting symptom complex rather than just one of these symptoms. In fact, when one symptom alone was present, it was most likely to be increasing spasticity. In no patient was there evidence of brain stem dysfunction or the sudden worsening of the patients' neurological status to suggest hemorrhage into a cyst.

We investigated the time interval within which the symptoms of a PTSCC develop and related this to the location and severity of the original injury. Although Barnett and Jousse (3) found the cyst symptoms appeared more rapidly in patients with severe cord injuries, we were unable to confirm this observation. In fact, in our patients with incomplete lesions, the time interval to new symptoms was one-half the time interval demonstrated by our patients with complete lesions. Although the number of patients within each category is small, there appears to be no relationship between severity of injury and the rapidity with which new symptoms develop. Concerning the location of the injury and the time interval to new symptoms, we agree with Williams et al. (7) that there is no positive correlation. Specifically the relatively rapid onset of new symptoms or the slowly progressive appearance of symptoms was as likely to occur with a thoracic injury as with a cervical injury.

Methods of treatment for PTSCCs have ranged from cordectomy (8) to shunting the cyst into either the peritoneal cavity (9) or into the subarachnoid space (6) to supportive, nonsurgical intervention (10). Our routine is to shunt those cysts which are of adequate size and in a suitable location into the adjacent subarachnoid space. Depending on the size and the number of cysts to be shunted, either a single level or a multiple level laminectomy is performed. Adhesions between the spinal cord and the dural/arachnoidal layers invariably are present at the old injury site and these are lysed before the cordotomy. The location of the incision on the cord surface and its depth depends on the position of the cyst as determined with MCT. A multiple side hole ventricular catheter is passed into the cyst and the catheter then is secured to the pial surface of the cord. The distal portion of the catheter is left in an area of subarachnoid space free of adhesions so that an effective drainage system from the cyst is established. If additional cysts are present, they may be shunted similarly as their size and location warrants. When bullet fragments are present, they are removed and fusion surgery is performed as deemed necessary. During surgery, somatosensory evoked potentials are monitored and we have noted a change in amplitude and latency after lysis of the adhesions and the after drainage of the cyst. More recently, our use of intraoperative real-time ultrasonography has allowed us to see both the cerebrospinal fluid CSF dynamics at the point of the tethered cord and the size of the cyst before and after shunting. The clinical results of this shunting procedure have been

gratifying. There have been no complications or permanent worsening of any patient's motor function as a result of this operation, although 1 patient had a decrease in motor strength for 72 hours whereas another experienced a subjective decrease in sensation and no improvement in his spasticity. The duration of the preoperative symptoms had no bearing on the outcome after shunting. All patients with symptoms of pain, hyperhidrosis, and motor/sensory loss showed improvement; however, complaints of increasing spasticity improved in only 50% of the cases. It must be added that a long-term follow-up (greater than 1 year) is available in only 2 patients, but in both we have noted no recurrence of the PTSCC symptoms.

A typical clinical history of one of our patients with a PTSCC follows and his MCT is shown in Figure 43.1. An

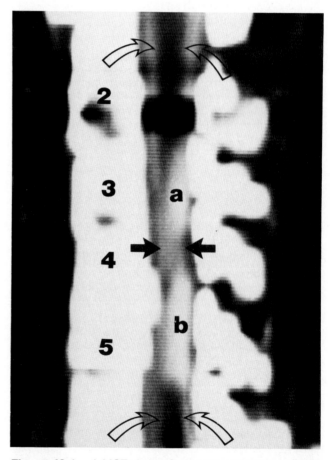

Figure 43.1. A MCT shows 2 separate cysts (a and b) 3½ years after a C5 fracture and a C4–5 subluxation. No cyst is identified between the 2 cysts, however that short area (*straight arrows*) is of increased density and may reflect a zone of altered spinal cord permeability. Both cysts reached the most dorsal portion of the cord and each was wide (greater than ½ width of the cord at its maximum width). The cord was normal in size below and above the cyst levels (*open curved arrows*). Note the predominate superior extension of the cysts from the site of injury. Based on these findings, 2 separate shunts were used for cyst decompression.

18-year-old male was involved in a motor vehicle accident suffering a C5 fracture with a C4–5 subluxation. He was a complete quadriplegic with a C5 motor and sensory level. No surgery was performed at his initial hospitalization. After a clinically stable period of 3½ years, he had the onset of increasing spasticity, hyperhidrosis, with loss of his C5 motor segment. Based on the MCT findings (Fig. 43.1), the patient had two shunts placed, each draining separate cysts. After the operation, there was increased strength in the C5 segment, decreased spasticity, and loss of hyperhidrosis.

RADIOGRAPHIC FEATURES

Metrizamide myelography via a C1–2 puncture with an average of 10 cc of contrast at a concentration of 220 mg/ml is used in the investigation of PTSCCs. If a complete block is present, we install additional contrast distal to the block. The rationale for this is to ensure that the entire spinal cord is bathed in metrizamide, increasing the chances of visualizing multilevel cysts, if present. It is necessary to use a water-soluble myelographic agent such as metrizamide rather than an oil-based agent (Pantopaque), because the diagnosis of a PTSCC can be made with Pantopaque myelography only on the basis of an enlarged spinal cord, and that happens only occasionally. Only a water-soluble agent such as metrizamide is able to penetrate through the cord substance to fill these cysts.

Because the cysts fill slowly, a delayed MCT is crucial in the diagnosis of PTSCCs. PTSCCs will be greatly underdiagnosed if Pantopaque is used because in 90% of the cases, the cord is either normal in size or atrophic (1). If MCT is performed immediately postmetrizamide myelography, intramedullary cysts may not have had sufficient time to fill and will not be detected with CT. We, therefore, advocate as close to a 4-hour delayed MCT as possible in order to maximize cyst opacification. Because of the demands of the clinical usage on our scanner we have not been able to perform a controlled study to determine how the time of scanning postmyelography relates to cyst opacification, however selection of a 4-hour delay corresponds well with experimental determination of time to maximum cord opacification in normal animals (11).

Careful scrutiny of the axial and reformatted images is necessary to exclude presence of multiple PTSCCs (Fig. 43.1). Although we have found that most patients (75%) have a single cyst (Figs. 43.2 and 43.3), multiplicity does occur (25%). Before the use of MCT, separate cysts had been demonstrated only on pathological specimens (4, 12, 13). In all cases, the cyst or cysts appear to have originated adjacent to the level of cord trauma. Radiographically PTSCCs are seen to vary in length from 0.5 cm to the entire length of the cord. As a general rule, the shorter cysts (2 cm or less) tend to expand superiorly (Fig. 43.3) wheras the longer cysts may have either a superior and inferior extension from the original injury site (Fig. 43.4)

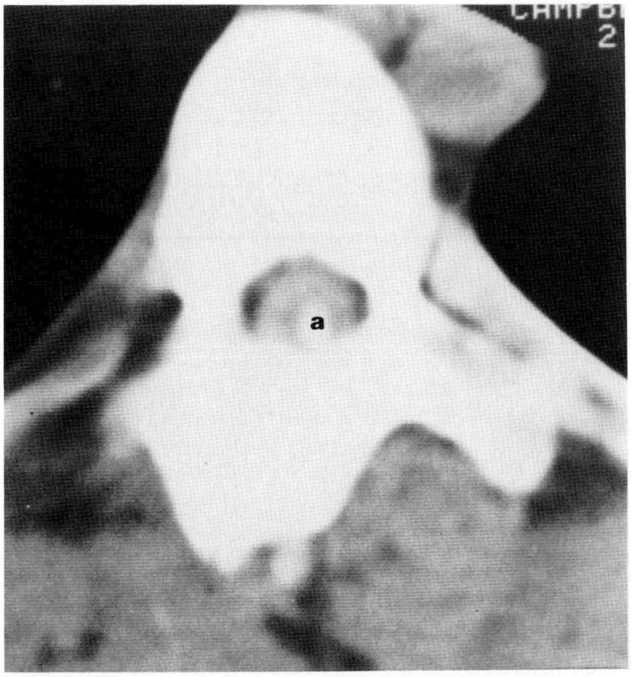

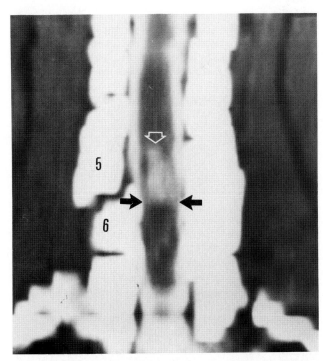

Figure 43.2. A single dorsal midline cyst (a) is seen in the midthoracic area. Note the remnant of noncystic cord tissue between the cyst and the contrast in the subarachnoid space. The fact that the cord is not enlarged means that if Pantopaque had been the myelographic agent used, the diagnosis in this case could not have been made.

Figure 43.3. Coronal reformatted MCT shows a relatively short (2 cm) but wide PTSCC. Note the facet subluxation between C5 and C6 and the fact that the cyst has extended superiorly from the lowest level of cord injury (*black arrows*). The tapering of the cyst at its most superior extent (*open arrow*) is a common feature of PTSCCs.

or a primary superior extension (Fig. 43.1). Because of these facts, it is necessary to scan both above and below the original injury site. Most concern clinically is directed toward the ascending cysts in patients with complete cord lesions; however, it is equally important to search for inferiorly expanding cysts particularly in patients with incomplete cord lesions because cyst expansion in that direction may rob them of important residual neurological function or be the source of pain.

The most common cyst location is dorsal (Fig. 43.2), however, central (Fig. 43.5) and ventral cysts (Fig. 43.6) do occur. Exact localization of cysts within the cord is important because ventral and central cysts are less acces-

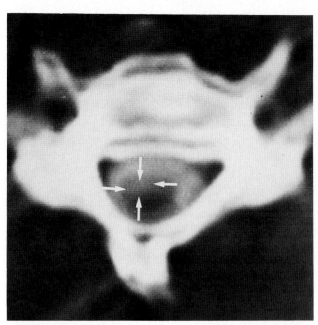

Figure 43.6 A narrow ventral cyst (*arrows*) is located eccentrically on the right side of the cervical cord. This short, narrow cyst measured only 0.5 cm in length. This along with the fact that in order to reach the cyst dissection through the cord would be required were factors which persuaded the surgeon not to operate.

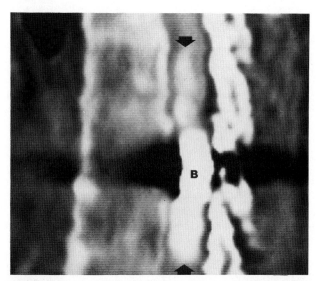

Figure 43.4. On this reformatted sagittal MCT, a 7-cm thoracic cord cyst is seen above and below (*arrows*) an intraspinal bullet fragment (B).

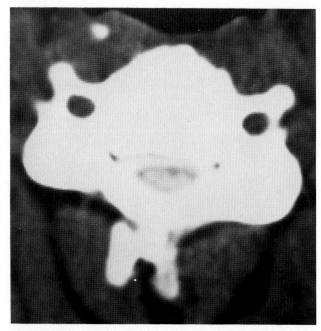

Figure 43.5 A large central cyst occupying more than half the width of the spinal cord is present in the midcervical area.

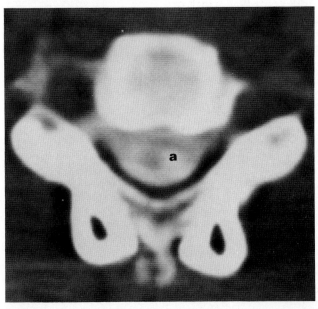

Figure 43.7. This cyst (a) is eccentrically located in the left dorsal portion of the cord. A paramidline incision was necessary in order to enter the middle of the cyst.

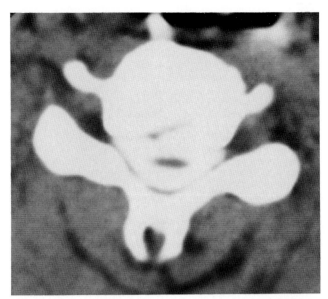

Figure 43.8.   A severely atrophied spinal cord is seen above the level of a PTSCC. This finding may be significant in a patient whose neurological findings cannot be explained by the level of the PTSCC. A prior anterior bony fusion accounts for the peculiar shape of the adjacent vertebral body.

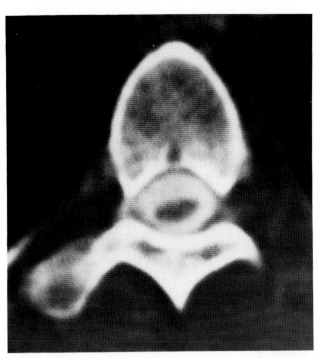

Figure 43.9.   The flattened ventral surface of thoracic cord indicates the presence of cord atrophy, which is less severe than the atrophy seen in Figure 43.8.

sible than those cysts which are dorsal and directly beneath the pial surface. The fact that most PTSCCs are dorsal correlates well with the known anatomical and histological features of the spinal cord. The dorsal gray matter has a rich capillary blood supply making that a primary site for posttraumatic hemorrhage (13). The poor connective tissue framework in that portion of the cord (14, 15), and the constraining effect of the posterior columns are factors which cause the initial enlargement of the cyst to occur in the dorsal portion of the cord in the majority of cases. As the cyst gets larger, it then may expand to areas outside of the dorsal cord. This relative ease of extension may explain why dorsal cysts tend to be longer than cysts in other locations. Besides the fact that most cysts are dorsal in location and spread most easily along that plane, pressure changes within the subarachnoid space and the adjacent cord account for changes in the cyst size. Crucial to PTSCC enlargement is the presence of fibrous adhesions at the injury site which tether the cord to the adjacent dura. In these injured patients, the constant rises and falls of CSF pressure attendant to everyday living (e.g., coughing, sneezing, straining) can not be dampened throughout the entire subarachnoid space as they would be in a normal person because of the presence of these adhesions. This means that the CSF pressure changes are funneled to the region where a small cyst has formed. The waves of pressure are transmitted to the cord substance itself forcing, over time, gradual but progressive cyst expansion. The source of the CSF equivalent fluid which fills the enlarging cyst is either produced by gliotic cells which line the cyst (13), or the fluid enters the cyst via abnormal Virchow-Robin spaces which have

enlarged as a consequence of the original injury (8, 16). In addition to a cyst's location along a ventral to dorsal plane, mention should be made of its midline (Fig. 43.2) or eccentric location (Figs. 43.6 and 43.7). The differentiation has clear surgical implications because a laterally located cyst would require a paramidline incision of the dura.

The majority of PTSCCs are wide, measuring greater than one-half the width of the cord at the same level (Figs. 43.2, 43.3, and 43.5). Narrow cysts are those less than one-half the cord width (Fig. 43.6) and cysts of this width, particularly when they are short and located in the ventral cord may persuade the surgeon not to operate.

Cord atrophy above (Fig. 43.8) or below (Fig. 43.9) a PTSCC may occur and this fact emphasizes the need to scan above and below the cyst level. Although we noted atrophy at a level removed from the cyst in only 25% of patients, it is conceivable that neurological signs and symptoms that are not attributable directly to a PTSCC may be explained by distant atrophy of the spinal cord. We presume that these atrophic changes and those that occur at the level of the cysts relate to compromise of either the perforating nutrient vessels or the major spinal arteries. Feigin et al. (12) described an autopsy of a PTSCC in which they found that degeneration of ascending tracts above the level of the cyst provides a pathological correlate to these MCT observations.

References

1. Quencer RM, Green BA, Eismont FJ: Posttraumatic spinal cord cysts: Clinical features and characterization with metri-

zamide computed tomography. *Radiology* 146:415–423, 1983.

2. Barnett HJM: Syringomyelia consequent on minor to moderate trauma. In: *Major Problems in Neurology, Syringomyelia.* Vol. I. London, W. B. Saunders, 1973, pp. 174–178.
3. Barnett HJM, Jousse AT: Syringomyelia as a late sequel to traumatic paraplegia and quadriplegia—clinical features. In: *Major Problems in Neurology, Syringomyelia.* Vol. I. London, W. B. Saunders, 1973, pp. 129–153.
4. Watson N: Ascending cystic degeneration of the cord after spinal cord injury. *Paraplegia* 19:89–95, 1981.
5. Rossier AB, Foo D, Shillito J, et al: Progressive late posttraumatic syringomyelia. *Paraplegia* 19:96–97, 1981.
6. Seibert CE, Dreisbach JM, Swanson WB, et al: Progressive posttraumatic cystic myelopathy. *AJNR* 2:115–119, 1981.
7. Williams B, Terry AF, Jones F, et al: Syringomyelia as a sequel to traumatic paraplegia. *Paraplegia* 19:67–80, 1981.
8. Durward QJ, Rice GP, Ball MJ, et al: Selective spinal cordectomy: Clinicopathological correlation. *J Neurosurg* 56:359–367, 1982.
9. Edgar RE: Surgical management of spinal cord cysts. *Paraplegia* 14:21–27, 1976.
10. Barnett HJM, Jousse AT: Nature, prognosis and management of posttraumatic syringomyelia. In: *Major Problems in Neurology, Syringomyelia.* Vol. I. London, W. B. Saunders, 1973, pp. 154–164.
11. Dubois PJ, Drayer BP, Sage M, et al: Intramedullary penetrance of metrizamide in the dog spinal cord. *AJNR* 2:313–317, 1981.
12. Feigen I, Ogata J, Bodzilovich G: Syringomyelia: the role of edema in its pathogenesis. *J Neuropathol Exp Neurol* 30:216–232, 1971.
13. Barnett HJM, Jousse AT, Ball MJ: Pathology and pathogenesis of progressive cystic myelopathy as a late sequel to spinal cord injury. In: *Major Problems in Neurology, Syringomyelia.* Vol. I. London, W. B. Saunders, 1973, pp. 179–219.
14. Turnbull IM, Breig A, Hassler O: Blood supply of the cervical spinal cord in man. A microangiographic cadaver study. *J Neurosurg* 24:951–965, 1966.
15. Gillilan LA: The arterial blood supply of the human spinal cord. *J Comp Neurol* 110:75–103, 1958.
16. Ball MJ, Dayan AD: Pathogenesis of syringomyelia. *Lancet* 2:794–801, 1972.

Index*

---

* Page numbers in italics denote figures; those followed by *t* or *f* denote tables or figures, respectively.

826 Index

828   Index

Traumatic injury—*continued*
  soft-tissue intraspinal lesions—*contin-ued*
    spinal cord atrophy, 780, 783, *794, 795*
    spinal cord edema, 227, 768, *778, 780*
    spinal cord fissures, 783, *792*
    spinal cord maceration, 783, *793*
    spinal cord transection, 780, 783, *793*
    subarachnoid hemorrhage, 786–787, *798*
  spondylolisthesis, 591
  stenosis, 551, 553, 556
    lateral, 557
  surgical complications, 781
Tuberculin skin test, 738
Tuberculoma, 743, 758
Tuberculosis
  active, 741
  age factors, 738
  bone destruction, 741, 744
  bone scanning, 739
  cervical, 756
  differential diagnosis, 741–743
  lumbar, 744
  paraplegia, 745–746
  paraspinal abscess, 741, 744, 746
  pyogenic infection, 741
  quiescent, 741
  treatment, 745–746
Tumors (*see also* specific tumors)
  benign, 661–665
  calcification, 367, 714–715
  characteristics, 704–713
  classification, 659
  congenital, 694
  diagnosis
    characterization, 714–715
    differential, 741
    localization, 713–714
  disc mimicry, 352–353, *358*
  epidural fat replacement, 318
  high-resolution CT, 245–259
  imaging protocol, 281
  in children, 271, 276–278, 279, 281, 694, 711
  incidence, 704
  intracranial, *250*, 258
  intradural
    extramedullary, 229, *233*, 234
    mimicry, 363
    relative frequency, 704
  intramedullary, 226–227, 246, *249–251,*
258
    intrathecal contrast, 246
  intraspinal, *376–378*
  intravenous contrast medium, 696–703
  malignant, 665–678
    primary, 665–676
    secondary, 676–678
  metastases, 111, *114*
    clinical features, 676
    differential diagnosis, 345, 349, 354
    epidural, 359, *370–371*
    origin sites, 704
    radiographic features, 676–678, 694, 712–713
    therapeutic goal, 712
    vertebral location, 712
  neural, 98–101
  paraspinal, 277, *376–378*
  pelvic, 741, *753*
  primary, 276–278
    differential diagnosis, 351–353, 357, 358, 367
    relative frequency, 704
  retroperitoneal, 741
  secondary, 278
  soft-tissue extensions, 706, *707, 708, 717, 728*
  spinal canal, 711–712
  spinal reconstruction, 720–727
  spinal resection
    blood loss control, 727, 730
    bowel management, 730–733
    margins, 727
    neural structure dissection, 733–735
    surgical approach, 727
    ureteral management, 730–733
  treatment
    chemotherapy, 716
    radiation therapy, 716
    surgical, 367, 716–735
    surgical planning, 727–735
  vascular, 352
Twining, method of, 59

Vacuum phenomenon, 379, 451, 452, 453, *454, 456, 457*
Varicosities, epidural, 379, *383*
Vascular disease, 260–261
Veins
  anterior external vertebral, *88*
  anterior radicular, *88*
  arterialization, 379

  ascending lumbar, *88*
  basivertebral, *88*, 92, 195, *199*
  epidural, *89*, 91–92, 345, 351, 358
  intervertebral, *88*, 92
  lateral anterior epidural, *88*
  medial anterior epidural, *88*
  posterior epidural vein, *88*
  posterior external vertebral plexus, *88*
  posterior radicular, *88*
  retrovertebral plexus, 92
  vertebral, anatomy, 5
Venography, epidural, 329, 334, 338–339, 461
Ventriculostomy, *207, 210,* 212, 214
Vertebrae
  anatomy, 3, 78
  anterior elements, 3
  cleft, 270
  defect segmentation, 270
  posterior elements, 3
  prosthetic, 725, 726
  rigidity, 547
  split, 349
Vertebral arch, posterior, anatomy, 3–4, *37–40, 42, 44*
Vertebral canal (*see* Spinal canal)
Vertebral column (*see* Spinal column)
Vertebrectomy, spinal reconstruction following, 721–723, 725–727
Virchow-Robin space, 813
Von Hippel-Lindau's disease, 689
Von Recklinghausen's disease
  neurofibroma-associated, 98, 680
  schwannoma-associated, 229, *233*
  surgical intervention, 681

Xenon, 245
X-ray
  detection, 122–124
  generation, 120–122
Xylocaine, 492, 493, 494

Zygapophyseal joints
  anatomy, 81
  asymmetry, 545
  capsular ruptures, 368
  degeneration, 510
  high-resolution CT, 510, 535, 545
  rheumatoid arthritis, 642, 649